Black's
Medical
Dictionary

Black's

Medical Dictionary

39th edition

Edited by Gordon Macpherson,
MB, BS

MADISON BOOKS
Lanham • New York • Oxford

© 1999 A & C Black (Publishers) Limited

In its earlier editions *Black's Medical Dictionary* was edited by:
J. D. Comrie, MD — first to seventeenth editions, 1906–42
H. A. Clegg, FRCP — eighteenth edition, 1944
W. A. R. Thomson, MD — nineteenth to thirty-fourth editions, 1948–84
C. W. H. Havard, FRCP — thirty-fifth to thirty-sixth editions, 1987–90
G. Macpherson, MB, BS — thirty-seventh to thirty-ninth editions, 1992–99

First published in the United States of America in 1999 by
MADISON BOOKS
4720 BOSTON WAY
LANHAM, MD 20706

Library of Congress Cataloging in Publication Data
ISBN 1–56833–129–0
Library of Congress Card Number 59–167

Distributed by National Book Network

Typeset in 9 on 10 pt Times New Roman by Ace Filmsetting Ltd, Frome, Somerset
Printed and bound in Great Britain by Butler & Tanner Ltd, Frome, Somerset

CONTENTS

PREFACE

Black's Medical Dictionary first appeared in 1906. In this, the 39th edition, many experts have contributed to reviewing and updating existing entries and preparing new ones. This edition has more than 5,500 entries and among new ones are those on information technology in medicine, medical ethics, preventive medicine, sports medicine, sex education, bovine spongiform encephalopathy and the safe use of medicines. Where appropriate, the texts provide a guide to treatments, but medicine evolves rapidly and the treatments described are based on current practice when the text was prepared.

New drugs are introduced regularly and in most cases I have covered particular groups of drugs and, though many individual drugs are included, I have not attempted to provide comprehensive lists of available drugs: these are the province of formularies and pharmacopoeias, just as dosages are the responsibility of the patient's doctors. Where specific drugs are mentioned I use the generic or official name as given in the *British Pharmacopoeia*.

Cross-references within the text of an entry are indicated by printing the subject of the reference in small capitals: the aim is to lead the reader to more information on the subject.

The number of appendices has been increased to provide some statistics on the National Health Service as well as addresses of many statutory, professional and international organizations connected with health care. Complementary medicine is increasingly popular with the public; the main text contains references to the many therapies available and I have compiled an appendix briefly describing the main ones.

Once again I am indebted to Ms Joanna Cameron for updating some existing illustrations and providing new ones with her customary skill.

I also thank the many experts without whose help the task of revising the dictionary would have been impossible: Dr K. A. Abbasi, MRCP; Ms N. Bates, BSc; Dr D. J. Carnall, MRCGP; Dr N. Craft, MRCGP; Dr P. H. Dangerfield, MD; Professor B. G. Gazzard, FRCP; Dr P. H. Groves, MRCPsych; Miss S. Hurley, BA; Miss A. J. Hutchinson, BA; Professor B. K. StJ. Livesley, FRCP; Dr S. R. Lowry, MB; Revd W. J. R. Morrison, MA; Dr N. D. L. Olsen, FRCP; Dr P. J. Rees, FRCP; Miss Ann Sommerville, BSc; Dr A. M. Tonks, FRCA; Mr J. H. Vickers, FRCS; Dr M. Weisz, FRCA.

I owe special thanks to Dr Lawrence Baker for revising many entries; to Dr Harvey Baker who updated the entries on dermatology; and to Dr R. E. Ferner who critically reviewed the entries on pharmacological medicine. I am indebted to Miss Anne Watts and Ms Tesni Hollands of A. & C. Black for their support and tolerance and to Miss Linda Beecham for her administrative help. Finally, I congratulate Miss Margaret Baker whose substantial skills have reshaped a mass of amended text into a comprehensible volume.

GORDON MACPHERSON

A

ABDOMEN The lower part of the trunk. Above, and separated from it by the diaphragm, lies the thorax or chest, and below lies the PELVIS, generally described as a separate cavity though continuous with that of the abdomen. Behind are the SPINAL COLUMN and lower ribs, which come within a few inches of the iliac bones. At the sides the contained organs are protected by the iliac bones and down-sloping ribs but in front the whole extent is protected only by soft tissues. The latter consist of the skin, a varying amount of fat, three layers of broad, flat muscle, another layer of fat, and finally the smooth, thin PERITONEUM which lines the whole cavity. These soft tissues allow the necessary distension when food is taken into the STOMACH, and the various important movements of the organs associated with digestion. The shape of the abdomen varies; in children it may protrude considerably, though if this is too marked it may indicate disease. In healthy young adults it should be either slightly prominent or slightly indrawn, and should show the outline of the muscular layer, especially of the pair of muscles running vertically (recti), which are divided into four or five

sections by transverse lines. In older people fat is usually deposited on and inside the abdomen.

Contents The principal contents of the abdominal cavity are the digestive organs, i.e. the stomach and INTESTINES, and the associated glands, the LIVER and PANCREAS. The position of the stomach is above and to the left when the individual is lying down, but may be much lower when standing. The liver lies above and

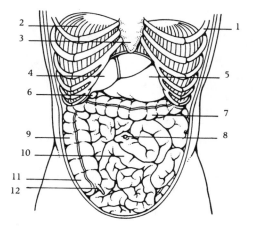

1	6th costal cartilage	7	transverse colon
2	diaphragm	8	position of umbilicus
3	xiphoid process	9	right flexure of colon
4	liver	10	small intestine
5	stomach	11	caecum
6	gall-bladder	12	appendix

Contents of abdomen in position.

to the right, largely under cover of the ribs, and occupying the hollow of the diaphragm. The two kidneys lie against the back wall on either side, protected by the last two ribs. From the kidneys run the URETERS, or urinary ducts, down along the back wall to the BLADDER in the pelvis. The pancreas lies across the spine between the kidneys, and on the upper end of each kidney is a SUPRARENAL gland. The spleen is positioned high up on the left and partly behind the stomach. The great blood vessels and nerves lie on the back wall, and the remainder of the space is taken up by the intestines or bowels (see INTESTINE). The large intestine lies in the flanks on either side in front of the kidneys, crossing below the stomach from right to left, while the small intestine hangs from the back wall in coils which fill up the spaces between the other organs. Hanging down from the stomach in front of the bowels is the OMENTUM, or apron, containing much fat, and helping to protect the bowels. In pregnancy the uterus, or womb, as it increases in

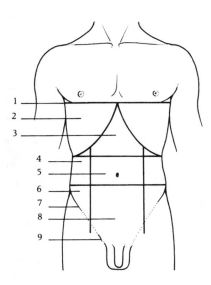

1	xiphisternal plane
2	hypochondriac region
3	epigastrium
4	right lumbar region
5	umbilical region
6	right iliac region
7	right anterior superior iliac spine
8	hypogastric region
9	inguinal region

Regions of the abdomen.

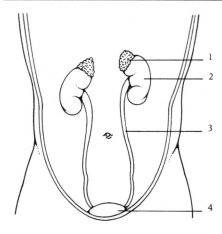

1 left adrenal gland
2 left kidney
3 left ureter
4 bladder

Position of renal system on rear wall of abdomen.

size, rises up from the pelvis into the abdomen, lifting the coils of the small intestine above it.

The PELVIS is the part of the abdomen within the bony pelvis (see BONE), and contains the rectum or end part of the intestine, the bladder, and, in the male the prostate, in the female the uterus, ovaries, and Fallopian tubes.

ABDOMEN, DISEASES OF (See under STOMACH, DISEASES OF; INTESTINE, DISEASES OF; DIARRHOEA; LIVER DISEASES; PANCREAS, DISEASES OF; GALL BLADDER, DISEASES OF; KIDNEYS, DISEASES OF; URINARY BLADDER, DISEASES OF; HERNIA; PERITONITIS; APPENDICITIS; TUMOUR.)
Various processes that can occur, include inflammation, ulceration, infection or tumour (see STOMACH, DISEASES OF). Abdominal disease may be of rapid onset, described as acute, or more long term when it is termed chronic. General symptoms of abdominal disease include:

Pain This is usually ill defined but can be very unpleasant and is termed visceral pain. Pain is initially felt near the mid line of the abdomen. Generally, abdominal pain felt high up in the mid line originates from the stomach and duodenum. Pain that is felt around the umbilicus arises from the small intestine, appendix and first part of the large bowel, and low mid-line pain comes from the rest of the large bowel. If the diseased organ secondarily inflames or infects the lining of the abdominal wall – the PERITONEUM – PERITONITIS occurs and the pain becomes more defined and quite severe, with local tenderness over the site of the diseased organ itself. Hence the pain of APPENDICITIS begins as a vague mid-line pain, and only later moves over to the right iliac fossa,

when the inflamed appendix has caused localized peritonitis. PERFORATION of one of the hollow organs in the abdomen – for example, a ruptured appendix or a gastric or duodenal ulcer (see STOMACH, DISEASES OF) eroding the wall of the gut – usually causes peritonitis with resulting severe pain.
The character of the pain is also important. It may be constant, as occurs in inflammatory diseases and infections, or colicky (intermittent) as in intestinal obstruction.

Swelling The commonest cause of abdominal swelling in women is pregnancy. In disease, swelling may be due to the accumulation of trapped intestinal contents within the bowel, the presence of free fluid (ascites) within the abdomen, or enlargement of one or more of the abdominal organs due to benign causes or tumour.

Constipation may be partial (only flatus can be passed), or complete (no faeces or flatus can be passed). It is often associated with abdominal swelling. In intestinal obstruction, the onset of symptoms is usually rapid with complete constipation and severe, colicky pain. In chronic constipation, the symptoms occur more gradually.

Nausea and vomiting may be due to irritation of the stomach, or intestinal obstruction, when it may be particularly foul and persistent. There are also important non-abdominal causes, such as in response to severe pain or motion sickness.

Diarrhoea may indicate serious disease, especially if it is persistent or contains blood.

Jaundice is a yellow discoloration of the skin and eyes, and may be due to disease in the liver or bile ducts.

Diagnosis and treatment Abdominal diseases are often difficult to diagnose because of the multiplicity of the organs contained within the abdomen, their inconstant position and the vagueness of some of the symptoms. Correct diagnosis usually requires experience, often supplemented by specialized investigations. For this reason, it is wise to consult an experienced practitioner at an early stage, particularly if the symptoms are severe, persistent, recurrent, or resistant to simple remedies.

ABDUCENT NERVE is the sixth nerve rising from the brain and controls the external rectus muscle of the eye, which turns the eye outwards. It is particularly liable to be paralysed in diseases of the nervous system, thus leading to an inward squint.

ABDUCT means to move a part of the body – for example, a limb – away from the mid line. (Opposite: adduct.)

ABLATION means the removal of any part of the body by a surgical operation.

ABORTIFACIENT is a drug which causes artificial abortion.

ABORTION is defined as the expulsion of a fetus showing no signs of life before the 28th week of pregnancy.

Spontaneous abortion, often called miscarriage, may occur at any time before 28 weeks, although it is commonest in the first 12 weeks of pregnancy. Of all diagnosed pregnancies 15–20 per cent end in spontaneous abortion.

The upper limit in the United Kingdom definition has recently been reduced to 24 weeks' gestation to take account of the fact that viability of a fetus is possible from 24 weeks' gestation onwards.

Spontaneous abortions occurring in early PREGNANCY are thought to be particularly associated with fetal defects such as chromosomal abnormalities. They have also been attributed to a lack of PROGESTERONE secretion during the developing pregnancy, abnormalities of the shape of the uterine cavity, and maternal disorders such as DIABETES MELLITUS, THYROID DISEASE and problems with the immune system. An incomplete response of the maternal immune system to pregnancy seems of particular importance in women who suffer recurrent miscarriages, defined as three or more spontaneous abortions.

Factors such as increased maternal age, a high number of previous pregnancies and smoking predispose to spontaneous abortion.

ULTRASOUND SCANS have altered the management of abortions. These make it possible to distinguish between threatened miscarriages, where the women have experienced some vaginal bleeding, but the fetus is alive; inevitable abortion, where the neck of the womb has started to open up; incomplete abortion, where part of the fetus or placenta is retained; and complete abortions. Whereas bed rest may be useful in treating threatened abortions, an inevitable or incomplete abortion will normally require the evacuation of the uterus and a complete miscarriage should require no treatment at all.

Evacuation of the uterus involves administering a general anaesthetic, gentle dilatation of the neck of the womb (cervix), and removal of the remaining products of the pregnancy.

Maternal factors are thought to account more often for late abortions. These include an inappropriately early opening of the neck of the womb (cervical incompetence), structural abnormalities and infections of the uterus.

Ultrasound scan is important to assess the condition of the intrauterine fetus. If the fetus appears normal uterine contractions may be suppressed with drugs.

In cases of cervical incompetence, it may be possible to close the cervical canal with a suture, which is removed at 38 weeks' gestation.

Therapeutic abortion Before this can take place, two doctors must agree that the continuation of the pregnancy would involve risk, greater than if the pregnancy were terminated, of injury to the physical or mental health of the mother or any existing child(ren). The legislation introduced in 1990 states that at the time of abortion the pregnancy should not have exceeded the 24th week.

There is no time limit on therapeutic abortion where the termination is done to save the mother's life, there is substantial risk of serious fetal handicap, or of grave permanent injury to the health of the mother.

About 175,000 terminations are performed a year on residents in England and Wales, under 1.5 per cent of them at over 20 weeks' gestation.

The mortality from therapeutic abortion is less than 1 per 100,000 women and, provided it is performed skilfully before 12 weeks of pregnancy, it is not associated with any reduction in fertility, increased rates of spontaneous abortion or preterm birth in subsequent pregnancies.

Methods of abortion A combination of two drugs, MIFEPRISTONE and a PROSTAGLANDIN, may be used to terminate a pregancy up to 63 days of gestation. If this treatment fails to expel the fetus within 48 hours, surgical termination can be done in 10 days or so. Up to 12 weeks vacuum curettage can be done under general or local anaesthesia. From that date it is probably safer, certainly after the fifteenth week, to induce abortion by administration of a prostaglandin into the woman's uterus, a procedure usually effective within 24 hours. A single termination rarely affects a woman's future fertility; multiple abortions may do so. In the United Kingdom illegal abortions are uncommon but in many countries this is not so; they carry a high risk of complications such as infection and perforation of the uterus and serious bleeding.

ABRASION means the rubbing off of the surface of the skin or of a mucous membrane due to some mechanical injury. Such injuries, though slight in themselves, are apt to allow entrance of dirt containing organisms and so to lead to an abscess or some severer form of inflammation.

Treatment The most effective form of treatment consists in the thorough and immediate cleansing of the wound with soap and water. An antiseptic such as 1 per cent cetrimide can then be applied, and a sterile dry dressing.

ABREACTION An emotional release caused by the recall of past unpleasant experiences. This is normally the result of psychoanalytical treatment in which psychotherapy, certain drugs, or hypnosis are used to effect the abreaction. The technique is used in the treatment of anxiety, hysteria, or other neurotic states.

ABRUPTIO PLACENTA Placental bleeding after the 24th week of pregnancy which may result in complete or partial detachment of the placenta from the wall of the womb. The woman may go into shock. The condition is sometimes associated with raised blood pressure and PRE-ECLAMPSIA.

ABSCESS is a localized collection of pus. A minute abscess is known as a pustule (see PUSTULE), a diffused production of pus is known as cellulitis or erysipelas (see ERYSIPELAS). An abscess may be acute or chronic. An acute abscess is one which develops rapidly within the course of a few days or hours. It is characterized by a definite set of symptoms.

Causes The direct cause is various bacteria. In a few cases the presence of foreign bodies, such as bullets or splinters, or contact with poisonous plants, such as poison ivy, may produce abscesses, but these foreign bodies may remain buried in the tissues without causing any trouble provided they are not contaminated with bacteria or other micro-organisms.

The micro-organisms most frequently found are STAPHYLOCOCCI, and next to these STREPTO-COCCI, though the latter cause more virulent abscesses. Other abscess-forming organisms are *Pseudomonas pyocyanea* and *Escherichia coli*, which lives always in the bowels, and under certain conditions wanders into the surrounding tissues and produces abscesses.

The presence of micro-organisms is not sufficient to produce suppuration (see IMMUNITY; and INFECTION); streptococci can often be found on the skin and in the skin glands of perfectly healthy individuals. Given the proper microorganisms in the tissues, whether they will produce abscesses or not depends upon the virulence of the organism and the individual's natural resistance.

When bacteria have gained access, for example, to a wound, they rapidly multiply, produce toxins, cause local dilatation of the blood-vessels, slowing of the blood-stream, and exudation of blood corpuscles and fluid. The LEUCOCYTES, or white corpuscles of the blood, collect around the invaded area, and destroy the latter either by consuming them (see PHAGO-CYTOSIS), or by forming a toxin that kills them. If the body's local defence mechanisms fail to do this, the abscess will spread and may in severe cases cause generalized infection or septicaemia.

Symptoms The classic symptoms of inflammation are redness, warmth, swelling, pain and fever. The lymph nodes in the neighbourhood may be swollen and tender in an attempt to stop the bacteria spreading to other parts of the body. Infection also causes an increase in the number of leucocytes in the blood (see LEUCOCYTOSIS). Immediately the abscess is opened, or bursts, the pain disappears, the temperature falls rapidly to normal, and healing proceeds rapidly. If, however, the abscess discharges into an internal cavity, such as the bowel or bladder, it may heal slowly and make the patient generally unwell.

Treatment Most local infections of the skin respond to antibiotics. If pus forms the abscess should be surgically opened and drained.

Abscesses can occur in any tissue in the body but the principles of treatment are broadly the same: use of an antibiotic and, where appropriate, surgery.

ABSORPTION Uptake by the body tissues of fluids or other substances. For example, food is absorbed from the digestive tract into the blood and lymph systems. Food is absorbed mainly in the small intestine (JEJUNUM and ILEUM), which is lined by multiple villi that increase its surface area.

ABSTRACT (1) A dry powder produced by extracting the active principles from a crude drug with strong alcohol, mixing with sugar of milk, and drying. Abstracts are standardized so as to be twice the strength of the crude drug. (2) Summary of scientific paper.

ACANTHOSIS NIGRICANS, is a darkly pigmented verrucous skin change, usually around the neck and axilla. It may be inherited but is most commonly acquired and is associated with adenocarcinoma, usually of the stomach (see CANCER), and certain hormonal disorders such as the POLYCYSTIC OVARY, ADDISON'S DISEASE and CUSHING'S SYNDROME.

ACARUS The group of animal parasites which includes *Sarcoptes scabiei*, the cause of the skin disease known as Itch, or Scabies. This parasite used to be known as *Acarus scabiei*. (See SCABIES.)

ACCIDENTAL DEATH In 1997 over 10,000 people died from accidents in England and Wales. Around 5,500 of the deaths occurred at home and over 3,000 in motor vehicle accidents. Many of these deaths would have been preventable, had appropriate safety measures been taken. A high proportion of deaths from accidents occur in males between 5 and 34 years of age. Alcohol is a significant factor. Since the introduction of compulsory use of car seat belts in the United Kingdom in the 1980s the incidence of deaths from driving has fallen. With employers more aware of the risks of injury and death in the work place – with legislation reinforcing education – the number of such incidents has fallen over the past 50 years or more. This group now comprises under 2 per cent of all accidental deaths. Accidental deaths in the elderly are mainly caused by falls, mostly at home. In infants choking is a significant cause of accidental death, food and small objects presenting the main hazards. Poisoning (often from drug overdose) and drowning are notable causes between the mid-twenties and mid-forties.

ACCIDENT PREVENTION IN THE HOME Every year 5,500 people are killed in accidents in British homes, a further 2.2 million need hospital treatment and 900,000 consult their GPs. Domestic accidents in England and Wales cost the health service several hundred million pounds a year. Many of these accidents happen to children or old people, and many of them are preventable.

Children's accidents can often be predicted by their stage of development. Small babies are most at risk of being dropped or having hot drinks spilled on them. As they learn to roll, crawl, and walk they are at risk of falls. As they become more inquisitive they are prone to poisoning from medicines and household chemicals. Older children are at risk from road traffic accidents. Boys are twice as likely to have accidents as girls, and children from deprived backgrounds are at particular risk. Sensible precautions will prevent many accidents. Small babies should not be left unattended on raised surfaces, and manufacturers' instructions should be followed when using all nursery equipment. Hot drinks should not be consumed anywhere near a baby or where a small child is running about. Heavy and dangerous objects should be moved out of children's reach, and parents should remember that children are quite capable of using toys as 'mounting blocks' to reach high shelves. All medicines and chemicals should be locked up. Bath water should be run from the cold tap first to ensure that a child does not get into a scalding running bath, and no child should be left unattended in a bath. Windows, especially on upper floors, should be fitted with locks that restrict the amount by which they can be opened, and stairgates can prevent many falls. By law all children's nightwear must be flameproof, but this does not remove the need for fireguards and care with naked flames and matches. Further information about preventing children's accidents can be obtained from the Child Accident Prevention Trust (see APPENDIX 2: ADDRESSES).

Old people may be frail and have impaired eyesight, hearing, and mobility that increase their risk of an accident. Special precautions, similar to those for children, may be needed for people suffering from dementia, but more general rules include ensuring adequate lighting (especially on stairwells), removing unnecessary furniture and other obstacles from main thoroughfares in the home, removing loose mats from hard floors, and wearing well-fitting shoes. Specific help like walking aids, grab rails, and bath aids may help some people.

Many aspects of home safety apply to people of all ages. Domestic fires account for three-quarters of the deaths and injuries in fires in Britain. Wiring should be checked every five years, and electrical equipment should be installed and maintained according to the manufacturers' instructions. Architectural glass is a major health hazard. Toughened glass is best as it breaks into cuboid pieces. Such safety glass should be used for domestic glazing (at least at low levels). Further information about accidents at home can be obtained from the Royal Society for the Prevention of Accidents (see APPENDIX 2: ADDRESSES).

Although many, if not all, accidents are potentially preventable, they continue to occur. Information on basic first aid can be found in APPENDIX 1: BASIC FIRST AID.

ACCOMMODATION The process by which the refractive power of the lens of the eye is increased by constriction of the ciliary muscle, producing an increased thickness and curvature of the lens. Rays of light from an object further than 6 metres away are parallel on reaching the eye. These rays are brought to a focus on the retina mainly by the cornea. If the eye is now directed at an object closer than 6 metres away, the rays of light from this near object will be diverging by the time they reach the eye. In order to focus these diverging beams of light, the refracting power of the lens must increase. In other words the lens must accommodate.

Diagram of eye in relaxed state (1) viewing a distant object and in an accommodated state; (2) with increased convexity of the lens for viewing a near object.

With age the lens loses its elasticity and thus becomes less spherical when tension in the zonule relaxes. This results in an increased long sightedness with age (presbyopia) requiring reading glasses for correction. (See AGEING.)

ACEBUTOLOL A BETA-ADRENORECEPTOR-BLOCKING (beta-blocking) drug which is used to treat HYPERTENSION and ANGINA. Like other beta-blockers, it slows the heart rate and may precipitate heart failure, so it should not be given to patients with incipient heart failure. Acebutolol can be used with caution in patients whose heart failure is satisfactorily controlled.

ACE INHIBITORS (see ANGIOTENSIN-CONVERTING ENZYME INHIBITORS).

ACETABULUM is the cup-shaped socket on the pelvis in which rests the head of the femur or thigh-bone, the two forming the hip joint. (See HIP-JOINT.)

ACETAZOLAMIDE is a drug which acts by inhibiting the enzyme carbonic anhydrase. This enzyme is of great importance in the production of acid and alkaline secretions in the body. Acetazolamide is sometimes used as a second-line drug for partial seizures in EPILEPSY. It also has a DIURETIC action and is used to treat GLAUCOMA. The drug has a range of side-effects. A topical derivative called dorzolamide, which is used as eye drops, has recently been introduced.

ACETOACETIC ACID is an organic acid produced by the liver when it is rapidly oxidizing fatty acids, a metabolic process which occurs, for example, during starvation. The acid produced is then converted to acetone, which is excreted.

ACETONE is a volatile, colourless organic compound of the ketone group produced by the partial oxidation of fatty acids. In some abnormal conditions, such as starvation, uncontrolled diabetes or prolonged vomiting, acetone and other ketones can accumulate in the blood (see KETONE). Acetone along with beta-hydroxybutyric and aceotacic acids may then appear in the urine, presaging developing coma.

ACETYLCHOLINE An acetic acid ester of the organic base choline, acetylcholine is one of the substances which mediates the transmission of nerve impulses from one nerve to another, or from a nerve to the organ it acts on such as muscles. It acts on both muscarinic receptors (blocked by ATROPINE and responsible for ganglionic and PARASYMPATHETIC transmission and also for SYMPATHETIC innervation of sweat glands) and nicotinic receptors (responsible for transmission of nerve impulses to muscles and blocked by curare, thus causing paralysis). Acetylcholine is rapidly destroyed by cholinesterase, an enzyme present in the blood. ANTICHOLINERGIC drugs such as PHYSOSTIGMINE prolong the action of acetylcholine.

ACETYLCYSTEINE is a drug that is used in the treatment of FIBROCYSTIC DISEASE OF THE PANCREAS and PARACETAMOL POISONING.

ACETYLSALICYCLIC ACID (see ASPIRIN).

ACHALASIA is another tem for spasm, but indicates not so much an active spasm of muscle as a failure to relax.

ACHALASIA OF THE CARDIA is a condition in which there is a failure to relax of the muscle fibres round the opening of the gullet, or oesophagus, into the stomach. (See OESOPHAGUS, DISEASES OF.)

ACHILLES TENDON A thick tendon that joins the calf muscles to the heel bone (calcaneus) and pulls up that bone. The tendon is prone to rupture in middle-aged people playing vigorous sports such as squash or tennis. Named after the classical Greek hero Achilles who was reputedly vulnerable to his enemies only in his heel.

ACHLORHYDRIA means an absence of hydrochloric acid from the stomach juice. If the condition persists after the administration of histamine, the person probably has atrophy of the stomach lining. Achlorhydria occurs in about 4 per cent of healthy people and in several conditions, including PERNICIOUS ANAEMIA, carcinoma of the stomach and GASTRITIS.

ACHONDROPLASIA The commonest form of retarded growth. It is a dominant hereditary disorder of endochondral ossification, in which the long bones of the arms and legs fail to grow properly, while the trunk and head develop normally. It affects both sexes and, while many infants are stillborn or die soon after birth, those who survive have normal intelligence, a normal expectation of life and good health.

ACICLOVIR is an antiviral drug that inhibits DNA synthesis in cells infected by HERPES viruses, although it does not eradicate them. It is only effective if started at the onset of infection; its uses include the systemic treatment of *VARICELLA-SIMPLEX* infections of the skin and mucous membranes (including genital herpes); it is also used topically in the eye. It is especially valuable for the treatment of herpes infections in those with IMMUNODEFICIENCY and may be required for the prevention of recurrence and prophylaxis – indeed, it may be life saving.

ACID BASE BALANCE The balance between the acid and alkaline elements present in the blood and body fluids. The normal hydrogen ion concentration of the plasma is a constant pH 7·4, and the lungs and kidneys have a crucial function in maintaining this figure. Changes in pH value will cause acidosis or alkalosis.

ACIDOSIS is a condition in which there is either (i) a production in the body of two abnormal acids – beta-hydroxybutyric and acetoacetic acids, or (ii) a diminution in the alkali reserve of the blood.

Causes The condition is usually due to faulty metabolism of fat which results in the production of beta-hydroxybutyric and acetoacetic acids. It occurs in DIABETES MELLITUS when this is either untreated or inadequately treated, starvation, persistent vomiting, and delayed anaesthetic vomiting. It also occurs in the terminal stages of glomerulonephritis (see KIDNEYS, DISEASES OF) when it is due to failure of the kidneys. A milder form of it may occur in severe fevers, particularly in children. (See also ACETONE.)

Symptoms General lassitude, vomiting, thirst, restlessness, and the presence of acetone in the urine form the earliest manifestations of the condition. In diabetes a state of coma may ensue and the disease end fatally.

Treatment The underlying condition must always be treated: e.g. if the acidosis is due to DIABETES MELLITUS insulin must be given. Sodium bicarbonate (see SODIUM) is rarely necessary for diabetic ketoacidosis; if it is used, it is invariably now given intravenously. Acidosis might be treated with oral sodium bicarbonate in cases of chronic renal failure. Anaesthetists dislike the administration of bicarbonate to acidotic patients, since there is some evidence that it can make intracellular acidosis worse. They almost always use hyperventilation of the artificially ventilated patient to correct acidosis.

ACINUS is the name applied to each of the minute sacs of which secreting glands are composed, and which usually cluster round the branches of the gland-duct like grapes on their stem. (See GLANDS.)

ACNE A common skin disease starting after puberty, and which may persist for many years. It arises from PILOSEBACEOUS (relating to hair-follicles and associated SEBACEOUS GLANDS) follicles on the face and neck and often trunk. SEBUM production is increased and bacterial proliferation causes inflammation with PAPULE and PUSTULE formation. Plugs of sebum and epidermal cells form blackheads (comedones).

Treatment Topical treatment with benzoyl peroxide gel, erythromycin or clindamycin lotions or retinoic acid may be effective. If not, long-term suppressive oral therapy with a TETRACYCLINE or ERYTHROMYCIN may be necessary. In females a combined oestrogen-antiandrogen 'pill' is an alternative. Severe resistant acne can be cleared by a 16-to-24-week course of oral isotretinoin, but this drug is TERATOGENIC and can cause many side-effects including depression, so its use requires specialist supervision.

ACNE ROSACEA (see ROSACEA).

ACOUSTIC NEUROMA A slowly growing benign tumour in the auditory canal arising from the Schwann cells of the acoustic cranial nerve. The neuroma, which accounts for about 7 per cent of all tumours inside the CRANIUM, may cause facial numbness, hearing loss, unsteady balance, headache, and tinnitus. It can usually be removed surgically, sometimes with microsurgical techniques that preserve the facial nerve.

ACRIFLAVINE An aniline derivative, this is an orange-red crystalline powder, readily soluble in water, with strong antiseptic powers.

ACROCYANOSIS A condition, occurring especially in young women, in which there is persistent blueness of hands, feet, nose and ears as a result of slow circulation of blood through the small vessels of the skin.

ACRODYNIA (see ERYTHROEDEMA).

ACROMEGALY A disorder caused by the increased secretion of growth hormone by an adenoma of the anterior PITUITARY GLAND. It results in excessive body growth of both the skeletal and the soft tissues. If it occurs in adolescence before the bony epiphyses have fused the result is gigantism. If it occurs in adult life the skeletal overgrowth is confined to the hands, feet, cranial sinuses and jaw. Most of the features are due to overgrowth of the cartilage of the nose and ear and the soft tissues which increase the thickness of the skin and lips. Viscera such as the thyroid and liver are also affected. The overgrowth of the soft tissues is gradual.

The local effects of the tumour commonly cause headache and, less frequently, impairment of vision, particularly of the temporal field of vision, as a result of pressure on the nerves to the eye. The tumour may damage the other pituitary cells giving rise to gonadal, thyroid or adrenocortical insufficiency. The diagnosis is confirmed by measuring the level of growth hormone in the serum and by an X-ray of the skull which usually shows enlargement of the pituitary fossa.

Treatment consists of removal or irradiation of the pituitary adenoma. This may have to be done via a craniotomy if the tumour is large but can often be done by an approach through the nose and sphenoid sinus. Deep X-ray therapy to the pituitary fossa is also effective treatment but it may take several years for irradiation to achieve its maximum effect. Drugs, such as bromocriptine, which are dopamine agonists, lower growth hormone levels in acromegaly and are particularly useful as an adjunct to radiotherapy.

ACROMION That part of the scapula, or shoulder blade, forming the tip of the shoulder and giving its squareness to the latter. It projects forward from the scapula, and, with the clavicle or collar-bone in front, forms a protecting arch of bone over the shoulder joint.

ACROPARAESTHESIA A disorder occurring predominantly in middle-aged women in which there is numbness and tingling of the fingers.

ACTH (ADRENOCORTICOTROPIC HORMONE) is the commonly used abbreviation for corticotrophin.

ACTINOMYCIN D (see DACTINOMYCIN).

ACTINOMYCOSIS A chronic infectious condition caused by an anaerobic micro-organism *Actinomyces israelii* that often occurs as a commensal on the gums, teeth, and tonsils. Commonest in adult men, the sites most affected are the jaw, lungs, and intestine, though the disease can occur anywhere. Suppurating granulomatous tumours develop which discharge an oily, thick pus containing yellowish ('sulphur') granules. A slowly progressive condition, actinomycosis usually responds to antibiotic drugs but improvement may be slow and surgery is sometimes needed to drain infected sites. Early diagnosis is important. Treatment is with antibiotics such as penicillin and tetracyclines. The disease occurs in cattle in which it is called woody tongue.

ACUPUNCTURE A traditional Chinese method of healing by inserting thin needles into certain areas beneath the skin and rotating them. Its rationale is that disease is a manifestation of a disturbance of Yin and Yang energy in the body, and that acupuncture brings this energy back into balance by what is described as 'the judicious stimulation or depression of the flow of energy in the various meridians'. What is still unclear to western doctors is why needling, which is the essence of acupuncture, should have the effect it is claimed to have. One theory is that the technique stimulates deep sensory nerves, promoting the production of pain-relieving ENDORPHINS. Of its efficacy in skilled Chinese hands, however, there can be no question, and in China the technique is an alternative to anaesthesia for some operations. The technique is increasingly used in the West, by medically qualified doctors as well as other complementary medicine practitioners. A survey in 1995 showed acupuncture to be the fourth most popular non-conventional therapy after osteopathy, chiropractic and homeopathy. The same survey reported that 80 per cent of those replying who had received acupuncture were satisfied with it (see APPENDIX 13: COMPLEMENTARY MEDICINE).

ACUTE A condition of short duration that starts quickly and has severe symptoms. It may also refer to a symptom, for example, severe pain. An 'acute' abdomen is a serious disorder of the abdomen requiring urgent treatment, usually surgery. Acute heart failure is the sudden stopping or defect in the action of the heart. Acute LEUKAEMIA is a rapid growth in the number of white blood cells, which is fatal if untreated. (Opposite: chronic.)

ACYCLOVIR (see ACICLOVIR).

ADACTYLY Absence of the digits.

ADDICTION Ideas about dependence and addiction have changed over the past two centuries. It was not until the mid 18th century that excessive drinking, or 'inebriety' as it was then known, came to be regarded as some sort of disease. Definitions of dependence have been produced using criteria which help experimental research. The emphasis has been on the observable behaviour of the user of the addictive substance or activity and how the addiction is learned, modified and reinforced. Some sociologists argue that consumption may be defined as abnormal (or deviant) if it exceeds the established norm of the community. The twenty-eighth report of the World Health Organization Expert Committee on Drug Dependence in 1993 defined drug dependence as 'a cluster of physiological, behavioural and cognitive phenomena of variable intensity, in which the use of a psychoactive drug (or drugs) takes on a high priority. The necessary descriptive characteristics are preoccupation with a desire to obtain and take the drug and persistent drug seeking behaviour. Determinants and the problematic consequences of drug dependence may be biological, psychological or social and usually interact.'

Drug dependence can have serious consequences for individuals, families, communities and even nations, with some countries' economies influenced by the production, export and consumption of addictive substances.

Different drugs cause different rates of dependence: tobacco is the commonest drug of addiction, heroin and cocaine cause high rates of addiction, whereas alcohol is much lower, with cannabis lower again. Smoking in the Western world reached a peak after the Second World War with almost 80 per cent of the male population smoking. The reports on the link between smoking and cancer in the early 1960s resulted in a decline that has continued to today when 26 per cent of the US population (28·1 per cent of men and 23·5 per cent of women) and in 1997 in England 28 per cent of men and 27 per cent of women were smoking cigarettes. Globally, tobacco consumption continues to grow, particularly in the developing world with multinational tobacco companies marketing their products aggressively.

Approximately 4 per cent of the population are dependent on alcohol and 2 per cent on other drugs, both legal and illegal, at any one time in Western countries. The way drugs are taken may vary from oral, nasal, inhalation or injection, and the route of use may influence the extent of reported dependence.

HIV and AIDS (see AIDS/HIV) have added another dimension to the effects of dependence. Major national variations occur in the prevalence of HIV among injecting drug users. In Northern Europe around 15 per cent of injectors are seropositive to HIV – namely, they are infected. More recent data on HEPATITIS C, a virus that is transmitted by similar means to HIV, show that 50–70 per cent of injectors in most countries are infected.

Over 40 distinct theories or models of drug misuse have been put forward. One is that the individual consumes drugs to cope with personal problems or difficulties in relations with others. The other main model emphasizes environmental influences such as drug availability, environmental pressures to consume drugs and sociocultural influences such as peer pressure. These complex multifactorial models are descriptive and clinical and are generally based on minimal experimental data.

By contrast to these models of why people misuse drugs, models of compulsive drug use, where individuals have a compulsive addiction, have been amenable to testing in the laboratory. Studies at cellular and nerve-receptor levels are attempting to identify mechanisms of tolerance and dependence for several substances. Classical behaviour theory is a key model for understanding drug dependence. This and current laboratory studies are being used to explain the reinforcing nature of dependent substances and are helping to provide an explanatory framework for dependence. Drug consumption is a learned form of behaviour. Numerous investigators have used conditioning theories to study why people misuse drugs. Laboratory studies are now locating the 'reward pathways' in the brain for opiates and stimulants where positive reinforcing mechanisms involve particular sectors of the brain. There is a consensus among experts in addiction that addictive behaviour is amenable to effective treatment and that the extent to which an addict complies with treatment makes it possible to predict a positive outcome. But there is a long way to go before the mechanisms of drug addiction are properly understood or ways of treating it generally agreed. Scientists, doctors, sociologists, law-enforcement agencies and governments will have to co-operate closely if solutions are to be found. (See also DRUG ADDICTION.)

Dependency can also develop in respect of physical activities such as gambling, computer games and use of the Internet.

ADDISON'S DISEASE   The cause of Addison's disease is a deficiency of the adrenocortical hormones CORTISOL, ALDOSTERONE and ANDROGENS due to destruction of the adrenal cortex. It occurs in about 1:25,000 of the population. Although the destruction of the adrenal cortex in Addison's original description was due to tuberculosis, a much more common cause today is auto-immune damage. Rare causes of Addison's disease include metastases from carcinoma, usually of the bronchus, granulomata and HAEMOCHROMATOSIS.

Symptoms The clinical symptoms appear slowly and depend on the severity of the underlying disease process. The patient usually complains of anorexia, nausea, weakness, tiredness and loss of weight. The skin becomes pigmented due to the increased production of ACTH. Faintness, especially on standing, is due to postural hypotension secondary to aldosterone deficiency. Women lose their axillary hair and both sexes are liable to develop mental symptoms such as depression. Acute episodes – Addisonian crises – may occur, brought on by

infection, injury or other stressful events; they are caused by a fall in aldosterone levels, leading to abnormal loss of sodium and water via the kidneys, dehydration, low blood pressure and confusion.

Diagnosis depends on demonstrating impaired serum levels of cortisol and inability of these levels to rise after an injection of ACTH.

Treatment consists in replacement of the deficient hormones – hydrocortisone is commonly used – and this enable patients to lead a completely normal life and to enjoy a normal life expectancy.

ADDUCT   To move a limb or any other part towards the midline of the body. (Opposite: abduct.)

ADENINE ARABINOSIDE A nitrogen-containing base compound that is a constituent of the nucleic acids deoxyribonucleic acid (see DNA) and ribonucleic acid (see RNA).

ADENITIS means inflammation of a gland. (See LYMPHATICS.)

ADENO-   A prefix denoting relation to a gland or glands.

ADENOCARCINOMA   A malignant growth of glandular tissue. This tissue is widespread throughout the body's organs and the tumours may occur, for example, in the stomach, ovaries, and uterus. Adenocarcinomas may be subdivided into those that arise from mucous or serous secreting glandular tissue.

ADENOIDS (see NOSE, DISEASES OF).

ADENOMA   A benign tumour composed of glandular tissue. It may arise in any part of the body in which glandular tissue occurs: e.g. the thyroid gland. It must be differentiated from an adenocarcinoma, which is a malignant tumour composed of glandular tissue. (See TUMOUR.)

ADENOSINE TRIPHOSPHATE (ATP)   A compound comprising the chemical substances adenine, ribose and phosphates. The chemical bonds of the phosphates contain energy needed for cell METABOLISM that occurs when muscle cells contract. This energy is made available when ATP breaks up to form other chemical groupings – adenosine diphosphate (ADP) and adenosine monophosphate (AMP). The energy needed for recombining AMP and ADP to form ATP is produced by the breakdown of carbohydrates or other constituencies of food.

ADENOVIRUSES   VIRUSES containing double-stranded DNA which cause around 5 per cent of clinically recognized respiratory illnesses. Of the 40 or so known types only a few have been properly studied to establish how they produce disease. Adenoviruses cause fever and inflammation of the respiratory tract and mucous membranes of the eyes, symptoms resembling those of the common cold. Infections are generally benign and self limiting and treatment is symptomatic and supportive, although the elderly and people with chronic chest conditions may develop secondary infections which require antibiotic treatment.

ADHESION   The abnormal union of two normally separate tissues. It may occur after inflammation or surgery. The result is often a fibrous band between the adjacent tissues. Examples are adhesions between joint surfaces – which reduce mobility of a joint – or, after operation, between loops of intestine, where the fibrous band may cause obstruction. Movement of the heart may be restricted by adhesions between the organ and its membranous cover, the pericardial sac.

ADIPOSE TISSUE or FAT is a loose variety of fibrous tissue, in the meshes of which lie cells, each of which is distended by several small drops, or one large drop, of fat. This tissue replaces fibrous tissue when the amount of food taken is in excess of the bodily requirements. (See DIET; OBESITY.)

ADIPOSIS DOLOROSA, also known as Dercum's disease, is a condition in which painful masses of fat develop under the skin. It is commoner in women than in men.

ADLER   Alfred Adler (1870–1937) was an Austrian psychiatrist who proposed psychoanalytical concepts based on individual psychology, his central thesis being that everyone is born with intrinsic feelings of inferiority. Thus life is a continuing struggle to overcome these feelings: failure results in neuroses.

ADOPTION (see CHILD ADOPTION).

ADRENAL GLANDS   Also known as SUPRARENAL GLANDS, these are two small triangular endocrine glands situated one upon the upper end of each kidney.

Structure Each suprarenal gland has an enveloping layer of fibrous tissue. Within this the gland shows two distinct parts: an outer, firm, deep-yellow, cortical (see CORTEX) layer, and a central, soft, dark-brown, medullary (see MEDULLA) portion. The cortical part consists of columns of cells running from the surface inwards, whilst in the medullary portion the cells are arranged irregularly and separated from one another by large capillary blood-vessels.

Functions Removal of the suprarenal glands in animals is speedily followed by great muscular

prostration and death in a few days. In human beings, disease of the suprarenal glands is apt to bring on Addison's disease, in which the chief symptoms are increasing weakness and bronzing of the skin. The medulla of the glands produces a substance – adrenaline – the effects of which closely resemble those brought about by activity of the SYMPATHETIC NERVOUS SYSTEM: dilated pupils, hair standing on end, quickening and strengthening of the heart-beat, immobilization of the gut, increased output of sugar from the liver into the blood-stream. Several hormones (called CORTICOSTEROIDS) are produced in the cortex of the gland and play a vital role in the metabolism of the body. Some (such as aldosterone) control the electrolyte balance of the body and help to maintain the blood pressure and blood volume. Others are concerned in carbohydrate metabolism, whilst others again are concerned with sex physiology. HYDROCORTISONE is the most important hormone of the adrenal cortex, controlling as it does the body's use of carbohydrates, fats and proteins. It also helps to suppress inflammatory reactions and has an influence on the immune system. (See ADRENALINE; ADDISON'S DISEASE; CORTISONE.)

ADRENALINE is the secretion of the adrenal medulla (see ADRENAL GLANDS). Its effect is similar to stimulation of the SYMPATHETIC NERVOUS SYSTEM as occurs when a person is excited, shocked or frightened. In the *United States Pharmocopoeia* it is known as epinephrine. It is also prepared synthetically. Among its important effects are raising of the blood pressure, increasing the amount of glucose in the blood, and constricting the smaller blood-vessels.

It has an important use when injected intramuscularly or intravenously in the treatment of ANAPHYLAXIS, and it may be applied directly to wounds, on gauze or lint, to check haemorrhage. Injected along with some local anaesthetic, it permits painless, bloodless operations to be performed on the eye, nose, etc. It is rarely, if ever, used nowadays hypodermically and is no longer given to treat asthma. In severe cardiac arrest adrenaline (1 in 10,000) by central intravenous injection is recommended.

ADRENERGIC RECEPTORS   The sites in the body on which ADRENALINE and comparable stimulants of the SYMPATHETIC NERVOUS SYSTEM act. Drugs which have an adrenaline-like action are described as being adrenergic. There are five different types of adrenergic receptors, known as alpha 1, alpha 2, beta 1, beta 2 and beta 3 respectively. Stimulation of alpha receptors leads to constriction of the bronchi, constriction of the blood vessels with consequent rise in blood pressure and dilatation of the pupils of the eyes. Stimulation of beta 1 receptors quickens the rate and output of the heart, while stimulation of beta 2 receptors dilates the bronchi. Beta 3 receptors are now known to mediate so-called non-shivering thermogenesis, a way of producing heat from specialized fat cells particularly relevant to the human infant.

For long it had been realized that in certain cases of ASTHMA adrenaline had not the usual beneficial effect of dilating the bronchi during an attack; rather it made the asthma worse. This was due to its acting on both the alpha and beta adrenergic receptors. A derivative, isoprenaline, was therefore produced which acted only on the beta receptors. This had an excellent effect in dilating the bronchi, but unfortunately also affected the heart, speeding it up and increasing its output – an undesirable effect which meant that isoprenaline had to be used with great care. In due course drugs were produced, such as salbutamol, which act predominantly on the beta 2 adrenergic receptors in the bronchi and have relatively little effect on the heart.

The converse of this story was the search for what became known as beta-adrenoceptor-blocking drugs, or beta-adrenergic-blocking drugs. The theoretical argument was that if such drugs could be synthesized, they could be of value in taking the strain off the heart – for example: stress → stimulation of the output of adrenaline → stimulation of the heart → increased work for the heart. A drug that could prevent this train of events would be of value, for example, in the treatment of ANGINA PECTORIS. Now there is a series of beta-adrenoceptor-blocking drugs of use not only in angina pectoris, but also in various other heart conditions such as disorders of rhythm, as well as high blood-pressure. They are also proving of value in the treatment of anxiety states by preventing disturbing features such as palpitations. Some are useful in the treatment of migraine. (see BETA-ADRENOCEPTOR-BLOCKING DRUGS).

ADRENOCORTICOTROPHIC HORMONE (ACTH)
A hormone which is released into the body during stress. Made and stored in the anterior pituitary gland, ACTH regulates the production of corticosteroid hormones from the adrenal gland. ACTH is vital for the growth and maintenance of the adrenal cortical cells. Its production is in part controlled by the amount of hydrocortisone in the blood and also by the hypothalmus. ACTH participates in the FEEDBACK MECHANISM of hormone production and actions involving particularly the hypothalamus and pituitary gland. The hormone is used to test adrenal function and treat conditions such as ASTHMA. (See CUSHING'S SYNDROME.)

ADRENOGENITAL SYNDROME or CONGENITAL ADRENAL HYPERPLASIA
An inherited condition, the adrenogenital syndrome or congenital adrenal hyperplasia is an uncommon disorder affecting about one baby in 7,500. The condition is present from birth and the victim suffers from various enzyme defects as well as a block on the production of HYDROCORTISONE

and ALDOSTERONE by the adrenal gland. In girls the syndrome produces virilization of the genital tract, which may become enlarged. The metabolism of salt and water is disturbed causing dehydration, low blood pressure, and loss of weight. Enlargement of the adrenal glands occurs and the affected individual may also develop excessive pigmentation in the skin. Treatment requires replacement of the missing hormones and, if started early, may lead to normal sexual development.

ADULT RESPIRATORY DISTRESS SYNDROME (ARDS)
A form of acute respiratory failure in which a variety of different disorders give rise to pulmonary injury by what is thought to be a common pathway. It has a high mortality (about 70 per cent).

The exact aetiology is unknown, but it is thought that, whatever the stimulus, activation of neutrophils (which may then be sequestered in the lungs) releases cytotoxic substances – substances that damage or kill cells – such as oxygen-free radicals and proteases which damage the alveolar capillary membranes. Once these are damaged protein-rich oedema fluid leaks into the alveoli and interstitial spaces. SURFACTANT is also lost. This impairs gas exchange and gives rise to the clinical and pathological picture of acute respiratory failure.

The typical patient with ARDS has rapidly worsening hypoxaemia (lack of oxygen in the blood), often requiring mechanical ventilation, which contrasts with the relative lack of physical signs. There are all the signs of respiratory failure (see TACHYPNOEA, TACHYCARDIA, CYANOSIS, etc.), though the chest may be clear apart from a few crackles. Radiographs show bilateral, patchy shadowing sparing the cardio and costophrenic angles. Blood gases will show a low PaO_2 (concentration of oxygen in pulmonary arterial blood) and usually a high $PaCO_2$ (concentration of carbon dioxide in pulmonary arterial blood). The lungs are 'stiff' – they are less effective because of the loss of surfactant and the non-cardiogenic pulmonary oedema.

Causes The causes of ARDS may be broadly divided into the following:

MICROBIOLOGICAL Pulmonary, distant, or generalized infection by bacteria, fungi, or viruses.

ACTIVATION OF HOST DEFENCE Massive transfusion, transfusion reaction, cardiopulmonary bypass, etc., may cause activation of NEUTROPHILS via complement pathways.

CHEMICAL This includes drugs, inhaled toxic gases and smoke, and metabolic disorders like URAEMIA and pancreatitis (see PANCREAS, DISEASES OF).

PHYSICAL Trauma to the lung, gastric aspiration, aspiration of water, etc.

Treatment The principles of management are supportive, with treatment of the underlying condition if that is possible. Oxygenation is improved by increasing inspired oxygen concentration and mechanical ventilation of the lungs. Attempts are made to reduce the formation of pulmonary oedema by careful management of fluid balance. Secondary infections are treated if they arise, as are the possible complications of prolonged ventilation with low lung compliance (e.g., PNEUMOTHORAX). There is some evidence that giving surfactant through a nebulizer or aerosol may help to improve lung effectiveness and reduce oedema. There is little evidence that steroids are of use. Some experimental evidence supports the use of free radical scavengers and ANTIOXIDANTS, but these are not commonly used. In severe cases extracorporeal gas exchange has been advocated as a supportive measure until the lungs have healed enough for adequate gas exchange. (See also RESPIRATORY DISTRESS SYNDROME and HYALINE MEMBRANE DISEASE.)

ADVANCE STATEMENTS ABOUT MEDICAL TREATMENT (see LIVING WILL).

ADVERSE REACTIONS TO DRUGS When a new drug is introduced, it has usually been studied only in relatively few patients – typically 1,500. If n patients have been studied, and no serious effects are observed, there is still a chance of a serious adverse effect's occurring in the general population as frequently as $3/n$ (1:500).

Adverse effects can be divided into types. First, those which are closely related to the concentration of the drug and accord with what is known of its PHARMACOLOGY. These so-called type-A (augmented pharmacological) effects are distinguished from type-B (bizarre) effects which are unpredictable, usually rare, and often severe. ANAPHYLAXIS is the most obvious of these, though bone-marrow suppression with CO-TRIMOXAZOLE, hepatic failure (see HEPATITIS) with SODIUM VALPROATE, or PULMONARY FIBROSIS with AMIODARONE would all be other examples. A more comprehensive classification includes reactions type C (chronic effects), D (delayed effects – such as teratogenesis or carcinogenesis) and E (end-of-dose effects – withdrawal effects). Examples of adverse reactions include nausea, skin eruptions, jaundice, sleepiness and headaches.

Patients should remind their doctors of any drug allergy, or adverse effect they have suffered in the past. Medical warning bracelets are easily obtained. Doctors should report adverse effects to the authorities, in the case of Britain to the Committee on Safety of Medicines (CSM), using the yellow-card reporting machinery.

AEDES AEGYPTI The scientific name of the mosquito which conveys to man (by biting) the viruses of yellow fever and of dengue or 'breakbone fever'. (See DENGUE; and YELLOW FEVER.)

AEGOPHONY The bleating or punchinello tone given to the voice as heard by AUSCULTATION with a stethoscope, when there is a small amount of fluid in the pleural cavity in the chest.

AEROBIC BACTERIA A bacterium that needs the presence of free oxygen for its life and multiplication (see also ANAEROBIC).

AEROPHAGY Swallowing abnormal quantities of air which can occur during rapid eating or drinking. Indigestion sufferers sometimes do this to relieve their symptoms.

AEROSOL (see INHALANTS).

AETIOLOGY That part of medical science dealing with the causes of disease.

AFFERENT An adjective to describe nerves, blood vessels, or lymphatic vessels that conduct their electrical charge or contents inwards to the brain, spinal cord or relevant organ. (Opposite: efferent.)

AFIBRINOGENAEMIA A condition in which the blood will not clot because FIBRIN is absent. It is characterized by haemorrhage. There are two forms: (*a*) a congenital form, and (*b*) an acquired form. The latter may be associated with advanced liver disease, or may occur as a complication of labour. Treatment consists of the intravenous injection of fibrinogen and blood transfusion.

AFTERBIRTH (see PLACENTA).

AFTERPAINS Pains similar to but feebler than those of labour, occurring in the two or three days following childbirth.

Causes are generally the presence of a blood-clot or retained piece of PLACENTA which the WOMB is attempting to expel.

AGAMMAGLOBULINAEMIA An inherited condition found in male infants, in which there is no GAMMA-GLOBULIN in the blood. These children are particularly susceptible to infections as they are unable to form antibodies to any infecting micro-organism. Acquired agammaglobulinaemia is a rare disorder occurring in both sexes in their twenties and forties, characterized by recurrent bacterial infections. The cause is a disturbance in the working of the immune system.

AGAR OR AGAR-AGAR A gelatinous substance prepared from seaweed. It is used in preparing culture-media for use in bacteriological laboratories. It is sometimes given for relieving constipation.

AGEING The result of a combination of natural, largely genetically programmed changes occurring in all body systems. Diseases or injuries may influence these changes, which impair the body's homeostatic mechanisms. A person's environment and lifestyle also affect the ageing process. The effects of ageing include: cessation of menstruation; wrinkling of the skin because of a loss of elastic tissue; failing memory (especially short term) and less ability to learn new skills along with slowed responses – changes caused by the loss of or less efficient working of nerve cells; the senses become less acute; the lungs become less efficient as does heart muscle, both causing a fall in exercise tolerance; arteries harden, which results in a rise in blood pressure and poor blood circulation; joints are less mobile, bones beome more brittle (OSTEOPOROSIS) and muscle bulk and strength are reduced; the lens of the eye becomes less elastic, resulting in poorer sight, and it may also become opaque (CATA-RACT).

In developed countries people are living longer, in part because infant and child mortality rates have dropped dramatically over the past 100 years or so. Improved standards of living and more effective health care have also contributed to greater longevity. The proportion of people over 65 years of age has greatly increased and that of the over 75s is still rising. In 1952, 255 people in the United Kingdom became cenenarians: by 1996 that figure had reached more than 5,200. This extreme longevity is attributed to a particular gene slowing the ageing process. Interestingly, those living to 100 often retain the mental faculties of people in their 60s and examination of centenarians' brains show that these are similar to those of 60-year-olds. (See MEDICINE OF AGEING.) (See also CLIMACTERIC.)

Help and advice can be obtained from Age Concern (see APPENDIX 2: ADDRESSES).

AGENESIS means incomplete development or the failure of any part or organ of the body to develop normally.

AGGLUTINATION Adherence together of small bodies in a fluid. Thus, blood corpuscles agglutinate into heaps (rouleaux) when added to the serum of a person belonging to an incompatible blood-group. Bacteria agglutinate into clumps and die when exposed to the presence of antibodies in the blood. This is important in regard to diagnosis of certain diseases due to bacteria. In typhoid fever, for example, the blood of an animal is immunized against typhoid bacilli by repeated injections of these. The blood-serum of the animal, known now as anti-typhoid serum, is issued to laboratories for use when bacilli are found in the excretions of a patient who is possibly suffering from typhoid fever. The bacilli are exposed to the action of a drop of the serum; if the serum shows the power of agglutinating these bacteria, this forms evidence that the bacteria in question are typhoid bacilli. The reaction may also be carried out in the contrary manner: that

is to say, the serum from the blood of a patient, who may be suffering from typhoid fever, but in regard to whom the diagnosis is still a matter of doubt, is added to a drop of fluid containing bacteria known to be typhoid bacilli; if these are agglutinated into clumps by the patient's serum, the patient is then known to be suffering from typhoid fever; if they do not agglutinate, his symptoms are due to some other condition. This reaction for typhoid fever is known as the Widal reaction. Comparable agglutination reactions, using an appropriate serum, are used in the diagnosis of a number of diseases, including glandular fever (when it is known as the Paul-Bunnell reaction), typhus fever (when it is known as the Weil-Felix reaction), undulant fever, and Weil's disease.

AGGRESSION A general term that covers a range of hostile behaviour, some beyond normal social behaviour. Some physical diseases cause aggressive outbursts, e.g. temporal lobe EPILEPSY and hypoglycaemia (see DIABETES). Certain mental disorders, such as antisocial personality disorders, alcohol or drug abuse and schizophrenia, may be associated with aggression.

Male sex hormones (ANDROGENS) appear to be linked to aggressive behaviour and aggression is commoner among adolescents and young adults than other sections of the population.

AGNOSIA The condition in which, in certain diseases of the brain, the patient loses the ability to recognize the character of objects through the senses – touch, taste, sight, hearing.

AGONIST (1) A muscle which contracts and causes a movement. Contraction of an agonist is complemented by relaxation of its antagonist. (2) A drug that acts through receptors on the surface of the cell or within the cell and provokes a biological response. As the body contains natural agonists that combine with cell receptors any 'occupation' of these cell receptors by drug molecules will have a pharmacological effect on the individual. The intensity of that pharmacological effect is believed to be directly proportional to the number of receptors on the cell that combine with the drug molecule. For example, the natural agonist noradrenaline contracts the smooth muscle of blood vessels; the drug agonist phenylnephrine has a similar effect.

Antagonists are drugs which will combine with the receptor site to prevent another agent from producing its greatest effect. If the drug has no efficacy of its own, but simply prevents the agonist acting at the receptor site, it is called a full antagonist. A partial antagonist is a drug that provokes some activity at the receptor site. An example of an antagonist is prazosin which acts against the natural agonist noradrenaline at the receptor site of the cells of blood-vessel muscle and prevents the vascular muscle contracting.

AGORAPHOBIA Sense of fear exper·enced in large open spaces and public places, and is a symptom of psychological disorder (see MENTAL ILLNESS) . There are said to be 300,000 victims of it in the United Kingdom. Those who suffer from what can be a most distressing condition can obtain help and advice from the Phobics Society (see APPENDIX 2: ADDRESSES).

AGRANULOCYTOSIS Condition in which the white cells (LEUCOCYTES) in the blood of the polynuclear or granular variety become greatly lessened in numbers or disappear altogether. It is usually caused by taking such drugs as amidopyrine, thiourea, sulphonamides, chloramphenicol and the immuno-suppressant drugs.

AGRAPHIA Loss of power to express ideas by writing. (See APHASIA.)

AGUE A traditional term for malaria and other (usually infectious disorders) in which the subject suffers alternating bouts of fever and cold shivering.

AIDS/HIV The Acquired Immune Deficiency Syndrome (AIDS) caused by infection with Human Immuno Deficiency Virus (HIV), a retrovirus, was first described in 1981 following the development of an unusual opportunistic infection (*PNEUMOCYSTIS CARINII PNEUMONIA*) and tumours (KAPOSI'S SARCOMA) associated with immune deficiency in a group of homosexuals. Transmission of HIV infection occurs by exchange of body fluids containing the virus, mainly blood, semen and breast milk. This may occur following sexual contact, during delivery or by exposure to needles contaminated with blood used medically or during illicit drug administration. In most of the world blood and donor organs for transplantation are now screened for HIV and transmission by this route has diminished substantially. Transmission by mosquitoes or by casual contact does not occur.

Epidemiology AIDS is a predominantly sexually transmitted disease and the distribution of infection varies greatly within risk groups between countries and even between regions and cities. The prevalence of HIV infection often parallels the frequency of other sexually transmitted diseases, particularly ulcerating conditions like chancroid. While the peak incidence of infection in the developed world, particularly in homosexuals, was in the early 1980s with a sharp decline subsequently, in resource-poor countries the epidemic, which is primarily heterosexual, continues unchecked. HIV predominantly affects the poor who may be ignorant about the means of transmission of HIV infection and in areas where women have little control over their sexuality. Part of the variation in the epidemic within resource-poor countries is explained by factors leading to poor

social cohesion which make it difficult to transmit simple health-education messages and where there may be little cultural inhibition to frequent partner change. The HIV pandemic still represents one of the greatest dangers to public health this century with approximately 20 million people being infected by 1996 (see table). While the heaviest burden presently falls upon sub-Saharan Africa, rapid increases in HIV infection are being seen in Asia which will have the greatest number of AIDS cases by the year 2000 because of the enormous population in this region.

Africa	14 million
Asia	5.2 million
North America and Europe	1.3 million
South America	1·5 million
Children with HIV	850,000
UK	30,000+

Estimated number of HIV-positive individuals worldwide in 1996 (WHO figures)

Transmission of HIV to children by infected mothers, both during delivery and via breast feeding, is particularly important. This occurs in up to 40 per cent of infected women but could be reduced very significantly by drug therapy (see below) and by changes, where necessary, in the WHO's policy about breast feeding.

Pathogenesis The cellular target of HIV infection is a subset of white blood cells called T-lymphocytes which carry the CD4 surface receptor. These so-called 'T-helper cells' are vital to the function of cell-mediated IMMUNITY. Infection of these cells leads to their destruction (HIV replicates at an enormous rate – 10^9) and over the course of several years the body is unable to generate sufficient new cells to keep pace and this leads to progressive destruction of the body's immune capabilities, evidenced clinically by the development of OPPORTUNISTIC infection and unusual TUMOURS.

Monitoring of clinical progression It is now possible to measure the number of viral particles present in the plasma. This gives an accurate guide to the likely progression rate which will be slow in those individuals with fewer than 10,000 particles per ml of plasma, but progressively more rapid above this figure. The main clinical monitoring of the immune system is through the numbers of CD4 lymphocytes in the blood. The normal count is around 850 cells per cc and, without treatment, eventual progression to AIDS is likely in those individuals whose CD4 count falls below 500 per cc and opportunistic infections occur most frequently when the count falls below 200 cells mm^{-3}. Most such opportunistic infections are treatable and death is only likely when the CD4 count falls below 50 cells per cc when infection is developed with organisms which are difficult to treat because of their low intrinsic virulence.

Simple, cheap and highly accurate tests are now available to detect HIV antibodies in the serum which normally occur within three weeks of infection and remain the cornerstone of the diagnosis.

Testing for HIV should only be done with the subject's INFORMED CONSENT because of the medical, legal, employment and insurance implications of a positive result; those tested should have appropriate counselling. However, in view of the markedly improved treatments (see below), many more individuals are coming forward for testing.

Early in the epidemic, when the pathogenesis was not clearly understood, a diagnosis of AIDS was important as this was a clinical marker of profound immune deficiency. In America the definition of AIDS has now been widened to include all those with a CD4 count below 200 cells per mm^{-3}, whether they suffered from an opportunistic infection or not.

Clinical features Most infected individuals have a viral illness some three weeks after contact with HIV. The clinical features are often non-specific and remain undiagnosed but include a fine red rash, large LYMPH NODES, an influenza-like illness, cerebral involvement and sometimes the development of opportunistic infections. The ANTIBODY test may be negative at this stage but there are usually high levels of virus particles in the blood. The antibody test is virtually always positive within three months of infection. HIV infection is often subsequently asymptomatic for a period of ten years or more, although in most patients progressive immune destruction is occurring during this time and a variety of minor opportunistic infections such as HERPES ZOSTER or oral THRUSH do occur. In addition, generalized LYMPHADENOPATHY is present in a third of patients and some suffer from severe malaise, weight loss, night sweats, mild fever, ANAEMIA or easy bruising due to THROMBOCYTOPAENIA.

The presentation of opportunistic infection is highly variable but most usually involves either the CENTRAL NERVOUS SYSTEM, the gastrointestinal tract or the LUNGS. Patients may present with a sudden onset of a neurological deficit or EPILEPSY due to a sudden onset of a STROKE-like syndrome or epilepsy due to a space-occupying lesion in the brain, most commonly TOXOPLASMOSIS. In late disease, HIV infection of the central nervous system itself may produce progressive memory loss, impaired concentration and mental slowness called AIDS DEMENTIA. A wide variety of opportunistic PROTOZOA or viruses produces DYSPHAGIA, DIARRHOEA and wasting. In the respiratory system the commonest opportunistic infection associated with AIDS, *Pneumocystis carinii* pneumonia, produces severe shortness of breath and sometimes CYANOSIS, usually with a striking lack of clinical signs in the chest.

Oesophageal, tracheal, bronchial or pulmonary candidiasis
Invasive cervical cancer
Extrapulmonary cryptococcosis
Disseminated or extrapulmonary coccidioidomycosis
Chronic cryptosporidiosis
Cytomegalovirus disease (other than liver, spleen or nodes)
HIV-related encephalopathy
Chronic or extensive *Herpes simplex* infection
Disseminated or extrapulmonary
Histoplasmosis
Kaposi sarcoma
Burkitt's lymphoma (or equivalent)
Immunoblastic lymphoma (or equivalent)
Cerebral lymphoma
Extrapulmonary *Mycobacterium avium-intracellulare* complex
Mycobacterium tuberculosis
Any other disseminated mycobacterial infection
Pneumocystis carinii pneumonia
Recurrent pneumonia
Progressive multifocal leucoencephalopathy (PML)
Recurrent salmonella septicaemia
Cerebral toxoplasmosis
HIV wasting syndrome

Important indicator conditions in HIV infection included in the AIDS Surveillance Case Definition.

In very late HIV infection, when the CD4 count has fallen below 50 cells per mm^{-3}, infection with CYTOMEGALOVIRUS may produce progressive RETINAL necrosis which will lead to blindness if untreated and a variety of gastrointestinal symptoms. At this stage, infection with atypical MYCOBACTERIA is also common, producing severe anaemia, wasting and fevers. The commonest tumour associated with HIV is Kaposi's sarcoma which produces purplish skin lesions. This and non-Hodgkins' lymphoma (see MALIGNANT LYMPHOMA), which is a hundred times more frequent than in the general population, are likely to be associated with or caused by opportunistic ONCOGENIC viral infections.

Treatment This includes rapid and adequate treatment of ulcerative sexually transmitted diseases and an appreciation that the spread of HIV is by sexual contact and that this can be reduced by using condoms. Over the past few years the treatment of HIV itself has been revolutionized as a result of understanding that drug failure is due to the development of quasi-viral species resistant to therapy and thus drugs should always be used in combination. Effective means of monitoring drug therapy using plasma viral load have been developed as have new potent proteinases against HIV. Three classes of drugs are currently in use. Nucleoside analogues, including ZIDOVUDINE and DIDANOSINE, interfere with the activity of the unique enzyme of the retrovirus reverse transcriptase which is essential for replication. Non-nucleoside reverse transcriptase inhibitors, such as nevirapine, act by a different mechanism on the same enzyme. The most potent single agents against HIV are the proteinase inhibitors which render a unique viral enzyme ineffective. These three classes of drugs are used in a variety of combinations in an attempt to reduce the plasma HIV viral load to below detectable limits, which is achieved in approximately 90 per cent of patients who have not previously received therapy. This usually also produces a profound rise in CD4 count. It is likely, however, that such treatments needs to be lifelong, they are associated with toxicities and long-term adherence is difficult. Thus the optimum time for treatment intervention remains controversial, some clinicians believing that this should be governed by the viral load rising above 10,000 copies and others believing that treatment is very difficult to take long term and should primarily be designed to prevent the development of opportunistic infections; thus initiation of therapy should be guided more by the CD4 count.

Recent studies have also shown that giving zidovudine during pregnancy can halve the rate of perinatal transmission of HIV infection and it is likely that similar combinations to those used above will, in the future, prove even more effective. Short regimes of treatment in late pregnancy in Thailand have been shown to be almost as efficacious as the more complex regimes currently used in the developed world.

AIR   The general constituents of air are:

	per cent
Oxygen	20·94
Nitrogen	78·09
Argon	0·94
Carbon dioxide	0·03

Besides these there are always ozone, minerals and organic matter in small and variable amounts, and more or less water vapour according to the weather. In the air of towns, sulphurous acid and sulphuretted hydrogen are important impurities derived from combustion. After air has been respired once, the oxygen falls by about 4 per cent and the carbonic acid rises to about 4 per cent, while organic matter and water vapour are greatly increased and the air rises in temperature. The cause of the discomfort felt in badly ventilated rooms and crowded halls is associated with the increase in the temperature and moisture of the air, but a high percentage of carbon dioxide may be present without causing any noticeable discomfort or appreciable quickening of the respiration. A combination of hot weather and emissions from vehicles and fossil fuel combustion produces pollutants linked to a rise in the incidence of asthma and other cardiorespiratory conditions. Falling levels of ozone in the upper atmosphere are also believed to contribute to global warming because ozone screens the earth from most of the sun's harmful ultraviolet radiation.

AIR EMBOLISM   A bubble of air in a blood vessel that affects the flow of blood from the heart. Air may enter the circulation after injury, infusions into the venous circulation, or surgery. The victim suffers breathlessness, chest discomfort, and acute heart failure.

AIR PASSAGES   These are the nose, pharynx or throat (the large cavity behind the nose and mouth), larynx, trachea or windpipe, and bronchi or bronchial tubes. The air, on entering the nose, passes through a high narrow passage on each side, the outer wall of which has three projections (the nasal conchae). It

1	airflow	5	eustachian tube
2	tongue	6	epiglottis
3	larynx	7	oesophagus
4	trachea		

Vertical section through the middle of the head and neck showing the upper air passages.

passes down into the pharynx where the food and air passages meet and cross. The larynx lies in front of the lower part of the pharynx and is the organ where the voice is produced (see VOICE AND SPEECH) by aid of the vocal cords. The opening between the cords is called the glottis, and shortly after passing this the air reaches the trachea or wind-pipe.

This leads into the chest and divides above the heart into two bronchi, one of which goes to each lung, in which it splits into finer and finer tubes (see LUNGS). The larynx is enclosed in two strong cartilages, the thyroid (of which the most projecting part, the Adam's apple, is a prominent point on the front of the neck) and the cricoid (which can be felt as a hard ring about an inch below). Beneath this, the trachea, which is stiffened by rings of cartilage, so that it is never closed in any position of the body, can be traced down till it disappears behind the breast-bone.

AIR-SICKNESS   This condition is very similar to sea-sickness. (See MOTION SICKNESS.)

AKINESIA   Loss, or impairment, of voluntary movement, or immobility. It is characteristically seen in PARKINSONISM.

ALASTRIM, or VARIOLA MINOR, is a form of smallpox which differs from ordinary smallpox in being milder and having a low mortality.

ALBENDAZOLE   A drug adjunct to surgery in the treatment of hydatid cysts caused by *Taenia echinococcus*, a small tapeworm (see TAENIASIS). If surgery is not possible, albendazole can be used on its own. The drug is also used to treat STRONGYLOIDIASIS.

ALBINISM   A group of inherited disorders characterized by absence or decrease of melanin in the skin, hair and eyes. The skin is pink, the hair white or pale yellow and the iris translucent. NYSTAGMUS, PHOTOPHOBIA, SQUINT and poor eyesight are common. Photoprotection of skin and eyes is essential. In the tropics, light-induced skin cancer may develop early.

ALBUMINS are water-soluble proteins. They enter into the composition of all the tissues of the body. Albumins are generally divided according to their source of origin, as muscle-albumin, milk-albumin, blood- or serum-albumin, egg-albumin, vegetable-albumin, etc. These differ both in chemical reactions and also physiologically. Serum albumin occurs in blood plasma where it is important in maintaining plasma volume.

When taken into the stomach they are all converted into a soluble form by the process of DIGESTION, and are then absorbed into the blood, whence they go to build up the tissues. Albumin is synthesized in the liver and in chronic liver disease this process is seriously affected. (See PROTEINURIA; KIDNEYS, DISEASES OF: glomerulonephritis.)

ALBUMINURIA (see PROTEINURIA).

ALCOHOL   A colourless liquid, also called ethanol or ethylalcohol, produced by the fermentation of carbohydrates by yeast. Medically, it is used as a solvent and an antiseptic. Recreationally, it is a widely used drug, taken in alcoholic drinks to give a pleasant taste and to relax, reduce inhibitions, and increase sociability. In moderate dose (see table) it seems to be safe and, indeed, research published in 1998 suggests that two or three standard drinks or units a day may reduce mortality from cardiovascular disease by 35 per cent and from cancer by 20 per cent. In larger doses, however, alcohol causes much mental and physical harm.

Alcohol depresses the central nervous system and disturbs both mental and physical functioning. Drunkenness causes slurred speech, muddled thinking, amnesia, drowsiness, erectile impotence, poor co-ordination, and dulled reactions – thereby making driving or operating machinery dangerous. Disinhibition may lead to extreme euphoria, irritability, misery, or aggression, depending on the underlying mood at the start of drinking. Severe intoxication may lead to coma and respiratory failure.

Persistent alcohol misuse leads to physical, mental, social, and occupational problems, as well as a risk of dependency. Misuse may follow several patterns – regular but controlled heavy intake, binge drinking, and dependence (alcoholism). The first pattern usually leads to mainly physical problems such as gastritis, peptic ulcer, liver disease, heart disease, and impotence. The second is commonest among young men and usually leads to mainly social and occupational problems – getting into fights, jeopardizing personal relationships, overspending on alcohol at weekends, and missing days off work because of hangovers. The third pattern – alcohol dependence – is the most serious, and can severely disrupt health and social stability.

Many researchers consider alcohol dependence to be an illness that runs in families, with a genetic component which is probably passed on as a vulnerable personality. But it is hard to disentangle genetic, environmental, and social factors in such families.

Alcohol causes tolerance and both physical and psychological dependence (see DRUG ADDICTION for definitions). Dependent drinkers classically drink early in the morning to relieve overnight withdrawal symptoms. These symptoms include anxiety, restlessness, nausea and vomiting, and tremor. Sudden withdrawal from regular heavy drinking can lead to life-threatening delirium tremens (DTs), with severe tremor, hallucinations (often visual – seeing spiders and monsters, rather than the pink elephants of romantic myth), and convulsions. This must be treated urgently with sedative drugs, preferably by intravenous drip. Similar symptoms, plus severe incoordination and double vision can occur in WERNICKE'S ENCEPHALOPATHY, a serious neurological condition due to lack of the B vitamin thiamine (whose absorption from the stomach is markedly reduced by alcohol). If not treated urgently with injections of thiamine and other vitamins, this can lead to an irreversible form of brain damage called Korsakoff's psychosis, with severe amnesia. Finally, prolonged alcohol misuse can cause a form of dementia.

In addition to these severe neurological disorders, the wide range of life-threatening problems caused by heavy drinking includes HEPATITIS, liver CIRRHOSIS, PANCREATITIS, gastrointestinal haemorrhage, fetal alcohol syndrome, and suicide. The social effects of alcohol misuse – such as marital breakdown, family violence, and severe debt – can be equally devastating.

Treatment of alcohol-related problems is only moderately successful. First, many of the physical problems are treated in the short term by doctors who fail to spot or never ask about heavy drinking. Second, attempts at treating alcohol dependence by detoxification or drying out (substituting a tranquillizing drug for alcohol and withdrawing it gradually over about a week) are not always followed up by adequate support at home, and drinking starts again. Home support by community alcohol teams comprising doctors, nurses, social workers and, when appropriate, probation officers is a recent development that may have better results. Many drinkers find the voluntary organization Alcoholics Anonymous (AA) and its related groups for relatives (Al-Anon) and teenagers (Alateen) helpful because total abstinence from alcohol is encouraged by intensive psychological and social support from fellow ex-drinkers.

---

1 standard drink = 1 unit
                 = ½ pint of beer
                 = 1 measure of spirits
                 = 1 glass of sherry or vermouth
                 = 1 glass of wine

Limits within which alcohol is believed not to cause long-term health risks:

Women up to 2 units a day, 14 a week

(Pregnant women should avoid alcohol completely. If this is too difficult, 1 unit a day seems to be safe for the baby.)

Men up to 3 units a day, 21 a week

Women absorb alcohol more quickly than men.

Useful contacts are Alcoholics Anonymous, Al-Anon Family Groups UK and Eire (including Alateen), Alcohol Concern, Scottish Council on Alcohol, and Accept (community services for problem drinkers and tranquillizer misusers) (see APPENDIX 2: ADDRESSES).

ALCURONIUM is a drug which relaxes voluntary muscles. Given by injection during anaesthesia to relax a patient undergoing surgery, the drug may delay the restart of spontaneous breathing.

ALDOSTERONE is a hormone secreted by the adrenal cortex (see ADRENAL GLANDS). It plays an important part in maintaining the electrolyte balance of the body by promoting the reabsorption of sodium and the secretion of potassium by the renal tubules. It is thus of primary importance in controlling the volume of the body fluids.

ALEXIA is another name for word-blindness. (See APHASIA; DYSLEXIA.)

ALFACALCIDOL is a synthetic form (or analogue) of vitamin D. (See APPENDIX 5: VITAMINS.)

ALGESIMETER is an instrument used in measuring the sensitiveness of areas of the skin.

ALGLUCERASE A drug used under specialist supervision for the rare hereditary disorder GAUCHER'S DISEASE.

ALIMENTARY CANAL (see GASTROINTESTINAL TRACT).

ALKALI A substance which neutralizes an acid to form a salt, and turns litmus and other vegetable dyes blue. Alkalis are generally oxides or carbonates of metals.

ALKALOIDS Substances found commonly in various plants. They are natural nitrogenous organic bases and combine with acids to form crystalline salts. Among alkaloids, morphine was discovered in 1805, strychnine in 1818, quinine and caffeine in 1820, nicotine in 1829, atropine in 1833. Only a few alkaloids occur in the animal kingdom, the outstanding example being adrenaline, which is formed in the medulla of the suprarenal, or adrenal, gland. Alkaloids are often used for medicinal purposes. The name of an alkaloid ends in 'ine' (in Latin *ina*).

Neutral principals are crystalline substances with actions similar to those of alkaloids but having a neutral reaction. The name of a neutral principal ends in 'in', e.g. digitalin, aloin.

The following are the more important alkaloids, with their source plants:

Aconite, *from Monkshood.*
Atropine, *from Belladonna* (juice of Deadly Nightshade).
Cocaine, *from Coca leaves.*
Hyoscine, *from Henbane.*
Morphine, Codeine, *from Opium* (juice of Poppy).
Thebaine, Nicotine, *from Tobacco.*
Physostigmine, *from Calabar bean.*
Pilocarpine, *from Jaborandi leaves.*
Quinidine, *from Cinchona or Peruvian bark.*
Strychnine, *from Nux Vomica seeds.*

ALKALOSIS means an increase in the alkalinity of the blood, or, more accurately, a decrease in the concentration of hydrogen ions in the blood. It occurs, for example, in patients who have had large doses of alkalis for the treatment of gastric ulcer. (see ACID BASE BALANCE; ACIDOSIS.)

ALKAPTONURIA (see OCHRONOSIS).

ALKYLATING AGENTS are so named because they alkylate or react with certain biochemical entities, particularly those concerned with the synthesis of NUCLEIC ACID. Alkylation is the substitution of an organic grouping in place of another grouping in a molecule.

The importance of the alkylating agents in medicine is that by interfering with the growth of cells they have proved of value in the treatment of various forms of malignant disease. Unfortunately they interfere with the growth of normal cells as well as malignant cells, and this restricts their use to a considerable extent.

Nevertheless several of them, including MUSTINE and THIOTEPA have proved of considerable value in the chemotherapy of malignant disease.

ALLANTOIN Prepared synthetically, this powder, which occurs naturally in comfrey root, has been used as an adjuvant in the treatment of skin ulcers. It has been thought to stimulate the formation of the surface epithelial layer of skin, but its therapeutic value is now more dubious

ALLANTOIS A vascular structure which, very early in the life of the embryo, grows out from its hind-gut. The end becomes attached to the wall of the womb. It spreads out at the end, becomes stalked, and develops later into the placenta and umbilical cord (see PLACENTA), which forms the only connection between the mother and embryo.

ALLELE or ALLELOMORPH A GENE which may exist in one or more forms, only one of which can occur in a given CHROMOSOME. Two alleles of a given gene are at the same relative positions on a pair of homologous (similarly structured) chromosomes. If the two alleles are identical the subject is homozygous for the gene – namely, the genes will exert a unaminous influence on a particular characteristic. If the alleles are different – with one having a dominant and the other a recessive influence – the subject is heterozygous. (See GENES.)

ALLERGEN Any substance, usually a protein, which, taken into the body, makes the body hypersensitive or 'allergic' to it. Thus in hay fever the allergen is pollen. (See ALLERGY).

ALLERGY A term generally used to describe an adverse reaction to any substance which the affected individual ingests, inhales, or touches. Strictly, allergy refers to reactions incited by an abnormal immunological response to an allergen. Susceptibility has a strong genetic component and is usually initiated by a high immunoglobulin E response (see IMMUNITY) to substances such as insect venom, egg proteins, peanuts, and grass pollen. Severe reactions are often termed ANAPHYLAXIS which may be local or systemic. Other immune mechanisms also contribute to allergic disorders. However adverse reactions to drugs, diagnostic materials, and other substances often do not involve recognized immunological mechanisms when the term 'hypersitivity' is preferable.

Adverse reactions may manifest themselves as URTICARIA wheezing or difficulty in breathing owing to spasm of the BRONCHIOLES, swollen joints, nausea and headaches. Severe allergic reactions may cause a person to go into SHOCK. Prevention is the best treatment with the sensitive individual avoiding the food or other factor such as pollen known to cause an allergic reaction. This may require extensive testing to establish the allergen. Sometimes an allergy may be cured by desensitizing the individual with small doses of the allergen (see IMMUNOTHERAPY). Severe allergic symptoms may require treatment with SYMPATHOMIMETIC DRUGS such as adrenaline, with ANTIHISTAMINES or with steroids. Expert medical attention is needed for patients with severe reactions.

ALLOCHEIRIA The name for a disorder of sensation in which sensations are referred to the wrong part of the body.

ALLOGRAFT A piece of tissue or an organ, such as the kidney, transplanted from one to another of the same species: e.g. from man to man. It is also known as a homograft.

ALLOPATHY A term applied sometimes by homoeopathists to the methods used by regular practitioners of medicine and surgery. The term literally means curing by inducing a different kind of action in the body, and is an erroneous designation.

ALLOPURINOL A drug used to treat gout. It acts by suppressing the formation of uric acid. It is also being used in treatment of uric acid stone in the kidney.

ALOPECIA means hair loss. It may be localized or total in the scalp. The commonest type, which is hereditary, is male baldness (androgenic alopecia). Female balding spares the anterior hair line, develops later, and is less severe than the male variety. Diffuse hair loss is common after childbirth, severe illness or infection (telogen alopecia). It begins 8 to 12 weeks after the causative event, and recovery is complete. Persistent diffuse hair loss may be caused by severe iron deficiency or hypothyroidism, or may be drug-induced.

Patchy localized hair loss is commonly caused by fungal infections (tinea capitis), especially in the tropics. It may also be due to trauma, e.g. hair pulling by children or disturbed adults, or hair-straightening by African or Afrocaribbean women (traction alopecia). Rarely, diseases of the scalp skin such as discoid lupus erythematosus (see LUPUS) or lichen planus (see LICHEN) may cause patchy alopecia with scarring which is irreversible. The long-term effects of radiotherapy may be similar.

Treatment depends on the cause. Specific antifungal drugs cure tinea capitis. Correction of THYROID or IRON deficiency may be dramatic. Male baldness may be modified slightly by long-term use of minoxidil lotion, or improved permanently by various types of hair-follicle grafting of transplants from the occipital scalp. Female balding may be amenable to anti-ANDROGEN/OESTROGEN regimens but severe forms require a wig.

ALOPECIA AREATA is a common form of reversible hair loss which may be patchy, total on the scalp, eyebrows or eyelashes, or universal on the body. The onset is sudden at any age and the affected scalp skin looks normal. The hair follicles remain intact but 'switched off' and usually hair growth recovers spontaneously. No consistently effective treatment is available but CORTICOSTEROID injections with a spray gun into the scalp may be useful. The regrown hair may be white at first but pigmentation recovers later.

ALPHA FETOPROTEIN A protein produced in the gut and liver of the fetus. Abnormality in the fetus, such as neural tube defect, may result in raised levels of alpha fetoprotein in the maternal blood. In DOWN'S SYNDROME levels may be abnormally low. In either case screening of the pregnancy should be done, including AMNIOCENTESIS to check the amount of alpha fetoprotein in the amniotic fluid. The protein may also be produced in some abnormal tissues in the adult, for example, in patients with liver cancer.

ALTERNATIVE MEDICINE (see COMPLEMENTARY MEDICINE).

ALTITUDE SICKNESS This condition, also known as mountain sickness, occurs in mountain climbers or hikers who have climbed too quickly to heights above 3000 m, thus failing to allow their bodies to acclimatize to altitude. The lower atmospheric pressure and shortage of oxygen result in hyperventilation – deep, quick breathing – and this reduces the amount of carbon dioxide in the blood. Nausea, anxiety, and exhaustion are presenting symptoms and seriously affected individuals may be acutely breathless because of pulmonary oedema (excess fluid in the lungs). Gradual climbing over two or three days should prevent mountain sickness. In serious cases the individual must be brought down to hospital as a matter of urgency. Most attacks, however, are mild.

ALVEOLITIS means inflammation of the alveoli (see ALVEOLUS) of the lungs caused by an allergic reaction. When the inflammation is caused by infection it is called PNEUMONIA and when by a chemical or physical agent it is called pneumonitis. It may be associated with systemic sclerosis or RHEUMATOID ARTHRITIS.

Extrinsic allergic alveolitis is the condition induced by the lungs becoming allergic (see ALLERGY) to various factors or substances. It includes BAGASSOSIS, FARMER'S LUNG, MUSHROOM-WORKER'S LUNG and BUDGERIGAR-FANCIER'S LUNG. It is characterized by the onset of shortness of breath, tightness of the chest, cough and fever. The onset may be sudden or gradual. Treatment consists of removal of the affected individual from the offending material to which he has become allergic. CORTICOSTEROIDS give temporary relief.

Fibrosing alveolitis In this disease there is diffuse fibrosis of the walls of the alveoli of the lungs. This causes loss of lung volume with both forced expiratory volume and vital capacity affected but the ratio between them remaining normal. The patient complains of cough and progressive dyspnoea. Typically the patient will be cyanosed, clubbed, and have crackles in the mid and lower lung fields. Blood gases will reveal HYPOXIA and, in early disease, hypocaphia (due to hyperventilation). There is an association with RHEUMATOID ARTHRITIS (about one-eighth of cases), systemic LUPUS ERYTHAMATOSUS, and systemic sclerosis. Certain drugs, e.g., bleomycin, busulphan, hexamethonium, high concentrations of oxygen, and inhalation of cadmium fumes may also cause this condition.

ALVEOLUS (1) The minute divisions of glands and the air sacs of the lungs. (2) The sockets of the teeth in the jawbone.

ALZHEIMER'S DISEASE is a progressive degenerating process of neural tissue affecting mainly the frontal and temporal lobes of the BRAIN in middle and late life. There is probably a genetic component to Alzheimer's disease, but early-onset Alzheimer's is linked to certain MUTATIONS in three particular genes. Examination of affected brains shows 'senile plaques' containing an AMYLOID-like material distributed throughout an atrophied CORTEX. Many remaining neurons show changes in their NEUROFIBRILS which thicken and twist into 'neurofibrillary tangles'. First symptoms are psychological with insidious impairment of recent memory and disorientation in time and space. This becomes increasingly associated with difficulties in judgment, comprehension and abstract reasoning. After very few years progressive neurological deterioration produces poor gait, immobility and death. After assessment has found no other organic cause for an affected individual's symptoms, treatment is primarily palliative. Recently, however, donepezil, a reversible inhibitor of anticholinesterase, has been introduced for the symptomatic treatment of mild to moderate dementia in patients with Alzheimer's. It helps about 4 in 10 sufferers (see DEMENTIA). See APPENDIX 2: ADDRESSES.

AMANTADINE A drug used to treat certain virus infections which is also of value in the prevention of some forms of influenza. It is also used to treat PARKINSONISM.

AMAUROSIS FUGAX Sudden transitory impairment, or loss of, vision. It usually affects only one eye, and is commonly due to circulatory failure. In its simplest form it occurs in normal people on rising suddenly from the sitting or recumbent position, when it is due to the effects of gravity. It also occurs in migraine. A not uncommon cause, particularly in elderly people, is transient ocular ischaemia (see ISCHAEMIA), resulting from blockage of the circulation to the retina (see EYE) by emboli (see EMBOLISM) from the common carotid artery or the heart. Treatment in this last group of cases consists of control of the blood pressure if this is raised, as it often is in such cases; the administration of drugs that reduce the stickiness of blood platelets such as aspirin. In some instances removal of the part of the carotid artery from which the emboli are coming may be indicated.

AMBIVALENCE   The psychological state in which a person concurrently hates and loves the same object or person.

AMBLYOPIA   Defective vision for which no recognizable cause exists in any part of the eye. It may be due to such causes as defective development or excessive use of tobacco or alcohol. The most important form is that associated with SQUINTING, or gross difference in refraction between the two eyes. It has been estimated that in Britain around 5 per cent of young adults have amblyopia due to this cause.

AMELIA   This is absence of the limbs, usually a congenital defect.

AMENORRHOEA   Absence of the menstrual flow during the time of life at which it should occur. (See MENSTRUATION.) If menstruation has never occurred the amenorrhoea is termed primary. If it ceases after having once become established it is known as secondary amenorrhoea. The only value of these terms is that some patients with either chromosome abnormalities or malformations of the genital tract fall into the primary category. Otherwise the age of onset of symptoms is more important.

The causes of amenorrhoea are numerous and treatment requires dealing with the primary cause. The commonest cause of amenorrhoea is pregnancy. HYPOTHALAMIC disorders such as psychological stress or ANOREXIA NERVOSA also cause amenorrhoea. Poor nutrition or loss of weight by dieting may cause it and any serious underlying disease such as tuberculosis or malaria may also result in the cessation of periods. The excess secretion of prolactin, whether this is the result of a micro-adenoma (see ADENOMA) of the PITUITARY GLAND or whether it is drug induced will cause amenorrhoea and possibly GALACTORRHOEA as well. Malfunction of the pituitary gland will result in a failure to produce the GONADOTROPHIC hormones with consequent amenorrhea. Excessive production of cortisol, as in CUSHING'S SYNDROME, or of androgens, as in the adreno-genital syndrome or the POLYCYSTIC OVARY syndrome, will result in amenorrhoea. Amenorrhoea occasionally

follows the use of the oral contraceptive pill and may be associated with both HYPOTHYROIDISM and obesity. It is thus important to take a careful history with emphasis on psychological factors, weight fluctuations and the use of drugs that may stimulate the release of PROLACTIN, and it is also important to look for evidence of VIRILIZATION.

A gynaecological examination is necessary in primary amenorrhoea to exclude malformations of the genital tract. Estimations of the gonadotrophic hormone levels will reveal whether the amenorrhoea is primary ovarian failure or secondary to pituitary disease. In view of the frequent psychosomatic origins of amenorrhoea, reassurance of the patient is of great importance, in particular with reference to marriage and the ability to conceive. When weight loss is the cause of amenorrhoea restoration of body weight alone can result in spontaneous menstruation. Patients with raised concentrations of serum GONADOTROPHIN hormones have primary ovarian failure. It is not amenable to treatment. Cyclical OESTROGEN/PROGESTOGEN therapy will usually establish withdrawal bleeding. If the amenorrhoea is due to mild pituitary failure menstruation may return after treatment with clomiphene. Clomiphene is a non-steroidal agent which competes for oestrogen receptors in the hypothalamus. The patients who are most likely to respond to clomiphene are those who have some evidence of endogenous oestrogen and gonadotrophin production.

AMENTIA   is the failure of the intellectual faculties to develop normally.

AMETHOCAINE   An effective local anaesthetic for topical application. Rapidly absorbed from mucous membranes, it should never be applied to inflamed, traumatized, or highly vascular surfaces. It should not be used when providing anaesthesia for bronchoscopy or cystoscopy. It is used in ophthalmology and in skin preparations. It may sensitize the skin. (see ANAESTHESIA.)

AMETROPIA (see REFRACTION).

AMIODARONE HYDROCHLORIDE   This drug is used to treat tachycardia associated with a congenital abnormality of heart rhythm known as the Wolff-Parkinson-White syndrome. It is used only under hospital or specialist supervision and has troublesome side-effects.

AMIKACIN   An AMINOGLYCOSIDE that is a semi-synthetic derivative of KANAMYCIN which is used to treat infections caused by micro-organisms resistant to GENTAMICIN and TOBRAMYCIN.

AMILORIDE   A diuretic that acts without causing excessive loss of potassium (see DIURETICS).

AMINES Substances derived from ammonia or AMINO-ACIDS which play an important part in the working of the body, including the brain and the circulatory system. They include ADRENALINE, NORADRENALINE and HISTAMINE. (See also MONOAMINE OXIDASE INHIBITORS.)

AMINO-ACIDS Chemical compounds that are the basic building blocks of all proteins. Each molecule consists of nitrogenous amino and acidic carboxyl groups of atoms joined to a group of carbon atoms. Polypeptides are formed by amino-acid molecules linking via peptide bonds. Many polypeptides link up in various configurations to form protein molecules. In humans proteins are made up from 20 different amino-acids. Eight of these are labelled essential amino-acids because the body cannot manufacture them and is dependent on the diet for their provision.

AMINOCAPROIC ACID A drug used to treat hereditary angioedema, a serious anaphylactic reaction of the skin and respiratory tract resulting from a deficiency in the body's immunological defence mechanisms. (See URTICARIA.)

AMINOGLUTETHIMIDE A drug that inhibits the synthesis of adrenal corticorteroids. It is proving of value in the treatment of cancer of the breast in post-menopausal women.

AMINOGLYCOSIDES A group of antibiotics usually reserved for use in patients with severe infections. They are effective against a wide range of BACTERIA including some gram-positive and many gram-negative organisms. Aminoglycosides must be used cautiously because they can damage the inner ear, thus affecting hearing, and the kidneys. Examples of this group are AMIKACIN and GENTAMICIN (effective against *Pseudomonas aeuriginosa*), neomycin (used only for topical administration for skin infections), and streptomycin (effective in combination with other drugs against *Mycobacterium tuberculosis*).

AMINOPHYLLINE A combination of theophylline and ethyl-enediamine. It is used in the treatment of bronchial asthma.

AMIODARONE A drug used under specialist supervision to control certain abnormal heart rhythms.

AMITRIPTYLINE (see ANTIDEPRESSANTS).

AMMONIA A compound of hydrogen and nitrogen that occurs naturally. The solution is colourless with a pungent smell; it is used in urine testing. In humans certain inherited defects in the metabolism of ammonia can cause neurological symptoms including mental retardation.

AMNESIA means loss of memory.

AMNIOCENTESIS A diagnostic procedure for detecting abnormalities of the FETUS. Usually done between the 16th and 18th weeks of pregnancy, amniocentesis is performed by piercing the amniotic sac in the pregnant uterus with a hollow needle and withdrawing a sample of AMNIOTIC FLUID for laboratory analysis. As well as checking for the presence of abnormal fetal cells the procedure can show the sex of the fetus. The risk of early rupture of the fetal membranes or of miscarriage is low (around 0.5 per cent).

AMNION is the tough fibrous membrane which lines the cavity of the womb during pregnancy, and contains from 0.5 to 1 litre (one to two pints) of fluid in which the embryo floats. It is formed from the ovum along with the embryo, and in labour the part of it at the mouth of the womb forms the 'bag of waters'. (See LABOUR.) When a child is 'born with a caul', the caul is a piece of amnion. (See CAUL.)

AMNIOSCOPY The insertion of a viewing instrument (amnioscope) through the abdominal wall into the pregnant uterus to examine the inside of the amniotic sac. The growing fetus can be viewed directly and its condition and sex assessed without disturbing the pregnancy. The amniotic sac may also be viewed late in pregnancy through the cervix or neck of the womb using an instrument called the fetoscope.

AMNIOTIC FLUID The clear fluid contained within the amnion that surrounds the fetus in the womb and protects it from external pressure. The fluid, mainly water, is produced by the amnion and is regularly circulated, being swallowed by the fetus and excreted through the kidneys back into the amniotic sac. By the 35th week of pregnancy there is about one litre of fluid but this falls to half a litre at term. The amniotic sac normally ruptures in early labour releasing the fluid or 'waters'.

AMNIOTIC SAC (see AMNION).

AMOEBA A minute protozoan organism consisting of a single cell, in which a nucleus is surrounded by protoplasm that changes its shape as the protozoon progresses or absorbs nourishment. Several varieties are found under different conditions within the human body. One variety, *Entamoeba coli*, is found in the large intestine of man without any associated disease; another, *Entamoeba gingivalis*, is found in the sockets of the teeth associated with pyorrhoea; another, *Entamoeba histolytica*, is the causative organism of amoebic dysentery (see DYSENTERY). Two, *Acanthamoeba* and *Naegleria fowleri*, cause the infection of the brain known as MENINGOENCEPHALITIS. *Enta-*

moeba histolytica may also cause meningoencephalitis. Other forms are found in the genital organs.

AMOEBIASIS (see DYSENTERY).

AMOXYCILLIN (see PENICILLIN, ANTIBIOTIC).

AMPHETAMINES A group of drugs closely related to adrenaline which act by stimulating the sympathetic nervous system. When taken by mouth they have a profound stimulating effect on the brain, producing a sense of well-being and confidence and seemingly increasing the capacity for mental work. They are, however, drugs of dependence and their medical use is now strictly limited, for example, to the treatment of narcolepsy.

Because they inhibit appetite, they rapidly achieved a reputation for slimming purposes, but they should not be used for this purpose. The dangers of amphetamines far outweigh their advantages.

AMPHORIC An adjective denoting the kind of breathing heard over a cavity in the lung. The sound is like that made by blowing over the mouth of a narrow-necked vase.

AMPHOTERICIN A highly toxic polygenic antifungal drug that must be given only under close medical supervision and for severe systemic fungal infections. It is not absorbed from the gut so is normally given PARENTERALLY. Oral and intestinal candidiasis (see candida) can, however, be treated with amphotericin tablets.

AMPICILLIN (see PENICILLIN, ANTIBIOTIC).

AMPOULE A small glass container having one end drawn out into a point capable of being sealed so as to preserve its contents sterile. It is used for containing solutions for hypodermic injection.

AMPULLA OF VATER The dilated section of the common bile duct when it is joined by the duct from the PANCREAS (see diagram on page 319).

AMPUTATION Severance of a limb, or part of a limb from the rest of the body. The leg is the most common site of amputation. It is usually performed as a controlled operation and may be required for a variety of reasons. In the young, severe injury is the most common cause, when damage to the limb is so extensive as to make it non-viable or functionally useless. In the elderly, amputation is more often the result of vascular insufficiency, resulting in gangrene or intractable pain.

The aim is to restore the patient to full mobility with a prosthetic (artificial) limb, which requires both a well-fitting PROSTHESIS and a well-healed surgical wound. If this is not

1 above knee
2 below knee
3 Syme's heel flap
4 midtarsal

Amputation sites of lower limb.

possible, the aim is to leave the patient with a limb stump that is still useful for balancing, sitting and transferring. Common types of lower-limb amputation are shown in the illustration. The Symes amputation can be walked upon without requiring a prosthesis. The below-knee amputation preserves normal flexion of the knee, and virtually normal walking can be achieved with a well-fitting artificial limb. Learning to walk is more difficult following an above-knee amputation, but some well-motivated patients can manage well. After any amputation it is not unusual for the patient to experience the sensation that the limb is still present. This is called a phantom limb and the sensation may persist for a long time. (See PROSTHESES, PHANTOM LIMB.)

AMSACRINE (see CYTOTOXIC).

AMYLASE An ENZYME in pancreatic juice which facilitates the conversion of starch to maltose. (See PANCREAS.)

AMYL NITRITE (Nitrate) A volatile, oily liquid prepared by the action of nitric and nitrous acids on amyl alcohol. It was used for many years to treat angina but has been superseded by other nitrate drugs such as glyceril trinitrate. The substance is misused by drug abusers to produce a 'high' and is referred to as 'poppers'.

AMYLOIDOSIS A rare condition in which deposits of complex protein, known as amyloid, are found in various parts of the body. It is a degenerative condition resulting from various causes such as chronic infection, including tuberculosis and rheumatoid arthritis.

AMYLOID PLAQUES Characteristic waxy deposits of amyloid found in primary amyloidosis, the cause of which is unknown.

AMYLOSE The name applied to any carbohydrate of the starch group.

ANABOLIC STEROIDS The nitrogen-retaining effect of androgen is responsible for the larger muscle mass of the male. This is called an anabolic effect. Attempts have been made to separate the anabolic effects of hormones from their virilizing effects. This is only partially successful. Thus anabolic steroids have the property of protein building so that when taken they lead to an increase in muscle bulk and strength. All the anabolic steroids have some androgenic activity but they cause less virilization than androgens in women. Androgenic side-effects may result from any of these anabolic compounds, especially if they are given for prolonged periods. All these compounds should therefore be used with caution in women, and are contra-indicated in men with prostatic carcinoma. Jaundice due to stasis of bile in the intrahepatic canaliculi is a hazard, and the depression of pituitary gonadotrophin production is a possible complication.

Anabolic steroids have been used to stimulate protein anabolism in debilitating illness and to promote growth in children with pituitary dwarfism and other disorders associated with interference of growth. Stimulation of protein anabolism may also be of value in acute renal failure, and the retention of nitrogen and calcium is of probable benefit to patients with OSTEOPOROSIS and to patients receiving corticosteroid therapy. Anabolic steroids may stimulate bone marrow function in hypoplastic anaemia.

They have been widely abused by athletes and body builders aiming to improve their strength, stamina, speed or body size. However, there are considerable doubts over their efficacy, with little experimental evidence that they work. Dangerous adverse effects include precocious MYOCARDIAL INFARCTION, DIABETES, liver disease, precocious carcinoma of the PROSTATE, acne, and severe psychiatric disorders. Anabolic steroids should not be used by athletes, who face bans from official competitions if they do.

The anabolic steroids in therapeutic use include nandrolone and stanozolol.

ANAEMIA The condition characterized by inadequate red blood cells and/or haemoglobin in the blood. It is considered to exist if haemoglobin levels are below 13 grams per 100 ml in males and below 12 grams per 100 ml in adult non-pregnant women. No simple classification of anaemia can be wholly accurate, but the most useful method is to divide anaemias into: (*a*) microcytic hypochromic or iron deficiency anaemia, (*b*) megaloblastic hyperchromic anaemia, (*c*) aplastic anaemia, (*d*) haemolytic anaemia, (*e*) inherited anaemias. In Britain, anaemia is much more common among women than in men. Thus, around 10 per cent of girls have anaemia at the age of 15, whilst in adult life the incidence is over 30 per cent between the ages of 30 and 40, around 20 per cent at 50, and around 30 per cent at 70. Among men the incidence is under 5 per cent until the age of 50, and it then rises to 20 per cent at the age of 70. Ninety per cent of all cases of anaemia in Britain are microcytic, 7 per cent are macrocytic, and 3 per cent are haemolytic or aplastic. Inherited anaemias include SICKLE-CELL ANAEMIA; and THALASSAEMIA.

Microcytic hypochromic anaemia This corresponds to a large extent with what used to be known as 'secondary anaemia'. It takes its name from the characteristic changes in the blood.
CAUSES
Loss of blood
- As a result of trauma. This is perhaps the simplest example of all, when, as a result of an accident involving a large artery, there is severe haemorrhage.
- Menstruation. The regular monthly loss of blood which women sustain as a result of menstruation always puts a strain on the blood-forming organs. If this loss is excessive, then over a period of time it may lead to quite severe anaemia.
- Child-birth. A considerable amount of blood is always lost at child-birth, and if this is severe, or if the woman was anaemic during pregnancy, a severe degree of anaemia may develop.
- Bleeding from the gastro-intestinal tract. The best example here is anaemia due to 'bleeding piles' (see PILES). Such bleeding, even though slight, if maintained over a long period of time, is a common cause of anaemia in both men and women. The haemorrhage may be more acute and occur from a duodenal or gastric ulcer, when it is known as haematemesis.
- Certain blood diseases, such as PURPURA and HAEMOPHILIA, which are characterized by bleeding.
Defective blood formation
- This is the main cause of anaemia in infections. The micro-organism responsible for the infection has a deleterious effect upon the blood-forming organs, just as it does upon other parts of the body.
- Toxins. In conditions such as chronic glomerulonephritis and uraemia there is a severe anaemia due to the effect of the disease upon blood formation.
- Drugs. Certain drugs, such as aspirin and the non-steroidal anti-inflammatory drugs, may cause occult gastro-intestinal bleeding.

Inadequate intake of iron The daily require-ment of iron for an adult is 12 mg, and 15 to 20 mg during pregnancy. This is well covered by an ordinary diet, so that by itself it is not a common cause. But if there is a steady loss of blood, as a result of heavy menstrual loss or 'bleeding piles', the intake of iron in the diet may not be sufficient to maintain adequate formation of haemoglobin.

Inadequate absorption of iron This may occur in diseases of intestinal malabsorption.

In many cases the anaemia is found to be due to a combination of two or more of these causes. A severe form of this anaemia in women, known as chlorosis, used to be com-mon, but it is seldom seen nowadays.

SYMPTOMS These depend upon whether the anaemia is sudden in onset, as in severe haem-orrhage, or gradual. In all cases, however, the striking sign is pallor, the depth of which depends upon the severity of the anaemia. The colour of the skin may be misleading, except in cases due to severe haemorrhage, as the skin of many people is normally pale. The best guide is the colour of the internal lining of the eyelid. When the onset of the anaemia is sudden the patient complains of weakness and giddiness, and he loses consciousness if he tries to stand or sit up. The breathing is rapid and distressed, the pulse is rapid, and the blood-pressure is low. In chronic cases the tongue is often sore (glossitis), and the nails of the fingers may be brittle and concave instead of convex (koilony-chia). In some cases, particularly in women, the Plummer-Vinson syndrome is present. This consists of difficulty in swallowing and may be accompanied by huskiness; in these cases GLOS-SITIS is also present. There may be slight en-largement of the spleen, and there is usually some diminution in gastric acidity.

CHANGES IN THE BLOOD The characteristic change is a diminution in both the haemo-globin and the red cell content of the blood. There is a relatively greater fall in the haemo-globin than in the red cell count. If the blood is examined under a microscope the red cells are seen to be paler and smaller than normal. These small red cells are known as microcytes.

TREATMENT consists primarily of giving suffi-cient iron by mouth to restore, and then maintain, a normal blood picture. The main iron preparation now used is ferrous sulphate, 200 mg, thrice daily after meals. When the blood picture has become normal, the dosage is gradually reduced. A preparation of iron is available which can be given intravenously, but this is only used in cases which do not respond to iron given by mouth, or in cases in which it is essential to obtain a quick response.

If, of course, there is haemorrhage, this must be arrested, and if the loss of blood has been severe it may be necessary to give a blood transfusion. Care must be taken to ensure that the patient is having an adequate diet. If there is any underlying metabolic, oncological, toxic or infective condition, this, of course, must be adequately treated after appropriate in-vestigations.

Megaloblastic hyperchromic anaemia There are various forms of anaemia of this type, such as those due to nutritional deficiencies but the most important is that known as pernicious anaemia.

PERNICIOUS ANAEMIA Up until about seventy years ago its cause was unknown and it was an invariably fatal disease. In 1926, two Ameri-cans, G. R. Minot and W. P. Murphy, reported that pernicious anaemia responded to treat-ment with liver. This discovery ranks in impor-tance with that of insulin in the treatment of diabetes mellitus. This form of treatment is based upon the now well-proved fact that pernicious anaemia is due to lack of what is known as the intrinsic factor. For the forma-tion of normal red blood corpuscles a sub-stance known as the extrinsic factor is necessary. The efficient absorption of this factor into the body is dependent on the presence of intrinsic factor which is produced normally by the mucosa lining the distal part of the stomach. It is the inability of the patient to produce the intrinsic factor that leads to the onset of pernicious anaemia. In a normal person with adequate amounts of intrinsic factor, approxi-mately 70 per cent of the extrinsic factor (which is vitamin B_{12} and is present in meat and other foods) in the daily diet is absorbed into the body. In patients with pernicious anaemia, however, less than 2 per cent is absorbed.

Symptoms Pernicious anaemia is a disease of middle age, being rare under the age of 40 years. It affects both men and women. The onset is usually insidious, so that the anaemia is usually well developed before medical advice is sought. In addition to the general symptoms and signs already described in the section on microcytic anaemia, the important features of pernicious anaemia are as follows. The patient, who is often prematurely grey-haired, has a characteristic lemon-yellow complexion. The tongue is often sore and appears thinner, smoother, and redder than usual. There is often soreness and excoriation of the corners of the mouth – a condition known as cheilosis. There may be slight enlargement of the spleen. There is a complete absence of free hydrochlo-ric acid in the stomach, even after the injection of histamine.

One of the most serious complications of pernicious anaemia is a disease with the cum-bersome title of SUBACUTE COMBINED DEGENERA-TION OF THE CORD. This, as the name indicates, is a degenerative condition of the spinal cord, and the importance of recognizing its onset is that it can be cured by adequate treatment of the anaemia. Its early manifestations are a sensation of tingling or 'pins and needles' in the legs, accompanied by stiffness. Later, if un-treated, the stiffness becomes progressively worse, finally leading to paralysis.

Changes in the blood The red cells are larger than normal, i.e. macrocytes and they appear to be redder than normal. They also vary in shape (poikilocytosis) and in size (anisocytosis). Occasionally a few primitive red cells (normoblasts) may be found. The total white cell count is diminished: i.e. there is leucopenia. The final diagnosis depends upon an examination of the bone marrow, which is found to contain megaloblasts.

Treatment consists of the administration of vitamin B_{12} in the form of hydroxocobalamin. It is given by injection. It must always be remembered that a patient with pernicious anaemia requires to take vitamin B_{12} for the rest of his or her life.

Aplastic anaemia is a disease in which the red blood corpuscles are very greatly reduced and in which no attempt appears to be made in the bone marrow towards their regeneration. It is more accurately called hypoplastic anaemia as the degree of impairment of bone marrow function is rarely complete. The cause in many cases is not known, but in rather less than half the cases the condition is due to some toxic substance, such as benzol or certain drugs, or ionizing radiations. The patient becomes very pale, with a tendency to haemorrhages under the skin and mucous membranes, and the temperature may at times be raised. The red blood corpuscles diminish steadily in numbers. Treatment consists primarily of regular blood transfusions. Although the disease is often fatal, the outlook has improved in recent years. About 25 per cent of patients recover when adequately treated, and others survive for several years. In severe cases promising results are being reported from the use of bone marrow transplantation.

Haemolytic anaemia results from the excessive destruction, or HAEMOLYSIS , of the red blood cells. This haemolysis may be due to undue fragility of the red blood cells, when the condition is known as congenital haemolytic anaemia, or acholuric jaundice.

ANAEROBE   The term applied to bacteria having the power to live without air. Such organisms are found growing freely, deep in the soil, as, for example, the tetanus bacillus.

ANAESTHESIA   The loss or absence of sensation or feeling. Commonly used to describe a reversible process which allows operations and painful or unpleasant procedures to be performed without distress to the patient.

The speciality of anaesthesia broadly covers the provision of anaesthesia for SURGERY, INTENSIVE THERAPY, chronic PAIN management, acute pain management and obstetric analgesia. Anaesthetists in Britain are trained specialists with a medical degree but in many countries some anaesthetists may be nurse practitioners working under the supervision of a medical anaesthetist.

The anaesthetist will assess the patient's fitness for anaesthesia, choose and perform the appropriate type of anaesthetic while monitoring and caring for the patient's well-being and, after the anaesthetic, will supervise recovery and the provision of postoperative pain relief.

Anaesthesia may be broadly divided into general and local anaesthesia.

General anaesthesia is most often produced by using a combination of drugs to induce a state of reversible unconsciousness. 'Balanced' anaesthesia uses a combination of drugs to provide UNCONSCIOUSNESS, ANALGESIA and a greater or lesser degree of muscle relaxation.

A general anaesthetic comprises induction, maintenance and recovery. Historically, anaesthesia has been divided into four stages (see below) but these are only clearly seen during induction and maintenance of anaesthesia using only inhalational agents.
(1)   Onset of induction to unconsciousness.
(2)   Stage of excitement.
(3)   Surgical anaesthesia
(4)   Overdosage
Induction involves the initial production of unconsciousness. Most often this is by INTRAVENOUS injection of a short-acting anaesthetic agent such as PROPOFOL, THIOPENTONE, ETOMIDATE or METHOHEXITONE. Alternatively an inhalational technique may be used.

Maintenance of anaesthesia may be provided by continuous or intermittent use of intravenous drugs but is commonly provided by administration of OXYGEN and NITROUS OXIDE containing a volatile anaesthetic agent. Anaesthetic machinery is capable of providing a constant concentration of these and has failsafe mechanisms and monitors which guard against the patient's receiving a gas mixture with inadequate oxygen (HYPOXIC). The gases are adminstered to the patient via a breathing circuit either through a MASK, a laryngeal mask or an ENDOTRACHEAL tube. For some types of surgery the patient is paralysed using muscle relaxants and is then artificially ventilated by machine (a VENTILATOR). Patients are closely monitored during anaesthesia by the anaesthetist using a variety of machines. Minimal monitoring includes ECG, BLOOD PRESSURE, PULSE OXIMETRY, inspired oxygen and end-tidal carbon-dioxide concentration – the amount of carbon dioxide in expired air when the lungs are at the 'empty' stage of the breathing cycle. Analgesic drugs and local or regional anaesthetic blocks are often given to supplement general anaesthesia.

Volatile anaesthetics are either halogenated hydrocarbons (HALOTHANE, CHLOROFORM) or halogenated ethers (isoflurane, enflurane, desflurane and sevoflurane). The most recently introduced agents (isoflurane, desflurane and sevoflurane) have the most rapid induction and recovery and undergo the least metabolism, though on a worldwide basis halothane, ether and chloroform are still widely used.

Despite several theories the mode of action of these agents is not fully understood. Their efficacy is related to the solubility of the anaesthetic gases in the LIPID substances in nerve cells and it is thought that they act at more than one site within the brain, probably at the cell membrane. By whatever method, they reversibly depress the conduction of impulses within the CENTRAL NERVOUS SYSTEM and thereby produce unconsciousness.

At the end of surgery any residual muscle relaxant in the body is reversed, the volatile agent is turned off and the patient breathes oxygen or oxygen-enriched air. This is the reversal or recovery phase of anaesthesia. Once the anaesthetist is satisfied with the degree of recovery patients are transferred to a recovery area within the operating-theatre complex where they are cared for by specialist staff, under the supervision of an anaesthetist, until they are ready to return to the ward.

Local anaesthetics are drugs which reversibly block the conduction of impulses in nerves. They therefore produce anaesthesia (and muscle relaxation) only in those areas of the body served by the nerve(s) affected by these drugs. Many drugs have some local anaesthetic action but the drugs used specifically for this purpose are all amide or ester derivatives of aromatic acids. Variations in the basic structure produces drugs with different speeds of onset, duration of action and preferential SENSORY rather than MOTOR blockade (stopping the activity in the sensory or motor nerves respectively that supply a part of the body).

The use of local rather than general anaesthesia will depend on the type of surgery and in some cases the unsuitability of the patient for general anaesthesia. It is also used to supplement general anaesthesia, relieve pain in LABOUR and in the treatment of pain. Several commonly used techniques are listed below:

LOCAL INFILTRATION An area of anaesthetized skin is produced by injecting small quantities of anaesthetic subcutaneously. This technique is used for SUTURING skin and removing small superficial lesions.

NERVE BLOCKS Local anaesthetic is injected close to a NERVE or nerve plexus, often using a peripheral nerve stimulator to identify the correct point. The anaesthetic diffuses into the nerve, blocking it and producing anaesthesia in the area supplied by it.

SPINAL ANAESTHESIA Small volumes of local anaesthetic are injected into the cerebrospinal fluid through a small-bore needle which has been inserted posteriorly through the tissues of the back and the dura matter. A dense motor and sensory blockade is produced in the lower half of the body. The upper limit is dependent on the volume and dose of anaesthetic, the patient's position and individual variation. If the block is too high, then respiratory-muscle paralysis and therefore respiratory arrest may occur. Hypotension may occur becaue of peripheral vasodilation caused by sympathetic-nerve blockade. Occasionally spinal anaesthesia is complicated by a headache, perhaps caused by continuing leakage of cerebrospinal fluid from the dural puncture point.

EPIDURAL ANAESTHESIA Spinal nerves are blocked in the epidural space with local anaesthetic injected through a fine plastic tube which is introduced into the space using a special needle (Tuohy needle). It can be used as a continuous technique either by intermittent injections, an infusion or by patient-controlled pump. This makes it ideal for surgery in the lower part of the body, the relief of pain in labour and for postoperative analgesia. Complications include HYPOTENSION, spinal headache (less than 1:100), poor efficacy, nerve damage (1:12,000) and spinal cord compression from CLOT or ABSCESS (extremely rare).

ANALEPTIC A restorative medicine, or one which acts as a stimulant of the central nervous system: for example caffeine.

ANALGESIA (see PAIN).

ANALGESICS Drugs which relieve or abolish pain. Unlike local anaesthetics they are usually given SYSTEMICALLY and produce no SENSORY or MOTOR blockade stopping the activity in the sensory or motor nerves respectively that supply a part of the body. The many different types of analgesics have varying modes of action. The choice of drug and method of administration will depend upon the type and severity of pain being treated.

Mild and moderate pain is treated with simple analgesics such as PARACETAMOL, ASPIRIN or one of the many NON-STEROIDAL ANTI-INFLAMMATORY (NSAIDs) group of drugs.

Paracetamol, which also has an ANTIPYRETIC effect, acts within the central nervous system by inhibition of PROSTAGLANDINS. It is often combined with other analgesics, e.g. aspirin or CODEINE, in proprietary compunds and has few side-effects. In overdosage it can cause liver damage.

The NSAIDs (including aspirin) inhibit prostaglandin synthesis. PROSTAGLANDINS are released by tissues that are inflamed and may cause pain at peripheral pain sensors or sensitize nerve endings to painful stimuli. By inhibiting their production, pain and inflammation are reduced. They are particularly effective for pain produced by inflammation – e.g. ARTHRITIS. Side-effects include gastrointestinal bleeding (caused by mucosal erosions particularly in the stomach), inhibition of PLATELET aggregation and potential for RENAL damage.

Severe pain is often treated with OPIOID drugs. The original drugs were naturally occurring plant ALKALOIDS (e.g. MORPHINE), whilst newer drugs are man-made. They mimic the action of naturally occurring compounds (ENDORPHINS and ENCEPHALINS) which are found within the brain and spinal cord and act on receptors to reduce the transmission of painful stimuli within the central nervous system (and possibly peripherally). They tend to produce side-effects of euphoria, respiratory depression, vomiting, constipation and itching. Chronic use or abuse of these drugs may give rise to addiction.

ANALYSIS means a separation into component parts by determination of the chemical constituents of a substance. The process of analysis is carried out by various means: e.g chromatographic analysis by means of the adsorption column; colorimetric analysis by means of various colour tests; densimetric analysis by estimation of the specific gravity; gasometric analysis by estimating the different gases given off in some process; polariscope analysis by means of the polariscope; volumetric analysis by measuring volumes of liquids. Analysis is also sometimes used as an abbreviation for PSYCHO-ANALYSIS.

ANAPHYLAXIS An immediate (and often unpleasant) hypersensitivity reaction produced by the body's immunoglobulin E (IgE) antibodies to a foreign substance (antigen); the affected tissues release histamine which causes local or systemic attack. An example is the pain, swelling, eruption, fever and sometimes collapse that may occur after the injection of tetanus antitoxin or immunization against diseases such as diphtheria or measles. The serum used in such injections is the trigger. Some people may suffer from anaphylaxis as a result of allergy to a particular food or substance such as animal hair or plant leaves. On rare occasions a person may be so sensitive that anaphylaxis may lead to profound shock and collapse which, unless the affected person receives urgent medical attention, may cause death. (See IMMUNITY.)

ANAPLASIA The state in which a body cell loses its distinctive characters and takes on a more primitive form; it occurs, for example, in cancer, when cells proliferate rapidly.

ANASTOMOSIS Direct intercommunication of the branches of two or more veins or arteries without any intervening network of capillary vessels. The term also describes the surgical joining of two hollow vessels, nerves or organs to form an intercommunication

ANATOMY The science which deals with the structure of the bodies of men and animals. Brief descriptions of the anatomy of each important organ are given under the headings of the various organs. It is studied by dissection of bodies bequeathed for the purpose or of the bodies of those who die in hospitals and similar institutions, unclaimed by relatives.

ANCROD An enzyme present in the venom of the Malayan pit viper which destroys the FIBRINOGEN in blood and thereby prevents the blood clotting. In other words it is an ANTICO-AGULANT.

ANCYLOSTOMIASIS A parasitic infection caused by the nematodes *Ancylostoma duodenale* and *Necator americanus* which results in hook-worm disease. These infections are exceedingly common in tropical and developing countries – millions of people being affected. Classically, *A. duodenale* occurred in the Far East, Mediterranean littoral, and Middle East, and *N. americanus* in tropical Africa, Central and South America, and the Far East; however, in recent years, geographical separation of the two human species is less distinct. In areas where standards of hygiene and sanitation are unsatisfactory, larvae (embryos) enter via intact skin, usually the feet. 'Ground itch' occasionally occurs as larvae enter the body. They then undergo a complex life-cycle, migrating through the lungs, trachea, and pharynx. Adult worms are 5–13 (mean 12) mm in length; their normal habitat is the small intestine – especially jejunum – where they adhere to the mucosa by hooks, thus causing seepage of blood into the lumen. A worm-pair produces large numbers of eggs, which are excreted in faeces; when deposited on moist soil they remain viable for many weeks or months. Clinical manifestations include microcytic hypochromic anaemia, hypoalbuminaemia (low serum protein) and, in a severe case, oedema. A chronic infection in childhood can give rise to physical, mental, and sexual retardation. Treatment is with one of the benzimidazole compounds, usually mebendazole or albendazole; however, in developing countries, cheaper preparations are used, including tetrachloroethylene, bephenium hydroxynaph-thoate, and pyrantel embonate. Anaemia usually responds to iron supplements; blood transfusion is rarely indicated.

Ancylostoma braziliensis A nematode infection of dogs, which in humans causes local disease (larva migrans) only, usually on the soles of the feet. It is usually acquired by walking on beaches contaminated with dog faeces in places such as the Caribbean.

ANDROGEN Is the general term for any one of a group of HORMONES which govern the development of the sexual organs and the secondary sexual characteristics of the male. TESTOSTERONE, the androgenic hormone formed in the interstitial cells of the testis, controls the development and maintenance of the male sex organs and secondary sex characteristics. In small doses it increases the number of SPERMATOZOA produced, but in large doses it inhibits the gonadotrophic activity of the anterior PITUITARY GLAND and suppresses the formation of the spermatozoa. It is both androgenic and anabolic in action. The anabolic effect includes the ability to stimulate protein synthesis and to diminish the catabolism of amino acids, and this is associated with retention of nitrogen, potassium, phosphorus and calcium. Doses in excess of 10 mg daily to the female may produce virilism.

Unconjugated testosterone is rarely used clinically because its derivatives have a more powerful and prolonged effect, and testosterone itself requires implantation into the subcutaneous fat, using a trocar and cannula for maximum therapeutic benefit. Testosterone propionate is prepared in an oily solution, as it is insoluble in water. It is effective for three days and is therefore administered intramuscularly twice weekly. Testosterone phenylpropionate is a long-acting micro-crystalline preparation, which, when given by intramuscular or subcutaneous injection, is effective for two weeks. Methyl-testosterone is only weakly active by mouth though it is absorbed sublingually. It does however produce a cholestatic jaundice in a significant proportion of patients and is therefore better avoided. Mesterolone is an effective oral androgen and is less hepatoxic. It does not inhibit pituitary gonadotrophic production and hence spermatogenesis is unimpaired. Testosterone undecanoate has recently been introduced and may well prove to be the oral androgen of choice.

The androgens in therapeutic use which can be given by mouth include: mesterolone, methyltestosterone, testosterone, testosterone undecanoate. Those that can be given by injection include: testosterone propionate, testosterone phenylpropionate, testosterone enanthate, testosterone esters and drostanolone.

ANENCEPHALY The term given to the condition in which a child is born with a defect of the skull and absence of the brain. Anencephaly is the most common major malformation of the central nervous system. It has an incidence of 0·65 per 1,000 live births. There is complete absence of the cerebral hemispheres and overlying skull and the brain stem and cerebellum are atrophic. If the pregnancy goes to term the infants rapidly die but in 50 per cent of pregnancies associated with anencephaly spontaneous abortion occurs. It is possible to detect the presence of anencephaly in the fetus by measuring the level of alpha foeto protein in the mother's serum or in the amniotic fluid. (See SPINA BIFIDA.)

ANEUPLOIDY The state in which there is an abnormal number of CHROMOSOMES: e.g. DOWN'S SYNDROME and TURNER SYNDROME.

ANEURINE is an alternative name for vitamin B_1. (See THIAMINE.)

ANEURYSM A localized swelling or dilatation of an artery due to weakening of its wall. The commonest sites are the aorta, the arteries of the legs, the carotids and the subclavian arteries. Aneurysms may also form in the arteries at the base of the brain usually due to an inherited defect of the arterial wall. Aneurysms usually arise in the elderly, with men affected more commonly than women. The commonest cause is degenerative atheromatous disease, but other rarer causes include trauma, inherited conditions such as MARFAN'S SYNDROME, or acquired conditions such as

SYPHILIS or POLYARTERITIS NODOSA. Once formed, the pressure of the circulating blood within the aneurysm causes it to increase in size. At first, there may be no symptoms or signs, but as the aneurysm enlarges it becomes detectable as a swelling which pulsates with each heartbeat. It may also cause pain due to pressure on local nerves or bones. Rupture of the aneurysm may occur at any time, but is much more likely when the aneurysm is large. Rupture is usually a surgical emergency, because the bleeding is arterial and therefore considerable amounts of blood may be lost very rapidly, leading to collapse, shock and even death. Rupture of an aneurysm in the circle of Willis causes subarachnoid haemorrhage.

Treatment Treatment is usually surgical. Once an aneurysm has formed the tendency is for it to enlarge progressively regardlessof any medical therapy. The surgery is often demanding and is therefore usually undertaken only when the aneurysm is large and the risk of rupture is therefore increased. The patient's general fitness for surgery is also an important consideration. The surgery usually involves either bypassing or replacing the affected part of the artery using a conduit made of either vein or a manmade fibre which has been woven or knitted into a tube.

ANGINA A feeling of constriction or suffocation often accompanied by pain (see ANGINA PECTORIS).

ANGINA PECTORIS Pain in the centre of the chest. Usually exercise – sometimes acute anxiety – brings it on and pain may be severe and felt also in the arms and the jaw. The condition, which is aggravated by cold weather, is the result of the heart's demand for blood being greater than the coronary arteries can provide. This failure is usually due to narrowing of the coronary arteries by atheroma; rarely, it may be caused by congenital defects in the arteries rendering them incapable of carrying sufficient blood to meet increased demands from the body. Angina may be relieved or prevented by such drugs as glyceryl trinitrate and propanolol. If drug treatment does not work, surgery on the coronary arteries such as angioplasty or bypass grafts may be necessary. People who suffer from angina pectoris need advice on their lifestyle, in particular about diet, exercise and avoidance of smoking or excessive alcohol consumption. They may have high blood pressure, which will also require medical treatment (see HYPERTENSION).

ANGIOCARDIOGRAPHY Radiography of the heart after injection into it of a radio-opaque substance.

ANGIOGENESIS INHIBITORS Two drugs, endostatin and angiostatin, that inhibit the blood supply to tumours are being tested in clinical trials in humans. The United States

National Cancer Institute has put a high priority on the research into these drugs. Tumours require a good blood supply and new blood-vessel formation – angiogenesis – triggers this. If angiogenesis is prevented, tumours will not grow or may even regress. Endostatin and angiostatin have eliminated brain, breast, colon and prostate cancers in mice with no apparent short-term effects. It may be several years, however – even if clinical trials proceed satisfactorily – before the use of these drugs to combat human cancers can be officially authorized.

ANGIOGRAPHY Radiography of blood vessels made visible by injecting into them a radio-opaque substance. In the case of arteries this is known as arteriography; the corresponding term for veins being venography or phlebography. This procedure demonstrates whether there is any narrowing or ballooning of the lumen of the vessel, changes usually caused by disease or injury.

ANGIOMA A tumour composed of blood-vessels. (See TUMOUR and NAEVUS.)

ANGIO-OEDEMA (see URTICARIA).

ANGIOPLASTY A method of treating blockage or narrowing of a blood vessel by recanalizing the vessel by inserting a balloon into the constriction to reopen it. The technique is used to treat a narrowed artery in the heart or a limb. About 65 per cent of patients treated benefit, but when symptoms persist or recur the procedure may be repeated. There is a small risk of damage to the vessel or valve. New procedures under development include the use of lasers, cutting drills and suction to remove the deposits of ATHEROMA blocking the arteries.

ANGIOTENSIN is a peptide that occurs in two forms I and II. The former results from the action of the enzyme RENIN on alpha globulin (a protein) produced by the liver and passed into the blood. During passage of the blood through the lungs angiotensin I is converted into an active form, angiotensin II, by an enzyme. This active form constricts the blood vessels and stimulates the release of two hormones VASOPRESSIN and ALDOSTERONE which raise the blood pressure. (See ANGIOTENSIN-CONVERTING ENZYME (ACE) INHIBITORS).

ANGIOTENSIN-CONVERTING ENZYME (ACE) INHIBITORS The enzyme that converts angiotensin I to angiotensin II is called angio-tensin-converting enzyme. Angiotensin II controls the blood pressure and is the most potent endogenous pressor substance produced in the body; angiotensin I has no such pressor activity. Inhibition of the enzyme that converts angiotensin I to angiotensin II will thus have marked effects on lowering the blood pressure and ACE inhibitors have a valuable role in treating heart failure when thiazides and beta-blockers cannot be used or fail to work. Captopril was the first ACE inhibitor to be synthesized. It lowers peripheral resistance by causing arteriolar dilatation and thus lowers blood pressure. Other drugs such as enalapril, lisinopril, cilazapril, quinapril and ramipril have since been developed. Some kidney disorders increase the production of angiotensin II and so cause hypertension.

ANGITIS, or ANGIITIS, means inflammation of a vessel such as a blood-vessel, lymph-vessel, or bile-duct.

ÅNGSTRÖM UNIT (called after the Swedish physicist) is a measurement of length and equals 1/10000 micrometre, or one-hundred-millionth of a centimetre. It is represented by the symbol Å and is used to give the length of electro-magnetic waves.

ANHIDROSIS is an abnormal diminution in the secretion of sweat. This may be caused by diseases or a congenital defect.

ANISOCYTOSIS This means inequality in the size of erythrocytes (red blood cells); it occurs in many forms but is prominent in megaloblastic anaemia.

ANKLE The joint between the leg bones (TIBIA and FIBULA) above, and the talus (the Roman dice-bone) below. It is a very strong joint with powerful ligaments binding the bones together at either side, and bony projections from the leg bones, which form large bosses on either side, called the outer and inner malleoli, extending about 12 mm (half an inch) below the actual joint. Two common injuries near the ankle are a sprain, on the inner side, consisting of tearing of the internal ligament; and fracture of the fibula (Pott's fracture) on the outer side. (See also JOINTS, DISEASES OF.)

ANKYLOSING SPONDYLITIS (see SPINE AND SPINAL CORD, DISEASES AND INJURIES OF).

ANKYLOSIS The condition of a joint in which the movements are restricted by fibrous bands, or by malformation, or by actual union of the bones. (See JOINTS, DISEASES OF.)

ANKYLOSTOMA (see ANCYLOSTOMIASIS).

ANODYNES Any drug or treatment that eases pain. These may range from opium – the oldest and most powerful anodyne but a highly addictive substance – through ANALGESICS to warmth and massage.

ANOPHELES Generic name of a widely distributed group of mosquitoes, certain species of which transmit to man the parasitic protozoa *Plasmodium*, the agent that causes malaria. *Anopheles maculipennis* and *A. bifurcatus* are both found in England and can both transmit the malaria parasite.

ANOREXIA Loss of appetite. (See APPETITE.)

ANOREXIA NERVOSA (see EATING DISORDERS).

ANOSMIA Loss of sense of smell. (See NOSE, DISEASES OF.)

ANOVULAR Absence of ovulation. Anovular menstruation occurs when a woman takes the contraceptive pill.

ANOXAEMIA Reduction of the oxygen content of the blood below normal limits.

ANOXIA That state in which the body tissues have an inadequate supply of oxygen. This may be because the blood in the lungs does not receive enough oxygen, or because there is not enough blood to receive the oxygen, or because the blood stagnates in the body. (See OXYGEN.)

ANTABUSE (see DISULFIRAM).

ANTACIDS Drugs traditionally used to treat gastrointestinal disorders, including peptic ulcer. They neutralize the hydrochloric acid secreted in the stomach's digestive juices and relieve pain and the discomfort of indigestion. A large number of proprietary preparations are on sale to the public and most contain compounds of aluminium or magnesium or a mixture of the two. Other agents include activated dimethicome – an antifoaming agent aimed at relieving flatulence, alginates, which protect against reflux oesophagitis and surface anaesthetics. Antacids commonly prescribed by doctors include aluminium hydroxide, magnesium carbonate and magnesium trisilicate. Sodium bicarbonate and calcium and bismuth compounds are also used, though the latter is best avoided as it may cause neurological side-effects.

ANTAGONIST (1) A muscle the contraction of which opposes that of another muscle called the AGONIST. When the agonist contracts the antagonist relaxes. For a fuller explanation see AGONIST. (2) The action of one drug in opposing the action of another.

ANTE- Prefix meaning before or forwards.

ANTEFLEXION The abnormal forward curvature of an organ in which the upper part is sharply bent forward. The term is especially applied to forward displacement of the UTERUS.

ANTENATAL CARE The protocol which doctors and midwives follow to ensure that the pregnant mother and her fetus are kept in good health and that the pregnancy and birth have a satisfactory outcome. The pregnant mother is seen regularly at a clinic where, for example, her blood pressure is checked and the growth and development of her child-to-be are carefully assessed and any problem or potential problems dealt with. Most antenatal care deals with normal pregnancies and is supervised by general practitioners and midwives in primary-care clinics. If any serious problems are identified the mother can be referred to specialists' clinics in hospitals. (See PREGNANCY.)

ANTEPARTUM An adjective describing an event before labour starts in pregnancy.

ANTERIOR An adjective that describes or relates to the front part of the body, limbs, or organs.

ANTERIOR TIBIAL SYNDROME (see MUSCLE).

ANTEVERSION The term applied to the forward tilting of an organ, especially of the UTERUS.

ANTHELMINTICS Substances which cause the death or expulsion of parasitic worms.

ANTHRACOSIS The change which takes place in the lungs and bronchial glands of coal miners, who inhale coal dust constantly. The lungs are amazingly efficient in coping with this problem. During a working lifetime a coalminer may inhale around 5000 grams of dust, but at post-mortem examination it is rare to find more than about 40 grams in his lungs. The affected tissues change in colour from greyish pink to jet black, owing to loading with minute carbon particles. (See PNEUMOCONIOSIS.)

ANTHRAX A serious disease occurring in sheep and cattle, and in those who tend them or handle the bones, skins and fleeces, even long after removal of the latter from the animals. It is sometimes referred to as malignant pustule, wool-sorters' disease, splenic fever of animals or murrain. It is now a rare condition in the United Kingdom. The cause is a bacillus (*B. anthracis*) which grows in long chains and produces spores of great vitality. These spores retain their life for years, in dried skins and fleeces; they are not destroyed by boiling, freezing, 5 per cent carbolic lotion, or, like many bacilli, by the gastric juice. The disease is communicated from a diseased animal to a crack in the skin, e.g. of a shepherd or butcher, or from contact with contaminated skins or fleeces. Nowadays skins are handled wet, but if they are allowed to dry so that dust laden with spores is inhaled by the workers an internal form of the disease results. Instances have occurred of the disease being conveyed on shaving brushes made from bristles of diseased animals. A few countries are believed to have developed anthrax as a weapon of war to be delivered by shells or rockets, despite international agreements to ban such weapons.

Symptoms

EXTERNAL FORM   This is the 'malignant pustule'. After inoculation of some small wound, a few hours or days elapse, and then a red, inflamed swelling appears, which grows larger till it covers half the face or the breadth of the arm, as the case may be. Upon its summit appears a bleb of pus, which bursts and leaves a black scab, perhaps 12 mm (half an inch) wide. At the same time there is great prostration and fever. The inflammation may last ten days or so, when it slowly subsides and the patient recovers, if surviving the fever and prostration.

INTERNAL FORM   This takes the form of pneumonia with haemorrhages, when the spores have been drawn into the lungs, or of ulcers of the stomach and intestines, with gangrene of the spleen, when they have been swallowed. It is usually fatal in two or three days.

Prevention is most important by disinfecting all hides, wool and hair coming from areas of the world. An efficient vaccine is now available. Treatment consists of the administration of large doses of penicillin or of one of the tetracyclines.

ANTI   Prefix meaning against.

ANTIBACTERIAL DRUGS   A group of drugs, which include ANTIBIOTICS, used to treat infections caused by BACTERIA. Drugs include CEPHALOSPORINS and cephamycins, TETRACYCLINES, AMINOGLYCOSIDES, MACROLIDES, SULPHONAMIDES and antituberculous compounds.

ANTIBIOTIC is the term used to describe any antibacterial agent derived from micro-organisms, though most of them are now prepared synthetically. Such agents destroy or inhibit the growth of other micro-organisms. Examples are penicillin, cephalosporin, aminoglycosides, streptomycin, and tetracycline.

Penicillin was the first antibiotic to be discovered and used in the 1940s. The discovery and isolation in 1958 of the penicillin nucleus, 6-amino penicillanic acid (6-PNA) allowed many new penicillins to be synthesized. These are now the largest single group of antibiotics used in clinical medicine. Most staphylococci have now developed resistance to benzylpenicillin, the early form of the drug, because they produce penicillinases, enzymes which break down the drug. Other types of penicillin such as cloxacillin and flucoxacillin are not affected and are used against penicillin-resistant staphylococci.

The cephalosporins are derived from the compound cephalosporin C which is obtained by fermentation of the mould cephalosporium. The cephalosporin nucleus 7 Amino cephalosporanic (7-ICA) acid has been the basis for the production of the semi-synthetic compounds of the cephalosporin nucleus. The first semi-synthetic cephalosporin, cephalothin, appeared in 1962; it was followed by cephaloridine in 1964. The original cephalosporins had to be given by injection but more recent preparations can be given by mouth. The newer preparations are less readily destroyed by beta lactamases and so they have a much broader spectrum of anti-bacterial activity. The newer cephalosporins include cephalexin, cefazolin, cephacetrile, cephapirin, cefamandole, cefuroxine, cephrodine, cefodroxil and cefotaxine. Inactivation of beta lactamase is the basis of bacterial resistance to both the penicillins and the cephalosporins so that attempts to prepare these antibiotics with resistance to beta lactamase is of great importance. A synthetic inhibitor of beta lactamase called clavulanic acid has recently been synthesized. This is used in combination with the penicillins and cephalosporins to prevent resistance. The cephamycins are a new addition to the beta lactam antibiotics. They are similar in structure to the cephalosporins but are produced, not by fungi, but by actinomycetes.

Overuse and misuse of antibiotics have resulted in many bacteria becoming resistant to them. Hospitals, in particular, have problems with METHICILLIN-RESISTANT *STAPHYLOCOCCUS AUREUS*, MRSA. Combinations of antibiotics are needed to combat resistant strains of bacteria.

ANTIBODIES are substances in the blood which destroy or neutralize various toxins or 'bodies' (e.g. bacteria), known generally as antigens. The antibodies are formed, usually, as a result of the introduction into the body of the antigens to which they are antagonistic, as in all infectious diseases.

ANTICHOLINERGIC   An action or drug that inhibits the activity of ACETYLCHOLINE.

ANTICOAGULANTS   Drugs which inhibit coagulation of the blood. The main ones now in use are HEPARIN, PHENINDIONE and WARFARIN. Heparin is a natural anticoagulant, acting quickly and directly on the blood-clotting process. The other two are synthetic agents and take longer to act; they affect blood coagulation factors. Anticoagulants prevent the extension of blood clots in EMBOLISM and THROMBOSIS. Patients who are on anticoagulants require to be carefully monitored under medical supervision, and should carry an Anticoagulant Card with instructions about the use of whatever drug they may be taking.

ANTICONVULSANT   A drug that reduces or prevents the severity of an epileptic convulsion or seizure. The nature of the fit and the patient's reaction influences the type of anticonvulsant used. Anticonveulsants inhibit the high level of electrical activity in the brain that causes the fit. Among regularly used anticonvulsants are carbamazepine, clonazepam, diazepam, phenobarbitone, phenytoin, primidone, and sodium valporate. The newer drugs gabentin, lamotrigine and vigabatrin are now available where control is hard to achieve. They are effective in partial seizures with or without secondary generalization (see EPILEPSY).

ANTIDEPRESSANT DRUGS   These widely used drugs include a wide range of different preparations which relieve depressed mood. They are quite distinct from the tranquillizers like diazepam – widely known by its trade name, Valium – and are not addictive. All the antidepressants available at the time of writing are more or less equally effective. In studies where patients agree to take either antidepressants or identical dummy PLACEBO pills (without knowing which), at least two-thirds of those who get antidepressants feel much better within three months. Fewer than one-third of those on placebo recover naturally in the same period.

The most widely prescribed type of antidepressants are the trycyclics, so called because their molecular structure includes three rings. The other commonly used types are named after the actions they have on chemicals in the brain: the specific serotonin reuptake inhibitors (SSRIs) and the monoamine oxidase inhibitors (MAOIs). All types of antidepressant work in similar ways. Tricyclic antidepressants have cured depression in millions of people. But they can cause unpleasant side-effects, particularly in the first couple of weeks. These include SEDATION, dry mouth, excessive sweating, CONSTIPATION, URINARY problems, and IMPOTENCE (inability to get an erection). Up to half of all people prescribed tricyclic drugs cannot tolerate the side-effects and stop treatment before their depression is properly treated. More seriously, tricyclics can upset the HEART rhythm in susceptible people and should never be given in the presence of heart disease.

The SSRIs are much newer, coming into wide use in the late 1980s. They increase the levels in the brain of the chemical messenger SEROTONIN or 5HT, which is thought to be depleted in depression. Indeed, the SSRIs are as effective as tricyclics and, although they can cause nausea and excessive sweating at first, they generally have fewer side-effects. Their main disadvantage, however, is that they cost a hundred times more than the most commonly used tricyclic, amitriptyline. On the other hand, they are more acceptable to many patients and they cause fewer drop-outs from treatment – up to a quarter rather than a half. The money saved by completed, successful treatment, may outweigh the prescribing costs.

The last group of antidepressants, the MAOIs, have been in use since the late 1950s. They are stimulants, rather than sedatives, and are particularly helpful for people who are physically and mentally slowed by depression. They work well but have one big disadvantage, a dangerous interaction with certain foods and other drugs, causing a sudden and very dangerous increase in BLOOD PRESSURE. People taking them have to carry round an information card explaining the risk and listing the things to avoid. Because of this risk MAOIs are not used much now, except when other treatments have failed. A new MAOI, moclobemide, which does not cause high blood pressure, is now available.

In general, antidepressants work by restoring the balance of chemicals in the brain. Improved sleep and lessening anxiety are usually the first signs of improvement, particularly among people taking the more sedative tricyclic drugs. Improvement in other symptoms follow, with the mood starting to lift after about two weeks of treatment. Most people feel well by three months, although a few residual symptoms, such as slowness in the mornings, may take longer to clear up. People taking antidepressants usually want to stop them as soon as they feel better. But the risk of relapse is high for up to a year and most doctors recommend continuing the drugs for around four to six months after recovery, with gradual reduction of the dose after that.

LITHIUM CARBONATE is a powerful antidepressant used for intractable depression. It should be used under specialist supervision as the gap between an effective dose and a toxic one is narrow.

ANTIDIURETIC HORMONE (ADH) (see VASOPRESSIN).

ANTIDOTES   An antidote is a therapeutic substance used to counteract the toxic action(s) of a specific substance. Very few substances have an antidote.

ANTIEMETIC   A drug that counteracts nausea and sickness. Some antihistamines and anticholinergics have an antiemetic effect. They are used to combat motion sickness or nausea and vomiting brought on by other drugs.

ANTIGEN   A substance which causes the formation of antibodies: it is usually a protein that is foreign to the body.

ANTIHISTAMINE DRUGS antagonize the action of HISTAMINE and are therefore of value in the treatment of certain allergic conditions. They may be divided into those with a central action (e.g. flupheniramine and cyclizine) and the new drugs, such as astemizole, loratidine and terfenadine with almost no central action. Antihistamines are also of some value in the treatment of vasomotor RHINITIS. They reduce rhinorrhoea and sneezing but are usually less effective in relieving nasal congestion. All antihistamines are also useful in the treatment of urticaria and certain allergic skin rashes, insect bites and stings. They are also used in the treatment of drug allergies. Chlorpheniramine or promethazine injections are useful in the emergency treatment of angio-oedema and anaphylaxis.

There is little evidence that any one antihistamine is superior to another and patients vary considerably in their response to them. The antihistamines differ in their duration of action and in the incidence of side-effects such as drowsiness. Most are short-acting, but some (such as promethazine) work for up to twelve hours. They all cause sedation but promethazine, trimeprazine and dimenhydrinate tend to be more sedating while chlorpheniramine and cyclizine are less so, as are astemizole, oxatomide and terfenadine. Patients should be warned that their ability to drive or operate machinery may be impaired and that the effects of alcohol may be increased.

ANTIHYPERTENSIVE DRUGS A group of drugs which are used to treat high blood pressure (HYPERTENSION). Untreated hypertension leads to strokes, heart attacks and heart failure. The high incidence of hypertension in western countries has led to intensive research to discover antihypertensive drugs and many have been marketed. The drugs may work by reducing the power of the heart beat, by dilating the blood vessels or by increasing the excretion of salts and water in the urine (diuresis). Antihypertensive treatment has greatly improved the prognosis of patients with high blood pressure by cutting the frequency of heart and RENAL FAILURE, STROKE, and CORONARY THROMBOSIS. Drugs used for treatment can be classified as follows: diuretics; vasodilator antihypertensives; centrally acting antihypertensives; adrenergic neurone-blocking drugs; alpha-adrenoreceptor-blocking drugs; drugs affecting the renin–angiotensin system; ganglion-blocking drugs; and tyrosine hydroxylase inhibitors. The drugs prescribed depend on many factors including the type of hypertension being treated. Treatment can be difficult because of the need to balance the effectiveness of a drug in reducing blood pressure against its side-effects. (See HYPERTENSION.)

ANTIMETABOLITES A group of drugs which have been introduced for the treatment of certain forms of malignant disease. Chemically, they closely resemble substances (or metabolites) which are essential for the life and growth of cells. When introduced into the body they are 'mistaken', so to speak, by the cell for the corresponding metabolite, thereby preventing the cell from making use of the metabolite, or substance, which is essential for its growth. By this means the life of the cell is affected and it ultimately dies.

ANTIMONY is the name applied to a metal and also to its sulphide, a black powder found in nature. The tartrate of potassium and antimony is commonly known as tartar emetic in reference to its chief property. The preparations of antimony, some of which are used in the treatment of tropical diseases such as kala-azar, are all irritants; hence in large doses they are poisons.

ANTIMUSCARINE A pharmacological effect where the action of ACETYLCHOLINE, a chemical neurotransmitter released at the junctions (synapses) of PARASYMPATHETIC and ganglionic nerves, is inhibited. The junctions between nerves and skeletal muscles have nicotinic receptors.

ANTIOXIDANT A compound that can neutralize oxygen-free radicals in the body; these are atoms and chemical groups that can damage cells. Free radicals are the product of various disease processes as well as of such agents as poisons, radiation and smoking. Natural antioxidants also occur in the body.

ANTIPERISTALSIS A movement in the bowels and stomach by which the food and other contents are passed upwards, instead of in the proper direction. (See PERISTALSIS.)

ANTIPSYCHOTIC DRUGS (see NEUROLEPTICS).

ANTIPYRETICS Measures used to reduce temperature in fever.

Varieties Cold-sponging, wet-pack, baths and diaphoretic drugs such as quinine, salicylates and aspirin.

Uses (see under above headings).

ANTISEPTICS prevent the growth of disease-causing micro-organisms without damaging living tissues.

Among chemicals used are boric acid, carbolic acid, hydrogen peroxide and products based on coal tar, such as cresol. Chlorhexidines, iodine, formaldehyde, flavines, alcohol and hexachlorophane are also used. Antiseptics are applied to prevent infection – for example, in preparing the skin before operation. They are also used to treat infected wounds.

ANTISPASMODICS These are ANTIMUSCARINIC drugs which have the property of relaxing smooth muscle. Along with other antimuscarinic drugs, antispasmodics may be helpful supportive treatment for patients with non-ulcer DYSPEPSIA, IRRITABLE BOWEL SYNDROME and DIVERTICULAR DISEASE. Examples of antispasmodic drugs are ATROPINE sulphate, dicyclomine bromide and PROPANTHELINE (a synthetic ANTIMUSCARINIC drug used as a treatment adjunct in gastrointestinal disorders and also for controlling urinary frequency), bromide, alverine, mabervine and pepermint oil. With the arrival of more powerful and specific antisecretory drugs, such as the histamine H_2-receptor antagonists – examples are CIMETIDINE and RANITIDINE – the use of antispasmodics has declined.

ANTITOXIN Any one of various preparations that contain ANTIBODIES which combine and neutralize the effects of a particular TOXIN released into the blood stream by BACTERIA. Examples are the toxins produced by DIPHTHERIA and TETANUS. Antitoxins are produced from the blood of humans or animals that have been exposed to a particular toxin – whether by INFECTION or by INOCULATION – and thus produced antibodies against it. They are usually given by intramuscular injection.

ANTIVENOM A therapeutic substance used to counteract the toxic action(s) of a specific animal TOXIN or venom. They are normally sterilized, proteinaceous GLOBULINS extracted from the SERUM of animals, usually horses, immunized against the specific toxin/venom. Most are given by intravenous or intramuscular injection and are most effective when given shortly after the bite or sting has occurred. Some antivenoms may be effective against the venoms of several closely related animal species.

ANTROSTOMY is the operation in which an opening is made through the nose into the maxillary antrum. (See ANTRUM.)

ANTRUM means a natural hollow or cavity. The maxillary antrum is now known as the maxillary sinus (see SINUS). The mastoid antrum is situated in the mastoid process, the mass of bone felt behind the ear. It may become the seat of an abscess in cases of suppuration of the middle ear (see EAR, DISEASES OF). The pyloric antrum is the part of the stomach immediately preceding the PYLORUS.

ANURIA is a condition in which no urine is voided. (See KIDNEYS, DISEASES OF: glomerulonephritis; URINE.)

ANUS is the opening at the lower end of the bowel. It is kept closed by two muscles, the external and internal sphincters. The latter is a muscular ring which extends about 25 mm (1 inch) up the bowel, is nearly 6 mm (¼ inch) thick, and is kept constantly contracted by the action of a nerve centre in the spinal cord. In disease of the spinal cord the muscle may be paralysed, and inability to retain the motions results.

ANUS, DISEASES OF (see RECTUM, DISEASES OF).

ANXIETY STATE (see NEUROSIS).

ANXIOLYTICS Drugs for the relief of anxiety. They will induce sleep when given in large doses at night and so are hypnotics as well. Conversely most hypnotics will sedate when given in divided doses during the day. Prescription of these drugs is widespread but physical and psychological dependence occurs as well as tolerance to their effects, especially among those with personality disorders or who abuse drugs and alcohol. This is particularly true of the BARBITURATES which are now limited in their use, but also applies to the BENZODIAZEPINES. Withdrawal syndromes may occur if drug treatment is stopped too abruptly. Hypnotic sedatives and anxiolytics should therefore not be prescribed indiscriminately, but reserved for short courses. Among the anxiolytics are the widely used benzodiazepines, the rarely used barbiturates, and the occasionally prescribed drugs such as BUSPIRONE and beta-blockers like PROPANOLOL and OXPRENOLOL.

AORTA The large vessel which opens out of the left ventricle of the heart and carries blood to all the body. It is about 45 cm (1½ feet) long and 2·5 cm (1 inch) wide. Like other arteries it possesses three coats, of which the middle one is much the thickest. This consists partly of muscle fibre, but is mainly composed of an elastic substance, called elastin. The aorta passes first to the right, and lies nearest the surface behind the end of the second right rib-cartilage; then it curves backwards and to the left, passes down behind the left lung close to the backbone, and through an opening in the diaphragm into the abdomen, where it divides, at the level of the navel, into the two common iliac arteries, which carry blood to the lower limbs. Its branches, in order, are: two coronary arteries to the heart wall; the brachiocephalic, left common carotid, and left subclavian arteries to the head, neck and upper limbs; several small branches to the oesophagus, bronchi, and other organs of the chest; nine pairs of intercostal arteries which run round the body between the ribs; one pair of subcostal arteries which is in series with the intercostal arteries; four (or five) lumbar arteries to the muscles of the loins; coeliac trunk to the stomach, liver and pancreas; two mesenteric arteries to the bowels; and suprarenal, renal and testicular arteries to the suprarenal body, kidney, and testicle on each side. From the termination of the aorta rises a small branch, the median sacral artery, which runs down into the pelvis. In the female the ovarian arteries replace the testicular.

The chief diseases of the aorta are atheroma and aneurysm. (See ARTERIES, DISEASES OF; ANEURYSM; and COARCTATION OF THE AORTA.)

AORTIC INCOMPETENCE or REGURGITATION The back flow of blood through the aortic valve of the heart into the left ventricle caused by an incompetent valve. The failure to close may be caused by a congenital defect or by damage from disease. The defect may be cured by surgical replacement of the damaged valve with an artificial valve. (See HEART DISEASES.)

AORTIC STENOSIS Narrowing of the aortic valve which obstructs the flow of blood through it with serious effects on the heart and the circulation. The muscle in the left ventricle works harder to compensate for the obstruction and thickens as a result. Stenosis is usually caused by the deposition of calcium on the valve and is commonly associated with atheroma. Untreated, the condition leads to heart failure, but nowadays the stenosis can be treated surgically.

AORTIC VALVE The valve that controls the flow of blood from the aorta to the left ventricle of the heart. (See HEART.)

AORTITIS A rare degenerative condition of the lining of the aorta. It may be the result of arteritis (inflammation of the arteries) or a consequence of untreated SYPHILIS. Aortitis may lead to thinning of the aorta's wall and development of an ANEURYSM.

AORTOGRAPHY is the technique of rendering the aorta visible in an X-ray film by injecting a radio-opaque substance into it. The procedure is used to detect the presence of an ANEURYSM. (See also ANGIOGRAPHY.)

APERIENTS Medicines which produce a natural movement of the bowels. (See CONSTIPATION; PURGATIVES.)

APEX The pointed portion of any organ which has a conical shape. The apex of each lung reaches about 3·5 to 5 cm (1½ or 2 inches) above the collar-bone into the neck. In health the apex of the heart can be felt below the fifth rib immediately inside the nipple.

APEX BEAT This is the beat of the apex of the heart, which can be felt through the skin to the left of the breastbone between the fifth and sixth ribs.

APGAR SCORE A method of assessing a baby's condition at birth, in which a value of 0, 1 or 2 is given to each of five signs: colour, heart-rate, muscle tone, respiratory (or breathing) effort, and the response to stimulation. A total score of 10 indicates that the newborn child is in excellent condition.

APHAKIA Absence of the lens of the eye.

APHASIA Loss of the power of speech, due to injury to the centres which govern this act in the BRAIN. The higher of these centres, which

1 medulla oblongata	7 central sulcus
2 lateral sulcus	8 sensation
3 speech	9 memories of written
4 movements of tongue	words
5 movements of trunk	10 sight
6 movements of leg	11 cerebellum

Areas on the left surface of cerebrum associated with definite functions.

have to do with forming the ideas of speech, putting words together in sentences, and governing the movements of MOUTH, TONGUE and LARYNX, lie on the surface of the cerebral hemispheres, especially of the left. The lower centres which control the muscles responsible for voice production.

Causes The cause is destruction of a portion of the brain, including one of these higher centres, owing to rupture of a blood-vessel, and haemorrhage into the brain tissue; or owing to blocking of a blood-vessel by an embolus (see EMBOLISM), or by clotting of the blood on the diseased wall of a vessel (see THROMBOSIS), any one of which cuts off the supply of blood to the part concerned. The causes are thus the same as in a stroke, and aphasia may be one of the symptoms of a stroke, especially when the right side of the body is paralysed, or may occur by itself, according to the extent of brain involved. Other diseases, such as tumours, may also be the cause, the important factor being interference with the functions of certain definite areas of the brain.

Symptoms The disorder generally follows a stroke and exists along with some paralysis on the right side of the body. Aphasia may come on suddenly and last only a few hours or days, being due then to a temporary circulatory disturbance in the brain. Generally it is permanent. Sometimes he or she is absolutely without the power of speech. When the condition is one of sensory aphasia – loss of perception of speech and its production – the individual forgets names of persons, of places, even of the commonest household articles.

Treatment This is as in stroke, of which the condition often forms a part (see STROKE). In some patients improvement is achieved by teaching the afflicted person to read and speak.

APHONIA Loss of voice, usually sudden. Commonly caused by emotional stress with no detectable physical abnormality in the larynx. Damage or disease of the larynx usually results in dysphonia (partial voice loss). Where no physical cause can be identified, reassurance and, if the voice does not quickly return, PSYCHOTHERAPY are the treatment.

APHTHOUS ULCER Single or multiple (and often recurrent) transiently painful ulcers in the oral mucous membrane that are usually self limiting. The cause is unknown and treatment is symptomatic.

APICECTOMY is the minor operation carried out to try to save a tooth which has an abscess on it or which does not respond to root treatment. In this the abscess and the apex of the tooth are removed.

APLASIA The complete or partial failure of tissue or an organ to develop.

APNOEA A general term meaning the cessation of breathing. Apnoea is a medical emergency. Death soon follows if breathing is not quickly restored. Apnoea may be caused by an obstruction to the airway, for example by the tongue during general anaesthesia, or by a disturbance of the mechanisms that control breathing. Rapid heavy breathing reduces the blood levels of carbon dioxide and can lead to a brief period of apnoea.

Neonatal apnoeic attacks may represent a serious emergency, being caused by prematurity, milk aspiration, heart failure, infection, hypoxia, hypoglycaemia or hypocalcaemia. If stimulation of the baby does not immediately restore breathing then bag and mask ventilation should be used.

APO- is a prefix implying separation or derivation from.

APODIA Absence of the foot.

APONEUROSIS is the term applied to the white fibrous membrane which serves as an investment for the muscles and which covers the skull beneath the scalp.

APOPLEXY (see STROKE).

APPENDICECTOMY, or appendectomy, is the operation for the removal of the appendix vermiformis.

APPENDICITIS This is an inflammatory condition of the appendix, and is a common surgical emergency, affecting mainly adolescents and young adults. It is usually due to a combination of obstruction and infection of the appendix, and has a variable clinical course ranging from episodes of mild self-limiting abdominal pain to life-threatening illness. Abdominal pain beginning in the centre of the abdomen but which later shifts position to the right iliac fossa is the classical symptom. The patient usually has accompanying fever and sometimes nausea, vomiting, loss of appetite, diarrhoea, or even constipation. The precise symptoms vary with the exact location of the appendix within the abdomen. In some individuals the appendix may 'grumble' with repeated mild attacks which resolve spontaneously. In an acute attack, the inflammatory process begins first in the wall of the appendix but, if the disease progresses, the appendix can become secondarily infected and pus may form within it. The blood supply may become compromised and its wall may become gangrenous. Eventually the appendix may rupture, giving rise to a localized abscess in the abdomen or, more rarely, free pus within the abdomen which causes generalized PERITONITIS. Rupture of the appendix is a serious complication and the patient may be severely unwell.

Treatment The best treatment is prompt surgical removal of the diseased appendix, usually with antibiotic cover. If performed early, before rupture occurs, the procedure is normally straightforward and recovery swift. If the appendix has already ruptured and there is abscess formation or free intra-abdominal pus, surgery is still the best treatment but postoperative complications are more likely, and full recovery may be slower. (See PERITONITIS.)

APPENDIX A term applied to the appendages of several hollow organs: for example, the larynx has two pouches called appendices, and the epiploic appendices are the tags of fat that hang from the exterior part of the large intestine. The commonest application, however, is to the vermiform appendix of the large intestine. This is a short, slim, blind-ended tube up to 10 cm long attached to the caecum (a pouch at the start of the large intestine). Its function is unknown, though it may once have had one in ancestral humans. It is, however, prone to inflammation and infection (see APPENDICITIS).

APPETITE is the craving for the food necessary to maintain the body and to supply it with sufficient energy to carry on its functions. The ultimate cause of appetite is a question of supply and demand in the muscles and various organs, but the proximate cause is doubtful. Unlike hunger, it is probably an acquired, rather than an inborn, sensation. Whatever other factors may be concerned, the tone of the stomach is of importance. Important factors in stimulating appetite are anticipation and the sight and smell of well-cooked food. Individuals who eat unsuitable substances such as faeces are described as suffering from pica, which occurs sometimes during pregnancy, in children, in hysteria, and often in mental disorders. The two chief disorders, however, are excessive increase of appetite and diminution or loss of appetite.

Excessive appetite may be simply a bad habit, due to habitual over-indulgence in good food, and resulting in gout, obesity, etc., according to the other habits and constitution of the person. It may also be a sign of diabetes mellitus or thyrotoxicosis. (See EATING DISORDERS.)

Diminished appetite is a sign common to almost all diseases causing general weakness, because the activity of the stomach and the secretion of gastric juice fail early when vital power is low. It is the most common sign of dyspepsia due to gastritis (see DYSPEPSIA) and of cancer of the stomach. In some cases it is a manifestation of stress or strain such as domestic worry or difficulties at work. Indeed, appetite seems to be particularly susceptible to emotional disturbances, as is evidenced by the linked conditions of bulimia (pathological overeating) and anorexia nervosa (pathological dieting). These are dealt with under their respective headings.

APPROVED NAMES is the term used for names devised or selected by the British Pharmacopoeia Commission for new drugs. (see PROPRIETARY NAMES; GENERIC DRUG; PATENT.)

APRAXIA Loss of power to carry out regulated movements. Although there is no muscle weakness or incoordination, there is difficulty in formulating movement patterns.

APYREXIA Absence of fever.

ARACHNODACTYLY, or MARFAN'S SYNDROME, is a congenital condition characterized by extreme length and slenderness of the fingers and toes and, to a lesser extent, of the limbs and trunk, laxity of the ligaments, and dislocation of the lens of the eye. The antero-posterior diameter of the skull is abnormally long, and the jaw is prominent. There may also be abnormalities of the heart.

ARACHNOID MEMBRANE is one of the membranes covering the brain and spinal cord (see BRAIN). Arachnoiditis is the name applied to inflammation of this membrane.

ARBOVIRUSES A group of around 200 viruses, which are transmitted to man by ARTHROPODS. They include the viruses of DENGUE and YELLOW FEVER which are transmitted by mosquitoes.

ARC EYE Damage to the corneal surface of the eye caused by ultraviolet light from arc welding. A painful condition, it usually heals if the eyes are covered with pads for a day or two. It can be prevented by the proper use of protective goggles. A similar condition occurs in snow blindness or when someone fails to protect the eyes when using sun-tan lamps.

ARCUS SENILIS (see EYE DISEASES).

ARENAVIRUSES A group of viruses, so called because under the electron microscope they have a sand-sprinkled (Latin, *arenosus*) appearance. Among the diseases in man for which they are responsible are LASSA FEVER in West Africa, Argentinian haemorrhagic fever (mortality rate 3 to 15 per cent), a similar disease in Bolivia (mortality rate 18 per cent), and lymphocytic choriomeningitis, in which deaths are uncommon.

AREOLA literally means a small space, and is the term applied to the red or dusky ring round the nipple, or round an inflamed part. Increase in the duskiness of the areola on the breast is an important early sign of pregnancy.

ARGYLL ROBERTSON PUPIL A condition (described originally by Dr Argyll Robertson) in which the pupils contract when the eyes converge on a near object, but fail to contract when a bright light falls on the eye. It is found in several diseases, especially in loco-motor ataxia and neurosyphilis, an advanced manifestation of SYPHILIS.

ARGYRIA, or ARGYRIOSIS means the effect produced by taking silver salts over a long period, and consists of a deep duskiness of the skin, especially of the exposed parts.

ARM That part of the upper limb between the shoulder and elbow, but is generally taken to include also the forearm and shoulder regions. The upper limb is attached to the body by the strong pectoral muscles in front and by several powerful muscles springing from the spine and ribs behind. The great mobility of the shoulder is largely due to the fact that the only contact with the bones of the trunk takes place between the collar-bone and the upper end of the sternum or breast-bone, the shoulder-blade sliding freely between the muscles of the back as the arm is raised and lowered. The bones of the arm are the clavicle or collar-bone and the scapula or shoulder-blade lying at the upper part of the chest, the humerus, a single bone in the upper arm, and the radius and ulna lying side by side in the forearm. Eight small bones compose the wrist (or carpus) and connect the hand with the lower end of the radius.

The shoulder-joint is a ball-and-socket joint formed by the head of the humerus rotating against the glenoid cavity of the scapula (shoulder blade). The elbow is a hinged joint formed at the lower end of the humerus above, while the ulna forms the chief part of the joint below, the radius resting lightly against the humerus. When the hand is rotated so as to lie palm up or back up, the radius in the first case lies alongside the ulna and in the latter crosses over it. The chief muscle which bends the elbow is the biceps in front of the upper arm, while the triceps lying behind straightens the limb. A group of muscles attached at the inner side of the elbow act to bend the wrist and fingers; another group of muscles attached to the outer side of the elbow have the general action of straightening and bending backwards the wrist and fingers.

One large artery (brachial artery) runs down the inner side of the upper arm dividing the elbow into two branches, the radial and ulnar arteries. The radial artery can be felt pulsating near the wrist. The ulnar artery lies to the inner side of the forearm, deeply imbedded in muscles. A large group of nerves lies at the inner side of the armpit, and these nerves run downwards to supply the muscles and skin of the arm. The ulnar nerve runs behind the inner side of the elbow, where it is exposed to trauma and is popularly known as the 'funny bone'. The large radial nerve runs down the back of the upper arm and the outer side of the forearm. At the back of the upper arm it is often damaged, leading then to the condition known as DROP-WRIST, in which the hand hangs helpless and cannot be raised.

The collar bone is commonly broken by falls on the shoulder, and the radius is often broken by falls on the palm of the hand. The highly mobile shoulder joint is liable to dislocate when the upper arm is sharply twisted, but the elbow-joint is seldom injured. A small bursa or cavity lies between the skin and the end of the ulna at the point of the elbow, and this is often inflamed as the result of injury, and in the same way as the bursa in front of the knee is affected in the condition known as housemaid's knee. (See BURSITIS.)

ARMPIT, or AXILLA, is the pyramidal hollow between the upper arm and chest, bounded in front by the pectoral or breast muscles, behind by the shoulder-blade and its muscles, and running up to a point beneath the collar-bone. It contains the axillary vessels and nerves which run to the arm, also much fatty tissue, many sweat glands and lymphatic glands. The latter are important, because in poisoned wounds of the arm they may become inflamed, resulting in abscess; and still more, because in cancer of the breast they may become infected with cancer, and have to be removed with the breast. Wounds in the armpit are dangerous on the outer, front, and back walls, because large blood vessels run there.

ARRHYTHMIA means any variation from the normal regular rhythm of the heart-beat. The condition is produced by some affection interfering with the mechanism which controls the beating of the heart, and includes the following disorders: sinus arrhythmia, atrial fibrillation, atrial flutter, heart block, extrasystole, pulsus alternans, and paroxysmal atrial tachycardia, ventricular tachycardia and ventricular fibrillation. (See HEART DISEASES and ELECTROCARDIOGRAM.)

ARSENIC A metalloid with industrial use in glass, wood preservative, herbicide, semiconductor manufacture, and as an alloy additive. It may be a component in alternative or traditional remedies both intentionally and as a contaminant. Common in the environment and in food, especially seafood, arsenic is odourless and tasteless and highly toxic by ingestion, inhalation and skin contact. It binds to sulphydryl groups inhibiting the action of many ENZYMES and also disrupts oxidative phosphorylation by substituting for PHOSPHORUS. Clinical effects of acute poisoning range from severe gastrointestinal effects, renal impairment or failure characterized by OLIGURIA, HAEMATURIA, PROTEINURIA and renal tubular necrosis. Shock, COMA and CONVULSIONS are reported, as are JAUNDICE and peripheral NEUROPATHY. Chronic exposures are harder to diagnose as effects are non-specific. They include gastrointestinal disturbances, hyperpigmentation and HYPERKERATOSIS of skin, localized OEDEMA, ALOPECIA, neuropathy, PARAESTHESIA, HEPATOMEGALY and JAUNDICE. Management is largely supportive, particularly ensuring adequate renal function. Concentrations of arsenic in urine and blood can be measured and CHELATION therapy instituted if needed. Several chelators are effective. These include DMPS (2, 3-dimercapto-1-propanesulphonate), penicillamine and dimercaprol; DMPS is now agent of choice.

ARTEFACT (See ARTIFACT).

ARTERIES are vessels which convey oxygenated blood away from the heart to the tissues of the body, limbs, and internal organs. In the case of most arteries, the blood has been purified by passing through the lungs, and is consequently bright red in colour, but in the pulmonary arteries which convey it to the lungs it is unoxygenated, dark, and like the blood in veins.

The arterial system begins at the left ventricle of the heart with the aorta (see AORTA), which gives off branches that subdivide into smaller and smaller vessels, the final divisions, called arterioles, being microscopic, and ending in a network of capillaries, which perforate the tissues like the pores of a sponge, and bathe them in blood that is collected and brought back to the heart by veins. (See CIRCULATION OF THE BLOOD.)

The chief arteries after the aorta and its branches (see AORTA) are: (1) the common carotid, running up each side of the neck and dividing into internal carotid to the brain, and external carotid to the neck and face; (2) the subclavian

1 external carotid
2 superior and inferior thyroid
3 brachiocephalic (innominate)
4 internal thoracic
5 lateral thoracic
6 brachial
7 superior mesenteric
8 inferior mesenteric
9 radial
10 ulnar
11 obturator
12 inferior gluteal
13 femoral
14 deep femoral
15 perforating
16 deep palmar arch
17 superficial palmar arch

18 digital
19 anterior tibial
20 peroneal (fibular)
21 arcuate
22 medial malleolar
23 plantar arch
24 superficial temporal
25 occipital
26 internal carotid
27 vertebral
28 common carotid
29 left subclavian
30 aortic arch
31 outline of heart
32 axillary
33 intercostal aortic
34 aorta
35 coeliac
36 left renal
37 spermatic
38 common iliac
39 internal iliac
40 external iliac
41 internal pudendal
42 descending genicular
43 popliteal
44 posterior tibial
45 dorsalis pedis

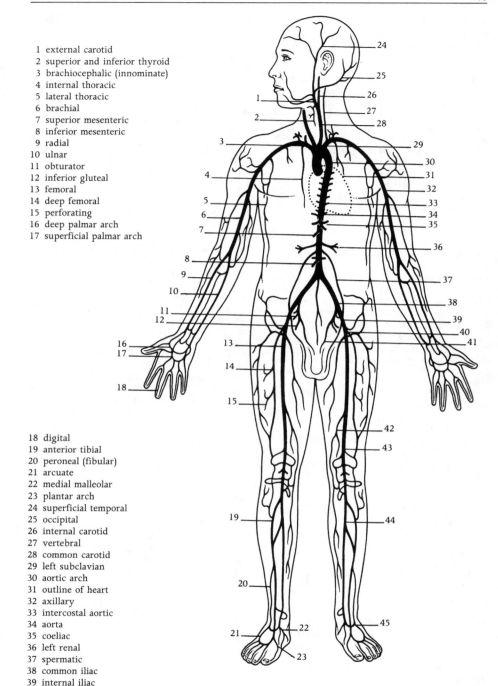

Diagram of body's arterial system.

1 adventitia
2 muscular coat or media
3 lumen

4 intima
5 elastic membrane
6 capillary supplying adventitia

Cross-sections showing structures of (left to right) artery, arteriole and vein.

to each arm, continued by the axillary in the armpit, and the brachial along the inner side of the arm, dividing at the elbow into the radial and the ulnar, which unite across the palm of the hand in arches that give branches to the fingers; (3) the two common iliacs, in which the aorta ends, each of which divides into the internal iliac to the organs in the pelvis, and the external iliac to the lower limb, continued by the femoral in the thigh, and the popliteal behind the knee, dividing into the anterior and posterior tibial arteries to the front and back of the leg. The latter passes behind the inner ankle to the sole of the foot, where it forms arches similar to those in the hand, and supplies the foot and toes by plantar branches.

Structure The arteries are highly elastic, dilating at each heart-beat as blood is driven into them, and forcing it on by their resiliency (see PULSE). Every artery has three coats: (a) the outer or adventitia, consisting of ordinary strong fibrous tissue; (b) the middle or media, consisting of muscular fibres supported by elastic fibres, which in some of the larger arteries form distinct membranes; and (c) the inner or intima, consisting of a layer of yellow elastic tissue on whose inner surface rests a layer of smooth plate-like endothelial cells, over which flows the blood. In the larger arteries the muscle of the middle coat is largely replaced by elastic fibres, which render the artery still more expansile and elastic. When an artery is cut across, the muscular coat instantly shrinks, drawing the cut end within the fibrous sheath that surrounds the artery, and bunching it up, so that a very small hole is left to be closed by blood-clot. (See HAEMORRHAGE.)

ARTERIES, DISEASES OF Arteries are the blood vessels that convey blood away from the heart to the tissues. The commonest cause of arterial disease is a degenerative condition known as atherosclerosis. Less commonly, inflammation of the arteries occurs. This inflammation is known as arteritis and occurs in a variety of conditions.

Atherosclerosis is due to the deposition of cholesterol into the walls of arteries. The process starts in childhood with the development of fatty streaks lining the arteries. In adulthood these progress, scarring and calcifying to form irregular narrowings within the arteries eventually leading to blockage of the vessel. The consequence of the narrowing or blockage depends on which vessels are involved – diseased cerebral vessels cause strokes, coronary vessels cause angina and heart attacks, renal vessels cause renal failure and peripheral arteries cause limb ischaemia (localized bloodlessness).

Risk factors predisposing individuals to atherosclerosis include age, male gender, raised plasma cholesterol concentration, high blood pressure, smoking, a family history of atherosclerosis, diabetes and obesity.

Arteritis occurs in a variety of conditions that produce inflammation in the arteries. Examples include syphilis – now rare in Britain – which produces inflammation of the aorta with subsequent dilatation (aneurysm formation) and risk of rupture; giant cell arteritis (temporal arteritis), a condition usually affecting the elderly, which involves the cranial arteries and leads to headache, tenderness over the temporal arteries and the risk of sudden blindness; Takayasau's syndrome, predominantly affecting young females, involves the aortic arch and its major branches, leading to the absence of pulses in affected vessels; polyarteritis nodosa is a condition causing multiple small nodules to form on the smaller arteries. General symptoms such as fever, malaise, weakness, anorexia and weight loss are accompanied by local manifestations of ischaemia (bloodlessness) in different parts of the body.

ARTERIOGRAPHY (see ANGIOGRAPHY).

ARTERIOLE is a small artery.

ARTERIO-VENOUS ANEURYSM is an abnormal communication between an artery and a vein. It is usually the result of an injury, such as a stab or a gunshot wound, which involves both a neighbouring artery and vein.

ARTERITIS means inflammation of an artery. (see ARTERIES, DISEASES OF.)

ARTHRALGIA Pain in a joint in which there is no swelling or other indications of arthritis.

ARTHRITIS refers to any condition of joints of the limbs or spine associated with inflammatory or structural change. It is distinguished from arthralgia which simply implies joint pain with or without any inflammatory or structural change. The two main categories of arthritis are osteoarthritis, in which the primary change is thought of as mechanical failure of articular cartilage, and rheumatoid arthritis, in which the primary problem is a chronic inflammation of the synovial lining, of joints, tendon sheaths and bursae. Other less common forms of inflammatory arthritis include psoriatic arthritis, Reiter's syndrome, colitic arthritis and Behçet's syndrome. Spondarthritis refers to an inflammatory arthritis with involvement of the spine and is often associated with the HLA B27 tissue type. (See OSTEOARTHRITIS; RHEUMATOID ARTHRITIS; RHEUMATIC FEVER.)

ARTHRODESIS is the operation for fixing a joint in a given position, from which it cannot be moved. It results in a pain-free, stable, strong joint in certain cases of joint disease such as osteoarthritis of the knee.

ARTHROPATHY is a term applied to any form of joint disease.

ARTHROPLASTY is the term applied to the operation for the making of a new joint as, for example, in advanced cases of osteoarthrosis of the hip, or the loosening of a fixed or stiff joint.

ARTHROPODS are segmented invertebrates with jointed legs. They include a wide range of organisms, such as scorpions, mites, ticks, spiders and centipedes (see ARBOVIRUSES).

ARTHROSCOPE: An endoscopic instrument that enables the operator to see inside a joint cavity and, if necessary, take a biopsy or carry out an operation.

ARTHROSCOPY Inspection of the interior of a joint (usually the knee) to diagnose any disorder there. The instrument used is a type of endoscope called an ARTHROSCOPE. The knee is often affected by conditions that are not easy to diagnose and are not revealed by X-ray examination. Surgery can be performed using arthroscopy and this reduces the time a patient has to be in hospital.

ARTICULAR means anything connected with a joint: e.g. articular rheumatism.

ARTICULATION is a term employed in two senses in medicine, either meaning the enunciation of words and sentences or meaning the type of contact between the surfaces of joints – these surfaces are called articular surfaces.

ARTIFACT (ARTEFACT) A foreign body found in living tissue viewed under a microscope. It is usually caused by faulty preparation of a specimen with the result that disease or abnormality seems to be present.

ARTIFICIAL INSEMINATION In this method of fertilization semen is collected either by the husband (AIH) or by a donor (AID) through masturbation and introduced into the cervix by means of an instrument around the time of ovulation.

AIH is thought to be particularly useful for men with retrograde ejaculation or erectile impotence.

AID may be considered when the partner's sperm count is either very low or zero. Insemination can be made with fresh or frozen semen. Donors should be tested for sexually transmitted diseases and their identity remain unknown to the infertile couple. The pregnancy rate over six months is 50–60 per cent. Artificial insemination is usually done at specially staffed centres with facilities to store semen and provide the individuals involved with appropriate counselling. Success rates are up to 70 per cent with fresh semen (used over a six-month period) and over 50 per cent with frozen semen.

ARTIFICIAL INTELLIGENCE The design and study of computer systems that have properties resembling human intelligence such as natural language, problem solving, and analysis of novel situations.

ARTIFICIAL KIDNEY (see DIALYSIS).

ARTIFICIAL LIMBS AND OTHER PARTS (see PROSTHESES).

ARTIFICIAL RESPIRATION (see APPENDIX 1: BASIC FIRST AID).

ARTIFICIAL VENTILATION OF THE LUNGS Normally, on inspiration, air is drawn into the lungs by a subatmospheric pressure within the pleural space. This is achieved by expanding the lungs using the intercostal muscles and the diaphragm. Expiration is achieved by reversing the process and, when breathing heavily, contracting the abdominal muscles. To produce ventilation artificially this cycle of air flowing in and out of the lungs must be reproduced (see LUNGS). This may be achieved using intermittent positive or negative pressure as described below.

Intermittent positive pressure (ITP) The simplest form of intermittent positive-pressure ventilation is mouth-to-mouth resuscitation (see APPENDIX 1: BASIC FIRST AID) where an individual blows his or her own expired gases into the lungs of an apnoeic person via the mouth or nose. Similarly gas may be blown into the lungs via a face mask (or down an endotracheal tube) and a self-inflating bag or an anaesthetic circuit containing a bag which is inflated by the flow of fresh gas from an anaesthetic machine, gas cylinder, or piped supply. In all these examples expiration is passive.

For more prolonged artificial ventilation it is usual to use a specially designed machine or ventilator to perform the task. The ventilators used in operating theatres when patients are anaesthetized and paralysed are relatively simple devices. Generally they consist of bellows which fill with fresh gas and which are then mechanically emptied (by means of a weight, piston, or compressed gas) via a circuit or tubes attached to an endotracheal tube into the patient's lungs. Adjustments can be made to the volume of fresh gas given with each breath and to the length of inspiration and expiration. Expiration is usually passive back to the atmosphere.

On the intensive-care unit, where patients are not usually paralysed, the ventilators are more complex. They have electronic controls which allow the user to programme a variety of pressure waveforms for inspiration and expiration. There are also programmes that allow the patient to breathe between ventilated breaths or to trigger ventilated breaths, or inhibit ventilation when the patient is breathing.

Indications for artificial ventilation are when the patient is unable to breathe adequately on his own. This may be due to injury or disease of the central nervous, cardiovascular, or respiratory systems or drug overdose. Artificial ventilation is performed to allow time for healing and recovery. Sometimes the patient is able to breathe but it is considered advisable to control ventilation – e.g. in severe head injury. Some operations require the patient to be paralysed for better or safer surgical access and this may require ventilation. With lung operations or very unwell patients ventilation is also indicated.

Artificial ventilation usually bypasses the physiological mechanisms for humidification of inspired air, so care must be taken to humidify inspired gases. It is important to monitor the efficacy of ventilation – e.g. by using blood gas measurement, pulse oximetry, and tidal carbon dioxide, and airways pressures.

Artificial ventilation is not without its hazards. The use of positive pressure raises the mean intrathoracic pressure. This can decrease venous return to the heart and cause a fall in CARDIAC OUTPUT and blood pressure. Positive-pressure ventilation may also cause PNEUMOTHORAX, but this is rare. While patients are ventilated, they are unable to breathe and so accidental disconnection from the ventilator may cause hypoxia and death.

Negative-pressure ventilation is seldom used nowadays. The chest or whole body, apart from the head, is placed inside an airtight box. A vacuum lowers the pressure within the box causing the chest to expand. Air is drawn into the lungs through the mouth and nose. At the end of inspiration the vacuum is stopped, the pressure in the box returns to atmospheric, and the patient exhales passively. This is the principle of the 'iron lung' which saved many lives during the polio epidemics of the 1950s. These machines are cumbersome and make access to the patient difficult. In addition, complex manipulation of ventilation is impossible.

Jet ventilation is a relatively modern form of ventilation which utilizes very small tidal volumes (see LUNGS) from a high-pressure source at high frequencies (20–100/min). First developed by physiologists to produce low stable intrathoracic pressures whilst studying CAROTID-BODY REFLEXES, it is sometimes now used in intensive therapy units for patients who do not achieve adequate gas exchanges with conventional ventilation. Its advantages are lower intrathoracic pressures (and therefore less risk of pneumothorax and impaired venous return) and better gas mixing within the lungs.

ARYTENOID The name applied to two cartilages in the larynx.

ASBESTOSIS A form of PNEUMOCONIOSIS, in which widespread fine scarring occurs in the lungs, leading to severe breathing disability. The main hazard, however, is the risk of cancer (MESOTHELIOMA) of the lung or PLEURA, or sometimes of the ovary. It is caused by the inhalation of mainly blue or brown asbestos dust, either during mining or quarrying, or in one of the many industries in which it is used: e.g. as an insulating material, in the making of paper, cardboard and brake linings. A person suffering from asbestosis is entitled to compensation as the disease is legally prescribed. About 900 people a year in the UK claim compensation, and 600 of these for mesothelioma; most patients with asbestosis now being diagnosed have it as a consequence of industrial practices used before 1970. The use of asbestos is now strictly controlled and, when blue asbestos is found in old buildings, skilled workmen are employed to dispose of it.

ASCARIASIS is the disease produced by infestation with the roundworm, *Ascaris lumbricoides*, also known as the maw-worm. Superficially it resembles a large earthworm. The male measures about 17 cm (7 inches) and the female 23 cm (9 inches) in length. It is a dirt disease, most prevalent where sanitation and cleanliness are lacking, particularly in the tropics and subtropics. Consumption of food contaminated by the ova (eggs), especially salad vegetables, is the commonest cause of infection. In children, infection is commonly acquired by crawling or playing on contaminated earth, and then sucking their fingers. After a complicated life-cycle in the body the adult worms end up in the intestines, whence they may be passed in the stools. A light infection may cause no symptoms. A heavy infection may lead to colic, or even obstruction of the gut. Occasionally a worm may wander into the stomach and be vomited up.

Treatment Mebendazole is the drug of choice in the UK, being given as a single dose. It should be combined with hygienic measures to break the cycle of autoinfection. All members of the family require treatment. Other anthelmintics include piperazine and pyrantel.

ASCITES An accumulation of fluid in the abdomen. The causes include heart failure, CANCER, CIRRHOSIS OF THE LIVER and infections.

ASCORBIC ACID (VITAMIN C) is a simple sugar found in living tissues, its highest concentrations being in the ADRENAL cortex and the eye. Stress and CORTICOTROPHIN lead to a loss of ascorbic acid from the adrenal cortex. Fresh fruit and vegetables, particularly blackcurrants, citrus fruits, berries and green vegetables are the richest dietary sources, or it may be synthetically prepared. Ascorbic acid is easily eliminated from the diet by traditional methods of cooking, being very soluble in water, and easily destroyed by heat, alkalis, traces of copper or by an oxidase released by damage to plant tissues. Ascorbic acid deficiency may lead to SCURVY, traditionally associated with sailors, among elderly people living alone or in poor communities living at subsistence level. It has been claimed that large doses (1–2g daily) will prevent the common cold, but few large controlled trials have been carried out and it is inadvisable for people to dose themselves with large quantities of ascorbic acid, which may result in the formation of oxalate stones in the urinary tract. (See VITAMIN.)

ASEPSIS A technique to produce a germ-free environment to protect patients from infection. It is used for any procedure that might introduce infection into the body and is essential for all surgery – even minor procedures. Asepsis is achieved by ensuring that all people who come into contact with the patient scrub their hands and wear sterilized gowns with disposable masks and gloves. Operating-theatre air and equipment must also be clean. An aseptic technique is also necessary when caring for patients whose IMMUNE SYSTEM is suppressed. An example is LEUKAEMIA, the treatment of which affects the immune system.

Asepsis is aimed at preventing infection, ANTISEPSIS is the use of chemicals to destroy germs already on the body or in a wound (see ANTISEPTICS).

ASH Action on Smoking and Health is a charity founded by the Royal College of Physicians in 1971 and supported by the Department of Health. It gathers information about the dangers of smoking which it disseminates to the public, commissions surveys on public attitudes to smoking and helps people to give up the habit. ASH has contributed substantially to the cut in the number of smokers: 6 out of 10 adults are now non-smokers, and an increasing number of public places are becoming smoke free. ASH has a small headquarters in London (see APPENDIX 2: ADDRESSES) from which further information may be obtained, with other national and regional branches in Scotland, Wales, and Northern Ireland.

ASPARAGINASE is an enzyme that breaks down the amino-acid, asparagine. This is of no significance to most cells in the body as they can make asparagine from simpler constituents. Certain tumours, however, are unable to do this and therefore, if they cannot receive ready-made supplies of the amino-acid, they die. It is on this basis that asparaginase is proving of promise in the treatment of tumours which, by the administration of asparaginase, are deprived of an essential metabolite – and perish.

ASPARTANE is an artificial sweetener 200 times as sweet as sugar but without the bitter after-taste of saccharine.

ASPERGILLOSIS is a disease caused by invasion of the lung by the fungus, *Aspergillus fumigatus*. The infection is acquired by inhalation of air-borne spores of the fungus which settle and grow in damaged parts of the lung such as healed tuberculous cavities, abscesses, or the dilated bronchi of BRONCHIECTASIS.

ASPERGILLUS A group of fungi including the common moulds. Several of these are capable of infecting the lungs and producing a disease resembling pulmonary tuberculosis.

ASPHYXIA means literally absence of pulse, but is the name given to the whole series of symptoms which follow stoppage of breathing and of the heart's action. Drowning is one cause but obstruction of the air passages may occur as the result of a foreign body or in some diseases, such as croup, diphtheria, swelling of the throat due to wounds or inflammation, asthma (to a partial extent), tumours in the chest (causing slow asphyxia), and the external conditions of suffocation and strangling. Placing the head in a plastic bag results in asphyxia and poisonous gases also cause asphyxia, for example, carbon monoxide gas, which may be given off by a stove or charcoal brazier in a badly ventilated room can kill people during sleep. (See CARBON MONOXIDE.) Several gases, such as sulphurous acid (from burning sulphur), ammonia, and chlorine (from bleaching-powder), cause involuntary closure of the entrance to the larynx, and thus prevent breathing. Other gases, such as nitrous oxide (or laughing-gas), chloroform, and ether, in poisonous quantity, stop the breathing by paralysing the respiration centre in the brain.

Symptoms In most cases death from asphyxia is due to insufficiency of oxygen supplied to the blood. The first signs are rapid pulse and gasping for breath. Next comes a rise in the blood pressure, causing throbbing in the head, with lividity or blueness of the skin, due to failure of aeration of the blood, followed by still greater struggles for breath and by general convulsions. The heart becomes over-distended and gradually weaker, a paralytic stage sets in, and all struggling and breathing slowly cease. When asphyxia is due to charcoal fumes, coal-gas, and other narcotic influences, there is no convulsive stage, and death ensues gently and may occur in the course of sleep.

Treatment So long as the heart continues to beat, recovery may be looked for with prompt treatment. The one essential of treatment is to get the impure blood aerated by artificial respiration. Besides this, the feeble circulation can be helped by various methods. (See APPENDIX 1: BASIC FIRST AID, choking, cardiac/respiratory arrest.)

ASPIRATION means the withdrawal of fluid or gases from the natural cavities of the body or from cavities produced by disease. It may be performed either for curative purposes, or, very often, a small amount is drawn off for diagnosis of the nature or origin of the fluid. An instrument called an aspirator is used to remove blood and fluid from a surgical operation site – for example, the abdomen or the mouth (in dentistry).

PLEURISY with effusion is a condition requiring aspiration, and a litre or more of fluid may be drawn off by an aspirator or a large syringe and needle. Chronic abscesses and tuberculous joints may call for its use, the operation being done with a small syringe and hollow needle. PERICARDITIS with effusion is another condition in which aspiration is sometimes performed. The spinal canal is aspirated by the operation of lumbar puncture. (See LUMBAR PUNCTURE.) In children the ventricles of the brain are sometimes similarly relieved from excess of fluid by piercing the fontanelle (soft spot) on the infant's head. (See HYDROCEPHALUS.)

ASPIRIN, or ACETYLSALICYLIC ACID A white crystalline powder which is used like sodium salicylate as a remedy for reducing inflammation and fever. It has some action in relieving pain and producing sleep and is therefore often used for headache and slighter degrees of insomnia. Daily doses are now used in the prevention of coronary thrombosis. The dose is 75 to 300 mg. Aspirin should be used with caution in children and in people with dyspepsia or gastric ulcers. (See ANALGESICS.)

ASPIRIN POISONING A commonly available ANALGESIC which is frequently taken in overdose. Clinical features of poisoning include NAUSEA, vomiting, TINNITUS, flushing, sweating, HYPERVENTILATION, DEHYDRATION, deafness and acid-base and ELECTROLYTE disturbances. In more severe cases individuals may be confused, drowsy and comatose. Rarely, RENAL failure, PULMONARY OEDEMA or cardiovascular collapse occur. Severe toxicity may be delayed as absorption of the drug may be prolonged due to the formation of drug concretions in the stomach. Treatment involves the repeated administration of activated CHARCOAL, monitoring of concentration of aspirin in blood and correction of acid-base and electrolyte imbalances. In more severely poisoned patients enhanced excretion of the drug may be necessary by alkalinizing the urine (by intravenous administration of SODIUM bicarbonate) or HAEMODIALYSIS.

ASSISTED CONCEPTION This technique is used when normal methods of conception or artificial insemination have failed. There are two types of assisted conception: in vitro fertilization (IVF), also known as zygote intrafallopian transfer (ZIFT), and gamete intrafallopian transfer (GIFT).

In vitro fertilization In this technique the female partner receives drugs to enhance ovulation. Just before ovulation several ripe eggs are collected under ultrasound guidance or through a laparoscope. The eggs are incubated with the prepared sperm. About 40 hours later, once the eggs have been fertilized, up to three embryos are transferred into the mother's uterus via the cervix. Pregnancy should then proceed normally. About one in five IFV pregnancies results in the birth of a child. The success rate falls rapidly if the female partner is aged 40 and over.

INDICATIONS In women with severely damaged fallopian tubes IVF offers the only chance of pregnancy. The method is also used in couples with unexplained infertility, male-factor infertility where the sperm count is only slightly abnormal, and in women who have suffered an early or surgical menopause. In these cases donor eggs are used.

Almost one quarter of pregnancies are multiple. Twin or triplet pregnancies are associated with many more problems such as premature labour. As the likelihood of multiple pregnancy increases with the number of eggs replaced into the uterus, legislation in the United Kingdom recommends that no more than three eggs are transferred in each IVF cycle.

It is also important to monitor the

preovulation phase in the woman by ultrasound scan so that not too many eggs develop, as this may lead to hyperstimulation of the ovaries which can cause the development of ovarian cysts.

Gamete intrafallopian transfer This method of fertilization may be used provided at least one fallopian tube is healthy and patent. As with IVF, ovulation is usually stimulated in the female partner. The woman then undergoes a laparoscopy just before ovulation during which the ripe eggs are picked up from the ovaries and injected into the fallopian tube together with prepared sperm from the husband. Fertilization then takes place as it does in natural conception.

GIFT is indicated in couples with unexplained infertility, minor male- or cervical-factor infertility. Associated problems are similar to IVF and are mainly related to an increased rate of multiple pregnancies.

The success rate for GIFT is about 17 per cent. (See ARTIFICIAL INSEMINATION.)

ASTEREOGNOSIS means the loss of the capacity to recognize the nature of an object by feeling it, and indicates a lesion (e.g. tumour) of the brain.

ASTHENIA A traditional term meaning want of strength.

ASTHENOPIA means a sense of weakness in the eyes, coming on when they are used. As a rule it is due to long-sightedness, slight inflammation, or weakness of the muscles that move the eyes. (See VISION.)

ASTHMA Asthma is a disorder of breathing characterized by widespread narrowing of airways within the lung. The main symptom is shortness of breath. A major feature of asthma is the reversibility of the airway narrowing and, consequently, the breathlessness. This variability in the obstruction may occur spontaneously or in response to treatment.

Cause There is a strong familial association of asthma and a great deal of interest in the genetic basis of the condition. Several GENES seem to be associated with the condition of ATOPY in which subjects have a predisposition to form ANTIBODIES of the IgE class against ALLERGENS they encounter, especially inhaled allergens. This leads to allergic RHINITIS (often manifest as hayfever), to asthma and ECZEMA.

The allergic response in the lining of the airway leads to an inflammatory reaction. Many cells are involved in this inflammatory process, including LYMPHOCYTES, EOSINOPHILS, NEUTROPHILS and MAST CELLS. The cells are attracted and controlled by a complex system of inflammatory mediators. The inflamed airway wall produced in this process is then sensitive to further allergic stimuli or to non-specific challenges such as dust, smoke or drying from the increased respiration during exercise. Recognition of this inflammation has concentrated attention on anti-inflammatory aspects of treatment.

Continued inflammation with poor control of asthma can result in permanent damage to the airway wall such that reversibility is reduced and airway narrowing becomes permanent. Appropriate anti-inflammatory therapy may help to prevent this damage.

Many allergens can be important triggers of asthma. House-dust mite, grass pollen and animal dander are the commonest problems. Occupational factors such as grain dusts, hard-metals fumes and chemicals in the plastic and paint industry are important in some adults. Viral infections are another common trigger.

The prevalence of asthma appears to be on the increase in most countries. Several factors have been linked to this increase. Most important may be the vulnerability of the immature IMMUNE SYSTEM in infants. High exposure to allergens such as house-dust mite early in life may prime the immune system while reduced exposure to common viral infections may delay the maturation of the immune system. In addition maternal smoking in pregnancy and infancy increases the risk.

Clinical course The major symptoms of asthma are breathlessness and cough. Occasionally cough may be the only symptom, especially in children, where night-time cough may be mistaken for recurrent infection and treated inappropriately with antibiotics.

The onset of asthma is usually in childhood, but it may begin at any age. In childhood boys are affected more often than girls but by adulthood the sex incidence is equal. Children who have mild asthma are more likely to grow out of the condition as they go through their teenage years, although symptoms may recur later.

The degree of airway narrowing, and its change with time and treatment, can be monitored by measuring the peak expiratory flow with a simple monitor at home, a peak-flow meter. The typical pattern shows the peak flow to be lowest in the early morning and this 'morning dipping' is often associated with disturbance of sleep.

Acute exacerbations of asthma may be provoked by infections or allergic stimuli. If they do not respond quickly and fully to medication, expert help should be sought urgently since oxygen and higher doses of drugs will be necessary to control the attack. In a severe attack the breathing rate and the pulse rate rise and the chest sounds wheezy. The peak-flow rate of air into the lungs falls. Patients may be unable to talk in full sentences without catching their breath, and the reduced oxygen in the blood in very severe attacks may produce the blue colour of cyanosis in the lips and tongue. Such acute attacks can be very frightening for the patient and family.

Treatment The first important consideration in the treatment of asthma is avoidance of precipitating factors. When this is a specific animal or occupational exposure, this may be possible. It is more difficult for house-dust mite or pollens. Exercise-induced asthma should be treated adequately rather than avoiding exercise.

Desensitization injections using small quanties of specific allergens are used widely in some countries but have limited value since most asthma is precipitated by many stimuli and controlled adequately with simple treatment.

There are two groups of main drugs for the treatment of asthma. The first are the bronchodilators which relax the smooth muscle in the wall of the airways, increase their diameter and relieve breathlessness. The most useful agents are the beta adrenergic agonists (see ADRENERGIC RECEPTORS) such as salbutamol and terbutaline. They are best given by inhalation into the airways since this reduces the general side-effects from oral use. These drugs are usually given to reverse airway narrowing or to prevent its onset on exercise. However, longer-acting inhaled beta agonists such as salmeterol and formoterol or the theophyllines given in tablet form can be used regularly as prevention. The beta agonists can cause TREMOR and PALPITATIONS in some patients.

The second group of drugs are the anti-inflammatory agents that act to reduce the airway inflammation.The main agents in this group are the CORTICOSTEROIDS. They must be taken regularly, even when symptoms are absent. Given by inhalation, they have few side-effects. In acute attacks short courses of oral steroids are used and in very severe disease regular oral steroids may be needed. Other drugs have a role in suppressing inflammation. Sodium cromoglycate has been available for some years and is generally less effective than inhaled steroids. Newer agents directed at specific steps in the inflammatory pathway such as leukotriene antagonists are alternative agents.

Treatment guidelines have been produced by various national and international bodies. Most have set out treatment in steps according to severity with objectives for asthma control based on symptoms and peak flow. Patients should have a management plan that sets out their regular treatment and their appropriate response to changes in their condition.

Advice and support for research into asthma is provided by the National Asthma Campaign (see APPENDIX 2: ADDRESSES).

ASTIGMATISM An error of refraction in the eye due to the cornea (the clear membrane in front of the eye) being unequally curved in different directions, so that rays of light in different meridians cannot be brought to a focus together on the retina. The curvature, instead of being globular, is egg-shaped, longer in one axis than the other. The condition causes objects to seem distorted and out of place, a ball for instance looking like an egg, a circle like an ellipse. The condition is remedied by suitable spectacles of which one surface forms part of a cylinder.

ASTROVIRUSES Small round viruses with no distinctive features, which have been isolated from the stools of infants with gastroenteritis (see DIARRHOEA).

ASYMPTOMATIC The lack of any symptoms of disease whether or not a disease is present.

ASYNERGIA The absence of harmonious and co-ordinated movements between muscles having opposite actions – e.g. the flexors and extensors of a joint – and is a sign of disease of the nervous system.

ASYSTOLE Arrest of the action of the heart.

ATAVISM The principle of inheritance of disease or bodily characters from grandparents or remoter ancestors, the parents not having been affected by these.

ATAXIA Loss of co-ordination, though the power necessary to make the movements is still present. Thus an ataxic person may have a good grip in each hand but be unable to do any fine movements with the fingers, or, if the ataxia be in the legs, he throws these about a great deal in walking, though he can lift the legs and take steps quite well. This is due to a sensory defect or to disease of the cerebellum. (See FRIEDREICH'S ATAXIA; LOCOMOTOR ATAXIA; APPENDIX 2: ADDRESSES.)

ATELECTASIS Collapse of a part of the lung, or failure of the lung to expand at birth.

ATENOLOL A drug that antagonizes beta ADRENERGIC RECEPTORS and is of value in the treatment of high blood-pressure, ANGINA and ARRHYTHMIAS. One of its practical advantages is that only one dose a day need be taken. Atenolol, being a beta-blocking drug, may precipitate ASTHMA, an effect that may be dangerous. Among the side-effects are fatigue and disturbed sleep. (See BETA-ADRENOCEPTOR-BLOCKING DRUGS.)

ATHEROMA Degenerative changes in the inner and middle coats of arteries. (See ARTERIES, DISEASES OF.)

ATHEROSCLEROSIS A form of arteriosclerosis, in which there is fatty degeneration of the middle coat of the arterial wall.   (See ARTERIES, DISEASES OF: arteriosclerosis.)

ATHETOSIS is the name for slow, involuntary, writhing, and repeated movements of the face, tongue, hands and feet, caused by disease of the brain. It is usually a manifestation of CEREBRAL PALSY. Drugs used to treat PARKINSON'S DISEASE can also cause athetosis.

ATHLETE'S FOOT A somewhat loose term applied to a skin eruption on the foot, usually between the toes. It is commonly due to RING-WORM, but may be due to other infections, or merely excessive sweating of the feet. It usually responds to careful foot hygiene and the use of antifungal powder.

ATLAS The first cervical vertebra. (See SPINAL COLUMN.)

ATONY Absence of tone or vigour in muscles and other organs.

ATOPY, meaning out of place, is a form of hypersensitivity characterized, amongst other features, by a familial tendency. It is due to the propensity of the affected individual to produce large amounts of reagin ANTIBODIES which stick to MAST cells in the mucosa so that when the ANTIGEN is inhaled histamine is released from the mast cell. It is the condition responsible for ASTHMA and HAY FEVER. (See also ALLERGY.) It is estimated that 10 per cent of the human race are subject to atopy. (See also DERMATITIS.)

ATRESIA The absence of a natural opening, or closure of it by a membrane. Thus atresia may be found in new-born infants preventing the bowels from moving, and, in young girls after puberty, absence of the menstrual flow may be due to such a malformation.

ATRIAL NATRIURETIC PEPTIDE The atria of the heart contain peptides with potent diuretic and vasodilating properties. It has been known since 1980 that extracts of human atria have potent diurectic and natriuretic effects in animals (see DIURETICS). In 1984 three polypeptide species were isolated from human atria and were called alpha, beta and gamma human atrial natriuretic peptides. Plasma concentration of immuno-reactive atrial natriuretic peptide can now be measured. The levels are low in healthy subjects and are increased in patients with congestive heart failure. Infusion of the peptides reduces blood pressure and causes a natriuresis and diuresis.

ATRIAL SEPTAL DEFECT (see HEART DISEASES, Congenital heart disease).

ATRIUM is the name now given to the two upper cavities of the heart. These used to be known as the auricles of the heart. The term is also applied to the part of the ear immediately internal to the drum of the ear. (Plural: atria.)

ATROPHY occurs when normal tissue or an organ wastes because the constituent cells die. Undernourishment, disease, injury, lack of use or ageing may cause atrophy. Muscular atrophy occurs in certain neurological diseases

such as poliomyelitis or muscular dystrophy. The ovary atrophies at the menopause. (See MUSCLES, DISEASES OF).

ATROPINE is the active principle of belladonna, the juice of the deadly nightshade. Because of its action in dilating the pupils it was at one time used as a cosmetic to give the eyes a full, lustrous appearance. It acts by antagonizing the action of the PARASYMPATHETIC NERVOUS SYSTEM. It temporarily impairs vision by paralysing accommodative power. (See ACCOMMODATION.) It inhibits the action of some of the nerves in the AUTONOMIC NERVOUS SYSTEM. The drug relaxes smooth muscle. It has the effect of checking the activity of almost all the glands of the body, including the SWEAT GLANDS of the skin and the SALIVARY GLANDS in the mouth. It relieves spasm by paralysing nerves in the muscle of the intestine, bile-ducts, bladder, stomach, etc. It has the power, in moderate doses, of markedly increasing the rate of the heart-beats, though by very large doses the heart, along with all other muscles, is paralysed and stopped.

Uses In eye troubles, atropine drops are used to dilate the pupil for more thorough examination of the interior of the eye, or to draw the iris away from wounds and ulcers on the centre of the eye; they also soothe the pain due to light falling on an inflamed eye, and are further used to paralyse the ciliary muscle and so prevent accommodative changes in the eye while the eye is being examined with the OPHTHALMOSCOPE. Atropine is used before general ANAESTHESIA to reduce secretions in the bronchial tree. It is given by injection. The drug can also be used to accelerate the heart rate in BRADYCARDIA as a result of coronary thrombosis.

ATROPINE POISONING (see BELLADONNA POISONING).

AUDIOMETRY The testing of hearing.

AUDITORY NERVE (see VESTIBULOCOCHLEAR NERVE).

AURA The peculiar feeling which persons, subject to epileptic seizures, have just before the onset of an attack. It may be a sensation of a cold breeze, a peculiar smell, a vision of some animal or person, an undefinable sense of disgust. Important for persons who experience it, an aura gives warning that a fit is coming and may enable a place of safety or seclusion to be reached.

AURAL Relating to the ear.

AURICLE A term applied both to the pinna or flap of the ear and also to the ear-shaped tip of the atrium of the heart.

AURISCOPE An instrument for examining the ear. The source of illumination may be incorporated in the instrument, as in the electric auriscope, or it may be an independent light which is reflected into the ear by means of a forehead mirror. (See EAR, DISEASES OF.)

AUSCULTATION The method used by physicians to determine, by listening, the condition of certain internal organs. The ancient physicians appear to have practised a kind of auscultation, by which they were able to detect the presence of air or fluids in the cavities of the chest and abdomen.

In 1819, the French physician, Laennec, introduced the method of auscultation by means of the stethoscope. Initially a wooden cylinder, the STETHOSCOPE has evolved into a binaural instrument consisting of a small expanded chest-piece and two flexible tubes, the ends of which fit into the ears of the observer. Various modifications of the binaural stethoscope have been introduced.

Conditions affecting the lungs can often be recognized by means of auscultation and the stethoscope. The same is true for the heart, in which disease can, by auscultation, often be identified with striking accuracy. But auscultation is also helpful in the investigation of ANEURYSMS and certain diseases of the OESOPHAGUS and STOMACH. The stethoscope is also a valuable aid in the detection of some forms of uterine tumours, especially in the diagnosis of pregnancy.

AUTISM The term autism was introduced by Kanner in 1943 to describe a development defect in which children are unable to mature socially despite excellent motor skill. Thus, despite their manual dexterity they are unable to form emotional bonds, even with their parents. Because of their disregard of other people they are refractory to discipline. Although they may acquire some language, they communicate little. The condition is rare, affecting up to four children in every 10,000, with more boys than girls affected. The causes are unknown but probably have a physical origin. A recent study suggests that MMR VACCINE (against mumps, measles and rubella) may occasionally cause autism but the risks of disability from having these infectious diseases are much higher than the risk of autism from MMR vaccination.

Advice and information on autism may be obtained from the National Autistic Society (see APPENDIX 2: ADDRESSES).

AUTO- Prefix meaning self.

AUTOANTIBODY An antibody produced by a person's immune system that acts against the body's own tissues resulting in AUTOIMMUNITY.

AUTOCLAVE This is a very effective way of ensuring that material, e.g. surgical dressings, is completely sterilized and that even the most resistant bacteria with which it may be contaminated, are destroyed. Its use is based upon the fact that water boils when its vapour pressure is equal to the pressure of the surrounding atmosphere. This means that if the pressure inside a closed vessel be increased, the temperature at which water inside the vessel boils, will rise above 100 °C. By adjusting the pressure, almost any temperature for the boiling of the water will be obtained.

AUTOGENOUS means self-generated and is the term applied to products which arise within the body. It is applied to bacterial vaccines manufactured from the organisms found in discharges from the body and used for the treatment of the person from whom the bacteria were derived.

AUTOIMMUNE DISORDERS A collection of conditions in which the body's immune system attacks its own tissues, identifying them as foreign substances. Genetic factors may play a part in this abnormal function but the causes are not clear. The disorder may affect one organ (organ-specific) or type of cell or several (non-organ-specific). Among the autoimmune disorders are ADDISON'S DISEASE; autoimmune haemolytic anaemia (see ANAEMIA); autoimmune chronic active HEPATITIS; DIABETES MELLITUS; MYASTHENIA GRAVIS; PERNICIOUS ANAEMIA; RHEUMATOID ARTHRITIS; and SYSTEMIC LUPUS ERYTHEMATOSUS. (See IMMUNITY.)

Treatment Any major deficiencies, such as thyroxin or insulin lack, should be corrected. Then the activity of the immune system should be reduced. CORTICOSTEROID drugs and, in more severe cases, strong immunosuppressant drugs – AZATHIOPRINE, CYCLOPHOSPHAMIDE or METHOTREXATE should be administered. Treatment is difficult because of the need to control the autoimmune condition without damaging the body's ability to combat other diseases.

AUTOIMMUNITY is a reaction to an individual's own tissues (self-antigens) to which tolerance has been lost (see IMMUNITY). Autoantibodies are not necessarily harmful and are commonly encountered in healthy persons. Autoimmune disease ensues when the immune system attacks the target cells of the autoimmune reaction.

AUTO-INTOXICATION means literally self-poisoning, and is any condition of poisoning brought about by substances formed in or by the body.

AUTOLYSIS The disintegration and softening of dead cells brought about by enzymes in the cells themselves.

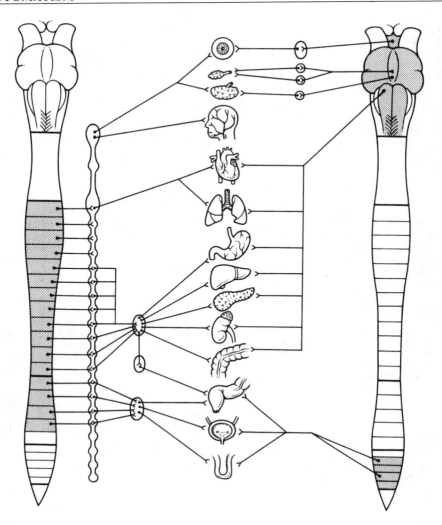

Schematic diagram of autonomic nervous system. (Left) Sympathetic nerves leaving middle section of spinal cord to connect via the vertebral ganglion (sympathetic trunk) to organs. (Right) Parasympathetic nerves leaving the brain and lower spinal cords to connect to organs.

AUTOMATISM The performance of acts without conscious will, as, for example, after an attack of epilepsy or concussion of the brain. In such conditions the person may perform acts of which he is neither conscious at the time nor has any memory afterwards. It is especially liable to occur when persons suffering from epilepsy, mental subnormality, or concussion consume alcoholic liquors. It may also occur following the taking of barbiturates or PSYCHEDELIC DRUGS. There are, however, other cases in which there are no such precipitatory factors. Thus it may occur following hypnosis, mental stress or strain, or conditions such as FUGUES or somnambulism (see SLEEP). The condition is of considerable importance from a legal point of view, because acts done in this state, and for which the person committing them is not responsible, may be of a criminal nature. According to English law, however, it entails complete loss of consciousness, and only then is it a defence to an action for negligence. A lesser impairment of consciousness is no defence.

AUTONOMIC NERVOUS SYSTEM Part of the nervous system which regulates the bodily functions that are not under conscious control. These include regulating the heart beat, intestinal movements, salivation, sweating, etc. It consists of two main divisions – the SYMPATHETIC and the PARASYMPATHETIC SYSTEMS. The smooth muscles, heart and most glands are connected to nerve fibres from both systems and their proper functioning depends on the balance between these two. (See NERVES.)

AUTOPSY   A post-mortem examination, or the examination of the internal organs of a dead body. (See NECROPSY.)

AUTO-SUGGESTION   A self-induced receptive, hypnotic state which is believed to improve the body's ability to help itself. Doctors have long realized that if they suggested to a patient that a particular treatment would work, it often did – a type of placebo effect. Some techniques now make use of this idea. For instance, people can be taught muscular relaxation to control their anxiety states – the biofeedback principle.

AVASCULAR   Without a blood supply. Avascular necrosis is the death of a tissue because the blood supply has been cut off.

AVERSION THERAPY   A form of psychological treatment in which such an unpleasant response is induced to his psychological aberration that the patient decides to give it up. Thus the victim of alcoholism is given a drug that makes the subsequent drinking of alcoholic liquors so unpleasant by inducing nausea and vomiting that he decides to give up drinking. (See ALCOHOL; and DISULFIRAM.) Aversion therapy may help in the treatment of alcoholism, drug addiction, sexual deviations, such as transvestism, and compulsive gambling.

AVITAMINOSIS   The condition of a human being or an animal deprived of one or more vitamins.

AVULSION   Forcible tearing away of one tissue from another. For example, a tendon may be avulsed from the bone to which it is attached or a nerve may be injured and torn away from the tissue in which it runs.

AXILLA   Anatomical name for the armpit. (See ARMPIT.)

AXIS   The name applied to the second cervical vertebra. (See SPINAL COLUMN.)

AXON   Nerve fibre: an elongated projection of a nerve cell or neurone that carries an electrical impulse to the tissue at the end of the axon. Large axons are covered by a sheath of insulating myelin which is interrupted at intervals by nodes of Lanvier, where other axons branch out. An axon may be more than a metre long. It ends by branching into several filaments called telodendria and these are in contact with muscle or gland membranes and other nerves. (See NERVES.)

AZATHIOPRINE   A CYTOTOXIC and an IMMUNOSUPPRESSIVE drug. In the first of these capacities it is proving of value in the treatment of acute leukaemia. As an immunosuppressive agent, by reducing the ANTIBODY response of the body it is proving of value in facilitating the success of transplant operations by reducing the chances of the transplanted organ, e.g. the kidney, being rejected by the body. It is also proving of value in the treatment of auto-immune disorders. (See CYTOTOXIC.)

AZOOSPERMIA   The condition characterized by lack of SPERMATOZOA in the SEMEN.

AZOTAEMIA means the presence of urea and other nitrogenous bodies in greater concentration than normal in the blood. The condition is generally associated with advanced types of kidney disease.

B

BABINSKI REFLEX is an abnormal response of the plantar reflex. When a sharp body is drawn along the sole of the foot, instead of the toes bending down towards the sole as usual, the great toe is turned upwards and the other toes tend to spread apart. This response may be obtained in normal infants, but after the age of about two years its presence indicates some severe disturbance in the upper part of the central nervous system. The Babinski reflex may occur in transient form during temporary states such as coma or after an epileptic fit and need not indicate permanent damage.

BACILLUS   This is a big group (genus) of GRAM-POSITIVE (see GRAM'S STAIN) rodlike bacteria. Found widely in the air and soil – commonly as spores – they feed on dead organic matter. As well as infecting and spoiling food, some are pathogenic to humans, causing, for example, anthrax, conjunctivitis and dysentery. They are also the source of some antibiotics (See under MICROBIOLOGY.)

BACITRACIN   A polypeptide antibiotic, with a spectrum similar to penicillin. It is not absorbed if taken orally but is valuable topically as an ointment in conjunction with neomycin or polymyxin.

BACK   The back consists mainly of the spinal column and hinder parts of the ribs, and the wide-spreading iliac or haunch bones with the sacrum below. The bones are covered by thick and powerful muscles, which above support and move the head and which below pass round the flanks and downwards into the lower limbs. The skin covering the back is not very sensitive and is not greatly subject to painful conditions. The powerful muscles, of which the chief is the erector spinae, are vulnerable to minor injuries, the result of twists and strains, and also to rheumatic affections (see LUMBAGO). Diseases and injuries of the spinal column and spinal cord are of a very serious nature (see SPINAL COLUMN; SPINAL CORD).

BACKACHE Most people suffer from backache at times during their lives; much of this has no identifiable cause – non-specific back pain, a diagnosis that is one of the biggest single causes of sickness absence in the UK's working population. Certain occupations, such as those involving long periods of sedentary work, lifting, bending and awkward physical work are especially likely to cause backache. Back pain is commonly the result of sporting activities. Non-specific back pain is probably the result of mechanical disorders in the muscles, ligaments, and joints of the back: torn muscles, sprained LIGAMENTS, and FIBROSITIS. These disorders are not always easy to diagnose, but mild muscular and ligamentous injuries are usually relieved with symptomatic treatment: warmth, gentle massage, analgesics, etc. Sometimes back pain is caused or worsened by muscle spasms, which may call for the use of antispasmodic drugs. STRESS and DEPRESSION (see MENTAL ILLNESS) can sometimes result in chronic backache and should be considered if no clear physical diagnosis can be made.

If back pain is severe and/or recurrent, possibly radiating round to the abdomen or down the back or a leg (sciatica), or is accompanied by weakness or loss of feeling in the leg(s), it may be caused by a prolapsed intervertebral (slipped disc) pressing on a nerve. The patient needs prompt investigation, including X-ray examination. Resting on a firm bed or board can relieve the symptoms but the patient may need a surgical operation to remove the disc and relieve pressure on the affected nerve.

Other local causes of back pain are osteoarthritis of the vertebral joints, ankylosing spondylitis (an inflammatory condition which can severely deform the spine), cancer (usually secondary cancer deposits spreading from a primary tumour elsewhere), osteomyelitis, osteoporosis, and PAGET'S DISEASE. Fractures of the spine – compressed fracture of a vertebra or a break in one of its spinous processes – are painful and potentially dangerous.

Backache can also be caused by disease elsewhere such as infection of the kidney or gall bladder (see LIVER), inflammation of the PANCREAS, disorders in the UTERUS and PELVIS or osteoarthritis of the HIP. Treatment is affected by tackling the underlying cause. Manipulation (by chiropractors, doctors, osteopaths, and physiotherapists) is often used to treat backache. It can effectively relieve pain but the practitioner doing the manipulation should have previously eliminated the possibility of a serious disorder – for instance, a fracture or cancer – before starting treatment. Among the many known causes of back pain are:

Mechanical and traumatic causes
Muscular tenderness and ligament strain.
Fractures of the spine.
Prolapsed intravertebral disc.
Spondylosis.
Congenital anomalies.

Inflammatory causes
Osteomyelitis.
Tuberculosis.
Brucellosis.
Paravertebral abscess.
Spondyloarthropathy.
Ankylosing spondylitis.
Reiter's syndrome.
Psoriatic arthropathy.

Neoplastic causes
Primary benign tumours.
Primary malignant tumours.
Metastatic disease.

Metabolic bone disease
Osteoporosis.
Osteomalacia.
Paget's disease.

Referred pain
Posterior duodenal ulcer.
Carcinoma of the pancreas.
Pelvic disease
Prolapse of the womb.
Ovarian inflammation and tumours.

Psychogenic causes
Anxiety.
Depression.

People with backache can obtain advice from the National Back Pain Association (see APPENDIX 2: ADDRESSES).

BACLOFEN A powerful muscle-relaxant used for patients with chronic severe spasticity – increased muscle rigidity – resulting from disorders such as MULTIPLE SCLEROSIS or traumatic partial section of the SPINAL CORD. Important adverse effects include SEDATION, HYPOTONIA and DELIRIUM.

BACTERAEMIA is the condition in which bacteria are present in the bloodstream.

BACTERIA are micro-organisms of a simple primitive form, though somewhat larger and more complex than viruses (see MICROBIOLOGY). Although responsible for a large number of human INFECTIONS, many of these may be successfully treated with ANTIBIOTICS, though resistant strains of bacteria do develop – increasingly so with the extensive use of antibiotics.

BACTERICIDE Anything which kills bacteria; the term is, however, usually applied to drugs and antiseptics which do this. Hence bactericidal.

BACTERIOLOGY (see MICROBIOLOGY).

BACTERIOPHAGE A VIRUS which has a BACTERIUM as its host. Containing either single-stranded or double-stranded DNA or RNA, a particular phage generally may infect one or a limited number of bacterial strains or species. After infection, once phage nucleic acid has entered the host cell, a lytic or a lysogenic cycle may result, depending on the phage and host types. Some (virulent) phages always induce a lytic cycle, whereby the bacterial synthetic machinery is programmed to produce viral components, which are assembled into virus particles and released on bacterial lysis (disintegration). Other (temperate) phages induce a non-lytic, or lysogenic, state, in which phage nucleic acid integrates stably into and replicates with the bacterial chromosome. The relationship can revert to a lytic cycle and production of new phages. In the process the phage may carry small amounts of donor bacterial DNA which may be expressed in a new host individual during lysogeny: the production of diphtheria toxin by *Corynebacterium diphtheriae* and of erythrogenic toxin by *Streptococcus pyogenes* are well-known examples of the effects of lysogeny.

BACTERIOSTATIC A term applied to substances that stop bacterial growth and cell division.

BACTERIURIA The presence of unusual bacteria in the urine, usually a sign of infection in the kidneys, bladder or urethra. Normal urine usually contains some harmless bacteria but, if bacterial numbers exceed 100,000 in each millilitre, that is abnormal. Investigation is necessary to establish the cause and enable treatment to start.

Men have longer urethras and fewer urinary tract infections (UTIs) than women. Risk factors include diabetes mellitus, pregnancy, impaired voiding and genitourinary malformations. Over 70 per cent of UTIs are due to *E. coli*, but of UTIs in hospital patients only 40 per cent are caused by *E. coli*.

Treatment Patients should be encouraged to drink plenty of water, with frequent urination. Specific antibiotic therapy with trimethoprim or amoxycillin is needed.

BACUP stands for the British Association of Cancer United Patients and their families and friends. It was founded by Dr Vicky Clement-Jones after she was treated for ovarian cancer and it became fully operational on 31 October 1985. The aim of the association is to provide an information service to cancer patients who want to know more about their illness or who need practical advice on how to cope with it. It does not seek to replace the traditional relationship between the doctor and patient, nor does it recommend specific treatment for particular patients; but its aim is to help patients to understand more about their illness so that they can communicate more effectively and freely with their medical advisors and their families and friends.

For full details of information and counselling services see APPENDIX 2: ADDRESSES.

BAGASSOSIS An industrial lung disease occurring in those who work with bagasse, which is the name given to the broken sugar cane after sugar has been extracted from it. Bagasse, which contains 6 per cent silica, is used in board-making. The inhalation of dust causes an acute lung affection, and subsequently in some cases a chronic lung disease. (See ALVEOLITIS.)

BAL is the abbreviation for British Anti-Lewisite. (See DIMERCAPROL.)

BALANCE The ability to balance is essential for a person to stand, walk, and run. Maintaining this ability is a complex exercise of coordination dependent on the brain, sensory and motor nerves and joints. There is a regular supply of information to the brain about the positions of various parts of the body and it responds with relevant instructions to the motor parts of the body. Eyes, the inner ear, skin and muscles all provide information. The cerebellum (part of the brain) collates all the information and initiates action. Balance may be affected by disorders in the balancing mechanism of the inner EAR (semicircular canals) such as MENIERE'S DISEASE and inflammation of the labyrinth (LABYRINTHITIS). Infection of the middle ear (OTITIS MEDIA) can also disturb the ability to balance, which may be accompanied by dizziness or VERTIGO. If the cerebellum is affected by disease – for instance a tumour or a stroke – the result will be faulty muscular coordination leading to clumsiness and inability to walk properly.

BALANITIS Inflammation of the GLANS PENIS. Acute balanitis is associated with allergic DERMATITIS and HERPES GENITALIS. Diabetics are at increased risk of non-specific secondary infections; if recurrent balanitis occurs, circumcision is usually indicated.

BALANTIDIASIS A form of dysentery caused by a protozoon known as *Balantidium coli*, a common parasite in pigs, which are usually the source of infection. It responds to metronidazole.

BALDNESS (See ALOPECIA.)

BALLOTTEMENT The technique of examining a fluid-filled part of the body for the presence of a floating object. For example, a fetus can be pushed away by a finger inside the mother's vagina. The fetus floats away from the examining finger and then bounces back on to it.

BALSAMS Substances which contain resins and benzoic acid. Balsam of Peru, balsam of tolu, and Friars' balsam (compound tincture of benzoin) are the chief. They are traditional remedies given internally for colds, and aid expectoration, while locally they are used to cover abrasions and stimulate ulcers.

BANDAGES Pieces of material used to support injured parts or to retain dressings in position. They come in various forms including elastic materials and plaster of Paris.

For more detailed information about bandaging the reader is referred to *First Aid Manual*, the authorized manual of the St John's Ambulance Association, St Andrew's Ambulance Association and British Red Cross Society.

BARAGNOSIS The inability on the part of a patient to recognize that an object placed in the hand has weight, a condition due to disease of the brain.

BARANY'S TEST A test for gauging the efficiency of the balancing mechanism (the vestibular apparatus) by applying hot or cold air or water to the external ear.

BARBER'S ITCH (see SYCOSIS).

BARBITURATES A group of drugs which are based on the structure of barbituric acid. Substitutions or alterations within the basic structure produce drugs which reversibly depress the central nervous system by inhibiting the transmission of impulses between certain neurones. Thus they cause drowsiness or unconsciousness (depending on dose), reduce the cerebral metabolic rate for oxygen and depress respiration but may accentuate pain in small doses. Their use as sedatives and hypnotics has largely been superseded by more modern drugs with more suitable pharmacological properties. Some members of this group of drugs, for instance, phenobarbitone, have selective anticonvulsant properties and are used in the treatment of GRAND MAL convulsions and status epilepticus (see EPILEPSY). The short-acting drugs thiopentone and methohexitone are widely used to induce general anaesthesia. Barbiturates are metabolized by the cytochrome P450 enzyme system in the liver. They are potent hepatic enzyme inducers and may therefore increase the metabolism of other drugs. This characteristic is used therapeutically in hyperbilirubinaenia (raised concentration of bile salts in the blood) and KERNICTERUS. Their use is contraindicated in PORPHYRIA (See also DRUG ADDICTION.)

BARIUM SULPHATE A radio-opaque white powder used in X-ray examinations of the stomach and gastrointestinal tract. The barium sulphate may be swallowed to enable the oesophagus, stomach and small and large intestines to be assessed for disorders such as ulceration, tumours, DIVERTICULAR DISEASE and polyps. It may also be inserted into the RECTUM or descending COLON to investigate for possible disease. These procedures are usually done after endoscopy examinations have been carried out.

BARORECEPTOR Specialized nerve ending which acts as a stretch receptor in the carotid sinus, aortic arch, atria, pulmonary veins, and left ventricle. Increased pressure in these structures increases the rate of discharge of the baroreceptors. This information is relayed to the medulla and is important in the control of blood pressure.

BARRIER CREAMS Substances, usually silicone based, applied to the skin before work to prevent damage by irritants. They are also used in medicine: e.g. for the prevention of bedsores and napkin rashes.

BARRIER NURSING The nursing of a patient suffering from an infectious disease in such a way that the risk of his passing on the disease to others is effectively reduced. Thus, precautions are taken to ensure that all infective matter, such as stools, urine, sputum, discharge from wounds, and anything that may be contaminated by such infective matter, such as nurses' uniforms, bedding and towels are so treated that they will not convey the infection. (See NURSING.)

BARTHOLIN'S GLANDS Two small glands opening either side of the external vaginal orifice. Their secretions help to lubricate the vulva, when a woman is sexually aroused. The glands may become infected and very painful; sometimes an abscess develops when local surgery is required. Otherwise antibiotics, analgesics and warm baths are usually effective.

BASAL CELL CARCINOMA The most common form of skin cancer, its main cause is cumulative exposure to ultraviolet light, and most tumours develop on exposed sites, chiefly the face and neck. It grows very slowly, often enlarging with a raised, pearly edge. The centre may ulcerate (rodent ulcer). It does not METASTASIZE and can be cured by surgical excision or RADIOTHERAPY. Small lesions can also be successfuly treated by curettage and CAUTERIZATION (see ELECTROCAUTERY) or CRYOSURGERY.

BASAL GANGLION Grey matter near the base of the cerebral hemispheres, consisting of the corpus striatum (caudate nucleus and lenticular nucleus (globus pallidus and putamen)), claustrum, and amygdaloid nucleus (see BRAIN). The basal ganglia are involved in the subconscious regulation of voluntary movement, and disorders in this region cause DYSKINESIAS.

BASAL METABOLISM (see METABOLISM).

BASILIC VEIN The prominent vein which runs from near the bend of the elbow upwards along the inner side of the upper arm.

BASOPHIL A type of white cell or LEUCOCYTE which has coarse granules in its CYTOPLASM that stain purple-black with certain chemicals. Basophils contain HISTAMINE and HEPARIN and have the ability to ingest foreign particles.

BASOPHILIA The blueish appearance under the microscope of immature red blood corpuscles when stained by certain dyes. This appearance, with the blue areas collected in points, is seen in lead poisoning and the condition is called punctate basophilia. The term basophilia may also mean an increase in the numbers of basophil cells in the blood.

BAT EARS The term commonly applied to prominent ears. The condition may be familial, but this is by no means the rule. Strapping the ears firmly back has no effect and is merely a waste of time and an embarrassment to the child. In cases in which the condition is proving a definite embarrassment to the child, it can be rectified by plastic surgery.

BATHER'S ITCH, also called SWIMMER'S ITCH, WATER ITCH, and SCHISTOSOME DERMATITIS, is the term given to a blotchy rash on the skin occurring in those bathing in water which is infested with the larvae of certain trematode worms known as Schistosomes (see SCHISTOSOMIASIS). The worm is parasitic in snails. The skin rash is caused by penetration of the skin by the free-swimming larval cercaria. Bather's itch is common in many parts of the world.

BCG VACCINE BCG (Bacillus Calmette-Guérin) vaccine, which was introduced in France in 1908, is the only vaccine that has produced significant immunity against the tubercle bacillus and at the same time has proved safe enough for use in human subjects. BCG vaccination is usually considered for five main groups of people. (1) Schoolchildren: the routine programme in schools usually covers children aged between 10 and 14. (2) Students, including those in teacher training colleges. (3) Children and new-born infants of Asian origin because of the high incidence of tuberculosis in this ethnic group. (4) Health workers, such as nurses, and others likely to be exposed to infection in their work. (5) Household contacts of people known to have active tuberculosis and new-born infants in households where there is a history of tuberculosis. A pre-vaccination tuberculin test is necessary in all age-groups except new-born infants, and only those with negative tuberculin reactions are vaccinated. Complications are few and far between. A local reaction at the site of vaccination usually occurs between two and six weeks after vaccination, beginning as a small papule that slowly increases in size. It may produce a small ulcer. This heals after around two months, leaving a small scar. (See IMMUNITY; TUBERCULIN.)

BECLOMETHASONE DIPROPIONATE is a CORTICOSTEROID used as an aerosol inhalant. It must be used regularly for its best effect. Unlike systemic corticosteroids inhaled forms are much less likely to suppress adrenal-gland activity and have fewer side-effects.

BED Nursing sick or injured patients can be greatly helped by the use of specially designed beds which may be used in hospitals, nursing homes, or at home. They must be easy to disinfect, to move, to adjust for height and to tilt. They should also have a firm mattress. Some beds, for instance, are designed with frames so that patients can be turned; others, like water beds, air and ripple beds, are used to prevent bedsores (see DECUBITUS ULCER) by providing uniform support for the whole body.

BED BATH A procedure for thoroughly washing a patient confined to bed.

BED BUG, or *Cimex lectularius*, is a wingless, blood-sucking insect, parasitic on man. It is a flat, rusty brown insect, 5 mm long and 3 mm wide, with an offensive, never forgotten smell, which cannot fly. The average life is 3 to 6 months, but it can live for a year without food. The bed bug remains hidden during the day in cracks in walls and floors, and in beds. It does not transmit any known disease. Eggs hatch out into larvae in 6 to 10 days, which become adult within about 12 weeks. A temperature of 44 °C kills the adult in an hour. Various agents have been used to disinfect premises, such as sulphur dioxide, ethylene oxide mixed with carbon dioxide, hydrogen cyanide and heavy naphtha, but insecticide is the most effective disinfecting agent.

BEDPAN A container made of metal, fibre, or plastic into which a person confined to bed can defaecate and, in the case of a female, urinate. Men use a urinal – a flask-shaped container – to urinate. Hospitals have special cleaning and sterilizing equipment for bedpans. They are much less used than in the past because patients are encouraged to be mobile as soon as possible and also because bedside commodes are preferred where this is practical.

BED SORES   (see DECUBITOUS ULCER).

BED WETTING (see ENURESIS).

BEER (see ALCOHOL).

BEE STINGS (see BITES AND STINGS).

BEHAVIOUR THERAPY A form of psychiatric treatment based on learning theory. Symptoms are considered to be conditioned responses, and treatment is aimed at removing them, regardless of the underlying diagnosis. Desensitization, operant conditioning, and aversion therapy are examples of behaviour therapy.

BEHÇET'S SYNDROME This is a syndrome of unknown aetiology. It is characterized by oral and genital ulceration, iridocyclitis and arthropathy. THROMBOPHLEBITIS is a common complication and involvement of the central nervous system may occur.

BELCHING (see ERUCTATION).

BELLADONNA POISONING *Atropa belladonna* (deadly nightshade) is a relatively rare plant and severe poisoning is not common. The berries, which are black, ripen from August to October and are the most commonly ingested part of the plant. However, all parts of the plant are toxic. The berries contain ATROPINE and other unidentified ALKALOIDS, the leaves HYOSCINE and atropine and the roots hyoscine. All these alkaloids have ANTICHOLINERGIC effect which may cause a dry mouth, dilated pupils with blurred vision, TACHYCARDIA, HALLUCINATIONS and PYREXIA. There may also be ATAXIA, agitation, disorientation and confusion. In severe cases there may be CONVULSIONS, COMA, respiratory depression and ARRHYTHMIAS. Clinical effects may be delayed in onset up to 12 hours and prolonged for several days. Treatment is supportive.

BELL'S PALSY refers to the isolated paralysis of the facial muscles on one or both sides, of unclear cause, though damage to the seventh cranial, or FACIAL NERVE, possibly of viral origin, is thought likely. Occurring in both sexes at any age, it presents with a facial pain on the affected side, followed by an inability to close the eye or smile. The mouth appears to be drawn over to the opposite side, and fluids may escape from the angle of the mouth. Lines of expression, are flattened and the patient is unable to wrinkle the brow.

Treatment Oral steroids, if started early, increase the rate of recovery, which occurs in over 90 per cent of patients, usually starting after two or three weeks and complete within three months. Permanent loss of function with facial contractures occurs in about 5 per cent of patients. Recurrence of Bell's palsy is unusual.

B ENDORPHIN A naturally occurring painkiller which is produced by the PITUITARY GLAND as part of a prohormone (pre-pro-opianomelanocortin). It is an agonist at opioid receptors, and its release is stimulated by pain and stress. (See ENDORPHINS.)

BENDS (see COMPRESSED AIR ILLNESS).

BENIGN Not harmful. Used especially to describe tumours that are not malignant.

BENNETT'S FRACTURE, so-called after an Irish surgeon, Edward Hallaran Bennett (1837–1907), is a longitudinal fracture of the first metacarpal bone, which also involves the carpometacarpal joint.

BENZEDRINE Proprietary name for amphetamine sulphate (see AMPHETAMINES).

BENZHEXOL One of the ANTIMUSCARINIC group of drugs used to treat PARKINSONISM. Acting by correcting the relative central cholinergic excess resulting from DOPAMINE deficiency, the drug has a moderate effect, reducing tremor and rigidity, but with little action on bradykinesia. It has a SYNERGISTIC effect when used with LEVODOPA and is useful in reducing SIALORRHOEA. Valuable in treating cases of Parkinsonian side-effects occurring with neuroleptic drugs. Tardive DYSKINESIA is not improved and may be made worse.

There are few significant differences between the various antimuscarinic drugs available, but some patients may tolerate one drug better than another or find that they need to adjust their drug regimen in relation to food.

BENZOCAINE Weak local anaesthetic found in some throat lozenges, rubefacient creams and gels. It may cause allergic hypersensitivity.

BENZODIAZEPINES A large family of drugs used as HYPNOTICS, ANXIOLYTICS, TRANQUILLIZERS, ANTICONVULSANTS, premedicants, and for intravenous sedation. They differ in their duration of action, metabolites, and lipid solubility. Short-acting ones are used as HYPNOTICS, longer acting ones as hypnotics and tranquillizers, and those with high lipid solubility act rapidly if given intravenously. They act at a specific central-nervous-system receptor or by potentiating the action of inhibitory neurotransmitters. They have advantages over other sedatives by having some selectivity for anxiety rather than general sedation. They do not induce hepatic enzymes and are safer in overdose. Unfortunately they may cause aggression, amnesia, excessive sedation, or confusion in the elderly. Those with long half lives or with metabolites having long half lives may produce a hangover effect, and dependence on these is now well recognized. Unlike barbiturates, they do not induce liver microsomal enzymes and they are safer in overdosage. Commonly used benzodiazepines include nitrazepam, flunitrazepam, loprazolam, temazepam, chloral hydrate and chlormethiazole.

BENZOTHIADIAZINES, or THIAZIDES, are a group of moderately potent DIURETICS which are effective when taken by mouth. They act by inhibiting the reabsorption of sodium and chloride in the renal tubules. They also have a blood-pressure-lowering effect. Chlorothiazide was the first member of this group to be introduced. Their main use is to relieve oedema in heart failure.

All thiazides are active by mouth with an onset of action within one to two hours, and a duration of twelve to twenty-four hours. Chlorthalidone is a thiazide-related compound that has a longer duration of action and only requires to be given on alternate days. The other thiazide drugs available include bendrofluazide, chlorthalidone, cyclopenthiazide, hydrochlorothiazide, hydroflumethiazide, indapamide, mefruside, methyclothiazide, metolazone, polythiazide and xipamide.

The loop diuretics are more potent than the thiazides. They are so called because they inhibit re-absorption from the ascending loop of Henle in the renal tubules. Frusemide, bumetanide, and ethacrynic acid are the three most important loop diuretics. (See DIURETICS.)

BENZYL BENZOATE An emulson that was widely used as a treatment for scabies but has been superseded by less irritant scabicides.

BENZYLPENICILLIN (see PENICILLIN).

BEREAVEMENT The normal mental state associated with the death and slow coming to terms with the death of a loved one. The well-recognized stages of the bereavement reaction are: denial, bargaining, anger and acceptance. If bereavement symptoms are severe or prolonged expert counselling may help.

BERIBERI (Singhalese: beri = extreme weakness.) Formerly a major health problem in many Asian countries, beriberi is a nutritional deficiency disease, resulting from prolonged deficiency of the water-soluble vitamin thiamine (vitamin B_1). It is often associated with deficiencies of other members of the the vitamin B complex (see APPENDIX 5: VITAMINS). A major public health problem in countries where highly polished rice constitutes the staple diet, beriberi also occurs sporadically in alcoholics (Wernicke's encephalopathy) and in people suffering from chronic malabsorptive states. Clinical symptoms include weakness, paralysis – involving especially the hands and feet (associated with sensory loss, particularly in the legs) – and 'burning sensations' in the feet (dry beriberi). Alternatively, it is accompanied by oedema, palpitations, dilated heart, and cardiac involvement (wet beriberi). Death usually results from cardiac failure. Thiamine deficiency can be confirmed by estimating erythrocyte transketolase concentration; blood and urine thiamine levels can be measured BY high-pressure liquid chromatography. Treatment consists of large doses of vitamin B_1 – orally or intramuscularly – a diet containing other vitamins of the B group, and rest.

Infantile beriberi This is the result of maternal thiamine deficiency; although the mother is not necessarily affected, the breast-fed baby may develop typical signs (see above). Optic and third cranial, and recurrent laryngeal nerves may be affected; encephalopathy can result in convulsions, coma, and death.

BERYLLIOSIS A disease of the lungs caused by the inhalation of particles of beryllium oxide.

BETA ADRENOCEPTOR (SEE ADRENERGIC RECEPTORS).

BETA-ADRENOCEPTOR-BLOCKING DRUGS antagonize the beta effects of the sympathetic nervous system, particularly affecting the heart, bronchi, pancreas, liver and peripheral vasculature. Various drugs are available (including ATENOLOL, metoprolol, and PROPRANOLOL), differing in their cardiac selectivity. Used mainly to control HYPERTENSION, ANGINA, TACHYDYSRHYTHMIAS, and MYOCARDIAL reinfarction, they slow the heart and have a hypotensive action, with a risk of inducing cardiac failure. Beta blockers cause bronchoconstriction and they should be avoided in patients with a history of ASTHMA or chronic obstructive airways disease, in whom brochospasm may be induced. They should be used cautiously in diabetics, as they may interfere with the metabolic and autonomic responses to hypo-glycaemia.

BETA BLOCKERS (see BETA-ADRENOCEPTOR-BLOCKING DRUGS).

BETAMETHASONE A CORTICOSTEROID which has an action comparable to that of PREDNISOLONE, but in much lower dosage. In the form of betamethasone valerate it is used as an application to the skin as an ointment or cream.

BETATRON (see RADIOTHERAPY).

BEZOAR A mass of ingested foreign material found in the stomach, usually in children or people with psychiatric illnesses. It may cause gastric obstruction and require surgical removal. The commonest type consists of hair and is known as a trichobezoar.

BICARBONATE OF SODA, or BAKING SODA, is an alkali, sometimes used as a home remedy for indigestion or soothing insect bites.

BICEPS A term used for a muscle that has two heads. The biceps femoris flexes the knee and extends the hip and the biceps brachii supinates the forearm and flexes the elbow and shoulder.

BICUSPID Having two cusps. The premolars are bicuspid teeth, and the mitral valve is a bicuspid valve.

BIFID Split into two parts.

BIFOCAL LENS A spectacle lens in which the upper part is shaped to assist distant vision and the lower part is for close work such as reading.

BIFURCATION The point at which a structure (for example, a blood vessel) divides into two branches.

BIGUANIDES are a group of oral HYPOGLY-CAEMIC drugs, of which METFORMIN is the only one available for treatment, used to treat non-insulin-dependent diabetics, when strict dieting and treatment with SULPHONYLUREAS have failed. It acts mainly by reducing GLUCONEOGENESIS and by increasing peripheral utilization of glucose. Hypoglycaemia is unusual, unless taken in overdose. Gastro-intestinal side-effects such as anorexia, nausea, vomiting, and transient diarrhoea are common initially, and may persist, particularly if large doses are taken. Metformin should not be given to patients with renal failure, in whom there is a danger of inducing lactic acidosis. (See DIABETES.)

BILATERAL Occurring on both sides of the body.

BILE A thick, bitter, greenish-brown fluid, secreted by the liver and stored in the gall-bladder (see LIVER: gall bladder). Consisting of water, mucus, bile pigments including BILIRUBIN, and various salts, it is discharged through the bile ducts into the intestine a few centimetres below the stomach. This discharge is increased shortly after eating, and again a few hours later. It helps in the digestion and absorption of food, particularly fats, and is itself reabsorbed, passing back through the blood of the liver. In JAUNDICE, obstruction of the bile ducts prevents discharge, leading to a build-up of bile in the blood and deposition in the tissues. The skin becomes greenish-yellow, while the stools become grey or white and the urine dark. Vomiting of bile is a sign of intestinal obstruction, but may occur in any case of persistent retching or vomiting, and should be fully investigated.

BILE DUCT The channel running from the GALL BLADDER to the DUODENUM that carries bile.

BILHARZIASIS is another name for schistosomiasis.

BILIARY COLIC Severe pain caused by the attempted (and sometimes successful) expulsion of a gallstone from the gall bladder via the BILE DUCT. The pain, which is felt in the upper right quadrant of the abdomen, may last for an hour or more. Strong ANALGESICS are required to subdue the pain and the patient may need hospital admission for examination and eventual surgery. Attacks may recur and the pain is sometimes mistakenly diagnosed as signalling a heart attack.

BILIRUBIN The chief pigment in human bile. It is derived from HAEMOGLOBIN which is the red pigment of the red blood corpuscles. The site of manufacture of bilirubin is the RETICULO-ENDOTHELIAL system. When bile is passed into the intestine from the GALL-BLAD-DER, part of the bilirubin is converted into stercobilin and excreted in the FAECES. The remainder is reabsorbed into the blood-stream, and of this portion the bulk goes back to the liver to be re-excreted into the bile, whilst a small proportion is excreted in the urine as urobilinogen.

BINAURAL Relating to both ears.

BINOCULAR Relating to both eyes. Binocular vision involves focusing on an object with both eyes simultaneously and is important in judging distance.

BINOVULAR TWINS Twins who result from the fertilization of two separate ova. (See MULTIPLE BIRTHS.)

BIO-AVAILABILITY refers to the proportion of a drug reaching the systemic circulation after a particular route of administration. The most important factor is first-pass metabolism – that is, pre-systemic metabolism in either the intestine or the liver. Many lipid soluble drugs such as beta blockers, some tricyclic ANTI-DEPRESSANTS, and various opiate ANALGESICS are severely affected. Food may affect bio-availability by modifying gastric emptying, thus slowing drug absorption. Ingested calcium may chelate with drugs such as tetracyclines, further reducing their absorption.

BIOFEEDBACK A technique whereby an auditory or visual stimulus follows on from a physiological response. Thus, a subject's ELEC-TROCARDIOGRAM may be monitored, and a signal passed back to the subject indicating his heart rate: e.g. a red light if the rate is between fifty and sixty beats a minute; a green light if it is between sixty and seventy a minute. Once the subject has learned to discriminate between these two rates he can then learn to control his heart rate. How this is learned is not clear, but by utilizing biofeedback some subjects can control heart rate and blood-pressure, relax spastic muscles, and even bring migraine under control.

BIOMECHANICAL ENGINEERING The joint utilization of engineering and biological knowledge to illuminate normal and abnormal functions of the human body. Blood flow, the reaction of bones and joints to stress, the design of kidney dialysis machines and the development of artificial body parts are among the practical results of this collaboration.

BIOPSY means the removal and examination of tissue from the living body for diagnostic purposes. For example, a piece of a tumour may be cut out and examined to determine whether it is cancerous.

BIOTIN One of the dozen or so vitamins included in the vitamin B complex. It is found in liver, eggs, and meat, and it is also synthesized by bacteria in the gut. Absorption from the gut is prevented by avidin, a constituent of egg-white. The daily requirement is small: a fraction of a milligram daily. Gross deficiency results in disturbances of the skin, a smooth tongue and lassitude. (See APPENDIX 5: VITAMINS.)

BIPOLAR DISORDER A type of mental illness typified by mood swings between elation and depression (see MENTAL ILLNESS).

BIRD FANCIER'S LUNG, or PIGEON BREED-ER'S LUNG as it is sometimes known, is a form of extrinsic allergic alveolitis resulting from sensitization to birds. In bird fanciers skin tests sometimes show sensitization to birds' drop-pings, eggs, protein and serum, even through there has been no evidence of any illness. (See ALVEOLITIS).

BIRTH CANAL The passage that extends from the neck of the womb (UTERUS), known as the CERVIX, to the opening of the VAGINA. The baby passes along this passage during childbirth.

BIRTH CONTROL (see CONTRACEPTION).

BIRTH DEFECTS (see CONGENITAL).

BIRTH-MARKS are of various kinds. The most common are port-wine marks (see NAE-VUS). Pigment spots are found, very often raised above the surface and more or less hairy, being then called moles (see MOLE).

BIRTH POOL A pool of warm water in which a woman can give birth to her baby. The infant is delivered into the water. The method was introduced during the 1980s and was claimed to make delivery less painful and upsetting. It has provoked controversy and so far is not widely available in the UK.

BIRTH RATE In 1996 614,184 live births were registered in England, a 0.2 per cent rise

on 1995. Of these 36 per cent occurred outside marriage. Overall, total fertility is falling slowly. The number of births per 1,000 women aged 40–44 years has been rising and in 1996 was 6.9 per cent. In 1995 nearly 148,000 abortions were performed under the Abortion Act 1967 in England, a fall of 1 per cent compared with 1994.

BISACODYL is a laxative which acts by stimulation of the nerve endings in the colon by direct contact with the mucous lining.

BISEXUAL Having the qualities of both sexes. The term is used to describe people who are sexually attracted to both men and women. A person's sexual preference may, however, vary during his or her lifetime.

BISMUTH Various bismuth chelates effec-tive in healing gastric and duodenal ulcers are available. They may act by a direct toxic effect on gastric HELICOBACTER PYLORI, or by stimulat-ing mucosal PROSTAGLANDIN or bicarbonate secretion. Healing tends to be longer than with H-RECEPTOR ANTAGONISTS and relapse still oc-curs. New regimens are being developed in-volving co-administration with antibiotics. ENCEPHALOPATHY, described with older high-dose bismuth preparations, has not been re-ported.

BISPHOSPHONATES, of which disodium etidronate is one, are a group of drugs used mainly in the treatment of PAGET'S DISEASE of bone and in established vertebral OSTEOPOROSIS. Their advantage over CALCITONIN (which has to be given by subcutaneous or intramusclar in-jection) is that they can be taken orally. They act by slowing both the rate of growth and dissolution, hence reducing the increased rate of bone turnover associated with the disease. Disodium etidronate is used with calcium car-bonate in a 90-day cycle (duration of therapy up to 3 years) in the treatment of osteoporosis.

BITES AND STINGS Animals' bites are best treated as puncture wounds which should simply be washed and dressed. ANTIBIOTICS may be given to minimize the risk of infection, and TETANUS toxoid given if appropriate. Should RABIES be a possibility, then further treatment must be considered. Bites and stings of venom-ous reptiles, amphibians, scorpions, snakes, spiders, insects and fish may result in clinical effects characteristic of that particular poison-ing. In some cases specific ANTIVENOMS may be administered to reduce morbidity and mortal-ity.

Many snakes are non-venomous (e.g. py-thons, garter snakes, king snakes, boa constric-tors) but may still inflict painful bites and cause local swelling. Most venomous snakes belong to the viper and cobra families and are com-mon in Asia, Africa, Australia, and South

America. Victims of bites may experience various effects including swelling, PARALYSIS of bitten area, blood-clotting defects, PALPITATIONS, respiratory difficulty, CONVULSIONS and other NEUROTOXIC and cardiac effects. Victims should be treated as for shock, i.e. kept at rest, warm, and given oxygen if required but nothing by mouth. The bite site should be immobilized but a TOURNIQUET must not be used. All victims require prompt transfer to a medical facility. When appropriate and available, antivenoms should be administered as soon as possible.

Similar management is appropriate for bites and stings by spiders, scorpions, sea-snakes, venomous fish and other marine animals and insects.

UK bites and stings: The adder (*Vipera berus*) is the only venomous snake native to Britain and is a timid animal that bites only when provoked. Fatal cases are rare. Only 14 deaths have been recorded in the UK since 1876, the last of these in 1975. Adder bites may result in marked swelling, weakness, collapse, shock, and in severe cases HYPOTENSION, non-specific changes in the electrocardiogram and peripheral leucocytosis. Victims of adder bites should be transferred to hospital quickly but passively, even if asymptomatic, with the affected limb being immobilized and the bite site left alone. Local incisions, suction, use of tourniquets, ice packs or permanganate must not be used. Hospital management may include use of a specific antivenom, Zagreb®.

The weever fish is found in the coastal waters of the British Isles, Europe, the eastern Atlantic, and the Mediterranean Sea. It possesses venomous spines in its dorsal fin. Stings and envenomation commonly occur when an individual treads on the fish. The victim may experience a localized but increasing pain over two hours. As the venom is heat-labile, immersion of the affected area in water at approximately 40 °C or as hot as can be tolerated for 30 minutes should ease the pain. Cold applications will worsen the discomfort. Simple ANALGESICS and ANTIHISTAMINES may be given.

Bees, wasps and hornets are insects of the Order Hymenoptera and the females possess stinging apparatus at the end of the abdomen. Stings may cause local pain and swelling but rarely cause severe toxicity. ANAPHYLACTIC reactions can occur in sensitive individuals which may be fatal. Deaths caused by upper-airway blockage as a result of stings in the mouth or neck regions are reported. In victims of stings the stinger should be removed as quickly as possible by flicking, scraping or pulling. The site should be cleaned. ANTIHISTAMINES and cold applications may bring relief. For ANAPHYLACTIC reactions ADRENALINE, by intramuscular injection, may be required.

BLACK DEATH An old name for plague. (See PLAGUE.)

BLACKHEADS (see ACNE).

BLACKWATER FEVER Acute intravascular haemolysis and renal failure, associated with severe *Plasmodium falciparum* infection. The complication is frequently fatal. It is associated with haemoglobinuria, jaundice, fever, vomiting, and severe anaemia. in an extreme case the patient's urine appears black. Tender enlarged liver and spleen are usually present. The precise aetiology remains obscure, but the disease is clearly triggered by quinine usage at subtherapeutic dosage in the presence of *P. falciparum* infection, especially in the nonimmune individual. Now that quinine is rarely used for chemoprophylaxis of this infection (it is reserved for treatment), blackwater fever has become very unusual. Treatment is as for severe complicated *P. falciparum* infection with renal impairment; dialysis and blood transfusion are usually indicated. When inadequately treated, the mortality rate may be over 40 per cent but, with satisfactory intensive therapy, this should be reduced substantially.

BLADDER, DISEASES OF (see URINARY BLADDER, DISEASES OF and GALL-BLADDER, DISEASES OF; see also URINE).

BLADDERS Sacs formed of muscular and fibrous tissue and lined by a mucous membrane, which is united loosely to the muscular coat, so as freely to allow increase and decrease in the contained cavity. Bladders are designed to contain some secretion or excretion, and communicate with the exterior by a narrow opening through which their contents can be discharged. In man there are two, the gall-bladder and the urinary bladder.

Gall-bladder This is situated under the liver in the upper part of the abdomen, and its function is to store the bile, which it discharges into the intestine by the bile duct. For further details, see LIVER.

Urinary bladder This is situated in the pelvis, in front of the last part of the bowel. The bladder, in the full state, rises up into the abdomen and holds about 570 ml (a pint) of urine. Two fine tubes, called the ureters, lead into the bladder, one from each kidney; and the urethra, a tube as wide as a lead pencil when distended, leads from it to the exterior, a distance of 4 cm (1½ inches) in the female and 20 cm (8 inches) in the male.
STRUCTURE The wall of the bladder is similar in structure to that of the bowels, and consists of four coats. The inner surface is lined by a soft MUCOUS MEMBRANE covered by EPITHELIAL cells of irregular shape. This is attached to the muscular coat by a loose, fibrous, sub-mucous coat, in which run numerous blood-vessels. In the muscular coat the muscle fibres are arranged in several layers, and run in various directions, thereby adding greatly to the strength of the wall. On its upper and back part, the bladder possesses a covering of serous membrane, formed by part of the general PERITONEAL lining of the ABDOMINAL

CAVITY, but this outermost coat does not extend down to the base of the bladder, where the latter lies in close contact with the other pelvic organs. The bladder is suspended in position by numerous ligaments, four of which are fibrous bands, while the remaining five are formed by thickened portions of the peritoneum. The base of the bladder is directed downwards and backwards, and in this part are the three openings of the URETERS and URETHRA. The exit from the bladder is kept closed by a muscular ring, which is relaxed every time water is passed.

BLEEDING (see HAEMORRHAGE; and VENESECTION).

BLENORRHOEA An excessive discharge of mucus or slimy material from a surface, such as that of the eye, nose, bowel, etc. The word catarrh is used with the same meaning, but also includes the idea of inflammation as the cause of such discharge.

BLEOMYCIN A cytotoxic antibiotic, obtained from *Streptomyces verticillus*, that is being used to treat solid cancerous tumours of the upper part of the gut and genital tract and lymphomas. Like other cytotoxic drugs it can have serious side-effects, and bleomycin may cause pulmonary fibrosis and skin pigmentation. (See CYTOTOXIC.)

BLEPHARITIS Inflammation of the eyelids. (See EYE DISEASES.)

BLEPHAROSPASM (see EYE DISEASES.)

BLINDNESS, INABILITY TO SEE The statutory definition for the purposes of registration as a blind person under the National Assistance Act, 1948, is that the person is 'so blind as to be unable to perform any work for which eyesight is essential'. Generally this is vision worse than 6/60 in the better eye, or with better acuity than this but where 'the field of vision is markedly contracted in the greater part of its extent'. Partial sight has no statutory definition but there are official guidelines for registering a person partially sighted. Generally these are a corrected visual acuity of 3/60 or less in the better eye with some contraction of the peripheral field, or better with gross field defects. In the UK over 100,000 people are registered as legally blind and some 50,000 as partially sighted. The World Health Organization has estimated that there are over 40 million binocularly blind people in the world. The causes of blindness vary with age and degree of development of the country. In Western society the commonest causes are 'other retinal disease, glaucoma, diabetic retinopathy and senile cataract'. (See also VISION.)

Any blind person, or his or her relatives, can obtain help and advice from the Royal National Institute for the Blind (see APPENDIX 2: ADDRESSES).

Night blindness (NYCTALOPIA) An inability to see in the dark. It can be associated with retinitis pigmentosa or Vitamin A deficiency. (See EYE DISEASES.)

BLIND SPOT (see VISION, FIELD OF).

BLISTERS AND COUNTER-IRRITANTS Formerly used to treat inflammatory skin conditions, these substances are rarely employed nowadays, having been largely superseded by topical steroids.

BLOOD consists of cellular components suspended in plasma. It circulates through the blood vessels carrying oxygen and nutrients to the organs and removing carbon dioxide and other waste products for excretion. In addition, it is the vehicle by which hormones and other humoral transmitters reach their sites of action.

Composition The cellular components are red cells or corpuscles (ERYTHROCYTES), white cells (LEUCOCYTES and LYMPHOCYTES.), and platelets.

The cells are biconcave discs with a diameter of 7.5μm. They contain haemoglobin, which is an iron containing porphyrin compound, which takes up oxygen in the lungs and releases it to the tissue.

The white cells are of various types – nomenclature depending on their morphology. They can leave the circulation to wander through the tissues. They are involved in combating infection, wound healing, and rejection of foreign bodied. Pus consists of the bodies of dead white cells.

Platelets are the smallest cellular components and play an important role in blood coagulation.

Erythrocytes are produced by the bone marrow in adults and have a life span of about 120

1 red blood cell (erythrocyte): (a) side view (b) plan view
2 platelets
3 white blood cells (leucocytes):(a) neutrophil or granular leucocyte; (b) lymphocyte

Red and white blood cells and platelets.

days. White cells are produced by the bone marrow and lymphoid tissue. Plasma consists of water, ELECTROLYTES, and plasma proteins. It comprises 48-58 per cent of blood volume. Plasma proteins are produced mainly by the liver and certain types of white cells. Blood volume and electrolyte composition are closely regulated by complex mechanisms involving the KIDNEYS, ADRENAL GLANDS, and HYPOTHALAMUS.

Haemoglobin		
concentration:	men	14–18 g/dl
	women	12–16 g/dl
Erythrocyte count:	men	$4.5–6.0 \times 10^{12}/l$
	women	$3.5–5.0 \times 10^{12}/l$
Mean corpuscular volume		76–96 fl.
Mean corpuscular		
haemoglobin concentration		31–35 g/dl
Mean corpuscular haemoglobin		27–32 pg
White cell count:		$4–10 \times 10^9/l$
Neutrophils		40–75%
Eosinophils		1–6%
Basophils		0–1%
Monocytes		2–10%
Lymphocytes		20–50%
Platelet count:		$150–400 \times 10^9/l$
Packed cell volume:	men	42–52%
	women	37–47%

Range of normal blood count.

BLOOD BANK A department in which blood products are prepared, stored, and tested prior to transfusion into patients.

BLOOD BRAIN BARRIER A functional semi-permeable membrane separating the brain and cerebrospinal fluid from the blood. It allows small and lipid soluble molecules to pass freely but is impermeable to large or ionized molecules and cells.

BLOOD CLOT A blood clot arises when blood comes into contact with a foreign surface, for example, damaged blood vessels, or when tissue factors are released from damaged tissue. An initial PLATELET plug is converted to a definitive clot by the deposition of FIBRIN, which is formed by the clotting cascade and erythrocytes.

BLOOD CORPUSCLE (see ERYTHROCYTE and LEUCOCYTE).

BLOOD COUNT The number of each of the cellular components per litre of blood. It may be calculated using a microscope or by an automated process.

BLOOD, DISEASES OF (see ANAEMIA; LEUKAEMIA).

BLOOD DONOR An individual who donates his or her own blood for use in patients of compatible blood group who require transfusion.

BLOOD GASES Specifically this describes the measurement of the tensions of oxygen and carbon dioxide in blood. However, it is usually used to describe the analysis of a sample of heparinized arterial blood not only for gases but for acid base assessment. This includes measurement of oxygen, carbon dioxide, oxygen saturation, pH, bicarbonate, and base excess (the amount of acid required to return a unit volume of the blood to normal pH).

BLOOD GROUPS People are divided into four main groups in respect of a certain reaction of the blood. This depends upon the capacity of the serum of one person's blood to agglutinate the red blood cells (erythrocytes) of another's in certain circumstances. The reaction depends on antigens, known as agglutinogens, in the erythrocytes and antibodies, known as agglutinins, in the serum. There are two of each, the agglutinogens being known as A and B. Anyone's erythrocytes may have (1) no agglutinogens, (2) agglutinogen A, (3) agglutinogen B, (4) agglutinogens A and B: these are the four groups. Since the identification of the ABO and Rhesus factors (see below) factors around 400 other antigens have been discovered, but they cause few problems over transfusions.

In blood transfusion, the person giving and the person receiving the blood must belong to the same blood group, or a dangerous reaction will take place from the agglutination that occurs when blood of a different group is present.

Group	Agglutinogens in the erythrocytes	Agglutinins in the plasma	Frequency in Great Britain
AB	A and B	None	2 per cent
A	A	Anti-B	46 per cent
B	B	Anti-A	8 per cent
O	Neither A nor B	Anti-A and Anti-B	44 per cent

The four main blood groups

Rhesus factor In addition to these A and B agglutinogens (or antigens) there is another one known as the Rhesus (or Rh) factor, so named because there is a similar antigen in the red blood corpuscles of the Rhesus monkey. About 84 per cent of the population have this Rh factor in their blood and are therefore known as 'Rh-positive'. The remaining 16 per cent who do not possess the factor are known as 'Rh-negative'.

The practical importance of the Rh factor is that, unlike the A and B agglutinogens, there are no naturally occurring Rh antibodies, but such antibodies may develop in an Rh-negative person if the Rh antigen is introduced into his or her circulation. This can occur (*a*) if an Rh-negative person is given a transfusion of Rh-positive blood, (b) if an Rh-negative mother married to an Rh-positive husband becomes pregnant and the fetus is Rh-positive. If this happens, the mother develops Rh antibodies which can pass into the fetal circulation, where they react with the baby's Rh antigen and cause HAEMOLYTIC DISEASE of the fetus and newborn. This means that the child may be stillborn or become jaundiced shortly after birth (see HAEMOLYTIC DISEASE OF THE NEWBORN).

As about one in six expectant mothers is Rh-negative a blood-group examination is now considered an essential part of the antenatal examination of a pregnant woman. All such Rh-negative expectant mothers are now given a 'Rhesus card' showing that they belong to the rhesus-negative blood group. This card they should always carry with them. Rh-positive blood should never be transfused to an Rh-negative girl or woman.

BLOOD-LETTING (see VENESECTION).

BLOOD-POISONING (see SEPTICAEMIA)

BLOOD-PRESSURE is that pressure which must be applied to an artery in order to stop the pulse beyond the point of pressure. It may be roughly estimated by feeling the pulse at the wrist, or more accurately measured using a SPHYGMOMANOMETER. It is dependent on the pumping force of the heart, together with the volume of blood, and on the elasticity of the blood vessels. The blood pressure is biphasic, being greatest (systolic pressure) at each heartbeat and falling (diastolic pressure) between beats. The average systolic pressure is around 100 mm HG in children, 120 mm Hg in young adults, and generally rises with age as the arteries get thicker and harder. Diastolic pressure in a healthy young adult is about 80 mm Hg, and a rise in diastolic pressure is often a more sure indicator of hypertension than a rise in systolic pressure. The latter is more labile and sensitive to changes of body position and emotional mood. HYPERTENSION has various causes, most important of which are KIDNEY DISEASE and mental stress. Systolic pressure may well be over 200 mm Hg. Abnormal hypertension is often accompanied by ARTERIAL DISEASE, with an increased risk of strokes, heart attacks, and heart failure (see HEART DISEASES). Various ANTIHYPERTENSIVE drugs are available; they should be carefully evaluated, considering the patient's full clinical history, before use.

HYPOTENSION may result from superficial vasodilation (for example, after a bath, or in fevers) and in weakening diseases or heart failure. The blood pressure generally falls on standing, leading to temporary postural hypotension – a particular danger in elderly people.

BLOOD TEST Removal of venous, capillary, or arterial blood for haematological,

microbiological, or biochemical laboratory investigations.

BLOOD TRANSFUSION (see TRANSFUSION OF BLOOD).

BLOOD VESSEL Tubes through which blood is conducted from or to the heart. Blood from the heart is conducted via arteries and arterioles through capillaries and back to the heart via venules and then veins. (See ARTERIES and VEINS).

BODY MASS INDEX (BMI) provides objective criteria of size to enable an estimation to be made of an individual's level or risk of morbidity and mortality. The BMI, which is derived from the extensive data held by life insurance companies, is calculated by dividing a person's weight by the square of his or her height (kilograms/metres^2). Acceptable BMIs range from 20–25 and any figure above 30 characterizes obesity. The index may be used (with some modification) to assess children and adolescents. (See OBESITY.)

BOILS (FURUNCULOSIS). A skin infection caused by *Staphylococcus aureus* beginning in adjacent FOLLICLES. As the folliculitis becomes confluent, a tender red lump develops which becomes NECROTIC centrally with pus formation. A cluster of boils becoming confluent is called a CARBUNCLE. Release of the pus and an oral antibiotic lead to rapid healing.

Recurrent boils are usually due to a reservoir of STAPHYLOCOCCAL bacteria in a nostril or elsewhere, but underlying DIABETES MELLITUS should always be excluded.

BOLUS A lump of food prepared for swallowing by chewing and mixing with saliva. The term is also used to describe the rapid intravenous injection of fluid or a drug, as opposed to a slower infusion.

BONDING The formation of a close selective attachment between two individuals, as in the relationship between a mother and her baby.

BONE The framework upon which the rest of the body is built up. The bones are generally called the skeleton, though this term also includes the cartilages which join the ribs to the breast- bone, protect the larynx, etc.

Structure of bone Bone is composed partly of fibrous tissue, partly of bone matrix comprising phosphate and carbonate of lime, intimately mixed together. As the bones of a child are composed to the extent of about two-thirds of fibrous tissue, whilst those of the aged contain one-third, the toughness of the former and the brittleness of the latter are evident. The shafts of the limb bones are composed of dense bone, the bone being a hard tube surrounded by a membrane, the periosteum, and enclosing a fatty substance, the marrow; and of cancellous bone, which forms the short bones and the ends of long bones, in which a fine lace-work of bone fills up the whole interior, enclosing marrow in its meshes. The marrow (see BONE MARROW) of the smaller bones is of great importance. It is red in colour, and in it red blood corpuscles are formed. Even the densest bone is tunnelled by fine canals (Haversian canals) in which run small blood-vessels, nerves and lymphatics, for the maintenance and repair of the bone. Round these Haversian canals the bone is arranged in circular plates called lamellae, the lamellae being separated from one another by clefts, known as lacunae, in which single bone-cells are contained. Even the lamellae are pierced by fine tubes known as canaliculi lodging processes of these cells. Each lamella is composed of very fine interlacing fibres.

GROWTH OF BONES Bones grow in thickness from the fibrous tissue and lime salts laid down by cells in their substance; while the long bones grow in length from a plate of cartilage (epiphyseal cartilage) which runs across the bone about 1·5 cm or more from its ends, and which on one surface is also constantly forming bone till the bone ceases to lengthen about the age of sixteen or eighteen. The existence of this cartilage is important to bear in mind, because in children an injury to it may lead to diminished growth of the limb.

REPAIR OF BONE is effected by cells of microscopic size some called osteoblasts, elaborating the materials brought by the blood, and laying down strands of fibrous tissue, between which bone earth is later deposited; while other cells, known as osteoclasts, dissolve and break up dead or damaged bone. When a fracture has occurred, and the broken ends have been brought into contact, these are surrounded by a mass of blood at first; this is partly absorbed and partly organized by these cells, first into fibrous tissue and later into bone. The mass surrounding the fractured ends is called the callus, and for some months it forms a distinct thickening, which is gradually smoothed away, leaving the bone as before the fracture. If the ends have not been brought accurately in contact a permanent thickening results.

VARIETIES OF BONES Apart from the structural varieties, bones fall into four classes: (*a*) long bones like those of the limbs; (*b*) short bones composed of cancellous tissue like those of the wrist and the ankle; (*c*) flat bones like those of the skull; (*d*) irregular bones like those of the face or the vertebrae of the spinal column (or backbone).

The skeleton consists of over 200 bones. It is divided into an AXIAL part, consisting of the skull, the vertebral column, the ribs with their cartilages, and the breast-bone; and an APPENDICULAR portion consisting of the four limbs. The hyoid bone in the neck, together with the cartilages protecting the larynx and windpipe, may be described as the VISCERAL skeleton.

AXIAL SKELETON The skull consists of the cranium, which has eight bones, viz. occipital, two parietal, two temporal, one frontal, ethmoid, and sphenoid; and of the face, which has fourteen bones, viz. two maxillae or upper jaw-bones, one mandible or lower jaw-bone, two malar or cheek bones, two nasal, two lacrimal, two turbinal, two palate bones, and one vomer bone. (For further details, see SKULL.) The vertebral column consists of seven vertebrae in the cervical or neck region, twelve dorsal vertebrae, five vertebrae in the lumbar or loin region, the sacrum or sacral bone (a mass formed of five vertebrae fused together and forming the back part of the pelvis, which is closed at the sides by the haunch-bones), and finally the coccyx (four small vertebrae representing the tail of lower animals). The vertebral column has four curves: the first forwards in the neck, the second backwards in the dorsal region, the third forward in the loins, and the lowest, involving the sacrum and coccyx, backwards. These are associated with the erect attitude, develop after a child learns to walk, and have the effect of diminishing jars and shocks before these reach internal organs. This is still further aided by discs of cartilage placed between each pair of vertebrae. Each vertebra has a solid part, the body in front, and behind this a ring of bone, the series of rings one above another forming a bony canal, up which runs the spinal cord to pass through an opening in the skull at the upper end of the canal and there join the brain. (For further details, see SPINAL COLUMN.) The ribs, twelve in number, on each side, are attached behind to the twelve dorsal vertebrae, while in front they end a few inches away from the breast-bone, but are continued forwards by cartilages. Of these the upper seven reach the breast-bone, these ribs being called true ribs, the next three are joined each to the cartilage above it, while the last two have their ends free and are called floating ribs. The breast-bone, or sternum, is shaped something like a short sword, about 15 cm (6 inches) long, and rather over 2·5 cm (1 inch) wide.

APPENDICULAR SKELETON The upper limb consists of the shoulder region and three segments – the upper arm, the forearm, and the wrist with the hand, separated from each other by joints. In the shoulder lie the clavicle or collar-bone (which is immediately beneath the skin, and forms a prominent object on the front of the neck), and the scapula or shoulder-blade behind the chest. In the upper arm is a single bone, the humerus. In the forearm are two bones, the radius and ulna; the radius, in the movements of alternately turning the hand palm up and back up (called, respectively, supination and pronation), rotating round the ulna, which remains fixed. In the carpus or wrist are eight small bones – the scaphoid, lunate, triquetral, pisiform, trapezium, trapezoid, capitate, and hamate. In the hand proper are five bones called metacarpals, upon which are set the four fingers, each containing the three bones known as phalanges, and the thumb with two phalanges.

The lower limb consists similarly of the region of the haunch and three segments – the thigh, the leg, and the foot. The haunch-bone is a large flat bone made up of three – the ilium, the ischium, and the pubis, fused together, and forms the side of the pelvis or basin which encloses some of the abdominal organs. The thigh contains the femur, and the leg contains two bones – the tibia and fibula. In the tarsus are seven bones: the talus (which forms part of the ankle joint), the calcaneus or heel-bone, the navicular, the lateral, intermediate, and medial cuneiforms, and the cuboid. These bones are so shaped as to form a distinct arch in the foot both from before back and from side to side. Finally, as in the hand, there are five metatarsals and fourteen phalanges, of which the great toe has two, the other toes three each.

Besides these named bones there are others sometimes found in sinews, called sesamoid bones, while the numbers of the regular bones may be increased by extra ribs or diminished by the fusion together of two or more bones.

BONE, DISEASES OF

Bone is not an inert scaffolding for the human body. It is a living, dynamic organ, being continuously remodelled in response to external mechanical and chemical influences and acting as a large reservoir for calcium and phosphate. It is as susceptible to disease as any other organ but responds in a way rather different from the rest of the body.

Osteoporosis In economic terms this is the most important disease of bone in the elderly, a gradual loss of bone mass with age. Its cause is not known but it is more common in women, especially after the menopause. It may be responsible in a large part for the epidemic of fractured neck of femur currently occurring in the developed world. Its course may be slowed by calcium supplements, exercise, and hormone-replacement therapy, but there is no known cure.

Osteomalacia or rickets is the loss of mineralization of the bone rather than simple loss of bone mass. It is caused by vitamin D deficiency and is probably the most important bone disease in the Third World. In sunlight the skin can synthesize vitamin D (see APPENDIX 5: VITAMINS), but normally rickets is caused by a poor diet, or a failure to absorb food normally (malabsorbtion). In rare cases vitamin D cannot be converted to its active state due to the congenital lack of the specific enzymes and the rickets will fail to respond to treatment with vitamin D. Malfunction of the parathyroid gland or of the kidneys can disturb the dynamic equilibrium of calcium and phosphate in the body and severely deplete the bone of its stores of both calcium and phosphate.

Congenital diseases These are rare but may produce certain types of dwarfism or a susceptibility to fractures (osteogenesis imperfecta).

Infection of bone (osteomyelitis) occurs most commonly after an open fracture, or in newborn babies. Once established it is very difficult to eradicate. The bacteria appear capable of lying dormant in the bone for the life of the patient and are not easily destroyed with antibiotics. At any time the infection can break out again causing further damage.

Paget's disease (see also separate entry) is a common disease of bone in the elderly, caused by overactivity of the osteoclasts (cells concerned with removal of old bone, before new bone is laid down by osteoblasts). The bone affected thickens and bows and may become painful. Treatment with calcitonin and diphosphonates may slow down the osteoclasts, and so hinder the course of the disease, but there is no cure.

If bone loses its blood supply (avascular necrosis) it eventually fractures or collapses. If the blood supply does not return, bone's normal capacity for healing is severely impaired.

For the following diseases see separate articles RICKETS; ACROMEGALY; OSTEOMALACIA; OSTEOPOROSIS; OSTEOGENESIS IMPERFECTA.

Tumours of bone These can be benign (noncancerous) or malignant (cancerous). Primary bone tumours are rare, but secondaries from carcinoma of the breast, prostate and kidneys are relatively common. They may form cavities in a bone, weakening it until it breaks under normal load (a pathological fracture). The bone eroded away by the tumour may also cause problems by causing high levels of calcium in the plasma.

OSTEOID OSTEOMA is a harmless small growth which can occur in any bone. Its pain is typically removed by aspirin.

EWING'S TUMOUR is a malignant growth affecting long bones, particularly the tibia (calf bone). The presenting symptoms are a throbbing pain in the limb and a high temperature. Treatment is combined surgery, radiotherapy and chemotherapy.

OSTEOSARCOMA is a malignant tumour of bone with a peak incidence between the ages of 10 and 20. It typically involves the knees, causing a warm tender swelling. Removal of the growth with bone conservation techniques can often replace amputation as the definitive treatment. Chemotherapy can improve long-term survival.

MYELOMA is a generalized malignant disease of blood cells which produces tumours in bones which have red bone marrow such as the skull and trunk bones. These tumours can cause pathological fractures.

BONE GRAFT (see BONE TRANSPLANT).

BONE MARROW

is the soft substance occupying the interior of bones. There are two kinds: yellow marrow, which contains a large amount of fat, is found within the shaft of long limb bones; while red marrow, which has a highly cellular structure, occupies the space within the RIBS, STERNUM, VERTEBRAL bodies, and the ends of the long bones. Bone marrow is the site of formation of the ERYTHROCYTES, granular LEUCOCYTES, and PLATELETS.

BONE MARROW TRANSPLANT The procedure by which malignant or defective bone marrow in a patient is replaced with normal bone marrow. Sometimes the patient's own marrow is used (when the disease is in remission); after storage using tissue-freezing technique (cryopreservation) it is reinfused into the patient after the diseased marrow has been treated (autologous transplant). More commonly, an allogeneic transplant is done, using marrow from a donor whose tissue has been matched for compatibility. The recipient's marrow is destroyed with cytotoxic drugs before transfusion. The recipient is initially nursed in an isolated environment to reduce the risk of infection.

BONE TRANSPLANT The insertion of a piece of bone from another site or from another person to fill a defect, provide supporting tissue, or encourage the growth of new bone.

BORAX, or BIBORATE OF SODA, acts in much the same ways as boric acid, but without its acid reaction.

Uses Its chief use is in the form of a lotion (about 1 part to 30 of water) in all forms of itching and chapping of the skin. In THRUSH and other forms of irritation about the mouth in children the honey of borax, smeared on several times a day, is very soothing. To clean the mouth as well as soothe it, borax in honey wiped over the gums and tongue is very efficient. As in the case of boric acid, it should not be used in infants and young children.

BORBORYGMUS Flatulence in the bowels.

BORNHOLM DISEASE, also known as devil's grip, and epidemic myalgia, is an acute infective disease due to COXSACKIE VIRUSES, and characterized by the abrupt onset of pain around the lower margin of the ribs, headache, and fever. It occurs in epidemics, usually during warm weather, and it is more common in young people than the old. The illness usually lasts seven to ten days. It is practically never fatal. The disease is named after the island of Bornholm in the Baltic, where several epidemics have been described.

BOTULINUM TOXIN The toxin of the anaerobic bacterium *CLOSTRIDIUM BOTULINUM* is now routinely used to treat focal DYSTONIAS in adults. These include blepharospasm (see EYE DISEASES), SPASMODIC TORTICOLLIS, muscular spasms of the face, squint and some types of tremor. Injected close to where the nerve enters the affected muscles, the toxin blocks nerve transmissions for up to four months, so relieving symptoms. The toxin is also being tried out in cerebral palsies, and research is continuing.

BOTULISM A rare type of food poisoning with a mortality greater than 50 per cent, caused by the presence of the exotoxin of the anaerobic bacterium *Clostridium botulinum*, usually in contaminated tinned or bottled food. Symptoms develop a few hours after ingestion.

The toxin has two components, one having haemaglutinin activity and the other neurotoxic activity which produces most of the symptoms. It has a lethal dose of as little as 1 mg/kg and is highly selective for cholinergic nerves. Thus the symptoms are those of autonomic parasympathetic blockade (dry mouth, constipation, urinary retention, mydriasis, blurred vision) and progress to blockade of somatic cholinergic transmission (muscle weakness). Death results from respiratory muscle paralysis. Treatment consists of supportive measures and 4 aminopyridine and 3, 4 diaminopyridine, which may antagonize the effect of the toxin.

BOUGIES Solid instruments for introduction into natural passages in the body either in order to apply medicaments which they contain or with which they are coated, or, more usually, in order to dilate a narrow part or stricture of the passage. Thus we have, for example, urethral bougies, oesophageal bougies, rectal bougies, made usually of flexible rubber or, in the case of the urethra, of steel.

BOVINE SPONGIFORM ENCEPHALO-PATHY (BSE) Known colloquially as 'mad cow disease', this fatal and so far untreatable degenerative disease of cattle that causes severe neurological disabilities appeared in the UK in the mid 1980s. The first case is believed to have been identified in Kent in 1984, but the disease may have been gestating in some animals well before that date. Along with scrapie in sheep and CREUTZFELDT-JACOB DISEASE (CJD) in humans, BSE belongs to a class of unusual degenerative diseases of the brain known as transmissible spongiform encephalopathies, the diagnosis of which cannot be confirmed until post-mortem, though the recent finding of the infective agent in the appendix tissue of an infected man suggests it might be possible to diagnose the disease in living victims. The disease is thought to be caused by infectious proteins or prions about which little has so far been discovered. Prions are also the cause of another degenerative disease of the brain called KURU, or trembling disease, affecting only members of a cannibalistic tribespeople living in New Guinea. The incubation period for Kuru has been estimated at 12 to 15 years. The rare human disease CJD was identified many years ago and occurs throughout the world. In Britain about 50 cases a year occur. Its mode of transmission is ill understood but it does not usually affect people until they are in their fifties.

Since the BSE epidemic in cattle developed in the UK, however, a new variant of CJD has been identified in over 20 people in Britain and is believed to be the result of their consuming the meat of BSE-infected cattle. Though producing similar symptoms to classical CJD, the new variant has been affecting much younger people and may have a shorter incubation period. If this incubation time turns out to be the same as for classical CJD, however, it could be 2005–2010 before the peak of this outbreak is reachged

The appearance of BSE in cattle is believed to have been the result of their being fed animal offal, probably including that from scrapie-infected sheep. Before 1996 it is thought that at least 710,000 infected cattle entered the human food chain. A bovine offal ban was put in place in 1989 – all neurological tissue such as brain and spinal cord had to be removed from animals killed for consumption – but there have been doubts about its effective policing, at least until 1996. In 1997 the British government spent £1.5bn paying for cattle to be destroyed. Because of the lack of knowledge about BSE and its ability to jump the species barrier it is impossible to forecast how many people might develop new variant CJD. Research into BSE and CJD has been stepped up, and a government inquiry about the epidemic was started in March 1998. Meanwhile, a ban on the export of British beef and restrictions on the type of meat and products made from beef that can be sold to the public remain in place.

BOWELS (see INTESTINE).

BOWEN'S DISEASE An uncommon chronic localized skin disease presenting as a solitary chronic fixed irregular plaque mimicking eczema or psoriasis. It is a fairly benign form of CARCINOMA in situ in the EPIDERMIS but can occasionally become invasive. It is curable by CRYOTHERAPY or surgical excision.

BOW LEGS, or GENU VARUM: A deformity of the legs which comprises outward curvature between knee and ankle. It may be normal in infancy and occurs in osteoarthrosis, rickets, and other metabolic bone disease. In early childhood it may correct with growth, but in other cases surgical correction by osteotomy or ephiphyseal stapling is possible.

BOXING INJURIES rank eighth in frequency among sports injuries. According to the 'Report on the Medical Aspects of Boxing' issued by the Committee on Boxing of the Royal College of Physicians of London in October 1969, of 224 ex-professional boxers examined, 37 showed evidence of brain damage which was disabling in thirteen.

The first type of damage occurs as an acute episode in which one or more severe blows leads to loss of consciousness and occasionally to death. Death in the acute phase is usually due to intracranial haemorrhage and this carries a mortality of 45 per cent even with the sophisticated surgical techniques currently available. The second type of damage develops over a much longer period and is cumulative, leading to the atrophy of the cerebral cortex and brain stem. The repair processes of the brain are very limited and even after mild concussion it may suffer a small amount of permanent structural damage. Brain scanning techniques now enable brain damage to be detected during life. Brain damage of the type previously associated with the punch-drunk syndrome is now being detected before obvious clinical signs have developed. Evidence of cerebral atrophy has been found in relatively young boxers including amateurs and those whose careers have been considered successful. The tragedy is that brain damage can only be detected after it has occurred. Many doctors are opposed to boxing, even with the present stricter medical precautions taken by those responsible for running the sport.

BRACHIAL means 'belonging to the upper arm'. There are, for example, a brachial artery, and a brachial plexus of nerves through which run all the nerves to the arm. The brachial plexus lies along the outer side of the armpit, and is liable to be damaged in dislocation at the shoulder.

BRACHYCEPHALIC means short-headed and is a term applied to skulls the breadth of which is at least four-fifths of the length. Brachycephaly is a characteristic of the Alpine race.

BRACHYDACTYLY The conditions in which the fingers or toes are abnormally short.

BRADYCARDIA Slowness of the beating of the heart with corresponding slowness of the pulse (below 60 per minute). (See HEART DISEASES.)

BRADYKINESIA refers to the slow, writhing movements of the body and limbs that may occur in various brain disorders (see ATHETOSIS).

BRADYKININ is a substance derived from plasma proteins, which plays an important role in many of the reactions of the body, including INFLAMMATION. Its prime action is in producing dilatation of arteries and veins. It has also been described as 'the most powerful pain-producing agent known'.

BRAILLE A system of printing or writing for the blind using tangible dots or points to represent the characters.

BRAIN The brain and spinal cord together form the central nervous sytem, the twelve nerves passing on each side from the brain, and

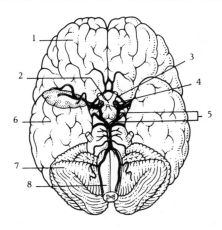

1 frontal lobe of cerebrum
2 optic chiasma
3 anterior cerebral artery
4 internal carotid artery
5 circle of Willis
6 temporal lobe of cerebrum
7 cerebellum
8 medulla oblongata (leading to spinal cord)

Brain viewed from below showing arterial
network (circle of Willis).

the thirty-one from the cord being called the
peripheral nervous system, while the complex
chains of nerves and ganglia lying within the
chest and abdomen, and acting to a large
extent independently of the other two systems,
though closely connected with them, make up
the autonomic system, and govern the activity
of the viscera.

Divisions The brain in its simplest form in
lowly vertebrate animals is a thickened part at
the front end of the spinal cord, developed in
order to govern the organs of special sense, viz.
smell, sight, hearing, and taste, lodged near at
hand. Higher in the scale, in fishes for example,
there are marked bulgings of nervous matter
forming the fore-brain, the mid-brain, and the
hind-brain, and that part connected with the
nerves of the eyes appears to be the highest
governing part. In man, however, the part in
front of this is specially developed, and not
only forms the great bulk of the entire brain,
but governs the activities of the rest. This part
is called the cerebrum.
CEREBRUM This forms the great bulk of the
brain in amount and consists of two cerebral
hemispheres which occupy the entire vault of
the cranium and are incompletely separated
from one another by a deep median cleft, the
longitudinal cerebral fissure. At the bottom of
this cleft the two hemispheres are united by a
thick band of some 200 million transverse
nerve fibres: the corpus callosum. Other clefts
or fissures, or sulci as they are known, make
deep impressions, dividing the cerebrum into

lobes. Of these the chief are the lateral sulcus
and the central sulcus. The lobes of the cerebrum are the frontal lobe in the forehead
region, the parietal lobe on the side and upper
part of the brain, the occipital lobe to the back,
and the temporal lobe lying just above the
region of the ear.
Numbers of shallower infoldings of the surface called furrows or sulci separate raised
areas called convolutions or gyri. The outer 3
mm or thereabouts of the cerebral hemispheres
consists of grey matter largely made up of
ganglion cells, while in the deeper part the
white matter consists of medullated nerve fibres connecting different parts of the surface
and passing down to the lower parts of the
brain. Among the white matter lie several
rounded masses of grey matter, the lentiform
and caudate nuclei. In the centre of each
cerebral hemisphere is an irregular cavity, the
lateral ventricle, each of which communicates
with that on the other side and behind with the
3rd ventricle through a small opening, the
inter-ventricular foramen, or foramen of Monro.
BASAL NUCLEI Two large masses of grey matter imbedded in the base of the cerebral hemispheres in man, but forming the chief part of
the brain in many animals. Between these
masses lies the 3rd ventricle, from which the
infundibulum, a funnel-shaped process, projects
downwards into the pituitary body, and above
lies the pineal gland. This region includes the
important hypothalamus.
MID-BRAIN, or mesencephalon A stalk about
20 mm long connecting the cerebrum with the
hind-brain. Down its centre lies a tube, the
cerebral aqueduct, or aqueduct of Sylvius,
connecting the 3rd and 4th ventricles. Above
this aqueduct lie the corpora quadrigemina,
and beneath it are the crura cerebri, strong
bands of white matter in which important
nerve fibres pass downwards from the cerebrum.
PONS A mass of nerve fibres, some of which
run crosswise and others as the continuation
of the crura cerebri downwards.
CEREBELLUM This lies towards the back, underneath the occipital lobes of the cerebrum.
MEDULLA OBLONGATA The lowest part of the
brain, in structure resembling the spinal cord,
with white matter on the surface and grey
matter in its interior. This is continuous through
the large opening in the skull, the foramen
magnum, with the spinal cord. Between the
medulla, pons, and cerebellum lies the 4th
ventricle of the brain.

Structure The brain is made up of grey and
white matter. In the cerebrum and cerebellum
the grey matter is arranged mainly in a layer
on the surface, though both have certain grey
masses imbedded in the white matter. In the
other parts the grey matter is found in definite
masses called nuclei, from which the nerves
spring. The grey matter consists mainly of
cells in which all the activities of the brain
begin. These cells vary considerably in size
and shape in different parts of the brain,

1 frontal lobe
2 frontal pole
3 lateral (sylvian) sulcus
4 temporal pole
5 superior temporal sulcus
6 temporal lobe
7 preoccipital notch

8 occipital lobe
9 angular gyrus
10 supramarginal gyrus
11 parietal lobe
12 postcentral gyrus
13 central sulcus
14 precentral gyrus

Side view of the brain.

1 sulcus of corpus callosum
2 uncus
3 hippocampal sulcus
4 lingual gyrus
5 calcarine sulcus
6 cuneus

7 precuneus
8 subparietal sulcus
9 paracentral lobule
10 thalamus
11 basal ganglion

Vertical section through the middle of the brain.

though all give off a number of processes, some of which form nerve fibres. The cells on the surface of the cerebral hemispheres, for example, are very numerous, being set in layers five or six deep. In shape these cells are pyramidal, giving off processes from the apex, from the centre of the base, and from various projections elsewhere on the cell. The grey matter is everywhere penetrated by a rich supply of blood-vessels, and the nerve cells and blood- vessels are supported in a fine network of fibres, known as neuroglia. The white matter consists of nerve fibres, each of which is attached, at one end, to a cell in the grey matter, while, at the other end, it splits up into a tree-like structure round another cell in another part of the grey matter in the brain or spinal cord. The fibres have insulating sheaths of a fatty material, which, in the mass, gives the white matter its colour, and they convey messages from one part of the brain to the other (association fibres), or, grouped into bundles, leave the brain as nerves, or pass down into the spinal cord, where they end near, and exert a control upon, cells from which in turn spring the nerves to the body. Both grey and white matter are bound together by a felt-work called neuroglia. The general arrangement of fibres can be best understood by describing the course of a motor nerve fibre. Arising in a cell on the surface in front of the central sulcus, such a fibre passes inwards towards the centre of the cerebral hemisphere, the collected mass of fibres as they lie between the lentiform nucleus and optic thalamus being known as the internal capsule. Hence the fibre passes down through the crus cerebri, giving off various small connecting fibres as it passes downwards. After passing through the pons it reaches the medulla, and at this point crosses to the opposite side (decussation of the pyramids). Entering the spinal cord, it passes downwards to end finally in a series of branches (arborization) which meet and touch (synapse) similar branches from one or more of the cells in the grey matter of the cord (see SPINAL CORD).

SIZE The weight of the average male brain is 1·4 kg, ranging from 1·24 to 1·68 kg, of the female brain 1·25 kg, ranging from 1·13 to 1·51 kg, but brains have been found as heavy as 1·8 kg, or, in exceptional cases, even more. The maximum mass of brain tissue is reached at the age of 20, and then decreases steadily.

MEMBRANES The brain is separated from the skull by three membranes: the dura mater, a thick fibrous membrane; the arachnoid mater, a more delicate structure; and the pia mater, adhering to the surface of the brain, and containing the blood- vessels which nourish it. Between each pair is a space containing fluid on which the brain floats as on a water-bed. The fluid beneath the arachnoid membrane mixes with that inside the ventricles through a small opening in the 4th ventricle, called the median aperture, or foramen of Magendie.

These fluid arrangements have a great influence in preserving the brain from injury.

NERVES Twelve nerves come off the brain:

I.	Olfactory, to the nose (smell).	
II.	Optic, to the eye (sight).	
III.	Oculomotor	
IV.	Trochlear	to eye-muscles.
V.	Abducent	
VI.	Trigeminal, to skin of face.	
VII.	Facial, to muscles of face.	
VIII.	Vestibulocochlear, to hear (hearing and balancing).	
IX.	Glossopharyngeal, to tongue (taste).	
X.	Vagus, to heart, larynx, lungs, and stomach.	
XI.	Spinal accessory, to muscles in neck.	
XII.	Hypoglossal, to muscles of tongue.	

BLOOD-VESSELS Four vessels carry blood to the brain: two internal carotid arteries in front, and two vertebral arteries behind. These communicate to form a circle (circle of Willis) inside the skull, so that if one is blocked the others, by dilating, take its place. The chief branch of the internal carotid artery on each side is the middle cerebral, and this gives off a small but very important branch which pierces the base of the brain and supplies the region of the internal capsule with blood. The chief importance of this vessel lies in the fact that the blood in it is under specially high pressure, owing to its close connection with the carotid artery, so that haemorrhage from it is liable to occur and thus give rise to apoplexy. Two veins, the internal cerebral veins, bring the blood away from the interior of the brain, but most of the small veins come to the surface and open into large venous sinuses, which run in grooves in the skull, and finally pour their blood into the internal jugular vein that accompanies the carotid artery on each side of the neck.

Functions The cerebrum is associated with the intellectual faculties in man, and also exerts a guiding influence over the rest of the nervous system. It is not, however, necessary to actual life. If the cerebrum of a frog is destroyed it still breathes and its heart beats, it can hop if pinched, and swim if put in water, but when left alone it sits still till it perishes. If the same happens to a pigeon it can fly when thrown in the air, and can alight, but it does not fly away when threatened, nor will it take food, having lost even the instinct to preserve life. If, on the other hand, the cerebellum of a pigeon is destroyed, the bird cannot maintain its balance, the cerebellum being concerned in the regulation of muscular movements and in preserving the equilibrium of the body.

Plato recognized three mental faculties, which he placed, respectively, in the liver, heart, and brain, these organs being supposed to secrete the 'animal spirits' appropriate to each faculty; and this view was accepted by the medical writers of antiquity. In the Middle Ages the

Arabian physicians, however, following Galen's opinion, placed the different mental faculties in the several ventricles of the brain, this theory being adopted by Duns Scotus, Thomas of Aquino, and referred to by Burton in his *Anatomy of Melancholy*.

Descartes (1596–1650) had the fanciful idea that the pineal body was the seat of the mind. After his time it was thought that the whole brain must act together in every process, from the fact that, in cases of severe injury to the head, much substance can be lost from some parts of the brain without impairment of any one definite function or memory.

But it is now known that definite areas of the surface are associated with definite functions. The earliest systematic attempt to localize the functions of the brain to certain areas was made by Gall and Spurzheim, who founded the system of phrenology in the first quarter of the nineteenth century. Although this system was proved to be wrong both as regards the functions of the brain and the philosophic analysis of mental processes, the criticism it called forth gave a great impetus to the attempt to localize the functions of the brain in definite spots. Between 1820 and 1840 it became established that, in people who have lost the power of speech during life, the brain shows some disease in the left frontal lobe after death, and in 1861 Broca made the first definite discovery in cerebral localization by proving that the faculty of speech is governed by a centre in the region of the inferior frontal gyrus, named (after him) Broca's convolution. His discovery was followed later by the important observation of Hughlings Jackson that certain forms of epilepsy, associated with movements beginning in a definite limb, are caused by disease affecting the part of the brain that borders on the central sulcus, and this discovery was confirmed and extended by many experimenters and physicians. Fritsch, Hitzig, Ferrier, Sherrington, Grünbaum and others have shown that definite areas near the central sulcus are associated with the movement of definite parts. Further, the occipital lobes are associated with the sense of sight, the temporal lobe with hearing, and the inner surface of the same lobe with taste and smell. The purely intellectual faculties are probably associated with the frontal lobes, which seem to govern nothing else. The cerebellum has to do with the powers of balancing and of regulating movements. The medulla and pons have important functions, governing many of the processes most essential to life, e.g. those of respiration, rate of the heart, swallowing, vomiting, and giving off all the nerves which arise from the brain, except the first four.

BRAIN, DISEASES OF
The human brain is a highly complex network of nerve cells and their interconnecting 'wires' or axons. Its diseases consist of either expanding masses (lumps or tumours); or of areas of shrinkage (atrophy) due to degeneration, or to loss of blood supply, usually from blockage of an artery.

Tumours All masses cause varying combinations of headache and vomiting – symptoms of raised pressure within the inexpansible bony box formed by the skull; general or localized epileptic fits; weakness of limbs or disordered speech; and varied mental changes. Tumours may be primary, arising in the brain, or secondary deposits from tumours arising in the lung, breast or other organs. Some brain tumours are benign and curable by surgery; examples include meningiomas and pituitary tumours. The symptoms depend on the size and situation of the mass. Abscesses, or blood clots (HAEMATOMAS) on the surface or within the brain may resemble tumours. Some are removable. GLIOMAS are primary malignant tumours, which despite surgery and radiotherapy usually have a bad prognosis.

Clinical examination and brain scanning (CT, or COMPUTED TOMOGRAPHY; MAGNETIC RESONANCE IMAGING (MRI)) are safe, accurate methods of demonstrating the tumour, its size, position and treatability.

Strokes When a blood vessel, usually an artery, is blocked by a clot, thrombus or embolism, the local area of the brain fed by that artery is damaged (see STROKE). The resulting infarct (softening) causes a stroke. The cells die and a patch of brain tissue shrinks. The obstruction in the blood vessel may be in a small artery in the brain, or a larger artery in the neck. Aspirin, anti-clotting, and other drugs reduce recurrent attacks, and a small number of people benefit if a narrowed neck artery is cleaned out by an operation, endarterectomy. Similar symptoms develop abruptly if a blood vessel bursts, causing a cerebral haemorrhage. The symptoms of a stroke are sudden weakness or paralysis of the arm and leg on the opposite side to the damaged area of brain (HEMIPARESIS); and sometimes loss of half of the field of vision to one side (HEMIANOPIA). The speech area is in the left side of the brain controlling language in right-handed people. In 60 per cent of left handers, the speech area is on the left side and in 40 per cent on the right side. If the speech area is damaged, difficulties in both understanding words, and in saying them, develops (see DYSPHASIA).

Degenerations (atrophy) For reasons often unknown, various groups of nerve cells degenerate prematurely. The illness resulting is determined by which groups of nerve cells are affected. If those in the deep basal ganglia are affected, a movement disorder occurs, such as Parkinson's disease, hereditary Huntington's chorea, or, in children with birth defects of the brain, athetosis and dystonias. Modern drugs, such as DOPAMINE drugs in PARKINSON'S DISEASE, and other treatments can improve the symptoms and reduce the disabilities of some of these diseases.

Drugs and injury Alcohol in excess, the abuse of many sedative drugs and artificial brain stimulants – such as cocaine, LSD and heroin (see DRUG ADDICTION) can damage the brain;

the effects can be reversible in early cases. Severe head injury can cause localized or diffuse brain damage (see HEAD INJURY).

Cerebral palsy Damage to the brain in children can occur in the uterus during pregnancy or can result from rare hereditary and genetic diseases. Stiff spastic limbs, movement disorders and speech defects are common. Some of these children are mentally backward. Physical and rehabilitation therapies may be beneficial.

Dementias In older people, a diffuse loss of cells, mainly at the front of the brain, causes Alzheimer's disease, the main feature being loss of memory, attention and reasoned judgement (dementia). It affects about 5 per cent of the over-80s, but is not simply due to ageing processes. Most patients require routine tests and brain scanning to indicate other treatable causes of dementia. Response to current treatments is poor. Like Parkinson's disease it progresses slowly over many years. It is uncommon for these diseases to run in families. Rarely, multiple strokes can cause dementia.

Infections in the brain are uncommon. Viruses such as measles, mumps, herpes, AIDS, and, rarely, immunization cause encephalitis: a diffuse inflammation (see AIDS/HIV; and ENCEPHALITIS). Bacteria may infect the membrane covering the brain causing meningitis. Antibiotics have allowed a cure or good control of symptoms in most cases of meningitis, but early diagnosis is essential. Severe headaches, fever, vomiting and increasing sleepiness are the principal symptoms which demand urgent advice from the doctor, and usually admission to hospital. If infection spreads from an unusually serious sinusitis or from a chronically infected middle ear, or from a penetrating injury of the skull, an abscess may slowly develop. Brain abscesses cause insidious drowsiness, headaches and at a late stage weakness of the limbs or loss of speech; a high temperature is seldom present. Early diagnosis, confirmed by brain scanning, is followed by antibiotics and surgery in hospital, but the outcome is good in only half the patients.

Another infection is caused by PRIONS. These infective agents cause the rare CREUTZFELDT-JAKOB disease (CJD) and its new variant form transmitted from cattle with bovine spongiform encephalopathy (BSE). CJD has an incubation period of up to 20 years and is typified by brain degeneration which leads to severe neurological disabilities and death. It can be diagnosed for certainty only at post-mortem and there is no cure. KURU or trembling disease is a similar disorder occurring in a cannabilistic tribe in New Guinea.

BRAIN INJURIES Most blows to the head cause no loss of consciousness and no brain injury. If someone is knocked out for a minute or two, there has been a brief commotion of the brain cells (CONCUSSION), but no after-effects. Most leave hospital within 1 to 3 days, have no organic signs, recover and return quickly to work without further complaints.

Severe head injuries cause unconsciousness for hours or many days, followed by loss of memory before and after that period of unconsciousness. The skull may be fractured, there may be fits in the first week, and there may develop a blood clot in the brain (intracerebral haematoma), or within the membranes covering the brain (extradural, and subdural haematomata). These clots compress the brain and the pressure inside the skull rises with urgent life-threatening consequences. They are identified by neurologists and neurosurgeons, confirmed by brain scans (see COMPUTED TOMOGRAPHY, MAGNETIC RESONANCE IMAGING), and require urgent surgical removal. Recovery may be complete, or in very severe cases can be marred by physical disabilities, epilepsy, and by changes in intelligence, rational judgement, and behaviour. Symptoms generally improve in the first two years.

A minority of those with minor head injuries have complaints and disabilities which seem disproportionate to the injury sustained. Referred to as the post-traumatic syndrome, this is not a diagnostic entity. The complaints are headaches, forgetfulness, irritability, slowness, poor concentration, fatigue, dizziness (usually not vertigo), intolerance of alcohol, light and noise, loss of interests and initiative, depression, anxiety, and impaired libido. Reassurance and return to light work help these symptoms to disappear, in most cases within three months. Psychological illness and unresolved compensation claims feature in many with implacable complaints.

People who have had brain injuries, and their relatives, can obtain help and advice from Headway National Head Injuries Association (see APPENDIX 2: ADDRESSES).

BRAIN-STEM DEATH Brain damage, resulting in the irreversible loss of brain function, renders the individual incapable of life without the aid of a ventilator. Criteria have been developed to recognize that 'death' has occurred and allow ventilation to be stopped. The UK criteria require the patient to be irreversibly unconscious and unable to regain the capacity to breathe spontaneously.

All reversible pharmacological, metabolic, endocrine and physiological causes must be excluded, and there should be no doubt that irreversible brain damage has occurred. Two senior doctors carry out diagnostic tests to confirm that brain-stem REFLEXES are absent. These tests must be repeated after a suitable interval before death can be declared. Imaging techniques are not required for death to be diagnosed. The test for brain-stem death are:

- Fixed dilated pupils of the eyes
- Absent CORNEAL REFLEX
- Absent VESTIBULO-OCULAR REFLEX
- No cranial motor response to somatic (physical) stimulation

- Absent gag and cough reflexes
- No respiratory effort in response to apnoea and adequate concentrations of CARBON DIOXIDE in the arterial blood.

BRAN The meal derived from the outer covering of a cereal grain. It contains little or no carbohydrate, and is mainly used to provide ROUGHAGE in the control of bowel function and the prevention of constipation.

BRANCHIAL CYST A cyst arising in the neck from remnants of the embryological branchial clefts. They are usually fluid filled and will therefore transilluminate.

BREASTBONE (see STERNUM).

BREASTS, or MAMMARY GLANDS, occur only in mammals and provide milk for feeding the young. These paired organs are usually fully developed only in adult females, but are present in rudimentary form in juveniles and males. In women, the two breasts overlie the second to sixth ribs on the front of the chest. On the surface of each breast is a central pink disc called the areola, which surrounds the nipple. Inside, the breast consists of fat, supporting tissue and glandular tissue, which is the part that produces milk following childbirth. Each breast consists of twelve to twenty compartments arranged radially around the nipple. Each compartment opens on to the tip of the nipple via its own duct through which the milk flows. The breast enlargement that occurs in pregnancy is due to development of the glandular part in preparation for lacation. In women beyond childbearing age, the glandular part of the breasts reduces (called involution) and the breasts become less firm and contain relatively more fat.

BREASTS, DISEASES OF The female breasts may be expected to undergo hormone-controlled enlargement at puberty, and later in pregnancy, and the glandular part of the breast undergoes evolution (shrinkage) after the menopause. The breast can also be affected by many different diseases, with common symptoms being pain, nipple discharge or retraction, and the formation of a lump within the breast.

Benign disease is much more common than cancer, particularly in young women, and includes acute inflammation of the breast (mastitis); abscess formation; and benign breast lumps, which may be fibroadenosis – diffuse lumpiness also called chronic mastitis or fibrocystic disease – in which one or more fluid-filled sacs (cysts) develop.

Women who are breastfeeding are particularly prone to mastitis, as infection may enter the breast via the nipple. The process may be arrested before a breast abscess forms by prompt treatment with antibiotics. Non-bacterial inflammation may result from mammary duct ectasia (dilatation), in which abnormal or blocked ducts may overflow. Initial treatments should be with antibiotics, but if an abscess does form it should be surgically drained.

Duct ectasia, with or without local mastitis, is the usual benign cause of various nipple complaints, with common symptoms being nipple retraction, discharge and skin change.

Breast lumps form the chief potential danger and may be either solid or cystic. Simple examination may fail to distinguish the two types, but aspiration of a benign cyst usually results in its disappearance. If the fluid is blood stained, or if a lump still remains, malignancy is possible, and all solid lumps need histological (tissue examination) or cytological (cell examination) assessment. As well as having their medical and family history taken, any women with a breast lump should undergo triple assessment: a combination of clinical examination, imaging – mammography for the over 35s and ultrasonagraphy for under 35s – and fine-needle aspiration. The medical history should include details of any previous lumps, family history (up to 10 per cent of breast cancer in Western countries is due to genetic disposition), pain, nipple discharge, change in size related to menstrual cycle and parous state, and any drugs being taken by the patient. Breasts should be inspected with the arms up and down, noting position, size, consistency, mobility, fixity, and local lymphadenopathy (glandular swelling). Nipples should be examined for the presence of inversion or discharge. Skin involvement (peau d'orange) should be noted, and, in particular, how long changes have been present. Fine-needle aspiration and cytological examination of the fluid are essential with ULTRASOUND, MAMMOGRAPHY and possible BIOPSY being considered, depending on the patient's age and the extent of clinical suspicion that cancer may be present. The commonest solid benign lump is a fibroadenoma, particularly in women of childbearing age, and is a painless, mobile lump. If small, it is usually safe to leave it alone, provided that the patient is warned to seek medical advice if its size or character changes or if the lump becomes painful. Fibroadenosis (diffuse lumpiness often in the upper, outer quadrant) is a common (benign) lump. Others include periductal mastitis, fat NECROSIS, GALACTOCELE, ABSCESS and non-breast lumps, e.g. LIPOMAS (fatty tissue) or SEBACEOUS CYSTS. A woman with breast discharge should have a mammograph, ductograph, or total duct excision until the cause of any underlying duct ectasia is known. Appropriate treatment should then be given.

Malignant disease most commonly – but not exclusively – occurs in postmenopausal women, classically presenting as a slowly growing, painless, firm lump. A blood-stained nipple discharge or eczematous skin change may also be suggestive of cancer.

The most commonly used classification of invasive cancers has split them into two types: ductal and lobular, but this is no longer suitable. There are also weaknesses in the tumour node mestastases (TNM) system and the International Union Against Cancer (UICC) classification.

The TNM system – which classifies the lump by size, fixity and presence of affected axillary glands and wider metastatic spread – is best combined with a pathological classification, when assessing the seriousness of a possibly cancerous lump. Risk factors for cancer include nulliparity (see NULLIPARA), first pregnancy over the age of 30 years, early MENARCHE, late MENOPAUSE and positive family history. The danger should be considered in women who are not breast feeding or with previous breast cancer, and must be carefully excluded if the woman is taking any contraceptive steroids or is on hormone-replacement therapy.

Screening programmes involving mammography are well established, the aim being to detect more tumours at an early and curable stage. Pick-up rate is 5 per 1,000 healthy women over 50 years. Yearly two-view mammograms could reduce mortality by 40 per cent but may cause alarm because there are 10 false positive mammograms for each true positive result. In premenopausal women breasts are denser, making mammograms harder to interpret, and screening appears not to save lives. About a quarter of women with a palpable breast lump turn out to have cancer.

TREATMENT This remains controversial, and all options should be carefully discussed with the patient and, where appropriate, with her partner. Locally contained disease may be treated by local excision of the lump, but sampling of the glands of the armpit of the same side should be performed to check for additional spread of the disease, and hence the need for CHEMOTHERAPY or RADIOTHERAPY. Depending on the extent of spread, simple mastectomy or modified radical mastectomy (which removes the lymph nodes draining the breast) may be required. Follow-up chemotherapy, for example, with TAMOXIFEN (an oestrogen antagonist), much improves survival (it saves 12 lives over 100 women treated), though it may occasionally cause endometrial carcinoma. Analysis in the mid 1990s of large-scale international studies of breast-cancer treatments showed wide variations in their effectiveness. As a result the NHS has encouraged hospitals to set up breast-treatment teams containing all the relevant health professional experts and to use those treatments shown to be most effective.

As well as the physical treatments provided, women with suspected or proven breast cancer should be offered psychological support because up to 30 per cent of affected women develop an anxiety state or depressive illness within a year of diagnosis. Problems over body image and sexual difficulties occur in and around one quarter of patients. Breast conservation and reconstructive surgery can improve the physical effects of mastectomy, and women should be advised on the prostheses and specially designed brassieres that are available. Specialist nurses and self-help groups are in-valuable in supporting affected women and their partners with the problems caused by breast cancer and its treatment. Breast Cancer Care, British Association of Cancer United Patients (BACUP), Cancerlink, and Cancer Relief Macmillan Fund are among voluntary organizations providing support (see APPENDIX 2: ADDRESSES).

BREAST FEEDING This is the natural way to feed a baby from birth to weaning. Human milk is an ideal food, containing a proper balance of nutrients, as well as an essential supply of antibodies to protect the infant against infections. Breast feeding also strengthens the physical bond between mother and child. For the first few weeks feeding should be on demand. Difficulties over breast feeding and the pressures of modern life, especially for working mothers, can, however, make it hard to continue breast feeding for more than a few weeks, or even to breast feed at all. Sometimes infections occur, producing soreness and even an abscess. Mothers should seek advice from health professionals about breast feeding, especially if problems arise.

BREAST RECONSTRUCTION (see MAMMOPLASTY).

BREAST REDUCTION (see MAMMOPLASTY).

BREAST SCREENING A set of investigations aimed at the early detection of breast cancer. It includes self-screening by monthly examination of the breasts and formal programmes of screening by palpation and mammography in special clinics. In the UK the NHS offers regular mammography examinations to all women between 50 and 64 years of age and in 1995–6 1.1 million women were screened, 76 per cent of those invited. Over 5,500 cancers were detected, 5.3 per 1,000 women screened.

BREATH-HOLDING Breath-holding attacks are not uncommon in infants and toddlers. They are characterized by the child's suddenly stopping breathing in the midst of a bout of crying evoked by pain, some emotional upset, or loss of temper. The breath may be held so long that the child goes blue in the face. The attack is never fatal and the condition disappears spontaneously after the age of 3 to 5 years, but once a child has acquired the habit it may recur quite often.

The attacks require no treatment other than reassurance as recovery is spontaneous and rapid. Parents should avoid dramatizing the attacks.

BREATHING (see RESPIRATION).

BREATHLESSNESS or DYSPNOEA may be due to any condition which renders the blood impure or deficient in oxygen, and which therefore produces excessive involuntary efforts to gain more air. Exercise is a natural cause and acute anxiety may provoke breathlessness in otherwise healthy people. Deprivation of oxygen – for example, in a building fire – will also cause the victim to raise his breathing rate. Disorders of the lung may diminish the area available for breathing: e.g. ASTHMA, PNEUMONIA, TUBERCULOSIS, EMPHYSEMA, BRONCHITIS, collections of fluid in the pleural cavities, and pressure by a TUMOUR or ANEURYSM.

- Pleurisy causes short, rapid breathing to avoid the pain of deep inspiration.
- Narrowing of the air passages may produce sudden and alarming attacks of difficult breathing, especially among children: e.g. in croup, asthma, and diphtheria (see these headings).
- Most cardiac disorders (see HEART DISEASES) cause breathlessness, especially when the person undergoes any special exertion.
- Anaemia is a frequent cause.
- Obesity is often associated with shortness of breath.

Mountain climbing may cause breathlessness because, as altitude increases, the amount of oxygen in the air falls (see ALTITUDE SICKNESS).

BREATH SOUNDS The transmitted sounds of breathing, heard when a stethoscope is applied to the chest. Normal breath sounds are described as vesicular. Abnormal sounds may be heard when there is increased fluid in the lungs or fibrosis (crepitation or crackles), when there is bronchospasm (rhonchi or wheezes), or when the lung is consolidated (bronchial breathing). Absent breath sounds occur with pleural effusion, pneumothorax, or after pneumonectomy.

BREECH DELIVERY (see BREECH PRESENTATION).

BREECH PRESENTATION By the 32nd week of pregnancy most babies are in a head-down position in the womb. Up to 4 per cent of them, however, have their buttocks (breech) presenting at the neck of the womb. If the baby is still a breech presentation at the 34th–35th week, the obstetrician may, by external manipulation, try to turn it to the head-down position. If this is not successful, the fetus is left in the breech position. Breech deliveries are more difficult for mother and baby because the buttocks are less efficient than the head at dilating the cervix and vagina. An EPISIOTOMY is usually necessary to assist delivery and obstetric FORCEPS may also have to be applied to the baby's head. If the infant and/or the mother become unduly distressed, the obstetrician may decide to deliver the baby by CAESAREAN SECTION; some obstetricians prefer to deliver most breech-presentation babies using this method.

BRIGHT'S DISEASE (see KIDNEYS, DISEASES OF: glomerulonephritis).

BRITISH DENTAL ASSOCIATION (see APPENDIX 10: PROFESSIONAL ORGANIZATIONS).

BRITISH MEDICAL ASSOCIATION (SEE APPENDIX 10: PROFESSIONAL ORGANIZATIONS).

BRITISH NATIONAL FORMULARY (BNF) is a pocket book for those concerned with the prescribing, dispensing and administration of medicines in Britain. It is produced jointly by the Royal Pharmaceutical Society and the British Medical Association and is revised twice yearly. The BNF is also available in electronic form.

BRITTLE BONE DISEASE is another name for OSTEOGENESIS IMPERFECTA.

BROMIDES introduced in 1857 as the first effective treatment for EPILEPSY, have been largely superseded by BARBITURATES and more recently ANTICONVULSANTS. They are also obsolete in their use as general SEDATIVES and HYPNOTICS. Bromide is notoriously cumulative in the body and is potentially poisonous.

BROMOCRIPTINE A drug that stimulates DOPAMINE receptors in the brain. It inhibits production of the hormone PROLACTIN and is used to treat GALACTORRHOEA (excessive milk secretion) and also to suppress normal LACTATION. The drug is helpful in treating premenstrual breast engorgement and also ACROMEGALY.

BRONCHIAL TUBES (see AIR PASSAGES; BRONCHUS; LUNGS).

BRONCHIECTASIS A condition characterized by dilatation of the bronchi. This is the result as a rule of infection of the bronchial tree leading to obstruction of the bronchi. As a result of the obstruction the affected individual cannot get rid of the secretions in the bronchi beyond the obstruction. This accumulates and becomes infected. The initial infection may be due to bacterial or viral pneumonia or the infection of the lungs complicating measles or whooping-cough. Once a common disease, immunization of infants against infectious diseases and the use of antiobiotics have greatly reduced its incidence.

Treatment consists of postural drainage of excessive lung secretions and antibiotics.

BRONCHIOLES The term applied to the finest divisions of the bronchial tubes.

BRONCHIOLITIS The name sometimes applied to bronchitis affecting the finest bronchial tubes, also known as capillary bronchitis.

BRONCHITIS Inflammation of the bronchial tubes. This may occur as an acute transient illness or as a chronic condition.

Acute bronchitis is due to an acute infection, viral or bacterial, of the bronchi. This is distinguished from pneumonia by the anatomical site involved – bronchitis affects the bronchi whilst pneumonia affects the lung tissue. The infection causes a productive cough, and fever. Secretions within airways sometimes lead to wheezing. Sometimes the specific causative organism may be identified from the sputum. The illness is normally self limiting but, if treatments are required, bacterial infections respond to a course of antibiotics.

Chronic bronchitis is a clinical diagnosis applied to patients with chronic cough and sputum production. For epidemiological studies it is defined as cough productive of sputum on most days during at least three consecutive months for not less than two consecutive years.

In the past industrial workers regularly exposed to heavily polluted air commonly developed bronchitis. The main aetiological factor is smoking. This leads to an increase in size and number of bronchial mucous glands. These are responsible for the excessive mucus production within the bronchial tree causing a persistent productive cough. The increased number of mucous glands along with the influx of inflammatory cells may lead to airway narrowing. When airway narrowing occurs, it slows the passage of air producing breathlessness. Other less important causative factors include exposure to pollutants and dusts. Infections do not cause the disease but frequently produce exacerbations with worsening of symptoms.

Treatments involve the use of antibiotics to treat the infections that produce exacerbations of symptoms. Bronchodilators (drugs that open up the airways) help to reverse the airway narrowing that causes the breathlessness. Cessation of smoking reduces the speed of progression.

BRONCHODILATOR This type of drug reduces the tone of smooth muscle in the bronchioles and therefore increases their diameter. Such drugs are used in the treatment of asthma and other causes of bronchoconstriction. As bronchiolar tone is a balance between sympathetic and parasympathetic activity, most bronchodilators are either B2 receptor agonists or cholinergic receptor antagonists, although theophyllines are also useful.

BRONCHOGRAPHY A radiographic procedure using a radio-opaque substance injected into the bronchial tree to show its outline. This is a simple procedure carried out under general anaesthesia and allows the accurate location of, for example, a lung ABSCESS, BRONCHIECTASIS, or a TUMOUR in the lung.

BRONCHOPHONY The resonance of the voice as heard by auscultation over the site of the large bronchial tubes, and, in diseased conditions, conveyed beyond these by cavities or solidification of parts of the lung.

BRONCHOPLEURAL FISTULA An abnormal communication between the tracheo-bronchial tree and the pleural cavity (see LUNGS). Most commonly occurring from breakdown of the bronchial stump following pneumonectomy, it may also be caused by trauma, neoplasia, or inflammation.

BRONCHO-PNEUMONIA (see PNEUMONIA).

BRONCHOSCOPE An instrument constructed on the principle of the telescope, which on introduction into the mouth is passed down through the larynx and TRACHEA and enables the observer to see the interior of the larger bronchial tubes. The bronchoscope has largely been superseded by fibreoptic bronchoscopy. (See ENDOSCOPE.)

BRONCHOSCOPY The use of a bronchoscope to visualize the interior of the bronchial tubes,

BRONCHUS, or bronchial tube, is the name applied to tubes into which the TRACHEA divides, one going to either lung. The name is also applied to the divisions of these tubes distributed throughout the lungs, the smallest being called bronchioles.

BRUCELLOSIS, also known as UNDULANT FEVER, MALTA FEVER, MEDITERRANEAN FEVER.

Causes In Malta and the Mediterranean littoral the causative organism is the *Brucella melitensis* which is conveyed in goat's milk. In Great Britain, the USA, and South Africa, the causative organism is the *Brucella abortus*, which is conveyed in cow's milk. This is the organism which is responsible for contagious abortion in cattle. In Great Britain brucellosis is largely an occupational disease and is now prescribed as an industrial disease (see OCCUPATIONAL DISEASES), and insured persons who contract the disease at work can claim industrial injuries benefit. The incidence of brucellosis in the UK has fallen from over 300 cases a year in 1970 to single figures in the 1990s.

Symptoms The characteristic features of the disease are undulating fever, drenching sweats, pains in the joints and back, and headache. There are, however, many atypical cases, and the diagnosis may be difficult. The liver and spleen may be enlarged. The diagnosis is confirmed by the finding of *Br. abortus*, or antibodies to it, in the blood. Recovery and convalescence tend to be slow.

Treatment Treatment is directed towards relieving the symptoms. The condition responds well to one of the tetracycline antibiotics, and also to gentamicin and co-trimoxazole, but relapse is all too common. In chronic cases a combination of streptomycin and one of the tetracyclines is often more effective.

Prevention It can be prevented by boiling or pasteurizing all milk used for human consumption. In Scandinavia, the Netherlands, Switzerland and Canada the disease has disappeared following its eradication in animals. Brucellosis has been eradicated from farm animals in the United Kingdom.

BRUISES, or CONTUSIONS, result from injuries to the deeper layers of the skin or underlying tissues, with variable bleeding, but without open wounds. Bruises range from a slight bluish discoloration, due to minimal trauma and haemorrhage, to a large black swelling in more severe cases. Diseases such as HAEMO-PHILIA and SCURVY, which reduce COAGULATION, should be suspected when extensive bruises are produced by minor injuries. Bruises change colour from blue-black to brown to yellow, gradually fading as the blood pigment is broken down and absorbed. Bruising in the abdomen or in the back in the area of the kidneys should prompt the examining doctor to assess whether there has been any damage to internal tissues or organs. Bruising in children, especially repeated bruising, may be caused by physical abuse. Adults, too, may be subjected to regular physical abuse.

BRUIT and **MURMUR** Abnormal sounds heard in connection with the heart, arteries, and veins on AUSCULTATION.

BRUXISM or TOOTH GRINDING Arrhythmic habit of grinding the teeth, usually while asleep and without being aware of it. The teeth may feel uncomfortable on wakening. It is common in children and is usually of no significance, although more severe forms, even during the waking period, may occur in the mentally handicapped. In adults it may be associated with stress or a malpositioned tooth or an overfilled tooth. The underlying cause should be treated but, if unsuccessful, a plastic splint can be fitted over the teeth.

BUBO A swelling of a lymphatic gland in the groin in venereal disease or in plague. (See PLAGUE.)

BUCCAL Relating to the mouth or inside of the cheek.

BUDGERIGAR-FANCIER'S LUNG is a form of extrinsic allergic alveolitis, resulting from sensitization to budgerigars, or parakeets as they are known in North America. Skin tests have revealed sensitization to the birds' droppings and/or serum. As it is estimated that budgerigars are kept in 5–6 million homes in

Britain, current figures suggest that anything up to 900 per 100,000 of the population are exposed to the risk of developing this condition. (See ALVEOLITIS.)

BUERGER'S DISEASE (see THROMBOANGIITIS OBLITERANS).

BULBAR PARALYSIS (see PARALYSIS; MOTOR NEURONE DISEASE).

BULIMIA means insatiable appetite of psychological origin. This eating disorder symptom may be of psychological origin or be the result of neurological disease, for example, a lesion of the HYPOTHALAMUS, Bulimia nervosa is linked to anorexia nervosa and is sometimes called the binge and purge syndrome. Bulimia nervosa is characterized by overpowering urges to eat large amounts of food followed by induced vomiting or abuse of laxatives to avoid any gain in weight. Most of the victims are prone to being overweight and all have a morbid fear of obesity. They indulge in bouts of gross overeating, or 'binge rounds' as they describe them, to 'fill the empty space inside'. By their bizarre behaviour, most of them manage to maintain a normal weight. It is most common in women in their 20s. The condition is accompanied by irregular menstruation, often amounting to amenorrhoea. Although there are many similarities to anorexia nervosa, it differs in that there is no attempt at deceit, and it is freely admitted that there is an eating disorder and there is distress about the symptoms it produces. In spite of this, the response to treatment, which is as in anorexia nervosa, is far from satisfactory. (See EATING DISORDERS.)

BULLA An air- or fluid-filled bubble occurring in the skin or lungs. The latter may be congenital or the result (in adults) of EMPHYSEMA. Skin bullae are really blisters.

BUMETANIDE is a strong loop diuretic which is active when taken by mouth. It acts quickly – within half-an-hour – and its action is over in a few hours. (See BENZOTHIADIAZINES, DIURETICS.)

BUNDLE BRANCH BLOCK An abnormality of the conduction of electrical impulses through the ventricles of the heart, resulting in delayed depolarization of the ventricular muscle. The electrocardiograph (see ELECTROCARDIOGRAM) shows characteristic widening of the QRS complexes. Abnormalities of the right and left bundle branches cause delayed contraction of the right and left ventricles respectively.

BUNDLE OF HIS, or atrioventricular bundle, is a bundle of special muscle fibres which pass from the atria to the ventricles of the heart and which form the pathway for the impulse which makes the ventricles contract, the impulse originating in the part of the atria known as the sinuatrial node.

BUNIONS (see CORNS AND BUNIONS).

BUPIVACAINE A local anaesthetic, about four times as potent as LIGNOCAINE. It has a slow onset of action (up to 30 minutes for full effect), but its effect lasts up to eight hours, making it particularly suitable for continuous epidural analgesia in LABOUR. It is commonly used for spinal anaesthesia, particularly lumbar epidural blockade (see ANAESTHESIA). It is contra-indicated in intravenous regional anaesthesia.

BURKITT'S LYMPHOMA Malignant LYMPHOMA in children previously infected with EPSTEIN BARR virus. It occurs mainly in the jaw and abdominal organs. It is common in parts of Africa where malaria is endemic.

BURNING FEET A SYNDROME characterized by a burning sensation in the soles of the feet. It is rare in temperate climes but widespread in India and the Far East. The precise cause is not known, but it is associated with malnutrition, and lack of one or more components of the vitamin B complex is the likeliest cause.

BURNS AND SCALDS Burns are injuries caused by dry heat, scalds by moist heat, but the two are similar in symptoms and treatment. Severe burns are also caused by contact with electric wires, and by the action of acids and other chemicals. The burn caused by chemicals differs from a burn by fire only in the fact that the outcome is more favourable, because the chemical destroys the bacteria on the part, so that less suppuration follows.

Severe and extensive burns are most frequently produced by the clothes, for example, of a child, catching fire. This applies especially to cotton garments, which blaze up quickly. It should be remembered that such a flame can immediately be extinguished by making the individual lie on the floor so that the flames are uppermost, and wrapping him in a rug, mat, or blanket. As prevention is always better than cure, particular care should always be exercised with electric fires and kettles or pots of boiling water in houses where there are young children or old people. Equally important is it that children's night-clothes and frocks be made of non-inflammable material. Pyjamas are also much safer than nightdresses. Severe scalds are usually produced by escape of steam in boiler explosions. Cigarettes are a common cause of fires and therefore of burns. People who have fallen asleep in bed or in a chair while smoking may set fire to the bed or chair. Discarded, unextinguished cigarettes are another cause.

Degrees of burns The French surgeon Dupuytren divided burns into six degrees, according to their depth. In practice, however, today burns are referred to as either superficial (or partial thickness) burns when there is sufficient skin tissue left to ensure regrowth of skin over the burned site; and deep (or full thickness) when the skin is totally destroyed and grafting will be necessary.

Symptoms Whilst many domestic burns are minor and insignificant, more severe burns and scalds can prove to be very dangerous to life. The main danger is due to SHOCK. This arises as a result of loss of fluid from the circulating blood at the site of the burn. This loss of fluid leads to a fall in the volume of the circulating blood. As the maintenance of an adequate blood volume is essential to life, the body attempts to compensate for this loss by withdrawing fluid from the uninjured areas of the body into the circulation. This, however, in turn, if carried too far begins to affect the viability of the body cells. As a sequel, essential body cells, such as those of the liver and kidneys, begin to suffer, and the liver and kidneys cease to function properly. This will show itself by the development of JAUNDICE and the appearance of albumin in the urine. (See PROTEINURIA.) In addition, the circulation begins to fail with a resultant lack of oxygen (see ANOXIA) in the tissues, and the victim becomes cyanosed (see CYANOSIS), restless and collapsed and, in some cases, death ensues. In addition, there is a strong risk of infection occurring. Particularly is this the case with severe burns which leave a large raw surface exposed and very vulnerable to any micro-organisms. The combination of shock and infection can all too often be life-threatening unless expert treatment is immediately available.

The immediate outcome of a burn is largely determined by its extent. This is of more significance than the depth of the burn. To assess the extent of a burn in relation to the surface of the body, what is known as the Rule of Nine has been evolved. The head and each arm cover 9 per cent of the body surface, whilst the front of the body, the back of the body, and each leg each cover 18 per cent, with the perineum (or crutch) accounting for the remaining 1 per cent. The greater the extent of the burn, the more seriously ill will the victim become from loss of fluid from his circulation, and therefore the more prompt should be his removal to hospital for expert treatment. The depth of the burn, unless this is very great, is mainly of import when the question arises as to how much surgical treatment, including skin grafting, will be required.

Treatment This depends upon the severity of the burn. In the case of quite minor burns or scalds, all that may be necessary if they are seen immediately is to hold the part under cold running water until the pain is relieved. Cooling is one of the most effective ways of relieving the pain of a burn. If the burn involves the distal part of a limb, e.g. the hand and forearm, one of the most effective ways of relieving pain is to immerse the burned part in lukewarm water and add cold water until the pain disappears. As the water warms and pain returns more cold water is added. After some three to four hours, pain will not reappear on warming, and the burn may be dressed in the usual way. Thereafter a simple dressing – e.g. a piece of sterile gauze covered by cotton-wool, and on top of this a bandage or adhesive dressing – should be applied. The part should be kept at rest and the dressing kept quite dry until healing takes place. Blisters should be pierced with a sterile needle, but the skin should not be cut away. No ointment or oil should be applied, and an antiseptic is not usually necessary.

In slightly more severe burns or scalds, it is probably more advisable to use some antiseptic dressing. These are the cases which should be taken to a doctor – whether a general practitioner, a factory doctor, or a casualty officer in hospital. There is still no general consensus of expert opinion as to the best 'antiseptic' to use. Among those recommended are CHLORHEXIDINE, and antibiotics such as BACITRACIN, NEOMYCIN and polymixin. An alternative is to use a Tulle Gras dressing which has been impregnated with a suitable antibiotic.

In the case of severe burns and scalds, the only sound rule is immediate removal to hospital. Unless there is any need for immediate resuscitation, such as artificial respiration, or attention to other injuries there may be, such as fractures or haemorrhage, nothing should be done on the spot to the patient except to make sure that he is as comfortable as possible and to keep him warm, and to cover the burn with a sterile (or clean) cloth such as a sheet, pillowcases, or towels wrung out in cold water. If pain is severe, morphine should be given – usually intravenously. Once the victim is in hospital, the primary decision is as to the extent of the burn, and whether or not a transfusion is necessary. If the burn is more than 9 per cent of the body surface in extent, a transfusion is called for. The precise treatment of the burn varies, but the essential is to prevent infection if this has not already occurred, or, if it has, to bring it under control as quickly as possible. The treatment of severe burns has made great advances, with quick transport to specialized burns units, modern resuscitative measures, the use of skin grafting and other artificial covering techniques and active rehabilitation programmes, offering victims a good chance of returing to normal life.

Chemical Burns   Phenol or lysol can be washed off promptly before they do much damage. Acid or alkali burns should be neutralized by washing them repeatedly with sodium bicarbonate or 1 per cent acetic acid, respectively. Alternatively, the following buffer solution may be used for either acid or alkali burns: monobasic potassium phosphate (70 grams), dibasic sodium phosphate (70 grams) in 850 millilitres of water. (See also PHOSPHORUS BURNS.)

BURSAE   Natural hollows in the fibrous tissues, lined by smooth cells and containing a little fluid. They are situated at points where there is much pressure or friction, and their purpose is to allow free movement without stretching or straining the tissues: for example, on the knee-cap or the point of the elbow, and, generally speaking, where one muscle rubs against another or against a bone. They develop also beneath corns and bunions, or where a bone comes to press in an unwonted manner on the skin.

BURSITIS   Inflammation within a bursa. Acute bursitis is usually the result of injury, injury especially on the knee or elbow, when the prominent part of the joint becomes swollen, hot, painful, and red.

Chronic bursitis is due to too much movement of, or pressure on, a bursa, with fluid building up in the bursa. Fluid may need to be drained and the affected area rested. Excision of a chronically inflamed bursa is sometimes necessary. For example, the condition of housemaid's knee is a chronic inflammation of the patellar bursa in front of the knee, due to too much kneeling.

Chronic bursitis about the sinews round the wrist and ankle is generally called a ganglion. (See GANGLION.)

BUTYROPHENONES are a group of drugs, including haloperidol used to treat psychotic illness (see MENTAL ILLNESS).

BYPASS OPERATION   A technique by which narrowing or blockage of an ARTERY, VEIN or a section of the GASTROINTESTINAL tract is bypassed using surgery. Arterial blockages usually caused by ATHEROSCLEROSIS, in the carotid, coronary or iliofemoral arteries, are bypassed utilizing sections of artery or vein taken from elsewhere in the patient. Tumour growths in the intestines are sometimes too large to remove and can be bypassed by linking up those parts of the intestines on each side of the growth.

BYSSINOSIS   Chronic inflammatory thickening of the lung tissue, due to the inhalation of dust in textile factories. It is found chiefly among cotton and flax workers and, to a lesser extent, among workers in soft hemp. It is rare or absent in workers in jute and the hard fibres of hemp and sisal. With much improved working conditions in the UK where byssinosis is a PRESCRIBED DISEASE, the disease is rare, but it is still common in some Asian countries where textiles are manufactured.

C

CACHET means an oval capsule, generally made of rice paper, for enclosing a dose of unpleasant medicine. Cachets are softened by moistening with water prior to swallowing.

CACHEXIA Severe weight loss and listlessness produced by serious disease such as cancer or tuberculosis or by prolonged starvation.

CADAVER A dead body.

CADMIUM POISONING is a recognized hazard in certain industrial processes, such as the manufacture of alloys, cadmium plating and glass blowing. Sewage sludge, which is used as fertilizer, may be contaminated by cadmium from industrial sources. Such cadmium could be taken up into vegetable crops and cadmium levels in sewage are carefully monitored. Cadmium, a tinlike metal, accumulates in the body. Long-term exposure can lead to EMPHYSEMA, RENAL failure and URINARY-TRACT CALCULI. Acute exposure causes GASTROENTERITIS and PNEUMONITIS. Cadmium contamination of food is the most likely source of poisoning. The EEC Directive on the Quality of Water for Human Consumption lays down 5 milligrams per litre as the upper safe level.

CAECUM The dilated commencement of the large intestine lying in the right lower corner of the abdomen. Into it the small intestine and the appendix vermiformis open, and it is continued upwards through the right flank as the ascending colon.

CAESAREAN SECTION The operation used to deliver a baby through its mother's abdominal wall. It is performed when the risks to mother or child of vaginal delivery are thought to outweigh the problems associated with operative delivery. One of the commonest reasons for Caesarean section is 'disproportion' between the size of the fetal head and the maternal pelvis. The need for a Caesarean should be assessed anew in each pregnancy. It is no longer true that a woman who has had a Caesarean section in the past will automatically have one for subsequent deliveries. Caesarean section rates vary dramatically from hospital to hospital, and especially between countries, emphasizing that the criteria for operative delivery are not universally agreed. Nearly 16 per cent of the 608,000 or so deliveries in England in 1995 were by Caesarean section compared with 10.4 per cent of 616,000 deliveries in 1985. In the USA the latest figure is about 25 per cent.

The operation is usually performed through a low, horizontal 'bikini line' incision. A general anaesthetic in a heavily pregnant woman carries increased risks, and nowadays the operation is often performed under regional – epidural or spinal – anaesthesia. This also allows the mother to see her baby as soon as it is born, and the baby is not exposed to agents used for general anaesthesia. If a general anaesthetic is needed (usually in an emergency), exposure to these agents may make the baby drowsy for some time afterwards.

Another problem with delivery by Caesarean section is, of course, that the mother must recover from the operation whilst coping with the demands of a small baby. (See LABOUR.)

CAESIUM-137 An artificially produced radioactive element that is used in RADIOTHERAPY TREATMENT.

CAFFEINE A white crystalline substance obtained from coffee, of which it is the active principle. Its main actions are as a cerebral stimulant, a cardiac stimulant, and as a diuretic. It is also of value in some cases of asthma. It is a constituent of many tablets for the relief of headache, usually combined with aspirin and paracetamol.

CAISSON DISEASE (see COMPRESSED AIR ILLNESS).

CALAMINE, or CARBONATE OF ZINC, is a mild astringent used, as calamine lotion, to soothe and protect the skin in many conditions such as eczema and urticaria.

CALCANEUS The heelbone or os calcis and the largest bone in the FOOT.

CALCICOSIS is the term applied to disease of the lung caused by the inhalation of marble dust by marble-cutters.

CALCIFEROL This is an outdated term for ergocaliciferol or vitamin D_2 (see Vitamin D in APPENDIX 5: VITAMINS).

CALCIFICATION The deposition of calcium salts in body tissues, normally BONES and TEETH, though abnormal deposits can occur in damaged muscles or the walls of arteries.

CALCITONIN A hormone, produced by the THYROID GLAND which is involved in the metabolism of bone. Acting to lower the CALCIUM and PHOSPHATE concentrations in the blood, calcitonin is given by injection in the treatment of some patients with HYPERCALCAEMIA (especially when associated with malignant disease). In severe cases of PAGET'S DISEASE it is used mainly for pain relief, but also relieves some of the neurological complications such as deafness. Long-term therapy with porcine calcitonin (obtained from pigs) may lead to the production of neutralizing antibodies and should therefore be replaced by synthetic salmon calcitonin which is less IMMUNOGENIC.

CALCIUM The metallic element present in chalk and other forms of lime. The chief preparations used in medicine are calcium carbonate (chalk), calcium chloride, calcium gluconate, calcium hydroxide (slaked lime), liquor of calcium hydroxide (lime-water), calcium lactate, and calcium phosphate (see LIME). Calcium gluconate is freely soluble in water and is used in conditions in which calcium should be given by injection. Calcium chloride is sometimes used in the resuscitation of patients with cardiopulmonary collapse.

Calcium is a most important element in diet; the chief sources of it are milk and cheese. Calcium is especially needed by the growing child and the pregnant and nursing mother. The uptake of calcium by the baby is helped by vitamin D (see APPENDIX 5: VITAMINS). A deficiency of calcium may cause TETANY and an excess result in the development of CALCULI (stones) in the KIDNEYS or GALL-BLADDER.

The recommended daily intakes of calcium are: 500 mg for children, 700 mg for adolescents, 500–900 mg for adults and 1200 mg for pregnant or nursing mothers.

CALCIUM-CHANNEL BLOCKERS, OR CALCIUM ANTAGONISTS, inhibit the inward flow of calcium through the specialized slow channels of cardiac and arterial smooth-muscle cells. By thus relaxing the smooth muscle, they have important applications in the treatment of HYPERTENSION and ANGINA. They should generally be avoided in heart failure, however, as further cardiac depression may cause clinical deterioration. Sudden withdrawal may exacerbate angina. Various types of calcium-channel blockers are available in the United Kingdom. These differ in their sites of action, leading to notable differences in their therapeutic effects. All the drugs are rapidly and completely absorbed, but extensive first-pass metabolism in the liver reduces bio-availability to around one fifth. Their hypotensive effect is additive with that of BETA-BLOCKERS; they should, therefore, be used with great caution, if at all, together. They are particularly useful when beta-blockers are contraindicated, for example, in asthmatics. However, calcium-channel blockers should be prescribed for hypertension only when THIAZIDES and beta blockers have failed, are contraindicated or not tolerated.

Verapamil, the longest available, is used to treat angina and hypertension. It is the only calcium-channel blocker effective against cardiac arrhythmias and it is the drug of choice in terminating supraventricular tachycardia. It may precipitate heart failure, and cause HYPOTENSION at high doses; it should never be used with beta-blockers. Nifedipine and diltiazem act more on the vessels and less on the myocardium than verapamil; they have no anti-arrhythmic activity. They are used in the prophylaxis and treatment of angina, and in hypertension. Nicardipine and similar drugs act mainly on the vessels, but are valuable in the treatment of hypertension and angina. Important differences exist between different calcium-channel blockers so their use must be carefully assessed.

CALCULI The general name given to concretions in, for example, the BLADDER, KIDNEYS, GALL-BLADDER.

CALIBRE A talking book service which is available to all blind and handicapped people who can supply a doctor's certificate certifying that they are unable to read printed books in the normal way. Its catalogue contains over 370 books for adults and over 250 for children, and additions are being made at the rate of around three a week. Full details can be obtained from Calibre (see APPENDIX 2: ADDRESSES).

CALLIPER A two-pronged instrument with pointed ends, for the measurement of diameters, such as that of the pelvis in obstetrics.

CALLIPER SPLINT This is applied to the broken leg in such a way that in walking the weight of the body is taken by the hip bone and not by the foot.

CALLOSITIES Areas of gross thickening of the epidermis in response to trauma. They usually occur on a foot due to bony deformity or ill-fitting footwear. (See CORNS AND BUNIONS.)

CALLUS The new tissue formed round the ends of a broken bone. (See FRACTURES.)

CALORIC TEST A test for vestibular function (see EAR). It is performed by irrigating the external auditory meatus of the ear with either cold or hot water. This usually stimulates the vestibular apparatus, causing NYSTAGMUS. If the vestibular apparatus is affected by disease, the response may be absent or reduced.

CALORIE A unit of energy. Two units are called by this name. The small calorie, or gram calorie, is the amount of heat required to raise one gram of water one degree centigrade in temperature. The large Calorie or kilocalorie, which is used in the study of dietetics and physiological processes, is the amount of heat required to raise one kilogram of water one degree centigrade in temperature. The number of Calories required to carry on the processes necessary for life and body warmth, such as the beating of the heart, the movements of the chest in breathing, and the chemical activities of the secreting glands, is, for an adult person of ordinary weight, somewhere in the neighbourhood of 1600 Calories. For ordinary sedentary occupations an individual requires about 2500 Calories, for light muscular work slightly over 3000 Calories, and for hard continuous labour about 4000 Calories daily.

Under the International System of Units (SI)

(see APPENDIX 6: MEASUREMENTS IN MEDICINE) the kilocalorie has been replaced by the joule, the abbreviation for which is J (1 kilocalorie=4186·8 J). As the term calorie, however, is so well established in medical writing, it has been retained in this edition. Conversion from Calories (or kilocalories) is made by multiplying by 4·186, but a factor of 4·2 is simpler and accurate enough for all practical purposes.

CALYX means a cup-shaped cavity, the term being especially applied to the recesses of the pelvis of the kidney.

CAMPYLOBACTER A species of microorganism found in farm and pet animals, and there is increasing evidence of its transmission from such sources to man. Outbreaks of infection with it have occurred following the drinking of unpasteurized milk from infected cows and eating undercooked meat and poultry. It causes diarrhoea, and remains the most commonly isolated bacterium associated with acute gastroenteritis. In 1995 almost 44,000 cases were identified in England and in 1996 this had fallen to a little over 43,300.

CANALICULUS means a small channel, and is applied to (*a*) the minute passage leading from the lacrimal pore on each eyelid to the lacrimal sac on the side of the nose; (*b*) any one of the minute canals in bone.

CANCELLOUS A term applied to loose bony tissues as found in the ends of the long bones.

CANCER The general term used to refer to a malignant tumour, irrespective of the tissue of origin. 'Malignancy' indicates that (i) the tumour is capable of progressive growth, unrestrained by the capsule of the parent organ and/or (ii) capable of distant spread via lymphatics or the blood stream resulting in development of secondary deposits of tumour known as 'metastases'. Microscopically, cancer cells appear different from the equivalent normal cells in the affected tissue. In particular they may show a lesser degree of differentiation (i.e. they are more 'primitive'), features indicative of a faster proliferative rate and disorganized alignment in relationship to other cells or blood vessels. The diagnosis of cancer usually depends upon the observation of these microscopic features in biopsies, i.e. tissue removed surgically for such examination.

Cancers are classified according to the type of cell from which they are derived as well as the organ of origin. Hence cancers arising within the bronchi, often collectively referred to as 'lung cancer', include both ADENOCARCINOMAS (derived from glandular EPITHELIUM) and squamous CARCINOMAS (derived from squamous epithelium). Sarcomas are cancers of connective tissue, including bone and cartilage. The behaviour of cancers and their response to therapy vary widely depending on this classification as well as on numerous other factors such as growth rate, differentiation in cell and characteristics and size at the time of presentation. It is entirely wrong to see cancer as a single disease entity with a universally poor prognosis.

Incidence In most western countries cancer is the second most important cause of death after heart disease and accounts for 20–25 per cent of all deaths. In the United Kingdom in 1995 nearly 157,000 people died of malignant disease. There is wide international variation in the most frequently encountered types of cancer, reflecting the importance of environmental factors in the development of cancer. In the UK as well as the USA, carcinoma of the BRONCHUS is the most common. Since it is usually inoperable at the time of diagnosis, it is even more strikingly the leading cause of cancer deaths. In women, breast cancer is most common, accounting for a quarter of all cancers; nevertheless, fewer than a half of women in whom breast cancer is discovered will die from the disease. Other common sites are as follows: males – colon and rectum, prostate and bladder; females – colon and rectum, uterus, ovary and pancreas.

In England and Wales in 1991 (the last year for which official figures are available) 212,000 people were registered as suffering from cancers of all types. Over 36,500 of them had lung cancer, over 27,700 had large bowel cancer, nearly 30,000 breast cancer and more than 8,000 uterine cancer. The incidence of cancer varies with age, the older a person is the more likely is he or she to develop the disease: the over 85s have an incidence about nine times greater than those in the 25–44 age group. There are also differences in incidence between sexes, for example, more men than women develop lung cancer, though the incidence in women is rising as the effects of smoking work through.

Causes of cancer In most cases the causes of cancer remain unknown. Rapid advances have, however, been made in the past two decades in understanding the differences between cancer cells and normal cells at the genetic level. It is now widely accepted that cancer results from acquired changes in the genetic make-up of a particular cell or group of cells which ultimately lead to a failure of the normal mechanisms regulating their growth. It appears that in most cases a cascade of changes is required for cells to behave in a truly malignant fashion; the critical changes affect specific key GENES, known as oncogenes, which are involved in growth regulation.

Since small genetic errors occur within cells at all times, most but not all of which are repaired, it follows that some cancers may develop as a result of an accumulation of random changes which cannot be attributed to environmental or other causes. The environmental factors known to cause cancer such as radiation and chemicals (including tar from tobacco, asbestos, etc.) do so by increasing the overall rate of acquired genetic damage.

Certain viral infections can induce specific cancers (e.g. HEPATITIS B virus and HEPATOMA, EPSTEIN BARR virus and LYMPHOMA) probably by inducing alterations in specific genes. HORMONES may also be a factor in the development of certain cancers such as those of the prostate and breast. Where there is a particular family tendency to certain types of cancer, it now appears that one or more of the critical genetic abnormalities required for development of that cancer may have been inherited. Where environmental factors such as tobacco smoking or asbestos are known to cause cancer, then health education and preventive measures can reduce the incidence of the relevant cancer. Cancer can also affect the white cells in the blood and is called LEUKEMIA.

Treatment Many cancers can be cured by surgical removal if they are detected early, before there has been spread of significant numbers of tumour cells to distant sites. Important within this group are breast, colon and skin cancer (melanoma). The probability of early detection of certain cancers can be increased by SCREENING PROGRAMMES in which (ideally) all people at particular risk of development of such cancers are examined at regular intervals. Routine screening for CERVICAL CANCER and BREAST CANCER is currently practised in the UK.

If complete surgical removal of the tumour is not possible because of its location or because spread from the primary site has occurred, an operation may nevertheless be helpful to relieve symptoms (e.g. pain) and to reduce the bulk of the tumour remaining to be dealt with by alternative means such as RADIOTHERAPY or CHEMOTHERAPY. In some cases radiotherapy is preferable to surgery and may be curative, for example, in the management of tumours of the larynx or of the uterine cervix. Certain tumours are highly sensitive to chemotherapy and may be cured by the use of chemotherapeutic drugs alone. These include testicular tumours, LEUKAEMIAS, LYMPHOMAS and a variety of tumours occurring in childhood. These tend to be rapidly growing tumours composed of primitive cells which are much more vulnerable to the toxic effects of the chemotherapeutic agents than the normal cells within the body.

Unfortunately neither radiotherapy nor currently available chemotherapy provides a curative option for the majority of common cancers if surgical excision is not feasible. New effective treatments in these conditions are urgently needed. Nevertheless the rapidly increasing knowledge of cancer biology will almost certainly lead to novel therapeutic approaches – including probably genetic techniques utilizing the recent discoveries of oncogenes (genes that can cause cancer) – at least by the early twenty-first century. Where cure is not possible, there often remains much that can be done for the cancer-sufferer in terms of control of unpleasant symptoms such as pain. Many of the most important recent advances in cancer care relate to such 'palliative' treatment, and include the establishment in the UK of palliative care hospices.

Families and patients can obtain valuable help and advice from Marie Curie Cancer Care, Cancer Relief Macmillan Fund, or the British Association of Cancer United Patients (see APPENDIX 2: ADDRESSES).

CANCRUM ORIS, also called WATER CANKER or NOMA, is a gangrenous ulcer about the mouth which affects weakly children, especially after some severe disease, such as measles. It is due to the growth of bacteria in the tissues.

CANDIDA Candidosis (moniliasis) is an oportunistic infection with the yeast, *Candida albicans*. It is encouraged by pregnancy, diabetes mellitus, prolonged wide-spectrum ANTIBIOTIC or CORTICOSTEROID therapy, and is also seen in debilitated infants, the elderly and immunocompromised patients, e.g. those with HIV or AIDS. It may cause white patches in the mouth or vulvovaginal area (THRUSH) and a red vesicular and scaly rash in the finger clefts, submammary folds or anogenital folds. Fingernail fold infection causes chronic PARONYCHIA with secondary nail DYSTROPHY and may complicate RAYNAUD'S phenomenon. CLOTRIMAZOLE and similar 'azoles' as creams, oral gels or vaginal pessaries are rapidly effective but severe systemic infections require oral itraconazole or even intravenous AMPHOTERICIN B.

CANINE TEETH, or EYE-TEETH (see TEETH).

CANKER The name applied to small ulcers which form about the mouth and lips as the result of some local irritation, e.g. a jagged tooth, or in dyspepsia or general poor health. (See MOUTH, DISEASES OF.)

CANNABIS Psychoactive substances obtained from *Cannabis sativa* or Indian Hemp, they are the oldest euphoriants. Also called marijuana, these substances do not usually result in physical dependence but abuse leads to passivity, apathy and inertia. Acute adverse effects include transient panic reactions and toxic psychoses. The panic reactions are characterized by anxiety, helplessness and loss of control and may be accompanied by florid paranoid thoughts and hallucinations. The toxic psychoses are characterized by the sudden onset of confusion and visual hallucinations. Even at lower doses cannabis products can precipitate functional psychoses in vulnerable individuals. The acute physical manifestations of short-term cannabis abuse are conjunctival suffusion and tachycardia.

The chopped leaves are usually smoked as a reefer or joint. They can, however, be eaten in food or taken as tea. The active ingredient is tetrahydrocannibol. There is much public debate in Western countries over the social use of cannabis. It is illegal to possess or supply the substance in the United Kingdom but cannabis is quite widely used. Cannabis is classified as a Schedule 1 drug under the Misuse of Drugs Act

1971 and is not used medicinally – despite some claims that it is helpful in ameliorating painful symptoms in certain serious chronic diseases such as multiple sclerosis. However, the British Medical Association has recently called on the government to amend the legislation to allow cannabinoids to be prescribed for a range of medical conditions, urging that controlled clinical trials be set up.

CANNULA A tube for insertion into the body, designed to fit tightly round a trocar, a sharp pointed instrument which is withdrawn from the cannula after insertion, so that fluid may run out through the latter.

CANTHARIDIN The active principle of cantharides or Spanish fly, a powder made of the body and wings of a dried beetle, *Cantharis vesicatoria*, which inhabits Spain, Italy, Sicily and Southern Russia.

Action It is an irritant, first, to the part with which it is brought in contact, and, secondly, to the genital and urinary organs by which it is discharged from the body.

Uses Cantharidin is a dangerous substance and was formerly used in veterinary practices for blistering.

CANTHUS The name applied to the angle at either end of the aperture between the eyelids.

CAPILLARIES The minute vessels which join the ends of the arteries to the commencement of the veins. Their walls consist of a single layer of fine, flat transparent cells, bound together at the edges, and the vessels form a meshwork all through the tissues of the body, bathing the latter in blood with only the thin capillary wall interposed, through which gases and fluids readily pass. These vessels are less than 0·025 mm in width. (See CIRCULATION OF THE BLOOD.)

CAPSULE A term used in several senses in medicine. The term is applied to a soluble case, usually of gelatine, for enclosing small doses of unpleasant medicine.

Enteric-coated capsules, which have been largely superseded by enteric-coated tablets, are capsules treated in such a manner that the ingredients do not come in contact with the acid stomach contents but are only released when the capsule disintegrates in the alkaline contents of the intestine.

The term is also applied to the fibrous or membranous envelope of various organs, as of the spleen, liver or kidney. It is also applied to the ligamentous bag surrounding various joints and attached by its edge to the bones on either side.

CAPTOPRIL An ACE-inhibitor drug introduced for the treatment of patients with severe HYPERTENSION. It acts by lowering the concentration in the blood of angiotensin II which is one of the factors responsible for high blood-pressure. (See ANGIOTENSIN; RENIN.)

CAPUT MEDUSAE is the term describing the abnormally dilated veins that form round the umbilicus in cirrhosis of the liver.

CAPUT SUCCEDANEUM The temporary swelling which is sometimes found on the head of the new-born infant. It is due to oedema in and around the scalp, caused by pressure on the head as the child is born. It is of no significance and quickly disappears spontaneously.

CARBACHOL A drug which stimulates the parasympathetic nervous system for example, for relieving GLAUCOMA and retention of urine due to ATONY.

CARBAMAZEPINE A drug used to treat TRIGEMINAL NEURALGIA and certain cases of epilepsy.

CARBARYL An insecticide effective against head-louse and pubic-louse infestations (see INSECTS IN RELATION TO DISEASE). Some louse resistance has emerged. As a result of this, and fears of possible carcinogenicity, it is now little used.

CARBENOXOLONE A derivative of glycyrrhizinic acid, the active principle of liquorice, which is sometimes used to treat ulceration of the oesophagus, stomach and duodenum, but its side-effects necessitate careful monitoring.

CARBIMAZOLE One of the most widely used drugs in the treatment of HYPERTHYROIDISM. It acts by interferring with the synthesis of THYROID hormone in the thyroid gland.

CARBOHYDRATE The term applied to an organic substance in which the hydrogen and oxygen are usually in the proportion to form water. Carbohydrates are all, chemically considered, derivatives of simple forms of sugar and are classified as monosaccharides (e.g. glucose), disaccharides (e.g. cane sugar), polysaccharides (e.g. starch). Many of the cheaper and most important foods are included in this group, which comprises sugars, starches, celluloses and gums. When one of these foods is digested, it is converted into a simple kind of sugar and absorbed in this form. Excess carbohydrates, not immediately needed by the body, are stored as glycogen in the liver and muscles. DIABETES MELLITUS, the most marked feature consists of an inability on the part of the tissues to assimilate and utilize the carbohydrate material. Each gram of carbohydrate is capable of furnishing slightly over 4 Calories of energy. (See DIET.)

CARBOLIC ACID, or PHENOL, was the precursor of all ANTISEPTICS. It paralyses and then destroys most forms of life, particularly organisms such as bacteria. It has been superseded by less penetrative and harmful antiseptics, though it is still used in calamine lotion for its anaesthetic effect.

CARBON DIOXIDE, or CARBONIC ACID, is formed by the body during metabolism and is exhaled by the lungs (see AIR, VENTILATION). Seen in sparkling waters and wines, it is also used in baths as a stimulant to the skin. Combined with oxygen in cylinders, it is used to control breathing in anaesthesia and in the treatment of victims of carbon monoxide poisoning.

CARBON MONOXIDE (CO) This is a colourless, odourless tasteless, non-irritating gas formed on incomplete combustion of organic fuels. Exposure to CO is frequently due to defective gas, oil or solid-fuel heating appliances. CO is a component of car exhaust fumes and deliberate exposure to these is a common method of suicide. Victims of fires often suffer from CO poisoning. It used to be a major component of coal gas but, since the introduction of natural gas as a fuel source in the UK, successful suicide by inhalation of gas from unlit household sources has fallen. CO combines reversibly with oxygen-carrying sites of HAEMOGLOBIN (Hb) molecules with an affinity 200 to 300 times greater than oxygen itself. The carboxyhaemoglobin (COHb) formed becomes unavailable for oxygen transportation. In addition the partial saturation of the Hb molecule results in tighter oxygen binding, impairing delivery to the tissues. CO also binds to MY-OGLOBIN and respiratory cytochrome ENZYMES. Exposure to CO at levels of 500 parts per million (ppm) would be expected to cause mild symptoms only and exposure to levels of 4,000 ppm would be rapidly fatal.

Clinical effects of acute exposure resemble those of atmospheric HYPOXIA. Tissues and organs with high oxygen consumption are affected to a great extent. Common effects include headaches, weakness, fatigue, flushing, nausea, vomiting, irritability, dizziness, drowsiness, disorientation, incoordination, visual disturbances, TACHYCARDIA and HYPERVENTILATION. In severe cases drowsiness may progress rapidly to COMA. There may also be metabolic ACIDOSIS, HYPOKALAEMIA, CONVULSIONS, HYPOTENSION, RESPIRATORY DEPRESSION, ECG changes and cardiovascular collapse. Cerebral OEDEMA is common and will lead to severe brain damage and focal neurological signs. Significant abnormalities on physical examination include impaired short-term memory, abnormal Rhomberg's test (standing unsupported with eyes closed) and unsteadiness of gait including heel–toe walking. Any one of these signs would classify the episode as severe. Victims' skin may be coloured pink, though this is very rarely seen even in severe incidents. The venous blood may look

'arterial'. Patients recovering from acute CO poisoning may suffer neurological sequelae including TREMORS, personality changes, memory impairment, visual loss, inability to concentrate and PARKINSONISM. Chronic low-level exposures may result in nausea, fatigue, headache, confusion, VOMITING, DIARRHOEA, abdominal pain and general malaise. They are often misdiagnosed as influenza or food poisoning.

First-aid treatment is to remove the victim from source of exposure, ensure an effective airway and give 100-per-cent oxygen by tight-fitting mask. In hospital, management is largely suppportive, with oxygen administration. A blood sample for COHb level determination should be taken as soon as practicable and, if possible, before oxygen is given. Ideally, oxygen therapy should continue until the COHb level falls below 5 per cent. Patients with any history of unconsciousness, a COHb level greater than 20 per cent on arrival, any neurological signs, any cardiac arrhythmias or anyone who is pregnant should be referred to a HYPERBARIC oxygen chamber for continued care where possible. Hyperbaric oxygen therapy shortens the half-life of COHb, increases PLASMA OXYGEN TRANSPORT and reverses the clinical effects resulting from acute exposures. Carbon monoxide is also an environmental poison and a component of cigarette smoke. Normal body COHb levels due to ENDOGENOUS CO production are 0.4 to 0.7 per cent. Non-smokers in urban areas may have level of 1–2 per cent as a result of environmental exposure. Smokers may have a COHb level of 5 to 6 per cent.

CARBOXYHAEMOGLOBINAEMIA The term applied to the state of the blood in carbon monoxide poisoning, in which this gas combines with the haemoglobin, displacing oxygen from it. (See CARBON MONOXIDE.)

CARBUNCLE (see BOIL).

CARCINOGENESIS is the means or method whereby the changes responsible for the induction of CANCER are brought about.

CARCINOGENS Agents, such as certain chemicals, asbestos fibres, high-powered radiation and tobacco smoke that have the property of causing cancer.

CARCINOMA A type of CANCER developing from cells found in the surface layer of an organ in the body.

CARCINOMATOSIS The spread of cancer cells from their original site of growth to other tissues in the body. Such a spread of cancer, which takes place mainly via blood and lymph vessels, is usually fatal. CHEMOTHERAPY and RADIOTHERAPY may, however, check the spread or sometimes destroy the cancerous growth.

CARDIA is a term applied to the upper opening of the stomach which lies immediately behind the heart.

CARDIAC ARREST occurs when the pumping action of the heart stops. This may be because the heart stops beating (see ASYSTOLE) or because the heart muscle starts contracting too fast to pump effectively (ventricular systole, the period when the heart contracts). Coronary thrombosis is the most frequent cause of arrest. Irreversible brain damage and death result without prompt treatment. Heart massage, defibrillation and artificial respiration, are customary treatment. Other causes of cardiac arrest are respiratory arrest, anaphylactic shock, and electrocution. Up to one third of patients treated in hospital whose heart rhythm is restored recover to an extent that enables them to return home. (See APPENDIX 1: BASIC FIRST AID: cardiac/respiratory arrest.)

CARDIAC CATHETERIZATION A diagnostic procedure in which a tube is inserted into a blood vessel under local anaesthetic and threaded through to the chambers of the heart to monitor blood flow, blood pressure, blood chemistry, and the output of the heart, and to take a sample of heart tissue. The technique is used to diagnose congenital heart disease and coronary artery disease. Another application is in the diagnosis and treatment of valvular disease in the heart. Catheterization should be reserved for life-threatening disorders as the procedure carries some risk.

CARDIAC CYCLE The various sequential movements of the heart that comprise the rhythmic relaxation and expansion of the heart muscles as first the atria contract and force the blood into the ventricles (diastole) which then contract (systole) to pump the blood round the body. (See ELECTROCARDIOGRAM.)

CARDIAC DISEASE (see HEART DISEASES).

CARDIAC GLYCOSIDES Drugs whose main actions are to increase the force of MYOCARDIAL contraction and reduce the conductivity of the NERVE fibres in the atrioventricular node of the HEART. They are useful in treating supraventricular tachycardias (rapid heart rhythm) and some forms of heart failure. Glycosides are a traditional group of cardiac drugs, originally derived from the leaves of foxglove plants and used as digitalis. The active principle has long been synthesized and used as DIGOXIN and DIGITOXIN.

CARDIAC MASSAGE is the procedure used to restart the action of the heart if it is suddenly arrested. For long the only recognized method of doing this was by opening the chest wall and massaging the heart directly by hand. This is perfectly feasible if the heart stops beating during an operation. Elsewhere, however, it is seldom a practicable proposition.

In many cases the arrested heart can be made to start beating again by rhythmic compression of the chest wall. This is done by placing the patient on a hard surface – a table or the floor

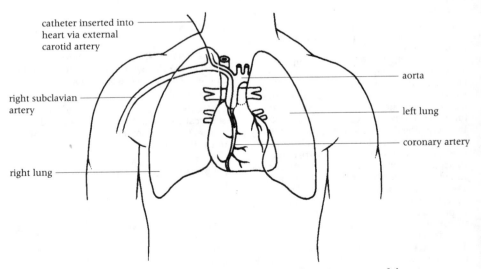

catheter inserted into heart via external carotid artery

right subclavian artery

right lung

aorta

left lung

coronary artery

Catherization of coronary artery, a diagnostic procedure to determine patency of the artery.

– and then placing the heel of the hand over the lower part of the sternum and compressing the chest wall firmly, but not too forcibly, at the rate of 60 to 80 times a minute. At the same time artificial respiration must be started by the mouth-to-mouth method. (See APPENDIX 1: BASIC FIRST AID.)

CARDIAC MUSCLE The muscle, unique to the heart, which comprises the walls of the atria and ventricles. It consists of long broadening cells (fibres) with special physiological characteristics which enable them to keep contracting and expanding indefinitely.

CARDIAC NEUROSIS Obsessional fear about the state of the heart. It tends to occur after a heart attack and may result in the patient's reproducing the symptoms of another attack.

CARDIAC OUTPUT The volume of blood pumped out by the ventricles during each cardiac cycle.

CARDIAC PACEMAKER The natural pacemaker is the sinuatrial node, found at the base of the HEART. The heart normally controls its rate and rhythm; heart block occurs when impulses cannot reach all parts of the heart. This may lead to ARRHYTHMIA, or even cause the heart to stop (see HEART DISEASES). Artificial pacemakers may then be used; in the United Kingdom these are required for around one person in every 2,000 of the population. Usually powered by mercury or lithium batteries, lasting up to ten years, they are either fixed to the outside of the chest or implanted in the armpit, and connected by a wire passing through a vein in the neck to the heart. Normally adjusted to deliver 65 to 75 impulses a minute, they also ensure a regular cardiac rhythm. Patients with pacemakers may be given a driving licence provided that their vehicle is not likely to be a source of danger to the public, and that they are receiving adequate and regular medical supervision from a cardiologist.

Although there are numerous possible sources of electrical interference with pacemakers, the overall risks are slight. Potential sources include anti-theft devices, airport weapon detectors, surgical diathermy, ultrasound, and short-wave heat treatment. Nevertheless, many pacemaker patients lead active and fulfilling lives, achieving high standards in many sports.

CARDIAC TAMPONADE Compression of the heart due to abnormal accumulation of fluid within the fibrous covering of the heart (PERICARDIUM). The result is irregular rhythm and death if the fluid is not removed.

CARDIOANGIOGRAPHY Rendering the outline of the heart visible on an X-ray film by injecting a radio-opaque substance into it.

CARDIOLOGY That branch of medical science devoted to the study of the diseases of the heart.

CARDIOMEGALY Enlargement of the heart (see HEART DISEASE).

CARDIOMYOPATHIES Diseases of heart muscle of unknown cause. There are three distinct varieties:

Hypertrophic cardiomyopathy is characterized by massive ventricular hypertrophy. This hypertrophied muscle is not efficient and cannot relax adequately so that the ventricles do not fill properly during diastole.

Congestive cardiomyopathy is characterized by dilatation of both ventricles causing severe impairment of contraction.

Restrictive cardiomyopathy – organic material collects around the endocardium and myocardium which restricts the inflow of blood to the ventricles.

The disorder usually presents with congestive cardiac failure for which there does not appear to be a known cause. (See HEART DISEASES.)

CARDIOPLEGIA A procedure whereby the heart is stopped by reducing its temperature (hypothermia), by injecting the muscle with a solution of salts or by electrostimulation. This enables surgeons to operate safely on the heart.

CARDIOPULMONARY BYPASS A procedure in which the body's circulation of blood is kept going when the heart is intentionally stopped to enable heart surgery to be carried out. A HEART-LUNG MACHINE substitutes for the heart's pumping action and the blood is oxygenated at the same time.

CARDIOSPASM means the spasmodic contraction of the muscle surrounding the opening of the oesophagus into the stomach: also termed achalasia of the cardia. (See OESOPHAGUS, DISEASES OF.)

CARDIOVASCULAR SYSTEM This refers to the whole circulatory system: the heart, the systemic circulation (the arteries and veins of the body) and the pulmonary circulation (the arteries and veins of the lungs). Blood circulates throughout the cardiovascular system bringing oxygen and nutrients to the tissues and removing carbon dioxide and other waste products.

CARDIOVERSION or DEFIBRILLATION is indicated in patients with ventricular fibrillation or tachycardia, fast or irregular heart beat, if other treatments have failed. A general anaesthetic is given if the patient is conscious, following which a carefully timed direct-current shock is applied to the patient's chest wall using a

DEFIBRILLATOR. The patient's ECG rhythm should then be monitored and anticoagulants considered, as the risk of EMBOLI is increased. (See DEFIBRILLATION.).

CARE IN COMMUNITY (see COMMUNITY CARE).

CARIES, dental decay, is the material remaining after the calcified structure of the tooth has been removed in dental disease. This is probably initiated by bacteria. As the decay is removed a hole develops and the tooth may collapse.

CARMINATIVES Preparations to relieve FLATULENCE, and any resulting griping, by the bringing up of wind, or ERUCTATION. Their essential constituent is an aromatic volatile oil, usually of vegetable extraction.

CARNEOUS MOLE An ovum which has died in the early months of pregnancy. It usually requires no treatment and evacuates itself.

CAROTENE A colouring matter of carrots, other plants, butter and yolk of egg, and is the precursor of vitamin A, which is formed from carotene in the liver. (See VITAMIN and APPENDIX 5: VITAMINS.)

CAROTID BODY A small reddish-brown structure measuring 5 to 7 × 2·5 to 4 millimetres, situated one on each side of the neck, where the carotid artery divides into the internal and external carotid arteries. Its main function is in controlling breathing so that an adequate supply of oxygen is maintained to the tissues of the body. Oxygen levels are controlled by a reflex operating between the carotid body and the respiratory centre in the brain.

CARPAL TUNNEL SYNDROME A condition characterized by attacks of pain and tingling in the first three or four fingers of one or both hands, which usually occur at night. It is caused by pressure on the median nerve as it passes under the strong ligament that lies across the front of the wrist. The condition may respond to use of a night splint on the hand. Otherwise a corticosteroid injection under the ligament may help. If not, pressure is relieved by surgical division of the compressing ligament.

CARPUS The Latin term for the wrist, composed of eight small bones firmly joined together with ligaments, but capable of a certain amount of sliding movement over one another. (See WRIST.)

CARRIERS OF DISEASE (see INFECTION).

CARTILAGE A hard but pliant substance forming parts of the skeleton, e.g. the cartilages of the ribs, of the larynx and of the ears. Microscopically, cartilage is found to consist of cells arranged in twos or in rows, and embedded in a ground-glass-like material devoid of blood-vessels and nerves. The end of every long bone has a smooth layer of hyaline cartilage on it where it forms a joint with other bones (articular cartilage), and in young persons up to about the age of sixteen there is a plate of cartilage (epiphyseal cartilage) running right across the bone about 12 mm (half an inch) from each end. The latter, by constantly thickening and changing into bone, causes the increase in length of the bone. (See BONE.) In some situations there is found a combination of cartilage and fibrous tissue, as in the discs between the vertebrae of the spine. This fibrocartilage, as it is known, combines the pliability of fibrous tissue with the elasticity of cartilage. (For cartilages of the knee, see KNEE.)

CARUNCLE Any small fleshy eminence, whether normal or abnormal.

CASEATION A process which takes place in the tissues in tuberculosis and some other chronic diseases. The central part of a diseased area, instead of changing into pus and so forming an abscess, changes to a firm cheese-like mass which may next be absorbed or may be converted into a calcareous deposit and fibrous tissue, and so healing results with the formation of a scar.

CASEIN That part of milk which forms cheese or curds. It is produced by the union of a substance, caseinogen, dissolved in the milk, with lime salts also dissolved in the milk, the union being produced by the action of rennin, a ferment from the stomach of the calf. The same change occurs in the human stomach as the first step in the digestion of milk, and therefore when milk is vomited curdled it merely shows that digestion has begun.

CASTRATION This is literally defined as deprivation of the power of generation. In practical terms this involves surgical removal of both OVARIES or TESTICLES. Such an operation is most commonly associated with the treatment of malignant lesions. In women who have reached the menopause, bilateral oophorectomy is routinely performed during HYSTERECTOMY, especially in cases of uterine carcinoma, and is usually performed when removing an ovarian tumour or malignant cyst. It is essential that the surgeon discusses with a woman before an operation when it might prove beneficial to remove her ovaries in addition to carrying out the main procedure. In men, orchidectomy is routine for testicular tumours, and is common when treating prostatic cancer. It is no longer performed on young boys as a means of preserving the alto voice, the 'castrato' role having been superseded by the countertenor.

CASTS of hollow organs are found in various diseases. Membranous casts of the air passages are found in diphtheria and in one form of bronchitis, and are sometimes coughed up entire. Casts of the interior of the bowels are passed in cases of mucous colitis associated with constipation, and casts of the microscopic tubules in the kidneys passed in the urine form one of the surest signs of glomerulonephritis.

CATALEPSY   A physical condition in which part or all of the body becomes rigid. Often associated with SCHIZOPHRENIA, it is character- ized by the adoption of strange – often statue- like – poses (CATATONIA), which may pass off within a few minutes, or may last for several hours or, rarely, days. Typically brought on by a sudden mental trauma, it may occur with prolonged depression or some other serious MENTAL ILLNESS, and occasionally with EPILEPSY. Successful treatment must depend upon due recognition of all precipitating factors and circumstances.

CATAPLEXY is a condition in which the patient has a sudden attack of muscular weak- ness affecting the whole body. (See also NAR- COLEPSY.)

CATARACT   An opacity of the lens sufficient to cause visual impairment.

Causes   Frequently there is no specific cause. Lens opacities become commoner with increas- ing age and probably 90 per cent of people over 75 have them. A smaller proportion of people suffer visual impairment, when the term cata- ract is usually applied. Apart from age, other risk factors for cataract development include DIABETES, high myopia (see REFRACTION), use of CORTICOSTEROIDS, renal failure, eye trauma, eye surgery and UVEITIS. There are also associations with DYSTROPHIA MYOTONICA, atopic DERMATI- TIS, infrared radiation and X-rays and sus- pected relationships with smoking, heavy alcohol consumption, diet and exposure to ULTRAVIO- LET RAYS. Cataracts are rarely found in infancy or childhood. In these age groups possible causes include hereditary factors, metabolic disorders and infections transmitted to the fetus in pregnancy.

Symptoms   No symptoms are specific to cata- ract. Patients commonly complain of blurred or misty vision and sometimes excessive glare from car head-lamps or sunlight.

Diagnosis   The diagnosis of cataract should be approached with caution because of the vari- able relationship of lens opacities to symptoms and the possibility of mistakenly attributing the cause of visual disturbance to cataract.

Treatment   The subject's lens is surgically re- moved and usually replaced by a synthetic intra-ocular lens implant. Several different operating techniques can be used depending on the patient's condition. This can be performed as a day case with the patient receiving a local anaesthetic. There is usually no need to per- form surgery in adults unless they request it. Occasionally a cataract is removed for other reasons: to improve the view into the eye for the doctor (e.g. in diabetes), or when one of the very rare complications of cataract occurs (GLAUCOMA or uveitis).

CATARRH   Inflammation of the mucous membranes, particularly those of the air pas- sages, associated with a copious secretion of mucus. Commonly the result of infection or local allergy, catarrh can affect the nose, middle ear and sinuses. The condition is usually self limiting but, if persistent, may need antibiotic treatment.

CATATONIA   A condition in which an indi- vidual takes up odd postures often accompa- nied by muteness or semicoma. The arms and legs may be moved passively by someone else into positions that the sufferer then holds for many hours. Catatonia occurs in SCHIZOPHRE- NIA. It may also be associated with organic brain disease such as encephalitis lethargica (see ENCEPHALITIS), tumours and carbon mon- oxide intoxication.

CATECHOLAMINES   Substances produced in the body from the dietary AMINO-ACIDS, PHENYLALANINE and TYROSINE. They include ADRENALINE, NORADRENALINE and DOPAMINE which have varying functions, usually as NEUROTRANSMITTERS, in the SYMPATHETIC and CENTRAL NERVOUS SYSTEMS. Their chemical struc- ture is based on a benzene ring with hydroxyl and amine side-chains.

CATGUT   This is used in surgery for tying cut arteries and stitching wounds. It is made from the fibrous coat of the intestines of animals, espe- cially of the sheep, requires very careful purifica- tion, and in the tissues is gradually absorbed – in about five to ten days – as it is itself an animal substance. Hardened catgut is catgut which has been treated with a suitable hardening agent to prolong the time taken for it to be absorbed; catgut hardened by treatment with chromium compounds is known as chromicized catgut.

CATHARTICS   Substances which produce an evacuation of the bowels. (See PURGATIVES.) The term 'cathartic' also means possessing the power to cleanse.

CATHERIZATION   Use of a CATHETER.

CATHETERS   Hollow tubes used for passing into various organs of the body, either for investigational purposes or to give some form of treatment. They are used under strict sterile conditions.

Cardiac catheters are introduced through a vein in the arm and passed into the heart in order to diagnose some of the more obscure forms of congenital heart disease, and often as a preliminary to operating on the heart.

Endotracheal catheters are used to pass down the TRACHEA into the lungs, usually in the course of administering ANAESTHETICS.

Eustachian catheters are small catheters that are passed along the floor of the nose into the EUSTACHIAN TUBE in order to inflate the ear.

Nasal catheters are tubes passed through the nose into the stomach to feed a patient who cannot swallow: so-called nasal feeding.

Rectal catheters are passed into the rectum in order to give injections.

Suprapubic catheters are passed into the bladder through an incision in the lower abdominal wall just above the pubis, either to allow urine to drain away from the bladder, or to wash out an infected bladder.

Ureteric catheters are small catheters that are passed up the ureter into the pelvis of the kidney, usually to determine the state of the kidney, either by obtaining a sample of urine direct from the kidney or to inject a radio-opaque substance preliminary to X-raying the kidney. (See PYELOGRAPHY.)

Urethral catheters are catheters that are passed along the urethra into the bladder, either to draw off urine or to wash out the bladder.

It is these last three types of catheters that are most extensively used.

'CAT SCANNER' (see CT SCANNER).

CAT-SCRATCH FEVER is a disease, probably due to a virus, which is characterized by enlargement of the glands. In spite of the name, there is a history of a cat scratch in only about half the cases; in others the infection is acquired through a puncture of the skin by a splinter or thorn. The glandular swelling is usually slight and of short duration, but in some cases may go on to abscess formation which requires aspiration. The infection is not controlled by penicillin.

CAUDA A tail or a tail-like structure. For example, the cauda equina is a collection of nerve roots from the lumbar sacral and coccygeal spinal nerves that runs down inside the spinal column until it leaves it through their respective openings.

CAUL The piece of AMNION which sometimes covers a child when he or she is born.

CAULIFLOWER EAR The term applied to the distortion of the external ear produced by repeated injury in sport. Initially it is due to a HAEMATOMA in the auricle (see EAR). To prevent deformity the blood should be drawn off from this haematoma as soon as possible, and a firm

pressure bandage then applied. Subsequent protection can be given to the ear by covering it with a few layers of two-way stretch strapping wound round the head.

CAUSALGIA A severe burning pain in a limb in which the sympathetic and somatic nerves have been damaged.

CAUSTICS AND CAUTERIES are used to destroy tissues, the former by chemical action, the latter by their high temperature. (See ELECTROCAUTERY.)

CAVERNOUS BREATHING A peculiar quality of the respiratory sounds heard on auscultation over a cavity in the lung.

CAVERNOUS SINUS A channel for venous blood placed either side of the SPHENOID bone at the base of the SKULL behind the eye sockets. Blood drains into it from the eye, the nose, the brain and part of the cheek and leaves via the internal jugular and facial veins. Sometimes the sinus becomes blocked by a blood clot (thrombus), usually a complication of a nearby bacterial infection. A potentially serious condition, it should be treated with antibiotics.

CEFOXITIN is a semi-synthetic antibiotic, given by injection, which is used in the treatment of infections due to Gram-negative micro-organisms such as *Proteus* which are resistant to many other antibiotics.

CELLS The basic structural unit of body tissues. There are around 10 billion in the human body and they are structurally and functionally linked to carry out the body's many complex activities.

Every cell consists essentially of a cell-body of soft albuminous material called cytoplasm, in which lies a kernel or nucleus which seems to direct all the activities of the cell. Within the nucleus may be seen a minute body, the nucleolus; and there may or may not be a cell-envelope around all. (See also MITOCHONDRIA.) Each cell nucleus carries a set of identical CHROMOSOMES, the body's genetic instructions.

Cells vary much in size, ranging in the human body from 0·0025 mm to about 0·025 mm.

All animals and plants consist at first of a single cell (the egg-cell, or ovum), which begins to develop when fertilized by the sperm-cell derived from the opposite sex. Development begins by a division into two new cells, then into four, and so on till a large mass is formed. These cells then arrange themselves into layers, and form various tubes, rods, and masses which represent in the embryo the organs of the fully developed animal. (See FETUS.)

When the individual organs have been laid down on a scaffolding of cells, these gradually change in shape and in chemical composition. The cells in the nervous system send out long

1 smooth endoplasmic reticulum
2 free ribosomes
3 nucleolus
4 rough endoplasmic reticulum
5 Golgi apparatus
6 microbody
7 cell membrane

8 exocytosis of secretory product
9 nuclear envelope
10 chromatin
11 glycogen granule
12 lysosome
13 mitochondrion
14 centrosomes (at right-angles to each other)

(Top left) Liver cell. (Top right) Bone cell. (Bottom) Diagrammatic representation of cell structure.

processes to form the nerves, those in the muscles become long and striped in appearance, and those which form fat become filled with fat droplets which distend the cells. Further, they begin to produce, between one another, the substances which give the various tissues their special character. Thus, in the future bones, some cells deposit lime salts, and others form cartilage; while, in tendons, they produce long white fibres of a gelatinous substance. In some organs the cells change little: thus the liver consists of columns of large cells packed together, while many cells, like the white blood corpuscles, retain their primitive characters almost entire.

Thus cells are the active agents in forming the body, and they have a similar function in repairing its wear and tear. TUMOURS, and especially malignant tumours, have a highly cellular structure, the cells being of an embryonic type, or, at best, forming poor imitations of the tissues in which they grow.

CELLULITIS Inflammation taking place in cellular tissue and usually refers to infection in the subcutaneous tissue. The word is erroneously used in the slimming business to refer to excess fatty tissue in the arms, buttocks and thighs. (See ABSCESS; ERYSIPELAS.)

CELLULOSE A carbohydrate substance forming the skeleton of most plant structures. It is colourless, transparent, insoluble in water and is practically unaffected by digestion. In vegetable foods it therefore adds to the bulk, but it is of no value as a food-stuff. It is found in practically a pure state in cotton-wool.

CEMENT (see TEETH).

CEMENT BURNS The result of prolonged contact of the skin with builders' cement. They are due to quicklime which constitutes 65 per cent of cement. As they are chemical, and not thermal, burns, the victim feels no immediate pain and therefore allows the contact to persist. The precautions that should be taken include adequate protection of the hands and feet, and avoidance of prolonged contact of the skin with cement. Cement, especially varieties containing chromium compounds, is a common cause of contact dermatitis (see SKIN DISEASES).

CENSOR   A term applied to the mental influence which prevents certain subconscious thoughts and wishes from coming into consciousness unless they are disguised so as to be unrecognizable.

CENTRAL NERVOUS SYSTEM   This comprises the nervous tissue of the brain and spinal cord but does not include the cranial and spinal nerves and the autonomic nervous system. This latter group makes up the peripheral nervous system. (See BRAIN and SPINAL CORD).

CENTRAL VENOUS PRESSURE   The pressure of blood within the right atrium of the HEART as measured by a catheter and manometer.

CENTRE   A term applied to a collection of nerve cells which give off nerve fibres and control some particular function: e.g. the speech centre and the vision centre in the brain.

CEPHALOSPORINS   These are broad-spectrum antibiotics'. Most are semi-synthetic derivatives of cephalosporin C, an antibiotic originally derived from a sewage outfall in Sardinia.

First-generation examples still in use include cephalexin and cefadroxil. They are orally active and, along with second-generation cefaclor, have a similar antimicrobial spectrum. They are used for 'resistant' urinary infections and urinary infections in pregnancy. Cephalosporins have a similar pharmacology to that of penicillin and about 10 per cent of patients allergic to penicillin will also be hypersensitive to cephalosporins. They are effective in treating SEPTICAEMIA, PNEUMONIA, MENINGITIS, biliary-tract infections and PERITONITIS.

Second-generation cefuroxime and cefamandole are less vulnerable to penicillinases and are useful for treating 'resistant' bacteria and *HAEMOPHILUS INFLUENZAE* and *NEISSERIA GONORRHOEA*. Third-generation cephalosporins include cefotaxime, ceftazidime and others; these are more effective than the second-generation in treating some Gram-negative infections.

CEREAL   Any grasslike plant bearing an edible seed. The important cereals are wheat, oats, barley, maize, rice and millet. Along with these are usually included tapioca (derived from the cassava plant), sago (derived from the pith of the sago palm) and arrowroot (derived from the root of a West Indian plant), all of which consist almost entirely of starch. Semolina, farola and macaroni are preparations of wheat.

	per cent
Water	10 to 12
Protein	10 to 12
Carbohydrate	65 to 75
Fat	0·5 to 8
Mineral matter	2

Composition of cereals

Cereals consist predominantly of carbohydrate. They are therefore an excellent source of energy. On the other hand, their deficiency in protein and fat means that to provide a balanced diet, they should be supplemented by other foods rich in protein and fat.

	Water	Protein	Fat	Carbo-hydrate	Cellu-lose	Ash
Wheat	12·0	11·0	1·7	71·2	2·2	1·9
Oatmeal	7·2	14·2	7·3	65·9	3·5	1·9
Barley	12·3	10·1	1·9	69·5	3·8	2·4
Rye	11·0	10·2	2·3	72·3	2·1	2·1
Maize	12·5	9·7	5·4	68·9	2·0	1·5
Rice (polished)	12·4	6·9	0·4	79·4	0·4	0·5
Millet	12·3	10·4	3·9	68·3	2·9	2·2
Buck-wheat	13·0	10·2	2·2	61·3	11·1	2·2

Composition of certain cereals.

CEREBELLAR ATAXIA   Uncoordinated movements, including an unsteady gait, caused by damage to or disease of the CEREBELLUM. Brain tumours, MULTIPLE SCLEROSIS and stroke can result in ataxia as can excessive consumption of alcohol. Degeneration of the cerebellum as a result of an inherited disease can also cause ataxia. Affected victims may have slurred speech, hand tremors and NYSTAGMUS.

CEREBELLUM AND CEREBRUM (see BRAIN).

CEREBRAL PALSY   The term used to describe a group of conditions characterized by varying degrees of paralysis and occurring in infancy or early childhood. In some 80 per cent of cases this takes the form of spastic paralysis: hence the old-fashioned lay description of them as 'spastics'. The incidence is believed to be around 2 or 2·5 per 1000 of the childhood community. In the majority of cases the abnormality dates from before birth or occurs during birth. Among the pre-natal factors are some genetic malformation of the brain, a congenital defect of the brain, or some adverse effect on the fetal brain as by infection during pregnancy. Among the factors during birth that may be responsible are trauma to the child or prolonged lack of oxygen such as can occur during a difficult labour. This last factor is considered by some to be the most important single factor. In some 10 to 15 per cent of cases the condition is acquired after birth, when it may be due to KERNICTERUS, infection of the brain, cerebral thrombosis or embolism, or trauma. The congenital form is commoner in boys than girls, and a high proportion of the cases are first-born children.

The disease manifests itself in many ways, though it may not be recognized until the infant is several months old. The victim may be spastic or flaccid, or the slow, writhing involuntary movements, known as athetosis, may be the predominant feature. These involuntary movements often disappear during sleep and may be controlled, or even abolished, in some cases by training the child to relax. The paralysis varies tremendously. It may involve the limbs on one side of the body (hemiplegia), both lower limbs (paralegia), or all four limbs (DIPLEGIA and QUADRIPLEGIA). Mental handicap (with an IQ under 70) is present in around 75 per cent of all children but children with diplegia or athetoid symptoms may have normal or even high intelligence.

The outlook for life is good, only the more severely affected cases dying in infancy. Although there is no cure, much can be done to help these disabled children, particularly if the condition is detected at an early stage. Little can be done to help those who have severe mental subnormality, but much can be done for those with normal intelligence by team work, giving attention to education, physiotherapy, occupational therapy and speech training. In this way many of these handicapped children are now reaching adult life as useful members of the community. Much help in dealing with these children can be obtained from SCOPE (formerly the Spastics Society), and the Scottish Council for Spastics (see APPENDIX 2: ADDRESSES).

CEREBROSPINAL FLUID   The fluid within the ventricles of the brain and bathing its surface and that of the spinal cord. Normally a clear, colourless fluid, its pressure when an individual is lying on one side is 50 to 150 mm water. A LUMBAR PUNCTURE should not be done if the intracranial pressure is raised (see HYDRO-CEPHALUS).

The cerebrospinal fluid provides useful information in various conditions and is invaluable in the diagnosis of acute and chronic inflammatory diseases of the nervous system. Bacterial MENINGITIS results in a large increase in the number of polymorphonuclear LEUCOCYTES, while a marked lymphocytosis is seen in viral meningitis and encephalitis, tuberculous meningitis and neurosyphilis. The total protein content is raised in many neurological diseases, being particularly high with NEUROFIBROMAS and Guillan-Barré syndrome, while the immunoglobulin G fraction is raised in MULTIPLE SCLEROSIS, neurosyphilis, and connective-tissue disorders. The glucose content is raised in DIABETES, but may be very low in bacterial MENINGITIS, when appropriately stained

smears or cultures often define the infecting organism.

CEREBROVASCULAR ACCIDENT (see STROKE.)

CERUMEN   The name for the wax-like secretion found in the external ear.

CERVICAL means anything pertaining to the neck, or to the neck of the womb.

CERVICAL CANCER   Cancer of the cervix, the neck of the womb, is one of the most common cancers affecting women throughout the world. In some areas its incidence is increasing. This cancer has clearly identifiable precancerous stages with abnormal changes occurring in the cells on the surface of the cervix. These changes can be detected by a cervical smear test. Early cancer can be cured by diathermy, laser treatment, electrocoagula-tion or cryosurgery. If the disease has spread into the body of the cervix or beyond, more extensive surgery and possibly radiotherapy may be needed. The cure rate is 95 per cent if treated in the early stages but may fall as low as 10 per cent in some severe cases. About 4,500 patients are diagnosed as having cervical cancer every year in the United Kingdom and about 1,900 die from it. Latest figures in England (1993) show that the incidence rates have fallen to 11.2 per 100,000 women, while death rates fell by over 30 per cent between 1988 and 1995 (see CERVICAL SMEAR). The sexual behaviour of a woman and her male partners influences the chances of getting this cancer. The earlier a woman has sexual intercourse and the more partners she has, the greater is the risk of developing the disease.

CERVICAL SMEAR   This screening test detects abnormal changes in the cells of the CERVIX and this enables an affected woman to have early treatment. The National Health Service has arrangements to check women regularly. A woman's first test should be within six months of her first experience of intercourse and thereafter at three-yearly intervals for the rest of her life. The test is simple, with some cells being scraped off the cervix with a spatula and the tissue then being examined microscopically.

CERVICAL VERTEBRAE   The seven bones of the top end of the backbone that form the neck. The first cervical vertebra is the atlas and this articulates with the base of the skull. The axis is the second vertebra, which contains a shaft of bone that allows the atlas to rotate on it, thus permitting the head to turn. (See SPINAL COLUMN.)

CERVICITIS   Inflammation of the cervix uteri or neck of the womb.

CERVIX UTERI The neck of the womb or uterus, placed partly above and partly within the vagina. (See UTERUS.)

CETRIMIDE (also known as CETAVLON) is the official name for a mixture of alkyl ammonium bromides. It is a potent antiseptic, and as a 1-per-cent solution is used for cleaning and disinfecting wounds, and in the first-aid treatment of burns. As it is also a detergent, it is particularly useful for cleaning the skin, and also for cleansing and disinfecting greasy and infected bowls and baths.

CHAFING OF THE SKIN, commonly seen in infants and elderly people, is caused by the constant rubbing of two moist surfaces, typically at the natural folds such as the groins, armpits, and elbows. Clothes and ill-fitting shoes may also cause friction and pressure. It is best prevented by keeping the skin clean and dry.

CHAGAS' DISEASE, or American trypanosomiasis, is a disease widespread in Central and South America, and caused by the *Trypanosoma cruzi*. The disease is transmitted by the biting bugs, *Panstrongylus megistus* and *Triatoma infestans*. It occurs in an acute and a chronic form. The former, which is most common in children, practically always affects the heart, and the prognosis is poor. The chronic form is commonest in adolescents and young adults and the outcome depends upon the extent to which the heart is involved. There is no effective drug treatment. It has been suggested that Charles Darwin acquired the disease during his historic voyage on *The Beagle* and that it was the chronic form that turned him into an invalid for 40 years of his life after his return home and ultimately was responsible for his death in 1882. (See also SLEEPING SICKNESS.)

CHALAZION (see EYE DISEASES).

CHALICOSIS A disorder of the lungs found among stonecutters, and due to the inhalation of fine particles of stone.

CHALK-STONES (see GOUT).

CHANCRE The primary lesion of syphilis.

CHANCROID A soft or non-syphilitic venereal sore. It is caused by a micro-organism known as *Haemophilus ducreyi*. It is usually acquired by sexual contact, and responds well to treatment with antibiotic. The disease is rare in the UK.

CHANGE OF LIFE (see CLIMACTERIC; MENSTRUATION).

CHAPPED HANDS occur in cold weather, when reduced sweat and sebaceous activity leads to decreased natural protection of the skin. Prolonged immersion in soapy water, followed by exposure to cold air, results in cracking of the skin.

Prevention consists of minimizing exposure to detergents and soapy water, and wearing rubber gloves for all routine household duties.

CHAPPED LIPS (see LIPS).

CHARCOAL Activated charcoal is a finely powdered material with a huge surface area ($1000m^2/g$) prepared from vegetable matter by carbonization and activated. It is capable of binding a variety of drugs and chemicals and is commonly used in the treatment of poisoning as a method of gastric decontamination. It is not systemically absorbed. It is also used occasionally for flatulence and as a deodorant for skin ulcers.

CHARCOT'S JOINT The name given to a painless swelling and disorganization of the joints resulting from damage to the pain fibres that occurs in DIABETIC NEUROPATHY, LEPROSY, SYRINGOMYELIA and SYPHILITIC INFECTION OF THE SPINAL CORD.

CHEILOSIS Inflammation of the lips. It is common at the angles of the lips (angular stomatitis) which is usually a consequence of sagging facial muscles or ill-fitting dentures producing folds at the corners of the mouth which retain food debris and allow proliferation of bacteria and candida. Atopic eczema (see SKIN DISEASES) is a common cause of cheilosis of the whole of the lips.

CHEIROPOMPHOLYX Pompholyx is an old name for vesicular eczema (see DERMATITIS) on the palms and fingers (cheiropompholyx) or soles of the feet (podopompholyx).

CHELATING AGENTS are compounds that will render an ion (usually a metal) biologically inactive by incorporating it into an inner ring structure in the molecule. (Hence the name from the Greek *chele*=claw.) When the complex formed in this way is harmless to the body and is excreted in the urine, such an agent is an effective way of ridding the body of toxic metals such as mercury. The main chelating agents are DIMERCAPROL, PENICILLAMINE and sodium calciumedetate.

CHEMOSIS Swelling of the conjunctiva of the EYE, usually caused by inflammation from injury or infection.

CHEMOTAXIS The ability of certain cells to attract or repel others.

CHEMOTHERAPY The prevention or treatment of disease by chemical substances. The term is generally used in two senses: the use of antibacterial and other drugs to treat infections, and the administration of ANTIMETABOLITES and other drugs to treat cancer. The discovery by Paul Ehrlich in 1910 of the action of Salvarsan in treating syphilis led to the introduction of SULPHONAMIDES in 1935, followed by PENICILLIN during World War II, which revolutionized the treatment of common infections. Many ANTIBACTERIAL drugs have been developed since then. These include CEPHALOSPORINS, cephamycins, TETRACYCLINES, AMINOGLYCOSIDES, MACROLIDES and CLINDAMYCIN as well as antituberculous drugs such as STREPTOMYCIN and METRONIDAZOLE. Unfortunately, overuse of chemotherapeutic drugs in medicine and in animal husbandry has stimulated widespread resistance among pathogenic micro-organisms previously susceptible. Chemotherapy also plays an important role in treating tropical diseases, especially MALARIA, SLEEPING SICKNESS and LEPROSY.

Recently chemotherapy has become increasingly effective in the treatment of cancer. Numerous drugs, generally CYTOTOXIC, are available; great care is required in their selection and to minimize side-effects. Certain tumours are highly sensitive to chemotherapy – especially TESTICULAR tumours, LEUKAEMIAS, LYMPHOMAS and various tumours, e.g. Wilms' tumour (see NEPHROBLASTOMA), occurring in childhood – and may even be cured.

CHENODEOXYCHOLIC ACID One of the bile acids (see BILE), which is used in the treatment of cholesterol gall-stones for patients with mild symptoms when other modern techniques are unsuitable. (See GALL-BLADDER, DISEASES OF.)

CHEST, or THORAX, is the upper part of the trunk. It is enclosed by the breast-bone(sternum) and the twelve ribs which join the sternum by way of cartilages and are attached to the spine behind. At the top of the thorax the opening in between the first ribs admits the windpipe (TRACHEA), the gullet (OESOPHAGUS) and the large blood vessels. The bottom of the thorax is separated from the abdomen below by the muscular DIAPHRAGM which is the main muscle of breathing. Other muscles of respiration, the intercostal muscles, lie in between the ribs. Overlying the ribs are layers of muscle and soft tissue including the breast tissue.

Contents The trachea divides into right and left main bronchi which go to the two LUNGS. The left lung is slightly smaller than the right. The right has three lobes (upper, middle and lower) and the left lung has two lobes (upper and lower). Each lung is covered by two thin membranes lubricated by a thin layer of fluid. These are the pleura and similar structures cover the heart (pericardium). The heart lies in the middle, displaced slightly to the left. The oesophagus passes right through the chest to enter the stomach just below the diaphragm. Various nerves, blood vessels and lymph channels run through the thorax. The thoracic duct is the main lymphatic drainage channel emptying into a vein on the left side of the root of the neck. (For diseases affecting the chest and its contents see HEART DISEASES; LUNGS, DISEASES OF; CHEST, DEFORMITIES OF.)

CHEST, DEFORMITIES OF The healthy chest is gently rounded all over, its contour being more rounded in women by the breast tissue. In cross section it is oval shaped with a longer dimension from side to side than back to front.

Barrel chest is found in long-standing asthma or chronic bronchitis and emphysema when the lungs are chronically enlarged. The anterioposterior dimension of the chest is increased and the ribs are near horizontal. In this position they can produce little further expansion of the chest and breathing often relies on accessory muscles in the neck lifting up the whole thoracic cage on inspiration.

Pigeon chest is one in which the cross-section of the chest becomes triangular with the sternum forming a sort of keel in front. It may be related to breathing problems in early life.

Rickety chest is uncommon now and is caused by rickets in early life (see RICKETS). There is a hollow down each side caused by the pull of muscles on the softer ribs in childhood. The line of knobs produced on each side where the ribs join their costal cartilages is known as the rickety rosary.

Pectus excavatum, or funnel chest, is quite a common abnormality where the central tendon of the diaphragm seems to be too short so that the lower part of the sternum is displaced inwards and the lower ribs are prominent. When severe it may displace the heart further to the left side.

Local abnormalities in the shape of the chest occur when there is a deformity in the spine such as scoliosis which alters the angles of the ribs. The chest wall may be locally flattened when the underlying lung is reduced in size locally over a prolonged period. (See SPINE AND SPINAL CORD, DISEASES AND INJURIES OF.) This may be seen over a scarred area of lung such as that seen in pulmonary TUBERCULOSIS.

CHEYNE-STOKES BREATHING A type of breathing seen in some serious neurological disorders, such as brain tumours and stroke, and also in the case of persons with advanced disease of the heart or kidneys. When well marked it is a sign that death is impending, though milder degrees of it do not carry such a serious implication in elderly patients. The breathing gets very faint for a short time, then gradually deepens till full expirations are taken for a few seconds, and then gradually dies away to another quiet period, again increasing in depth after a few seconds and so on in cycles.

CHIASMA This is an X-shaped crossing. The optic chiasma is where the nerve fibres from the nasal half of each retina cross over the mid line to join the optic tract from the other side.

CHICKENPOX or VARICELLA An acute contagious disease predominantly of children, though it may occur at any age, characterized by feverishness and an eruption on the skin. The name, chickenpox, is said to be derived from the resemblance of the eruption to boiled chick-peas.

Causes The disease occurs in epidemics affecting especially children under the age of ten years. It has no connection with smallpox, to which it bears a superficial resemblance. It is due to the varicella zoster virus, and the condition is an extremely infectious one from child to child. Although an attack confers lifelong immunity, the virus may lie dormant and manifest itself in adult life as herpes zoster or shingles (see HERPES ZOSTER).

Symptoms There is an incubation period of fourteen to twenty-one days after infection, and then the child becomes feverish or has a slight shivering, or may feel more severely ill with vomiting and pains in the back and legs. Almost at the same time, an eruption consisting of red pimples which quickly change into vesicles filled with clear fluid appears on the back and chest, sometimes about the forehead, and less frequently on the limbs. These vesicles appear over several days and during the second day may show a change of their contents to turbid, purulent fluid and within a day or two they burst, or, at all events, shrivel up and become covered with brownish crusts. The small crusts have all dried up and fallen off in little more than a week and recovery is almost always complete.

Treatment The fever can be reduced with paracetamol and the itching soothed with calamine lotion. If the child is very unwell, an antiviral drug, aciclovir, can be used at an early stage.

CHIGGER Another name for *Trombicula autumnalis*, popularly known as the harvest mite (see BITES AND STINGS).

CHILBLAIN, or ERYTHEMA PERNIO An inflamed condition of the hands or feet, or occasionally of the ears, and should not be confused with cracked or CHAPPED HANDS. Most commonly found in childhood and old age, it may be associated with generally poor health, though there may also be a genetic predisposition. Prevention with good food, warm clothing, a warm environment, and regular exercise to maintain the circulation, is the best treatment.

CHILD ABUSE The physical or emotional mistreatment of a child. Neglect, physical injury, and sexual abuse are all forms of child abuse and they may be caused by parents, relatives, or carers. Greater awareness of the problem has led to an increase in reported incidents. And some experts believe that proved cases of child abuse increased four- or fivefold over the past decade. In England around 35,000 children are on child-protection registers. The definition of abuse is that a child is treated in a way that is unacceptable in a given culture at a given time. Physical abuse or non-accidental injury is the most easily recognized form. Victims of sexual abuse may not reveal their experiences until adulthood and often not at all. Where child abuse is suspected, full investigation of the circumstances is necessary, and this may mean admitting a child to hospital or to local authority care. Abuse may be the result of impulsive action by adults or it may be premeditated, for example, the continued sexual exploitation of a child over several years. Premeditated physical assault is rare but is liable to cause serious injury to a child and requires urgent action when identified. Adults will go to some lengths to cover up persistent abuse. The child's interests are paramount but the parents may well be under severe stress and also require sympathetic handling.

In recent years persistent child abuse in some children's homes has come to light, with widespread publicity following offenders' appearances in court. Local communities have also protested about convicted paedophiles, released from prison, coming to live in their communities.

In the United Kingdom local-government social services departments are central in the prevention, investigation and management of cases of child abuse. They have four important protection duties laid down in the Children Act 1989. They are charged (1) to prevent children sufering ill treatment and neglect; (2) to safeguard and promote the welfare of children in need; (3) when requested by a court, to investigate a child's circumstances; (4) to investigate information – in concert with the NSPCC (National Society for the Prevention of Cruelty to Children) – that a child is suffering or is likely to suffer significant harm and to decide whether action is necessary to safeguard and promote the child's welfare.

When anyone suspects that child abuse is occurring, contact should be made with the relevant social services department.

CHILD ADOPTION Adoption was relatively uncommon until the Second World War with only 6,000 adoption orders annually. This peaked at nearly 25,000 in 1968 as adoption became more socially acceptable and the numbers of babies born to lone mothers rose in a climate hostile to single parenthood.

Adoption declined as the availability of babies fell with the introduction of the Abortion

Act, 1968, improving contraceptive services and increasing acceptability of single parenthood.

However, with 10 per cent of couples suffering infertility, the demand continued, leading to the adoption of those previously perceived as difficult to place, i.e. physically, intellectually and/or emotionally disabled children and adolescents, those with terminal illness and children of ethnic-minority groups.

Recent controversies regarding homosexual couples as adoptive parents, adoption of children with or at high risk of HIV/AIDS, transcultural adoption and the increasing use of intercountry adoption to fulfil the needs of childless couples have provoked urgent consideration of the ethical dilemmas of adoption and its consequences for the children, their adoptive and birth families and society generally.

Detailed statistics have been unavailable since 1984 but in general there has been a downward trend with relatively more older children being placed. Detailed reasons for adoption (i.e. interfamily, step-parent, intercountry, etc.) are not available but approximately one-third are adopted from local-authority care.

In the UK all adoptions (including interfamily and step-parent adoption) must take place through a registered adoption agency which may be local-authority based or provided by a registered voluntary agency. All local authorities must act as agencies, the voluntary agencies often providing specialist services to promote and support the adoption of more difficult-to-place children. Occasionally an adoption allowance will be awarded.

Adoption orders cannot be granted until a child has resided with its proposed adopters for 13 weeks. In the case of new-born infants the mother cannot give formal consent to placement until the baby is 6 weeks old, although informal arrangements can be made before this time.

In the UK the concept of responsibility of birth parents to their children and their rights to continued involvement after adoption are acknowledged by the Children Act, 1989. However, in all discussions the child's interests remain paramount. The Act also recognizes adopted children's need to have information regarding their origins.

BAAF – British Agencies for Adoption and Fostering – is the national organization of adoptive agencies, both local authority and voluntary sector. The organization promotes and provides training service, development and research, has several specialist professional subgroups (i.e. medical, legal, etc.) and produces a quarterly journal.

PPIAS – Parent to Parent Information Service on Adoptive Services – is an effective national support network of adoptive parents who offer free information, a 'listening ear' and, to members, a quarterly newsletter.

National Organization for Counselling Adoptees and their parents (NORCAP), is concerned with adopted children and birth parents who wish to make contact.

The Registrar General operates an Adoption Contact Register for adopted persons and anyone related to that person by blood, half blood or marriage. Information can be obtained from the Office of Population Censuses and Surveys. For the addresses of these organizations see APPENDIX 2: ADDRESSES.

CHILDBIRTH (see LABOUR).

CHILD DEVELOPMENT Children develop new skills in predictable patterns which can be observed as series of milestones along the road to maturity. Up to the age of 3 years milestones are traditionally charted in four areas:

(1) motor – a reflection of physical strength;
(2) social interaction with parents and strangers;
(3) language – including hearing;
(4) fine co-ordination – including vision.

Health-care professionals use these milestones to assess overall developmental progress and as an aid to pinpoint specific problems. Whilst the sequence is generally similar, the age at which a child reaches a given milestone is variable, even within one family, and reflects the child's physical health, environment and personality. If a child has a limited disability, one area of development may lag behind the others. A deaf child will have delayed language but will smile, walk and build towers at the expected time. A mild delay in all areas may reflect personality, chronic hospitalization or poor environmental stimulation, but a severe generalized delay suggests major brain dysfunction.

A child should be able at 6 months to:
● roll over from front to back.
● reach for and shake a rattle.
● look round to see where noises are coming from.
● transfer a cube from one hand to the other.

at 1 year
● walk holding on to furniture.
● hold and drink from a cup.
● use four words with meaning.
● pick up a small object between thumb and forefinger.

at 18 months
● climb on to furniture.
● pull socks off.
● attempt to join in rhymes.
● build a tower of three bricks.

at 2 years
● kick a ball.
● tell about experiences.
● name five toys.
● copy vertical and horizontal lines.

at 3 years
● hop on one foot.
● wash hands.
● know first name.
● copy a circle.

After the age of 3 the discovery of major developmental problems is unlikely. However, deafness and learning disabilities may go unappreciated until the child is much older.

CHILDREN ACT The Children Act 1989 (Children Act) introduced major reforms of child-care law. It encourages negotiation and cooperation between parents, children and professionals to resolve problems affecting children. The aim is to enable children to stay within their own families with appropriate backup from local-authority and professional resources. The emphasis is on empowering families rather than paternalistic control. The Act set up a court made up of three tiers, the High Court, county court and magistrates' court, each with concurrent jurisdiction. The Act has been broadened, clarified and interpreted by subsidiary legislation, rules, case law and official guidance.

CHILLS AND COLDS, though generally trivial, may serve as a prelude to serious disease. The 'common cold' is caused by a virus, transmitted by sneezing or coughing between members of families, schools, or people working together. It may be precipitated by breathing in damp and chilly air, though some people – particularly the elderly – are at greater risk.

Symptoms Nasal catarrh with a frontal headache is common, while inflammation of the SINUSES, sometimes spreading to the middle ear with mild fever, may occur. Rarely lasting more than a few days, it may be followed by TONSILLITIS or LARYNGITIS, while secondary respiratory infections such as BRONCHITIS, or even PNEUMONIA, may occur in predisposed individuals. Although mild, a cold often causes a short period of immuno-depression, which may lead to more serious diseases such as measles, whooping cough, influenza and tuberculosis.

Treatment A couple of days' bedrest provides relief for the sufferer, while also reducing the exposure of others to his infection. Vaccines seem to be ineffectual in the prevention of colds. Prompt medical advice should be sought in cases of prolonged or severe secondary infections.

CHIMERA is an organism, whether plant, animal or human being, in which there are at least two kinds of tissue differing in their genetic constitution.

CHINESE AVIAN INFLUENZA A variety of influenza in chickens occurring in southern China that in 1997 appeared to jump the species barrier and infect humans. Some cases of the human version of the infection occurred in Hong Kong. There were fears of a serious epidemic which, because of a lack of natural resistance among humans, might have led to its worldwide spread. This has not so far occurred.

CHIROPODY is that part of medical science which is concerned with the health of the FEET. The modern chiropodist is a specialist capable of providing a fully comprehensive foot-health service. This includes the palliation of established deformities and dysfunction both as short-term treatment for immediate relief of painful symptoms and long-term management to secure optimum results. This requires the backing of effective appliances and footwear services. It also involves curative footcare, including the use of various therapeutic techniques, including minor surgery and the prescription and provision of specialized and individual appliances. Among conditions routinely treated are walking disorders in children, injuries to the feet of joggers and athletes, corns, bunions and hammer toes, ulcers and foot infections. Chiropody also has a preventive role which includes inspection of children's feet and the detection of foot conditions requiring treatment and advice and also foot- health education. The chiropodist is trained to recognize medical conditions which manifest themselves in the feet, such as circulatory disorders, diabetes mellitus and diseases causing ulceration.

The scope of practice of chiropodists is defined by the Society of Chiropodists and Podologists as comprising the maintenance of the feet in healthy condition and the treatment of their disabilities by methods covered by the syllabus of training hitherto approved by the Department of Health. The only course of training in the United Kingdom recognized for the purpose of state registration by the Chiropodists Board of the Council for Professions Supplementary to Medicine is the Society of Chiropodists 3-year full-time course. The course includes instruction and examination in the relevant aspects of anatomy and physiology, local analgesia, medicine and surgery, as well as in podology and therapeutics. For the registered address of the Society of Chiropodists and Podologists see APPENDIX 2: ADDRESSES.

CHIROPRACTOR A person who practises chiropractic. It is mainly a system of physical manipulations of minor displacements of the spinal column. These minor displacements, or SUBLUXATIONS of the spine are believed to affect the associated or neighbouring nerves and so cause malfunctions of the muscles throughout the body. By manipulating the affected part of the spinal column the patient's complaint, whatever it may be – for example, backache – is relieved. Information can be obtained from the Chiropractic Advancement Association (see APPENDIX 2: ADDRESSES).

CHLAMYDIA A genus of micro-organisms which include those responsible for NON-SPECIFIC URETHRITIS, ORNITHOSIS, PSITTACOSIS, and TRACHOMA. They are also widespread in birds and animals. Chlamydia can be sexually transmitted and in developed countries *Chlamydia trachomatis* is the most significant cause of non-specific urethritis (NSU). In 1995 in England over 39,000 new cases of chlamydia were diagnosed.

CHLOASMA This is an increase in the melanin pigment of the skin as a result of hormonal stimulation. It is commonly seen in pregnancy and sometimes in women on the contraceptive pill. It mainly affects the face.

CHLORAL HYDRATE This drug is now rarely used but chloral betaine (Welldorm) is occasionally used in the elderly.

CHLORAMBUCIL One of several ALKYLATING AGENTS widely used in cancer chemotherapy, chlorambucil is an oral drug commonly used to treat chronic lymphocytic LEUKEMIA, non-Hodgkin's lymphomas, HODGKIN'S DISEASE and OVARIAN CANCER. Apart from suppression of bone-marrow activity, side-effects are few.

CHLORAMPHENICOL is an antibiotic derived from a soil organism, *Streptomyces venezuelae*. It is also prepared synthetically. It is active against a wide range of organisms, but its most striking feature is its activity against certain RICKETTSIAS. It has proved effective in the treatment of typhus, scrub typhus, Rocky Mountain spotted fever, typhoid and paratyphoid fevers. Its activity against certain organisms not susceptible to the sulphonamides and penicillin is proving of value. Particularly is this true of its use in the treatment of meningitis due to *H. influenzae*. It is given by mouth. The drug is also used (as drops) to treat infections of the external ear and for superficial eye infections.

It is an antibiotic, however, that must be administered with discrimination because in certain individuals it may cause aplastic anaemia (see ANAEMIA), particularly if given for too long a period or in repeated courses.

CHLORDANE An insecticide which has been used sucessfully against flies and mosquitoes resistant to DDT, and for the control of ticks and mites. It requires special handling as it is toxic to man when applied to the skin.

CHLORDIAZEPOXIDE A widely used antianxiety drug. (See TRANQUILLIZERS, BENZODIAZEPINES.)

CHLORHEXIDINE, also known as HIBITANE, is an antiseptic which has a bacteriostatic action against many bacteria.

CHLORINATED LIME, also known as CHLORIDE OF LIME, is a white powder made by passing chlorine gas over slaked lime. It is a powerful bleaching agent and disinfectant, useful for household tasks, and effective in the disinfection of swimming pools and drinking water.

When mixed with acidulated water, it gives off chlorine, a greenish gas with a pungent, choking smell, and highly toxic to all forms of bacterial life. Because of the adverse effects of chlorine on the environment, its use is strictly controlled.

CHLORINE (see CHLORINATED LIME, and SODIUM HYPOCHLORITE).

CHLORMETHIAZOLE A useful hypnotic particularly for elderly patients because of its freedom from hang-over effect. It is particularly useful in the acute withdrawal symptoms of alcoholism and is used to treat STATUS EPILEPTICUS. The drug's sedative effects are a useful adjunct to regional anaesthesia and may also be of help in ECLAMPSIA. Dependence may occur occasionally and therefore the length of period for which the drug is used should be limited. Side-effects include sneezing, conjunctival irritation and occasional headache.

CHLOROFORM A colourless, volatile liquid, half as heavy again as water, and, unlike ether, non-inflammable. It was discovered by Liebig in 1831, and is a compound of carbon, hydrogen, and chlorine ($CHCl_3$). It does not dissolve to a large amount in water, but mixes readily with alcohol or ether. It dissolves sulphur, phosphorus, fats, resins, and most substances which contain a large proportion of carbon; it is therefore very useful as a cleansing agent. It was introduced into medicine in 1847 by Sir J. Y. Simpson, who was then in search of a substance which could produce unconsciousness for operative purposes more conveniently than ether, introduced a short time previously by Morton in America. (See ANAESTHESIA.)

Uses Chloroform is used as a solvent of fats, resins, etc., in many chemical processes. It is now rarely used in medicine.

CHLOROMA, or GREEN CANCER, is the name of a disease in which greenish growths appear under the skin, and in which a change takes place in the blood resembling that in leukaemia.

CHLOROPHYLL The green colouring matter of plants. Its main use is as a colouring agent, principally for soaps, oils and fats. It is also being found of value as a deodorant dressing to remove, or diminish, the unpleasant odour of heavily infected sores and wounds.

CHLOROQUINE, which is a 4-aminoquinoline, was introduced during the 1939–45 War for the treatment of MALARIA. The drug is also used for PROPHYLAXIS against malaria where the risk of chloroquine-resistant falciparum is still low. It has also been found of value in the treatment of the skin condition known as chronic discoid lupus erythematosus, and of rheumatoid arthritis.

CHLOROTHIAZIDE A potent BENZOTHIA-DIAZINE diuretic which is active when taken by mouth. It has also a blood-pressure- lowering effect when used in conjunction with other hypotensive drugs.

CHLOROXYLENOL An antiseptic used for treating cuts, abrasions and wounds. It is also widely used in obstetric practice. It is only slightly soluble in water (1 in 3,000).

CHLORPROMAZINE is chemically related to the antihistamine drug, promethazine. One of the first antipsychotic drugs to be marketed, it is used extensively in psychiatry on account of its action in calming psychotic activity without producing undue general depression or clouding of consciousness. The drug is used particularly in schizophrenia and mania. It carries a risk of contact sensitization, so should be handled with care, and the drug has a wide range of side-effects.

CHLORPROPAMIDE An oral hypoglycae-mic agent. It is a sulphonamide derivative and acts by stimulating the release of insulin from the pancreas. As it has a prolonged action, it need only be given once a day. Those taking chlorpropamide should bear in mind that in around 10 per cent of people it causes undue sensitivity to alcohol, resulting in severe flush-ing of the face, headache and a feeling of intoxication. (See also DIABETES MELLITUS, SULPHONYLUREAS.)

CHLORTETRACYCLINE (See TETRA-CYCLINES.)

CHOKING is the process which results from an obstruction to breathing situated in the larynx (see AIR PASSAGES). It may occur as the result of disease causing swelling round the glottis (the entrance to the larynx), or of some nervous disorders that interfere with the regulation of the muscles which open and shut the larynx, but generally it is due to the irritation of a piece of food or other substance introduced by the mouth, which provokes coughing but only partly interferes with breathing. As the mucous membrane lining the upper part of the latter is specially sensitive, coughing results in order to expel the cause of irritation. At the same time, if the foreign body is of any size, lividity of the face appears, due to partial suffocation (see ASPHYXIA).

Treatment The choking person should take slow, deep inspirations, which do not force the particle further in (as sudden catchings of the breath between the coughs do), and which produce more powerful coughs. If the coughing is weak, one or two strong blows with the palm of the hand over either shoulder blade, timed to coincide with coughs aid the effect of the coughing. In the case of a baby, sit down with left forearm resting on thigh. Place the baby chest down along the forearm, holding its head and jaw with the fingers and thumb. The infant's head should be lower than its trunk. Gently deliver three or four blows between the shoulder blades with the free hand. The resus-citator should not attempt blind finger sweeps at the back of the mouth; these can impact a foreign body in the larynx.

If normal breathing (in adult or child) cannot be quickly restored seek urgent medical help. Sometimes an emergency TRACHEOSTOMY is nec-essary to restore the air supply to the lungs. (See APPENDIX 1: FIRST AID.).

CHOLAGOGUES Substances which increase the flow of bile by stimulating evacuation of the gall-bladder. The great majority of these act only by increasing the activity of the digestive organs, and so producing a flow of bile already stored up in the gall-bladder. Substances which stimulate the liver to secrete more bile are known as CHOLERETIC.

CHOLANGIOGRAPHY The process whereby the bile ducts and the gall-bladder are rendered radio-opaque and therefore visible on an X-ray film.

CHOLANGITIS Inflammation of the bile ducts.

CHOLECYSTECTOMY Removal of the gall-bladder by operation.

CHOLECYSTITIS Inflammation of the gall-bladder (see GALL-BLADDER, DISEASES OF).

CHOLECYSTOGRAPHY The process whereby the gall-bladder is rendered radio-opaque and therefore visisble on an X-ray film.

CHOLECYSTOKININ The HORMONE re-leased from the lining membrane of the DUODE-NUM when food is taken, and which initiates emptying of the gall-bladder.

CHOLELITHIASIS The presence of gall-stones in the bile- ducts and/or in the gall-bladder. (See GALL-BLADDER, DISEASES OF.)

CHOLELITHOTOMY The removal of gall-stones from the gall-bladder or bile ducts, when CHOLECYSTECTOMY or LITHOTRIPSY are inappro-priate or not possible. It involves a cholecystomy, an operation to open the gall-bladder.

CHOLERA Bacterial infection caused by *Vibrio cholerae*. This comma-shaped bacterium produces a toxin which results in a net flux of water and electrolytes towards the small-intes-tinal lumen. The patient suffers profuse watery diarrhoea, and resultant dehydration and elec-trolyte imbalance. The small intestine is not affected structurally. Formerly known as the Asiatic cholera, the disease has occurred in epidemics and pandemics for many centuries. In 1823, it broke out of Asia, and extended into Asia Minor and Russia. It traversed Europe, arriving at Sunderland, England, in October 1831; London was affected in January 1832. It subsequently spread through much of North and Central America. The second pandemic originated in 1841 in India and China and extended in a similar direction to that of the first. The third began, also in the east, in 1850 and entered Europe in 1853; it was a major problem in North and South America. During this epidemic, Dr John Snow, a London anaesthetist, carried out seminal epidemiological work in Soho, London, which established that the source of infection was contaminated drinking water derived from the Broad Street pump. Several smaller epidemics involved Europe in the latter years of the 19th century, but none has arisen in Britain or the United States for many years. In 1971, the El Tor biotype of *V. cholerae* emerged and replaced much of the classical infection in Asia and, to a much lesser extent, Europe; parts of Africa were seriously affected. Recently a non-01 strain has arisen and is causing much disease in Asia. Cholera remains a major health problem (this is technically the seventh pandemic) in many countries of Asia, Africa and South America. It is one of three quarantinable infections.

Incubation period varies from a few hours to 5 days. Watery diarrhoea may be torrential and the resultant dehydration and electrolyte imbalance complicated by cardiac failure commonly causes death. The victim's skin elasticity is lost, the eyes are sunken, and the radial pulse may be barely perceptible. Urine production may be completely suppressed. Diagnosis is by detection of *V. cholerae* in a faecal sample. Treatment consists of rapid rehydration. Whereas the intravenous route may be required in a severe case, in the vast majority of patients oral rehydration (using an appropriate solution containing sodium chloride, glucose, sodium bicarbonate, and potassium) gives satisfactory results. Proprietary rehydration fluids do not always contain adequate sodium for rehydration in a severe case. ANTIBIOTICS, e.g. tetracycline and doxycycline, reduce the period during which *V. cholerae* is excreted (in children and pregnant women, furazolidone is safer); in an epidemic, rapid resistance to these, and other antibiotics has been clearly demonstrated. Prevention consists of improving public health infrastructure – in particular, the quality of drinking water. When supplies of the latter are satisfactory, the infection fails to thrive. Although a vaccine was first produced by Haffkine in 1893, immunization techniques remain unsatisfactory; they should not be mandatory for entry to any country. Improved vaccines are currently undergoing development and clinical trial.

CHOLERETIC The term applied to a drug that stimulates the flow of BILE.

CHOLESTASIS A reduction or stoppage in the flow of BILE into the intestine caused either by a blockage such as a stone in the bile duct or by liver disease disturbing the production of bile. The first type is called extrahepatic biliary obstruction and the second intrahepatic cholestasis. The patient develops jaundice and itching and passes dark urine and pale faeces.

CHOLESTEROL A LIPID that is an important constituent of body cells and so widely distributed throughout the body. It is especially abundant in the brain, nervous tissue, adrenal glands and skin. It is also found in egg yolk and gall-stones. It plays an important role in the body, being essential for the production of the sex hormones, as well as the repair of membranes. It is also the source from which bile acids are manufactured. The total amount in the body of a man weighing 70 kilograms (10 stones) is around 140 grams, and the amount present in the blood is 3·6 to 7·8 m.mol per litre or 150 to 250 milligrams per 100 millilitres.

A high blood-cholesterol level – that is, one over 6 m.mol per litre or 238 mg per 100 ml – is undesirable as there appears to be a correlation between a high blood cholesterol and ATHEROMA, the form of arterial degenerative disease associated with coronary thrombosis and high blood-pressure. This is well exemplified in DIABETES MELLITUS and HYPOTHYROIDISM, two diseases in which there is a high blood cholesterol, sometimes going as high as 20 m.mol per litre; patients with these diseases are known to be particularly prone to arterial disease. There is also a familial disease known as hypercholesterolaemia, in which members of affected families have a blood cholesterol of around 18 m.mol per litre, or more, and are particularly liable to premature degenerative disease of the arteries.

Cholesterol exists in two forms in the blood: high-density lipoproteins (HDLs) which are believed to protect against arterial disease, and a low-density version (LDLs) and very low-density type (VLDLs), these latter two being risk factors.

The rising incidence of arterial disease in western countries in recent years has drawn attention to this relationship between high levels of cholesterol in the blood and arterial disease. The available evidence indicates that there is a relationship between blood-cholesterol levels and the amount of fat consumed. However, the blood-cholesterol level bears little relationship with the amount of cholesterol consumed, most of the cholesterol in the body being produced by the body itself.

On the other hand, diets high in saturated fatty acids, chiefly animal fats such as red meat, butter and dripping, tend to raise the blood-cholesterol level; while foods high in unsaturated fatty acids, chiefly vegetable products such as olive and sunflower oils, and oily fish such as mackerel and herring, tend to lower it. There is a tendency in Western society to eat too much animal fat, and current health recommendations are for everyone to decrease saturated-fat intake, increase unsaturated-fat intake, increase daily exercise, and avoid obesity. This advice is particulary important for people with high blood-cholesterol level, with DIABETES MELLITUS, or a history of CORONARY THROMBOSIS.

CHOLESTYRAMINE A drug of value in the treatment of the PRURITUS, or ITCHING, which occurs in association with JAUNDICE. This it does by 'binding' the bile salts in the gut and so preventing their being reabsorbed into the bloodstream, where their excess in jaundice is responsible for the itching. It is also proving useful in reducing the level of cholesterol and triglycerides in the blood and thereby, like CLOFIBRATE, helping to reduce the incidence of coronary artery heart disease. (See CORONARY THROMBOSIS; HYPERLIPIDAEMIA.)

CHOLINE One of the many constituents of the vitamin B complex. Lack of it in the experimental animal produces a fatty liver. It is found in egg-yolk, liver, and meat. The probable daily human requirement is 500 mg, an amount amply covered by the ordinary diet. Choline can be synthesized by the body (see APPENDIX 5: VITAMINS).

CHOLINERGIC A description of nerve fibres that release ACETYLCHOLINE as a NEUROTRANSMITTER.

CHONDROMA A tumour composed in part of cartilage. (See TUMOUR.)

CHORDA A nerve fibre, tendon or cord.

CHOREA, or ST VITUS'S DANCE, is the occurrence of short, purposeless involuntary movements of the face, head, hands and feet. Movements are sudden, but the affected person may hold the new posture for several seconds. Chorea is often accompanied by ATHETOSIS when it is termed choreoathetosis. Choreic symptoms are often due to disease of the basal ganglion in the brain. The withdrawal of phenothiazines may cause the symptoms, as can the drugs used to treat PARKINSON'S DISEASE. Types of chorea include HUNTINGTON'S, SYDENHAM'S, which affects children, and senile.

CHORIOCARCINOMA A form of cancer affecting the CHORION, in the treatment of which particularly impressive results are being obtained from the use of methotrexate.

CHORION This is the more external of the two fetal membranes. (See PLACENTA.)

CHORIONIC GONADOTROPHIC HORMONE A hormone produced by the PLACENTA during pregnancy. It is similar to the pituitary GONADOTROPHINS, which are blocked during pregnancy. Large amounts appear in a woman's urine when she is pregnant and are used as the basis for pregnancy tests. Human gonadotrophins are used to treat delayed puberty and premenstrual tension.

CHOROID (see EYE).

CHOROIDITIS (see UVEITIS).

CHOROID PLEXUS An extensive web of blood vessels occurring in the ventricles of the brain and producing the cerebrospinal fluid. (See BRAIN.)

CHRISTMAS DISEASE A hereditary disorder of blood coagulation which can only be distinguished from HAEMOPHILIA by laboratory tests. It is so called after the surname of the first case reported in this country. About one out of every ten patients clinically diagnosed as haemophiliac has in fact Christmas disease. It is due to lack in the blood of Factor IX (see COAGULATION).

CHROMAFFIN A term applied to certain cells and organs in the body, such as part of the adrenal glands, which have a peculiar affinity for chrome salts. These cells and tissues generally are supposed to secrete substances which have an important action in maintaining the tone and elasticity of the blood-vessels and muscles.

CHROMIC ACID is used in several industries, particularly in chromium plating. Unless precautions are taken it may lead to dermatitis of the hands, arms, chest and face. It may also cause deep ulcers, especially of the nasal septum and knuckles.

CHROMOSOMES The rod-shaped bodies to be found in the nucleus of every cell in the body. They contain the GENES, or hereditary elements, which establish the characteristics of an individual. Composed of a long double coiled filament of DNA, they occur in pairs – one from the maternal, the other from the paternal – and human beings possess forty-six, made up of twenty-three pairs. The number of chromosomes is specific for each species of animal. Each chromosone can duplicate an exact copy of itself between each cell division. (See GENETIC CODE; GENETICS; HEREDITY; MEIOSIS; SEX CHROMOSOMES.)

CHRONIC A persistent or recurring condition. The disease, which may or may not be severe, often starts gradually and changes will be slow. Opposite: acute.

CHRONIC OBSTRUCTIVE PULMONARY DISEASE (COPD) An umbrella title that includes smoking-related lung diseases such as BRONCHITIS, chronic airway-flow limitation,

EMPHYSEMA and some cases of chronic ASTHMA. The disease is underdiagnosed, with only a quarter of sufferers being identified. Early warning signs may be passed off by the victim as 'smoker's cough'. Symptoms include cyanosis – blue tinge to the skin because of oxygen shortage – and breathlessness. Patients may develop HEART failure and OEDEMA. Treatment is of the underlying disease and, most importantly, cessation of smoking. The British Thoracic Society has recently prepared guidelines for primary health-care teams on management of COPD.

CHYLE   The milky fluid which is absorbed by the lymphatic vessels of the intestine. The absorbed portion consists of fats in very fine emulsion, like milk, so that these vessels receive the name of lacteals (L. *lac*, milk). This absorbed chyle mixes with the lymph and is discharged into the thoracic duct, a vessel, which passes up through the chest to open into the jugular vein on the left side of the neck, where the chyle mixes with the blood.

CHYLURIA   The passage of CHYLE in the urine. This results in the passing of a milky-looking urine. It is one of the manifestations of FILARIASIS, where it is due to obstruction of the LYMPHATICS by the causative parasite.

CHYME   Partly digested food as it issues from the stomach into the intestine. It is very acid and grey in colour, containing salts and sugars in solution, and the animal food softened into a semi-liquid mass. It is next converted into chyle.

CHYMOPAPAIN   An ENZYME obtained from the paw-paw, which is being used in the treatment of prolapsed INTERVERTEBRAL DISCS. When injected into the disc it dissolves it.

CHYMOTRYPSIN   An ENZYME produced by the PANCREAS which digests protein. It is used as an aid in operations for removal of a cataract (see ZONULOLYSIS), and also by inhalation to loosen and liquefy secretions in the windpipe and bronchi.

CICATRIX   Another word for scar.

CILIA   A term applied to minute, lash-like processes which are seen with the aid of the microscope upon the cells covering certain mucous membranes: e.g. the TRACHEA (or windpipe) and nose and which maintain movement in the fluid passing over these membranes. They are also found on certain bacteria which have the power of rapid movement.

CILIARY BODY   That part of the eye that connects the IRIS and the CHOROID. The ciliary ring is next to the choroid, the ciliary proc-

esses comprise many ridges behind the iris, to which the lens's suspensory ligament is attached, and the ciliary muscle, which contracts to change the curvature of the lens and so adjust the accommodation of the eye. (See EYE.)

CIMETIDINE is a drug (known as an H_2 ANTAGONIST) that is widely used in the treatment of PEPTIC ULCER. It acts by reducing the hyperacidity of the gastric juice by antagonizing histamine receptors in the stomach.

CIMEX LECTULARIUS (see BED BUG).

CINCHONA   The general name for several trees in the bark of which quinine is found. This bark is also known as Jesuit's bark, having been brought first to notice by Spanish priests in South America and brought to Europe first by the Countess of Cinchon, wife of the Viceroy of Peru, in 1640. The red cinchona bark is that which contains most quinine, and from which it is usually prepared. (See QUININE.) Various extracts and tinctures are made direct from cinchona bark, and used in place of quinine.

CINNAMON   The bark of *Cinnamomum zeylanicum*, a species of laurel grown in Sri Lanka (Ceylon). It has a stimulating action upon the stomach, and assists digestion; hence its use as a condiment. It is also an antispasmodic.

CIRCLE OF WILLIS, or CIRCULUS ARTERIOSUS, is a circle of arteries at the base of the brain, which is formed by the junction of the basilar, posterior cerebral, internal carotid and anterior cerebral arteries. Congenital defects may occur in these arteries and lead to the formation of ANEURYSMS. (See diagram, BRAIN.)

CIRCULATION OF THE BLOOD   This principle was demonstrated for the first time by William Harvey in 1628. Harvey proved, first of all, mainly by the examination of living animals, that the arteries contain only blood. Secondly, he showed by three main propositions that this blood must go round from arteries to veins in a continuous circuit. (1) The quantity of blood passing from the veins into the heart in the course of a whole day is so great that it is quite impossible it could all be manufactured from the food. (2) The blood in the arteries passes in a constant stream to all the members of the body, and does not return by the same route. (3) The blood in the veins flows incessantly to the heart, and does not ebb and flow, as is shown by the valves in veins and in the heart, and by the fact that veins when pressed on do not fill from above. Having proved these points, he assumed there must be 'pores in the flesh' through which the blood 'percolated' from the ends of the arteries to the commencements of the veins. The last link in the evidence was supplied some thirty years later by Malpighi, an Italian scientist, who with the help of the microscope showed these 'pores' to be the minute vessels now called capillaries.

The course of the circulation is as follows   The veins pour their blood, coming from the head, trunk, limbs and abdominal organs, into the right atrium of the heart. This contracts and drives the blood into the right ventricle, which then forces the blood into the lungs by way of the pulmonary artery. Here it is contained in thin-walled capillaries, over which the air plays freely, and through which gases pass readily out

1 aorta	8 bloodflow to body
2 superior vena cava	9 left pulmonary artery
3 bundle of His	10 pulmonary veins
4 right atrium	11 left atrium
5 right ventricle	12 left ventricle
6 inferior vena cava	13 course of electroneural
7 bloodflow from body	impulses

Diagram of the heart and attendant blood vessels opened from the front to show the flow of blood.

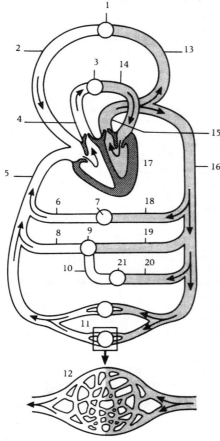

1 head and neck	12 capillary bed
2 superior vena cava	13 carotid artery
3 lungs	14 pulmonary vein
4 pulmonary artery	15 aorta
5 inferior vena cava	16 descending aorta
6 renal vein	17 heart
7 kidney	18 renal artery
8 hepatic vein	19 hepatic artery
9 liver	20 mesenteric and
10 hepatic portal vein	gastric artery
11 limbs	21 gut

Schematic plan of the body's circulation

and in. The blood gives off carbon dioxide (CO_2) and takes up oxygen (see RESPIRATION), and passes on by the pulmonary veins to the left atrium of the heart. The left atrium expels it into the left ventricle, which forces it on into the aorta, by which it is distributed all over the body. Passing through capillaries in the various tissues, it enters the veins, which ultimately unite into two great veins, the superior and the inferior vena cava, these emptying into the right atrium. This complete circle is accomplished by any particular drop of blood in about half a minute.

In one part of the body there is a further complication. The veins coming from the bowels, charged with food material and other products, split up, and their blood undergoes a second capillary circulation through the liver. Here it is relieved of some food material and purified, and then passes into the inferior vena cava, and so to the right atrium. This is known as the portal circulation.

The circle is maintained always in one direction by four valves, situated one at the outlet from each cavity of the heart. (See HEART.)

The blood in the arteries going to the body generally is bright red, that in the veins dull red in colour, owing to the former being charged with oxygen, the latter with carbon dioxide (see RESPIRATION). For the same reason the blood in the pulmonary artery is dark, that in

1 brachiocephalic trunk
2 aortic arch
3 superior vena cava
4 right pulmonary artery
5 right atrium
6 right superior and inferior pulmonary veins
7 right coronary artery
8 right ventricle
9 inferior vena cava

10 descending aorta
11 left common carotid artery
12 left subclavian artery
13 left pulmonary artery
14 left superior and inferior pulmonary veins
15 left atrium
16 branches of left coronary artery
17 left ventricle

Anterior view of heart showing main blood vessels including coronary arteries.

the pulmonary veins bright. There is no direct communication between the right and left sides of the heart, the blood passing from the right ventricle to the left atrium through the lungs.

In the embryo, before birth, the course of circulation is somewhat different, owing to the fact that no nourishment comes from the bowels nor air into the lungs. Accordingly, two large arteries pass out of the navel, and convey blood to be changed by contact with maternal blood (see PLACENTA), while a large vein brings this blood back again. There are also communications between the right and left atria, and between pulmonary artery and aorta. The latter is known as the ductus arteriosus. At birth all these extra vessels and connections close and rapidly shrivel up.

CIRCUMCISION A surgical procedure to remove the prepuce of the penis in males and a part or all of the external genitalia in females. Circumcision is mainly done for religious or ethnic reasons. There is virtually no medical or surgical reason for circumcision in the male new-born infant. The prepuce is not normally retractable in infancy so this is not an indication for circumcision. By the age of one the prepuce is retractable in most boys. The Americans are more enthusiastic about circumcision, and the reason offered is that cancer of the penis occurs only when a foreskin is present.

This is however a rare disease. In the uncircumcised adult there is an increased transmission of herpes and cytomegaloviruses during the reproductive years but this can be reduced by adequate cleansing. PHIMOSIS is an indication for circumcision. Haemorrhage, infection and meatal stenosis are rare complications of circumcision.

Circumcision in women is a damaging procedure, involving the removal of all or parts of the clitoris, labia majora and labia minora, sometimes combined with narowing of the entrance to the vagina. The result may be psychological and sexual problems and complications in child-birth, with no known benefit to the woman's health, though cultural pressures have resulted in its continuation in some Muslim and African countries, despite widespread condemnation of the practice and campaigns to stop it. It has been estimated that over 80 million women in 30 countries have been circumcised.

CIRRHOSIS, or FIBROSIS, is a diseased condition, in which the proper tissue is replaced by fibrous tissue similar to scar tissue. The name cirrhosis was originally given by Laennec to the disease as occurring in the liver, because of its yellow colour. (See LIVER DISEASES.)

CIRSOID ANEURYSM The condition in which a group of arteries become abnormally dilated and tortuous.

CISPLATIN A toxic drug with an alkylating action that gives it useful anti-tumour properties, especially against solid tumours such as ovarian and testicular cancers (see CYTOTOXIC).

CITRIC ACID This is responsible for the sharp taste associated with citrus fruits, such as lemons and limes, and other fruits such as currants and raspberries. Although chemically different, it is similar in action and appearance to tartaric acid, obtained from grapes and other fruits, and similar to malic acid, found in apples and pears.

Uses These acids stimulate the flow of saliva, and hence act to allay thirst and create a feeling of coolness, valuable in the treatment of fever.

CLAUDICATION A cramplike pain that occurs in the legs on walking. It may cause the sufferer to limp or, if severe, stop him or her from walking. The usual cause is narrowing or blockage of the arteries in the legs due to atherosclerosis. Intermittent claudication occurs when a person has to stop every so often to let the pain, caused by the build-up of waste products in the muscles, to subside. The condition may be improved by the patient's walking for an hour a day (resting when the pain starts). Oxpentifylline, a vasodilator, may help, as may calcium-channel-blocking drugs. Patients must avoid all tobacco products.

CLAUSTROPHOBIA Fear of being in a confined space, or the fear experienced while in it.

CLAVICLE The bone which runs from the upper end of the breast- bone towards the tip of the shoulder across the root of the neck. It supports the upper limb, keeps it out from the side, and gives breadth to the shoulders. The bone is shaped like an 'f' with two curves, which give it increased strength. It is, however, liable to be broken by falls on the hand or on the shoulder, and is the most frequently fractured bone in the body. (See FRACTURES.)

CLAW-FOOT, or PES CAVUS, is a familial deformity of the foot characterized by an abnormally high arch of the foot accompanied by shortening of the foot, clawing of the toes and inversion, or turning inwards, of the foot and heel. Its main effect is to impair the resilience of the foot resulting in a stiff gait and aching pain. Milder cases are treated with special shoes fitted with a sponge rubber insole. More severe cases may require surgical treatment.

CLAW-HAND A (contraction) deformity of the hand and fingers, especially of the ring and little fingers. The condition is generally due to paralysis of the ulnar nerve. A somewhat similar condition is produced by contraction of the fibrous tissues in the palm of the hand, partly due to rheumatic changes and partly to injury caused by the constant pressure of a tool against the palm of the hand. (See DUPUYTREN'S CONTRACTURE.)

CLAW-TOES (see CLAW-FOOT).

CLEFT FOOT A rare congenital abnormality characterized by the absence of one or more toes and a deep central cleft that divides the foot into two. It is sometimes known as lobster foot or lobster claw. It may be accompanied by other congenital defects, such as cleft hand, absent permanent teeth, cleft lip and palate, absence of the nails, and defects of the eye.

CLEFT HAND A rare congenital abnormality characterized by the absence of one or more fingers and a deep central cleft that divides the hand into two. It is sometimes known as lobster hand. It may be accompanied by other congenital defects, such as cleft foot, absent permanent teeth, cleft lip and palate, absence of the nails and defects of the eye.

CLEFT PALATE A fissure in the roof of the mouth (palate) and/or the lip which is present at birth. It is found in varying degrees of severity in about 1 in 700 children. Modern plastic surgery can greatly improve the appearance of the baby and often further cosmetic surgery later will not be necessary. The parent of the child who has cleft lip and/or palate will be given detailed advice specific to his case. In general the team of specialists involved are the paediatrician, plastic surgeon, dentist or orthodontic specialist, and speech therapist. (See PALATE, MALFORMATIONS OF.)

CLICKING FINGER A condition usually occurring in middle-aged people in which the victim finds on wakening in the morning that he or she cannot straighten the ring or middle finger spontaneously, but only by a special effort, when it suddenly straightens with a painful click. Hence the name. In due course the finger remains bent at all times unless a special effort is made to straighten it with the other hand. The condition is due to a swelling developing in one of the tendons of the affected finger. If the tendon sheath is slit open surgically, the condition is relieved. Many cases recover spontaneously if the patient is prepared to wait.

CLIMACTERIC This was a word originally applied to the end of certain epochs or stages in the life of an individual, at which some great change was supposed to take place. (See also MENOPAUSE.)

CLINDAMYCIN An antibiotic used in the treatment of serious infections. It is active against GRAM-POSITIVE cocci, including penicillin-resistant STAPHYLOCOCCI and also many ANAEROBES, especially *Bacteroides fragilis*. It is recommended for staphylococcal bone and joint infections such as OSTEOMYELITIS and intra-abdominal sepsis, as well as ENDOCARDITIS prophylaxis. Clindamycin has only limited use because of its adverse effects; patients should discontinue immediately if diarrhoea or colitis develops.

CLINICAL means literally 'belonging to a bed', but the word is used to denote anything associated with the practical study or observation of sick people, as clinical medicine, clinical thermometers.

CLINICAL GOVERNANCE A concept, introduced in a UK government White Paper in 1997, aimed at 'ensuring that all NHS organizations have in place proper processes for continuously monitoring and improving clinical audit'. All clinicians and managers will be expected to understand their individual and collective responsibilities for assuring accountability for the quality of patient care. Clinical governance will be included in the NHS legislation based on the 1997 White Paper. (See also MEDICAL AUDIT.)

CLINICAL GUIDELINES Systematically developed statements which assist clinicians and patients to decide on appropriate treatments for specific conditions. The guidelines are attractive to health managers and patients because they are potentially able to standardize clinical practice around an appropriate norm. This helps to ensure that patients receive the right treatment of an acceptable standard. In the United Kingdom the NHS Executive has with advice from doctors been developing and adopting high-quality national guidelines to improve clinical effectiveness of NHS care. Some doctors have reservations about guidelines because (1) health-care managers might use them primarily to contain costs; (2) inflexibility would discourage clinical innovations; (3) they could encourage litigation by patients.

CLINICAL PSYCHOLOGY Psychology is the scientific study of behaviour. It may be applied in various settings including education, industry and health care. Clinical psychology is concerned with the practical application of research findings in the fields of physical and mental health. Training in clinical psychology involves a degree in Psychology followed by postgraduate training. Clinical psychologists are specifically skilled in applying theoretical models and objective methods of observation and measurement and in therapeutic interventions aimed at changing patient's dysfunctional behaviour, including thoughts and feelings as well as actions. Dysfunctional behaviour is explained in terms of normal processes and modified by applying principles of normal learning, adaption and social interaction.

Clinical psychologists are involved in health care in the following ways: (1) Assessment of thoughts, emotions and behaviour using standardized methods. (2) Treatment based on theoretical models and scientific evidence about behaviour change. Behaviour change is considered when it contributes to physical, psychological or social functioning. (3) Consultation with other health-care professionals about problems concerning emotions, thinking and behaviour. (4) Research on a wide variety of topics including the relationship between stress, psychological functioning and disease, the aetiology of problem behaviours, methods and theories of behaviour change. (5) Teaching other professionals about normal and dysfunctional behaviour, emotions and functioning.

Clinical psychologists may specialize in work in particular branches of patient care, including surgery, psychiatry, geriatrics, paediatrics, mental handicap, obstetrics and gynaecology, cardiology, neurology, general practice and physical rehabilitation. Whilst the focus of their work is frequently the patient, at times it may encompass the behaviour of the health-care professionals.

CLINICAL RISK MANAGEMENT Initially driven by anxiety about the possibility of medical negligence cases, clinical risk management has evolved into the study of iatrogenic disease. The first priority of risk managers is to ensure that all therapies in medicine are as safe as possible. Allied to this is a recognition that errors may occur even when error-prevention strategies are in place. Lastly, any accidents that occur are analysed, allowing a broader understanding of their cause. Risk management is generally centred on single adverse events. The threat of litigation is taken as an opportunity to expose unsafe conditions of practice and to put pressure on those with the authority to implement change. These might include senior clinicians, hospital management, the purchasing authorities, and even the secretary of state for health. Attention is focused on organizational factors rather than the individuals involved in a specific case.

CLINICAL SIGNS The physical manifestations of an illness elicited by a doctor when examining a patient, e.g. a rash, lump, swelling or fever.

CLINICAL TRIALS Voltaire defined medical treatment as the act of pouring drugs, of which one knew nothing, into a patient, of whom one knew less. This derisive appraisal of the therapeutics of his time was nearly true as there were virtually no drugs of significant therapeutic value and any benefit the patient received was usually a placebo effect.

The development of effective medical treatment only dates back 50 years or so. When useful drugs did become available in the 1940s and the 1950s doctors realized the importance of evaluating their effectiveness. This lead to the introduction of the so-called clinical trials. Systematic measures were introduced to assess the efficacy initially of new medicines and, later, of surgical operations. This is now done by controlled, randomized clinical trials which compare the new treatment under evaluation either with a placebo or the previous standard treatment. If possible this is done on a double blind basis when neither the patient nor the doctor knows at the time whether the test treatment or the control is being administered: this enables bias to be removed. Such trials have to be done to recognized ethical standards with the procedure properly explained to the participating subjects. (See EVIDENCE-BASED MEDICINE.)

CLINICS (see MATERNITY AND CHILD WELFARE).

CLITORIS   A small sensitive organ comprising erectile tissue at the top of the female genitalia where the labial folds meet below the pubic bone. Clitoral tissue extends into the anterior roof of the vagina. During sexual excitement the clitoris enlarges and hardens and may be the focus of orgasm. (See CIRCUMCISION.)

CLOFAZIMINE   A drug used in the treatment of LEPROSY.

CLOFIBRATE (see HYPERLIPIDAEMIA).

CLOMIPHENE   A drug that stimulates ovulation, or the production of ova, through the medium of the pituitary gland. When used in the treatment of female infertility, one of its hazards is that, if given in too big doses, it may produce multiple births.

CLOMIPRAMINE   A tricyclic antidepressant drug. (See ANTIDEPRESSANTS.)

CLONAZEPAM   A drug to treat EPILEPSY and MYOCLONUS. (See TRANQUILLIZER.)

CLONE   A group of cells genetically identical to each other that have arisen from one cell by asexual reproduction (see CLONING).

CLONIC   A word applied to short spasmodic movements.

CLONIDINE   A drug originally introduced for the treatment of high blood-pressure. It is an alpha$_2$ adrenoreceptor agonist. It may also help in the prevention of attacks of migraine. If it is used in the treatment of high blood-pressure, its use must not be stopped abruptly as this may result in a sudden rise of blood-pressure within a matter of hours to a dangerously high level.

CLONING, from the Greek *klon* meaning a cutting such as is used to propagate plants, is essentially a form of asexual reproduction. The initial stages have been successfully achieved in rabbits. In essence the technique consists of destroying the nucleus of the egg and replacing it with the nucleus from a body cell of the same species – either a male or a female. This provides the egg with a full complement of CHROMOSOMES and it starts to divide and grow just at it would if it had retained its nucleus and been fertilized with a spermatozoon. The vital difference is that the embryo resulting from this cloning process owes nothing genetically to the female egg. It is identical in every respect with the animal from which the introduced nucleus was obtained.

In 1997 the first mammal to be cloned from the tissue of an adult animal was born. A technique that scientists have been trying to perfect for decades, the success of the Roslin Institute, near Edinburgh, in producing 'Dolly', a cloned sheep, has profound implications. Already some scientists are talking of cloning humans, though this seems a distant prospect and one with great medical, legal and ethical consequences. The key to the scientists' success in producing Dolly was the ability to coordinate the fusion of a donor cell (from an adult) containing all its DNA with a recipient egg from which DNA had been removed. The difficulty of the technique is shown by the fact that, out of 277 fused pairs of cells where the donor cell was from adult tissue, Dolly was the only survivor.

CLONUS   A succession of intermittent muscular relaxations and contractions usually resulting from a sustained stretching stimulus. An example is the clonus stimulated in the calf muscle by maintaining sustained upward pressure on the sole of the foot. The condition is often a sign of disease in the brain or spinal cord.

CLOSTRIDIUM   The genus, or variety, of micro-organisms that produce spores which enable them to survive under adverse conditions. They normally grow in soil, water and decomposing plant and animal matter, where they play an important part in the process of PUTREFACTION. Among the important members of the group, or genus, are *Clostridium welchii*, *Cl. septicum* and *Cl. oedematiens*, the causes of gas gangrene (see GANGRENE); *Cl. tetani*, the cause of TETANUS; and *Cl. botulinum*, the cause of BOTULISM.

CLOT   The term applied to any semi-solid mass of blood, lymph or other body fluid. Clotting in the blood is due to the formation of strings of fibrin produced by the action of a ferment. Milk clots in a similar manner in the stomach when exposed to the action of the ferment rennin. Clotting occurs naturally when blood is shed and comes in contact with tissues outside the blood-vessels. It occurs also at times in diseased vessels (thrombosis), producing serious effects upon the tissues supplied or drained by these vessels. Clots also form sometimes in the heart when the circulation is feeble and irregular. (See COAGULATION; EMBOLISM; THROMBOSIS.)

CLOTRIMAZOLE   A drug of the IMIDAZOLE group used to treat fungal infections of the skin and vagina.

CLOTTING TIME (see COAGULATION).

CLOXACILLIN   An ANTIBIOTIC used to treat infections caused by penicillinase-producing STAPHYLOCOCCI. (See PENICILLIN, ANTIBIOTIC.)

CLOZAPINE   A recently introduced antipsychotic drug used to treat schizophrenic patients who have not responded to other treatments or have suffered serious side-effects from them. Improvement is gradual and it may be several weeks before severe symptoms are relieved. The drug can cause AGRANULOCYTOSIS and so it is given under close hospital supervision.

CLUBBING   The term applied to the thickening and broadening of the finger tips and, less commonly, the tips of the toes, that occurs in certain chronic diseases of the lungs and heart. It is due to interstitial oedema especially at the nail bed leading to a loss of the acute angle between the nail and the skin of the finger. It is associated with lung cancer, empyema, bronchietasis and congenital cyanotic heart disease.

CLUB-FOOT (see TALIPES).

CLUSTER HEADACHES   This is a distinct entity separate from migraine, although it is sometimes referred to as migrainous neuralgia. The name derives from the fact that the headaches cluster in periods of six to twelve weeks at certain times of the year. The headache is usually on one side and often around the eye. Lacrimation and running of the nose are frequently associated. A chronic form in which attacks persist for more than six months exists. Prophylactic treatment with LITHIUM CARBONATE is usually effective.

COAGULATION of the blood is the process whereby bleeding (or haemorrhage) is normally arrested in the body. Blood starts to clot as soon as the skin (or other tissue) has been cut. Coagulation is part of the process of HAEMOSTASIS which is the arrest of bleeding from an injured or diseased blood vessel. Haemostasis depends on the combined activities of vascular, PLATELET and PLASMA elements which are offset by processes to restrict the accumulation of platelets and FIBRIN to the damaged area. The

three-stage process of coagulation is complex, involving many different substances. It is simply summarized in the following diagram:

$$\text{prothrombin + calcium + thromboplastin}$$
$$\downarrow$$
$$\text{thrombin + fibrinogen}$$
$$\downarrow$$
$$\text{fibrin}$$

Prothrombin and calcium are normally present in the blood. Thromboplastin is an enzyme which is normally found in the blood platelets and in tissue cells. When bleeding occurs from a blood-vessel there is always some damage to tissue cells and to the blood platelets. As a result of this damage, thromboplastin is released and comes in contact with the prothrombin and calcium in the blood. In the presence of thromboplastin and calcium prothrombin is converted into thrombin, which in turn interacts with fibrinogen, a protein always present in the blood, to form fibrin. Fibrin consists of needle-shaped crystals, which, with the assistance of the blood platelets, form a fine network in which the blood corpuscles become enmeshed. This meshwork, or clot as it is known, gradually retracts until it forms a tight mass which, unless the tissue injury is very severe or a major artery has been damaged, prevents any further bleeding. It will thus be seen that clotting, or coagulation, does not occur in the healthy blood-vessel because there is no thromboplastin present. There is now evidence suggesting that there is an anti-thrombin substance present in the blood in small amounts, and that this substance antagonizes any small amounts of thrombin that may be formed as a result of small amounts of thromboplastin being released. The clotting or coagulation time is the time taken for blood to clot and can be measured under controlled conditions to ensure that it is normal (three to eight minutes). In certain diseases – HAEMOPHILIA, for example – clotting time is greatly extended.

COARCTATION OF THE AORTA   A narrowing of the aorta in the vicinity of the insertion of the ductus arteriosus. It is a congenital abnormality. Satisfactory results are now obtained from surgical treatment.

COBALAMINS   A group of substances which have an enzyme action (see ENZYME) and are essential for normal growth and nutrition. (See also CYANOCOBALAMIN; HYDROXOCOBALAMIN.)

COBALT-60 is a radioactive isotope of the metallic element cobalt (Co). It is used in the treatment of malignant disease. (See RADIOTHERAPY.)

COCAINE   Coca leaves are obtained from two South American plants, *Erythroxylum coca* and *Erythroxylum truxillense*, and contain an alkaloid, cocaine, which has marked effects as a stimulant, and, locally applied, as an anaesthetic by paralysing nerves of sensation. The dried leaves have been used from time immemorial by the South American Indians, who chew them mixed with a little lime. Their effect is to dull the mucous surfaces of mouth and stomach, with which the saliva, produced by chewing them, comes into contact, thus blunting, for long periods, all feeling of hunger. The cocaine, being absorbed, produces on the central nervous system a stimulating effect, so that all sense of fatigue and breathlessness vanishes for the time. It was by the use of coca that the Indian post-runners of South America were able to achieve their extraordinary feats of endurance. The continued use of the drug, however, results in emaciation, loss of memory, sleeplessness and general breakdown. Addiction to cocaine or a derivative, 'crack', is now a serious social problem in many countries. (See DRUG ADDICTION.)

Uses Before the serious effects that result from its habitual use were realized, the drug was sometimes used by hunters, travellers and others to relieve exhaustion and breathlessness in climbing mountains and to dull hunger. The chief use in medicine has been by local application to dull pain. Now it is used only in the treatment of diseases of the ear, nose and throat. A 5-per-cent spray solution is used to anaesthetize the throat and nose. Because of its serious side-effects and the risk of addiction, cocaine is now a carefully controlled drug.

COCCI Spherical bacteria that cause a variety of infections. STAPHYLOCOCCI, STREPTOCOCCI and MENINGOCOCCI are examples.

COCCYDYNIA, or COCCYGODYNIA, means the sensation of severe pain in the coccyx.

COCCYX The lower end of the SPINAL COLUMN, resembling a bird's beak and consisting of four fused nodules of bone, which represent vertebrae, and correspond to the tail in lower animals. Above the coccyx lies a much larger bone, the SACRUM, and together they form the back wall of the PELVIS, which protects the organs in the lower ABDOMEN.

COCHLEA That part of the inner ear concerned with hearing. (See EAR.)

COCHLEAR INPLANTS A cochlear implant is an electronic device, inserted under a general anaesthetic, which stimulates the auditory system, restoring partial hearing in profound sensory deafness. Although there are many types of cochlear implant, they all consist of a microphone, a signal processor, a signal coupler (transmitter and receiver), and an array of electrodes. Most are multi-channel implants. The microphone and signal processor are worn outside the body, like a conventional hearing aid. They receive sound and convert it into an electronic signal which is transmitted through the skin to the receiver. Here the signal is transmitted to the array of electrodes which stimulates the cochlear nerve. Although cochlear implants do not provide normal hearing, most profoundly deaf patients who receive a cochlear implant are able to detect a variety of sounds, including environmental sounds and speech. The duration of hearing loss and age at implantation are among the many factors which influence the results.

CODEINE One of the active principles of OPIUM, it is an ANALGESIC which in the form of codeine phosphate is used to suppress persistent coughs and to relieve pain such as headaches and musculoskeletal discomfort. Side-effects include constipation, nausea and sleepiness. Dependence is rare.

COD-LIVER OIL is derived from the fresh liver of the cod (*Gadus callarius*). It is a rich source of vitamin D, used in the prevention and treatment of rickets, and vitamin A. Human milk contains more than enough vitamin D for the breast-fed baby, provided the mother has a balanced diet, with adequate exposure to sunlight, or is taking vitamin supplements during pregnancy and lactation if considered necessary. All baby foods in the UK contain added vitamins, and therefore supplementation is unnecessary until weaning begins, and the baby starts taking cow's milk, which contains less vitamin D than human milk. (See APPENDIX 5: VITAMINS.)

COELIAC DISEASE A wasting disease of childhood in which there is inability to absorb fat from the intestines; there is therefore an excess of fat in the stools. It is the result of a constitutional intolerance of GLUTEN (a constituent of wheat flour) which damages the lining membrane of the SMALL INTESTINE. This in turn interferes with the absorption of fat. Treatment is by means of a gluten-free diet. People with coeliac disease, or parents or guardians of coeliac children can obtain help and guidance from the Coeliac Society of the United Kingdom, (see APPENDIX 2: ADDRESSES). (See also GLUTEN; MALABSORPTION SYNDROME; SPRUE.)

COELIOSCOPY A method of viewing the interior of the abdomen in patients in whom a tumour or some other condition requiring operation may be present but cannot with certainty be diagnosed. The examination is carried out by making a minute opening under local anaesthesia, and inserting an ENDOSCOPE, a long flexible instrument bearing an electric lamp and telescopic lenses like that for examining the bladder (cystoscope), into the abdominal cavity. Certain of the abdominal organs can then be directly inspected in turn.

COGNITION The mental processes by which a person acquires knowledge. Among these are reasoning, creative actions and solving problems.

COGNITIVE BEHAVIOURAL THERAPY A technique for the treatment of mental disorders that is based on the concept that how people perceive the world and themselves influences their behaviour and emotions. A depressed individual may think that all untoward events are his or her fault, while good events occur by chance. The therapist points out the falsity of this perception and urges the patient to think more positively.

COHORT STUDY A systemized follow-up study of people for a specific time or until the occurrence of a defined event such as a particular illness or death. The aim is to follow the disease course and/or the reasons for the participants' deaths. Different cohorts may be compared and conclusions drawn about a particular disease or drug treatment.

COITUS is sexual intercourse.
Coitus interruptus (see CONTRACEPTION).

COLCHICUM The bulb of *Colchicum autumnale*, or meadow-saffron, has long been used as a remedy for gout. How it acts is not quite certain.

Uses Its main use is in gout, for which colchicine, the active principle of colchicum, in doses of 0·5 mg every one or two hours until the pain is relieved, followed by 0·5 mg thrice daily for about a week, is the form generally employed.

COLD, INJURIES FROM (see CHILBLAIN; FROSTBITE; HYPOTHERMIA; also CHILLS AND COLDS).

COLD SORES (see HERPES SIMPLEX).

COLD WEATHER ITCH is a common form of itchiness that occurs in cold weather. It is characterized by slight dryness of the skin, and is particularly troublesome in the legs of old people. The dryness may be accompanied by some mild inflammation of the skin. Treatment is by the application of emollients such as aqueous cream or zinc ointment.

COLDS (see CHILLS AND COLDS).

COLECTOMY The operation for removing the colon.

COLIC This term is generally used for an attack of spasmodic pain in the abdomen.

Simple colic often results from the build-up of indigestible material in the alimentary tract, leading to spasmodic contractions in the muscular lining. Other causes include habitual constipation, with accumulation of faecal material; and as an accompaniment of neurological disorders. Major risks include sudden obstruction of the bowel from twisting, intussusception, or as a result of a tumour or similar condition. (See INTESTINE, DISEASES OF; INTUSSUSCEPTION.)

Lead colic (also known as painter's colic, colica Pictonum, Devonshire colic, dry belly-ache) is due to the absorption of lead into the system. (See LEAD POISONING.)

Biliary colic and **renal colic** are the terms applied to that violent pain which is produced, in the one case where a biliary calculus or gall-stone passes down from the gall-bladder into the intestine, and in the other where a renal calculus descends from the kidney along the ureter into the bladder. (See GALL-BLADDER, DISEASES OF; and KIDNEYS, DISEASES OF.)

Treatment This consists of means to relieve the spasmodic pain with warmth and analgesics, and removal where possible, of the underlying cause.

COLIFORM Description of a gram negative bacterium found in the faeces. It covers the bacterial groups *Enterobacter*, *Escherichia*, and *Klebsiella*.

COLISTIN A polymyxin antibiotic (see POLYMYXIN) active against many Gram-negative organisms, including *Pseudomonas aeruginosa*. It is not absorbed by mouth and therefore needs to be given by injection to obtain a systemic effect; this is rarely indicated, however, as it has serious adverse effects. Colistin is used by mouth in bowel-sterilization regimens before surgery in NEUTROPENIC patients. It is given by inhalation of a nebulized solution as an adjunct to some standard antibiotic therapy, and is included in some topical preparations, chiefly for skin, eye and ear infections.

COLITIS Inflammation of the colon, the first part of the large intestine. The subject suffers from diarrhoea, usually passing blood and mucus, abdominal pain or discomfort and fever. Colitis can be caused by various micro-organisms: for example, CAMPYLOBACTER and SHIGELLA bacteria, viruses or amoeba. Anxiety and antibiotic drugs may also cause colitis, the latter by directly irritating the lining of the gut.

Ulcerative colitis, the most important form, is an acute condition of unknown cause. Suggested causes include an abnormal immune response, possibly to bacteria or certain foods. Amoebiasis (see DYSENTERY) should be excluded. Predominantly a disease of young adults, it is very liable to relapse and the rectum is always affected. There is a strong familial tendency, with an association between ulcerative colitis, ankylosing spondylitis and Crohn's disease.

SYMPTOMS The onset may be sudden or insidious. In the acute form there is severe diarrhoea and the patient may pass up to twenty stools a day. The stools, which may be small in quantity, are fluid and contain blood, pus and mucus. There is always fever, which runs an irregular course. In other cases the patient first notices some irregularity of the movement of the bowels, with the passage of blood. This becomes gradually more marked. There may be pain but usually a varying amount of abdominal discomfort. The constant diarrhoea leads to emaciation, weakness and anaemia. As a rule the acute phase passes into a chronic stage. The chronic form is liable to run a prolonged course, and most patients suffer relapses for many years. SIGMOIDOSCOPY, BIOPSY, abdominal X-RAY and BARIUM ENEMA are essential diagnostic procedures.

TREATMENT Non-specific, though complete bedrest is essential during the acute stage, with a high-protein, low-residue diet. Corticosteroids, given by mouth or enema, help to control the diarrhoea. Intravenous nutrition may be required. The anaemia is treated with iron supplements, with blood infusions if necessary. Blood cultures should be taken, repeatedly if the fever persists. If septicaemia is suspected, broad-spectrum antibiotics should be given. Surgery to remove part of the affected colon may be necessary. After recovery, the patient should remain on a low-residue diet, with regular follow-up by the physician, Mesalazine and SULPHASALAZINE are helpful in the prevention of recurrences.

Patients and their relatives can obtain help and advice from the National Association for Colitis and Crohn's Disease (see APPENDIX 2: ADDRESSES).

COLLAGEN The most abundant protein in the body. It is the major structural component of many parts of the body and occurs in many different forms. Thus it exists as thick fibres in skin and tendons. It is also an important constituent of the heart and blood vessels. With calcium salts it provides the rigid structure of bone. It also occurs as a delicate structure in the cornea of the eye, and in what is known as the basement membrane of many tissues including the glomeruli of the kidneys and the capsule of the lens of the eye. It plays a part in many diseases, hereditary and otherwise. Among the inherited abnormalities of collagen are those responsible for aneurysms of the CIRCLE OF WILLIS and for OSTEOGENESIS IMPERFECTA. On boiling it is converted into gelatin.

COLLAGEN DISEASES A general term for a group of diseases, including acute rheumatism and rheumatoid arthritis, characterized by changes in the tissue collagen. This group of diseases can be split into true collagen disorder – an uncommon, usually inherited condition resulting in abnormal development of collagen fibres – and connective tissue diseases in which the body's immune system reacts against its own tissues and organs, known as autoimmune disease.

COLLAPSE (see SHOCK).

COLLAR-BONE (see CLAVICLE).

COLLES'S FRACTURE is a fracture of the lower end of the radius close to the wrist, caused usually by a fall forwards on the palm of the hand, in which the lower fragment is displaced backwards. (See FRACTURES.)

COLLODIONS consist basically of a thick, colourless, syrupy liquid, made by dissolving gun-cotton (pyroxylin) in a mixture of ether and alcohol or with acetone. When painted on the skin the solvent evaporates, leaving a tough protective film behind that is useful for covering wounds. Flexible collodion, or collodion as it is often referred to, contains 1·6 per cent of pyroxylin, with colophony, castor oil and alcohol (90 per cent) in solvent ether. It should be kept in a well-sealed container. Being relatively elastic, it does not crack through the movements of the skin.

COLLOID A type of suspension, for instance milk, in which insoluble particles are suspended in a fluid. In medical parlance a colloid preparation is one containing PLASMA PROTEINS and is used to treat patients in SHOCK. The follicles of the thyroid gland also contain a colloid substance.

COLOBOMA simply means a defect, but its use is usually restricted to congenital defects of the eye. These may involve, the lens, the iris, the retina or the eyelid.

COLON The first part of the large intestine. (See INTESTINE.)

COLONIC IRRIGATION Washing out the large bowel with an enema of water or other medication.

COLONOSCOPE An ENDOSCOPE for viewing the interior of the colon. It is made of fibre glass which ensures flexibility, and incorporates a system of lenses for magnification and a lighting system.

COLOSTOMY The operation for the establishment of an artificial opening into the colon. This acts as an artificial anus. The operation is carried out when there is an obstruction in the colon or rectum that cannot be overcome, or in cases, such as cancer of the rectum in which the rectum and part of the colon have to be removed. Such a colostomy opening can be trained to function in such a way that the patient can carry on a normal life, eating a more or less normal diet. Anyone wishing help or advice in the practical management of a colostomy should get in touch with the British Colostomy Association (See APPENDIX 2: ADDRESSES.) (See STOMA.)

COLOSTRUM The first fluid secreted by the mammary glands for two or three days after childbirth. It contains less casein and more albumin than ordinary milk.

COLOUR BLINDNESS (see VISION, Defective colour vision).

COLPORRHAPHY An operation designed to strengthen the pelvic floor in cases of prolapse of the UTERUS. The surgeon excises redundant tissue from the front vaginal wall (anterior colporrhaphy) or from the rear wall (posterior colporrhaphy), thus narrowing the vagina and tightening the muscles.

COLPOSCOPY The method of examining the VAGINA and CERVIX by means of the binocular instrument known as the colposcope. It is used to screen for cancer of the cervix.

COMA A state of profound unconsciousness, in which the patient cannot be roused, and reflex movements are absent. Signs include long, deep, sighing respirations, a rapid, weak pulse, and low blood pressure. Usually the result of a STROKE, it may also be due to high fever, DIABETES MELLITUS, GLOMERULONEPHRITIS, alcohol, EPILEPSY, cerebral TUMOUR, MENINGITIS, injury to the head, overdose of INSULIN, CARBON MONOXIDE POISONING, poisoning from OPIUM and other NARCOTIC drugs. Though usually of relatively short duration, and terminating in death, unless yielding to treatment, it may occasionally last for months or even years. (See UNCONSCIOUSNESS.)

COMA POSITION (see RECOVERY POSITION and APPENDIX 1: BASIC FIRST AID).

COMEDONES (see ACNE).

COMMENSAL Micro-organisms which live in or on the body (e.g. in the gut or respiratory tract, or on the skin) without doing any harm to the individual.

COMMINUTED FRACTURE A break in a bone in which the broken ends splinter into pieces. It is usually the result of a crushing force which also damages surrounding tissues such as nerves, blood vessels and muscles. Such a fracture is harder to set than a simple (clean) break. (See FRACTURES.)

COMMISSURE means a joining, and is a term applied to strands of nerve fibres which join one side of the brain to the other, to the band joining one optic nerve to the other, to the junctions of the lips at the corners of the mouth, etc.

COMMITTEE ON SAFETY OF MEDICINES (CSM) An independent advisory committee – launched in 1971 in the United Kingdom – composed of doctors, pharmacists and other specialists. It advises the Medicines Control Agency in the United Kingdom on the safety, efficacy and pharmaceutical quality of MEDICINES for which licences are sought and also reviews reports of ADVERSE REACTIONS to licensed medicines, including spontaneous 'Yellow Card' reports from doctors or pharmacists who suspect that a patient has suffered an adverse reaction from a medicine. Its predecessor, the Committee for Safety of Drugs, was set up in 1963 in response to the THALIDOMIDE disaster.

COMMON COLD (see CHILLS AND COLDS).

COMMUNICABLE DISEASE This is an infectious or contagious disease, which can be passed from one person to another. Direct physical contact, the handling of an infected object or the transfer by droplets coughed or breathed out are all ways in which microorganisms can be transmitted. The government produces a list of NOTIFIABLE DISEASES, which includes all the dangerous communicable diseases.

COMMUNITY CARE Community care is intended to enable people to lead independent lives at home or in local residential units for as long as they are able to do so. For many years there has been a trend in Britain for care for elderly people and those with mental or physical problems to be shifted from hospitals and into community settings. In 1988 Sir Roy Griffiths's report to the Secretaries of State for Social Services, *Community Care: Agenda for Action*, advised on the best use of public funds to provide effective community care. The White Paper *Caring for People*, published in 1989, outlined the government's ideas for developing these proposals further. The plans were then enshrined in law with the National Health Service and Community Care Act of 1990.

Since April 1993 local social services departments have been responsible for assessing what help people need from community care services. These can include home helps, meals on wheels, sheltered housing, etc. Recipients of these services are means tested and make variable contributions towards the costs. Policies on charging vary from one area to another and there are wide geographical variations in the range of services provided free and the charges levied for others. Some changes are likely as the result of policy initiatives on the organization of the benefits system from the Labour Government.

People with complex needs may be assigned a case manager to coordinate the care package and ensure that appropriate responses are made to changing circumstances. The success of community care hinges on effective coordination of the services of an often large number of providers from the health and social services sectors. Poor communication between sectors and inadequate coordination of services have been among the most common complaints about the community care reforms.

At the time of writing health care for people being cared for in the community remains largely free under the NHS arrangements, although there are regular debates about where the boundaries should be drawn between free health services and means-tested social care.

As care has shifted more and more into the community previous hospital facilities have become redundant. Vast numbers of beds in long-stay geriatric hospitals and in-patient psychiatric wards have been closed. There is now concern that too few beds remain to provide essential emergency and respite services. In some areas delay in setting up community services for elderly people who have been admitted to hospital has caused 'bed blocking' in acute units by people who are ready for discharge to community settings.

Community care, if correctly funded and coordinated, is an excellent way of caring for people with long-term needs, but considerable work is still needed in Britain to ensure that all patients have access to high-quality community care when they need it. Problems in providing such are are not confined to the UK.

COMMUNITY HEALTH COUNCIL A local group of people appointed to represent the views of the local community on services provided by Britain's National Health Service. The councils are funded by the state, have no executive powers, but publish an annual report. Members have access to hospitals and the public can contact them about local services and ways of making complaints about hospital care. (see NATIONAL HEALTH SERVICE).

COMMUNITY PHYSICIAN A doctor who works in the specialty that encompasses PREVENTIVE MEDICINE, EPIDEMIOLOGY and PUBLIC HEALTH.

COMPATIBILITY The extent to which a person's defence systems will accept invading foreign substances, for example, an injection of a drug, a blood transfusion or an organ transplant. When incompatibility occurs there is usually a rapid antibody attack on the invading antigen with a severe local or system reaction in the individual receiving the antigenic substance. (See IMMUNITY.)

COMPENSATION In medical parlance a term applied to the counterbalancing of some defect of structure or function by some other special bodily development. The body possesses a remarkable power of adapting itself to even serious defects, so that disability due to these passes off after a time. The term is most often applied to the ability possessed by the heart to increase in size, and therefore in power, when the need for greater pumping action arises in consequence of a defective valve or some other abnormality in the circulation. A heart in this condition is, however, more liable to be prejudicially affected by strains and diseased processes, and the term 'failure of compensation' is applied to the symptoms that result when this power becomes temporarily insufficient.

Compensation also refers to the financial compensation awarded to an individual who has been injured or been made ill as a result of wrongful action or inaction by another individual or organization. Doctors and other therapists are increasingly being sued for compensation because patients believe that they have had unsatisfactory or damaging treatment. Compensation neurosis or 'traumatic' neurosis is a psychological reaction to the prospects of compensation. It is a condition about which specialists disagree. Sufferers complain of a range of symptoms that may be a genuine consequence of their condition or an exaggerated response.

COMPLEMENT is a normal constituent of blood serum which plays an important part in the antibody-antigen reaction which is the basis of many immunity processes. (See IMMUNITY.)

COMPLEMENTARY MEDICINE, COMPLEMENTARY THERAPY or NON-CONVENTIONAL MEDICINE The term complementary therapy or medicine is often used as a synonym for alternative therapy. However, those treatments which can be used alongside conventional Western-oriented, science-based medical care are best described as complementary. They cover a wide range of practices ranging from YOGA, HEALING, HOMEOPATHY and MASSAGE to OSTEOPATHY and CHIROPRACTIC.

Alternative therapies replace conventional treatments. The accompanying table describes a range of different treatments. Because terms such as complementary, fringe, natural, non-conventional, unorthodox and alternative medicine are used interchangeably, it is probably best to use the non-pejorative title non-conventional therapies. This solution is suggested in *Complementary Medicine: New Approaches to Good Practice* produced by the British Medical Association (Oxford University Press, 1993). That report usefully provides a working definition of non-conventional therapies as follows: 'Those forms of treatment which are not widely used by orthodox health care professionals, and the skills of which are not taught as part of the undergraduate curriculum of orthodox medical and paramedical health care courses.' Readers wanting a helpful source of information on non-conventional therapy should refer to this publication and also to *The Which? Guide to Complementary Medicine* (Barbara Rowlands, Consumer's Association, 1997). (See APPENDIX 13: COMPLEMENTARY MEDICINE.)

COMPLEMENT SYSTEM This is part of the body's defence mechanism that comprises a series of 20 serum PEPTIDES that are sequentially activated to produce three significant effects. These are the release of small peptides which provoke inflammation and attract PHAGOCYTES; secondly, a substance (component C3b) is deposited on the membranes of invading bacteria or viruses and attracts phagocytes to destroy the microbes; thirdly, the activation of substances that damage cell membranes – called lytic components – which hasten the destruction of 'foreign' cells.

COMPLEX The term applied to a combination of various actions or symptoms. The term is particularly applied to a set of symptoms occurring together in mental disease with such regularity as to receive a special name.

COMPLEXION (see ACNE; SKIN DISEASES; SUNBURN).

COMPLIANCE The extent to which a patient follows the advice of a doctor or other health professional, especially in respect of drug or other treatments. This is generally increased if the patient understands the condition, and the basis for the proposed treatment.

COMPRESS is the name given to a pad of linen or flannel wrung out of water and bound to the body. It is generally wrung out of cold water, and may be covered with a piece of waterproof material. It is used to subdue pain or inflammation. A hot compress is generally called a fomentation. (See FOMENTATION.)

COMPRESSED AIR ILLNESS or CAISSON DISEASE This affects workers operating in compressed-air environments, such as underwater divers and workers in caissons (i.e., an ammunition wagon, a chest of explosive materials, or a strong case for keeping out the water while the foundations of a bridge are being built; derived from the French *caisse*, meaning case or chest). Its chief symptoms are pains in the joints and limbs (bends), pain in the stomach, headache and dizziness, and paralysis. Sudden death may occur. The condition is caused by the accumulation of bubbles of nitrogen in different parts of the body, usually because of too rapid decompression when the worker returns to normal atmospheric presure, a change that must be made gradually.

COMPRESSION SYNDROME (see MUSCLES, DISEASES OF).

COMPUTED TOMOGRAPHY or COMPUTERIZED TOMOGRAPHY Tomography is an X-ray examination technique in which only structures in a particular plane produce clearly focused images. Whole-body computed tomography was introduced in 1977 and has already made a major impact in the investigation and management of medical and surgical disease. The technique is particularly valuable where a mass distorts the contour of an organ, e.g. a pancreatic tumour, or a lesion which has a density different from that of surrounding tissue, e.g. a metastasis in the liver. Computed tomography can distinguish soft tissues from cysts or fat, but in general soft tissue masses have similar appearances, so that distinguishing an inflammatory mass from a malignant process may be impossible. Computed tomography is particularly useful in patients with suspected malignancy. It can also define the extent of the cancer by detecting enlarged lymph nodes, indicating lymphatic spread. The main indications for computed tomography of the body are: mediastinal masses, suspected pulmonary metastases, adrenal disease, pancreatic masses, retroperitoneal lymph nodes, intra-abdominal abscesses, orbital tumours and the staging of cancer.

CONCEPTION signifies the complex set of changes which occur in the ovum and in the body of the mother at the beginning of pregnancy. The precise moment of conception is that at which the male element, or spermatozoon, and the female element, or ovum, fuse together. Only one-third of these conceptions survive to birth, whilst 15 per cent are cut short by spontaneous abortion or stillbirth. The remainder – over one half – are lost very early during pregnancy without trace. (See FETUS.)

CONCUSSION OF THE BRAIN (see BRAIN INJURIES).

CONDITIONED REFLEX The development of a specific response by an individual to a specific stimulus. The best-known conditioned reflex is the one described by Ivan Pavlov in which dogs that became accustomed to being fed when a bell was sounded salivated on hearing the bell even if no food was given. The conditioned reflex is an important part of behavioural theory.

CONDOM A thin rubber or plastic sheath placed over the erect penis before sexual intercourse. It is the most effective type of barrier contraception and is also valuable in preventing the transfer between sexual partners of pathogenic organisms such as gonococci, which cause gonorrhoea, and human immuno-deficiency virus, which may lead to AIDS. Sheaths are most effective when properly used and with spermicides. The female condom might be suitable for contraception when a woman misses a day or two of her contraceptive pill, if there is DYSPAREUNIA, when the perineum needs protection, e.g. after childbirth, or in cases of latex allergy to traditional condoms. Used properly with spermicide, they provide an effective barrier both to infections and spermatozoa. Failure may result if the penis goes alongside it, if it gets pushed up into the vagina or falls out.

CONDYLE A rounded prominence at the end of a bone: for example, the prominences at the outer and inner sides of the knee on the thigh-bone (or FEMUR). The projecting part of a condyle is sometimes known as an epicondyle, as in the case of the condyle at the lower end of the HUMERUS where the epicondyles form the prominences on the outer and inner side of the elbow.

CONDYLOMA A localized, rounded swelling of mucous membrane about the opening of the bowel, and the genital organs, sometimes known as 'genital warts' or 'ano-genital warts'. There are two main forms of them: condyloma latum, which is syphilitic in origin, and condyloma acuminatum, which often occurs in association with sexually transmitted disease, but is only indirectly due to it, being primarily a virus infection.

CONE (1) A light-sensitive cell in the retina of the eye that can also distinguish colours. The other type of light-sensitive cell is called a rod. There are around six million cones in the human retina and these are thought to comprise three types that are sensitive to the three primary colours of red, blue, and green. (2) A cone biopsy is a surgical technique in which a conical or cylindrical section of the lower part of the neck of the womb is excised.

CONFIDENTIALITY The ethical principle that doctors do not reveal information to other people (or to organizations) that their patients have given to them in confidence. Normally the doctor must get permission to release confidential information to an employer (or other authoritative body), insurance company or lawyer. The doctor does have to provide such information if required by a court of law (see ETHICS).

CONGENITAL deformities, diseases, etc., are those which are either present at birth, or which, being transmitted direct from the parents, show themselves some time after birth.

CONGENITAL ADRENAL HYPERPLASIA (see ADRENOGENITAL SYNDROME and GENETIC DISORDERS).

CONGESTION The accumulation of blood or other body fluid in a particular part of the body. The condition may be due to some failure in the circulation (see CIRCULATION, DISORDERS OF), but as a rule is one of the early signs of inflammation (see ABSCESS; INFLAMMATION).

CONJUGATE DEVIATION The term for describing the persistent and involuntary turning of both eyes in any one direction, and is a sign of a lesion in the brain.

CONJUNCTIVA (see EYE).

CONJUNCTIVITIS (see EYE DISEASES).

CONNECTIVE TISSUE This tissue holds together the different structures in the body. It comprises a matrix of substances called mucopolysaccharides in which are embedded a variety of specialist tissues and cells. These include elastic (yellow), collagenous (white) and reticular fibres as well as fibroblasts, macrophages and MAST CELLS. This variety is assembled in differing proportions to provide structures with varying functions: bone, cartilage, tendons and ligaments as well as fatty and elastic tissues.

CONSANGUINOUS A relationship by blood: siblings are closely consanguinous, cousins, and grandparents and grandchildren less so.

CONSERVATIVE TREATMENT Medical treatment which involves the minimum of active interference by the practitioner. For example, a disc lesion in the back might be treated by bed rest in contrast to surgical intervention to remove the damaged disc.

CONSOLIDATION A term applied to solidification of an organ, especially of a lung. The consolidation may be of a permanent nature due to formation of fibrous tissue, or may be temporary, as in acute pneumonia.

CONSTIPATION A condition in which the bowels are opened infrequently or incompletely, as a result of which the motions are dry and hard. Although one daily movement of the bowels is most common in health, the exact frequency may vary, though less than three times a week is generally regarded as constipation. It is a chronic condition, and must be distinguished from acute obstruction, a much more severe condition. (See INTESTINE, DISEASES OF.) The stools may vary considerably in colour, consistency, and amount, according to the nature and quantity of food and drink taken.

Causes The most common causes are (1) habit, (2) 'a greedy colon', which absorbs water too quickly, (3) a spastic colon, in which the muscles remain in a state of spasm, (4) lack of tone in the muscle, (5) a low-roughage diet. Of these, poor habit is the most important. The condition is usually aggravated by the use of aperients and purgatives. Uncommon causes, such as tumour, result in stricture of the bowel, leading to obstruction.

Symptoms and effects The stools are dark, hard, and passed with difficulty, and in small amount. In severe, persistent cases there may be swelling of the abdomen, from the retention of large masses of the remnants from digestion. Colic may occur in long-standing cases. Piles, which are a cause of increasing constipation, are often brought on by inattention to the bowels to begin with.

Treatment If there is no organic cause, such as tumour or other source of mechanical obstruction, attention to daily habit is the most important matter. Daily exercise, regular opening of the bowels at the same time each day, should be cultivated. A high-roughage diet is important, with plenty of fruit and vegetables. A cereal rich in bran is helpful, and wholemeal bread should be preferred.

CONSTITUTION, or DIATHESIS, means the general condition of the body, especially with reference to its liability to certain diseases.

CONSULTANT In Britain's health service a consultant is the senior career post for a fully qualified specialist. He or she normally sees patients referred by general practitioners – hence the historical term 'consultant' – or emergency cases admitted direct to hospital. NHS consultants are also allowed to do a certain amount of private practice. A consultant has to undergo several years of specialist training in hospital as a 'junior' doctor or dentist and pass higher examinations. There were over 21,000 consultants in Great Britain in 1996 and over 32,000 GPs for a population of more than 54 million (See APPENDIX 7: UK HEALTH STATISTICS.

CONSUMPTION (see TUBERCULOSIS).

CONTACT LENSES are lenses worn in contact with the eye, behind the eyelids and in front of the cornea. They may be worn for cosmetic, optical or therapeutic reasons. The commonest reason for wear is cosmetic, many short-sighted people preferring to wear contact lenses instead of glasses. Optical reasons for contact-lens wear include cataract surgery (usually unilateral extraction) and the considerable improvement in overall standard of vision experienced by very short-sighted people by wearing contact lenses instead of glasses. Therapeutic lenses are those used in the treatment of eye disease, 'bandage lenses' are used in certain corneal diseases: contact lenses can be soaked in a particular drug and then put on the eye so that the drug slowly leaks out on to the eye. Contact lenses may be hard, soft or gas permeable. Hard lenses are more optically accurate (because they are rigid), cheaper and more durable than soft. The main advantage of soft lenses is that they are more comfortable to wear. Gas-permeable lenses are so called because they are more permeable to oxygen than other lenses, thus allowing more oxygen to reach the cornea.

CONTAGION means the principle of spread of disease by direct contact with the body of an affected person.

CONTINUED FEVERS are typhus, typhoid and relapsing fevers, so called because of their continuing over a more or less definite space of time.

CONTINUOUS POSITIVE AIRWAYS PRESSURE A method for treating babies who suffer from alveolar collapse in the lung as a result of HYALINE MEMBRANE DISEASE (RESPIRATORY DISTRESS SYNDROME).

CONTRACEPTION A means of avoiding pregnancy despite sexual activity. There is no ideal contraceptive, and the choice of method depends on balancing considerations of safety, effectiveness, and acceptability. The best choice for any couple will depend on their ages and personal circumstances and may well vary with time. Contraceptive techniques can be classified in various ways, but one of the most useful is into 'barrier' and 'non-barrier' methods.

Barrier methods These involve a physical barrier which prevents sperm from reaching the cervix. Barrier methods reduce the risk of spreading sexually transmitted diseases, and the sheath is the best protection against HIV infection (see AIDS/HIV) for sexually active people. The efficiency of barrier methods is improved if they are used in conjunction with a spermicidal foam or jelly, but care is needed to ensure that the preparation chosen does not damage the rubber barrier.
CONDOM (SHEATH) This is the most commonly used barrier contraceptive. It consists of a rubber sheath which is placed over the erect penis before intromission and removed after ejaculation. The failure rate, if properly used, is about 4 per cent.
DIAPHRAGM or CAP A rubber dome that is inserted into the vagina before intercourse and fits snugly over the cervix. It should be used with an appropriate spermicide and is removed six hours after intercourse. A woman must be measured to ensure that she is supplied with the correct size of diaphragm, and the fit should be checked annually or after more than about 7 lbs. change in weight. The failure rate, if properly used, is about 2 per cent.

Non-barrier methods These do not provide a physical barrier between sperm and cervix and so do not protect against sexually transmitted diseases, including HIV.
COITUS INTERRUPTUS This involves the man's withdrawing his penis from the vagina before ejaculation. Because some sperm may leak before full ejaculation, the method is not very reliable.
SAFE PERIOD This involves avoiding intercourse around the time when the woman ovulates and is at risk of pregnancy. The safe times can be predicted using temperature charts to identify

the rise in temperature before ovulation or by careful assessment of the quality of the cervical mucus. This method works best if the woman has regular menstrual cycles. If used carefully it can be very effective and is free from side-effects, but it requires a highly motivated couple to succeed. It is approved by the Catholic church.

SPERMICIDAL GELS, CREAMS, PESSARIES, ETC. These are supposed to prevent pregnancy by killing sperm before they reach the cervix, but they are unreliable and should be used only in conjunction with a barrier method.

INTRAUTERINE CONTRACEPTIVE DEVICE (COIL) This is a small metal or plastic shape placed inside the uterus that prevents pregnancy by disrupting implantation. Some people regard it as a form of abortion, so it is not acceptable to all religious groups. There is a significantly increased risk of pelvic infection and eventual infertility in women who have used coils, and in many countries their use has declined substantially. They must be inserted by a specially trained health worker, but once in place they permit intercourse at any time with no prior planning. Increased pain and bleeding may be caused during menstruation, but, if severe, these may indicate that the coil is incorrectly sited, and that its position should be checked.

HORMONAL METHODS These include the combined oestrogen and progesterone and progesterone-only contraceptive pills, as well as longer-acting depot preparations. They modify the woman's hormonal environment and prevent pregnancy by disrupting various stages of the menstrual cycle, especially ovulation. The combined oestrogen and progesterone pills are very effective and are the most popular form of contraception. A wide range of preparations is available and the *British National Formulary* contains details of the commonly used varieties.

The main side-effects are an increased risk of cardiovascular disease. The lowest possible dose of oestrogen should be used, and many preparations use phasic preparations in which the dose of oestrogen varies with the time of the cycle. The progesterone- only or 'mini' pill does not contain any oestrogen and must be taken at the same time every day. It is not as effective as the combined pill, but failure rates of less than 1-per-100 woman years can be achieved. It has few serious side-effects, but may cause menstrual irregularities. It is suitable for use by mothers who are breast feeding. Depot preparations include intramuscular injections, subcutaneous implants, and intravaginal rings. They are useful in cases where the woman cannot be relied on to take a pill regularly but needs effective contraception. Their main side-effect is their prolonged action, which means that users cannot suddenly decide that they would like to become pregnant.

Contraceptive pills for use by men are under development.

STERILIZATION Permanent contraception can be achieved by sterilizing either the male or female partner. The operation on men is easier and safer. Although sterilization can sometimes be reversed, this cannot be guaranteed and couples should be counselled in advance that the method is irreversible. There is a small but definite failure rate with sterilization, and this should also be made clear before the operation is performed.

POST-COITAL CONTRACEPTION This is, in effect, a high dose of the combined oral contraceptive given within 72 hours of unprotected intercourse. It can cause nausea and vomiting. It is useful in an emergency, e.g. if a sheath splits during intercourse or after rape, but, if a woman requests it repeatedly because she is forgetting to use her usual method of contraception, further counselling and a change of regular method is indicated.

Mifepristone is a medical alternative to surgical termination of intrauterine pregnancy of up to 63 days' gestation but its use is controversial. (See APPENDIX 2: ADDRESSES.)

CONTRACTURE The permanent shortening of a muscle or of fibrous tissue. Contraction is the name given to the temporary shortening of a muscle.

CONTRAST MEDIUM A material that is used to increase the visibility of the body's tissues and organs during radiography. A common example is the use of barium which is given by mouth or as an enema to show up the alimentary tract.

CONTRE-COUP An injury in which a bone, generally the skull, is fractured, not at the spot where the violence is applied, but at the exactly opposite point.

CONTROLLED DRUGS In the United Kingdom controlled drugs are those preparations referred to under the Misuse of Drugs Act, 1971. The act prohibits activities related to the manufacture, supply and possession of these drugs and they are classified into three groups which determine the penalties for offences involving their misuse. For example, class A includes COCAINE, DIAMORPHINE, MORPHINE, LSD and PETHIDINE. Class B includes AMPHETAMINES, BARBITURATES, CANNABIS, CODEINE and PENTAZOCINE. Class C includes drugs related to amphetamines such as diethylpropion and chlorphentermine, meprobamate and most BENZODIAZEPINES.

The Misuse of Drugs Regulations, 1985, define the classes of person authorized to supply and possess controlled drugs and lay down the conditions under which these activities may be carried out. In the Regulations drugs are divided into five schedules specifying the requirements for supply, possession, prescribing and record-keeping. Schedule 1 contains drugs, such as cannabis, which are not used as medicines. Schedules 2 and 3 contain drugs which are subject to the prescription requirements of the Act (see below). They are distinguished in the *British National Formulary*

(BNF) by the symbol CD and they include morphine, diamorphine (heroin), other opioid analgesics, barbiturates, amphetamines, cocaine and diethylpropion. Schedules 4 and 5 contain drugs such as the benzodiazepines which are subject to minimal control. A full list of the drugs in each schedule can be found in the BNF.

Prescriptions for drugs in schedules 2 and 3 must be signed and dated by the prescriber, who must give his address. The prescription must be in the prescriber's own handwriting and provide the name and address of the patient and the total quantity of the preparation in both words and figures. The pharmacist is not allowed to dispense a controlled drug unless all the information required by law is given on the prescription.

The Misuse of Drugs (Notification and Supply of Addicts) Regulations, 1973, govern the notification of addicts. This is required in respect of the following commonly used drugs: cocaine, dextromoramide, diamorphine, dipipanone, hydrocodeine, hydromorphone, levorphanol, methadone, morphine, opium, oxycodone, pethidine, phenazocine and piritranide.

Any doctor who suspects that his patient may be addicted to one of these drugs must notify the Chief Medical Officer at the Home Office in writing within seven days. Notification in writing must be confirmed annually if the patient is still being treated by the doctor. The Home Office maintains an Index of Addicts which is available to doctors on a confidential basis.

CONTUSION (see BRUISES).

CONVALESCENCE   The condition through which a person passes after having suffered from some acute disease, and before complete health and strength are regained.

CONVERGENCE   (1) Inward turning of the eyes to focus on a near point with the result that a single image is registered by both retinas. (2) The coming together of various nerve fibres to form a nerve tract that provides a single pathway from different parts of the brain.

CONVOLUTIONS (see BRAIN).

CONVULSIONS   Rapidly alternating contractions and relaxations of the muscles, causing irregular movements of the limbs or body generally, usually accompanied by unconsciousness. Generally a symptom of some other trouble, often of a minor nature in children, they are rarely a danger to life. Nevertheless a cause of alarm, they should always be taken seriously.

Causes   The most common cause of convulsions in adults is EPILEPSY, and it can also cause them in infants and children. The relative frequency of non-epileptic convulsions in infants and young children is probably due to an instability of the immature nervous system. An American investigation showed that in a large group of otherwise normal children, some 6 per cent had had one or more convulsions.

In young infants convulsions may be due to birth injuries, usually the result of a difficult labour. The convulsions in these cases are due to damage of the brain, either by bleeding from torn blood-vessels or concussion of the brain. In older infants convulsions may be due to the irritability of the brain often associated with rickets, a condition known as tetany. Other metabolic causes include hypoglycaemia and hypokalaemia. A sudden rise of temperature, such as may occur in any infection, may induce convulsions in an infant and young child.

Diseases of the brain, such as meningitis, encephalitis and tumours, or any disturbance of the brain due to bleeding, blockage of a blood-vessel, or irritation of the brain by a fracture of the skull, may also be responsible for convulsions.

Asphyxia, such as may occur in a young child during a paroxysm of whooping-cough, may also bring on convulsions.

Treatment   Tepid sponging may help if there is fever, and a spoon or spatula should be put between the child's teeth if there is a possibility of his biting his tounge. Unless particularly severe, the movements seldom need be restrained. If the convulsions persist, it may be necessary to give parenteral BENZODIAZEPINES. As a rule a sedative, or an injection of one of the barbiturates, controls the convulsions. Once these are under control, the cause of the convulsions must be sought and the necessary treatment given

COOLEY'S ANAEMIA (see THALASSAEMIA).

COOMB'S TEST   A sensitive test that detects ANTIBODIES to the body's red cells (see ERYTHROCYTE). There are two methods: one, the direct, identifies those antibodies that are bound to the cells; the other, indirect, method identifies those circulating unattached in the serum.

CO-ORDINATION   The governing power exercised by the brain as a whole, or by certain centres in the nervous system, to make various muscles contract in harmony, and so produce definite actions, instead of meaningless movements. It is bound up intimately with the complex sense of localization, which enables a person with his eyes shut to tell, by sensations received from the bones, joints and muscles, the position of the various parts of his body. The power is impaired in various diseases, such as locomotor ataxia. It is tested by making the patient shut his eyes, moving his hand in various directions, and then telling him to bring the point of the forefinger steadily to the tip of the nose, or by other simple movements.

COPPER is an essential nutrient for man, and all tissues in the human body contain traces of it. The total amount in the adult body is 100 to 150 mg. Many essential enzyme systems are dependent on traces of copper. On the other hand, there is no evidence that dietary deficiency of copper ever occurs in man. Infants are born with an ample store, and the normal diet for an adult contains around 2 mg of copper a day. It is used in medicine as the two salts, sulphate of copper (blue stone) and nitrate of copper. The former is, in small doses, a powerful astringent, and in larger doses an irritant. Both are caustics when applied externally. Externally, either is used to rub on unhealthy ulcers and growths to stimulate the granulation tissue to more rapid healing.

COPROLALIA An inherited condition, usually beginning in childhood, it presents with motor tics, with irrepressible, explosive, occasionally obscene, verbal ejaculations. (See GILLES DE LA TOURETTE'S SYNDROME).

COPULATION The act of coitus or sexual intercourse when the man inserts his erect penis into the woman's vagina and after a succession of thrusting movements ejaculates his semen.

CORDOTOMY, or CHORDOTOMY, is the surgical operation of cutting the antero-lateral tracts of the SPINAL CORD to relieve otherwise intractable pain. It is also sometimes known as tractotomy.

CORNEA (see EYE).

CORNEAL GRAFT (KERATOPLASTY) If the cornea becomes damaged or diseased and vision is impaired, it can be removed and replaced by a corneal graft. The graft is taken from the cornea of a human donor. Some of the indication for corneal grafting include keratoconus, corneal dystrophies, severe corneal scarring following herpes simplex, alkali burns or injury. Because the graft is a foreign protein, there is a danger that the recipient's immune system may set up a reaction causing rejection of the graft. Rejection results in oedema of the graft with subsequent poor vision. Once a corneal graft has been taken from a donor, it should be used as quickly as possible. Corneas can be stored for days in tissue-culture medium at low temperature. A small number of grafts are autografts in which a patient's cornea is repositioned.

The Department of Health has drawn up a list of suitable eye-banks to which people can apply to bequeath their eyes, and an official form is now available for the bequest of eyes. (See also DONORS; TRANSPLANTATION.)

CORNEAL REFLEX Instinctive closing of eyelids when the surface of the CORNEA is lightly touched with a fine hair.

CORNS AND BUNIONS A corn is a localized thickening of the cuticle or epidermis, of a conical shape, the point of the cone being directed inwards and being known as the 'eye' of the corn. A general thickening over a wider area is called a callosity. Bunion is a condition found over the joint at the base of the great toe, in which not only is there thickening of the skin, but the head of the metatarsal bone becomes prominent. Hammer-toe is a condition of the second toe, often caused by short boots, in which the toe becomes bent at its two joints in such a way as to resemble a hammer.

Corns and bunions are caused by badly fitting shoes, hence the importance of children and adults wearing properly fitted footwear. Corns can be pared after softening in warm water or painted with salicylic acid collodion or other proprietary preparations. Bad corns may need treatment by a CHIROPODIST. Bunions may require surgical treatment. Regular foot care is important in patients with DIABETES MELLITUS.

CORONARY A term applied to several structures in the body encircling an organ in the manner of a crown. The coronary arteries are the arteries of supply to the heart which arise from the aorta, just beyond the aortic valve, and through which the blood is delivered to the muscle of the heart. Disease of the coronary arteries is a very serious condition producing various abnormal forms of heart action and the disease, angina pectoris.

CORONARY ANGIOPLASTY A technique of dilating atheromatous obstructions in coronary arteries by inserting a catheter with a balloon on the end into the affected artery. It is passed through the blockage (guided by X-ray FLUOROSCOPY) and inflated.

CORONARY ARTERIES The right coronary artery arises from the right sinus of the valsalva and passes into the right atrio-ventricular groove to supply the right ventricle, part of the intraventricular septum and the inferior part of the left ventricle. The left coronary artery arises from the left sinus and divides into an anterior descending branch which supplies the septum and the anterior and apical parts of the heart, and the circumflex branch which passes into the left antrio-ventricular groove and supplies the lateral posterior surfaces of the heart. Small anastomoses exist between the coronary arteries and they have the potential of enlarging if the blood flow through a neighbouring coronary artery is compromised. (See CIRCULATION for diagram of heart and coronary arteries.) Coronary artery disease is damage to the heart caused by the narrowing or blockage of these arteries. It commonly presents as ANGINA PECTORIS or acute myocardial infarction (see CORONARY THROMBOSIS).

CORONARY ARTERY VEIN BYPASS GRAFTING (CAVBG) When coronary arteries, narrowed by disease, cannot supply the heart muscle with sufficient blood the cardiac circulation may be improved by grafting a section of vein from the leg to bypass the obstruction. Around 10,000 people in the United Kingdom have this operation annually and the results are usually good. It is a major procedure that lasts several hours and necessitates temporarily stopping the heart with blood circulation and oxygenation taken over by a HEART-LUNG MACHINE.

CORONARY THROMBOSIS is the acute, dramatic manifestation of ischaemic heart disease, one of the major killing diseases of western civilization. In 1988, ischaemic heart disease was responsible for about 153,000 deaths in England and Wales, a figure that fell to 133,000 in 1995. The alternative name for ischaemic heart disease is coronary artery disease. The underlying cause is disease of the coronary arteries which carry the blood supply to the heart muscle (or myocardium). This results in narrowing of the arteries until finally they are unable to transport sufficient blood for the myocardium to function efficiently. One of three things may happen. If the narrowing of the coronary arteries occurs gradually, then either the individual concerned will develop ANGINA PECTORIS or he will develop signs of a failing heart. (See HEART DISEASES.)

If the narrowing occurs suddenly or leads to complete blockage, or occlusion, of a major branch of one of the coronary arteries, then the victim collapses with acute pain and distress. This is the condition commonly referred to as a coronary thrombosis because it is usually due to the affected artery suddenly becoming completely blocked by THROMBOSIS. More correctly, it should be described as coronary occlusion, because the final occluding factor need not necessarily be thrombosis. Alternatively, it is sometimes referred to as myocardial infarction, this describing the destructive changes produced in the myocardium by lack of its blood supply. (See INFARCTION.)

Causes The precise cause is not known, but there is a wide range of factors which play a part in inducing coronary artery disease. Heredity is an important factor. It is commoner in men than in women. It is more common in those in sedentary occupations than in those who lead a more physically active life and the disease is more likely to occur in those with high blood-pressure than in those with normal blood-pressure. Obesity is a contributory factor. The disease is more common among smokers than non-smokers. It is often associated with a high level of CHOLESTEROL in the blood. This in turn has been linked with an excessive consumption of animal, as opposed to vegetable, fats. In this connection the important factors seem to be the saturated fatty acids of animal fats which would appear to be more likely to lead to a high level of cholesterol in the blood than the unsaturated fatty acids of vegetable fats. As more research on the subject is carried out the arguments continue about the relative influ-

ence of the different factors. (See APPENDIX 2: ADDRESSES.)

Symptoms The presenting symptom is the sudden onset, often at rest, of acute, agonizing pain in the front of the chest. This rapidly radiates all over the front of the chest and often down over the abdomen. It is often accompanied by nausea and vomiting, so that suspicion may be aroused of some acute abdominal condition such as gall-stone colic or a perforated peptic ulcer. The victim soon goes into SHOCK, with a pale, cold sweating skin, rapid pulse and difficulty in breathing. There is usually some rise in temperature.

Treatment is immediate relief of the pain by injections of diamorphine. Thrombolytic drugs should be given as soon as possible and ARRHYTHMIAS corrected. Subsequent treatment includes the continued administration of drugs to relieve the pain, the administration of drugs that may be necessary to deal with the heart failure that commonly develops and the irregular action of the heart that quite often develops, and the administration of oxygen. Patients are usually admitted to coronary care units, where they receive constant supervision. Such units maintain an emergency, skilled, round-the-clock staff of doctors and nurses, as well as all the necessary resuscitation facilities that may be required.

The outcome varies considerably. The first hour is when the patient is at greatest risk of death. If he or she is treated, then there is a 50-per-cent reduction in mortality compared with waiting until hospital admission. As each day passes the prognosis improves with a first coronary thrombosis, provided the patient does not have a high blood-pressure and is not overweight. Following recovery, there should be a gradual return to work, care being taken to avoid any increase in weight, unnecessary stress and strain, and to observe moderation in all things. Smoking should be stopped. At one time, patients who had had a coronary thrombosis were kept in bed for prolonged periods. Today, however, in uncomplicated cases the aim is to get them up and about as soon as possible. Most patients are in hospital for a week to ten days and back at work in three months or sooner.

CORONAVIRUSES, so called because in electron micrographs the spikes projecting from the virus resemble a crown, are a group of viruses which have been isolated from people with common colds, and have also been shown to produce common colds under experimental conditions. Their precise significance in the causation of the common cold is still undetermined.

CORONER An independent legal officer of the Crown who is responsible for deciding whether to hold a postmortem and an inquest in cases of sudden or unexpected or unnatural death. He presides over an inquest, if held, sometimes with the help of a jury. Coroners are usually lawyers or doctors – some are double qualified – who have been qualified for at least five years. In Scotland the coroner is known as the procurator fiscal.

CORPULENCE (see OBESITY).

COR PULMONALE is another name for pulmonary heart disease, which is character- ized by hypertrophy and failure of the right VENTRICLE of the heart as a result of disease of the LUNGS or disorder of the pulmonary circu- lation.

CORPUSCLE means a small body. (See BLOOD.)

CORPUS LUTEUM The mass of cells formed in the ruptured Graafian follicle in the OVARY from which the ovum is discharged about fifteen days before the onset of the next men- strual period. When the ovum escapes the follicle fills up with blood. This is soon replaced by cells which contain a yellow fatty material. The follicle and its luteal cells constitute the corpus luteum. The corpus luteum begins to disappear after ten days, unless the discharged ovum is fertilized and pregnancy ensues. In pregnancy the corpus luteum persists and grows and secretes the hormone, progesterone.

CORRIGAN'S PULSE The name applied to the collapsing pulse found with incompetence of the heart's aortic valve. It is so called after Sir Dominic John Corrigan (1802–80), the fam- ous Dublin physician, who first described it.

CORROSIVES are poisonous substances which corrode or eat away the mucous surfaces of mouth, gullet and stomach with which they come in contact. Examples are strong mineral acids like sulphuric, nitric and hydrochloric acids, caustic alkalis, and some salts like chlo- rides of mercury and zinc. (See POISONS.)

CORROSIVE SUBLIMATE, or PERCHLORIDE OF MERCURY, is a powerful antiseptic and an irritant poison. It is not to be confounded with subchloride of mercury or calomel. (See ANTI- SEPTICS; MERCURY.)

CORSET A support device worn around the trunk to help in the treatment of backache and spinal injuries or disorders.

CORTEX The tissues that form the outer part of an organ and which are positioned just below the capsule or outer membrane. Exam- ples are the cerebal CORTEX of the BRAIN and the renal cortex of the KIDNEY.

CORTICOSTEROIDS The generic term for the group of hormones with a CORTISONE-like action. Many chemical modifications of the cortisone molecule have been prepared in an attempt to dissociate therapeutic action from side effects. Analogues are already available with no mineralo-corticoid effects and steroids with a gluco-corticoid activity and no inflam- matory action have been synthesized. The main corticosteroid hormones currently available are cortisone, hydrocortisone, prednisone, pred- nisolone, methyl prednisolone, triam-cinolone, dexamethasone, beta-methasone and paramethasone. They are used clinically in three quite distinct circumstances. First they constitute replacement therapy in states of adrenocortical insufficiency or hypopituitar- ism. In this situation the dose is physiological, namely the equivalent of the normal adrenal output under similar circumstances, and it is not associated with any side effects. Secondly, steroids are used to depress secretory activity of the adrenal cortex in conditions where this is abnormally high or where the adrenal cortex is producing abnormal hormones, as occurs in some hirsute women. The third application for corticosteroids is in suppressing the manifesta- tions of disease in a wide variety of inflamma- tory and allergic conditions and in reducing antibody production in a number of auto- immune diseases. The inflammatory reaction is normally part of the body's defence mechanism and is to be encouraged rather than inhibited. However, in the case of those diseases in which the body's reaction is disproportionate to the offending agent, the steroid hormones can inhibit this undesirable response and although the underlying condition is not cured as a result it may resolve spontaneously. When such com- pounds are used for anti-inflammatory proper- ties, the dose must be pharmacological; that is it must exceed the normal physiological re- quirement. Indeed, the necessary dose may exceed the normal maximum output of the healthy adrenal gland, which is about 250 to 300 mg cortisol per day. When doses of this order are used there are inevitable risks and side effects. A drug-induced Cushing's syndrome will result.

Corticosteroid treatment of short duration, as in angioneurotic oedema of the larynx or other allergic crises, may at the same time be life-saving and without significant risk. Pro- longed therapy of such connective-tissue disor- ders, such as polyarteritis with its attendant hazards, is generally accepted because there are no other agents of therapeutic value. Similarly the absence of alternative medical treatment for such conditions as auto-immune haemolytic ANAEMIA and auto-immune THROMBOCYTOPENIA PURPURA establishes steroid therapy as the treatment of choice, which few would dispute. The place of steroids in such chronic conditions as RHEUMATOID ARTHRITIS, ASTHMA and ECZEMA, is more debatable.

Although one must be aware of the side- effects, it is possible to become so obsessed with the risks of therapy as to underestimate the misery and danger of unrelieved chronic asthma or the incapacity, frustration and psychological trauma of rheumatoid arthritis. On the other hand, a form of treatment with the hazards of steroid therapy should never be undertaken lightly or until other established remedies have failed.

The incidence and severity of side-effects are related to the dose and duration of treatment. Prolonged daily treatment with 15 mg of prednisolone, or more, will cause hyper-cortisonism. Less than 10 mg prednisolone a day may be tolerated by most patients indefinitely. When used in pharmacological doses, steroid therapy is associated with certain side-effects which are so common as to be almost invariable but are not usually of serious consequence. These include gain in weight, fat distribution of the cushingoid type, acne and hirsutism, amenorrhoea, striae and increased bruising tendency. The more serious complications which fortunately occur much less frequently include infection, dyspepsia and peptic ulceration, gastrointestinal haemorrhage, adrenal suppression, osteoporosis, psychosis, diabetes mellitus, myopathy and potassium depletion.

CORTICOTROPHIN is the *British Pharmacopoeia* name for the adrenocorticotrophic hormone of the pituitary gland, also known as ACTH. It is so called because it stimulates the functions of the cortex of the suprarenal glands. This results, among other things, in an increased output of cortisone, Although first isolated from the pituitary gland in 1933, it was not until the discovery, in 1949, of the effect of cortisone and corticotrophin in rheumatoid arthritis that it came into general use. No means of synthesis has yet been discovered, and the only available sources are the pituitary glands of animals. It is only active when given by intravenous or intramuscular injection, but there are preparations available, which give a more prolonged action and which are given subcutaneously. As its action is predominantly the same as that of cortisone, the action of the two is discussed together in the section on CORTISONE.

CORTISOL Another name for HYDROCORTISONE.

CORTISONE, originally known as Compound E, was isolated from beef adrenal glands in 1936 by workers at the Mayo Clinic. Its chemical name is 11-dehydro-17-hydroxycorticosterone. Mainly because of difficulties in obtaining adequate amounts, little interest was taken in it until, in 1949, Hench and Kendall and their colleagues demonstrated its dramatic, if transitory, effect in RHEUMATOID ARTHRITIS. The precise mode of action of cortisone is still not known. Among other things, it prevents (or delays) the proliferative changes in the tissues which are the normal response to infection and in allergic conditions. Among the conditions which have been shown to benefit from cortisone are rheumatoid arthritis, RHEUMATIC FEVER, GOUT, certain eye conditions, certain skin conditions and ADDISON'S DISEASE.

Cortisone has two disadvantages which will always tend to restrict its use. One is that in chronic conditions such as rheumatoid arthritis the effect of cortisone is merely temporary, and tends to stop when administration is stopped. The other is that cortisone has serious side-effects, and therefore it must only be used under medical supervision.

For all practical purposes CORTICOTROPHIN and cortisone have the same action. (See also BETAMETHASONE; DEXAMETHASONE; HYDROCORTISONE; PREDNISOLONE; AND TRIAMCINOLONE.)

CORYNEBACTERIA A genus of aerobic and anaerobic gram-positive bacteria widely distributed and best known as parasites and pathogens in humans. *C. diphtheria*, a prime example, causes diphtheria.

CORYZA is the technical name of a 'cold in the head'.

COSTAL Anything pertaining to the ribs.

COSTALGIA Pain in the ribs.

COT DEATH (see SUDDEN INFANT DEATH SYNDROME).

CO-TRIMOXAZOLE This drug – a mixture of trimethoprim and the sulphonamide sulphamethoxazole – is now regarded as so unsafe that it should be used only in the prophylaxis or treatment of pneumocystis PNEUMONIA, and in acute exacerbations of chronic BRONCHITIS, urinary tract infections and OTITIS MEDIA, where indicated.

COTTON WOOL, or ABSORBENT COTTON as it is now technically named by the *British Pharmacopoeia*, is a downy material made from the hairs on cotton plant seeds (Gossypium herbaceum). It is used in medicine for a great variety of purposes.

COUGH A sudden indrawing of air with the GLOTTIS wide open. This is followed by a blowing out of air against a closed glottis. The glottis then suddenly opens and the air in the lungs is expelled under high pressure – up to 300 millimetres of mercury and at a speed of 960 kilometres (600 miles) an hour. Its purpose is to rid the air passages and windpipe of what are colloquially known as foreign bodies, including the excessive mucus and other secretions produced in infections of the lungs and upper air passages, such as bronchitis and sore throat. As such secretions contain many micro-organisms, it is clear what an important part coughing plays in spreading the common cold and other infections of the nose, throat and lungs. It is a REFLEX action produced by stimulation of nerve endings in the air passages and may therefore be induced by irritation of these nerve endings by inflammation without any secretion. This results in the dry irritable cough which can be such a troublesome feature of the early and late stages of acute bronchitis, TRACHEITIS and LARYNGITIS. Conversely the inability to cough in inflammatory conditions of the lungs, such as bronchitis and broncho-pneumonia, especially in old folk, is an ominous sign, and every effort must be made to stimulate coughing so far as this is possible.

COUGH SYNCOPE Temporary loss of consciousness that may be induced by a severe spasm of coughing. This is the result of the high pressure that may be induced in the chest – over 200 millimetres of mercury – by such a spasm. This prevents the return of blood to the heart, the veins in the neck begin to bulge and the blood-pressure falls. This may so reduce the blood flow to the brain that the individual feels giddy and may then lose consciousness. (See FAINTING.)

COUNSELLING Psychological support and advice provided by a trained therapist or health professional. The aim is to help an individual manage a particular personal or family problem. This may be a diagnosis of cancer, mental and physical trauma following an accident or assault or a bereavement. Counselling can help people cope with a wide range of demanding circumstances. It is usually done on a one-to-one basis – sometimes in small groups – and needs to be provided with skill and sensitivity or there is a risk of worsening the individual's difficulties. There has been rapid growth in counselling services and it is vital that those providing them have been properly trained.

COWPER's GLANDS Also known as the bulbourethral glands, these are a pair of glands whose ducts open into the urethra at the base of the PENIS. They secrete a fluid that is one of the constituents of the SEMEN which carries the spermatozoa and is ejaculated into the vagina during coitus.

COWPOX is a disease affecting the udders of cows, on which it produces vesicles. It is communicable to man, and there has for centuries been a tradition that persons who have caught this cowpox from cows do not suffer afterwards from SMALLPOX. This formed the basis for Jenner's experiments on vaccination. (See VACCINATION.)

COXALGIA or COXODYNIA means pain in the hip-joint.

COXA VARA A condition in which the neck of the thigh-bone is bent so that the lower limbs are turned outwards and lameness results.

COXSACKIE VIRUSES A group of viruses so-called because they were first isolated from two patients with a disease resembling paralytic poliomyelitis, in the village of Coxsackie in New York State. Thirty distinct types have now been identified. They constitute one of the three groups of viruses included in the family of ENTEROVIRUSES. They are divided into two groups: A and B. Despite the large number of types of group A virus (24) in existence, evidence of their role in causing human disease is limited. Some, however, cause aseptic meningitis, and others cause a condition known as HERPANGINA. HAND, FOOT AND MOUTH DISEASE is another disease caused by the A group. All 6 types of group B virus have been associated with outbreaks of aseptic meningitis, and they are also the cause of BORNHOLM DISEASE. Epidemics of type B_2 infections tend to occur in alternate years.

CRAB-LOUSE Another name for *Pediculus pubis*, a louse that infests the pubic region. (See PEDICULOSIS.)

CRACKED-POT SOUND A peculiar resonance heard sometimes on percussion of the chest over a cavity in the lung, resembling the jarring sound heard on striking a cracked pot or bell. It is also heard on percussion over the skull in patients with diseases of the brain such as haemorrhages and tumours, and in certain cases of fracture of the skull.

CRADLE A cage which is placed over the legs of a patient in bed, in order to take the weight of the bed-clothes off the legs.

CRADLE CAP or CRUSTA LACTEA as it is technically known, is the form of seborrhoea of the scalp which is not uncommon in nursing infants. It usually responds to a daily shampoo with cetrimide solution. Warm olive oil gently massaged into the scalp and left overnight, after which the scales can be washed off, also helps with the condition.

CRAMP A painful spasmodic contraction of muscles, most commonly occurring in the limbs, but also apt to affect certain internal organs.

Night cramp is most common in the elderly, during pregnancy, in diabetics and in those with peripheral vascular disease. It comes on suddenly, often during sleep, the patient being aroused by an agonizing feeling of pain in the calf of the leg or back of the thigh. This painful disorder can be relieved by firmly grasping or briskly rubbing the affected part with the hand.

Swimmer's cramp includes usually spasm of the arteries as well as of the muscles, due to cold and exertion. The limbs should be massaged and the victim kept warm.

Writer's cramp is painful spasms in hand muscles. These make writing, typing or delicate hand activities impossible. Sometimes resting the hand for several weeks will cure the condition but it tends to recur.

Heat cramps are painful contractions of muscles occurring in men (e.g. stokers) working in high temperatures. The cramps are due to excessive loss of salt in the sweat, and can be cured, and prevented, by giving salt water to drink. (See also HEATSTROKE.)

CRANIAL NERVES are those arising from the brain. (See BRAIN.)

CRANIUM The part of the skull enclosing the brain as distinguished from the face.

CREAM The oily or fatty part of milk from which butter is prepared. Various medicinal preparations are known also as cream, e.g. cold cream, which is a simple ointment containing rose-water, beeswax, borax, and almond oil scented with oil of rose.

CREATINE A nitrogenous substance, methyl-guanidine-acetic acid. In the adult human body there are about 120 grams of it, and 98 per cent of this is present in the muscles. Much of the creatine in muscle is combined with phosphoric acid as phosphocreatine, which plays an important part in the chemistry of muscular contraction.

CREATINE KINASE An ENZYME which is proving of value in the investigation and diagnosis of muscular dystrophy (see MYOPATHY), in which it is found in the blood in greatly increased amounts.

CREATININE is the anhydride of creatine and is derived from it. It is purely a waste product.

CREATININE CLEARANCE A method of assessing the function of the kidney by comparing the amount of creatinine – a product of body metabolism which is normally excreted by the kidneys – in the blood with the amount appearing in the urine.

CREEPING ERUPTION is a skin condition caused by the invasion of the skin by the larvae of various species of nematode worms. It owes its name to the fact that as the larva moves through and along the skin it leaves behind it a long creeping thin red line. (See STRONGYLOIDIASIS.)

CREMATION (see DEAD, DISPOSAL OF THE).

CRENATION Abnormal microscopic appearance of blood cells in which their usually smooth margins appear irregular. It usually occurs after a blood specimen has been stored for a long time but occasionally it may indicate a blood disorder.

CREOSOTE A clear, yellow liquid, of aromatic smell and burning taste, prepared by distillation from pine-wood or from beech-wood. It mixes readily with alcohol, ether, chloroform, glycerin, and oils.

It is a powerful antiseptic and disinfectant. Creosote is an ingredient of some disinfectant fluids.

CREPITATIONS Certain sounds which occur along with the breath sounds, as heard by AUSCULTATION, in various diseases of the lungs. They are signs of the presence of moist exudations in the lungs or in the bronchial tubes, are classified as fine, medium, and coarse crepitations, and resemble the sound made by bursting bubbles of various sizes.

CREPITUS means a grating sound. It is found in cases of fractured bones when the ends rub together; also in cases of severe chronic arthritis by the rubbing together of the dried internal surfaces of the joints.

CRESOL An oily liquid obtained from coal tar. It is a powerful antiseptic and disinfectant.

Uses It is used combined with soap to form a clear saponaceous fluid known as lysol, which can be mixed with water in any proportions. For the disinfection of drains it is used at a dilution of 1 in 20; for heavily infected linen 1 in 40; for floors and walls 1 in 100.

CRETINISM An out-of-date name for congenital hypothyroidism, a disease caused by defective thyroid function in fetal life or early in infancy.

CREUTZFELDT-JAKOB DISEASE (CJD) A slowly progressive fatal disease caused by an infectious agent called a prion, an altered form of normal protein about which little is known. The incidence of classical CJD is rare and has primarily affected adults in their late 50s. The incubation period is around 20 years and symptoms are dementia, seizures, focal signs in the central nervous system, MYOCLONUS and visual disturbances. The mode of transmission is unclear but some people have been infected by inadvertent transmission during corneal transplantation and, possibly, during neurosurgery. An inherited form has also been identified. A few patients treated with human growth hormone obtained from cadaveric pituitary glands have also developed CJD. There is no treatment.

The prions accumulate in the brain, damaging NEURONS and producing small cavities. Definite diagnosis can be made only by pathological examination of brain tissue after the victim's death. Prions are unusually resistant to inactivation by chemicals, heat, X-RAYS, or ULTRAVIOLET light. The infectious agent is similar to the agent that causes scrapie in sheep and BOVINE SPONGIFORM ENCEPHALOPATHY (BSE) in cattle. The agent can transfer from one animal species to another and since the mid 1980s in the United Kingdom some cases of 'human' (known as new variant) CJD have occurred as a result, it is believed, of consumption of meat from cattle with BSE. Recently there have been suggestions that scrapie in sheep may cause new CJD and urgent research is being done to clarify the position.

The epidemic of BSE had resulted, most experts believed, from cattle being fed with offal from infected cattle. Sheep, too, were fed cattle offal. Up to early 1998, 23 people in Britain (and one in France) had been diagnosed as having new variant CJD, a small number of them at a young age, which suggests that this form of the disease has a much shorter incubation time than classical CJD. It is, however, impossible to forecast how many individuals may be incubating the disease.

The development of new variant CJD has led to a programme of slaughtering infected and suspect animals, the tightening up of regulations covering the slaughter of cattle for consumption, an end to feeding animal offal to cattle, and strict registration of the provenance of all cattle. As a result, the incidence of BSE among cattle has declined sharply. Research suggests that the new variant CJD is more infectious than the classical variety and scientists are urgently seeking a reliable method of early identification of individuals carrying the infectious agent. The BSE epidemic among cattle in Britain led to a ban on the export of beef and cattle products and a restriction on the use of cattle products in Britain.

A ban was also imposed on the use of UK-sourced human serum in blood products such as plasma because the serum is pooled from a large number of donors making it impossible to track suspect samples. Blood for transfusion, which comes from identifiable donors and is not pooled, can still be used.

CRISIS is a word used with several distinct meanings. (1) The traditional meaning is that of a rapid loss of fever and return to comparative health in certain acute diseases. For example, pneumonia, if allowed to run its natural course, ends by a crisis, usually on the eighth day, the temperature falling in twenty-four hours to normal, the pulse and breathing becoming slow and regular, and the patient passing from a partly delirious state into natural sleep. The opposite mode of ending to crisis is by lysis: for example, in typhoid fever, where the patient slowly improves during a period of a week or more, without any sudden change. (2) A current use of the word crisis, and still more frequently of critical, is to signify a dangerous state of illness in which it is uncertain whether the sufferer will recover or not.

CROHN'S DISEASE is a chronic inflammatory disease that may occur in any part of the gut. The terminal ileum, colon and junction between the anus and rectum are particularly vulnerable. ULCERS, FISTULAE and granulomatous tissue develop and the whole bowel may be affected. The cause is unknown, though the disorder may have an immunological origin. Steroids, given systematically and locally, may improve symptoms. Metronidazole and azathioprine may help. The aim of treatment is to control the patient's symptoms. (See APPENDIX 2: ADDRESSES: Colitis and Crohn's Disease.)

CROTAMITON A topical cream used to treat pruritus.

CROUP is a household term for a group of diseases characterized by swelling and partial blockage of the entrance to the larynx, occurring in children and characterized by crowing inspiration. There are various causes including diphtheritic laryngitis (see DIPHTHERIA) and acute laryngitis. It is an account of this last condition which will be given here. (See also LARYNGO-TRACHEO-BRONCHITIS.)

Croup tends to occur in epidemics, particularly in autumn and early spring, and is almost exclusively viral in origin, commonly due to influenza or other respiratory viruses. It is always potentially dangerous, particularly in young children and infants, in whom the relatively small laryngeal airway may easily be blocked, leading to suffocation.

Symptoms Attacks generally come on at night, following a cold caught during the past couple of days. The breathing is hoarse and croaking (croup), with a barking cough and harsh respiratory noise. The natural tendency for the laryngeal airway to collapse is increased by the child's desperate attempts to overcome the obstruction. Parental anxiety, added to child's, only exacerbates the situation. After struggling for up to several hours, the child finally falls asleep. The condition may recur.

Treatment Most children with croup should be looked after at home if the environment is suitable. Severe episodes may require hospital treatment including tracheostomy or intubation to prevent brain damage or even death. There is little evidence that putting the child in a cold mist tent or giving antibiotics or corticosteroids is of any value. Of greater importance is the reassurance of the child, and careful observation for signs of deterioration.

CRUCIATE LIGAMENTS Two strong ligaments in the interior of the knee-joint, which cross one another like the limbs of the letter X. They are so attached as to become taut when the lower limb is straightened, and they prevent over-extension or bending forwards at the knee. They are sometimes strained or torn as a result of sporting injuries or vehicle accidents. Surgery may be needed to repair the damage.

CRURAL means something connected with the leg.

CRUSH SYNDROME A condition in which kidney failure occurs in patients who have been the victims of severe crushing accidents. The fundamental injury is damage to muscle. The limb swells. The blood volume falls. Blood UREA rises; there is also a rise in the POTASSIUM content of the blood. Urgent treatment in an intensive therapy unit is required and renal dialysis may well be necessary. The patient may survive; or he dies with renal failure. Post-mortem examination shows degeneration of the tubules of the kidney, and the presence in them of pigment casts.

CRUTCH-PALSY (see DROP-WRIST).

CRYOANALGESIA The induction of ANAL-GESIA by the use of cold produced by means of a special probe. The use of cold for the relief of pain dates back to the early days of man. Two millennia ago, Hippocrates was recommending snow and ice packs as a preoperative analgesic. The modern probe allows a precise temperature to be induced in a prescribed area. Among its uses is in the relief of chronic pain which will not respond to any other form of treatment. This applies particularly to chronic facial pain.

CRYOPRECIPITATE When frozen plasma is allowed to thaw slowly at 4 °C, a proportion of the plasma protein remains undissolved in the cold thawed plasma and stays in this state until the plasma is warmed. It is this cold insoluble precipitate that is known as cryoprecipitate. It can be recovered quite easily by centrifuging. Its value is that it is a rich source of Factor VIII, which is used in the treatment of HAEMOPHILIA.

CRYOPRESERVATION Maintenance at very low temperatures of the viability of tissues or organs that have been excised from the body.

CRYOSCOPY The method of finding the concentration of blood, urine, etc., by observing their freezing-point.

CRYOSURGERY The use of cold in surgery. Its advantages include little associated pain, little or no bleeding, and excellent healing with little or no scar formation. Hence its relatively wide use in eye surgery. The coolants used include liquid nitrogen with which temperatures as low as -196 °C can be obtained, carbon dioxide (-78 °C) and nitrous oxide (-88 °C).

CRYOTHERAPY The treatment of disease by refrigeration. The two main forms in which it is now used are HYPOTHERMIA and refrigeration anaesthesia.

CRYPTOCOCCOSIS is a rare disease due to infection with a yeast known as *Cryptococcus neoformans*. Around 5 to 10 cases are diagnosed annually in the United Kingdom. It usually involves the lungs in the first instance, but may spread to the meninges and other parts of the body; including the skin. It responds well as a rule to treatment with AMPHOTERICIN B, clotrimazole, and flucytosine.

CRYPTOCOCCUS A genus of yeasts. *Cryptococcus neoformans* is widespread in nature and present in particularly large numbers in the faeces of pigeons. It occasionally infects man, as a result of the inhalation of dust contaminated by the faeces of pigeons, causing the disease known as cryptococcosis.

CRYPTORCHIDISM An undescended testis. The testes normally descend into the scrotum during the seventh month of gestation. Until then the testis is an abdominal organ. If the testes do not descend before the first year of life they usually remain undescended until puberty and even then descent is not achieved in some instances. Fertility is impaired when one testis is affected and is usually absent in the bilateral cases. The incidence of undescended testis in full-term children at birth is 3·5 per cent, falling to less than 2 per cent at one month and 0·7 per cent at one year. Because of the high risk of infertility undescended testes should be brought down as early as possible and at the latest by the age of two. Sometimes medical treatment with human chorionic gonadotrophin is helpful but frequently surgical interference is necessary. This is the operation of orchidopexy.

CT SCANNER The machine which combines the use of a computer and X-rays to produce cross-sectional images of the body (see COMPUTED TOMOGRAPHY).

CULDOSCOPY is a method of examining the pelvic organs in women by means of an instrument comparable to a CYSTOSCOPE inserted into the pelvic cavity through the vagina. The instrument used for this purpose is known as a culdoscope.

CUPPING A traditional practice, now very rarely used, for treating cases of deep-seated congestion by drawing blood to the surface. It causes sudden dilatation of the superficial blood-vessels, and so probably contracts those of underlying organs. But whatever the explanation, it seems to offer relief in difficulty of breathing due to asthma, bronchitis and pleurisy and soothes in lumbago and various forms of rheumatic pain.

CUPRUM is the Latin word for copper.

CURARE, known also as CURARA, WOORALI, WOURARI, URARI, and TICUNAS, is a dark-coloured extract from some trees of the Strychnos family. It is used by the South American Indians as an arrow poison, and is extremely potent, its action depending upon a crystalline ALKALOID: *d*-tubocurarine chloride. This alkaloid paralyses the nerve endings in muscle. For many years it was considered to be much too dangerous for use in man, but research has shown that the pure alkaloid can be used with safety. Its main use is in ANAESTHESIA, where the muscular relaxation it produces is of invaluable assistance to the surgeon. With the aid of tubocurarine adequate muscular relaxation can be obtained with a lesser degree of anaesthesia than would be required were the drug not being used. It is a drug, however, that should only be used by a skilled anaesthetist. Its action is antagonized by neostigmine. It has also been used in the treatment of spastic conditions.

CURDLED MILK (see CASEIN).

CURETTE   Spoon-shaped instrument with a cutting edge used for scooping out the contents of any body cavity, e.g. the uterus or for removing certain skin lesions, such as verrucae.

CUSHING'S SYNDROME   Described in 1932 by Harvey Cushing, the American neurosurgeon, it is due to the excess production of CORTISOL. It can thus result from an ADRENAL tumour secreting cortisol or from a pituitary tumour secreting ACTH and stimulating both adrenal cortexes to hypertrophy and secrete excess cortisol. It is sometimes the result of ectopic production of ACTH from non-endocrine tumours in the LUNG and PANCREAS. The patient gains weight and the obesity tends to have a characteristic distribution over the face, neck and shoulder and pelvic girdles. Purple striae develop over the abdomen and there is often increased hairiness or hirsutism. The blood pressure is commonly raised and the bone softens as a result of OSTEOPOROSIS. The best test to establish the diagnosis is to measure the amount of cortisol in a 24-hourly specimen of urine. Once the diagnosis has been established it is then necessary to undertake further tests to determine the cause.

CUTANEOUS means belonging to the skin. (See SKIN; SKIN DISEASES.)

CUTICLE (see SKIN).

CUTS (see WOUNDS).

CYANIDE POISONING   Cyanide inhibits cellular RESPIRATION by binding rapidly and reversibly with the ENZYME cytochrome oxidase. Effects of poisoning are due to tissue hypoxia. It is toxic by inhalation, ingestion and prolonged skin contact. Cyanide acts extremely quickly once absorbed. Following inhalation of hydrogen cyanide gas, deaths can occur within minutes. Ingestion of inorganic cyanide salts may produce symptoms within 10 minutes, again proceeding rapidly to death. On a full stomach effects may be delayed for an hour or more. Signs of cyanide poisoning are headache,

dizziness, vomiting, weakness, ATAXIA, HYPERVENTILATION, DYSPNOEA, HYPOTENSION and collapse. Loss of vision and hearing may occur, then COMA and CONVULSIONS. Other features include cardiac ARRHYTHMIAS and PULMONARY OEDEMA. Patients may have a lactic ACIDOSIS. Their arterial oxygen tension is likely to be normal but venous oxygen tension high and similar to that of arterial blood. Administration of oxygen when available is the most important first-aid management. Rescuers should be trained, must not put themselves at risk and should use protective clothing and breathing apparatus. In unconscious victims establish a clear airway and give 100-per-cent oxygen. If breathing stops and oxygen is unavailable, initiate expired air resuscitation. If cyanide salts were ingested, mouth-to-mouth contact must be avoided and a mask with a one-way valve employed instead. Some commercially available first-aid kits contain AMYL NITRATE as an antidote which may be employed if oxygen is unavailable.

Once in hospital, or if a trained physician is on the scene, then antidotes may be administered. There are several different intravenous antidotes that may be used either alone or in combination. In mild to moderate cases sodium thiosulphate is usually given. In more severe cases either dicobalt edetate, sodium nitrite, or cyanocobalamin may be used, followed by sodium thiosulphate. Cyanocobalamin is currently unlicensed in the UK. Some of these (e.g. dicobalt edetate) should be given only where diagnosis is certain, otherwise serious adverse reations or toxicity due to the antidotes may occur.

CYANIDES   Salts of hydrocyanic or prussic acid. They are highly poisonous, and are also powerful antiseptics. (See CYANIDE POISONING; WOUNDS.)

CYANOCOBALAMIN   The name given by the British Pharmacopoeia Commission to vitamin B_{12}. It is a red cobalt-containing substance, and it owes its name to the fact that it contains cyanide and cobalt. Vitamin B_{12} was first isolated in 1948 and was found to be an effective substitute for liver in the treatment of pernicious anaemia. (See ANAEMIA.) It has now been replaced by HYDROXOCOBALAMIN as the standard treatment for this condition. (See COBALAMINS.)

CYANOSIS   A condition of in which the skin, usually of the face and extremities, turns a bluish tinge. It accompanies states in which the blood is not properly oxygenated in the lungs. It appears earliest through the nails, on the lips, and the tips of the ears, and over the cheeks. It may be due to blockage of the air passages, or to disease in the lungs, or to a feeble circulation, as in heart disease. (See CHRONIC OBSTRUCTIVE PULMONARY DISEASE; METHAEMOGLOBINAEMIA.)

CYBERNETICS The science of communication and control in the animal and in the machine.

CYCLAMATES Artificial sweetening agents which are about 30 times as sweet as cane sugar. After being in use since 1965, they were banned by Government decree in 1969 because of adverse reports received from the USA.

CYCLICAL OEDEMA This is a syndrome in women characterized by irregular intermittent bouts of generalized swelling. Sometimes the fluid retention is more pronounced before the menstrual period. The eye lids are puffy and the face and fingers feel stiff and bloated. The breasts may feel swollen and the abdomen distended and ankles may swell. The diurnal weight gain may exceed 4 kg. The underlying disturbance is due to increased loss of fluid from the vascular compartment, probably from leakage of protein from the capillaries increasing the tissue osmotic pressure. Recent evidence suggests a decrease in the urinary excretion of dopamine may contribute as this catecholamine has a natriuretic action. This may explain why drugs that are dopamine antagonists, such as chlorpromazine, may precipitate or aggravate cyclical oedema. Conversely bromocriptine, a dopamine agonist, may improve the oedema.

CYCLIZINE HYDROCHLORIDE An AN-TIHISTAMINE DRUG which is mainly used for the prevention of sickness, including sea-sickness.

CYCLOPHOSPHAMIDE A NITROGEN MUS-TARD derivative used to treat various forms of malignant disease, including Hodgkin's disease and chronic lymphocytic leukaemia. (See CYTO-TOXIC.)

CYCLOPLEGIA Paralysis of the ciliary muscle of the eye, which results in the loss of the power of accommodation in the eye. (See ACCOMMODATION.)

CYCLOPROPANE One of the most potent of the anaesthetics given by inhalation. Its advantages are that it acts quickly, causes little irritation to the lungs, and its effects pass off quickly.

CYCLOSERINE An antibiotic derived from an actinomycete, used to treat certain infections of the genito-urinary tract, and and in combination with other drugs to treat tuberculosis.

CYCLOSPORIN A A drug used to prevent the rejection of transplanted organs such as the heart and kidneys. (See TRANSPLANTATION.)

CYCLOTHYMIA The state characterized by extreme swings of mood from elation to depression, and vice versa.

CYCLOTRON A machine in which positively charged atomic particles are so accelerated that they acquire energies equivalent to those produced by millions of volts. From the medical point of view its interest is that it is a source of neutrons. (See RADIOTHERAPY.)

CYESIS Another term for pregnancy.

CYPROTERONE ACETATE An anti-androgen. It inhibits the effects of androgens at receptor level and is therefore useful in the treatment of prostate cancer, acne, hirsutism in women and in the treatment of severe hypersexuality and sexual deviation in men. (See OESTROGEN.)

CYSTECTOMY The surgical excision of the bladder. When this is done, usually to treat cancer of the bladder, an alternative means of collecting urine from the kidneys must be arranged. The URETERS of the kidney can be transplanted into a loop of bowel which is brought to the surface of the abdomen to form a STOMA that exits into an externally worn pouch. The latest surgical technque is to fashion a substitute bladder from a section of intestine and to implant the ureters into it, thus allowing the patient to void urine through the urethra as normal.

CYSTEINE An AMINO-ACID containing SUL-PHUR that is an essential constituent of many of the body's ENZYMES.

CYSTIC DUCT The tube that runs from the gall bladder and joins up with the hepatic duct (formed from the bile ducts) to form the common bile duct. The bile produced by the liver cells is drained through this system and enters the small intestine to help in the digestion of food.

CYSTICERCOSIS This disease rarely occurs except in Central Europe, Ethiopia, South Africa, and part of Asia. It results from ova being swallowed or regurgitated into the stomach from an adult pork tapeworm in the intestine. In the stomach the larvae escape from the eggs and are absorbed. They are carried in the blood to various parts of the body, most commonly the subcutaneous tissue and skeletal muscle, where they develop and form cysticerci. When superficial, they may be felt under the skin as small pea-like bodies. Although they cause no symptoms here, cysts may also develop in the brain. Five years later the larvae die, and the brain-tissue reaction may result in epileptic fits, obscure neurological disorders, and personality changes. The cysts calcify at this stage, though to a greater degree in the muscles than the brain, allowing them to be seen radiologically. Epilepsy starting in adult life, in anyone who has previously lived in an endemic area, should suggest the possibility of cysticercosis.

Treatment Most important is prevention of the initial tapeworm infection, by ensuring that pork is well cooked before eating it. Nurses and others attending to a patient harbouring an adult tapeworm must be careful to avoid ingesting ova from contaminated hands. The tapeworm itself can be destroyed with NICLOSAMIDE. Brain infections are treated with sedatives and anti-convulsants, surgery rarely being necessary. Most patients make a good recovery.

CYSTIC FIBROSIS This is the commonest serious genetic disease in Caucasian children, with an incidence of about 1 per 2000 births. It is an autosomal recessive disorder of the mucus-secreting glands of the lungs, the pancreas, the mouth, and the gastro-intestinal tract, as well as the sweat glands of the skin. The defective GENE is sited on CHROMOSOME 7. Individuals who inherit the gene only on one set of chromosomes can, however, carry the defect into successive generations. Where parents have a child with cystic fibrosis, they have a one-in-four chance of subsequent children having the disease. They should seek GENETIC COUNSELLING.

The disorder is characterized by failure to gain weight in spite of a good appetite, by repeated attacks of bronchitis, and the passage of loose, foul-smelling and slimy stools. A simple, cheap, reliable test for detecting the disease by examination of the stools has now been evolved, which permits the early diagnosis of the disease. Amniocentesis, which yields amniotic fluid along with cells shed from the foetus's skin, can be used to diagnose cystic fibrosis prenatally. The levels of various enzymes can be measured in the fluid and are abnormal when the fetus is affected by cystic fibrosis. A useful diagnostic test on the postnatal infant is the sweat test. This detects the abnormal amount of salt that is excreted via the sweat glands when cystic fibrosis is present.

Treatment This consists basically of regular physiotherapy and postural drainage, antibiotics and the taking of pancreatic enzyme tablets and vitamins. The earlier treatment is started, the better the results. Whereas two decades ago, only 12 per cent of affected children survived beyond adolescence, today 75 per cent survive into adult life, and an increasing number are surviving into their 40s. Parents of children with cystic fibrosis, seeking help and advice, can obtain this from the Cystic Fibrosis Trust (see APPENDIX 2: ADDRESSES).

CYSTITIS Inflammation of the bladder. The presenting symptom is usually dysuria; that is, a feeling of discomfort when urine is passed and frequently a stinging or burning pain in the urethra. There is also a feeling of wanting to pass water much more often than usual and yet there is very little urine present when the act is performed. Cystitis may be associated with a dragging ache in the lower abdomen. The urine usually looks dark or stronger than normal. It is frequently associated with haematuria, which means blood in the urine and is the result of the inflammation. It is a common problem; over half the women in Britain suffer from it at some time in their life. The cause of the disease is a bacterial infection of the bladder, the germs having entered the urethra and ascended into the bladder. The most common organism responsible is called ESCHERACHIA COLI. This organism normally lives in the bowel where it causes no harm. It is therefore likely to be present on the skin around the anus so that there is always a potential for infection. The disease is much more common in women because the urethra, vagina and anus are very close together and the urethra is much shorter in the female than it is in the male. It also explains why women commonly suffer cystitis after sexual intercourse and honeymoon cystitis is a very common presentation of bladder inflammation. In most cases the inflammation is more of a nuisance than a danger but the infection can spread up to the kidneys and cause PYELITIS which is a much more serious disorder.

In cases of cystitis the urine should be cultured to grow the responsible organism. The relevant antibiotic can then be prescribed. Fluids should be taken freely not only for an acute attack of cystitis but also to prevent further attacks, because if the urine is dilute the organism is less likely to grow. Bicarbonate of soda is also helpful as this reduces the acidity of the urine and helps to relieve the burning pain, and inhibits the growth of the bacteria. Careful hygiene, in order to keep clean down below, is also important. (See URINARY BLADDER, DISEASES OF.)

CYSTOCOELE A prolapse of the base of the bladder in a woman. The pelvic floor muscles may be weakened after childbirth and, when the woman strains, the front wall of the vagina bulges. Stress incontinence often accompanies a cystocoele and surgical repair is then advisable (see COLPORRHAPHY).

CYSTOGRAM An X-ray picture of the urinary bladder.

CYSTOMETER An instrument for measuring the pressure in the urinary bladder.

CYSTOSCOPE An instrument for viewing the interior of the bladder. It consists of a narrow tube carrying a small electric lamp at its end, a small mirror set obliquely opposite an opening near the end of the tube, and a telescope which is passed down the tube and by which the reflection of the brightly illuminated bladder wall in the mirror is examined. It is of great value in the diagnosis of conditions like ulcers and small tumours of the bladder.

Fine catheters can be passed along the cystoscope, and by the aid of vision can be inserted into each ureter and pushed up to the kidney, so that the urine from each kidney may be obtained and examined separately in order to diagnose which of these organs is diseased.

CYSTS Hollow tumours, containing fluid or soft material. They are almost always simple in nature.

Varieties

RETENTION CYSTS In these, in consequence of irritation or other cause, some cavity which ought naturally to contain a little fluid becomes distended or the natural outlet from the cavity becomes blocked. Wens are caused by the blockage of the outlet from sebaceous glands in the skin, so that an accumulation of fatty matter takes place. RANULA is a clear swelling under the tongue, due to a collection of saliva in consequence of an obstruction to a salivary duct. Cysts in the breasts are, in many cases, the result of blockage in milk ducts, due to inflammation; they should be assessed to exclude cancer (see BREASTS, DISEASES OF). Cysts also form in the kidney as a result of obstruction to the free outflow of the urine.

DEVELOPMENTAL CYSTS Of these, the most important are the huge cysts that originate in the ovaries. The cause is doubtful, but the cyst probably begins at a very early period of life, gradually enlarges, and buds off smaller cysts from its wall. The contents are usually a clear gelatinous fluid. Very often both ovaries are affected, and the cysts may slowly reach a great size, often, however, taking a lifetime to do so.

A similar condition sometimes occurs in the kidney, and the tumour may have reached a great size in an infant even before birth (congenital cystic kidney).

Dermoid cysts are small cavities, which also originate probably early in life, but do not reach any great size till fairly late in life. They appear about parts of the body where clefts occur in the embryo and close up before birth, such as the corner of the eyes, the side of the neck, the middle line of the body. They contain hair, fatty matter, fragments of bone, scraps of skin, even numerous teeth.

HYDATID CYSTS are produced in many organs, particularly in the liver, by a parasite which is the larval stage of a tapeworm found in dogs. They occur in people who keep dogs and allow them to contaminate their food. (See TAENIASIS.)

CYTARABINE An antimetabolite substance that interferes with cellular division (see CYTOTOXIC).

CYTO- A prefix meaning something connected with a cell or cells.

CYTOGENETICS The study of the structure and functions of the cells of the body, with particular reference to the CHROMOSOMES.

CYTOLOGY The study of cells.

CYTOMEGALOVIRUSES A group of viruses belonging to the herpesvirus group. They are so-called from the swollen appearance of infected cells ('cytomegalo' = large cell). Their importance is that they are responsible for the condition of cytomegalic disease of the newborn. The virus is transmitted from the mother either to her unborn baby while still in the uterus or to the baby during birth. In some cases the baby may show no evidence of infection, but in others it may cause a fatal disease characterized by jaundice and an enlarged liver and spleen. In those who recover from this severe form of the disease, there may be permanent mental retardation. In England and Wales, around 400 babies a year are born mentally retarded because the mother was infected with the virus in pregnancy.

CYTOMETER An instrument for counting and measuring cells.

CYTOPLASM The PROTOPLASM of the cell body. (See CELLS.)

CYTOTOXIC means being destructive to cells. Many cytotoxic drugs are now available for the treatment of cancer and to suppress the immune system to prevent rejection of organ transplants. In some patients with cancer the treatment with cytotoxic drugs, or CHEMOTHERAPY, is given with the aim of curing the disease. Under these circumstances some degree of drug-related toxicity is acceptable. Patients with acute LEUKAEMIA and LYMPHOMAS as well as some carcinomas can be be cured with cytotoxic drugs. They are frequently used in combination because of the enhanced response achieved when given in this way.

The cytotoxic drugs include: (1) the alkylating agents which act by damaging DNA, thus interfering with cell reproduction. Cyclophosphamide, ifosfamide, chlorambucil, kelphalan, busulphan, thiotepa and mustine are examples of alkylating agents.

(2) There are a number of cytotoxic antibiotics used in the treatment of cancer – doxorubicin, bleomycin, actinomycin D, mithramycin and amsacrine are examples. They are used primarily in the treatment of acute leukaemia and lymphomas.

(3) Antimetabolites – these drugs combine irreversibly with vital enzymes systems of the cell and hence prevent normal cell division. Methotrexate, cytarabine, fluorouracil, mercaptopurine and azathioprine are examples.

(4) Another group of cytotoxic drugs are the vinca alkaloids such as vincristine, vinblastine and vindesima.

(5) Some newer cytotoxic drugs have been introduced, such as cisplatin. This cytotoxic agent is particularly useful in the treatment of carcinoma of the ovary and teratomas of the testis.

Carboplatin, a derivative of cisplatin, is given intravenously in ovarian cancer and small-cell lung cancer. Better tolerated than cisplatin, the drug causes less nausea and vomiting, nephrotoxicity, neurotoxicity and ototoxicity.

Where platinum-containing therapy has failed, intravenous treatment with paclitaxel may be tried. With only a limited success rate, it is relatively toxic and should be carefully supervised; responses, however, are sometimes prolonged.

Also of increasing importance in treating cancer are interferons. These are naturally occurring proteins with complex effects on immunity and cell function. Although toxic, with numerous adverse effects, they have shown some antitumour effect against certain lymphomas and solid tumours.

D

DACRYOCYSTITIS (see EYE DISEASES).

DACTINOMYCIN A cytotoxic antibiotic drug principally used for treating cancers such as acute LEUKAEMIAS and LYMPHOMAS in children. It is given intravenously and treatment normally takes place in hospital. The drug was previously known as actinomycin D. Side-effects are potentially serious.

DACTYLITIS Inflammation of a finger or toe.

DANAZOL This drug inhibits pituitary gonadotrophin secretion and is used in the treatment of ENDOMETRIOSIS, MENORRHAGIA and GYNAE-COMASTIA. The dose is usually of the order of 100 mg twice daily and side-effects may include nausea, dizziness, flushing and skeletal muscle pain. It is mildly androgenic.

D and C (DILATATION AND CURETTAGE): Scraping the lining of the uterus using a curette after opening up the cervix using a series of dilators. Incomplete ABORTIONS and uterine POLYPS may be treated by this procedure, but it is usually used to obtain tissue samples to assist in diagnosis of uterine disorders.

DANDRUFF or SCURF The white scales shed from the scalp. The disorder is caused by increased production of epidermal surface cells. Treatment is regular washing with an antidandruff shampoo. (See SEBORRHOEA.)

DANGEROUS DRUGS (see CONTROLLED DRUGS).

DANTROLENE A muscle-relaxing drug, indicated for chronic severe spasticity of voluntary muscle such as may occur after a stroke or in cerebral palsy and multiple sclerosis. Unlike most other relaxants, it acts directly on the muscle, thus producing fewer central-nervous-system side-effects. It is contraindicated if liver function is impaired and is not recommended for children or for acute muscle spasm. It may cause drowsiness, resulting in impaired performance at skilled tasks and driving.

DAPSONE One of the most effective drugs in the treatment of LEPROSY. An antibacterial drug, its use may cause nausea, vomiting and, occasionally, it may harm nerves, the liver and red blood cells. During treatment blood tests are done to check on liver function and the number of red cells in the blood.

The drug is also used to treat dermatitis herpetiformis, a rare skin disorder.

DARTOS The thin muscle just under the skin of the scrotum which enables the scrotum to alter its shape.

DAY BLINDNESS A condition in which the patient sees better in a dim light or by night than in daylight. It is only found in conditions in which the light is very glaring, as in the desert and on snow, and is relieved by resting the retina, for example by wearing coloured glasses for a time.

DAYDREAMS occur when an individual during waking hours imagines enjoyable or exciting events or images. Most people daydream at some stage during their lives but it tends to occur when someone is stressed or unhappy. Children and teenagers in particular may sometimes daydream a lot. This should not usually worry their parents or teachers unless their work suffers or it affects the individual's personal relationships.

In those circumstances professional advice should be sought from a doctor or counsellor.

DAY SURGERY Surgery done in a clinic or a hospital without an overnight stay either before or after the operation. Improvements in surgery, especially the introduction of MINI-MALLY INVASIVE SURGERY, as well as more effective methods of anaesthesia, have simplified many procedures and reduced the physical and mental stress on patients. Patients undergoing day surgery should be accompanied home by a friend or relative. Occasionally a patient may develop complications that require a post-operative stay in hospital.

DDT or DICHLORODIPHENYL TRICHLORETHANE is the generally used abbreviation for the compound which has been given the official name of dicophane. It was first synthesized in 1874, but it was not until 1940 that, as a result of research work in Switzerland, its remarkable toxic action on insects was discovered. This work was taken up and rapidly expanded in Great Britain and the USA, and one of its first practical applications was in controlling the spread of TYPHUS. This disease is transmitted by the louse, one of the insects for which DDT is most toxic. Its toxic action against the mosquito has also been amply proved, and it thus rapidly became one of the most effective measures in controlling MALARIA. DDT is toxic to a large range of insects in addition to the louse and the mosquito; these include house-flies, bed-bugs, clothes-moths, fleas, cockroaches, and ants. It is also active against many agricultural and horticultural pests, including weevils, flour beetles, pine sawfly, and most varieties of scale insect.

DDT has thus had a wide use in medicine, public health, veterinary medicine, horticulture, and agriculture. Unfortunately, the indiscriminate use of DDT is potentially hazardous, and its use is now restricted or banned in several countries, including the United Kingdom.

The danger of DDT is that it enters the biological food chain with the result that animals at the end of the food chain such as birds or predators may build up lethal concentrations of the substance in their tissues.

In any case an increasing number of species of insects were becoming resistant to DDT. Fortunately, newer insecticides have been introduced which are toxic to DDT-resistant insects, but there are doubts whether this supply of new insecticides can be maintained as insects develop resistance to them.

DEAD, DISPOSAL OF THE Practically, only three methods have been used from the earliest times: burial; embalming; cremation. BURIAL is perhaps the earliest and most primitive method. It was customary to bury the bodies of the dead in consecrated ground around the churches till the earlier half of the nineteenth century, when the utterly insanitary state of churchyards led to legislation for their better control. Burials in Britain take place usually upon production of a certificate from a registrar of deaths, to whom notice of the death, accompanied by a medical certificate, must be given without delay by the nearest relatives.

Embalming is still used occasionally. The process consists in removing the internal organs by small openings and filling the body cavities with various aromatics of antiseptic power, the skin being swathed in bandages or otherwise protected from the action of the air. Bodies are also preserved by injecting the blood-vessels with strong antiseptics like perchloride of mercury.

Cremation or incineration of the body is now the commonest method of disposal of the dead in the UK, where land for burials is increasingly scarce. The process of incineration takes between one and two hours. About 2·3 to 3·2 kg (5 to 7 pounds) of ash result from the combustion of the body, and there is no admixture with that from the fuel.

In order to prevent any abuse, special certificates are required, and the necessary forms for these are obtained from the cremating authority.

DEAD FINGERS (see RAYNAUD'S DISEASE).

DEADLY NIGHTSHADE The popular name of *Atropa belladonna*, from which atropine is procured. Its poisonous black berries are sometimes eaten by children. (See ATROPINE.)

DEAD SPACE Gas exchange only occurs in the terminal parts of the pulmonary airways. That portion of each breath that is taken into the lungs but does not take part in gas exchange is known as dead space. Anatomical dead space describes air in the airways up to the terminal bronchioles. Physiological dead space also includes gas in alveoli which are unable to take part in gas exchange because of structural abnormalities or disease.

DEAFNESS Impairment of hearing, which affects about 2 million adults in the UK. In infants permanent deafness is much less common: about 1–2 per 1000. It is essential, however, that deafness is picked up early so that appropriate treatment and support can be given to improve hearing and/or ensure that the child can learn to speak.

In most people, deafness is a result of sensorineural hearing impairment, commonly known as nerve deafness. This means that the abnormality is located in the inner ear (the cochlea), the auditory nerve or in the brain itself. The prevalence of this type of hearing impairment rises greatly in elderly people to the extent that over 50 per cent of the over-70s have a moderate hearing impairment. In most cases, no definite cause can be found, but excessive exposure to noise, either at work (e.g. shipyards and steelworks) at lesiure (loud music). Anyone, such as service personnel, exposed to gunfire or explosions, is also likely to develop some hearing impairment.

Conductive hearing impairment is the other main classification. Here there is an abnormality of the external or middle ear preventing the normal transmission of sound waves to the inner ear. This is most commonly due to chronic otitis media where there is inflammation of the middle ear, often with a perforation of the ear drum. It is thought that in the majority of cases this is a sequela of childhood middle-ear disease. Wax does not interfere with hearing unless it totally obstructs the ear canal or is impacted against the tympanic membrane.

Treatment Conductive hearing impairment can, in many cases, be treated by an operation on the middle ear or by the use of a hearing aid. Sensorineural hearing impairments can be treated only with a hearing aid. In the UK hearing aids are available free on the NHS. Most NHS hearing aids are ear-level hearing aids, that is, they fit behind the ear with the sound transmitted to the ear via a mould in the external ear. Smaller hearing aids are becoming available which fit within the ear itself and people can wear such aids in both ears. The use of certain types of hearing aid may be augmented by fittings incorporated into the aid which pick up sound directly from television sets or from telephones, and from wire loop systems in halls, lecture theatres and classrooms. More recently bone-anchored hearing aids have been developed where the hearing aid is attached directly to the bones of the skull using a titanium screw. This type of hearing aid is particularly useful in children with abnormal or absent ear canals who cannot therefore wear conventional hearing aids. People with hearing impairment should seek medical advice before purchasing any of the many types of hearing aid available commercially. Those people with a hearing impairment which is so profound ('stone deaf') that they cannot be helped by a hearing aid can sometimes now be fitted with an electrical implant in their inner ear (a cochlear implant).

Congenital hearing loss accounts for a very small proportion of the hearing-impaired population. It is important to detect at an early stage as, if undetected and unaided, it may lead to delayed or absent development of speech. The commonest cause of hearing difficulties in childhood is otitis media with effusion (glue ear). This usually resolves spontaneously, though if it persists, surgical intervention may be required usually involving insertion of a ventilation tube (see GROMMET) into the ear drum, often combined with removal of the adenoids (see NOSE, DISEASES OF). Recent studies, however, suggest that in many children this operation is not effective and the extent of its use is controversial.

Advice and information on deafness and hearing aids may be obtained from the Royal National Institute for Deaf People (see APPENDIX 2: ADDRESSES).

DEAMINATION The process of removal of the amino group, NH$_2$, from amino-acids not required for building up body protein. This is carried out mainly in the liver by means of an enzyme, deaminase. The fatty acid residue is either burnt up to yield energy, or is converted into glucose.

DEATH, CAUSES OF Although the final cause of death is usually failure of the vital centres which govern the beating of the heart and the act of breathing, the practical question is the disease or injury which leads to this failure.

The principal causes of death in England in 1995 were ischaemic heart disease (133,000) and cerebrovascular disease (59,600). Cancer of the respiratory organs accounted for 31,500 deaths and cancer of the stomach for 7,000.

Nearly 12,600 women died from cancer of the breast and over 1,330 from uterine cancer. Overall in 1995, just over 139,000 people died from malignant disease.

DEATH CERTIFICATE A certificate required by law to be signed by a medical practitioner stating the main and any contributary causes of a person's death.

DEATH RATE In 1995, the death rate in the UK was 11·1 per thousand, a fall from the figure of 11·7 in 1985.

DEATH, SIGNS OF There are some minor signs, such as relaxation of the facial muscles, which produces the staring eye and gaping mouth of the 'Hippocratic countenance', as well as a loss of the curves of the back, which becomes flat by contact with the bed or table; discoloration of the skin, which becomes of a wax-yellow hue, and loses its pink transparency at the finger-webs; absence of blistering and redness if the skin is burned (Christison's sign); and failure of a ligature tied round the finger to produce, after its removal, the usual change of a white ring, which, after a few seconds, becomes redder than the surrounding skin in a living person.

The only certain sign of death, however, is that the heart has stopped beating. To ensure that this is permanent, it is necessary to listen over the heart with a stethoscope, or directly with the ear, for at least five minutes. Permanent stoppage of breathing should also be confirmed by observing that a mirror held before the mouth shows no haze, or that a feather placed on the upper lip does not flutter. An important sign is that if a cut is made in the skin or blood vessel after death no bleeding takes place.

In the vast majority of cases there is no difficulty in ensuring that death has occurred. The introduction of organ transplantation, however, and of more effective mechanical means of resuscitation, such as respirators, whereby an individual's heart can be kept beating almost indefinitely, has raised difficulties in a minority of cases. To solve the problem in these cases the concept of 'brain death' has been introduced. In this context it has to be borne in mind that there is no legal definition of death. Death has traditionally been diagnosed by the irreversible cessation of respiration and heart-beat. In the Code of Practice drawn up in 1983 by a Working Party of the Health Departments of Great Britain and Northern Ireland, however, it is stated that 'death can also be diagnosed by the irreversible cessation of brain-stem function'. This is described as 'brain death'. The brain-stem consists of the mid-brain, pons and medulla oblongata which contain the centres controlling the vital processes of the body such as consciousness, breathing and the beating of the heart (see BRAIN). This new concept of death, which has been widely accepted in medical and legal circles throughout the world, means that it is now legitimate to equate brain death with death, that the essential component of brain death is death of the brain-stem, and that a dead brain-stem can be reliably diagnosed at the bedside.

Four points are important in determining the time that has elapsed since death. HYPOSTASIS, or congestion, begins to appear as livid spots on the back, often mistaken for bruises, three hours or more after death. It is due to the blood running into the vessels in the lowest parts. Loss of heat begins at once after death, and the body has become as cold as the surrounding air after 12 hours, though this is delayed by hot weather, death from asphyxia, and some other causes. Rigidity, or rigor mortis, begins in six hours, takes another six to become fully established, remains for twelve hours and passes off during the succeeding twelve hours. It comes on quickly when extreme exertion has been indulged in immediately before death. Conversely it is slow in onset and slight in death from wasting diseases. It is slight or absent in children. It begins in the small muscles of the eyelid and jaw and then spreads over the body. Putrefaction is variable in time of onset, but usually begins in 2 or 3 days, as a greenish tint over the abdomen. (See PUTREFACTION.)

DEATH, SUDDEN   If death from accidents is excluded, this means the death of an apparently healthy person. This most commonly occurs as a result of cardiac arrest and among those over 35 the reason is most often the result of CORONARY ARTERY DISEASE leading to a MYOCARDIAL INFARCTION. Other causes of sudden death include ANAPHYLACTIC shock, ASTHMA, MYOCARDITIS, PNEUMONIA, stroke and suicide. A ruptured aortic aneurysm or an ANEURYSM in a cerebral artery can also cause sudden death. Sudden deaths must be reported to the coroner.

DEBILITY   A state of weakness.

DEBRIDEMENT   The surgical removal of foreign material and damaged tissue from a wound.

DECAY, DENTAL   (see CARIES).

DECIBEL   The unit of hearing. One decibel is the least intensity of sound at which a given note can be heard. The usual abbreviation for decibel is dB.

DECIDUA   The soft coat which lines the interior of the womb during pregnancy and which is cast off at birth.

DECOCTION   A preparation made by boiling various plants in water and straining the fluid.

DECOMPENSATION   A failing condition of the heart in a case of valvular disease.

DECONGESTANTS   Drugs which relieve nasal congestion and stuffiness. They may be given orally or by nasal spray, and most are sympathomimetics which cause vasoconstriction in the nasal mucosa. Too frequent use reduces their effectiveness. Examples are sodium chloride nasal drops or ephedrine drops. Warm moist air is also a traditional effective decongestant.

DECUBITUS refers to the positions taken up in bed by patients suffering from various conditions such as pneumonia, peritonitis, or severe exhaustion. Such patients are liable to develop BED SORES, or ULCER DECUBITUS.

DECUSSATION   Any point in the nervous system at which nerve fibres cross from one side to the other: e.g. the decussation of the pyramidal tracts in the medulla, where the motor fibres from one side of the brain cross to the other side of the spinal cord.

DEFAECATION   Opening the bowels. (See CONSTIPATION; DIARRHOEA.)

DEFIBRILLATION   If a heart is fibrillating (see VENTRICULAR FIBRILLATION) the application of a large electric shock via paddles applied to the chest wall causes simultaneous electrical depolarization of all the cardiac cells and may allow the pacemaker to re-establish sinus rhythm. One paddle is placed below the right clavicle and the other over the cardiac apex. Care must be taken that no one is in contact with the patient or the bed when the shock is given, to avoid electrocution.

DEFICIENCY DISEASE   Any disease resulting from the absence from the diet of any substance essential to good health: e.g. one of the vitamins.

DEFORMITIES   Malformations or distortions of part of the body. They may be present at birth, or they may be the result of injuries, or disease, or simply produced by bad posture, like the curved spine occasionally found in children. (See BURNS; CHEST, DEFORMITIES OF; CLUB-FOOT; FINGERS; FLAT-FOOT; KNOCK-KNEE; LEPROSY; PALATE, MALFORMATIONS OF; PARALYSIS; RICKETS; SCAR; SKULL; SPINE AND SPINAL CORD, DISEASES AND INJURIES OF; JOINTS, DISEASES OF.)

DEGENERATION   A change in structure or in chemical composition of a tissue or organ by which its vitality is lowered or its function interfered with. Degeneration is of various kinds, the chief being fatty, fibroid (see CIRRHOSIS), calcareous, waxy, colloid, and mucoid.

Causes of degeneration are, in many cases, very obscure. In some cases heredity plays a part, particular organs, for example the kidneys, tending to show fibroid changes in successive generations. Fatty, fibroid, and calcareous degenerations are part of the natural change in old age. Defective nutrition may bring them on prematurely, as may excessive and long-continued strain upon an organ like the heart. Various poisons, like alcohol, play a special part in producing the changes, and so do the poisons produced by various diseases, particularly syphilis and tuberculosis.

DEGENERATIVE DISORDERS An umbrella description for a wide variety of conditions in which there is increased deterioration of the structure or function (or both) of the body. Ageing causes a steady degeneration of many tissues and organs – for example, wrinkling of the skin, cataract and poor neuromuscular coordination. In degenerative disorders the changes occur earlier in life. The nervous system, muscles, arteries, joints and eyes are all susceptible. Specialized tissues are replaced by CONNECTIVE TISSUE. The commonest example in the nervous system is ALZHEIMER'S DISEASE, which causes dementia, while in HUNTINGTON'S CHOREA, a genetic disorder, dementia is accompanied by incoordination of movements.

DEGLUTITION means the act of swallowing. (See CHOKING.)

DEHISCENCE The breaking open of a wound that is partly healed, usually after surgery.

DEHYDRATION Removal of water. A reduction in the water content of the body. It may be caused by an inadequate intake or abnormal losses through sweating, vomiting, diarrhoea, or diuresis. The initial symptom is thirst which progresses to confusion and exhaustion. Rehydration may be produced by drinking, but in severe cases intravenous treatment may be necessary.

DÉJÀ VU A feeling of having already experienced an event which the person is doing or seeing at the moment. French for 'already seen', déjà vu is quite common but no satisfactory explanation for the phenomenon has been discovered.

DELHI BOIL is a form of chronic sore occurring in Eastern countries, caused by a protozoan parasite, *Leishmania tropica*. (See LEISHMANIASIS.)

DELINQUENCY Behaviour by a young person that would be judged a crime if carried out by an adult. Delinquency may also include noncriminal activies – for example, running away from home, missing school lessons, drug or alcohol abuse, and unruly behaviour in public places.

DELIRIUM A condition of altered consciousness in which there is disorientation (as in a confusional state), incoherent talk and restlessness but with hallucination, illusions or delusions also present.

Delirium (confusion) The *milieu intérieur* of some old people is so fragile that acute confusion is a common effect of physical illness. Elderly people are often referred to as being 'confused'; unfortunately this term is often inappropriately applied to a wide range of eccentricities of speech and behaviour as if it were a diagnosis. It can be applied to a patient with the early memory loss of DEMENTIA, forgetful, disorientated and wandering; to the dejected old person with depression, often termed pseudo-dementia; to the patient whose consciousness is clouded in the delirium of acute illness; to the paranoid deluded sufferer of late-onset SCHIZOPHRENIA or even to the patient presenting with the acute DYSPHASIA and incoherence of a stroke.

Delirium tremens is the form of delirium most commonly due to withdrawal from alcohol, if dependent on it. There is restlessness, fear or even terror accompanied by vivid, usually visual, hallucinations or illusions. The level of consciousness is impaired and the patient may be disorientated for time, place and person.

Treatment is, as a rule, the treatment of causes. (See also ALCOHOL.) As the delirium in fevers is due partly to high temperature this should be lowered by tepid sponging. Careful nursing is one of the keystones of successful treatment, which includes ensuring that ample fluids are taken and nutrition is maintained.

DELIVERY The final expulsion of the child in the act of birth. (See LABOUR.)

DELTA WAVES Abnormal electrical waves observed in the electroencephalogram. (See ELECTROENCEPHALOGRAPHY.) The frequency of the normal alpha waves is ten per second. That of the delta waves is seven or less per second. They occur in the region of tumours of the brain, and in the brains of patients with EPILEPSY.

DELTOID The powerful triangular muscle attached above to the collar-bone and shoulder-blade, and below, by its point, to the humerus, nearly half-way down the outer side of the upper arm. Its action is to raise the arm from the side, and it covers and gives roundness to the shoulder. (See MUSCLE.)

DELUSIONS An irrational *idée fixe* peculiar to individuals. They fail to respond to reasonable argument and the delusion is often paranoid in character with a belief that a person or persons are persecuting them. The existence of a delusion, of such a nature as to influence donduct seriusly, is one of the most important signs in reaching a decision to arrange for the compulsory admission of the patient to hospital for observation. (See MENTAL ILLNESS.)

DEMENTIA An acquired and irreversible deterioration in intellectual function. Around 10 per cent of people aged over 65 and 20 per cent of those aged 75 or more are affected to some extent. The disorder is due to progressive brain disease. It appears gradually as a disturbance in problem solving and agility of thought which may be considered to be due to tiredness, boredom or DEPRESSION. As memory failure develops, the affected person becomes bewildered, anxious and emotional when dealing with new surroundings and complex conversations. In professional skilled workers this is frequently first recognized by family and friends. Catastrophic reactions are usually brief but are commonly associated with an underlying depression which can be mistaken for progressive apathy. The condition progresses relentlessly with loss of recent memory extending to affect distant memory and failure to recognize even friends and family. Physical aggression, unsocial behaviour, deteriorating personal cleanliness and incoherent speech commonly develop. Similar symptoms to those in dementia can occur in curable conditions including depression, INTRACRANIAL tumours, SUBDURAL haematoma, SYPHILIS, VITAMIN B_1 deficiency and repeated episodes of cerebral ischaemia. This last may lead to multi-infarct dementia.

Treatment If organic disease is identified, it should, where possible, be treated. Otherwise the treatment of dementia is alleviation of its symptoms. The affected person must be kept clean and properly fed. Good nursing care in comfortable surroundings is important and sedation with appropriate drugs may be required. Patients may eventually need institutional care. (See ALZHEIMER'S DISEASE.)

DEMOGRAPHY The study of populations and factors affecting their health.

DE MORGAN'S SPOTS are small HAEMANGIOMAS which occur in the skin of middle-aged people. No more than 3 mm in diameter, they are rarely widespread and are not malignant.

DEMYELINATION Destruction of the fatty myelin sheath (see MYELIN) around nerve fibres (see NERVES) which interferes with the nerve function. It can occur after injury to the nerve, but is particularly associated with multiple sclerosis.

DENDRITIC ULCER A branching ulcer on the surface of the cornea caused by herpes simplex infection.

DENERVATION Interruption of the nerve supply to an organ or other structure.

DENGUE The term is Spanish, of African origin. The disease was first described by B. Rush in Philadelphia in 1780, and is also known as dengue fever, breakbone fever, and dandy fever, among others. Both endemic and epidemic in tropical and subtropical regions, it is also an acute arboviral infection caused by a flavivirus (family *togaviridae*) – of which there are four – transmitted by mosquitoes of the subgenus Stegomyia, genus *Aëdes* – especially *Aëdes aegypti*. Four serotypes are distinct. Incubation period is 5–8 days, and is followed by abrupt onset of symptoms; fever, facial erythema – with intense itching (which spreads throughout the body), sore throat, running eyes, and painful muscles and joints are common accompaniments. The symptoms subside within a few days and are frequently succeeded by a relapse similar to the first; this diphasic response is often accompanied by a typical 'saddle-back' temperature chart. Further relapses may occur, and joint pains continue for some months. In uncomplicated dengue the mortality rate is virtually zero. Diagnosis is by virus isolation or demonstration of a rising antibody-concentration in the acute phase of infection. There is no specific treatment, but mild analgesics can be used to relieve the pains, and calamine lotion the pruritus. Prevention can be achieved by reduction of the mosquito-vector population.

In 1997 more people than ever before were infected with dengue fever in the Americas, particularly Brazil and Cuba. In 1998 the fever has reached PANDEMIC levels in South-East Asia, with children the worst sufferers. Indonesia's official figures, which probably underestimate the problem, report that 400 people died in the first quarter of 1998, over twice the previous year's number. The increase is attributed to rapid urbanization and increasing human travel within and between countries. Urban areas provide many opportunities for mosquitoes to breed in standing pools and containers of water. The risk of dengue is higher than for nearly half a century.

Dengue haemorrhagic fever This is a more severe form of the disease which usually occurs in young children; it is largely confined to the indigenous population(s) of south-east Asia. It is accompanied by significant complications and mortality. Immunological status of the host is considered important in pathogenesis.

DENTINE (see TEETH).

DENTIST An individual trained to diagnose and treat disorders of the teeth and gums as well as to advise on preventive measures to ensure that these areas remain healthy. Dentistry is divided into several groupings.

General dental practitioner Concerned with primary dental care.

Community dental practitioner Part of the public-health team and is largely concerned with monitoring dental health and treating the young and the handicapped.

In the hospitals and dental schools are those who are involved in only one of the specialities.

Restorative dentist Concerned with the repair of teeth damaged by trauma and caries, and the replacement of missing teeth.

Orthodontist Correction of jaws and teeth which are misaligned or irregular. This is done with appliances which may be removable or fixed to the teeth which are then moved with springs or elastics.

Oral and maxillo-facial surgeons Surgery to the mouth and face. This not only includes removal of buried teeth but also treatment for fractured facial bones, removal of cancers and the repair of missing tissue and the cosmetic restoration of facial anomalies such as cleft palate or large or small jaws.

Most routine dental prevention and treatment take place in general dental practitioners' surgeries. Some of the costs are covered by the NHS but many patients have to pay or part-pay for the services provided. A small number of dental patients have complex problems that require hospital admission so that they can be treated by hospital dentists.

DENTITION (see TEETH).

DENTURE A plate or frame bearing false teeth. It may be complete (replacing all the teeth in one jaw) or partial.

DEODORANTS Substances which remove or lessen objectionable odours. Some, which have a powerful odour, simply cover other smells, but the most effective act by giving off oxygen, so as to convert the objectionable substances into simple and harmless ones.

Varieties Volatile oils of plants, such as eucalyptus and turpentine, chlorine water and chlorinated lime, peroxide of hydrogen and charcoal have been used as deodorants. There are now many commercial products available.

DEOXYRIBONUCLEIC ACID (see DNA).

DEPILATION The process of destroying hair; substances and processes used for this purpose being known as depilatories. The purpose may be effected in three ways: by removing the hairs at the level of the skin surface; by pulling the hairs out (epilation); by destroying the roots and so preventing the growth of new hairs.

Shaving is the most effective way of removing superfluous hairs. Rubbing morning and night with a smooth pumice-stone is said to be helpful. Electrolysis and diathermy are also used.

DEPRESSION A collection of psychological symptoms including sadness, depressive thoughts characterized by worry, poor self-image, self-blame, guilt and low self-confidence; downbeat views on the future; and a feeling of hopelessness. Sufferers may consider suicide and in severe depression may soon develop HALLUCINATIONS and DELUSIONS. Depression is a word that is regularly misused. Most people experience days or weeks when they feel low and fed up, feelings that may recur but generally they get over it without needing to seek medical help. Doctors make the diagnosis of depression when they believe a patient to be ill with a condition that may affect physical health and in some instances be life threatening. This form of depression is common, with up to 15 per cent of the population suffering from it at any one time, while about 20 per cent of adults have 'medical' depression at some time during their lives and it is one of the commonest presenting disorders in general practice. Women seem more liable to develop depression than men, with one in six of the former and one in nine of the latter seeking medical help.

Manic depression is a serious form of the disorder that recurs throughout life and is manifested by bouts of abnormal elation – the manic stage. Both the manic and depressive phases are commonly accompanied by psychotic symptoms such as delusions, hallucinations and a loss of sense of reality. This combination is sometimes termed a manic-depressive psychosis or bipolar affective disorder because of the illness's division into two parts. Another psychiatric description is the catch-all term 'affective disorder'.

Symptoms These vary with the illness's severity. Anxiety and variable moods are the main symptoms in mild depression. The sufferer may cry without any reason or be unresponsive to relatives and friends. In its more severe form, depression presents with a loss of appetite, sleeping problems, lack of interest in and enjoyment of social activities, tiredness for no obvious reason, an indifference to sexual activity and a lack of concentration. The individual's physical and mental activities slow down and he or she may contemplate suicide. Symptoms may vary during the 24 hours, being less troublesome during the latter part of the day and worse at night. Some people get depressed during the winter months, probably as a consequence of the long hours of darkness: this disorder – SEASONAL AFFECTIVE DISORDER SYNDROME (SADS) – is thought to be more common in populations living in areas with long winters and limited daylight. Untreated, a person with depressive symptoms may steadily worsen, even withdrawing to bed for much of the time, and allowing his personal appearance, hygiene and environment to deteriorate. Children and adolescents may also suffer from depression and the disorder is not always recognized.

Causes A real depressive illness rarely has a single obvious cause, though sometimes the death of a close relative, loss of employment or a broken personal relationship may trigger a bout. Depression probably has a genetic background, for instance, manic depression seems to run in some families. Viral infections sometimes cause depression and hormonal disorders, for example, hypothyroidism or postnatal hormonal disturbances (postnatal depression) will cause it. Difficult family or social relations can contribute to the development of the disorder. Depression is believed to occur because of chemical changes in the transmission of signals in the nervous system, with a reduction in the neurochemicals that facilitate the passage of messages throughout the system.

Treatment This depends on the type and severity of the depression. These are three main forms.

PSYCHOTHERAPY either on a one-to-one basis or as part of a group is valuable for those whose depression is the result of life style or personality problems. Various types of psychotherapy are available.

DRUG TREATMENT is the most common method and is particularly helpful for those with physical symptoms. ANTIDEPRESSANT drugs are divided into three main groups: TRICYCLICS (amitriptyline, imipramine and dothiepin are examples); MONOAMINE OXIDASE INHIBITORS (MAOIS) phenelzine, isocarboxazid and tranylcypromine are examples); and SELECTIVE SEROTONIN REUPTAKE INHIBITORS (SSRIS) (fluoxetine – well known as Prozac®, fluvoxamine and paroxetine are examples). For manic depression lithium carbonate is the main preventive drug and it is also used for persistent depression that fails to respond to other treatments. Long-term lithium treatment reduces the likelihood of relapse in about 80 per cent of manic depressives, but the margin between control and toxic side-effects is narrow, so the drug must be carefully supervised. Indeed, all drug treatment for depression needs regular monitoring as the substances have powerful chemical properties with consequential side-effects in some people. Furthermore the nature of the illness means that some sufferers forget or do not want to take the medication.

ELECTROCONVULSIVE THERAPY (ECT) If drug treatents fail, severely depressed patients may be considered for ECT. This treatment has been used for many years but is now only rarely recommended. Given under general anaesthetic, in appropriate circumstances, ECT is safe and effective and may even be life saving, though temporary impairment of memory may occur. Because the treatment was often misused in the past, it still carries a reputation that worries patients and relatives; hence careful assessment and counselling are essential before use is recommended.

Some patients with depression, particularly those with manic depression or who are a danger to themselves or the public, or who are suicidal, may need admission to hospital, or in severe cases to a secure unit, in order to initiate treatment. But as far as possible patients are treated in the community (see MENTAL ILLNESS).

DEPRESSOR The name given to a nerve by whose stimulation motion, secretion, or some other function is restrained or prevented: e.g. the depressor nerve of the heart slows the beating of this organ.

DEPRIVATION SCORE A measure of an individual or group's lack of normal social amenities such as proper housing, diet and warmth. It was devised by a GP (Jarman) in the 1980s to help assess the medical services needed by a socially deprived population.

DERBYSHIRE NECK A traditional name for goitre, which was fairly common in Derbyshire. (See GOITRE.)

DERMABRASION, or 'skin planing', is a method of removing the superficial layers of the skin, useful in the treatment of tattoos and acne scars.

DERMATITIS Synonymous with eczema in all respects; although the lay term 'eczema' usually refers to atopic or endogenous eczema, there are many other causes. Susceptibility to dermatitis is genetically determined in some cases, in others environmental irritants and allergens are implicated. Symptoms typically include itching, dryness or cracking and, occasionally, soreness of the skin. Physical signs include redness (erythema), scaling and vesiculation (tiny blisters just beneath the surface of the skin). (See ECZEMA.)

DERMATOFIBROMA (HISTIOCYTOMA) Firm, painless nodule in the skin, typically on a leg, due to excessive formation of collagen. A common disorder, it is often a slow response to an insect bite and persists indefinitely.

DERMATOGLYPHICS is the study of the patterns made by the ridges and crevices of the hands and the soles of the feet.

DERMATOLOGY In essence, this is the study of the skin. As well as being an organ in its own right, the skin is a stage on which other organs as well as the emotions most visibly play out their roles. Changes in its blood vessels – and hence blood flow through – the skin, may indicate a major immunological response to a range of potential factors (see SKIN DISEASES).

DERMATOME (1) Embryological tissue which has developed from the somites to become the dermis and subcutaneous tissue. The cutaneous area that is derived from each dermatome is supplied by a single dorsal spinal nerve root. (2) A surgical instrument for removing very thin slices of skin for grafting.

DERMATOMYOSITIS A rare disease, possibly caused by an autoimmune reaction, in which muscle inflammation and weakness is associated with a characteristic heliotrope ERYTHEMA of the face and backs of the hands. In adults it may be associated with underlying MALIGNANCY.

DERMATOPHYTES Fungi which can infect skin, hair and nails. About 30 species in three genera are PATHOGENIC to humans (see TINEA).

DERMOGRAPHISM (FACTITOUS URTICARIA) Transient ERYTHEMA and wealing caused by trauma to the skin.

DERMOID CYST (see CYSTS).

DESENSITIZATION In psychiatry a method for treating phobias used in behaviour therapy. The affected individual is slowly acclimatized to the cause of his or her fear. For desensitization against allergies see HYPOSENSITIZATION.

DESFERRIOXAMINE A chelating agent in the treatment of iron poisoning and thalassaemia.

DESIGNER DRUGS A group of chemical substances produced illegally whose properties and effects are similar to those of drugs of abuse. They may be derived from narcotic ANALGESIC drugs, AMPHETAMINES or HALLUCINOGENS. Ecstasy is a widely used designer drug and has caused deaths among teenagers. Designer drugs are potentially dangerous, especially if taken with alcohol.

DESQUAMATION The scaling off of the superficial layer of the epidermis.

DETACHED RETINA Separation of the retina from the choroid in the eye (see EYE). It may be due to trauma or be secondary to tumour or inflammation of the choroid and causes blindness in the affected part of the retina. It can be treated surgically using photocoagulation.

DETERGENTS Substances which clean the skin surface. This means that, strictly speaking, any soap, or soap-like substance used in washing, is a detergent. At the present day, however, the term is largely used for the synthetic detergents which are now used on such a large scale. These are prepared by the cracking and oxidation of high petroleum waxes with sulphuric acid. The commoner ones in commercial preparations are aryl alkyl sulphate or sulphonate and secondary alkyl sulphate.

In view of their widespread use they appear to cause relatively little trouble with the skin, but more trouble has been reported with the so-called 'biological' detergents. They are so named because they contain an ENZYME which destroys protein. As a result they are claimed to remove proteins – stains such as blood, chocolate, milk or gravy, which are relatively difficult for ordinary detergents to remove. Unfortunately these 'biological' detergents may cause dermatitis. In addition, they have been reported to cause asthma in those using them, and even more so in workers manufacturing them.

DETOXICATION Reduction or removal of the toxic properties of poisons or remedies. (See VACCINE.)

DEVIANCE Variation from normal. Often used to describe sexual behaviour.

DEVONSHIRE COLIC This is caused by drinking cider which has been stored in contact with lead, so that colic comes on as a result of lead poisoning.

DEXAMETHASONE A corticosteroid derivative. As an anti-inflammatory agent it is approximately 30 times as effective as cortisone and eight times as effective as prednisolone. On the other hand, it has practically none of the salt-retaining properties of cortisone.

DEXAMPHETAMINE A drug that stimulates the central nervous system. It can be used to treat NARCOLEPSY and hyperactive children but should not be used to combat obesity or treat depression. It is also a drug of abuse.

DEXTRAN The name given to a group of POLYSACCHARIDES which was first discovered in sugar-beet preparations which had become infected with certain bacteria. A homogenous preparation of it, with a consistent molecular weight and free from PROTEIN, is in appropriate clinical circumstances used as a substitute for plasma for transfusion purposes. Dextran is often used as an immediate transfusion measure to treat severe bleeding or certain types of shock until properly cross-matched blood is available for transfusion. A blood sample for cross-matching must be taken before giving intravenous dextran.

DEXTROCARDIA A condition in which a person's heart is situated on the right of the chest in a mirror image of its usual position. This may be associated with similar inversion of the abdominal organs – situs inversus.

DEXTROSE Another name for purified grape sugar or glucose.

DIA- is a prefix meaning through or thoroughly.

DIABETES INSIPIDUS A disease characterized by excessive thirst and the passing of large volumes of urine which have a low specific gravity and contain no abnormal constituents. It is either due to a lack of the antidiuretic hormone normally produced by the HYPOTHALAMUS and stored in the posterior PITUITARY GLAND, or to a defect in the renal tubules which prevents them responding to the antidiuretic hormone vasopressin. When the disorder is due to a VASOPRESSIN insufficiency, a primary or secondary tumour in the area of the pituitary stalk is responsible for one third of cases. In another one third of cases there is no apparent cause and such IDIOPATHIC cases are sometimes familial. A further one third of cases result from a variety of lesions including trauma, basal MENINGITIS and granulomatous lesions in the pituitary stalk area. When the renal tubules fail to respond to vasopressin this is usually because of a genetic defect transmitted as a sex-linked recessive characteristic and the disease is called nephrogenic diabetes insipidus. Metabolic abnormalities such as HYPERCALCAEMIA and potassium depletion render the renal tubule less sensitive to vasopressin and certain drugs such as lithium and tetracycline may have a similar effect.

If the disease is due to a deficiency of vasopressin, treatment should be with the analogue of vasopressin called desmopressin which is more potent than the natural hormone and has less pressor activity. It also has the advantage in that it is absorbed from the nasal mucosa and so does not require to be injected.

Nephrogenic diabetes insipidus cannot be treated with desmopressin. The urine volume can, however, usually be reduced by half by a THIAZIDE diuretic. Diabetes insipidus is a relatively rare condition and must be differentiated from DIABETES MELLITUS which is an entirely different disease.

DIABETES MELLITUS is a condition characterized by a raised concentration of glucose in the blood because of a deficiency in the production and/or action of INSULIN, a pancreatic hormone made in special cells called the islet cells of Langerhans.

Mering and Minkowski in 1889 found that diabetes followed removal of the pancreas from animals. In 1909 it was established that the defect was due to the failure of the pancreas to produce a hormone which was given the name insulin. However it was not until 1921 that two research workers, Banting and Best, first isolated insulin.

Insulin-dependent and non-insulin-dependent diabetes have a varied pathological pattern and are caused by the interaction of several genetic and environmental factors.

Symptoms Thirst, polyuria, GLYCOSURIA, weight loss despite eating, and recurrent infections, e.g. BALANITIS and VULVAL infections, are the main symptoms.

However, subjects with non-insulin-dependent diabetes may have the disease for several years without symptoms and diagnosis is often made incidentally or when presenting with a complication of the disease.

Classification

INSULIN-DEPENDENT DIABETES MELLITUS (IDDM) (juvenile-onset diabetes, Type I diabetes) describes subjects with a severe deficiency or absence of insulin production. Insulin therapy is essential to prevent KETOSIS – a disturbance of the body's acid/base balance and an accumulation of ketones in the tissues. The onset is most commonly during childhood, but can occur at any age. Symptoms are acute and weight loss is common.

NON-INSULIN-DEPENDENT DIABETES MELLITUS (NIDDM) (maturity-onset diabetes, Type II diabetes): this may be further sub-divided into obese and non-obese groups. This type usually occurs after the age of 40 years with an insidious onset. Subjects are often overweight and weight loss is uncommon. KETOSIS rarely develops. Insulin production is reduced but not absent.

DIABETES ASSOCIATED WITH OTHER CONDITIONS (a) Due to pancreatic disease, e.g. chronic PANCREATITIS; (b) secondary to drugs, e.g. GLUCOCORTICOIDS (see PANCREAS, DISEASES OF); (c) excess hormone production, e.g. growth hormone (ACROMEGALY); (d) insulin receptor abnormalities; (e) GENETIC syndromes (see GENETIC DISORDERS).

GESTATIONAL DIABETES Diabetes occurring in pregnancy and resolving afterwards.

Aetiology Insulin-dependent diabetes occurs as a result of autoimmune destruction of beta cells within the pancreas. Genetic influences are important and individuals with certain HLA tissue types (HLA DR3 and HLA DR4) are more at risk. However, the risks associated with the HLA genes are small. If one parent has IDDM, the risk of a child's developing IDDM by the age of 25 years is 1·5–2·5 per cent and the risk of a sibling of an IDDM subject's developing diabetes is about 3 per cent.

Non-insulin-dependent diabetes has no HLA association, but the genetic influences are much stronger. The risks of developing diabetes vary with different races. Obesity, decreased exercise and ageing increase the risks of disease development. The risk of a sibling of a NIDDM subject's developing NIDDM up to the age of 80 years is 30–40 per cent.

Treatment of diabetes aims to prevent symptoms, restore carbohydrate metabolism to as near normal as possible and to minimize complications. Concentration of glucose, fructosamine and glycated haemoglobin in the blood are used to give an indication of blood-glucose control.

Insulin-dependent diabetes requires insulin for treatment. Non-insulin-dependent diabetes may be treated with diet, oral HYPOGLYCAEMIC agents or insulin.

DIET Many NIDDM diabetics may be treated with diet alone. For those subjects who are overweight, weight loss is important, although often unsuccessful. A diet high in complex carbohydrate, high in fibre, low in fat and aiming towards ideal body weight is prescribed. Subjects taking insulin need to eat at regular intervals in relation to their insulin regime and missing meals may result in hypoglycaemia, a lowering of the amount of glucose in the blood. ORAL HYPOGLYCAEMICS are used in the treatment of non-insulin- dependent diabetes in addition to diet, when diet alone fails to control blood sugar levels. (a) SULPHONYLUREAS act mainly by increasing the production of insulin. (b) Biguanides, of which only Metformin is available, may be used alone or in addition to sulphonylureas. Its main actions are to lower the production of glucose by the liver and improve its uptake in the peripheral tissues.

INSULIN All insulin is injected – mainly by syringe but sometimes by insulin pump – because it is inactivated by gastrointestinal enzymes. There are three main types of insulin preparation: (a) short action (approximately 6 hours), with rapid onset; (b) intermediate action (approximately 12 hours); (c) long action, with slow onset and lasting for up to 36 hours. Human, porcine and bovine preparations are available. Much of the insulin now used is prepared by genetic engineering techniques from micro-organisms. There are many regimens of insulin treatment involving different combinations of insulin. Regimens vary depending on the requirements of the patients, most of whom administer the insulin themselves. Carbohydrate intake, energy expenditure and the presence of infection are important determinants of insulin requirements on a day-to-day basis.

Complications The risks of complications increase with duration of disease.

INCREASED RISKS are present of (a) heart disease, (b) peripheral vascular disease and (c) cerebrovascular disease.

DIABETIC EYE DISEASE (a) retinopathy, (b) cataract. Regular examination of the fundus enables any abnormalities developing to be detected and treatment given when appropriate to preserve eyesight.

NEPHROPATHY Subjects with diabetes may develop kidney damage which can result in renal failure.

NEUROPATHY (a) Symmetrical sensory polyneuropathy, damage to the sensory nerves that commonly presents with tingling, numbness of pain in the feet or hands. (b) Asymmetrical motor diabetic neuropathy presenting as progressive weakness and wasting of the proximal muscles of legs. (c) Mononeuropathy, individual motor or sensory nerves may be affected. (d) Autonomic neuropathy, which affects the autonomic nervous system, has many presentations, including IMPOTENCE, diarrhoea or constipation and postural HYPOTENSION.

SKIN LESIONS There are several skin disorders associated with diabetes including (a) Necrobiosis lipoidica diabeticorum characterized by one or more yellow atrophic lesions on the legs. (b) Ulcers, which most commonly occur on the feet due to peripheral vascular disease, neuropathy and infection. Foot care is very important.

DIABETIC KETOACIDOSIS occurs when there is insufficient insulin present to prevent KETONE production. This may occur before the diagnosis of IDDM or when insufficient insulin is being given. The presence of large amounts of ketones in the urine indicates excess ketone production and treatment should be sought immediately. Coma and death may result if the condition is left untreated.

DIABETIC HYPOGLYCAEMIA occurs when amounts of glucose in the blood become low. This may occur in subjects taking sulphonylureas or insulin. Symptoms usually develop when the glucose concentration falls below 2·5 mmol/l. They may, however, occur at higher concentrations in subjects with persistent hyperglycaemia – an excess of glucose – and at lower levels in subjects with persistent hypoglycaemia. Symptoms include confusion, hunger and sweating. Refined sugar followed by complex carbohydrate will return the glucose concentration to normal. If the subject is unable to swallow, glucagon may be given intramuscularly or glucose intravenously, followed by oral carbohydrate, once the subject is able to swallow.

Though it has been shown that careful control of the patient's metabolism prevents late complications in the small blood vessels, the risk of hypoglycaemia is increased and patients need to be well motivated to keep to their dietary and treatment regime. This regime is also very expensive. All risk factors for the patient's cardiovascular system – not simply controlling hyperglycaemia – may need to be reduced if late complications to the cardiovascular system are to be avoided.

Diabetes is one of the world's most serious health problems. Recent projections suggest that the disorder will affect nearly 240 million individuals worldwide by 2010, double its prevalence in 1994. The incidence of insulin-dependent diabetes is rising in young children; they will be liable to develop late complications.

Although there are complications associated with diabetes, many subjects live normal lives and survive to an old age. People with diabetes or their relatives can obtain advice from the British Diabetic Association (see APPENDIX 2: ADDRESSES).

DIAGNOSIS The skill of distinguishing one disease from another, and is essential to scientific and successful treatment. The name is also given to the opinion arrived at as to the nature of a disease. It is in diagnosis more than in treatment that the highest medical skill is required, and, for a diagnosis, the past and hereditary history of a case, the symptoms complained of, and the signs of disease found upon examination are all weighed. Many methods of laboratory examination are also used at the present day in aiding diagnosis.

DIALYSIS A procedure used to filter off waste products from the blood and remove surplus fluid from the body in someone who has KIDNEY failure. The scientific process involves separating crystalloid and COLLOID substances from a solution by interposing a semipermeable membrane, such as cellophane, between the solution and pure water. The crystalloid substances pass through the membrane into the water until a state of equilibrium, so far as the crystalloid substances are concerned, is established between the two sides of the membrane. The colloid substances do not pass through the membrane.

Dialysis is available as either haemodialysis or peritoneal dialysis.

Haemodialysis Blood is removed from the circulation either through an artificial arteriovenous fistula (junction) or a temporary or permanent internal catheter in the jugular vein. It then passes through an artificial kidney ('dialyser') to remove toxins (e.g. potassium and urea) by diffusion and excess salt and water by ultrafiltration from the blood into dialysis fluid prepared in a 'proportionator' (often referred to as a 'kidney machine'). Dialysers vary in design and performance but all work on the principle of a semipermeable membrane separating blood from dialysis fluid. Haemodialysis is undertaken two to three times a week for 4 to 6 hours a session.

Peritoneal dialysis uses the peritoneal lining as a semipermeable membrane. Approximately 2 litres of sterile fluid is run into the peritoneum through the permanent indwelling catheter, is left for 3 to 4 hours, and the cycle is repeated three to four times per day. Most patients undertake continuous ambulatory peritoneal dialysis (CAPD), a few use a machine overnight (continuous cycling peritoneal dialysis, CCPD) which allows greater clearance of toxins.

Disadvantages of haemodialysis include cardiovascular instability, hypertension, bone disease, anaemia and development of periarticular AMYLOIDOSIS. Disadvantages of peritoneal dialysis include peritonitis, poor drainage of fluid and gradual loss of overall efficiency as endogenous renal function declines. Haemodialysis is usually done in outpatient dialysis clinics by skilled nurses but some patients can carry out the procedure at home. Both haemodialysis and peritoneal dialysis carry a relatively high morbidity and the ideal treatment for patients with end-stage renal failure is successful renal TRANSPLANTION.

DIAMORPHINE and DIACETYLMORPHINE are other names for HEROIN.

DIAPHORESIS Another name for sweating. (See PERSPIRATION.)

DIAPHRAGM, or MIDRIFF, is the muscular partition which separates the cavity of the abdomen from that of the chest. It is very thin and is of a dome shape, extending up on the right side to the space beneath the fourth rib, on the left to that beneath the fifth. In contact with its lower surface are, on the right side, the liver, right kidney, and suprarenal body, and to the left the stomach, pancreas, left kidney, suprarenal body, and spleen; while upon its upper surface lies the heart, with a lung on either side. The diaphragm is attached by its edge to the lower margin of the chest all round, and consists of muscular fibres meeting round a trefoil-shaped piece of fibrous tissue in the centre. It completely shuts off the above-named cavities from one another, being pierced only by openings for the gullet, the aorta, and the inferior vena cava, with a few minute openings for nerves and small vessels. The diaphragm is of great importance in respiration, playing the chief part in filling the lungs. During deep respiration its movements are responsible for 60 per cent of the total amount of air breathed and in the horizontal posture, or in sleep, an even greater percentage.

The description 'diaphragm' is also used for the hemispherical rubber ('dutch') cap used in conjunction with a chemical spermicide as a contraceptive. It fits over the neck of the uterus (cervix) inside the vagina. (See CONTRACEPTION.)

DIAPHYSECTOMY The operation whereby a part of the shaft of a long bone (e.g. humerus, femur) is excised.

DIAPHYSIS The shaft of a long bone.

DIAPULSE A form of pulsed high-frequency electrical energy, consisting of pulsed shortwave bursts of energy of 1000 watts maximum, with an average input of 36 watts. It is used as a form of physiotherapy, particularly in the treatment of severe sprains.

DIARRHOEA or looseness of the bowels is increased frequency, fluidity or volume of bowel movements as compared to the person's customary pattern of bowel movements. Most people have occasional attacks of acute diarrhoea, usually caused by contaminated food or water. Such attacks normally clear up within a day or two, whether or not they are treated. Chronic diarrhoea, on the other hand, may be the result of a serious intestinal disorder or of more general disease.

The commonest cause of acute diarrhoea is food poisoning, the organisms involved usually being STAPHYLOCOCCUS, CLOSTRIDIUM BACTERIA, SALMONELLA or CAMPYLOBACTER. A person may also acquire infective diarrhoea as a result of droplet infections from adenoviruses or echoviruses. Interference with the bacterial flora of the intestine may cause acute diarrhoea: this often happens to someone who travels to another country and acquires unfamiliar intestinal bacteria. Other infections include bacillary dysentery, typhoid fever and paratyphoid fevers (see ENTERIC FEVERS). Drug toxicity, food allergy, food intolerance and anxiety may also cause acute diarrhoea, and habitual constipation may result in attacks of diarrhoea.

TREATMENT of diarrhoea in adults depends on the cause. The water and salts (see ELECTROLYTES) lost during a severe attack must be replaced to prevent dehydration. Ready-prepared mixtures of salts can be bought from a chemist. Antidiarrhoeal drugs such as codeine phosphate or loperamide should be used in infectious diarrhoea only if the symptoms are disabling. Antibacterial drugs may be used under medical direction. Persistent diarrhoea – longer than a week – or blood-stained diarrhoea must be investigated under medical supervision.

Diarrhoea in infants is such a serious condition that it requires separate consideration. One of its features is that it is usually accompanied by vomiting. Some 10 per cent of the cases in this country are due to the DYSENTERY organisms and will not be considered here. The remainder constitute the group of cases now usually referred to as infantile gastroenteritis. The condition is rare after the age of fifteen months, and the majority of cases occur between the ages of two and four months. The younger the infant, the higher the mortality rate. This is the type of diarrhoea which used to be known as 'summer diarrhoea' because of its high incidence in the late summer, but during recent years this seasonal incidence has tended to disappear. The precise cause is still obscure, but certain strains of the organism known as *ESCHERICHIA COLI (E. coli)* are responsible for some cases, whilst in others a virus, often the rotavirus, is the cause. One predisposing factor is artificial feeding. The condition is rare in breast-fed babies, and when it does occur in these it is usually less severe. The environment of the infant is also important. The condition is highly infectious and, if a case occurs in a maternity home or a children's hospital, it tends to spread quickly. This is why such an institution is closed to all further admissions if a case of infantile gastroenteritis occurs; and is not opened until the infection has been completely eradicated. A third factor is infection elsewhere in the body, particularly in the ear or the mastoid.

TREATMENT An infant with diarrhoea should not be fed milk but should be given an electrolyte mixture to replace lost water and salts. If the diarrhoea improves within 24 hours, milk can gradually be reintroduced. If diarrhoea continues beyond 36 to 48 hours, a doctor should be consulted. Any signs of dehydration require urgent medical attention; such signs include drowsiness, lack of response, loose skin, persistent crying, glazed eyes and a dry mouth and tongue.

DIASTASE A mixture of enzymes obtained from malt. These enzymes have the property of converting starch into sugar. It is used in the preparation of predigested starchy foods, and in the treatment of dyspepsia, particularly that due to inability to digest starch adequately. It is also used for the conversion of starch to fermentable sugars in the brewing and fermentation industries.

DIASTASIS A term applied to separation of the end of a growing bone from the shaft. The condition resembles a fracture, but is more serious because of the damage done to the growing cartilage through which the separation takes place, so that the future growth of the bone is considerably diminished.

DIASTOLE The relaxation of a hollow organ. The term is applied in particular to the heart, to indicate the resting period between the beats (systole), while blood is flowing into the organ.

DIASTOLIC PRESSURE The pressure exerted by the blood against the arterial wall during diastole. This is the lowest blood pressure in the cardiac cycle.

DIATHERMY A process by which electric currents can be passed into the deeper parts of the body so as to produce internal warmth and relieve pain; or, by using powerful currents, to destroy tumours and diseased parts bloodlessly. The form of electricity used consists of high-frequency oscillations, the frequency of oscillation ranging from 10 million to 25,000 million oscillations per second. The current passes between two electrodes placed on the skin.

The so-called ultra-short-wave diathermy (or short-wave diathermy, as it is usually referred to) has replaced the original long-wave diathermy, as it is produced consistently at a stable wave-length (11 metres) and is easier to apply. In recent years microwave diathermy has been developed, which has a still higher oscillating current (25,000 million cycles per second, compared with 500 million for short-wave diathermy).

When the current passes, a distinct sensation of increasing warmth is experienced and the temperature of the body gradually rises; the heart's action becomes quicker; there is sweating with increased excretion of waste products. The general blood-pressure is also distinctly lowered. The method is used in painful rheumatic conditions, both of muscles and joints, and in severe cases of neuritis, such as sciatica.

By concentrating the current in a small electrode, the heating effects immediately below this are very much increased. The diathermy knife utilizes this technique to coagulate bleeding vessels and cauterize abnormal tissue during surgery.

DIATHESIS A constitutional or inherited state giving an individual a predisposition towards a disease, a group of diseases or a structural or metabolic abnormality. An example is haemophilia, a bleeding disorder.

DIAZEPAM (see TRANQUILLIZERS, BENZO-DIAZEPINES).

DICEPHALUS The term applied to a fetal 'monster' having two heads.

DICHLORODIPHENYL TRICHLORO-ETHANE (see DDT).

DICROTISM A condition in which the pulse occurs as a beat each time the heart contracts. A dicrotic wave is naturally present in a tracing of any pulse as recorded by an instrument for the purpose, but in health it is imperceptible to the finger. In fevers, a dicrotic pulse is a serious sign in which the heart continues to beat violently while the small blood-vessels have lost their tone. (See PULSE.)

DIDANOSINE (ddI, DDI) A nucleoside reverse transcriptase inhibitor used to treat progressive or advanced HIV infection (see AIDS/HIV). Preferably it should be given in combination with other antiretroviral drugs. This drug has a range of potentially serious side-effects such as PANCREATITIS, peripheral NEUROPATHY, DIABETES MELLITUS and liver failure. Its use requires monitoring and patients taking it should receive counselling.

DIELDRIN An effective insecticide toxic to a wide range of insects. It is more toxic to man than DDT, and must therefore be handled with care. Its use in the UK is restricted.

DIENCEPHALON (see BRAIN).

DIENOESTROL A synthetic oestrogen closely related to STILBOESTROL. It is not as potent as stilboestrol, but is less toxic and is used as a cream to treat vaginal dryness.

DIET The mixture of food and drink consumed by an individual. Variations in morbidity and mortality between population groups are believed to be due, in part, to differences in diet. A balanced diet was traditionally viewed as one which provided at least the minimum requirement of energy, protein, vitamins and minerals needed by the body. However, since nutritional deficiencies are no longer a major problem in developed countries, it seems more appropriate to consider a 'healthy' diet as being one which provides all essential nutrients in sufficient quantities to prevent deficiencies but which also avoids health problems associated with nutrient excesses.

Major diet-related health problems in prosperous communities tend to be the result of dietary excesses, whereas in underdeveloped, poor communities problems associated with dietary deficiencies predominate. Excessive intakes of dietary energy, saturated fats, sugar, salt and alcohol, together with an inadequate intake of dietary fibre, have been linked to the high prevalence of OBESITY, cardiovascular disease, dental CARIES, HYPERTENSION, gall-stones (see GALL-BLADDER, DISEASES OF), non-insulin dependent DIABETES MELLITUS and certain CANCERS (e.g. breast, endometrium, intestine and stomach) seen in developed nations. Health-promotion strategies in these countries generally advocate a reduction in the intake of fat, particularly saturated fat, and salt, the avoidance of excessive intakes of alcohol and simple sugars, an increased consumption of starch and fibre and the avoidance of obesity by taking appropriate physical exercise. A maximum level of dietary cholesterol is sometimes specified.

Under-nutrition, including protein-energy malnutrition and specific vitamin and mineral deficiencies, is an important cause of poor health in underdeveloped countries. Priorities here centre on ensuring that the diet provides enough nutrients to maintain health.

In healthy people, dietary requirements depend on age, sex and level of physical activity. Pregnancy and lactation further alter requirements. The presence of infections, fever, burns, fractures and surgery all increase dietary energy and protein requirements and can precipitate under-nutrition in previously well-nourished people.

In addition to disease prevention, diet has a role in the treatment of certain clinical disorders, e.g. obesity, diabetes mellitus, HYPERLIPIDAEMIAS, inborn errors of metabolism, food intolerances and hepatic and renal diseases. Therapeutic diets increase or restrict the amount and/or change the type of fat, carbohydrate, protein, fibre, vitamins, minerals and/or water in the diet according to clinical indications. Additionally, the consistency of the food eaten may need to be altered. A commercially available or 'homemade' liquid diet can be used to provide all or some of a patient's nutritional needs if necessary. Although the enteral (by mouth) route is the preferred route for feeding and can be used for most patients, parenteral or intravenous feeding is occasionally required in a minority of patients whose gastrointestinal tract is unavailable or unreliable over a period of time.

DIETITIAN (see DIATETICS).

DIETETICS Dietitians apply dietetics, the science of nutrition, to the feeding of groups and individuals in health and disease. Their training requires a degree course in the nutritional and biological sciences. The role of the dietitian can be divided as follows.

Preventive By liaising with health education departments, schools and various groups in the community. They plan and provide nutrition education programs including in-service training and the production of educational material in nutrition. They are encouraged to plan and participate in food surveys and research projects which involve the assessment of nutritional status.

Therapeutic They advise patients who require specific dietary therapy as all or part of their treatment. They teach patients in hospitals to manage their own dietary treatment and ensure a supportive follow-up so that they and their families can be seen to be coping with the diet. They advise catering departments on the adaptation of menus for individual diets and on the nutritional value of the food supplied to patients and staff. They advise social services departments so that meals-on-wheels provision has adequate nutritional value.

Industry The advice of dietitians is sought by industry in the production of product information literature, data sheets and professional leaflets for manufacturers of ordinary foods and specialist dietetic food. They give advice to the manufacturers on nutritional and dietetic requirements of their products.

DIETHYLCARBAMAZINE CITRATE A filaricide derived from PIPERAZINE used to treat FILARIASIS – a group of diseases caused by parasitic worms called nematode filariae.

DIFFERENTIAL DIAGNOSIS A list of the possible diagnoses that might explain a patient's symptoms and signs and from which the correct diagnosis will be extracted after further investigations.

DIFFERENTIATION The gradual diversification of early embryonic cells into the specialized cells, tissues and organs that go to make up the fully developed organism.

DIGESTION, ABSORPTION, AND ASSIMILATION The three processes by which the body incorporates food are digestion, absorption, and assimilation. In digestion, food is softened and converted into a form soluble in the watery fluids of the body; or, in the case of fat, into minute globules. The substances formed are then absorbed from the bowels and carried throughout the body by the blood. In assimilation, these substances, deposited from the blood, are used by the various tissues for their growth and repair. In Britain, transit time through the digestive tract in young and middle-aged people averages two to four days (slightly longer in the elderly, and dependent on the amount of fibre in the diet). All but 12 hours of this is spent in the colon.

Digestion

SALIVARY DIGESTION occurs in the mouth with chewing, to break up the food, and thoroughly to mix the starchy ingredients – such as bread and potatoes – with SALIVA containing PTYALIN that changes them into sugar. After swallowing the salivary action is soon checked by the gastric acid in the STOMACH.

GASTRIC DIGESTION is facilitated by slow churning movements mixing the food with the gastric juice and rendering it soluble. The final product, CHYME, passes through the PYLORUS into the INTESTINE. Gastric digestion of a simple meal takes about one hour, and a heavy dinner up to seven hours.

INTESTINAL DIGESTION The softened food leaves the stomach and enters the intestine where four factors act on it: (a) BILE; (b) pancreatic juice (see PANCREATIN), (c) intestinal juice, and (d) bacteria. Intestinal juice contains enzymes which complete the breakdown of proteins into their constituent aminoacids, act on disaccharides, such as MALTOSE, SUCROSE and LACTOSE, converting them into the monosaccharide glucose and split fats into fatty acids and glycerin. Bacteria are normal ocupants of both small and large intestines. In the former they have a fermentive action, acting on carbohydrate to produce acetic, butyric and lactic acids. In the latter they have a putrefactive action, decomposing protein into its constituent parts. The intestinal bacteria have a key part in the manufacture of certain components of the vitamin B complex.

Absorption The only substance absorbed from the stomach to any extent is ALCOHOL. Water quickly passes through the stomach into the intestine, but it is only after several hours of intestinal digestion that the bulk of the food is taken into the system. Fats produced from the CHYLE leaving the stomach are taken up by lymph vessels called lacteals, ultimately reaching the blood, while sugars, salts and aminoacids formed from proteins pass directly into the small blood vessels of the intestine. The process is facilitated by the large number of microscopic villi which line the intestine. Food materials are mainly absorbed by the small intestine, water and salts by the large intestine or colon. The food is passed down the intestine by contractions of its muscular wall until finally the indigestible residue, together with various wastes excreted from the liver and intestinal walls, is expelled from the anus as stools or faeces.

Assimilation takes place more slowly as the blood circulates through the body and each organ extracts what is necessary for its own growth and repair. When the food supply exceeds immediate bodily requirements, it is stored up for future use, with fat being deposited in various sites, sugar being converted into GLYCOGEN in the LIVER. Muscles have the greatest requirements with sugar and aminoacids being assimilated for heat production and work. To function satisfactorily the body requires an adequate daily water intake of about 1.5 litres (3 pints), with a similar amount being discharged from the body in the urine, perspiration and other excretions such as saliva and tears.

DIGITALIS The leaf of the wild fox-glove, Digitalis purpurea, gathered when the flowers are at a certain stage, dried, and powdered. The leaf contains several active principles, which can be extracted in various ways. Its action is to strengthen involuntary muscular contraction, particularly that of the muscle fibres in the heart and blood-vessels. For many years it was used to treat heart disease associated with atrial fibrillation. Digitalis no longer appears in the *British National Formulary*; DIGOXIN is used instead. Digitalis has the double action of increasing the strength of each beat and of lengthening each intervening pause (diastole), so that the muscle of the damaged organ obtains longer periods for rest and repair. It promotes the excretion of sodium by the kidney and so has a diuretic effect.

DIGITOXIN   A cardiac glycoside similar to DIGOXIN but with a long half life and thus the need for fewer maintenance doses. Digoxin is more widely used.

DIGOXIN   One of a number of drugs known as cardiac glycosides. They increase myocardial contractility, depress the conducting tissue while increasing myocardial excitability, and increase activity of the VAGUS nerve. It is usually given orally for the treatment of atrial FIBRILLATION and heart failure. The adverse effects of overdosage (which occur more commonly in people with hypokalaemia, the elderly, and those with renal failure) are vomiting, DYS-RHYTHMIAS, muscle weakness, and visual disturbances. The ELECTROCARDIOGRAM has a characteristic appearance.

DIHYDROCODEINE   An analgesic drug with similar efficacy to codeine.

DILATATION AND CURETTAGE (D AND C)   A gynaecological operation to scrape away the lining of the uterus (endometrium). The procedure may be used to diagnose and treat heavy bleeding from the womb (endometriosis) as well as other uterine disorders. It can be used to terminate a pregnancy or to clean out the uterus after a partial miscarriage. D and C is increasingly being replaced with a technique using a hysteroscope, a type of ENDOSCOPE.

DILATOR   (1) A muscle which has the action of increasing the diameter of an organ or vessel. (2) A drug which usually acts by relaxing smooth muscle to increase the diameter of blood vessels, the bronchial tree, or other organs. (3) An instrument used to increase the diameter of an orifice or organ either to treat a stricture or allow surgical access.

DILUENTS   are watery fluids of a non-irritating nature, which are given to increase the amount of perspiration or of urine, and carry solids with them from the system. Examples are water, milk, barley-water, and solutions of alkaline salts.

DIMENHYDRINATE, or DRAMAMINE, is a drug, obtainable without prescription, to prevent and treat travel sickness.

DIMERCAPROL   Dimercaprol (British Anti-Lewisite, BAL)   A chelating agent used in the treatment of metal poisoning (e.g. arsenic, lead,

mercury). It has a high incidence of side-effects and is now only rarely used as it has been superseded by less toxic chelating agents.

DINOESTROL (see OESTROGEN).

DINOPROSTONE   A PROSTAGLANDIN given via the VAGINA into a pregnant UTERUS (outside the AMNION) to induce medically a late therapeutic abortion. It requires careful medical supervision.

DIOCTYL SODIUM SULPHOSUCCINATE   A faecal-softening agent used to treat constipation in old people. It can be given orally or as a rectal suppository.

DIODONE   A complex, radio-opaque organic, iodine-containing preparation, used for contrast radiography of parts of the body, in particular, the urinary tract (see PYELOGRAPHY).

DIOPTRE   A term used in the measurement of the refractive or focusing power of lenses; one dioptre is the power of a lens with a focal distance of one metre and is the unit of refractive power. As a stronger lens has a greater refractive power, this means that the focal distance will be shorter. The strength in dioptres therefore is the reciprocal of the focal length expressed in metres.

DIPHENHYDRAMINE   A widely used AN-TIHISTAMINE DRUG.

DIPHENOXYLATE   also known as CO-PHENOTROPE or LOMITIL© When mixed with ATROPINE sulphate, it is used as an adjunct to rehydration in patients with acute diarrhoea. It has no antibacterial properties but is sometimes used to treat traveller's diarrhoea.

DIPHTHERIA is an acute infectious disease of the respiratory tract. Rarely seen in the UK since the introduction of inoculation in 1940, it is still an important cause of disease in many parts of the world. The infection is caused by the *Corynebacterium diphtheriae*, of which there are three strains, and is spread by water droplets. It usually presents with a sore throat, and there is a slightly raised membrane on the tonsils surrounded by an inflammatory zone. There may be some swelling of the neck and lymph nodes, though the patient's temperature is seldom much raised. Occasionally the disease occurs in the eye or genital tract, or it may complicate lesions of the skin. More serious consequences follow the absorption of TOXINS which damage the heart muscle and the nervous system. The disease is notifiable, and has an average incubation period of two to four days. Patients are isolated until cultures from six daily nose and throat swabs are negative. Diphtheria may occur at all ages, though it is commonest in childhood. In the Schick test, a minute amount of toxin is injected into the skin of the arm, producing an area of inflammation in those with little resistance, who should then be immunized.

Treatment Provided the patient is not allergic to horse serum, an injection of the antitoxin is given immediately. A one-week course of penicillin is started (or erythromycin if the patient is allergic to penicillin). Diphtheria may cause temporary muscle weakness or paralysis, which should resolve without special treatment; if the respiratory muscles are involved, however, artificial respiration may be necessary.

All infants should be immunized against diptheria; for details see table under IMMUNIZATION.

DIPHYLLOBOTHRIUM LATUM A fish tapeworm which infests man and may cause a form of megaloblastic anaemia. (See ANAEMIA.)

DIPLEGIA Extensive paralysis on both sides of the body but affecting the legs more than the arms. (See PARALYSIS.)

DIPLO- A prefix meaning twofold.

DIPLOCOCCUS A group of bacterial organisms which have a tendency to occur in pairs: e.g. pneumococci.

DIPLOË The layer of spongy bone which intervenes between the compact outer and inner tables of the skull.

DIPLOID An adjective describing cells, nuclei or organisms in which every chromosome – apart from the Y sex one – is represented twice.

DIPLOPIA Double vision. It is due to some irregularity in action of the muscles which move the eyeballs, in consequence of which the eyes are placed so that rays of light from one object do not fall upon corresponding parts of the two retinae, and two images are produced. It is a symptom of several nervous diseases, and often a temporary attack follows an injury to the eye, intoxication, or some febrile disease like diphtheria.

DIPROSOPUS The term applied to a fetus which has two faces instead of one.

DIPSOMANIA A morbid and insatiable craving for alcohol. (See ALCOHOL.)

DIPYGUS A fetus with a double pelvis.

DISABILITY An observable mental or physical loss or impairment which is measurable and which may be permanent or temporary. If the

disability is serious enough to affect a person's normal function adversely, it is described as a handicap.

DISABLED PERSONS in the United Kingdom have a range of services and financial support available to help them to lead as normal and active a life as possible. Officially, the disabled include those with significant impairment of any kind, including impairment of sight and hearing, learning difficulties, and chronic illness as well as disablement due to accidents and the like.

Social services are provided by local authority social services departments. They include: practical help in the home (usually through home helps or aids to daily living), assistance in taking advantage of available educational facilities, help with adaptations to the disabled person's house, provision of meals ('Meals on Wheels' or luncheon centres), and help in obtaining a telephone. Many of these facilities will involve the disabled person in some expense, but full details can be obtained from the local social services department which will, if necessary, send a social worker to discuss the matter in the disabled person's home. Owing to lack of funds and staff, many local authority social service departments are unable to provide the full range of services.

Aids to daily living There is now a wide range of aids for the disabled. Full details and addresses of local offices can be obtained from: Disabled Living Foundation; British Red Cross; National Demonstration Centre, Pinderfields General Hospital; and Disability Scotland, Information Department. See APPENDIX 2: ADDRESSES.

Aids to mobility and transport Some car manufacturers make specially equipped or adapted cars, and some have official systems for discounts. Details can be obtained from local dealers. Help can be also obtained from Motability, which provides advice (see APPENDIX 2: ADDRESSES).

DISARTICULATION The amputation of a bone by cutting through the joint of which the bone forms a part.

DISC An anatomical term describing a rounded flattened structure. Examples are the cartilagenous disc positioned between two vertebrae (see SPINAL COLUMN) and the optic disc. (See EYE.)

DISCHARGE Abnormal emission or emissions from any part of the body. It usually applies to purulent material: e.g. the septic material which comes away from an infected ear, or nose.

DISCISSION The term applied to an operation for destroying a structure by tearing it without removal: e.g. the operation of needling the lens of the eye for cataract.

DISCOID LUPUS ERYTHEMATOSUS (DLE) (see LUPUS ERYTHEMATOSUS).

DISEASE Any abnormality of bodily structure or function, other than those arising directly from physical injury.

DISINFECTANTS Substances that destroy micro-organisms and prevent their causing infections. The name is usually applied to powerful chemicals that are also capable of destroying tissue and so are used only to sterilize inanimate surfaces. ANTISEPTICS are used to cleanse living tissues.

DISINFECTION Processes by which vegetative organisms, excluding spores, are killed in order to prevent the items disinfected from passing on infection. Equipment, bedlinen and hard surfaces may all be disinfected – the method chosen will depend on the material and size of the object. One of the most important procedures in preventing the spread of infection is the careful washing of hands before handling equipment and between treating different patients. Sterilization is different from disinfection in that the methods used kill all living organisms and spores.

Methods of disinfection (1) Skin, wounds etc. – chlorhexidine (with detergent or spirit); iodine (with detergent or spirit); cetrimide; ethyl alcohol; all must stay in contact with the skin for long enough for bacteria to be killed. (2) Hard surfaces (floors, walls etc.) – hypochlorites (i.e. bleaches) with or without detergent; cetrimide; iodine-containing solutions; ethyl alcohol. (3) Equipment – wet or dry heat (e.g. boiling for more than five minutes); submersion in liquid disinfectants for the appropriate time (e.g. glutaraldehyde 2·5 per cent, chlorhexidine in spirit 70 per cent, formaldehyde (irritant), chlorhexidine 0·1 per cent aqueous), hypochlorites.

DISINFESTATION The destruction of insect pests, especially lice, whether on the person or in dwelling-places.

DISLOCATIONS Injuries to joints of such a nature that the ends of the opposed bones are forced more or less out of connection with one another. Besides displacement of the bones, there is bruising of the tissues around them, and tearing of the ligaments which bind the bones together.

Dislocations, like fractures, are divided into simple and compound, the bone in the latter case being forced through the skin. This seldom occurs, since the round head of the bone has not the same power to wound as the sharp end of a broken bone. Dislocations are also divided

according as they are (1) congenital, i.e. present at birth in consequence of some malformation, or (2) acquired at a later period in consequence of injury, the great majority falling into the latter class. The reduction of a dislocated joint is a skilled procedure and should be done by an appropriately trained professional.

DISODIUM CROMOGLYCATE A drug used in the prophylactic treatment of allergic disorders, particularly ASTHMA, CONJUNCTIVITIS, nasal allergies, and food allergies, especially in children. Although inappropriate for the treatment of acute attacks of asthma, regular inhalations of the drug can reduce the incidence of asthma, and allow the dose of BRONCHODILATORS and oral CORTICOSTEROIDS to be cut.

DISORIENTATION Orientation in a clinical sense includes a person's awareness of time and place in relation to himself and others, the recognition of personal friends and familiar places and the ability to remember at least some past experience and to register new data. It is therefore dependent on the ability to recall all learned memories and make effective use of memory. Disorientation can be the presenting feature of both DELIRIUM (confusion) and DEMENTIA; delirium is reversible, developing dramatically, and accompanied by evidence of systemic disease, dementia is a gradually evolving, irreversible condition.

DISPLACEMENT A term used in psychological medicine to describe the mental process of attaching to one object painful emotions associated with another object.

DISSECTION (1) The cutting of tissue to separate the structural components for identification or removal during an operation or the study of anatomy. (2) Dissection of an artery involves tearing of the inner part of the wall allowing blood to track through the media occluding the origins of smaller arteries and often leading to vessel rupture.

DISSEMINATED Spread of disease from its original site throughout an organ or the body. Often used to describe the spread of cancer.

DISSEMINATED SCLEROSIS (see MULTIPLE SCLEROSIS).

DISSOCIATION A psychiatric term describing the process where an individual separates his or her ideas and thoughts from consciousness, thus allowing them to function independently. The result may be that the individual holds contrary views on the same subject.

DISSOCIATIVE DISORDER A collection of psychological disorders in which a particular mental function becomes cut off from a person's mind. Hysterical AMNESIA is one example when the person forgets his or her personal history but can still absorb and talk about new events. Other examples are FUGUE, depersonalization (detachment from self and environment) and MULTIPLE-PERSONALITY disorders.

DISTAL An adjective applied to a body part that is further away from another part with reference, for example, to the trunk.

DISTICHIASIS is the term applied to the condition in which there are two complete rows of eyelashes in one eyelid (or in both).

DISTOMA is a general term including various forms of trematodes, or fluke-worms, parasitic in the intestine, lung and other organs.

DISULFIRAM OR TETRAETHYLTHIURAM DI-SULPHIDE is used as an adjunct in the treatment of alcoholism. It is relatively non-toxic by itself, but when taken in conjunction with alcohol it produces most unpleasant effects: e.g. flushing of the face, palpitations, a sense of oppression and distress, and ultimately sickness and vomiting. The rationale of treatment therefore is to give the alcoholic subject a course of disulfiram and then demonstrate, by letting him take some alcoholic liquor, how unpleasant are the effects. If the patient is co-operative, the treatment may be effective, but there is some risk so it must be given under skilled medical supervision.

DISUSE ATROPHY The wasting of muscles after prolonged immobility. This can be seen after lengthy immobilization in a plaster cast and is particularly severe following paralysis of a limb through nerve injury. (See ATROPHY.)

DITHRANOL A drug used to treat PSORIASIS. It is usually very effective, being applied normally for short contact periods of up to 1 hour. Dithranol can cause severe skin irritation so must be used with care and at appropriate concentrations. Hands should be thoroughly washed after use.

DIURESIS An increase in the production of urine. This may result from increased fluid intake, decreased levels of antidiuretic hormone, renal disease, or the use of drugs (see DIURETICS).

DIURETICS Substances which increase urine and solute production by the KIDNEY. They are used in the treatment of heart failure, HYPERTENSION, and sometimes for ASCITES secondary to liver failure. They may work by extra-renal or renal mechanisms.

Extra-renal (a) Inhibiting release of antidiuretic hormone, e.g. water, alcohol. (b) Increased renal blood flow, e.g. dopamine in renal doses.

Renal (a) Osmotic diuretics act by 'holding' water in the renal tubules and preventing its reabsorption, e.g. mannitol. (b) Loop diuretics prevent sodium, and therefore water, reabsorption, e.g. frusemide. (c) Drugs acting on the cortical segment of the Loop of Henle prevent sodium reabsorption, but are 'weaker' than loop diuretics, e.g. thiazides. (d) Drugs acting on the distal tubule prevent sodium reabsorption by retaining potassium, e.g. spironalactone.

The potential side-effects of diuretics are HYPOKALAEMIA, dehydration, and GOUT (in susceptible individuals). (See KIDNEYS.)

DIVERTICULAR DISEASE The presence of numerous diverticula (sacs or pouches) in the lining of the colon accompanied by spasmodic lower abdominal pain and erratic bowel movements. The sacs may become inflamed causing pain (diverticulitis).

DIVERTICULITIS Inflammation of diverticula (see DIVERTICULUM) in the large intestine. It is characterized by pain in the left lower side of the abdomen, which has been aptly described as 'left-sided appendicitis' as it resembles the pain of appendicitis but occurs in the opposite side of the abdomen. The onset is often sudden, with fever and constipation. It may, or may not, be preceded by DIVERTICULOSIS. Treatment consists of rest, no solid food but ample fluid, and the administration of tetracycline. Complications are unusual but include abscess formation, perforation of the colon, and severe bleeding.

DIVERTICULOSIS The presence of diverticula (see DIVERTICULUM) or sacs in the large intestine. Such diverticula are not uncommon over the age of 40, increasing with age until over the age of 70 they may be present in one-third to one-half of the population. They mostly occur in the lower part of the colon, and are predominantly due to muscular hyperactivity of the bowel forcing the lining of the bowel through weak points in the bowel wall, just as the inner tube of a pneumatic tyre bulges through a defective tyre. There is increasing evidence that the low-residue diet of western civilization is a contributory cause. The condition may or may not produce symptoms. If it does, these consist of disturbance of the normal bowel function and pain in the left side in the lower abdomen. If it is causing symptoms, treatment consists of a high-residue diet (see CONSTIPATION) and an AGAR or METHYL-CELLULOSE preparation.

DIVERTICULUM A pouch or pocket leading off a main cavity or tube. The term is especially applied to protrusions from the intestine, which may be present either at the time of birth as a developmental peculiarity, or which develop in numbers upon the large intestine during the course of life. The process of formation of these intestinal pockets is known as diverticulosis, and inflammation of them as diverticulitis.

DIZYGOTIC TWINS Two people born at the same time to the same parents after fertilization of two separate oocytes. They may be of different sexes and are no more likely to resemble each other than any other sibling pairs.

DIZZINESS This is a vague symptom and it is important to establish what the individual means by dizziness. It may encompass a feeling of disequilibrium, it may be light-headedness, faintness, a sensation of swimming or floating, an imbalance or unsteadiness or episodes of mental confusion. It may be true vertigo which is an hallucination of movement (see VERTIGO). These symptoms may be due to diseases of the ear, eye, central nervous system, cardiovascular system, endocrine system or they may be a manifestation of psychiatric disease. It is a common symptom in the elderly and by the age of eighty two thirds of women and one third of men have suffered from the condition.

DMSA (see LEAD).

DNA is the abbreviation for deoxy-ribonucleic acid, one of the two types of NUCLEIC ACID that occur in nature. It is the fundamental genetic material of all cells, and is present in the nucleus of the CELL where it forms part of the CHROMOSOME and acts as the carrier of genetic information. The molecule is very large, with a molecular weight of several millions, and consists of two single chains of nucleotides (see NUCLEIC ACID) which are twisted round each other to form a double helix (or spiral). The genetic information carried by DNA is encoded along one of these strands. A GENE, which represents the genetic information needed to form protein, is a stretch of DNA containing, on average, around 1000 nucleotides paired in these two strands.

To allow it to fulfil its vitally important function as the carrier of genetic information in living cells, DNA has the following properties. It is stable so that successive generations of species maintain their individual characteristics, but not so stable that evolutionary changes cannot take place. It must be able to store a vast amount of information. For example, an animal cell contains genetic information for the synthesis of over a million proteins. It must be duplicated exactly before each cell division to ensure that both daughter cells contain an accurate copy of the genetic information of the parent cells (see CELLS; GENETIC CODE).

DOBUTAMINE A cardiac stimulant drug of the inotropic sympathomimetic group, it acts on sympathetic receptors in cardiac muscle and increases the contractility and hence improves the cardiac output but has little effect on the cardiac rate. It is particularly useful in cardiogenic shock. It must be given by intravenous infusion.

DOCTOR The academic title granted to someone who has a higher university degree than a master's degree. Some UK universities grant a medical doctorate (MD) for a research thesis of approved standard. In Britain 'doctor' is also the title given to a qualified medical practitioner registered by the General Medical Council, usually after he or she has obtained bachelor's degrees in medicine and surgery (MB, BS). (The conjoint boards of the Royal Colleges of Physicians and Surgeons (England and Scotland) or the Society of Apothecaries also award medical degrees or diplomas.) In the UK a doctor has to spend a year of supervised practice in a recognized hospital post before he or she is registered as a fully qualified doctor, but specialists have to obtain further training and degrees before they can practise as specialists in the NHS and general practitioners are expected to complete a three-year vocational training course before practising as an independent GP. In Britain surgical specialists are customarily addressed as 'Mr'. Other countries have different regulations.

DOG BITES (see BITES AND STINGS; RABIES).

DOLICHOCEPHALIC means long-headed and is a term applied to skulls the breadth of which is less than four-fifths of the length.

DONEPEZIL A drug that reversibly inhibits ANTICHOLINERASE. It is used for the symptomatic treatment of mild to moderate dementia only in ALZHEIMER's disease. Around four in ten patients may benefit by a reduction in the rate of cognitive and non-cognitive deterioration.

DONOR INSEMINATION Use of the semen of an anonymous donor to produce fertilization in cases of infertility where the male partner has oligospermia or impotence. The donor is chosen for ethnic and physiognomic similarity to the male partner and is screened for transmissible diseases (e.g. HIV, syphilis, hepatitis, gonorrhoea, and genetic disorders). Insemination is performed at the time of ovulation by introducing the semen into the upper vagina. Semen may be fresh or have been stored frozen in liquid nitrogen. (See ARTIFICIAL INSEMINATION.)

DONORS People who donate parts of their bodies for use in other people. Many organs and tissues can be donated. The commonest is blood; but skin, corneas, kidneys, livers, and hearts can all be used. Combined heart and lung transplants are being increasingly used for patients with severe lung diseases, and, if the recipients have a condition such as cystic fibrosis in which the heart is normal, it is sometimes possible for them to receive a heart and lungs from one donor and to donate their own heart to someone else. Recent work has explored the possibility of using pancreatic transplants. Apart from blood, it is unusual for tissue to be taken from living donors. Skin, small pieces of liver, and a kidney can, in theory, be obtained from living donors, but the ethics of this are hotly debated and the situations under which it may be done are tightly controlled. Because transplanted organs are seen by the receiving body as 'foreign bodies', careful cross-matching before transplantation is necessary to avoid rejection.

There are strict regulations about how death should be diagnosed before organs can be removed for transplantation, and potential donors must satisfy the BRAIN-STEM DEATH CRITERIA, performed twice by two doctors who are independent of the transplant team. There is a great shortage of suitable organs for donation – partly because they must be in excellent condition if the operation is to be a success. Some medical conditions or modes of death make people unsuitable as organ donors. This makes it all the more important that people should be encouraged to donate their organs. People who wish to do so can carry a special card indicating their willingness to become donors in the event of their death. These cards can be obtained from various sources, including hospitals, GPs' surgeries and many public buildings such as libraries.

Information about becoming a blood donor can be obtained by telephoning 0345-711 711. Those who wish to bequeath their bodies for dissection purposes should get in touch with HM Inspector of Anatomy. Other would-be organ donors may contact the British Organ Donor Society. (See APPENDIX 2: ADDRESSES.)

DOPA A precursor of DOPAMINE and NORADRENALINE. Levodopa is a drug used in the treatment of PARKINSON'S DISEASE. It can cross the blood-brain barrier and increase the concentration of dopamine in the basal ganglia. It also inhibits prolactin secretion and may be used to treat GALACTORRHEA.

DOPAMINE is a catecholamine and a precursor of noradrenaline. Its highest concentration is in that portion of the brain known as the basal nuclei (see BRAIN) where its function is to convey inhibitory influences to the extrapyramidal system. There is good evidence that dopamine deficiency is one of the causative factors in PARKINSONISM.

Dopamine is given by intravenous infusion as treatment for cardiogenic shock in cardiac infarction or cardiac surgery.

DORSAL ROOT GANGLIA These are swellings on the dorsal roots of spinal nerves just proximal to the union of the dorsal and ventral nerve roots. They are situated in the intervertebral formanina and contain the cell bodies of sensory neurones. (See SPINAL COLUMN and SPINAL CORD.)

DORSUM (adjective: dorsal) The back or posterior part of an organ or structure. The dorsum of the hand is the opposite surface to the palm.

DORZOLAMIDE A carbonic anhydrase-inhibitor drug restricted to use in patients with raised intra-ocular pressure in ocular hypertension or open-angle GLAUCOMA. It can be used alone or as an adjunct to a topical BETA-BLOCKER.

DOSAGE Many factors influence the activity with which drugs operate. Among the factors which affect the necessary quantity are age, weight, sex, idiosyncrasy, genetic disorders, habitual use, disease, fasting, combination with other drugs, the form in which the drug is given, and the route by which it is given. AGE is but one factor. Normally, a young child requires a smaller dose than an adult. There are, however, other factors to be taken into consideration. Thus, children are more susceptible than adults to some drugs such as morphine, whilst they are less sensitive to others such as atropine. Various methods have been introduced for calculating roughly and quickly appropriate doses. These may be based on age, body weight or body surface area, the latter being most reliable. For example, a formula based on the surface area of the child is:

$$\text{adult dose} \times \frac{\text{surface area in square metres}}{1 \cdot 82}$$

An approximate rule of thumb, based on children of average height and weight, and assuming an adult dose of 100 mg is:

Age years	Average weight kg	Dose mg
1	10	25
7	25	50
12	40	75
Adult	70	100

Old people, too, often show an increased susceptibility to drugs. This is probably due to a variety of factors, such as decreased weight in many old people; diminished activity of the tissues and therefore diminished rate at which a drug is utilized; and diminished activity of the kidneys resulting in decreased rate of excretion of the drug.

Weight and sex have both to be taken into consideration. Women require slightly smaller doses than men, probably because they tend to be lighter in weight. The effect of weight on dosage is partly dependent on the fact that much of the extra weight of a heavy individual is made up of fatty tissue which is not as active as other tissue of the body. In practice, the question of weight seldom makes much difference unless the individual is grossly overweight or underweight.

Idiosyncrasy occasionally causes drugs administered in the ordinary dose to produce unexpected effects. Thus, some people are but little affected by some drugs, whilst in others certain drugs, such as potassium iodide, or atropine, produce excessive symptoms in minute doses. In some cases this may be due to hypersensitiveness, or an allergic reaction, to the drug. This is a possibility that must always be borne in mind, particularly with penicillin. As a rule the individual has had the drug in question previously. An individual who is known to be allergic to penicillin is strongly recommended to carry a card to this effect.

Habitual use of a drug is perhaps the influence that causes the greatest increase in the dose necessary to produce the requisite effect. The classical example of this is opium and its derivatives. Arsenic is another example that was often encountered in the days when arsenical drugs were one of the great stand-bys in the Pharmacopoeia.

Disease may modify the dose of medicines. This can occur in several ways. Thus, in serious illnesses the patient may be more susceptible to drugs, such as narcotics, that depress tissue activity, and therefore smaller doses must be given. Again, absorption of the drug from the gut may be slowed up by disease of the gut, or its effect may be enhanced if there is disease of the kidneys, interfering with the excretion of the drug.

Fasting aids the rapidity of absorption of, and also makes the body more susceptible to the action of, drugs. Partly for this reason, as well as to avoid irritation of the stomach, it is usual to prescribe drugs to be taken after meals, and diluted with water.

Combination of drugs is to be avoided if possible as it is often difficult to assess what their combined effect may be. In some cases they may have a mutually antagonistic effect, which means that the patient will not obtain full benefit. Sometimes a combination may have a deleterious effect.

Form, route and frequency of administration are all important and doctors and pharmacists will advise a given patient on these. Drugs are now produced in many forms, though tablets are the most common and, usually, convenient. In Britain, medicines are given by mouth whenever possible, unless there is some degree of urgency, or because the drug is either destroyed in, or is not absorbed from, the gut. In these circumstances, it is given intravenously, intramuscularly or subcutaneously. In some cases, as in cases of ASTHMA or BRONCHITIS, the drug may be given in the form of an INHALANT, in order to get the maximum concentration at the point where it is wanted: that is, in the lungs. If a local effect is wanted, as in cases of diseases

of the skin, the drug is applied topically to the skin. In some countries there is a tendency to give medicines in the form of a suppository which is inserted in the rectum.

Recent years have seen developments whereby the assimilation of drugs into the body can be more carefully controlled. These include, for example, what are known as transdermals, in which drugs are built into a plaster that is stuck on the skin, and the drug is then absorbed into the body at a controlled rate. This method is now being used for the administration of GLYCERYL TRINITRATE in the treatment of ANGINA PECTORIS, and of hyoscine hydrobromide in the treatment of MOTION SICKNESS. Another is a new class of implantable devices. These are tiny polymers infused with a drug and implanted just under the skin by injection. They can be tailored so as to deliver drugs at virtually any rate – from minutes to years. A modification of these polymers now being investigated is the incorporation of magnetic particles which allow an extra burst of the incorporated drug to be released in response to an oscillating magnetic field which is induced by a magnetic 'watch' worn by the patient. In this way the patient can switch on an extra dose of drug when this is needed: insulin, for instance, in the case of diabetics. In yet another new development, a core of drug is enclosed in a semipermeable membrane and is released in the stomach at a given rate. (See also LIPOSOMES.)

DOTHIEPIN A drug used in the treatment of depression, particularly when the patient needs sedation. (See ANTIDEPRESSANTS.)

DOUBLE BLIND TRIAL A scientific study in which neither the investigators assessing the outcome nor the subjects being treated know which treatment the subject is receiving. The results are analysed after all the data has been collected and the code has been broken. (See INTERVENTION STUDY).

DOUBLE VISION (see SQUINT).

DOUCHE An application to the body of a jet of fluid via a pipe or tube. It may be used to clean any part of the body but is used most commonly with reference to the vagina. (Although used as a method of contraception it is ineffective.)

DOWN'S (DOWN) SYNDROME is a genetic disorder in which the affected person usually carries an extra chromosome – 47 instead of the normal 46 – resulting in a characteristic flat facial look with slanting eyes, hence its original description of Mongolism. A large tongue, a small round skull and short thick hands and feet are other manifestations. Many victims have varying degrees of mental handicap. The palm print is distinctive and those with the syndrome may also have heart defects, intestinal malformations, deafness and squints. The condition was named after Dr J. L. H. Down, the London doctor who first described it in 1866.

The incidence is approximately 1 per 600 births, but the incidence in the community is lower than this, as many Down's syndrome victims die in infancy. This high death-rate is due partly to the fact that these children have a much higher incidence of other congenital deformities, such as malformations of the heart, than other children, and partly to their lower resistance to infection.

It is much commoner in children born to older women. Thus, the risk of having a Down's child in women over 45 is more than 1 in 60, compared with less than 1 in 1000 in women under 30. Forty per cent of children with Down's syndrome are born to mothers over 40, 30 per cent to those aged 35 to 40. For mothers who give birth to a Down's child when they are younger the chances of a subsequent child being affected is relatively high. Precise figures in this respect can be misleading, and the best advice for a young mother who has had a Down's child, and who wishes to know the risk of her having another, is to go and discuss the matter with her family doctor. Despite the low risk of recurrences, particularly in young couples, diagnostic AMNIOCENTESIS is often advised in future pregnancies, especially if the mother is over 35. Other prenatal screening tests are chorionic villus sampling and the triple marker test. (See PRENATAL DIAGNOSIS.)

In 95 per cent of cases the cause is the presence of an extra CHROMOSOME in the ovum. The cause of this extra chromosome is not known. In the remaining cases the cause is a fault in the division of the germ cells known as translocation. There is an extra CHROMOSOME in the no. 21 group, hence the disease is referred to as trisomy 21. It is usually caused by an unequal distribution of chromosomes in the production of the egg cells. Occasionally it results from chromosomal rearrangements, or abnormal mitosis in the fertilized egg cell.

The degree of mental backwardness varies considerably. Up to a third of all severely mentally handicapped children of school age have Down's syndrome. It has been estimated that 6 per cent of Down's children are probably capable of profiting appreciably from attendance at schools for the educationally handicapped. Practically all who survive to school age gain some benefit. Most eventually acquire some degree of speech, and about 5 per cent learn to read. They practically never learn to write. Most learn to wash, dress and feed themselves, and many are able to run simple errands.

Although there is no known cure for the condition, there is much that can be done for the children, especially if they can be kept at home rather than sent to an institution, and a number of societies are very helpful. Parents will naturally feel a combination of strong emotions, including anger and guilt, and vigorous counselling can be very valuable. Contact:

The Down's Syndrome Association (see APPENDIX 2: ADDRESSES).

DOXORUBICIN A successful and widely used antitumour drugs. It is used in the treatment of acute LEUKAEMIA, LYMPHOMA, and various forms of SARCOMA and cancer, including cancer of the bladder. (See CYTOTOXIC.)

DOXYCYCLINE A wide-spectrum, long-acting antibiotic of the TETRACYCLINE GROUP, which is active against a wide range of micro-organisms, including the causative organisms of scrub TYPHUS, TRACHOMA, PSITTACOSIS, LYME DISEASE and some influenzas.

DPT VACCINATION Often called the triple vaccine, the injections produces immunity against DIPHTHERIA, whooping cough (PERTUSSIS) and TETANUS. The vaccine is given as a course of three injections to infants around the ages of two, three and four months, with a booster injection of diphtheria and tetanus at around 5 years of age (see schedule in IMMUNIZATION).

DRACONTIASIS or DRACUNCULIASIS A nematode infection caused by *Dracunculus medinensis* (guinea-worm). Although mentioned in ancient writings from the Middle East (it is arguably the oldest parasitic disease to have been documented), it is now confined to west and central Africa, and western parts of India. Infection is acquired by drinking water containing waterfleas (*Cyclops* spp.) – freshwater crustaceans – which carry infected larvae. These are freed by digestive enzymes following ingestion, and migrate to the body cavities, where they mature. The female attains a length of 60–120 cm and, when gravid, migrates to subcutaneous tissues, usually in the feet and legs. Secretion of enzyme(s) produces a papular (bullous) lesion in which larvae are formed; this bursts in fresh water, discharging a milky fluid, containing numerous larvae. These are ingested by water-fleas, thus completing the cycle. The major clinical problem is secondary infection of the worm track, causing cellulitis, synovitis, epididymo-orchitis, periarticular fibrosis, and arthritis; tetanus is a potentially lethal complication. Chemotherapy is unsatisfactory; metronidazole, mebendazole, thiabendazole, and niridazole have been used with some success, but the time-honoured method of extracting the female adult by winding it around a matchstick remains in use. Surgical treatment may be necessary. Ultimate prevention consists of removing *Cyclops* spp. from drinking water (in this sense, dracontiasis is probably unique); the World Health Organization is attempting to achieve this.

DRAMAMINE (see DIMENHYDRINATE).

DRAUGHT, or DRAFT, is a small mixture intended to be taken at one dose. It consists generally of two or four tablespoonfuls of fluid.

DREAMS (see SLEEP).

DREPANOCYTOSIS Another term for SICKLE-CELL ANAEMIA, which is characterized by the presence in the blood of red blood corpuscles sickle-like in shape. The anaemia is a severe one and afflicts black people.

DRESSINGS (see WOUNDS).

DROP ATTACKS A brief episode affecting the nervous system that causes the person to fall suddenly. There is no loss of consciousness. In some cases the loss of tone in the muscles, responsible for the fall, may persist for several hours. In such cases moving the patient or applying pressure to the soles of the feet may restore the tone to the muscles. In most cases, however, recovery is immediate. The cause is probably a temporary interference with the blood supply to the brain. In others there may be some disturbance of the vestibular apparatus which controls the balance of the body. (See EAR DISEASES OF; TRANSIENT ISCHAEMIC ATTACK.)

DROP-FOOT This is the inability to dorsiflex the foot at the ankle. The foot hangs down and has to be swung clear of the ground while walking. It is commonly caused by damage to the lateral popliteal nerve or the peroneal muscles.

DROP WRIST This is the inability to extend the hand at the wrist. It is usually due to damage to the radial nerve which supplies the extensor muscles.

DROWNING (see APPENDIX 1: BASIC FIRST AID).

DRUG ABSORPTION Drugs are usually administered distant to their site of action in the body. They must then pass across cell membranes to reach their site of action. For example – drugs given by mouth must pass across the gut membrane to enter the blood stream and then pass through the endothelium of vessel walls to reach the site of action in the tissues. This process is called absorption and may depend on lipid diffusion, aqueous diffusion, active transport, or pinocytosis – a process in which a cell takes in small droplets of fluid by cytoplasmic engulfment.

DRUG ADDICTION or DEPENDENCE is the compulsion to take a drug repeatedly. (See ADDICTION.) Psychological dependence occurs when the drug user craves the drug's desirable effects. Physical dependence occurs when the user has to continue taking the drug to avoid distressing withdrawal or abstinence symptoms. Drug misuse and dependence are surprisingly common, occurring with widely used drugs such as alcohol, caffeine, and nicotine as

well as with certain prescribed drugs such as benzodiazepine tranquillizers. Less socially acceptable but frequently misused drugs are described below.

Accurate figures for drug taking, whether among teenagers or adults, are hard to obtain but there seems little doubt that the incidence of substance misuse is rising, with younger children being drawn into the drug culture by dealers determined to create a bigger 'market' for their 'products'. Latest figures (for the period from 30 September 1993 to 31 March 1996) of users presenting to drug-misuse services for the first time show a rise from 16,810 to 23,313. Heroin users predominate (7,720 to 12,623), while for cannabis users the figures are from 1,078 to 1,623 and for Ecstasy from 186 to 335.

Cannabis, derived from the plant *Cannabis sativa*, is a widely used but illegal recreational drug that does not seem to be addictive. Its two main forms are marijuana – known in the 1960s as 'pot' – which comes from the dried leaves, and hashish which comes from the resin. Cannabis may be used in food and drink but is usually smoked in cigarettes called 'joints' or 'reefers' to induce relaxation and a feeling of well-being. Heavy use can cause apathy and vagueness and may even cause psychosis. Whether or not cannabis leads people to using harder drugs is debatable.

About 1 in 10 of Britain's teenagers misuses volatile substances such as toluene at some time, but only about 1 in 40 does so regularly. These substances are given off by certain glues, solvents, varnishes, and liquid fuels, all of which can be bought cheaply in shops, although their sale to children under 16 is illegal. They are often inhaled from plastic bags held over the nose and mouth. Central-nervous-system excitation, with euphoria and disinhibition, is followed by depression and lethargy. Unpleasant effects include facial rash, nausea and vomiting, tremor, dizziness, and clumsiness. Death from coma and acute cardiac toxicity is a serious risk. Chronic heavy use can cause peripheral neuropathy and irreversible cerebellar damage. (See SOLVENT ABUSE.)

The hallucinogenic or psychedelic drugs include lysergic acid diethylamide (LSD or acid), magic mushrooms, ecstasy (MDMA), and phencyclidine (PCP or 'angel' dust, mainly used in the USA). These drugs have no medicinal uses. Taken by mouth, they produce vivid 'trips', with heightened emotions and perceptions and sometimes with hallucinations. They are not physically addictive but can cause nightmarish bad trips during use and flashbacks (vivid reruns of trips) after use, and can probably trigger psychosis.

Stimulant drugs such as amphetamine and cocaine act like adrenaline and speed up the central nervous system, making the user feel confident, energetic, and powerful for several hours. They can also cause severe insomnia, anxiety, paranoia, psychosis, and even sudden death due to convulsions or tachycardia. Depression may occur on withdrawal of these drugs, and in some users this is sufficiently deterrent to cause psychological dependence. Amphetamine ('speed') is mainly synthesized illegally and may be eaten, sniffed, or injected. Related drugs such as dexamphetamine sulphate (Dexedrine) and diethylpropion hydrochloride (Tenuate, Dospan) are prescribed pills that enter the black market. ECSTASY is another amphetamine derivative that has become a popular recreational drug among young 'clubbers'. It may have fatal allergic effects. Cocaine and related drugs are used in medicine as local anaesthetics. Illegal supplies of cocaine ('snow' or 'ice') and its derivative, 'crack', come mainly from South America, where they are made from the plant *Erythroxylon coca*. Cocaine is usually sniffed ('snorted') or rubbed into the gums; crack is burnt and inhaled.

Opiate drugs are derived from the opium poppy, *Papaver somniferum*. They are described as narcotic because they induce sleep. Their main medical use is as potent oral or injectable analgesics such as morphine, diamorphine, pethidine, and codeine. The commonest illegal opiate is heroin, a powdered form of diamorphine that may be smoked, sniffed, or injected to induce euphoria and drowsiness. Regular opiate misuse leads to tolerance (the need to take ever larger doses to achieve the same effect) and marked dependence. The withdrawal syndrome is like a bout of severe gastric flu with painful abdominal cramps. A less addictive oral opiate, methadone, can be prescribed as a substitute that is easier to withdraw.

Some 75,000–150,000 Britons now misuse opiates and other drugs intravenously, and pose a huge public-health problem because injections with shared dirty needles can carry the blood-borne viruses that cause AIDS and hepatitis B. Many clinics now operate schemes to exchange old needles for clean ones, free of charge.

DRUG BINDING   The process of attachment of a drug to a receptor or plasma protein, fat, mucopolysaccharide or other tissue component. This process may be reversible or irreversible.

DRUG CLEARANCE   The volume of blood from which a drug is completely removed in one minute is known as clearance. Renal clearance of a drug is the amount of blood completely cleared of the drug by the kidney in one minute.

DRUG INTERACTIONS   Many patients are on several prescribed drugs, and numerous medicines are available over the counter, so the potential for drug interaction is large. A drug may interact with another by inhibiting its action, potentiating its action, or by simple summation of effects.

The interaction may take place: (1) Prior to absorption or administration, e.g. antacids bind tetracycline in the gut and prevent absorp-

tion. (2) By interfering with protein binding – one drug may displace another from binding sites on plasma proteins. The action of the displaced drug will be increased because more drug is now available, e.g. anticoagulants are displaced by analgesics. (3) During metabolism or excretion of the drug – some drugs increase or decrease the activity of liver enzymes which metabolize drugs, thus affecting their rate of destruction, e.g. barbiturates, nicotine, and alcohol all activate hepatic enzymes. Altering the pH of urine will affect the excretion of drugs via the kidney. (4) At the drug receptor – one drug may displace another at the receptor affecting its efficacy or duration of action.

DRUG METABOLISM   A process by which the body destroys and excretes drugs, so limiting their duration of action. Phase 1 metabolism consists of transformation by oxidation, reduction, or hydrolysis. In phase 2 this transformed product is conjugated (joined up) with another molecule to produce a water-soluble product which is easier to excrete.

DRUGS   These are natural products or synthetic chemicals that can alter the way the body works, or be used to prevent or treat disease. One or more drugs, combined with stabilizers, colourings, and other ingredients, makes up a medicine for practical use in treating patients. (See DRUG ADDICTION, MEDICINES.) In Britain the supply of drugs is controlled by the Medicines Act. Some drugs are available only on prescription, some both on prescription and over the counter, and some are not available on NHS prescription. When enquiring about drugs that a patient is taking, it is essential to ask about all items bought over the counter and any herbal or traditional remedies that might be used, as these can interact with other prescribed drugs or affect the patient's presenting complaints. Each drug has a single generic name, but many will also have several proprietary (brand) names. It is often much cheaper to prescribe the generic form of a drug, and many doctors do so. Many hospitals and general practices in the United Kingdom now provide a list of suggested drugs for doctors to prescribe. If a doctor wishes to use a drug not on the list he has to give a valid reason.

Prescriptions for drugs should be printed or written clearly in ink and signed and dated by the prescriber. They should include the patient's name, address and age (obligatory for children under 12), the name of the drug to be supplied, the dose and dose frequency, and the total quantity to be supplied. Any special instructions (e.g. 'after food') should be stated. There are special regulations about the prescription of drugs controlled under the Misuse of Drugs Regulations, 1985 (see CONTROLLED DRUGS). A pharmacist can advise about which drugs are available without prescription, and is able to recommend treatment for many minor complaints. Information about exemption from prescription charges in the NHS can be obtained from health visitors, general practitioners, or social security offices.

DRUGS IN PREGNANCY Unnecessary drugs during pregnancy should be avoided because of the adverse effect of some drugs on the fetus which have no harmful effect on the mother. Drugs may pass through the placenta and damage the fetus because their pharmacological effects are enhanced as the enzyme systems responsible for their degradation are undeveloped in the fetus. Thus, if the drug can pass through the placenta, the pharmacological effect on the fetus may be great whilst that on the mother is minimal. Warfarin may thus induce fetal and placental haemorrhage and thiazide administration may produce thrombocytopenia in the new born. Many progestogens have androgenic side effects and their administration to a mother for the purpose of preventing recurrent abortion may produce virilization of the female fetus. Tetracycline administered during the last trimester commonly stains the deciduous teeth of the child yellow.

The other dangers of administering drugs in pregnancy are the teratogenic effects. It is understandable that a drug may interfere with a mechanism essential for growth and result in arrested or distorted development of the fetus and yet cause no disturbance in the adult in whom these differentiation and organization processes have ceased to be relevant. Thus the effect of a drug upon a fetus may differ qualitatively as well as quantitatively from its effect on the mother. The susceptibility of the embryo will depend on the stage of development it has reached when the drug is given. The stage of early differentiation, that is from the beginning of the third week to the end of the tenth week of pregnancy, is the time of greatest susceptibility. After this time the risk of congenital malformation from drug treatment is less although the death of the fetus can occur at any time.

DRUNKENNESS (see ALCOHOL).

DUCHENNE MUSCULAR DYSTROPHY An X-linked recessive disorder, occurring almost exclusively in males. Characterized by progressive muscular weakness and wasting, it is symmetrical in nature. Tendon reflexes are preserved until a late stage and, there is no fasciculation and no sensory loss. It is the most common form of muscular dystrophy, ocurring in 30 per 100,000 live male births. Spontaneous mutations are common. The disease usually appears within the first three years of life, beginning in the pelvic girdle and lower limbs and later spreading to the shoulder girdle. The calf muscles become bulky (pseudohypertrophy). The weakness gives rise to a characteristic waddling gait and, when rising from the supine position, the child rolls on to his face and then uses his arms to push himself up. Death usually

occurs by the middle of the second decade from respiratory infections. Prenatal screening of female carriers using gene probes is increasingly available. Research is under way with a view to developing GENE therapy (see DYSTROPHY, MYOPATHY).

DUCT The name applied to a passage leading from a gland into some hollow organ, or on to the surface of the body, by which the secretion of the gland is discharged: e.g. the pancreatic duct and the bile duct opening into the duodenum, and the sweat ducts opening on the skin surface.

DUCTLESS GLAND Any one of certain glands in the body the secretion of which goes directly into the blood stream and so is carried to different parts of the body. These glands – the pituitary, thyroid, parathyroid, adrenal and reproductive – are also known as the ENDOCRINE GLANDS. Some glands may be both duct glands and ductless glands. For example, the pancreas manufactures a digestive juice which passes by a duct into the small intestine. It also manufactures, by means of special cells, a substance called insulin which passes straight into the blood.

DUCTUS ARTERIOSUS The blood-vessel in the fetus through which blood passes from the pulmonary artery to the aorta, thereby bypassing the lungs, which do not function during intra-uterine life. (See CIRCULATION OF THE BLOOD.) The ductus normally ceases to function soon after birth and within a few weeks is converted into a fibrous cord. Occasionally this obliteration does not occur: a condition known as patent ductus arteriosus. This is one of the more common congenital defects of the heart, and one which responds particularly well to surgical treatment. Closure of the duct can also be achieved in some cases by the administration of indomethacin. (See HEART DISEASES.)

DUCTUS DEFERENS, or VAS DEFERENS The tube which carries spermatozoa from the epididymis to the seminal vesicles. (See TESTICLE.)

DUMBNESS (see SPEECH DISORDERS).

DUMPING SYNDROME A sensation of weakness and sweating after a meal in patients who have undergone GASTRECTOMY. Rapid emptying of the stomach and the drawing of fluid from the blood into the intestine has been blamed, but the exact cause is debated.

DUODENAL ILEUS Dilatation of the duodenum due to chronic obstruction of the duodenum, caused by an abnormal position of arteries in the region of the duodenum pressing on it.

DUODENAL ULCER This disorder is related to gastric ulcer (see STOMACH, DISEASES OF), both being a form of chronic peptic ulcer. Although becoming less frequent in Western communities, peptic ulcers still affect around 10 per cent of the UK population at some time. The incidence of peptic ulcer is increasing in many developing countries. Duodenal ulcers are 10–15 times more common than gastric ulcers, and occur in people from 20 years onwards; gastric ulcers generally occur in those over 40 years, and are rare in women until after the menopause. The male to female ratio for duodenal ulcer varies between 4:1 and 2:1 in different communities, while that for gastric ulcer is less than 2:1. Social class and blood groups are also influential, with duodenal ulcer being more common among the upper social classes, and those of blood group O.

Causes Until recently there was no general consensus of expert opinion as to the precise cause of peptic ulcers. What probably happens is that there is some abrasion, or break, in the lining membrane (or mucosa) of the stomach and/or duodenum, and that it is gradually eroded and deepened by the gastric juice. What was not known, however, was why this only occurred in some people. It is now known that the bacterium HELICOBACTER PYLORI is present in the antrum of the stomach of people with peptic ulcers and that the ulcers heal if *H. pylori* is eradicated. Mental stress is also a probable provocative factor. Smoking seems to accentuate, if not cause, duodenal ulcer, and the drinking of alcohol is probably harmful. The apparent association with a given blood group, and the fact that relatives of a patient with a peptic ulcer are unduly likely to develop such an ulcer suggest that there is some constitutional factor.

Symptoms and signs Peptic ulcers may present in different ways, but chronic, episodic pain lasting several months or years is most common and medical treatment is recommended (see below). Occasionally, however, there may be an acute episode of bleeding or perforation, or obstruction of the gastric outlet, with little previous history. Most commonly, there is pain of varying intensity in the middle or upper right part of the abdomen. It tends to occur two or three hours after a meal, most commonly at night, and is relieved by some food, such as a glass of milk; untreated it may last up to an hour. Vomiting is unusual, but there is often tenderness and stiffness ('guarding') of the abdominal muscles. Confirmation of the diagnosis is made by radiological examination ('barium meal'), the ulcer appearing as a niche on the film, or direct endoscopic visualization of the ulcer (see FIBREOPTIC ENDOSCOPY). Chief complications are perforation of the ulcer, leading to the vomiting of blood, or HAEMATEMESIS; or less severe bleeding from the ulcer, the blood passing down the gut, resulting in dark, tarry stools (see MELAENA).

Treatment of a perforation involves initial management of any complications, such as shock, haemorrhage, perforation, or gastric outlet obstruction, usually involving surgery and blood replacement. Medical treatment of a chronic ulcer should include regular meals, avoidance of fatty foods, strong tea or coffee and alcohol. Patients should also stop smoking and try to reduce the stress in their lives. ANTACIDS may provide symptomatic relief. However, the mainstay of treatment involves 4-to-6-week courses with drugs such as CIMETIDINE and RANITIDINE. These are H_2 RECEPTOR ANTAGONISTS which heal peptic ulcers by reducing gastric-acid output. Of those relapsing after stopping this treatment 60–95 per cent have infection with *H. pylori*. A combination of BISMUTH chelate, AMOXYCILLIN and METRONIDAZOLE – 'triple regime' – should eliminate the infection: some physicians prefer the triple regime as first choice treatment. Surgery may be necessary if medical measures fail, but its use is less common than before effective medical treatments were developed.

DUODENUM The first part of the intestine immediately beyond the stomach, so named because its length is about twelve fingerbreadths. (See INTESTINE.)

DUPUYTREN'S CONTRACTURE A condition of unknown aetiology in which there is progressive thickening and contracture of the palmar fascia with adherence of the overlying skin. A clawing deformity of the fingers, particularly the little and ring fingers, develops. It is associated with liver disease, diabetes, epilepsy, and gout. Treatment is surgical to excise the affected fascia.

DURA MATER The outermost and strongest of the three membranes or meninges which envelop the brain and spinal cord. In it run vessels which nourish the inner surface of the skull. (See BRAIN.)

DWARF, or DWARFISM, is a term applied to under-development of the body. The causes are either developmental or due to food insufficient in quantity or unsuitable in quality, or to defects in some of the body secretions which can be corrected. The first-named group includes pituitary dwarfism, the subjects being very small people with normally proportioned parts, also achondroplasic dwarfs (see ACHONDROPLASIA) with large globular head and shortened limbs and stumpy fingers. It is now known that in a certain proportion of children of short stature this can be remedied by administration of the growth hormone of PITUITARY GLAND, provided this is given at an early enough age. All children who by the age of 5 years are at least what is technically known as 'three standard deviations below the mean' should be referred for examination by specialists to determine whether or not their lack of height is due to lack of growth hormone and therefore likely to respond to treatment with the hormone.

Where dwarfism is attributable to a primary defect of the THYROID GLAND, the condition may be treatable. In this class are also included various forms of defective growth associated with defects in the secretions of the digestive organs, especially the PANCREAS; this type of defect, often known as pancreatic infantilism, is mainly confined to a retardation of physical development, while the mental changes are little marked. Another form of dwarfism, associated with a deformity of the bones, is produced by RICKETS in early life.

DYNAMOMETER is an elliptical ring of steel to which is attached a dial and moving index. It is used to test the strength of the muscles of the forearm, being squeezed in the hand, and registering the pressure in pounds or kilograms.

DYS- A prefix meaning difficult or painful.

DYSARTHRIA A general term applied when weakness or incoordination of the speech musculature prevents clear pronunciation of words. The individual's speech may sound as if it is slurred or weak. It may be due to damage affecting the centres in the brain which control movements of the speech muscles or damage to the muscles themselves.

Examples of dysarthria may be found in strokes, CEREBRAL PALSY and the latter stages of PARKINSON'S DISEASE, MULTIPLE SCLEROSIS and MOTOR NEURONE DISEASE. Whatever the cause a speech therapist can assess the extent of the dysarthria and suggest exercises or an alternative means of communication.

DYSCALCULIA A condition commonly seen when the brain's PARIETAL LOBE is diseased or injured, in which an individual finds it hard to carry out simple mathematical calculations.

DYSCHEZIA Constipation due to retention of faeces in the rectum. This retention is the outcome of irregular habits, which damp down the normal reflex causing defaecation.

DYSDIADOCHOKINESIA Loss of the ability to perform rapid alternate movements, such as winding up a watch. It is a sign of a lesion in the cerebellum. (See BRAIN.)

DYSENTERY A clinical state arising from invasive colo-rectal disease; it is accompanied by abdominal colic, diarrhoea, and passage of blood/mucus in the stool. It is accompanied by fever. It is common throughout the tropics and subtropics. Although the two major forms are caused by Shigella spp. (bacillary dysentery) and Entamoeba histolytica (amoebic dysentery), other organisms including enterohaemorrhagic Escherichia coli (serotypes 0157:H7 and 026:H11) and Campylobacter spp. are also relevant. The condition(s) should be differentiated from inflammatory bowel disease (especially ulcerative colitis), which can present clinically for the first time in a traveller to a tropical/subtropical area. Other causes of dysentery include Balantidium coli and that caused by schistosomiasis (bilharzia) – Schistosoma mansoni and S. japonicum infection.

Shigellosis This form occurs both sporadically and endemically, and is usually caused by Shigella dysenteriae-1 (Shiga's bacillus), Shigella flexneri, Shigella boydii, and Shigella sonnei; the latter is the most benign and occurs in temperate climates also. It is transmitted by food and water contamination, direct contact, and by flies; the organisms thrive in the presence of overcrowding and insanitary conditions. The incubation is 1–7 days, and the severity of the clinical manifestations is dependent on the responsible strain. Duration of illness varies from a few days to two weeks. Disease is particularly severe in young, old, and malnourished individuals. Complications include perforation and haemorrhage from the colo-rectum, the haemolytic uraemic syndrome (which includes renal failure), and Reiter's syndrome. Diagnosis is dependent on demonstration of Shigella spp. in a faecal sample(s) – before or usually after culture. If dehydration is present, this should be treated accordingly, usually with an oral rehydration technique. Shigella spp. responds to many antimicrobial compounds, the first used being sulphonamides; trimethoprim-sulphamethoxazole, trimethoprim, ampicillin, and amoxycillin have also been used extensively. Recently, a widespread resistance to broad-spectrum antibiotics has developed, especially in Asia and southern America, and the agent of such choice is a quinolone compound, e.g., ciprofloxacin; nalidixic acid is also effective. Prevention depends on improved hygiene and sanitation, careful protection of food from flies, fly destruction, and garbage disposal. A Shigella spp. carrier must not be allowed to handle food.

***Entamoeba histolytica* infection** Although most cases occur in the tropics and subtropics, this is not always the case. Dysentery may be accompanied by weight loss, anaemia, and occasionally dyspnoea. E. histolytica contaminates food, e.g., uncooked vegetables, or drinking water. After ingestion of the cyst-stage, and following the action of digestive enzymes, the motile trophozoite emerges in the colon causing local invasive disease (amoebic colitis). On entering the portal system, these organisms may gain access to the liver, causing invasive hepatic disease (amoebic liver 'abscess'). Other sites of 'abscess' formation include the lungs (usually right) and brain. In the colo-rectum an amoeboma may be difficult to differentiate from a carcinoma. Clinical symptoms usually occur within a week, but can be delayed for months, or even years; onset may be acute – as for Shigella spp. infection. Perforation, colo-rectal haemorrhage, and appendicitis are unusual complications. Diagnosis is by demonstration of E. histolytica trophozoites in a fresh faecal sample; other amoebae affecting man do not invade tissues. Research techniques can be used to differentiate between pathogenic (*E. dysenteriae*) and non-pathogenic strains (*E. dispar*). Alternatively, several serological tests are of value in diagnosis, but only in the presence of invasive disease. Treatment consists of one of the 5-nitroimidazole compounds – metronidazole, tinidazole, and ornidazole; alcohol avoidance is important during their administration. A 5–10 day course should be followed by diloxanide furoate for 10 days. Other compounds – emetine, chloroquine, iodoquinol, and paromomycin – are now rarely used. Invasive disease involving the liver or other organ(s) usually responds favourably to a similar regimen; aspiration of a liver 'abscess' is now rarely indicated, as controlled trials have indicated a similar resolution rate whether this technique is used or not, provided a 5-nitro-imidazole compound is administered.

DYSIDROSIS Disturbance of sweat secretion.

DYSKINESIA Abnormal movements of the muscles resulting from disorder of the brain. Movements are uncoordinated and involuntary and occur in facial as well as limb muscles. They include athetosis (writhing movements), CHOREA (jerking movements predominate), choreoathetosis (a combined type), myoclonus (spasms), tics and tremors.

DYSLEXIA is difficulty in reading or learning to read. It is always accompanied by difficulty in writing, and particularly by difficulties in spelling. Reading difficulties might be due to various factors, for example, a general learning problem, bad teaching or understimulation, or a perceptive problem such as poor eyesight. Specific dyslexia ('word blindess'), however, affects 4–8 per cent of otherwise normal children to some extent. It is three times more common in boys than in girls, and there is often a family history.

Support and advice may be obtained from the British Dyslexia Association (see APPENDIX 2: ADDRESSES).

DYSMENORRHOEA Painful menstruation. (See MENSTRUATION.)

DYSPAREUNIA means painful or difficult coitus.

DYSPEPSIA This is another name for indigestion. It describes a sensation of pain or discomfort in the upper abdomen or lower chest following eating. There may be additional symptoms of heartburn, flatulence, or nausea. There are many causes of dyspepsia including oesophagitis, peptic ulcer, gallstones, hiatus hernia, malignancy of the stomach or oesophagus, and hepatic or pancreatic disease. Occa-

sionally it may be psychological in origin. Treatment depends on the underlying cause but, if there is no specific pathology, avoidance of precipitating foods may be helpful.

DYSPHAGIA Difficulty in swallowing. This may be caused by narrowing of the oesophagus because of physical disease such as cancer or injury. Disturbance to the nervous control of the swallowing mechanism – for example, in STROKE or MOTOR NEURONE DISEASE – can also cause dysphagia.

DYSPHASIA is the term used to describe the difficulties in understanding language and in self-expression, most frequently after stroke (see STROKE), or other brain damage. When there is a total loss in the ability to communicate through speech or writing, it is known as global aphasia. Many more individuals have a partial understanding of what is said to them. They are also able to put their own thoughts into words to some extent. The general term for this less severe condition is dysphasia. Individuals vary widely, but in general there are two main types of dysphasia. Some people may have a good understanding of spoken language but have difficulty in self-expression; this is called expressive or motor dysphasia. Others may have a very poor ability to understand speech, but will have a considerable spoken output consisting of jargon words; this is known as receptive or sensory dysphasia. Similar difficulties may occur with reading, and this is called DYSLEXIA (a term more commonly encountered in the different context of children's reading disability). Adults who have suffered a stroke or another form of brain damage may also have difficulty in writing, or dysgraphia. The speech therapist can assess the finer diagnostic points. (See SPEECH THERAPY.)

No case is too severe or too mild to be referred to a speech therapist for an assessment. The victim, his relatives and other visitors may be anxious about the effects of the stroke and may find it helpful to have the details of the dysphasic problem explained to them. The speech therapist can help them adjust to the effects of the stroke on communication.

Dysphasia may come on suddenly and last only for a few hours or days, being due to a temporary block in the circulation of blood to the brain. The effects may be permanent, but although the individual may have difficulty in understanding language and expressing himself, he will be quite aware of his surroundings and may be very frustrated by his inability to communicate with others.

Further information may be obtained from Action for Dysphasic Adults. (See APPENDIX 2: ADDRESSES.)

DYSPHONIA Abnormal vocal sounds when speaking. It is caused by injury or disease of the larynx or of the nerves suplying the laryngeal muscles.

DYSPLASIA Abnormal development of cells, tissues or structures in the body.

DYSPNOEA Difficulty in breathing (see BREATHLESSNESS; ORTHOPNOEA).

DYSRHYTHMIA Disturbance in the rhythmical contractions of the heart. It is also called ARRHYTHMIA.

DYSTOCIA Slow or painful birth of a child. This may occur because the baby is large and/or the mother's pelvis is small or wrongly shaped for the baby to pass through easily. Abnormal presentation of the baby is another cause (see LABOUR, BREECH PRESENTATION).

DYSTONIA refers to a type of involuntary movement characterized by a sustained muscle contraction, frequently causing twisting and repetitive movements or abnormal postures, and caused by inappropriate instructions from the brain. It is sometimes called torsion spasm, and may be synonymous with athetosis when the extremities are involved. Often the condition is of unknown cause (idiopathic), but an inherited predisposition is increasingly recognized among some cases. Others may be associated with known pathology of the brain such as CEREBRAL PALSY or Wilson's disease. The presentation of dystonia may be focal (usually in adults) causing blepharospasm (forceful eye closure), oromandibular dystonia (spasms of the tongue and jaw), cranial dystonia/Meige syndrome/Brueghel's syndrome (eyes and jaw both involved), spastic or spasmodic dysphonia/laryngeal dystonia (strained or whispering speech), spasmodic dysphagia (difficulty swallowing), spasmodic torti/latero/ante/retrocollis (rotation, sideways, forward or backward tilting of the neck), dystonic writer's cramp or axial dystonia (spasms deviating the torso). Foot dystonia occurs almost exclusively in children and adolescents. In adults, the condition usually remains focal or involves at most an adjacent body part. In children, it may spread to become generalized. The condition has always been considered rare, but commonly is either not diagnosed or mistakenly thought to be of psychological origin. It may, in fact, be half as common as multiple sclerosis. Similar features can occur in some subjects treated with major tranquillizing drugs, in whom a predisposition to develop dystonia may be present. (See APPENDIX 2: ADDRESSES.)

DYSTROPHIA MYOTONICA A type of muscular dystrophy (see MYOPATHY) in which the affected person has weakness and wasting of the muscles, particularly those in the face and neck. Other effects are CATARACT, ptosis (see EYE DISEASES), baldness and malfunctioning of the ENDOCRINE system. Both sexes may be affected by this inherited disorder.

DYSTROPHY means defective or faulty nutrition, and is a term applied to a group of developmental changes occurring in the muscles, independently of the nervous system (see MYOPATHY). The best-known form is progressive muscular dystrophy, a group of hereditary disorders characterized by symmetrical wasting and weakness, with no sensory loss. There are three types: Duchenne (usually occurring in boys within the first three years of life), limb girdle (occurring in either sex in the second or third decade), and facio-scapulo-humeral (either sex, any age). The three types have different prognoses, but may lead to severe disability and premature death, often from respiratory failure. The third type progresses very slowly, however, and is compatible with a long life.

Diagnosis may be confirmed by ELECTROMYOGRAPHY (EMG) or muscle biopsy. Although genetic research is pointing to possible treatment or prevention, at present no effective treatment is known, and deterioration may occur with excessive confinement to bed. Physiotherapeutic and orthopaedic measures may be necessary to counteract deformities and contractures, and may help in coping with some disabilities.

DYSURIA Difficulty or pain in urination. The condition is commonly associated with frequency and urgency of MICTURITION if caused by infection of the bladder (CYSTITIS) or URETHRA (see URETHRA, DISEASES OF). A burning feeling is common and relief is achieved by treating the underlying cause. Drinking large amounts of water may help to alleviate symptoms. If these persist, medical advice should be sought.

E

EAR The ear is concerned with two functions. The more evident is that of the sense of hearing; the other is the sense of equilibration and of motion. The organ is divided into three parts: (1) the external ear, consisting of the auricle on the surface of the head, and the tube which leads inwards to the drum; (2) the middle ear, separated from the former by the tympanic membrane or drum, and from the internal ear by two other membranes, but communicating with the throat by the Eustachian tube; and (3) the internal ear, comprising the complicated labyrinth from which runs the vestibulocochlear nerve into the brain.

External ear The auricle or pinna, shaped in man something like a crumpled-up funnel, is not essential to the sense of hearing, although in animals it appears to play an important part. It consists of a framework of elastic cartilage covered by skin, the lobule at the lower end

1 tragus   4 concha
2 lobule   5 antihelix
3 antitragus   6 helix

The auricle or pinna of the ear.

being a small mass of fat. From the bottom of the concha the external auditory (or acoustic) meatus runs inwards for 25 mm (1 inch), to end blindly at the drum. This passage is short in young children, in whom the drum is almost at the surface, and it lengthens as the skull bones develop. The outer half of the passage is surrounded by cartilage, lined by skin, on which are placed fine hairs pointing outwards, and glands secreting a small amount of wax. In the inner half, the skin is smooth and lies directly upon the temporal bone, in the substance of which the whole hearing apparatus is enclosed. The two parts meet at a slight angle, so as to give the whole passage a curve, which can be straightened by pulling the auricle upwards and backwards, when the drum can often be clearly seen by a good light.

Middle ear The tympanic membrane, forming the drum, is stretched completely across the end of the passage, being placed rather obliquely, so that it makes an angle of about 60° with the floor. It is about 8 mm (one-third of an inch) across, very thin, and white or pale pink in colour, so that it is partly transparent, and some of the contents of the middle ear shine through it. From this description it can be readily understood how easily it is torn, and how dangerous are blows on the side of the head, and rough manipulations to remove wax. The cavity of the middle ear is about 8 mm (one-third of an inch) wide and 4 mm (one-sixth of an inch) in depth from the tympanic membrane to the inner wall of bone. Although important structures, like the facial nerve which runs down behind it, lie close around, its only important contents are three small bones, the malleus (hammer), incus (anvil), and stapes (stirrup), collectively known as the auditory ossicles, with two minute muscles which regulate their movements, and the chorda tympani nerve which runs across the cavity. The audi-

tory ossicles are of great importance. The malleus has a long spicule of bone, the handle, embedded in the substance of the drum, while its head is in contact with the incus. The incus, suspended by one process of bone, has another affixed to the stapes, and the latter fits, by what would in a real stirrup be the footpiece, into one (fenestra vestibuli) of the two openings which lead through the inner wall of the middle ear into the internal ear. Accordingly these three bones form a chain across the middle ear, connecting the drum with the internal ear. Their function is to convert the air-waves, which strike upon the drum, into mechanical movements which can affect the fluid in the inner ear, because air-waves produce little effect upon fluid directly.

The middle ear has two connections which are of great importance as regards disease: in front, it communicates by a passage 37 mm (1½ inches) long, the Eustachian (or auditory) tube, with the upper part of the throat, behind the nose; behind and above, it opens into a cavity known as the mastoid antrum. The Eustachian tube admits air from the throat, and so keeps the pressure on both sides of the drum fairly equal. Serious deafness is produced by its closure, and it also, unfortunately, forms a channel by which acute inflammation, as in measles, can and does spread to the ear. The antrum occupies the interior of the projecting mass of bone, the mastoid process, which is felt on the surface of the head behind the ear; this cavity, along with the middle ear, is separated from the interior of the skull only by a thin plate of bone about the thickness of a playing card.

Internal ear This consists of a complex system of hollows in the substance of the temporal bone enclosing a membranous duplicate. Between the membrane and the bone is a fluid known as perilymph, while the membrane is distended by another collection of fluid known as endolymph. This membranous labyrinth, as it is called, consists of two parts. The hinder part, comprising a sac, the utricle, and three short semicircular canals opening at each end into it, is the part concerned with the balancing sense; the forward part consists of another

1 cochlear duct   4 semicircular canals
2 ductus reuniens   5 utricle
3 ductus endolymphaticus 6 saccule

Membranous labyrinth of internal ear (see diagram on page 163).

1 auricle cartilage
2 external acoustic meatus
3 mastoid process
4 facial nerve
5 styloid process
6 internal ear
7 stapes

8 incus
9 malleus
10 facial nerve
11 internal carotid artery
12 auditory tube
13 tympanic membrane

External and middle parts of the right ear from the front.

small bag, the saccule, and of a still more important part, the cochlear duct, and is the part concerned in hearing. In the cochlear duct is placed the spiral organ of Corti, on which the sound-waves are finally received and by which the sounds are communicated to the cochlear nerve, a branch of the vestibulocochlear nerve, which ends in filaments to this organ of Corti. The essential parts in the organ of Corti are a double row of rods and several rows of cells furnished with fine hairs of varying length. Different musical notes are perhaps appreciated by different rods and hair cells.

The act of hearing When sound-waves in the air reach the ear, the drum is alternately pressed in and pulled out, in consequence of which a to-and-fro movement is communicated to the chain of ossicles. The foot of the stapes communicates these movements to the perilymph. Finally these motions reach the delicate filaments placed in the organ of Corti, and so affect the nerve of hearing, which conveys impressions to the centre in the brain. There are two theories of hearing. The first is that of Helmholtz, who compared the organ of Corti to a piano and presumed that each sound caused a vibration of a corresponding part of Corti's organ. The second and later theory assumes that the entire organ of Corti is thrown into vibration by sounds, and that the nature of the sound is

analysed and perceived by the hearing-centre in the brain.

EAR, DISEASES OF Diseases may affect the ear alone or as part of a more generalized condition. The disease may affect the outer, middle or inner ear or a combination of these.

Assessment A full assessment, including detailed examination, is essential to enable the correct choice of treatment to be made.
EXAMINATION of the ear includes inspection of the external ear. An auriscope is used to examine the external ear canal and the ear drum. As the AURISCOPE is inserted, the auricle is pulled gently upwards and backwards to straighten the ear canal and allow a better view of the ear drum. If a more detailed inspection is required, a microscope may be used to improve illumination and magnification.
TUNING-FORK TESTS are routinely performed to identify the presence of deafness. They also help to differentiate between conductive and nerve deafness.
HEARING TESTS are carried out to determine the level of hearing. An audiometer is used to deliver a series of short tones of varying frequency to the ear, either through a pair of headphones or via a sound transducer applied directly to the skull. The intensity of the sound

Auriscope positioned in the ear for viewing external auditory meatus and ear drum.

is gradually reduced until it is no longer heard and this represents the threshold of hearing, at that frequency, through air and bone respectively. It may be necessary to play a masking noise into the opposite ear to prevent that ear from hearing the tones, enabling each ear to be tested independently.

General symptoms   The following are some of the chief symptoms of ear disease:

DEAFNESS (see DEAFNESS).

EARACHE is most commonly due to acute inflammation of the middle ear, but may also be due to acute or chronic inflammation of the external ear or neuralgia affecting the outer ear. Perceived pain in this region may be referred from other areas, such as the earache commonly experienced after tonsillectomy or that caused by carious teeth. The treatment will depend on the underlying cause.

TINNITUS, or ringing in the ear, is very common, often accompanying deafness but is sometimes the only symptom of ear disease. It is very distressing and affected patients may become clinically depressed. Even normal people sometimes experience tinnitus, particularly if put in soundproofed surroundings. It may be described as hissing, buzzing, the sound of the sea, or of bells. The intensity of the tinnitus usually fluctuates, sometimes disappearing altogether. It may occur in almost any form of ear disease, but is particularly troublesome in nerve deaf-

ness due to ageing and in noise-induced deafness.

The symptom seems to originate in the brain's subcortical regions, high in the central nervous system. It may be a symptom of general diseases such as anaemia, high blood pressure and arterial disease, in which cases it is often synchronous with the pulse, and may also be caused by drugs such as QUININE, SALICYLATES (SALICYLIC ACID and its salts, for example, aspirin) and certain ANTIBIOTICS. Treatment of any underlying ear disorder or systemic disease, including depression, may reduce or even cure the tinnitus, but unfortunately in many cases the noises persist. Management involves psychological techniques and initially an explanation of the mechanism and reassurance that tinnitus does not signify brain disease, or an impending stroke, may help the person. Cognitive psychological approaches can be effective and are used in tinnitus retraining therapy. Tinnitus maskers – which look like hearing aids – have long been used with a suitably pitched sound helping to 'mask' the condition.

Diseases of the external ear

WAX (cerumen) is produced by specialized glands in the outer part of the ear canal only. Impacted wax within the ear canal can cause deafness, tinnitus and sometimes disturbance of balance. Wax can sometimes be softened with olive oil,

5-per-cent bicarbonate of soda or commercially prepared drops and it will gradually liquefy and 'remove itself'. If this is ineffective, syringing by a doctor or nurse will usually remove the wax but sometimes it is necessary for a specialist (otologist) to remove it manually with instruments. Syringing should not be done if perforation of the tympanic membrane (eardrum) is suspected.

FOREIGN BODIES, such as peas, beads or buttons, may be found in the external ear canal, especially in children who have usually introduced them themselves. Live insects may also be trapped in the external canal causing intense irritation and noise, and in such cases spirit drops are first instilled into the ear to kill the insect. Except in foreign bodies of vegetable origin, where swelling and pain may occur, syringing may be used to remove some foreign bodies, but often removal by a specialist using suitable instrumentation and an operating microscope is required. In children a general anaesthetic may be needed.

ACUTE OTITIS EXTERNA may be a diffuse inflammation or a boil (furuncle) occurring in the outer ear canal. The pinna is usually tender on movement (unlike acute otitis media) and a serious discharge may be present (see below). Infection may be caused by bacteria or fungi. Initially treatment should be local, using magnesium sulphate paste or glycerine and 10-percent ichthaminol. Topical antibiotic drops can be used and sometimes systemic antibiotics are necessary, especially if infection is acute.

CHRONIC OTITIS EXTERNA, producing pain and discharge, can be caused by eczema, seborrheic dermatitis or psoriasis. Hair lotions and cosmetic preparations may trigger local allergic reactions in the external ear, and the chronic disorder may be the result of swimming or use of dirty towels. Aural toilet and topical antibiotic or antifungal agents – along with removal of any precipitating cause – are the usual treatments.

TUMOURS of the ear can arise in the skin of the auricle often as a result of exposure to sunlight and can be benign or malignant. Within the ear canal itself, the commonest tumours are benign outgrowths from the surrounding bone, said to occur in swimmers as a result of repeated exposure to cold water. Polyps may result from chronic infection of the ear canal and drum, particularly in the presence of a perforation. These polyps are soft and may be large enough to fill the ear canal, but may shrink considerably after treatment of the associated infection.

Diseases of the middle ear

OTITIS MEDIA, or infection of the middle ear, usually occurs, in its acute form, as a result of infection spreading up the Eustachian tubes from the nose, throat or sinuses. It may occur following a cold, tonsilitis or sinusitis, and may also be caused by swimming and diving where water and infected secretions are forced up the Eustachian tube into the middle ear. Primarily it is a disease of children with as many as 1.5 million cases occurring in Britain every year.

Pain is always present and it may be intense and throbbing or sharp in character. It is accompanied by deafness, fever and often TINNITUS.

In infants, crying may be the only sign that something is wrong, though this is usually accompanied by some localizing manifestation such as rubbing or pulling at the ear. Examination of the ear usually reveals redness, and sometimes bulging, of the ear drum. In the early stages there is no discharge, but in the later stages there may be a discharge from perforation of the ear drum as a result of the pressure created in the middle ear by the accumulated pus. This is usually accompanied by an immediate reduction in pain.

Treatment consists of the immediate administration of an antibiotic, usually one of the penicillins, e.g. amoxycillin. In the majority of cases, no further treatment is required, but if this does not quickly bring relief, then it may be necessary to perform a myringotomy, or incision of the ear drum, to drain pus from the middle ear. When otitis media is treated immediately with sufficient dosage of the appropriate antibiotic, the chances of any permanent damage to the ear or to hearing are reduced to a negligible degree, as is the risk of any complications such as mastoiditis (discussed later in this section).

CHRONIC OTITIS MEDIA WITH EFFUSION, or GLUE EAR, is the commonest inflammatory condition of the middle ear in children, to the extent that one in four children in the UK entering school has had an episode of 'glue ear'. It is characterized by a persistent sticky fluid in the middle ear (hence the name 'glue ear') which causes a conductive-type deafness (see DEAFNESS). It may be associated with enlarged adenoids which impair the function of the Eustachian tube. If the hearing impairment is persistent and causes problems, drainage of the fluid, along with antibiotic treatment, may be needed, possibly in conjunction with removal of the adenoids. The insertion of grommets (ventilation tubes) was once standard treatment, but results were variable and the operation is less popular than a decade or so ago.

MASTOIDITIS is a serious complication of inflammation of the middle ear, the incidence of which has been dramatically reduced by the introduction of antibiotics. Inflammation in this cavity usually arises by direct spread of acute or chronic inflammation from the middle ear. The signs of this condition include swelling and tenderness of the skin behind the ear, redness and swelling inside the ear, pain in the side of the head, high fever, and a discharge from the ear. The management of this condition in the first instance is with antibiotics, usually given intravenously but, if the condition fails to improve, surgical treatment is necessary. This involves draining any pus from the middle ear and mastoid, and removing diseased lining and bone from the mastoid.

Diseases of the inner ear

MENIERE'S DISEASE is a common idiopathic disorder of ENDOLYMPH control in the SEMICIRCU-

LAR CANALS (see EAR), characterized by the triad of episodic VERTIGO with deafness and tinnitus. The aetiology is unknown and usually one ear only is affected at first, but eventually the opposite ear is affected in approximately 50 per cent of cases. The onset of dizziness is often sudden and lasts for up to 24 hours. The hearing loss is temporary in the early stages, but with each attack there may be a progressive nerve deafness. Nausea and vomiting often occur. Treatment during the attacks includes rest and drugs to control sickness. Surgical treatment is sometimes required if crippling attacks of dizziness persist despite these measures.

OTOSCLEROSIS is a condition in which new bone grows in the middle ear to cause fixation of the stapes bone leading to impairment of the transmission of sound. The conductive-hearing loss is usually progressive, but may be partially overcome by a hearing aid. Surgical treatment involves bypassing the fixed bone with an artificial prosthesis.

EATING DISORDERS covers the terms OBESITY, feeding problems in childhood, ANOREXIA NERVOSA, and BULIMIA NERVOSA, of which the latter two are described here.

Anorexia nervosa, often called the slimmer's disease, is a syndrome characterized by loss of at least a quarter of normal weight, by fear of normal weight and, in women, by amenorrhea. An individual's body image may be distorted so that the sufferer cannot judge real weight and wants to diet even when already very thin.

Anorexia nervosa usually begins in adolescence, affecting about 1–2 per cent of teenagers and college students at any time. It is twenty times commoner among women than men and is commonest among daughters of professional couples. Up to 10 per cent of sufferers' sisters also have the syndrome. Anorexia may be linked with episodes of bulimia.

The symptoms result from secretive self-starvation, usually with excessive exercise, self-induced vomiting, and misuse of laxatives. An anorexic (or anorectic) person may wear layers of baggy clothes to keep warm and to hide the figure. Fine facial hair called lanugo may grow, perhaps as heat insulation. Starvation can cause serious problems such as ANAEMIA, low blood pressure, slow heart rate, swollen ankles, and OSTEOPOROSIS. Sudden death from heart arrythmias may occur, particularly if the sufferer misuses DIURETIC tablets to lose weight and also depletes the body's level of potassium.

There is probably no single cause of anorexia nervosa. Social pressure to be thin seems to be an important factor and has increased over the past 20–30 years, along with the incidence of the syndrome. Psychological theories include fear of adulthood and fear of losing parents' attention.

Treatment should start with the general practitioner who should first rule out other illnesses causing similar signs and symptoms. These include depression and disorders of the bowel, pituitary gland, thyroid gland, and ovaries.

If the diagnosis is clearly anorexia nervosa, the general practitioner may refer the sufferer to a psychiatrist or psychologist. Moderately ill sufferers can be treated by COGNITIVE BEHAVIOURAL THERAPY. A simple form of this is to agree targets for daily calorie intake and for acceptable body weight. The sufferer and the therapist (the general practitioner or a member of the psychiatric team) then monitor progress towards both targets by keeping a diary of food intake and measuring weight regularly. Counselling or more intensely personal PSYCHOTHERAPY may help too. Severe life-threatening complications will need urgent medical treatment in hospital, including rehydration and feeding using a nasogastric tube or an intravenous drip.

About half of anorectic sufferers recover fully within four years, a quarter improve, and a quarter remain severely underweight with (in the case of women) menstrual abnormalities. Recovery after ten years is rare and about 3 per cent die within that period, half of them by suicide.

Bulimia nervosa is a syndrome characterized by binge eating, self-induced vomiting and laxative misuse, and fear of fatness. There is some overlap between anorexia nervosa and bulimia but, unlike the former, bulimia may start at any age from about 16 to 40 and is probably more directly linked with ordinary dieting. Bulimic sufferers say that, although they feel depressed and guilty after binges, the 'buzz' and relief after vomiting and purging are addictive. They often respond well to cognitive behaviour therapy.

Bulimia nervosa does not necessarily cause weight loss because the binges – for example of a loaf of bread, a packet of cereal, and several cans of cold baked beans at one sitting – are cancelled out by purging, by self-induced vomiting and by brief episodes of starvation. The full syndrome has been found in about 1 per cent of women but mild forms may be much commoner. In one survey of female college students 13 per cent admitted to having had bulimic symptoms.

Bulimia nervosa rarely leads to serious physical illness or death. But repeated vomiting can cause oesophageal burns, salivary gland infections, small tears in the stomach, and occasionally dehydration and chemical imbalances in the blood. Inducing vomiting using fingers may produce two tell-tale signs – bite marks on the knuckles and rotten, pitted teeth.

Those suffering from this condition may obtain advice from the Eating Disorders Association, (see APPENDIX 2: ADDRESSES).

EBOLA VIRUS DISEASE is another name for VIRAL HAEMORRHAGIC FEVER. The ebola virus is one of the most virulent microorganisms known. Like the MARBURG virus, it belongs to the filovirus group which originates in Africa. Once predominantly confined to central Africa and

Sudan, increased population mobility and wars have meant that the infection occasionally occurs elsewhere, with air travellers developing symptoms on returning home. The disease can neither be prevented nor cured at present.

EBURNATION is a process of hardening and polishing which takes place at the ends of bones, giving them an ivory-like appearance. It is caused by the wearing away, in consequence of osteoarthrosis, of the smooth plates of cartilage which in health cover the ends of the bones.

ECCHYMOSIS The development of a discoloured skin patch resulting from escape of blood into the tissues just under the skin, often from bruising.

ECG (See ELECTROCARDIOGRAM.)

ECHINOCOCCUS The immature form of a small tapeworm, *Taenia echinococcus*, found in dogs, wolves, and jackals from which human beings become infected, so that they harbour the immature parasite in the form known as hydatid cyst. (See TAENIASIS.)

ECHOCARDIOGRAPHY The use of ultrasonics (see ULTRASOUND) for the purpose of examining the heart. By thus recording the echo (hence the name) from the heart of ultra-sound waves it is possible to study, for example, the movements of the heart valves (see HEART), as well as the state of the interior of the heart. Safe, reliable and painless, the procedures cut the need for the physically interventionist procedure of CARDIAC CATHETERIZATION.

ECHOLALIA is the meaningless repetition, by a person suffering from mental degeneration, of words and phrases addressed to him.

ECHOVIRUSES, of which there are more than 30 known types, occur in all parts of the world. Their full name is Enteric Cytopathogenic Human Orphan (hence the abbreviation, ECHO). They owe their cumbersome full name to the fact that they were originally found in the stools of children without disease. Practically all of them, however, have now been identified with definite diseases. They are more common in children than in adults, and have been responsible for outbreaks of meningitis, common-cold-like illnesses, gastro-intestinal infections, and infections of the respiratory tract. They are particularly dangerous when they infect premature infants, and there have been several outbreaks of such infection in neonatal units, in which premature infants and other seriously ill small babies are nursed. The virus is introduced to such units by mothers, staff and visitors who are unaware that they are carriers of the virus.

ECLAMPSIA A rare disorder in which convulsions occur during late pregnancy. This condition is said to occur in around 50 out of every 100,000 pregnant women. It occurs especially in the later months and at the time of delivery, but a few cases occur only after delivery has taken place. The cause is not known although cerebral oedema is thought to occur. In practically all cases the kidneys are profoundly affected. Effective antenatal care should identify most women at risk of developing eclampsia.

Symptoms There are several warning symptoms, such as dizziness, headache, oedema, vomiting, and the secretion of albumin in the urine. These are normally accompanied by a rise in blood pressure, sometimes severe. Pre-eclamptic symptoms may be present for some days or weeks before the seizure takes place, and, if a woman is found to have these during antenatal care, preventive measures must be taken. Untreated, convuslions and unconsciousness are very likely, with serious migrainelike frontal headache and epigastric pain the PRODROMAL symptoms.

Treatment Prevention of eclampsia by dealing with pre-eclamptic symptoms is the best management, but even this may not prevent convulsions. Hospital treatment is essential if eclampsia develops, preferably in a specialist unit. The treatment of the seizures is that generally applicable to convulsions of any kind, with appropriate sedatives given such as intravenous DIAZEPAM. HYDRALIZINE intravenously should also be administered to reduce the blood pressure. Magnesium sulphate given intramuscularly sometimes helps to control the fits. The baby's condition should be monitored throughout.

Urgent delivery of the baby, if necessary by CAESAREAN SECTION, is the most effective 'treatment' for a mother with acute eclampsia

Women who have suffered from eclampsia are liable to suffer a recurrence in a further preganancy. Careful monitoring is required. There is a self-help organization, Action on Pre-eclampsia (APEC), to advise on the condition: see APPENDIX 2: ADDRESSES.

ECSTASY refers to a morbid mental condition, associated with an extreme sense of well-being, with a feeling of rapture, and temporary loss of self-control. It often presents as a form of religious obsession, with a feeling of direct communication with God, saintly voices and images being perceived. In milder cases the patient may preach as though with a divine mission to help others. Ecstasy may occur in happiness psychosis, schizophrenia, certain forms of epilepsy, and abnormal personalities.

The term is also a slang drug name for an amphetamine derivative, 3, 4-methylenedioxymethamphetamine or MDMA, increasingly used as a 'recreational' drug. It is classified as a Class A drug under the Misuse of Drugs Act 1971. MDMA is structurally similar to endogenous CATECHOLAMINES and produces central and peripheral sympathetic stimulation of alpha and beta ADRENERGIC RECEPTORS. It is taken into nerve terminals by the serotonin transporter and causes release of the NEUROTRANSMITTER substances serotonin and dopamine. Following this, SEROTONIN depletion is prolonged. As serotonin plays a major part in mood control, this leads to the characteristic 'midweek depression' experienced by MDMA users. Several fatalities in young people have been attributed to adverse reactions resulting from MDMA use/abuse. The principal effects are increase in pulse, blood pressure, tem-perature and respiratory rate. Additional complications such as cardiac ARRHYTHMIAS, heatstroke-type syndrome, HYPONATRAEMIA and brain haemorrhage may occur. Management of patients who get to hospital is largely symptomatic and supportive but may include gastric decontamination, and use of DIAZEPAM as the first line of treatment as it reduces central stimulation which may also reduce TACHYCARDIA, HYPERTENSION and PYREXIA.

ECT (See ELECTROCONVULSIVE THERAPY.)

ECTASIA A term that means widening, usually referring to a disorder of a duct bearing secretions from a gland or organ. For example, mammary duct ectasia.

ECTHYMA In debilitated or immuno-depressed subjects, staphylococcal IMPETIGO or folliculitis (inflammation of hair follicles (see SKIN)) may become ulcerated. This is called ecthyma and is seen in vagrants, drug addicts, and individuals with HIV or uncontrolled DIABETES MELLITUS.

ECTO- is a prefix meaning on the outside.

ECTOPIC means out of the usual place. For example, the congenital displacement of the heart outside the thoracic cavity is said to be ectopic. An 'ectopic gestation' means a pregnancy outside of the womb (see ECTOPIC PREGNANCY).

ECTOPIC BEAT A heart muscle contraction that is outside the normal sequence of the cardiac cycle. The impulse is generated outside the usual focus of the SINOATRIAL NODE. Also known as extrasystoles, ectopic beats are called ventricular if they arise from a focus in the VENTRICLES and supraventricular if they arise in the ATRIA. They may cause no symptoms and the affected subject may be unaware of them. The beat may, however, be the result of heart disease or may be caused by nicotine or caffeine. If persistent, the individual may suffer from irregular rhythm or ventricular fibrillation and need treatment with anti-arrhythmic drugs.

ECTOPIC PREGNANCY An ectopic pregnancy most commonly develops in the FALLOPIAN TUBE. Occasionally it may occur in an OVARY, rarely in the uterine CERVIX or the abdominal cavity. Around 1 in 200 pregnant women have an ectopic gestation. As pregnancy proceeds, surrounding tissues may be damaged and, if serious bleeding happens, the woman may present as an 'abdominal emergency'. A life-threatening condition, this needs urgent surgery. Most women recover satisfactorily and can have further pregnancies despite the removal of one fallopian tube as a result of the ectopic gestation. Death is unusual. This disorder of pregnancy may occur because infection or a previous abdominal injury or operation may have damaged the normal descent of an ovum from the ovary to the womb. The first symptoms usually appear during the first two months of pregnancy, perhaps before the woman realizes she is pregnant. Severe lower abdominal pain and vaginal bleeding are common presenting symptoms.

ECTROMELIA means the absence of a limb or limbs, from congenital causes.

ECTROPION (see EYE DISEASES).

ECZEMA (see DERMATITIS).

EDENTULOUS Lacking teeth: this may be because teeth have not developed or because they have been removed or fallen out.

EDTA Ethylenediamine tetraacetic acid is used to treat poisoning with metals such as lead and strontium. A chelating agent EDTA is used in the form of sodium or calcium salts. The stable chelate compounds resulting from the treatment are excreted in the urine.

EDUCATION (see MEDICAL EDUCATION).

EEG (See ELECTROENCEPHALOGRAPHY.)

EFFERENT The term applied to vessels which convey away blood or a secretion from a part, or to nerves which carry nerve impulses outwards from the nerve-centres. (Opposite: AFFERENT.)

EFFORT SYNDROME Also known as Da Costa's syndrome, this is a condition in which symptoms occur, such as palpitations and shortness of breath, which are attributed by the patient to disorder of the heart. There is no evidence, however, of heart disease, and psychological factors are thought to be of importance. (See PSYCHOSOMATIC DISEASES.)

EFFUSION The passage of fluid through the walls of a blood vessel into a tissue or body cavity. It commonly occurs as a result of inflammation or damage to the blood vessel. A pleural effusion may occur in heart failure (as a result of increased blood pressure in the veins forcing out fluid) or as a result of inflammation in the lung tissue (pneumonia). Effusions may also develop in damaged joints.

EGG (see OVUM).

EGO A psychoanalytical term to describe that part of the mind which develops as a result of the individual's interactions with the outside world. FREUD describes the ego as reconciling the demands of the ID (a person's unconscious, instinctive mind), the superego (moral conscience) and the reality of the outside world.

EISENMENGER REACTION A condition in which the subject suffers from a defect in one of the dividing walls (septum) of the heart and this is accompanied by PULMONARY HYPERTENSION. The defect allows blood low in oxygen to flow from the right to the left side of the heart and be pumped into the aorta, which normally carries oxygenated blood to the body. The patient suffers from cyanosis and has a dusky blue appearance. There is an increase in red blood cells as the body attempts to compensate for the lowered oxygen delivery. The condition requires early surgical repair of the septal defect.

EJACULATION The expulsion of SEMEN from the penis during ORGASM. The stimulation of sexual intercourse or masturbation produces a spinal reflex action that causes ejaculation. The semen comprises several constituents arising from COWPER'S GLAND, the PROSTATE GLAND, the TESTICLES, and the SEMINAL VESICLES and these are discharged in sequence. (See also PREMATURE EJACULATION.)

ELASTIC TISSUE CONNECTIVE TISSUE which contains a profusion of yellow elastic fibres. Long, slender and branching, these fibres (made up of elastin, an albuminlike PROTEIN) ensure that the elastic tissue is flexible and stretchable. The dermis layer of the skin, arterial walls and the alveolar walls in the LUNGS all contain elastic tissue.

ELBOW The joint formed between the humerus above and the radius and ulna below. The humerus has at its lower end a rounded surface, against which the head of the radius moves, and a deep groove to which a saddle-shaped surface at the upper end of the ulna fits. The head of the radius rests upon a projection of the ulna and is bound to it by a stout annular ligament, within which it can rotate. Two important movements take place at this joint: a flail-like backward and forward movement of the radius and ulna moving together upon the humerus, and a rotary movement of

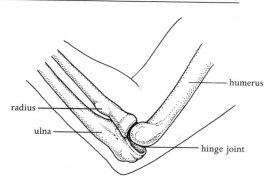

Right elbow joint: an example of a hinge joint.

the radius on the ulna, by which the lower end of the radius is crossed over the ulna and again brought side by side with it, according as the hand is turned palm downwards and palm upwards. The joint is secured at the sides by strong lateral ligaments, and at the back and front is covered by powerful muscles. The ulnar nerve as it passes down to the forearm has an exposed position behind the inner edge of the humerus at its lower end; this is popularly known as the 'funny-bone'. The elbow is seldom dislocated, but a not uncommon accident consists in the chipping off, through a fall on the elbow, of the olecranon process which forms the point behind the joint.

ELECTRICAL INJURIES These are usually caused by the passage through the body of an electric current of high voltage owing to accidental contact with a live wire or to a discharge of lightning. The general effects produced are included under the term electric shock, but vary greatly in degree. The local effects include spasmodic contraction of muscles, fracture of bones, and in severe cases more or less widespread destruction of tissues which may amount simply to burns of the skin or may include necrosis of masses of muscle and internal organs. Fright due to unexpectedness of the shock and pain due to the sudden cramp of muscles are the commonest symptoms and in most cases pass off in a few minutes or less. In more severe cases, especially when the person has remained in contact with a live wire for some time or has been unable to let go of the electrical contact owing to spasmodic contraction of his muscles, the effects are more pronounced and may include concussion or compression of the brain. (See BRAIN, DISEASES OF.) In still severer cases, death may ensue either from paralysis of the respiration or stoppage of the heart's action.If prompt measures are taken for treatment the victim can often be resuscitated.

In Britain there are an average of 110 deaths a year from electrocution, half of these occurring in the home.)

Treatment   No electrical apparatus or switch should be touched by anyone who is in metallic contact with the ground, such as through a metal pipe, especially, for example, from a bath. The first action is to break the current. This can sometimes be done by turning off a switch. If the victim is grasping or in contact with a live wire, the contact may be severed with safety only by someone wearing rubber gloves or rubber boots, but as these are not likely to be immediately available, his hands may be protected by a thick wrapping of dry cloth, or the live wire may be hooked or pushed out of the way with a long wooden stick. If the injured person is unconscious, and especially if breathing has stopped, artificial respiration should be applied as described in APPENDIX: BASIC FIRST AID, Electrocution. When the patient begins to breathe again, he must be treated for shock and professional help obtained urgently.

Patient connected via electrodes on chest to electrocardiograph (heart-monitoring machine).

ELECTROCARDIOGRAM (ECG)   A record of the variations in electric potential which occur in the heart as it contracts and relaxes. Any muscle in use produces an electric current, but when an individual is at rest the main muscular current in the body is that produced by the heart. This can be recorded by connecting the outside of the body by electrodes with an instrument known as an electrocardiograph. The patient is connected to the electrocardiograph by leads from either the arms and legs or different points on the chest. The normal electrocardiogram of each heart-beat shows one wave corresponding to the activity of the atria and four waves corresponding to

the phases of each ventricular beat (see illustration). Various readily recognizable changes are seen in cases in which the heart is acting in an abnormal manner, or in which one or other side of the heart is hypertrophied. This record therefore forms a useful aid in many cases of heart disease. The main applications of the electrocardiogram are in the diagnosis of myocardial infarction and of cardiac arrhythmias.

ELECTROCAUTERY or GALVANOCAUTERY. The use of an electrically heated needle or loop to destroy diseased or unwanted tissue. Benign growths, warts and polyps can be removed with this technique.

ELECTROCOAGULATION   A method of sealing blood vessels using heat generated by high-frequency electric current through fine needles or a surgical knife. The procedure is used during surgery to close newly cut vessels. It can also be used to stop nose bleeds and to remove vascular deformities such as naevi.

ELECTROCOCHLEOGRAPHY is a method of recording the activity of the cochlea, the part of the inner ear concerned with hearing. (See EAR.)

ELECTROCONVULSIVE THERAPY (ECT)   A controversial, although rapidly effective treatment for cases of severe depression, particularly where psychotic features are present (see PSYCHOSIS), or in high-risk patients such as suicidal or postpartum patients. ECT is only indicated after antidepressants have been tried and shown to be ineffective; the full procedure of treatment should be explained to the patient, whose consent must be obtained.

Before treatment, the patient will have been fasted for at least eight hours. After checking for any potential drug ALLERGIES or interac-

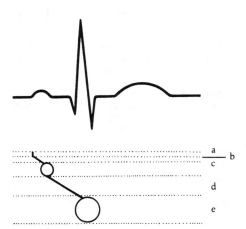

(a) origin of the sinus impulse
(b) conduction through the sino-atrial junction
(c) atrial activation
(d) conduction through the atrioventricular junction
(e) spread of activation within the ventricles

Tracing of normal electrical impulse that initiates heartbeat (after *The Cardiac Arrhythmias Pocket Book*, Boehrringer, Ingelheim).

tions, the patient is given a general anaesthetic and muscle relaxants. Depending on the side of the patient's dominance, either unilateral (on the side of the non-dominant hemisphere of the BRAIN) or bilateral (if dominance is uncertain, e.g. in left-handed people) positioning of electrodes is used. Unilateral ECT has the advantage of being associated with less anterograde AMNESIA. When the current passes the muscles will contract for approximately 10 seconds, with further tonic spasms lasting up to one minute. The patient should then be put in the COMA or recovery position and observed until fully conscious. Up to 12 treatments may be given over a month, improvement usually showing after the third session. Widely used at one time, the treatment is now given only rarely. It can be extremely frightening for patients and relatives and is not recommended for children.

ELECTROENCEPHALOGRAPHY (EEG)
In the brain there is a regular, rhythmical change of electric potential, due to the rhythmic discharge of energy by nerve cells. These changes can be recorded graphically and the 'brain waves' examined, a procedure introduced to medicine in the 1920s. These records – electroencephalograms – are useful in diagnosis. For example, the abnormal electroencephalogram occurring in epilepsy is characteristic of this disease. The normal waves, known as alpha waves, occur with a frequency of 10 per second. Abnormal waves, with a frequency of 7 or less per second, are known as delta waves and occur in the region of cerebral tumours and in the brains of epileptics. An electroencephalogram can assess whether an individual is awake, alert or asleep. It may also be used during surgery to monitor the depth of unconsciousness in anaesthetized patients.

ELECTROLYSIS
The use of shortwave electric currents to destroy the roots of hairs (see SKIN) and so remove unwanted hair from the skin surface. If used by a trained operator, the procedure is safe, but care must be taken in the vicinity of the eyes and, as electrolysis of hair on the legs is such a lengthy process, it is best avoided there.

ELECTROLYTES
Substances, for example, potassium chloride, whose molecules split into their constituent electrically charged particles, known as ions, when dissolved in fluid. In medicine the term is customarily used to describe the ion itself. The description 'serum electrolyte concentration' means the amounts of separate ions – for example, sodium and chloride in the case of salt – present in the serum of the circulating blood. Various diseases alter the amounts of electrolytes in the blood, either because more than normal are lost through vomiting or diarrhoea, or electrolytes may be retained because the kidney is not excreting them properly. Measurements of electrolytes are valuable clues to the type of disease and

provide a means of monitoring a course of treatment. Electrolyte imbalances can be corrected by administering appropriate substances orally or intravenously or by DIALYSIS.

ELECTROMYOGRAPHY (EMG)
The recording of electrical activity in a muscle using electrodes placed in the fibres. The procedure is used to diagnose muscle and nerve disorders and to assess recovery in certain types of paralysis.

ELECTRON is one of the subatomic particles. (See RADIOTHERAPY.)

ELECTRON MICROSCOPE (see MICROSCOPE).

ELECTRO-OCULOGRAPHY
A method of recording movements of the eyes, which is proving of value in assessing the function of the retina (see EYE.)

ELECTROPHORESIS
The migration of charged particles between electrodes. A simple method of electrophoresis, known as paper electrophoresis, has been introduced to analyse proteins in body fluids. This method consists in applying the protein-containing solution as a spot or a streak to a strip of filter paper which has been soaked in buffer solution and across the ends of which a potential difference is then applied for some hours. Comparison is made between filter strips of normal fluids and that of the patient under investigation. Identification and quantification of proteins in the blood are possible using this method.

ELECTRORETINOGRAM
An electroretinogram is the record of an electrical response of visual receptors in the retina (see EYE), which can be measured with corneal electrodes.

ELEPHANTIASIS
A clinical state characterized by chronically oedematous and thickened tissue, especially involving the lower extremities and genitalia, regardless of the cause. It arises from repeated attacks of inflammation of the skin and subcutaneous tissue, with concurrent obstruction of lymphatic vessels. In a tropical country, the usual cause is lymphatic filariasis; however, podoconiosis (resulting from silica particles which penetrate the intact skin of the feet) – which has a more limited geographical distribution – should also be considered.

FILARIAL ELEPHANTIASIS *Wuchereria bancrofti* and *Brugia malayi* are conveyed to man by a mosquito bite. Patrick Manson first delineated the man–mosquito component in the life-cycle at Amoy, China in 1875–9; G. C. Low (1900) was responsible for elucidation of the mosquito–man cycle. Resultant lymphatic obstruction gives rise to enlargement and disfiguration, with thickening of the skin (resembling that of an elephant) in one or both lower limbs and occasionally genitalia (involving particularly the scrotum). Elephantiasis affecting an upper limb is unusual; when it occurs, it is usually associated with *B. malayi* infection. Concurrent involvement of the abdominal lymphatics can give rise to chyluria. By the time the condition is clinically manifest, lymphatic damage is invariably irreversible, and evidence (including serology) of an active filarial infection is usually absent. However, when evidence of continuing activity exists, a course of diethylcarbamazine should be administered (see FILARIASIS). Relief can be obtained by using elastic bandaging, massage, rest, and elevation of the affected limb. Surgery is sometimes indicated. In prevention, destruction of mosquitoes is important.

ELISA   (See ENZYME-LINKED IMMUNO-SORBENT ASSAY.)

ELIXIR   A liquid preparation of a potent or nauseous drug made pleasant to the taste by the addition of aromatic substances and sugar. The name was specially applied to several preparations greatly used in the Middle Ages, which had the effect of acting as a tonic to the stomach and relieving constipation, and which were known, for example, as the elixir of Paracelsus, the elixir of long life. The main constituent of all of these was tincture of aloes.

EMACIATION   Pronounced wasting, and is a common symptom of many diseases, particularly of those which are associated with a prolonged or repeated rise of temperature, such as tuberculosis. It is also associated with diseases of the alimentary system in which digestion is inefficient, or in which the food is not fully absorbed: for example, in diarrhoea of long-standing, whatever its cause. It is also a marked feature of severe malnutrition and malignant disease.

EMBALMING (see DEAD, DISPOSAL OF THE).

EMBOLECTOMY   Surgical removal of a clot or embolus to clear an obstruction in an artery. The obstruction may be cleared by inserting a balloon (Fogarty) catheter into the blood vessel or by surgical incision through the arterial wall. Embolectomy may be a life-saving operation when a patient has a PULMONARY EMBOLISM.

EMBOLISM   The plugging of a small blood-vessel by an EMBOLUS which has been carried through the larger vessels by the blood stream. It is due usually to fragments of a clot which has formed in some vessel, or to small portions carried off from the edge of a heart-valve when this organ is diseased; but the plug may also be a small mass of bacteria, or a fragment of a tumour, or even a mass of air bubbles sucked into the veins during operations on the neck.

The result is usually more or less destruction of the organ or part of an organ supplied by the obstructed vessel. This is particularly the case in the brain, where softening of the brain, with aphasia or apoplexy, may be the result. If the plug is a fragment of malignant tumour, a new growth develops at the spot; and if it is a mass of bacteria, an abscess forms there. Air-embolism occasionally causes sudden death in the case of wounds in the neck, the air bubbles completely stopping the flow of blood. Fat-embolism is a condition which has been known to cause death, masses of fat, in consequence of such an injury as a fractured bone, finding their way into the circulation and stopping the blood in its passage through the lungs. (See also PULMONARY EMBOLISM.)

EMBOLUS   Substances – for example, air, AMNIOTIC FLUID, blood clot, fat or foreign body – that are carried by the blood from a vessel (or vessels) in one part of the body to another part where the matter lodges in a blood vessel causing a blockage (see EMBOLISM).

EMBROCATIONS are mixtures, usually of an oily nature, intended for external application in cases of rheumatism, sprains, and other painful conditions. Their action is due mainly to the massage employed in rubbing in the embrocations, in part to the counter-irritant action of the drugs which they contain. (See LINIMENTS.)

EMBRYO   The fetus in the womb prior to the end of the second month. (See FETUS.)

EMBRYOLOGY   The study of the growth and development of an EMBRYO and subsequently the FETUS from the fertilization of the OVUM by the SPERMATOZOON through the gestational period until birth. Embryology is valuable in the understanding of adult anatomy, how the body works and the occurrence of CONGENITAL deformities.

EMBRYO RESEARCH   When a woman is treated for infertility it is necessary to nurture human embryos for a few days (until the first cell divisions of the fertilized egg have occurred) in a specialized laboratory. More eggs are fertilized than are usually needed because not all fertilizations are successful. Surplus embryos may be frozen for use in later attempts to implant an embryo in the womb. Research has been done on very early embryos but the practice is controversial and some countries have either forbidden it or imposed tight restrictions.

EMBRYO TRANSFER is the process where by the initial stages of procreation are produced outside the human body and completed in the uterus or womb. The procedure is also known as 'embryo transplantation' and 'in vitro fertilization'. It consists of extracting an ovum (or egg) from the prospective mother's body and placing this in a dish where it is mixed with the male partner's semen and special nutrient fluids. After the ovum is fertilized by the sperm it is transferred to another dish containing a special nutrient solution. Here it is left for several days while the normal early stages of development (see FETUS) take place. The early EMBRYO) as it has then become, is then implanted in the mother's uterus, where it 'takes root' and develops as a normal fetus.

The first 'test-tube baby', to use the popular, and widely used, term for such a child was born by CAESAREAN SECTION in England on 25 July 1978. Many other children, conceived in this manner, have since been born, and, though only 10 per cent of women conceive at the first attempt, the overall success rate is improving. Embryo transplantation and research are controversial procedures and in many countries are controlled by legislation.

EMESIS means VOMITING.

EMETICS A substance which induces vomiting (emesis). They were previously used for gut decontamination in the treatment of posioning but are now considered obsolete. This is because the efficacy of emesis as a means of gut decontamination is unproved, there is a delay between administration and actual emesis during which time continued absorption of the poison may occur and some emetics have effects other than vomiting which may mask the clinical features of the ingested poison. The most commonly used emetic was syrup of ipecacuanha (ipecac). Salt (sodium chloride) water emetics were also used but there are many cases of fatal HYPERNATRAEMIA resulting from such use and salt water emetics should never be given. The most common method of gut decontamination currently used is the administration of activated CHARCOAL.

EMETINE The active principles of ipecacuanha. (See IPECACUANHA.)

EMG (see ELECTROMYOGRAPHY).

EMISSION A discharge. The term is commonly used to describe the orgasmic flow of semen from the erect penis that occurs during sleep. Described as a nocturnal emission or, colloquially, as a 'wet dream', it is a common event in late PUBERTY.

EMMETROPIA The normal condition of the eye as regards refraction of light rays. When the muscles in the eyeball are completely relaxed the focusing power is accurately adjusted for parallel rays, so that vision is perfect for distant objects.

EMOLLIENTS are substances which have a softening and soothing effect upon the skin. They include dusting powders such as French chalk, oils such as olive oil and almond oil, and fats such as the various pharmacopoeial preparations of paraffin, suet, and lard. Glycerin is also an excellent emollient.

Uses They are used in various inflammatory conditions such as eczema, when the skin becomes hard, cracked, and painful. They may be used in the form of a dusting powder, an oil or an ointment.

EMOTION Mental arousal that the individual may find enjoyable or unpleasant. The three components are subjective, physiological and behavioural. The instinctive fear and flee response in animals comprises physiological reaction – raised heart rate, pallor and sweating – to an unpleasant event or stimulus. The loving relationship between mother and child is another well-recognized emotional event. If this emotional bond is absent or inadequate the child may suffer emotional deprivation, which can be the trigger for behavioural problems ranging from attention craving to aggression. Emotional problems are common in human society, covering a wide spectrum of psychological disturbances. Upbringing, relationships or psychiatric illnesses such as anxiety and depression may all contribute to the development of emotional problems (see MENTAL ILLNESS).

EMPATHY The facility to understand and be sympathetic to the feelings and thoughts of another individual. Empathy in the therapist is an essential component of successful psychotherapy and is a valuable characteristic in anyone who is a member of a caring profession.

EMPHYSEMA means an abnormal presence of air in certain parts of the body. In its restricted sense, however, it is generally employed to designate an affection of the lungs, of which there are two forms. In one of these there is over-distension of the air-cells of these organs, and in parts destruction of their walls, giving rise to the formation of large sacs, from the rupture and running together of a number of contiguous air-vesicles. This is much the more common of the two forms and is the one which is usually meant when the term 'emphysema' is used. In the other form the air is infiltrated into the connective tissue beneath the pleura and between the pulmonary air-cells, constituting what is known as acute interstitial emphysema.

Causes Where a portion of the lung has become wasted, or its vesicular structure permanently obliterated by disease, without corresponding falling-in of the chest wall, the neighbouring air-vesicles, or some of them, undergo dilatation to fill the vacuum.

In cases of bronchitis, and especially of

bronchial asthma, where numbers of the smaller bronchial tubes become obstructed, the air in the pulmonary vesicles remains imprisoned, the force of expiration being insufficient to expel it; on the other hand, the stronger force of inspiration being adequate to overcome the resistance, the air-cells tend to become more and more distended, and permanent alterations in their structure, including emphysema, are the result.

Emphysema also arises from exertion involving expiratory efforts, during which the glottis is constricted, as in paroxysms of coughing, in straining, and in lifting heavy weights. Whooping-cough is well known as an exciting cause of emphysema.

Smoking is an important cause of emphysema. In the affected portions of the lungs there are loss of the natural elasticity of the air-cells, destruction of many of the pulmonary capillary blood-vessels, and diminution of aerating surface for the blood. As a consequence there is a strain on the heart and the venous system generally, leading to dilatation of the right side of the heart, and so to oedema.

Symptoms The chief symptom in this complaint is shortness of breath, more or less constant but greatly aggravated by exertion, and by attacks of bronchitis, to which people suffering from emphysema are specially liable. The respiration is of a wheezy character. In severe forms of the disease the patient comes to acquire a peculiar bluish and bloated appearance, and the configuration of the chest is altered, assuming the character known as the barrel-shaped chest.

Treatment The patient's general health should be improved and he or she should stop smoking and avoid polluted environments. Regular physiotherapy to drain the lungs of fluid and improve breathing is of great help. Emphysematous patients are prone to infection of the lungs and they should have annual immunization against influenza. During attacks of urgent breathlessness anti-spasmodic remedies should be given, while inhalation of oxygen will often afford marked and speedy relief.

Surgical emphysema is the term applied when air is present under the skin. It may get there, for example, if the lungs are wounded through the chest wall, or if the wind-pipe is pierced at any point in its path.

EMPIRICAL Method of treatment founded simply on experience. Because a given remedy has been successful in the treatment of a certain group of symptoms, it is assumed, by those who uphold this principle, that it will be successful in the treatment of other cases presenting similar groups of symptoms, without any inquiry as to the cause of the symptoms or reason underlying the action of the remedy. It is the contrary of 'rational' or 'scientific' treatment. Sometimes a course of treatment must perforce be empirical for want of knowledge.

EMPROSTHOTONOS The spasm of abdominal muscles that occurs in TETANUS, making the body arch forwards.

EMPYEMA An accumulation of pus within a cavity, the term being generally reserved for collections of pus within one of the pleural cavities. Since the advent of antibiotics, the condition is relatively uncommon in developed countries. The condition is virtually an abscess, and therefore gives rise to the general symptoms accompanying that condition; but, on account of the thick unyielding wall of the chest, it is unlikely to burst through the surface, and therefore it is of particular importance that the condition should be recognized early, and, as a rule, treated surgically.

The condition most commonly follows an attack of pneumonia. It may also occur in the advanced stage of pulmonary tuberculosis. Empyema also occurs at times through infection from some serious disease in neighbouring organs, such as cancer of the gullet, or follows upon wounds penetrating the chest wall.

EMULSIONS are oil-in-water or water-in-oil dispersions. Therapeutic emulsions (creams) require an added stabilizing substance.

ENAMEL (see TEETH).

ENCEPHALIN A naturally occurring brain PEPTIDE, the effects of which resemble those of MORPHINE or other opiates (see ENDORPHIN).

ENCEPHALITIS means inflammation or infection of the brain, usually caused by a virus but may also be the result of bacterial infection. It occurs throughout the world and affects all racial groups and ages. Rarely it occurs as a complication of common viral disease such as measles, mumps, glandular fever, or chicken-pox. It may occur with no evidence of infection elsewhere such as herpes simplex encephalitis, the most common form seen in Europe and America. Rabies is another form of viral encephalitis, and the HIV virus which causes AIDS invades the brain to cause another form of encephalitis. In some countries – North and South America, Japan and east Asia and Russia – there may be epidemics spread by the bite of mosquitoes or ticks.

The clinical features begin with symptoms like influenza – aches, temperature and wretchedness; then the patient develops a headache with drowsiness, confusion, and neck stiffness. Severely ill patients develop changes in behaviour, abnormalities of speech and deterioration to come with epileptic seizures. Some develop paralysis and memory loss. CT and MRI brain scans shows brain swelling, and damage to the temporal lobes if the herpes virus is involved. Electroencephalography, which records the brainwaves, is abnormal. Diagnosis is possible by an examination of the blood or other body fluids for antibody reaction to the virus, and modern laboratory techniques are very specific.

In general, drugs are not effective against viruses – antibiotics are of no use. Herpes encephalitis does respond to treatment with the anti-viral agent, acyclovir. Treatment is supportive: patients should be given painkillers, fluid replacement drugs to reduce brain swelling and to counter epilepsy if it occurs. Fortunately, most sufferers from encephalitis make a complete recovery but some are left severely disabled with physical defects, personality and memory disturbance and epileptic fits. Rabies is always fatal and the changes found in patients with AIDS are almost always progressive. Except in very specific circumstances, it is not possible to be immunized against encephalitis.

Encephalitis lethargica is one, now rare, variety that reached epidemic levels after the First World War. It was characterized by drowsiness and headache leading on to coma. The disease occasionally occurs as a complication after mumps and sometimes affected individuals subsequently develop postencephalitic PARKINSONISM.

ENCEPHALOID   A form of cancer which, to the naked eye, resembles the tissue of the brain.

ENCEPHALOMYELITIS   Inflammation of the substance of both brain and spinal cord.

ENCEPHALOPATHY   The term covering certain conditions in which there are signs of cerebral irritation without any localized lesion to account for them. The two best examples are hypertensive encephalopathy and lead encephalopathy. In the former, which occurs in the later stages of chronic GLOMERULONEPHRITIS, or URAEMIA, the headache, convulsions, and delirium which constitute the main symptoms are supposed to be due to a deficient blood-supply to the brain.

ENCHONDROMA   A tumour formed of cartilage. (See TUMOUR.)

ENCYSTED   Enclosed within a bladder-like wall. The term is applied to parasites, collections of pus, etc., which are shut off from surrounding tissues by a membrane or by adhesions.

ENDARTERECTOMY   Surgical reopening of an artery obstructed by ATHEROMA. If a blood clot is present the reboring process is called thromboendarterectomy. Restored patency allows arterial blood supply to restart. The CAROTID arteries and arteries to the legs are those most commonly operated on.

ENDARTERITIS   Inflammation of the inner coat of an artery. (See ARTERIES, DISEASES OF.)

ENDEMIC   Diseases which exist in particular localities or among certain races. Some diseases, which are at times epidemic over wide districts, have a restricted area where they are always endemic, and from which they spread. For example, both cholera and plague are endemic in certain parts of Asia.

ENDO-   Prefix meaning situated inside.

ENDOCARDITIS   Inflammation of the lining, valves and muscle of the heart. The main causes are bacterial and virus infections and rheumatic fever and the condition occurs most often in patients whose endocardium is already damaged by congenital deformities or whose immune system has been suppressed by drugs. Infection may be introduced into the bloodstream during dental treatment or surgical procedures, especially on the heart or on the gastrointestinal system. Treatment is with large doses of antibiotic drugs.

ENDOCRINE GLANDS   Organs whose function is to secrete into the blood or lymph substances known as HORMONES which play an important part in general changes or the activities of other organs at a distance. Some organs have a double function, such as the pancreas, which pours digestive secretions by a duct into the intestine, and, at the same time, has an endocrine or internal secretion (insulin) which is secreted direct into the blood. Various diseases arise as the result of defects or excess in the internal secretions of the different glands. The chief endocrine glands are:

Adrenal glands   These two glands, also known as SUPRARENAL GLANDS, lie immediately above the kidneys. The central or medullary portion of the glands forms the secretions known as adrenaline or epinephrine, and noradrenaline. Adrenaline acts upon structures innervated by sympathetic nerves; its action is therefore said to be sympathomimetic. Briefly, the blood-vessels of the skin and of the abdominal viscera (except the intestines) are constricted, and at the same time the arteries of the muscles and the coronary arteries are dilated; systolic blood-pressure rises; blood-sugar increases; the metabolic rate rises; muscle fatigue is diminished. The superficial or cortical part of the glands produce steroid-based substances such as aldosterone, cortisone, hydrocortisone, and deoxycortone acetate, for the maintenance of life. It is the absence of these substances, due to atrophy or destruction of the suprarenal cortex, that is responsible for the condition known as ADDISON'S DISEASE.

Ovaries and testicles   In addition to their main function of producing reproductive cells, these organs secrete substances which have a general effect upon the other bodily tissues.

The ovary secretes at least two hormones, known, respectively, as oestradiol (follicular hormone) and progesterone (corpus luteum hormone). Oestradiol develops (under the stimulus of the anterior pituitary lobe) each time an OVUM in the OVARY becomes mature, causes extensive proliferation of the ENDOMETRIUM lining the UTERUS, a stage ending with shedding of the ovum about 14 days before the onset of MENSTRUATION. The corpus luteum, which then forms, secretes both progesterone and oestradiol. Progesterone brings about great activity of the glands in the endometrium. The uterus is now ready to receive the ovum if it is fertilized. If fertilization does not occur, the corpus luteum degenerates, the hormones cease acting, and menstruation takes place.

The hormone secreted by the testicles is known as TESTOSTERONE. It is responsible for the growth of the male secondary sex characteristics.

Pancreas This gland is situated in the upper part of the abdomen and, in addition to the digestive enzymes it produces, a substance known as INSULIN is absorbed from it into the circulating blood. This controls carbohydrate metabolism and faulty or absent insulin production causes DIABETES MELLITUS.

Parathyroid glands These are four minute glands lying at the side of, or behind, the thyroid. They have a certain effect in controlling the absorption of lime salts by the bones and other tissues. When their secretion is defective, tetany occurs.

Pituitary gland This gland is attached to the base of the brain and rests in a hollow on the base of the skull. It is the most important of all endocrine glands and consists of two embryologically and functionally distinct lobes. The function of the anterior lobe depends on the secretion by the HYPOTHALAMUS of certain 'neuro-hormones' which control the secretion of the pituitary trophic hormones. The hypothalamic centres involved in the control of specific pituitary hormones appear to be anatomically separate. Through the pituitary trophic hormones the activity of the thyroid, adrenal cortex and the sex glands is controlled. The anterior pituitary and the target glands are linked through a feedback control cycle. The liberation of trophic hormones is inhibited by a rising concentration of the circulating hormone of the target gland and stimulated by a fall in its concentration. Six trophic (polypeptide) hormones are formed by the anterior pituitary. Growth hormone (GH) and prolactin are simple proteins formed in the acidophil cells. Follicle-stimulating hormone (FSH), luteinizing hormone (LH) and thyroid-stimulating hormone (TSH) are glycoproteins formed in the basophil cells. Adrenocorticotrophic hormone (ACTH), although a polypeptide, is derived from basophil cells.

The posterior pituitary lobe, or neuro-hypophysis, is closely connected with the hypothalamus by the hypothalamic-hypophyseal tracts. It is concerned with the production or storage of oxytocin and vasopressin (the antidiuretic hormone).

PITUITARY HORMONES Growth hormone, gonadotrophic hormone, adrenocorticotrophic hormone and thyrotrophic hormones can be assayed in blood or urine by radio-immunoassay techniques. Growth hormone extracted from human pituitary glands obtained at autopsy was available for clinical use until 1985 when it was withdrawn as it is believed to carry the virus responsible for CREUTZFELDT-JAKOB DISEASE. However growth hormone produced by DNA recombinant techniques is now available as somatropin.

Human pituitary gonadotrophins are readily obtained from post-menopausal urine. Commercial extracts from this source are available and are effective for treatment of infertility due to gonadotrophin insufficiency.

The adrenocorticotrophic hormone is extracted from animal pituitary glands and has been available therapeutically for many years. It is used as a test of adrenal function, and, under certain circumstances, in conditions for which cortico-steroid therapy is indicated. The pharmacologically active polypeptide of ACTH has been synthesized and is called tetracosactrin. Thyrotrophic hormone is also available but it has no therapeutic application.

HYPOTHALAMIC RELEASING HORMONES which affect the release of each of the six anterior pituitary hormones have been identified. Their blood levels are only one-thousandth of those of the pituitary trophic hormones. The release of thyrotrophin, adrenocorticotrophin, growth hormone, follicle-stimulating hormone and luteinizing hormone is stimulated whilst release of prolactin is inhibited. The structure of the releasing hormones for TSH, FSH-LH, GH and, most recently, ACTH is known and they have all been synthesized. Thyrotrophin-releasing hormone (TRH) is used as a diagnostic test of thyroid function but it has no therapeutic application. FSH-LH-releasing hormone provides a useful diagnostic test of gonadotrophine reserve in patients with pituitary disease and is now used in the treatment of infertility and amenorrhoea in patients with functional hypothalamic disturbance. As this is the commonest variety of secondary amenorrhoea the potential use is great. The therapeutic use of GH-releasing hormone and corticotrophin releasing hormone has yet to be established. Most cases of congenital deficiency of GH, FSH, LH and ACTH are due to defects in the hypothalamic production of releasing hormone and are not a primary pituitary defect, so that the therapeutic implication of this recently synthesized group of releasing hormones is considerable.

GALACTORRHOEA is frequently due to a microadenoma of the pituitary. Dopamine is the prolactin-release inhibiting hormone. Its duration of action is short so its therapeutic value is limited. However, BROMOCRIPTINE is a DOPAMINE agonist with a more prolonged action and is effective treatment for galactorrhoea.

Thyroid gland The functions of the thyroid gland are controlled by the pituitary gland (see above) and the HYPOTHALAMUS, situated in the brain. The thyroid, situated in the front of the neck below the LARYNX, helps to regulate the body's METABOLISM. It comprises two lobes each side of the TRACHEA joined by an isthmus. Two types of secretory cells in the gland, follicular cells (the majority) and parafollicular cells, secrete, respectively, the iodine-containing hormones THYROXINE (T_4) and TRI-IODOTHYRINE (T_3) and the hormone CALCITONIN. T_3 and T_4 help control metabolism and calcitonin, in conjunction with parathyroid hormone (see above), regulates the body's calcium balance. Deficiencies in thyroid function produce HYPOTHYROIDISM and, in children, retarded development. Excess thyroid activity causes THYROTOXICOSIS.

ENDOCRINOLOGY The study of the endocrine system, the substances (hormones) it secretes and its disorders (see ENDOCRINE GLANDS.)

ENDOGENOUS Coming from within the body. Endogenous depression, for instance, occurs as a result of causes inside a person.

ENDOLYMPH The fluid that fills the membranous labyrinth of the inner ear (see diagram on page 328).

ENDOMETRIOSIS The condition in which the endometrium (i.e. the cells lining the interior of the uterus) is found in other parts of the body. The most common site of such misplaced endometrium is the muscle of the uterus. The next most common site is the ovary, followed by the PERITONEUM lining the PELVIS, but it also occurs anywhere in the bowel. The cause is not known. It never occurs before puberty and seldom after the menopause. The main symptoms it produces are MENORRHAGIA, DYSPAREUNIA, painful menstruation and pelvic pain. Treatment is usually by removal of the affected area, but in some cases satisfactory results are obtained from the administration of PROGESTOGENS such as NORETHISTERONE, NORETHYNODREL and DANAZOL.

ENDOMETRITIS Inflammation of the mucous membrane lining the womb. (See UTERUS, DISEASES OF.)

ENDOMETRIUM The mucous membrane which lines the interior of the uterus.

END ORGAN A structure at the end of a peripheral nerve that acts as receptor for a sensation. For example, the olfactory nerves have end organs that pick up smells.

ENDORPHINS PEPTIDES produced in the brain which have a pain-relieving action. Hence their alternative name of opiate peptides. Their name is derived from *endo*genous mor*phine*. They have been defined as endogenous opiates or any naturally occurring substances in the brain with pharmacological actions resembling opiate alkaloids such as MORPHINE. There is some evidence that the pain-relieving action of ACUPUNCTURE may be due to the release of these opiate peptides. It has also been suggested that they may have an anti-psychotic action and therefore of value in the treatment of major psychotic illnesses such as SCHIZOPHRENIA.

ENDOSCOPE A tube-shaped instrument inserted into a cavity in the body to investigate

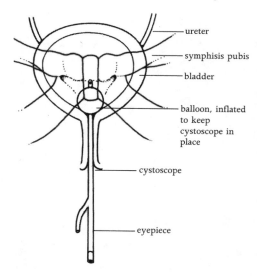

Cystoscope: an endoscope for examining inside the bladder.

Percutaneous nephroscope and stone forceps.

insertion tube

forceps (various types canbe attached)

control lever

eyepiece

A fibreoptic bronchoscope used to examine the larger bronchial tubes of the lungs to determine, for example, whether a tumour is present.

and treat disorders. It is flexible and equipped with lenses and a light source. Examples of endoscopes are the cystoscope for use in the bladder, the gastroscope for examining the stomach and the arthroscope for looking into joints. (See FIBREOPTIC ENDOSCOPY.)

ENDOSCOPY   Examination of a body cavity using an ENDOSCOPE in order to diagnose or treat a disorder in the cavity. The development of endoscopy has reduced the need for major surgery as many diagnostic procedures can be performed with an endoscope as can MINIMALLY INVASIVE SURGERY. The development of fibre optics (the transmission of light along bundles of glass or plastic fibres) has greatly advanced the practice of endoscopy and hospitals now routinely run endoscopy clinics on an outpatient basis.

ENDOTHELIUM   The membrane lining various vessels and cavities of the body, such as the

pleura, pericardium, peritoneum, lymphatic vessels, blood-vessels, and joints. It consists of a fibrous layer covered with thin flat cells, which render the surface perfectly smooth and secrete the fluid for its lubrication.

ENDOTOXIN   A poison produced by certain gram-negative bacteria that is released after the micro-organisms die. Endotoxins can cause fever and shock, the latter by rendering the walls of blood vessels permeable so that fluid leaks into the tissues, with a consequent sharp fall in blood pressure. (See EXOTOXIN.)

ENDOTRACHEAL INTUBATION   Insertion of a rubber or plastic tube through the nose or mouth into the trachea. The tube often has a cuff at its lower end which, when inflated, provides an airtight seal. This allows an anaesthetist to supply oxygen or anaesthetic gases to the lungs and know exactly how much the patient is receiving. Endotracheal intubation is necessary to undertake artificial ventilation of a patient (see ANAESTHESIA).

ENEMA   Introduction of fluid into the rectum via the anus. Enemas may be given to clear the intestine of faeces prior to intestinal surgery or to relieve severe constipation. They may also be used to give barium for diagnostic X-rays as well as drugs such as CORTICOSTEROIDS, used to treat ulcerative COLITIS. The patient is placed on his or her side with a support under the hips. A CATHETER with a lubricated end is inserted into the rectum and warmed enema fluid gently injected. Disposable enemas and miniature enemas, which can be self administered, are widely used; they contain preprepared solution.

ENGAGEMENT   The event during pregnancy when the presenting part of the baby, usually the head, moves down into the mother's pelvis.

ENKEPHALINS   PEPTIDES that have a pain-killing effect similar to that of ENDORPHINS. Produced by certain nerve endings and in the brain, enkephalins (also spelt encephalins) are also believed to act as a sedative and mood changer.

ENOPHTHALMOS   Abnormal retraction of the eye into its socket: for example, when the sympathetic nerve in the neck is paralysed.

ENTAMOEBA (see AMOEBA).

ENTERAL FEEDING   In severely ill patients the metabolic responses to tissue damage may be sufficient to cause a reduction of muscle mass and of plasma proteins. This state of catabolism may also impair the immune response to infection and delay the healing of wounds. It is probable that as many as one half of patients who have had a major operation a week previously show evidence of protein malnutrition. This can be detected clinically by a loss of weight and a reduction in the skinfold thickness and arm circumference. Biochemically the serum albumin concentration falls as does the lymphocyte count. The protein reserves of the body fall even more dramatically when there are sepsis, burns, acute pancreatitis or renal failure.

The purpose of enteral feeding is to give a liquid, low residue food through a naso-gastric feeding tube. It has the advantage over parenteral nutrition that the septic complications of insertion of catheters into veins are avoided. It is also much cheaper. Enteral feeding may either take the form of intermittent feeding through a large-bore naso-gastric tube or continuous gravity feeding through a fine-bore tube.

A number of proprietary enteral foods are available. Some contain whole protein as the nitrogen source. Others, and these are called elemental diets, contain free amino acids. Diarrhoea is the most common problem with enteral feeding and it tends to occur when enteral feeding is introduced too rapidly or with too strong a preparation.

ENTERALGIA   Another name for colic.

ENTERIC-COATED   A description of tablets covered in material that allows them to pass through the stomach and enter the intestine unaltered. Drugs coated in this way are those whose action is reduced or stopped by acid in the stomach.

ENTERIC FEVER   Enteric fever is caused by bacterial infection with either *Salmonella typhi* or *Salmonella paratyphi* A, B or C. These infections are called typhoid fever, or paratyphoid fever respectively. Unlike other salmonellas, *S. typhi* and *S. paratyphi* are primarily human pathogens – infections that attack humans – and humans are the main reservoir from person to person. Transmission usually occurs by ingestion of water or food that has been contaminated with human faeces, for example, by drinking water contaminated with sewage, or foods prepared by a cook infected with or carrying the organisms. Enteric fever is EN-DEMIC in many areas of the world, including Africa, Central and South America, the Indian subcontinent and south-east Asia. Infection occasionally occurs in southern and eastern Europe, particularly with *S. paratyphi* B. However, in northern and western Europe and North America most cases are imported.

Clinical course   The incubation period of enteric fever is 7–21 days. During this time ingested organisms penetrate the wall of the small intestine and replicate in local lymph nodes before invading the blood stream. They are dispersed around the body, settling particu-larly in the RETICULO-ENDOTHELIAL tissue of the liver, spleen and bone marrow, and also the gall bladder. Early symptoms include headache, malaise, dry cough, constipation and a slowly rising fever. Despite the fever the patient's pulse rate is often slow and he or she may have an enlarged spleen. In the second week of illness organisms invade the blood stream again and symptoms progress. In general, symptoms of typhoid fever are more severe than those of paratyphoid fever. Increasing mental slowness and confusion are common, and a more sustained high fever is present. In some individuals discrete red spots appear on the upper trunk (rose spots). By the third week of illness the patient may become severely toxic, with marked confusion and delirium, abdominal distension, MYOCARDITIS, and occasionally intestinal haemorrage and/or perforation. Such complications may be fatal, although are unusual if prompt treatment is given. Subsequently symptoms improve slowly into the fourth and fifth weeks, although may relapse.

Diagnosis   Enteric fever should be considered in any traveller or resident in an endemic area presenting with a febrile illness. The most common differential diagnosis is malaria. Diagnosis is usually made by isolation of the organism from cultures of blood in the first two weeks of illness. Later the organisms are found in the stools and urine. Serological tests for ANTIBODIES against *Salmonella typhi* ANTIGENS (the Widal test) are less useful due to cross-reactions with antigens on other bacteria, and difficulties with interpretation in individuals immunized with typhoid vaccines.

Treatment   Where facilities are available hospital admission is required. Antibiotic therapy with chloramphenicol or amoxycillin is effective. However, widespread resistance to these agents has emerged, and quinolone antibiotics, such as ciprofloxacin, are now recommended initial therapy for enteric fever in the UK and in areas where resistance is common. A few individuals become chronic carriers of the organisms after they have recovered from the symptoms. These people are a potential source of spread to others and should be excluded from occupations handling food or drinking water. Prolonged courses of antibiotic therapy may be required to eradicate carriage.

Prevention   Worldwide, the most important preventive measure is improvement of sanitation and maintenance of clean water supplies. Vaccination is available for travellers to endemic areas.

ENTERITIS means inflammation of the intestines. (See DIARRHOEA; INTESTINE, DISEASES OF.)

ENTEROBIASIS   Infection with Enterobius vermicularis, the threadworm, or pinworm as it is known in the USA. It is the most common of all the intestinal parasites in Britain and the least harmful. The male is about 6 mm (¼ inch) in length and the female about 12 mm (½ inch) in length. Each resembles a little piece of thread. These worms live in considerable numbers in the lower bowel, affecting children particularly. They cause great irritation round the anus, especially in the evening when the female worm emerges from the anus to lay its eggs and then die. Apart from this irritation around the anus, they seldom cause any symptoms. The most effective form of treatment is either viprynium embonate or piperazine citrate.

ENTEROCELE   A hernia of the bowel. (See HERNIA.)

ENTEROGASTRONE   A hormone derived from the mucosal lining of the small intestine which inhibits the movements and secretion of the stomach.

ENTEROKINASE   The ENZYME secreted in the DUODENUM and jejunum (see INTESTINE) which converts the enzyme, trypsinogen, secreted by the PANCREAS, into TRYPSIN. (See also DIGESTION.)

ENTEROPTOSIS   A condition in which, owing to a lax condition of the mesenteries and ligaments which support the bowels, the latter descend into the lower part of the abdominal cavity.

ENTEROSTOMY   An operation by which an artificial opening is formed into the intestine and joined to another part of the intestine or brought to the exterior via the abdominal wall.

ENTEROTOXIN   A type of TOXIN that causes inflammation of the intestinal lining and results in vomiting and diarrhoea (see FOOD POISONING).

ENT DISORDERS (see OTORHINOLARYNGOLOGY).

ENTEROVIRUSES   A family of viruses which include the POLIOMYELITIS, COXSACKIE and ECHO groups of viruses. Their importance lies in their tendency to invade the central nervous system. They receive their name from the fact that their mode of entry into the body is through the gut.

ENTOMOPHOBIA is excessive fear of insects, particularly spiders, mites and other anthropods.

ENTONOX   A proprietary analgesic drug taken by inhalation and comprising half nitrous oxide and half oxygen. It is valuable in providing relief to casualties who are in pain as it provides analgesia without making them unconscious. Entonox is also used in obstetric practice to ease the pains of childbirth.

ENTROPION (see EYE DISEASES).

ENURESIS   Bed wetting or the involuntary passage of urine at night. It can occur at all ages but is a particular problem with children and the elderly. Enuresis in children usually stops as they grow older but, when it persists, the child (and parents) need advice. Treatment is by positive reinforcement of bladder control, alarm systems such as the 'pad and bell', or ocasionally by drugs.

Constipation is a common cause of urinary incontinence – and hence bedwetting – in the elderly and should be treated. Enuresis in the elderly may also be due to organic disease or to mental deterioration and confusion. Appropriate investigation, treatment and nursing should be arranged. (See NOCTURNAL ENURESIS.)

ENVIRONMENTAL HEALTH OFFICER A local-authority health official specially qualified in aspects of environmental health such as clean air, food hygiene, housing, pollution, sanitation and water supplies. He or she is responsible for running the authority's environmental health department and, when EPIDEMIOLOGICAL advice is needed, the relevant public-health physician acts in a consultative capacity (see PUBLIC HEALTH).

ENVIRONMENTAL MEDICINE   The study of the consequences for people's health of the natural environment. This includes the effects of climate, geography, sunlight and natural vegetation.

ENZYME   A protein that acts as a catalyst for the body's metabolic processes. The body contains thousands of enzymes, with each cell producing several varieties. The first enzyme was obtained in a reasonably pure state in 1926. Since then several hundred enzymes have been obtained in pure crystalline form. Many more have been purified to less exacting standards and all have been proved to be proteins. They are present in the digestive fluids and in many of the tissues, and are capable of producing in small amount the transformation on a large scale of various compounds. Indeed, they are an integral, essential component of what might be described as the *modus operandi* of the body. Examples of enzymes are found in the PTYALIN of saliva and DIASTASE of pancreatic juice which split up starch into sugar, the PEPSIN of the gastric juice and the trypsin of pancreatic juice which break proteins into simpler molecules and eventually into the constituent amino-acids, the thrombin of the blood which causes coagulation.

ENZYME-LINKED IMMUNOSORBENT ASSAY (ELISA)   This is a sensitive, safe and cheap method for measuring the quantity of a substance. An antibody to the substance is prepared along with an enzyme which binds to the antibody and which can be accurately measured using colour changes that occur as a result of the chemical reaction.

EOSINOPHIL Any cell in the body with granules in its substance that stain easily with the dye eosin. About 2 per cent of the white cells of the blood are eosinophils.

EOSINOPHILIA means an abnormal increase in the number of eosinophils in the blood. It occurs in Hodgkin's disease, in asthma and hay fever, in some skin diseases, and in parasitic infestation.

EPHEDRINE An ALKALOID derived from a species of *Ephedra* or prepared synthetically. A BRONCHODILATOR, it was once widely used to treat asthma, but has now been superseded by the much safer (and more effective) selective beta-2-adrenoceptor stimulants (see ADRENERGIC RECEPTORS).

EPHELIS A freckle.

EPI- A prefix meaning situated on or outside of.

EPICANTHIC FOLD A vertical skinfold that runs from the upper eyelid to the side of the nose. These folds are normal in oriental races but uncommon in others, although babies may have a temporary fold that disappears. Folds are present in people with Down's Syndrome.

EPICONDYLE The protuberance above a CONDYLE at the end of a bone with an articulating joint – for example, at the bottom of the humerus, the bone of the upper arm.

EPIDEMIC is a term applied to a disease which affects a large number of people in a particular locality at one time. The term is, in a sense, opposed to endemic, which means a disease always found in the locality in question. A disease may, however, be endemic as a rule – for example, malaria in swampy districts, and may become at times epidemic, when an unusually large number of people are affected. The rapid expansion of air travel has extended the scope for the spread of epidemic and endemic disease.

An epidemic disease is usually infectious from person to person, but not necessarily so since many persons in a locality may simply be exposed to the same cause at one time; for example, outbreaks of lead-poisoning are epidemic in this sense.

The laws which govern the outbreak of epidemics are ill understood. Infected food supplies, such as drinking water contaminated by waste from people with cholera or typhoid fever, milk infected with tubercle bacillus, or 'fast food' products contaminated with salmonella. The migrations of certain animals, such

as rats, are in some cases responsible for the spread of plague, from which these animals die in great numbers. Certain epidemics occur at certain seasons: for example, whooping-cough occurs in spring, whereas measles produces two epidemics, as a rule, one in winter and one in March. Influenza, the common cold, and other infections of the upper respiratory tract, such as sore throat, occur predominantly in the winter.

There is another variation, both as regards the number of persons affected and the number who die in successive epidemics: the severity of successive epidemics rising and falling over periods of five or ten years.

EPIDEMIC ENCEPHALITIS Another term for encephalitis lethargica (see ENCEPHALITIS).

EPIDEMIOLOGY The study of disease as it affects groups of people. Originating in the study of epidemics of diseases like CHOLERA, PLAGUE and SMALLPOX, epidemiology is an important discipline which contributes to the control not only of infectious diseases but also of conditions such as heart disease and cancer. Their distributions in populations can provide important pointers to possible causes. The relation between the environment and disease is an essential part of epidemiology. (See PUBLIC HEALTH.)

EPIDERMIS The outer layer of the skin, which forms the protective covering of the body. (See SKIN.)

EPIDERMOPHYTON A fungus infection of the skin causing RINGWORM or TINEA.

EPIDURAL ANAESTHESIA (see ANAESTHESIA).

EPIDYDIMIS An oblong body attached to the upper part of each TESTICLE, composed of convoluted vessels and ducts, that connects the VASA EFFERENTIA to the vas deferens. Sperm cells produced in the testis pass along the epidydimis, maturing as they go, to be stored in the seminal vesicles until EJACULATION occurs. The epidydimis may be damaged by trauma or infection resulting sometimes in sterility. Cysts may also occur. (See TESTICLE.)

EPIGASTRIUM The region lying in the middle of the ABDOMEN over the stomach.

EPIGLOTTIS A leaf-like piece of elastic cartilage covered with mucous membrane, which stands upright between the back of the tongue and the glottis, or entrance to the larynx. In the act of swallowing, it prevents fluids and solids from passing off the back of the tongue into the larynx.

EPIGLOTTITIS Acute epiglottitis is an acute inflammatory oedema of the epiglottis, due to *Haemophilus influenzae*, which causes laryngeal obstruction due to swelling and immobilization of the epiglottis. It is a disease predominantly of children, occurs usually in the winter, and may prove rapidly fatal.

EPIGNATHUS   Maldevelopment of the fetus in which the deformed remains of one twin are united to the upper jaw of the other.

EPILATION   Removal of hair by the roots. (See DEPILATION.)

EPILEPSY (FITS, SEIZURES)   Epilepsy is a common symptom with a prevalence of 1 in 200 (0·5 per cent) of the population and an incidence of about 50/100,000 per year. In childhood up to 5 per cent of individuals have one or more fits before the age of 12, but in many children the prognosis is good.

It is a recurrent and paroxysmal disorder starting suddenly and ceasing spontaneously due to occasional sudden excessive rapid and local discharge of the nerve cells in the grey matter (cortex) of the brain. Epilepsy always arises as a disorder of the brain, commonly of microscopic size, but it is not itself a disease. Epilepsy should be diagnosed by the clinical symptoms based on the observations of witnesses. Its cause is established by laboratory tests, and brain scanning. Fits can be the first sign of a tumour, or follow a stroke, brain injury or infection.

A single epileptic fit is not epilepsy. Of those people who have a single seizure, a significant minority (20 per cent) have no further attacks. By definition, they are not epileptic.

Major (generalized) seizures   The salient features are a sudden, often unprovoked onset; the patient emits a cry, then falls to the ground, rigid, blue, and then twitching or jerking both sides of the body: the tonic-clonic convulsion. Drowsiness and confusion may last for some hours after recovering consciousness. Some experience a momentary warning (aura): a smell, or sensation in the head or abdomen, vision, or DÉJÀ VU.

Partial seizures: FOCAL MOTOR (JACKSONIAN) begin with twitching of the angle of the mouth, the thumb, or the big toe. If the seizure discharge then spreads, the twitching or jerking spreads gradually through the limbs. Consciousness is preserved unless the seizure spreads to produce a secondary generalized fit. In some attacks the eyes and head may turn, the arm may rise, and the body may turn, whilst some patients feel tingling in the limbs.

Temporal lobe seizures (complex partial seizures)   The patient usually appears blank, vacant and may be unable to talk or may mumble or chatter, though later he often has no memory of this period. He may be able to carry out complex tasks, taking off gloves or clothes and may smack his lips or, rub repeatedly on one limb (automatisms). A sense of strangeness supervenes: unreality, or a feeling of having experienced it all before (déjà vu). There may be

a sense of panic. Strange unpleasant smells and tastes are olfactory and gustatory hallucinations. The visual hallucinations evoke complex scenes. An initial rising sense of warmth or discomfort in the stomach, or 'speeding-up' of thoughts are common psychomotor symptoms. All these strange symptoms are brief, disappearing within a few seconds or up to 3 or 4 minutes.

Petit mal attacks start in childhood. They last a few seconds. The child ceases what he is doing, stares, looks a little pale, and may flutter the eyelids. The head may drop forwards. Attacks are commonly provoked by overbreathing. The child and parents may be unaware of the attacks – 'just daydreaming'. Major fits develop in one third of subjects. By contrast with other types of epilepsy, the ELECTROENCEPHALOGRAM (EEG) is diagnostic.

PRECAUTIONS   Children with epilepsy should take normal school exercises and games, and can swim under strict supervision. Adults must avoid working at heights, with exposed dangerous machinery and driving vehicles on public roads. Current legislation allows driving after two years' complete freedom from attacks during waking hours; those who for more than three years have had a history of attacks only whilst asleep may also drive.

TREATMENT identifies, and avoids where possible, any factors (such as shortage of sleep or excessive fluids) which aggravate or trigger attacks. Anti-epileptic drugs are usually necessary for several years under medical supervision. Carbamazepine, phenytoin and sodium valproate are the most frequently prescribed. The dose is governed by the degree of control of fits and some drug levels can be monitored by blood tests. Strict adherence to the drug schedule gives a good chance of total suppression of fits, especially in younger patients whose fits have started recently. The table summarizes anticonvulsant drugs in use. Interactions can occur between anti-epileptics and, if drug treatment is changed, the patient needs careful monitoring. In particular, abrupt withdrawal of a drug should be avoided as this may precipitate severe rebound seizures.

	Indications†
First-choice drugs:	
Ethosuximide	PM, JME
Phenobarbitone	M, P
Phenytoin	M, P, CP
Carbamazepine	M, P, CP
Valproate	M, PM, JME
Second-line drugs:	
Primidone	M, P, CP
Clobazam	M, CP
Vigabatrin	M, CP, P
Lamotrigine	M, CP, P
Gabapentin	M, CP, P
Topimirate	P

† M = major generalized tonic-clonic; P = partial or focal; CP = complex partial (temporal lobe); PM = petit mal; JME = juvenile myoclonic epilepsy.

Anticonvulsant drugs

Patients who have an epileptic seizure should not be restrained or have a gag or anything else placed in their mouths, nor should they be moved unless in danger of further injury. Any tight clothing around the neck should be loosened and, when the seizure has passed, the person should be placed in the recovery position to facilitate a return to consciousness (see APPENDIX 1: BASIC FIRST AID).

Patients with epilepsy and their relatives can obtain further advice and information from the British Epilepsy Association or the Epilepsy Association of Scotland (see APPENDIX 2: ADDRESSES).

EPILOIA (see TUBEROSE SCLEROSIS).

EPIPHORA Inadequate drainage of tears in the eyes with the result that they 'overflow' down the cheeks. The condition is caused by an abnormality of the tear ducts which drain away the normal secretions that keep the eyeball moist.

EPIPHYSIS The spongy extremity of a bone, attached to it for the purpose of forming a joint with the similar process of another bone. An epiphysis is covered on its surface by cartilage, is developed from a distinct centre of ossification, and in a young person is connected with the shaft of the bone by a plate of cartilage that disappears in the adult. Separation of an epiphysis is a form of fracture which sometimes occurs in children, and is apt to be more serious than a break through bony tissue because it involves damage to the plate of growing cartilage, so that, although union takes place readily, the subsequent growth of the bone may be interfered with and the full growth of the limb may afterwards fail to be attained.

EPIPHYSITIS Inflammation of an epiphysis.

EPISCLERA The most superficial layer of the sclera of the eye (see EYE). It sometimes becomes inflamed (episcleritis) but the condition usually clears without treatment.

EPISIOTOMY A cut made in the PERINEUM to enlarge the vaginal opening and facilitate childbirth. (See LABOUR.).

EPISTAXIS Bleeding from the nose. (See HAEMORRHAGE.)

EPITHELIOMA is a tumour of malignant nature arising in the epithelium covering the surface of the body. (See CANCER.)

EPITHELIUM is the cellular layer which forms the epidermis on the skin, covers the inner surface of the bowels, and forms the lining of ducts and hollow organs, like the bladder. It

Diagram of ciliated epithelium (1) and pseudostratified columnar ciliated epithelium (2).

1 squamous epithelium seen in section
2 squamous epithelium seen in face view
3 cuboidal and columnar epithelium in face view
4 stratified, squamous, non-keratinized epithelium
5 stratified, squamous, keratinized epithelium
6 transitional epithelium
7 columnar epithelium
8 cuboid epithelium

Diagram of various types of epithelium.

consists of one or more layers of cells which adhere to one another, and is one of the simplest tissues of the body. It is of several forms: for example, the epidermis is formed of scaly epithelium, the cells being in several layers and more or less flattened. (See SKIN.) The bowels are lined by a single layer of columnar epithelium, the cells being long and narrow in shape. The air passages are lined by ciliated epithelium: that is to say, each cell is provided with lashes which drive the fluid upon the surface of the passages gradually upwards.

EPIZOÖTIC Any disease in animals which diffuses itself widely. The term corresponds to the word epidemic as applied to human beings. In plague, for example, an epizoötic in rats usually precedes the epidemic in human beings.

EPSOM SALTS The popular name for magnesium sulphate, which is used as a saline purgative.

EPSTEIN BARR VIRUS The virus that causes GLANDULAR FEVER or infectious mononucleosis. It is similar to the viruses that cause herpes and is associated with BURKITT'S LYMPHOMA. It has been suggested that Epstein Barr virus is a cause of MYALGIC ENCEPHALOMYELITIS, also known as chronic fatigue syndrome.

EPULIS is a term applied to any tumour connected with the jaws. (See MOUTH, DISEASES OF.)

EQUINE OESTROGENS (see OESTROGEN).

ERB'S PARALYSIS is a form of paralysis of the arm due to stretching or tearing of the fibres of the brachial nerve plexus. Such damage to the brachial plexus may occur during birth, and it is found that the arm lies by the side of the body with elbow extended, forearm pronated, and the fingers flexed. The infant is unable to raise the arm.

ERCP (ENDOSCOPIC RETROGRADE CHOLANGIOPANCREATOGRAPHY) This is a procedure in which a catheter is passed via an ENDOSCOPE into the AMPULLA OF VATER of the common BILE DUCT. The duct is then injected with a radioopaque material to show up the ducts radiologically. The technique is used to diagnose pancreatic disease as well as obstructive jaundice.

ERECTION The rigid state of the PENIS when it responds to sexual stimulus. An erection is necessary for effective penetration of the vagina. As a result of sexual arousal the three cylinders of erectile tissue in the penis become engorged with blood, lengthening, raising and hardening the penis. Muscles surrounding the blood vessels contract and retain the blood in the penis. Erections also occur during sleep and in young boys. Inability to have or maintain an erection is one cause of impotence.

ERETHISM is the psychic disturbance that is one of the manifestations of chronic mercury poisoning (see MERCURY). It is characterized by irritability, self-consciousness, shyness, timidity, embarrassment, lack of concentration, depression and resentment of criticism. It was this condition that gave rise to the phrase, 'mad as a hatter', as chronic mercurial poisoning used to be one of the occupational hazards of the hat-making industry.

ERG- A prefix indicating activity or work.

ERGOMETRINE An active constituent of ergot, it has a powerful action in controlling the excessive bleeding from the uterus which may occur after childbirth. The official *British Pharmacopoeia* preparation is ergometrine maleate.

ERGONOMICS A broad science involving the application of psychological and physiological principles to the study of man in relation to his work and working surroundings. It includes the design of buildings, machinery, vehicles, and anything else with which man has contact in the course of his work.

ERGOSTEROL A sterol found in yeasts and fungi and in plant and animal fat. Under the action of sunlight or ultra-violet rays it produces vitamin D_2. The substance produced in this way is known as calciferol, and is used for the prevention and cure of rickets and osteomalacia. A similar change in the ergosterol of the skin is produced when the body is freely exposed to sunlight. Calciferol is probably not so active as, and differs chemically from, the vitamin D occurring in fish-liver oils. (See APPENDIX 5: VITAMINS.)

ERGOT The spawn of *Claviceps purpurea*, a fungus which grows in the grain of rye. It contains several active principles, including the alkaloids, ergometrine, ergotoxine and ergotamine. Ergot causes prolonged contraction of unstriped muscle fibres all over the body, particularly the muscle fibres of the blood-vessels and of the UTERUS. This action on the womb has made the drug of great value in midwifery since the 16th century until replaced by ERGOMETRINE.

ERGOTAMINE One of the alkaloids in ergot. In the form of ergotamine tartrate it is usually given orally to treat MIGRAINE. It is usually given by mouth. Ergotamine treatment carries a risk and should be medically supervised.

ERGOT POISONING or ERGOTISM occasionally results from eating bread made from diseased rye. Several terrible epidemics (St Anthony's Fire), characterized by intense pain and hallucinations, occurred in France and Germany during the Middle Ages (see ERYSIPELAS). Its symptoms are the occurrence of spasmodic muscular contractions, and the gradual production of gangrene in parts like the fingers, toes and tips of the ears.

EROGENOUS A term to describe those parts of the body – for example, the mouth, breasts and genitals – which, when stimulated, result in the individual's sexual arousal.

EROSION means a process of gradual wearing down of structures in the body. The term is applied to the effect of tumours, when they cause destruction of tissue in their neighbourhood without actually growing into the latter: for example, an aneurysm may erode bones in its neighbourhood. The term is also applied to minute ulcers, for example, erosions of the stomach, caused by extreme acidity of the gastric juice.

Dental erosion is the loss of tooth substance due to a cause other than decay or trauma. This is usually due to the presence of acid, e.g. frequent vomiting or the excessive intake of citrus fruits. The teeth appear very smooth and later develop saucer-shaped depressions.

EROTICISM   The emotional nature and characteristics of sexual arousal. This may occur as a result of visual, auditory or physical stimuli and also as a result of sexually oriented memories or imaginings.

ERUCTATION, or belching, is the sudden escape of gas or of portions of half-digested food from the stomach up into the mouth.

ERUPTION or RASH, means an outbreak, in a scattered form, upon the surface of the skin, usually raised and red, or it may be covered with scales, or crusts, or vesicles containing fluid. Eruptions differ in appearance: for example, the eruption of measles is always distinguishable from that of chickenpox. But the same disease may also produce different eruptions in different people or in the same person in different states of health, or even on different parts of the body at one time.

Eruptions may be acute or chronic. Most of the acute eruptions belong to the EXANTHE-MATA: i.e. they are bright in colour and burst out suddenly like a flower. These are the eruptions of SCARLET FEVER, MEASLES, GERMAN MEASLES, SMALLPOX and CHICKENPOX. In general the severity of these diseases can be measured by the amount of eruption. Some eruptions are very transitory, like nettle-rash, appearing and vanishing again in the course of a few hours. (See SKIN DISEASES.)

ERYSIPELAS   A STREPTOCOCCAL infection of the skin characterized by an acute onset with fever, malaise and a striking, usually unilateral, rash almost always on a lower leg or the face. Shivering, local pain and tenderness are associated with a sharply defined, spreading, bright red swollen zone of skin inflammation. On the leg, blistering and PURPURA may follow. The bacteria enter the skin through a fissure in a toe cleft (often associated with TINEA PEDIS) or via a crack in the skin behind an ear or in a nostril.

Treatment   PENICILLIN in full dosage should be given orally for ten days. In those allergic to penicillin, ERYTHROMYCIN can be substituted. Recurrent attacks are common and may cause progressive lymphatic damage leading to chronic OEDEMA. Such recurrences can be prevented by long-term prophylactic oral penicillin.

ERYTHEMA   Rednbess of the skin due to dilatation of dermal blood vessels. It may be transient or chronic, localized or widespread, and it can be blanched by pressure. Erythema may be caused by excessive exposure to heat or ultraviolet light, or by inflammation of the skin due to infection, dermatitis, and various allergic reactions, e.g. to drugs. It may be emotional (e.g. as in flushing), mediated by the autonomic nervous system.

Erythema ab igne is a fixed redness of the skin caused by chronic exposure to heat from a domestic fire or radiator.

Erythema pernio (see CHILBLAIN)   Redness induced by spasm of the skin arterioles due to cold. It affects the hands, feet or calves in winter. The red swollen areas are cooler than normal.

Erythema nodosum   A singular pattern of red, tender nodules occurring on the shins, often lasting several weeks. It may be caused by a streptococcal throat infection, primary tuberculosis, sarcoidosis or may be drug-induced.

Erythema multiforme is an acute allergic eruption of the extremities characterized by circular areas of erythema, purpura and blistering, which resolve over two or three weeks, caused by infections or drugs. In severe forms the mucous membranes of the eyes, mouth and genitalia may be involved.

Erythema infectiosum is an acute contagious disease of children caused by a parvovirus. In young children a bright erythema of the face gives a 'slapped cheek' appearance.

ERYTHRASMA   A superficial mild infection of the skin caused by CORYNEBACTERIA. It produces pink or slightly brown flaky areas of skin usually on the upper inner thighs or axillae. Toe clefts may be affected with thickened white macerated skin. The affected areas fluoresce coral pink under ultraviolet light. CLOTRIMAZOLE or KETOCONAZOLE cream clear the rash rapidly. Very extensive erythrasma responds to oral ERYTHROMYCIN given for seven days.

ERYTHROBLASTOSIS FETALIS (see HAEMOLYTIC DISEASE OF THE NEW-BORN).

ERYTHROBLASTS   A series of nucleated cells in the bone marrow that go through various stages of development until they form ERYTHROCYTES. They may appear in the blood in certain diseases.

ERYTHROCYTES   The biconcave red blood cells that carry oxygen from the lungs to the tissues, and return carbon dioxide. They have an excess of membrane, some of which may be lost in various disorders, as a result of which they become progressively more spherical and rigid. Erythrocytes, which have no nuclei, are formed during ERYTHROPOEISIS from ERYTHRO-BLAST cells in the BONE MARROW and each mm^3

of blood contains 5 million of them. They are by far the largest constituent among the blood cells and they contain large amounts of the oxygen carrier HAEMOGLOBIN. They have a life of about 120 days after which they are absorbed by MACROPHAGES, the blood's scavenging cells. Most components of the erythrocytes including the red pigment haemoglobin are reused, though some of the pigment is broken down to the waste product BILIRUBIN.

ERYTHROCYTE SEDIMENTATION RATE
(see ESR).

ERYTHRODERMA   A rare universal itching inflammation of the skin, which is red, thickened and scaly. It is also called generalized exfoliative dermatitis (see SKIN, DISEASES OF). It may complicate chronic ECZEMA or PSORIASIS, particularly in men, in the second half of life. It may also result from HYPERSENSITIVITY to a drug, such as gold injections used in RHEUMATOID ARTHRITIS. Rarely, it may be a manifestation of T-cell LYMPHOMA.

Universal inflammation of the skin may cause heart failure, particularly in elderly people with pre-existing heart disease. It may lead to hypothermia due to excessive heat loss from the skin and protein deficiency caused by the shedding of large quantities of scale containing keratin. Rarely, these complications can be fatal.

Treatment depends on the cause but in eczematous erythroderma oral CORTICOSTEROID (PREDNISOLONE) in full dosage may be needed.

ERYTHROEDEMA   Other terms for this condition are ACRODYNIA and PINK DISEASE. This is a rare disease of infants with the following features: restlessness, weakness, neuritis and swelling and redness of the face, fingers and toes and used to be a manifestation of mercurial poisoning because teething powders contained mercury, which is now banned in preparations for children.

ERYTHROMELALGIA, or RED NEURALGIA, is a condition in which the fingers or toes, or even larger portions of the limbs, become purple, bloated in appearance, and very painful. In people suffering from the condition, which is not a common one, the attacks come and go, being worse in summer (unlike chilblains), and worse on exertion or when the affected parts are warmed or allowed to hang down. The condition may appear without apparent cause, but is often associated with vascular diseases, such as hypertension and polycythaemia vera. It aso occurs in association with certain diseases of the central nervous system, and in cases of metallic poisoning: e.g. arsenic, mercury and thallium. Treatment is unsatisfactory but aspirin provides sympomatic relief.

ERYTHROMYCIN   One of the macrolides, it has an antibacterial spectrum similar to, but not identical to, that of penicillin. The drug is a valuable alternative for patients who are allergic to penicillin. Erythromycin is used for respiratory infections, including WHOOPING COUGH, CHLAMYDIA, LEGIONNAIRE'S DISEASE, SYPHILIS and enteritis caused by *campylobacter*. It is also used with neomycin as prophylaxis before bowel surgery. Though often active against penicillin-resistant staphylococci, these bacteria are now sometimes resistant to erythromycin. The drug may be given orally, intravenously or topically (for acne).

ERYTHROPOEISIS   The process by which erythrocytes or red blood cells are produced. The initiating cell is the haemopoietic stem cell from which an identifiable proerythroblast develops. This goes through several stages as a normoblast before losing its nucleus to become an erythrocyte. This process takes place in the blood-forming bone-marrow tissue.

ERYTHROPOIETIN   The protein, produced mainly in the kidney, that is the major stimulus for the production of erythrocytes, or red blood corpuscles. (See BLOOD.)

ESCHAR   Hard adherent crust caused by tissue killed by heat, chemicals or disease.

ESCHERICHIA   The generic name for the group of gram-negative, usually motile, rod-shaped bacteria that can ferment CARBOHYDRATES. They occur naturally in the intestines of man and some animals. *E. coli*, which ferments lactose, is not normally harmful but some varieties cause gastrointestinal infections which may be severe in old people. *E. coli* is also used in laboratory experiments for genetic and bacteriological research.

ESERINE   Another name for PHYSOSTIGMINE.

ESMARCH'S BANDAGE   A rubber bandage which is applied to a limb before surgery from below upwards in order to drive blood from it. The bandage is removed after an inflated pneumatic TOURNIQUET has been placed round the limb; the operation can then proceed.

ESR   The ESR or erythrocyte sedimentation rate is a test that measures the rate at which red blood cells settle out of suspension in blood plasma. In certain diseases, such as infection and malignancy, the amount of proteins in the plasma increases; the result is that red cells settle out more quickly and this test is used to show whether disease is present.

ESSENTIAL AMINO ACIDS are amino acids that are essential for the body to grow and develop normally but which the body is unable to produce. Nine essential amino acids exist – HISTIDINE, ISOLEUCINE, LEUCINE, LYSINE, METHIO-

NINE, PHENYLALANINE, THREONINE, TRYPTOPHAN, and VALINE – and they are present in foods rich in protein: dairy products, eggs, meat, and liver.

ESSENTIAL FATTY ACIDS Three acids – arachidonic, linolenic and tinoleic – essential for life which the body cannot produce. They are found in natural vegetable and fish oils and their functions are varied. EFAs have a vital function in fat metabolism and transfer and they are also precursors of PROSTAGLANDINS.

ESSENTIAL HYPERTENSION or BENIGN HYPERTENSION is the traditional name for the disorder which affects most people with high blood pressure. As many as 20 per cent of middle-aged people in the United Kingdom probably have hypertension. The systolic pressure of those with essential hypertension is raised but they have no other classic signs of high blood pressure – for example, changes in the fundus of the eye or protein in the urine. Research has not shown any identifiable cause but, untreated, the condition can lead to complications. Risk factors include obesity, tobacco smoking, excess alcohol consumption, stress and a sedentary life style (see HYPERTENSION).

ESTER An organic compound formed from an alcohol and an acid by the removal of water.

ETHACRYNIC ACID A potent DIURETIC, with a rapid onset, and a short duration (4 to 6 hours), of action. (See BENZOTHIADIAZINES, DIURETICS.)

ETHAMBUTOL is a synthetic drug, often included in the treatment regimen of TUBERCULOSIS when the infection is thought to be resistant to other drugs. The main side-effects are visual disturbances, chiefly loss of acuity and colour blindness. Such toxic effects are more common when excessive dosages are used, or the patient has some renal impairment, in which case the drug should be avoided, as it should be in young children.

ETHANOL is another name for ethyl alcohol. (See ALCOHOL.)

ETHER A colourless, volatile, highly inflammable liquid, formed by the action of sulphuric acid on alcohol. Ether boils below body temperature and therefore rapidly evaporates when sprayed over the skin. Dissolving many substances such as fats, oils and resins better than alcohol or water, it is used in the preparation of many drugs. Formerly used as an anaesthetic by inhalation, it is now largely replaced by safer and more efficient drugs. Side-effects: ether irritates the respiratory tract and may affect the circulation.

ETHICS Within most cultures, care of the sick has been seen as entailing special duties, codified as a set of moral standards governing professional practice. Although these duties have been articulated and interpreted in differing ways, a common factor is the awareness they reflect of an imbalance of power between doctor and patient and an acknowledgement of the vulnerability of the sick person. A function of medical ethics is to counteract the power imbalance by encouraging doctors to act in the best interests of their patients, refrain from taking advantage of them and use their skills in a manner which preserves the honour of their profession. It has always been accepted, however, that doctors cannot use their knowledge indiscriminately to fulfil patients' wishes. The deliberate ending of life, for example, even at a patient's request, has usually been seen as alien to the shared values inherent in medical ethics. It is, however, symptomatic of changing concepts of ethics and of the growing power of patient choice that legal challenges have been mounted in several countries to the prohibition of euthanasia. Thus ethics can be seen as regulating individual doctor–patient relationships, integrating doctors within a moral community of their professional peers and reflecting societal demands for change.

Medical ethics are embedded in cultural values which evolve. Acceptance of abortion within well-defined legal parameters in some jurisdictions is an example of how society influences the way in which perceptions about ethical obligations change. Because they are often linked to the moral views predominating in society, medical ethics cannot be seen as embodying uniform standards independent of cultural context. Some countries which permit capital punishment or female genital mutilation, for example, expect doctors to carry out such procedures. Some doctors would argue that their ethical obligation to minimize pain and suffering obliges them to comply, whereas others would deem their ethical obligations to be the complete opposite. The medical community attempts to address such variations by establishing globally applicable ethical principles through debate within bodies such as the World Medical Association (WMA) or World Psychiatric Association (WPA). Norm-setting bodies increasingly reflect accepted concepts of human rights and patient rights within professional ethical codes.

Practical changes within society may also affect the perceived balance of power within the doctor–patient relationship and therefore have an impact on ethics. In developed societies, for example, patients are increasingly well informed about treatment options. Media such as the Internet provide them with access to highly specialized knowledge. Social measures such as a well-established complaints system, procedures for legal redress and guarantees of rights such as those set out in the NHS's *Patient's Charter* appear to reduce the perceived imbalance in the relationship. Law as well as ethics emphasizes the importance of informed patient consent and the often legally binding nature of informed patient refusal of treatment. Ethics reflect the changing relationship by emphasizing skills such as effective communication and generation of mutual trust within a doctor–patient partnership.

In the past, however, medical ethics were frequently criticized for concentrating more on regulating relations between doctors and protecting them from competition rather than addressing the duties owed to patients. The so-called Hippocratic oath, which many see as the basis of modern ethical standards, begins by enumerating the obligations owed to teachers and their progeny before listing prohibitions relating to treatment. Some see this as having set the tone, in Western medicine at least, for later attempts to set ethical benchmarks for medicine. Modern medical ethics, however, has little concern with issues of professional etiquette which featured so prominently in English codes of medical ethics, such as that drawn up by Thomas Percival in 1792 and revisited without major amendments until well into the 20th century. A widely known modern code is the WMA's International Code of Medical Ethics which seeks to provide a modern restatement of the Hippocratic principles.

Traditionally, ethical codes have sought to establish absolutist positions. The WMA code, for example, imposes an apparently absolute duty of confidentiality which extends beyond the patient's death. Increasingly, however, ethics are perceived as a tool for making morally appropriate decisions in a sphere where there is rarely one 'right' answer. Many factors – such as current emphasis on autonomy and the individual values of patients, awareness of social and cultural diversity and the phenomenal advance of new technology which has blurred some moral distinctions about what constitutes a 'person' – have contributed to the perception that ethical dilemmas have to be resolved on a case-by-case basis. An approach adopted by American ethicists has been moral analysis of cases using four fundamental principles: autonomy, beneficence, non-maleficence and justice. The 'four principles' provide a useful framework within which ethical dilemmas can be teased out, but they are criticized for their apparent simplicity in the face of complex problems and for the fact that the moral imperatives implicit in each principle often conflict with some or all of the other three. As with any other approach to problem solving, the 'four principles' require interpretation. Enduring ethical precepts such as the obligation to benefit patients and avoid harm (beneficence and non-maleficence) may be differently interpreted in cases where prolongation of life is contrary to a patient's wishes or where sentience has been irrevocably lost. In such cases, treatment may be seen as constituting a 'harm' rather than a 'benefit'. Many regret the advance of ethical arguments based on the context of the relevant events and perceive these as undermining traditional absolutist values. There is little likelihood, however, of a return to the past tradition of enunciating a set of immutable responses which neither require

justification nor are susceptible to modification according to the circumstances.

The importance accorded to ethics in daily practice has greatly increased in the past 50 years. From being seen mainly as a set of values passed on from experienced practitioners to their students at the bedside, medical ethics have increasingly become the domain of lawyers, academic philosophers and professional ethicists with experienced practitioners retaining a central role. In the UK, law and medical ethics increasingly interact. Judges resolve cases on the basis of established medical ethical guidance and new ethical guidance draws in turn on common-law judgements in individual cases. Multidisciplinary practice has stimulated the growth of the new discipline of 'healthcare ethics' which seeks to provide uniformity across long-established professional boundaries. The trend is to set common standards for a range of health professionals and others who may have a duty of care, such as hospital chaplains and ancillary workers. Since a primary function of ethics is to find reasonable answers in situations where different interests or priorities conflict, managers and healthcare purchasers are increasingly seen as potential partners in the effort to establish a common approach. Widely accepted ethical values are increasingly applied to the previously unacknowledged dilemmas of rationing scarce resources.

In modern debate about ethics, two important trends can be identified. As a result of the increasingly high profile accorded to applied ethics, there is a trend for professions not previously subject to widely agreed standards of behaviour to adopt codes of ethical practice. Business ethics or the ethics of management are comparatively new. At the same time, there is some debate about whether professionals, such as doctors, traditionally subject to special ethical duties, should be seen as simply doing a job for payment like any other worker. As some doctors perceive their power and kudos eroded by top-down management decisions regarding rationing of care and bottom-up pressure for patients to exercise autonomy about treatment decisions, it is sometimes argued that realistic limits must be set on medical obligations. A logical implication of patient choice and rejection of medical paternalism would appear to be a concomitant reduction in the freedom of doctors to carry out their own ethical obligations. The concept of conscientious objection, incorporated to some extent in law (e.g. in relation to abortion) ensures that doctors are not obliged to act contrary to their own personal or professional values.

ETHICS COMMITTEES Various types of ethics committee operate in the UK, fulfilling four main functions: the monitoring of research, debate of difficult patient cases, establishing norms of practice and publishing ethical guidance. They were developed following an initiative from the Royal College of Physicians of London in 1967, when the college recommended that clinical research investigation should be subject to ethical review.

The commonest – Local Research Ethics Committees (LRECs) – have provided a monitoring system of research on humans since that time. Established by NHS health authorities, LRECs were primarily perceived as exercising authority over research carried out on NHS patients or on NHS premises or using NHS records. Their power and significance, however, developed considerably in the 1980s and 90s when national and international guidance made approval by an 'appropriately constituted' ethics committee obligatory for any research project involving humans or human tissue. The work of LRECs is supplemented by so-called 'independent' ethics committees usually set up by pharmaceutical companies and since 1997 by multi-centre research ethics committees (MRECs). Although initially criticized for variability in terms of training, expertise, balance of membership and rigour of analysis, LRECs have become indispensable to the conduct of research and are doubtless partly responsible for the lack of demand in the UK for legislation governing research. An important but critical survey published by the Kings' Fund Institute in 1992 produced 12 detailed recommendations concerning LRECs' composition and working practice. This, combined with pressure from the pharmaceutical industry for greater uniformity of standards, stimulated interest in the provision of training programmes for LRECs. A plethora of guidelines is available and LRECs which fail to comply with recognized standards could incur legal liability. They are increasingly governed by international standards of practice. In 1997, guidelines on 'Good Clinical Practice', produced by the International Committee on Harmonization (ICHP), were introduced into the UK and have almost the *de facto* status of law.

Other categories of ethics committee include Ethics Advisory Committees which debate difficult patient cases. Most are attached to specialized health facilities such as fertility clinics or children's care facilities. The 1990s have seen a greatly increased interest in professional ethics and the establishment of many new ethics committees, including some like that of the Palliative Care Association which cross professional boundaries. Guidance on professional and ethical standards is produced by these new bodies and by the well-established ethics committees of regulatory or representative bodies, such as the royal colleges of medicine and nursing, the General Medical Council, United Kingdom Central Council for Nursing, Midwifery and Health Visiting, British Medical Association (see APPENDIX 10: PROFESSIONAL ORGANIZATIONS) and bodies representing paramedics and professions supplementary to medicine. Their guidance ranges from general codes of practice to detailed analysis of single topics such as euthanasia or surrogacy.

Unlike many European countries, Britain does not have a national ethics committee, although the Nuffield Bioethics Committee, established in 1991 to consider ethical issues arising from biomedical and biological advances, fulfils this function in some respects. It has produced a series of reports on the ethics of procedures such as xenotransplantation, genetic screening and the use of human tissue.

ETHINYLOESTRADIOL A highly active OESTROGEN, which is about twenty times as active as STILBOESTROL. It is active when given by mouth. (See OESTROGEN.)

ETHISTERONE The name approved by the *British Pharmacopoeia* for the orally active analogue of progesterone. It is given in certain cases of menorrhagia and habitual abortion, where a deficient secretion of the corpus luteum is suspected. (See PROGESTERONE.)

ETHMOID A bone in the base of the skull which separates the cavity of the nose from the membranes of the brain. It is a spongy bone with numerous cavities or sinuses.

Suppuration in the ethmoidal sinuses is sometimes responsible for inflammation in neighbouring parts such as the eye.

ETHOSUXIMIDE A drug used in the treatment of the form of epilepsy known as petit mal. (See EPILEPSY.)

ETHYL CHLORIDE A flammable colourless liquid that is extremely volatile, and rapidly produces freezing of the surface, when sprayed upon it. Now used to produce insensibility to pain for small and short operations, ethyl chloride was once used as an inhalant general anaesthetic for brief operations, and to induce anaesthesia in patients in whom the anaesthesia is subsequently to be maintained by some other anaesthetic such as nitrous oxide or ether.

ETHYLENE A colourless flammable gas occasionally used as an inhalant anaesthetic.

ETHYLOESTRENOL (see ANABOLIC STEROIDS).

ETIDRONATE Also known as disodium etidronate, this is one of a group of substances called biphosphates used mainly to treat PAGET'S DISEASE of the bone. The drug is given orally and, when combined with calcium carbonate (Didrone®), it is used to treat OSTEOPOROSIS and to prevent bone loss in postmenopausal women, especially if hormone replacement therapy is not appropriate for a woman.

ETIOLOGY, or AETIOLOGY, means the group of conditions which form the cause of any disease.

ETOMIDATE An intravenous agent for inducing general ANAESTHESIA prior to surgery or other procedures that require patients to be unconscious. When the drug is injected intravenously, pain sometimes occurs, but this can be minimized by premedication with an OPIOID ANALGESIC.

EU- is a prefix meaning satisfactory or beneficial.

EUCALYPTUS, or BLUE-GUM (*Eucalyptus globulus*), is a tree, originally a native of Australia, and now grown all over the world. Its important constituent, oil of eucalyptus, is an oil of pleasant smell and spicy taste, which is obtained by distillation from the leaves of the tree. The oil may be used as a disinfectant and deodorant.

EUGENICS The study and cultivation of conditions that may improve the human race, in particular the detection and elimination of genetic disease.

EUNUCH A man whose testes have been removed or seriously damaged so that he is unable to produce male hormones and thus is sterile. A male castrated before puberty will have a feminine appearance and underdeveloped secondary sexual characteristics. The term was historically used to describe boys, castrated to make them suitable for working in harems, or boy singers, castrated to retain their higher-register voices (*castrati* singers).

EUSOL This stands for Edinburgh University Solution, a solution of 12·5 g of boric acid and 12·5 g of chlorinated lime in 1 litre of water. It was introduced during the 1914–18 War as an antiseptic for the treatment of wounds, and proved to be one of the most valuable antiseptics then available. It is now largely replaced by modern antiseptics, and the introduction of the antibacterial drugs.

EUPHORIA A feeling of well-being. This may occur normally, for instance, when someone has passed an examination. In some neurological or psychiatric conditions, however, patients may have an exaggerated and quite unjustified feeling of euphoria. This is then a symptom of the underlying condition. Euphoria may also be drug induced – by drugs of addiction or by therapeutic drugs such as corticosteroids.

EUPHORIANTS Drugs which induce a state of euphoria or well-being.

EUSTACHIAN TUBES The passages, one on each side, leading from the throat to the middle ear. Each is about 38 mm (1½ inches) long and is large at either end, though at its narrowest part it only admits a fine probe. The tubes open widely in the act of swallowing or yawning. The opening into the throat is situated just behind the lower part of the nose, so that a catheter can be passed through the corresponding nostril into the tube for inflation of the middle ear. (See also EAR; NOSE.)

EUTHANASIA The procuring of an easy and painless death. Whether a medical practitioner, with the consent of the patient or relatives, should have the power to put to death painlessly, using drugs or by deliberately withholding treatment, any person suffering from a painful, distressing and incurable disease, the outcome of which is inevitably fatal, is a contentious social, ethical, religious and moral issue. Various legal safeguards have been proposed, but there are obvious objections to the recognition of such a procedure. In the Netherlands voluntary euthanasia under strictly controlled criteria is legal. In the United Kingdom it is not. (See LIVING WILL.)

EVACUANT is a name for a purgative medicine.

EVALUATION   (see PUBLIC HEALTH).

EVIDENCE   (see EVIDENCE-BASED MEDICINE).

EVIDENCE-BASED MEDICINE The process of systematically finding, appraising and using the best available research findings as the basis for clinical decisions about individual patients. It has been developing internationally for the past twenty years, but since around 1990 its development has accelerated. The International Cochrane Collaboration exercise finds and reviews relevant research. Several other centres have been set up to look at the clinical application of research results, including the Centre for Evidence-Based Medicine, in Oxford.

The aim of evidence-based medicine is to encourage clinicians and managers to do the things which have been shown to be effective and to stop doing things which have been shown to be ineffective. The aim is to try to improve patient care. Critics of evidence-based practice question the emphasis on the use of randomized controlled trials. Some doctors are concerned that health-care managers might try to impose treatment protocols on clinicians as a method of containing costs: they emphasize the need to retain an individualized approach, which takes the views of each person receiving care into account.

EWING'S SARCOMA An uncommon but very malignant cancer of the bone in children and young adults, the condition was first identified as different from OSTEOSARCOMA by Dr J. Ewing in 1921. It usually occurs in the limbs or pelvis and soon spreads to other parts of the body. Treatment is RADIOTHERAPY and CYTOTOXIC drugs. Since the use of the latter the number of patients who survive for five years or more has much improved.

EX- (EXO-) Prefix meaning outer or outside.

EXANTHEM Rash caused by a systemic infection. Several childhood infections, e.g. MEASLES and RUBELLA, have characteristic exanthemata.

EXCHANGE TRANSFUSION A method of treating new-born infants with HAEMOLYTIC DISEASE. Blood is taken out of the baby through the umbilical vein and is replaced with the same quantity of blood from a donor that is compatible with the mother's blood. The procedure is repeated several times to get rid of damaged cells while maintaining the infant's blood volume and keeping its red cell (erythrocyte) count constant.

EXCIPIENT An inert substance added to a prescription in order to make the remedy as prescribed more suitable in bulk, consistence, or form for administration.

EXCISION A term applied to the removal of any structure from the body, when such removal necessitates a certain amount of separation from surrounding parts. For example, the excision of a tumour, of a gland, of a joint. When an opening is simply made into the body the term incision is used. When a limb, or part of one, is removed, the term amputation is employed.

EXCITEMENT (see DELIRIUM; ECSTASY; HYSTERIA; MENTAL ILLNESS).

EXCORIATION means the destruction of small pieces of the surface of skin or mucous membrane. (See CHAFING OF THE SKIN.)

EXCRETA Waste substances discharged from the body, in particular faeces.

EXERCISE An activity requiring physical exertion. Everyone should take regular exercise. This keeps MUSCLES in tone, maintains the CARDIOVASCULAR system in good shape, helps to keep weight at an optimum level and promotes relaxation and sleep. When an individual is at rest, the heart's output is 5 litres of blood per minute. When running at 12 km (7½ miles) per hour, this rises to around 25 litres, obliging the heart and lungs to operate more efficiently and speeding up the metabolism of food to provide the necessary energy. Lack of exercise by children may lead to faulty posture and flabby muscles; in adults it results in an increase in weight and poorly functioning respiratory and cardiovascular system, with an increased chance of heart disease later in life. Adolescents and adults, participating regularly in sporting activities, should train regularly, preferably under expert supervision, to ensure that they do not place potentially damaging demands on their cardiovascular, respiratory and musculoskeletal systems. Those wanting to participate in demanding sports would be wise to have a medical examination before embarking on training programmes (see SPORTING INJURIES).

EXFOLIATION The separation, in layers, of pieces of dead bone or skin.

EXOCRINE GLAND A gland that secretes its products through a duct to the surface of the body or of an organ. The sweat glands in the skin and the salivary glands in the mouth are examples. The secretion is set off by a HORMONE or a NEUROTRANSMITTER.

EXOGENOUS Arising outside the body. For example, exogenous depression is an illness caused by an outside factor such as the death of a close relative. Or an illness may occur because of something eaten in the diet.

EXOMPHALOS The term applied to a hernia formed by the projection of abdominal organs through the umbilicus.

EXOPTHTHALMIC GOITRE Sometimes called Graves' disease, this is a disorder in which there is overactivity of the thyroid gland, protrusion of the eyes, and other symptoms. (See HYPERTHYROIDISM.)

EXOPHTHALMOMETER or PROPTOMETER An instrument used to measure the extent of protrusion of the eyeball, a development that occurs in certain disorders such as GOITRE, TUMOURS, OEDEMA, injuries, orbital inflammation or cavernous venous thrombosis (a blood clot in the cavernous sinus in the base of the skull behind each eye). (See EXOPHTHALMOS.)

EXOPHTHALMOS, or PROPTOSIS, refers to forward displacement of the eyeball and must be distinguished from retraction of the eyelids, which causes an illusion of exophthalmos. Lid retraction usually results from activation of the autonomic nervous sytem. Exophthalmos is a more serious disorder caused by inflammatory and infiltrative changes in the retro-orbital tissues and is essentially a feature of GRAVES' DISEASE, though it has been described in chronic thyroiditis. Exophthalmos commonly starts shortly after the development of THYROTOXICOSIS but may occur months or even years after hyperthyroidism has been successfully treated. Only 3 per cent of patients with Graves' disease develop severe exophthalmos. The degree of exophthalmos is not correlated with the severity of hyperthyroidism even when their onset is simultaneous. Some of the worst examples of endocrine exophthalmos occur in the euthyroid state and may appear in patients who have never had thyrotoxicosis; this disorder is named ophthalmic Graves' disease. The exophthalmos of Graves' disease is due to auto-immunity (see IMMUNITY). Antibodies to surface antigens on the eye muscles are produced and this causes an inflammatory reaction in the muscle and retro-orbital tissues.

Exophthalmos may also occur as a result of oedema, injury, cavernous venous thrombosis or a tumour at the back of the eye, pushing the eyeball forwards. In this situation it is always unilateral.

EXOSTOSIS An outgrowth from a bone; it may be due to chronic inflammation, constant pressure or tension on the bone, or tumour-formation. (See BONE, DISEASES OF.)

EXOTOXIN A powerful poison produced by a bacterial cell and secreted into its surrounding environment. Exotoxins are often damaging to only few tissues and they are usually inactivated by chemicals, heat and light. Bacteria causing BOTULISM, DIPHTHERIA and TETANUS all produce exotoxins. (See ENDOTOXIN.)

EXPECTANT A form of treatment in which the cure of the patient is left mainly to nature, while the physician simply watches for any unsatisfactory developments or symptoms, and relieves them if they occur.

EXPECTORANTS Drugs which are claimed to help the removal of secretions from the air passages. There is, however, no clear evidence that they do this. A simple expectorant may, however, be a useful placebo. Most preparations are available without a doctor's prescription and pharmacists will advise on which might be helpful for particular patients with dry or congestive coughs.

EXPECTORATION means either material brought up from the chest by the air passages, or the act by which it is brought up.

EXPIRATION (1) Breathing out air from the lungs. (2) The act of dying.

EXPLORATION A surgical operation to investigate the cause of a patient's illness.

EXPOSURE (1) A term used in BEHAVIOUR THERAPY to describe a method of treating fears and phobias. The subject is confronted by the circumstances he or she fears, either gradually or suddenly, with the aim of defusing the fear or phobia. (2) The term is also a colloquialism for public exposure by a man of his genitals to achieve sexual relief.

EXSANGUINATE The removal of blood from the body. This may occur as the result of

a serious accident in which the victim bleeds extensively. Rarely it may happen that bleeding becomes uncontrollable during an operation.

EXTENSION is the process of straightening or stretching a limb. When used in the natural sense, it involves the contraction of the muscles opposing those used in FLEXION. In cases of fractured limbs, extension is employed during the application of splints, in order to reduce the displacement caused by the fracture, and prevent movement of the broken ends of bone. It is effected by gently and steadily pulling upon the part of the limb beyond the fracture. Extension of a more permanent type is used in the after-treatment of some fractures, as well as in diseases of the spine, by placing the patient upon an inclined bed and affixing weights to his lower limbs or to his head by means of adhesive plaster or of straps.

EXTIRPATION The total removal of a growth organ or tissue by surgery.

EXTRA- is the Latin prefix meaning outside of, or in addition, such as extra-capsular, meaning outside the capsule of a joint, and extrasystole, meaning an additional contraction of the heart.

EXTRACELLULAR An adjective that describes an object or event outside a cell. An example is extracellular fluid, the medium surrounding a cell.

EXTRACTS are preparations, usually of a semi-solid consistence, containing the active parts of various plants extracted in one of several ways. In the case of some extracts the juice of the fresh plant is simply pressed out and purified; in the case of others the active principles are dissolved out in water, which is then to a great extent driven off by evaporation; other extracts are similarly made by the help of alcohol, and in some cases ether is the solvent.

EXTRADURAL Outside the DURA MATER, the outermost of the three membranes that cover the BRAIN and SPINAL CORD. The extra-dural or epidural space is the space between the vertebral canal and the dura mater of the spinal cord (see ANAESTHESIA: epidural).

EXTRAPYRAMIDAL SYSTEM This is a complex part of the nervous system, extending from the cortex to the medulla, in the brain, from which emerge descending spinal pathways which influence voluntary motor activity throughout the body. Although the normal functions of the system are ill understood, there are characteristic signs of an extrapyramidal lesion. These include disturbance of voluntary movements, notably slowness and 'poverty' of movement; disturbance of muscular tone, which may be increased or decreased; and involuntary movements, such as a tremor, irregular jerking movements, or slow writing movements.

Diseases There are several diseases that result from lesions to the extrapyramidal system, of which the most common is PARKINSONISM. Others include WILSON'S DISEASE, KERNICTERUS, CHOREA and ATHETOSIS.

EXTRASENSORY PERCEPTION (ESP) An alleged way of perceiving current events (clairvoyance), future events (precognition) or the thoughts of other people (telepathy). ESP has never been scientifically proved and does not involve the use of any known senses.

EXTRASYSTOLE is a term applied to premature contraction of one or more of the chambers of the heart. A beat of the heart occurs sooner than it should do in the ordinary rhythm and is followed by a longer rest than usual before the next beat. In an extrasystole the stimulus to contraction arises in a part of the heart other than the usual. Extrasystoles often give rise to an unpleasant sensation as of the heart stumbling over a beat, but their occurrence is not usually serious. (See HEART.)

EXTRAUTERINE PREGNANCY (see ECTOPIC PREGNANCY).

EXTRAVASATION An escape of fluid from the vessels or passages which ought to contain it. Extravasation of blood due to tearing of vessel walls is found in strokes, and in the commoner condition known as a bruise. Extravasation of urine takes place when the bladder or the urethra is ruptured by a blow on the abdomen or on the crutch (or perineum), or torn in a fracture of the pelvis.

EXTRINSIC (1) Originating outside the body. (2) Extrinisc muscle is one whose origin is some way from the part of the body it acts on – for example, the muscles controlling the movement of the eyeball which are attached to the bony orbit in which the eye sits.

EXUDATION The process in which some of the constituents of the blood pass slowly through the walls of the small vessels in the course of inflammation, and also means the accumulation resulting from this process. For example, in pleurisy the solid, rough material deposited on the surface of the lung is an exudation.

EYE The eye is the sensory organ of sight. It is an elaborate photoreceptor detecting information, in the form of light, from the environment and transmitting this information by a series of electro-chemical changes to the brain. The visual cortex is the part of the brain that processes this information (i.e. the visual cortex is what 'sees' the environment). There are two eyes, each a roughly spherical hollow organ held within a bony cavity (the orbit). Each orbit is situated on the front of the skull, one on each side of the nose. The eye consists of an outer wall of three main layers and a central cavity divided into three.

1 fovea	11 lens
2 optic nerve	12 anterior chamber
3 sclera	13 vitreous humour
4 choroid	14 pigment cells
5 retina	15 cone
6 ora serrata	16 rod
7 ciliary muscle	17 felt-work of dendrons
8 conjunctiva	18 axon
9 iris	19 ganglion cells
10 cornea	20 axon to optic nerve

(Left) Horizontal section through the right eye. (Right) Cross-section of the retina of eye.

The **outer coat** consists of the opaque sclera posteriorly and the clear cornea anteriorly; their junction is called the limbus.

SCLERA This is white, opaque, and constitutes the posterior five-sixths of the outer layer. It is made of dense fibrous tissue. The sclera is visible anteriorly, between the eyelids, as the 'white of the eye'. Posteriorly and anteriorly it is covered by Tenons capsule, which in turn is covered by transparent conjunctiva. There is a hole in the sclera medial to the posterior pole of the eye through which nerve fibres from the retina leave the eye in the optic nerve. Other smaller nerve fibres and blood vessels also pass through the sclera at different points.

CORNEA This constitutes the transparent colourless anterior one-sixth of the eye. It is transparent in order to allow light into the eye and is more steeply curved than the sclera. Viewed from in front, the cornea is roughly circular. Most of the focusing power of the eye is provided by the cornea (the lens acts as the 'fine adjustment'). It has an outer epithelium, a central stroma and an inner endothelium. The cornea is supplied with very fine nerve fibres which make it exquisitely sensitive to pain. The central cornea has no blood supply – it relies mainly on aqueous humour for nutrition. Blood vessels and large nerve fibres in the cornea would prevent light entering the eye.

LIMBUS is the junction between cornea and sclera. It contains the trabecular meshwork, a sieve-like structure through which aqueous humour leaves the eye.

The **middle coat (uveal tract)** consists of the choroid, ciliary body and iris.

CHOROID A highly vascular sheet of tissue lining the posterior two-thirds of the sclera. The network of vessels provides the blood supply for the outer half of the retina. The blood supply of the choroid is derived from numerous ciliary vessels which pierce the sclera in front and behind.

CILIARY BODY A ring of tissue extending 6 mm back from the anterior limitation of the sclera. The various muscles of the ciliary body by their contractions and relaxations are responsible for changing the shape of the lens during accommodation. The ciliary body is lined by cells that secrete aqueous humour. Posteriorly the ciliary body is continuous with the choroid, anteriorly it is continuous with the iris.

IRIS A flattened muscular diaphragm that is attached at its periphery to the ciliary body and has a round central opening, the pupil. By contraction and relaxation of the muscles of the iris the pupil can be dilated or constricted (dilated in the dark or when aroused, constricted in bright light and for close work). The iris forms a partial division between the anterior chamber and the posterior chamber of the eye. It lies in front of the lens and forms the back wall of the anterior chamber. The iris is visible from in front, through the transparent cornea, as the 'coloured part of the eye'. The amount and distribution of iris pigment determine the colour of the iris. The pupil is merely a hole in the centre of the iris and appears black.

The **inner layer** The RETINA is a multi-layered tissue (ten layers in all) which extends from the edges of the optic nerve to line the inner surface of the choroid up to the junction of ciliary body and choroid. Here the true retina ends at the ora serrata. The retina contains light sensitive cells of two types: (i) cones: Cells that operate at high and medium levels of illumination. They subserve fine discrimination of vision and colour vision. (ii) rods: Cells that function best at low light intensity and subserve black and white vision.

The retina contains about 6 million cones and about 100 million rods. Information from them is conveyed by the nerve fibres which are in the inner part of the retina to leave the eye in the optic nerve. There are no photoreceptors at the optic disc (the point where the optic nerve leaves the eye) and therefore there is no light perception from this small area. The optic disc thus produces a physiological blind spot in the visual field.

The retina can be subdivided into several areas:

PERIPHERAL RETINA contains mainly rods and a few scattered cones. Visual acuity from this area is fairly coarse.

MACULA LUTEA, so called because histologically it looks like a yellow spot. It occupies an area 4·5 mm in diameter lateral to the optic disc. This area of specialized retina can produce a high level of visual acuity. Cones are abundant here but there are few rods.

FOVEA CENTRALIS: A small central depression at the centre of the macula. Here the cones are tightly packed, rods are absent. It is responsible for the highest levels of visual acuity.

The **chambers of the eye** There are three, anterior and posterior chambers and the vitreous cavity.

ANTERIOR CHAMBER Limited in front by the inner surface of the cornea, behind by the iris and pupil. It contains a transparent clear watery fluid, the aqueous humour. This is constantly being produced by cells of the ciliary body and constantly drained away through the trabecular meshwork. The trabecular meshwork lies in the angle between the iris and inner surface of the cornea.

POSTERIOR CHAMBER A narrow space between the iris and pupil in front and the lens behind. It too contains aqueous humour in transit from the ciliary epithelium to the anterior chamber, via the pupil.

VITREOUS CAVITY The largest cavity of the eye. In front it is bounded by the lens and behind by the retina. It contains vitreous humour.

Lens Transparent, elastic and biconvex in cross section, it lies behind the iris and in front of the vitreous cavity. Viewed from the front it is roughly circular and about 10 mm in diameter. The diameter and thickness of the lens vary with its accommodative state. The lens consists of:

CAPSULE a thin transparent membrane surrounding the cortex and nucleus.

CORTEX This is made up of newly made lens fibres that are relatively soft. It separates the capsule on the outside from the nucleus at the centre of the lens.

NUCLEUS   The dense central area of old lens fibres that have become compacted by new lens fibres laid down over them.

ZONULE   Numerous radially arranged fibres attached between the ciliary body and the lens around its circumference. Tension in these zonular fibres can be adjusted by the muscles of the ciliary body, thus changing the shape of the lens and altering its power of accommodation.

VITREOUS HUMOUR   A transparent clear jelly-like structure made up of a network of collagen fibres suspended in a viscid fluid. Its shape conforms to that of the vitreous cavity within which it is contained, i.e. it is spherical except for a shallow concave depression on its anterior surface. The lens lies in this depression.

Eyelids   These are multilayered curtains of tissue whose functions include spreading of the tear film over the front of the eye to prevent desiccation, protection from injury or external irritation and to some extent to control light entering the eye. Each eye has an upper and lower lid which form an elliptical opening (the palpebral fissure) when the eyes are open. The lids meet at the medial canthus and lateral canthus respectively. The inner medial canthus is fixed, the lateral canthus is more mobile. An epicanthus is a fold of skin which covers the medial canthus in oriental races. Each lid consists of several layers. From front to back they are: very thin skin, a sheet of muscle (orbicularis oculi whose fibres are concentric around the palpebral fissure and which produce closure of the eyelids), the orbital septum (modified near the lid margin to form the tarsal plates) and, finally, lining the back surface of the lid, the conjunctiva (known here as tarsal conjunctiva). At the free margin of each lid are the eyelashes, the openings of tear glands which lie within the lid and the lacrimal punctum. Toward the medial edge of each lid in an elevation known as the papilla. The lacrimal punctum opens into this papilla. The punctum forms the open end of the cannaliculus, part of the tear-drainage mechanism.

Orbit   The bony cavity within which the eye is held. The orbits lie one on either side of the nose, on the front of the skull. They afford considerable protection for the eye. Each is roughly pyramidal in shape, with the apex pointing backwards and the base forming the open anterior part of the orbit. The bone of the anterior orbital margin is thickened to protect the eye from injury. There are various openings into the posterior part of the orbit, namely the optic canal which allows the optic nerve to leave the orbit en route for the brain, the superior orbital fissure and inferior orbital fissure which allow passage of nerves and blood vessels to and from the orbit. The most important structures holding the eye within the orbit are the extra-ocular muscles, a suspensory ligament of connective tissue that forms a hammock on which the eye rests and which is slung between the medial and lateral walls of

the orbit. Finally, the orbital septum, a sheet of connective tissue extending from the anterior margin of the orbit into the lids, helps keep the eye in place. A pad of fat fills in the orbit behind the eye and acts as a cushion for the eye.

Conjunctiva   A transparent mucous membrane that extends from the limbus over the anterior sclera or 'white of the eye'. This is the bulbar conjunctiva. The conjunctiva does not cover the cornea. Conjunctiva passes from the eye on to the inner surface of the eyelid at the fornices and is continuous with the tarsal conjunctiva. The semilunar fold is the vertical crescent of conjunctiva at the medial aspect of the palpebral fissure. The caruncle is a piece of modified skin just within the inner canthus.

Eye muscles (extra ocular muscles)   There are six in all, the four rectus muscles (superior, inferior, medial and lateral rectus muscles) and two oblique muscles (superior and inferior oblique muscles). The muscles are attached at various points between the bony orbit and the eyeball. By their combined action they move the eye in horizontal and vertical gaze. They also produce torsional movement of the eye (i.e. clockwise or anticlockwise movements when viewed from the front).

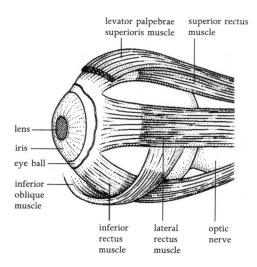

Extrinsic muscles of left eye.

Lacrimal apparatus   There are two components, a tear production system, namely the lacrimal gland and accessory lacrimal glands, and a drainage system.

LACRIMAL GLAND   Located below a small depression in the bony roof of the orbit. Numerous tear ducts open from it predominantly the upper lid. Accessory lacrimal glands are found in the conjunctiva and within the eyelids. The former open directly on to the surface of the conjunctiva, the latter on to the eyelid margin.

LACRIMAL DRAINAGE SYSTEM   This consists of

Punctum   An elevated opening toward the

medial aspect of each lid. Each punctum opens into a cannaliculus.

Cannaliculus A fine tube-like structure running within the lid, parallel to the lid margin. The cannaliculus from upper and lower lid join to form a common cannaliculus which opens into the lacrimal sac.

Lacrimal sac A small sac on the side of the nose which opens into the nasolacrimal duct. During blinking the sac sucks tears into itself from the cannaliculus. Tears then drain by gravity down the nasolacrimal duct.

Nasolacrimal duct A tubular structure which runs down through the wall of the nose and opens into the nasal cavity.

Tears keep the front of the eye moist; they also contain nutrients and various components to protect the eye from infection. Crying results from excess tear production. The drainage system cannot cope with the excess and therefore tears overflow on to the face. Newborn babies do not produce tears for the first three months of life.

Visual pathway Light stimulates the rods and cones of the retina. Electrochemical messages are then passed to nerve fibres in the retina and then via the optic nerve to the optic chiasm. Here information from the temporal (outer) half of each retina continues to the same side of the brain. Information from the nasal (inner) half of each retina crosses to the other side within the optic chiasm. The rearranged nerve fibres then pass through the optic tract to the lateral geniculate body, then the optic radiation to reach the visual cortex in the occipital lobe of the brain.

EYEBALL (see EYE).

EYE DISEASES

Arcus senilis The white ring or crescent which tends to form at the edge of the cornea with age. It is uncommon in the young when it may be associated with high levels of blood lipids.

Blepharitis A chronic inflammation of the lid margins. SEBORRHOEA and STAPHYLOCOCCAL infection are likely contributors. The eyes are typically intermittently red, sore and gritty over months or years. Treatment is difficult and prone to fail. Measures to reduce debris on the lid margins, intermittent courses of topical antibiotics, steroids or systemic antibiotics may help the sufferer.

Blepharospasm Involuntary closure of the eye. This may accompany irritation but may also occur without an apparent cause. It may be severe enough to interfere with vision. Treatment involves removing the source of irritation, if present. Severe and persistent cases may respond to injection of *Botulinum* toxin into the orbicularis muscle.

Chalazion A firm lump in the eyelid relating to a blocked MEIBOMIAN gland, felt deep within the lid. Treatment is not always necessary. A proportion spontaneously resolve. There can be associated infection when the lid becomes red and painful requiring antibiotic treatment. If troublesome, the chalazion can be incised under local anaesthetic.

Conjunctivitis Inflammation of the conjunctiva which may affect one or both eyes. Typically the eye is red, itchy, sticky and gritty but is not usually painful. Redness is not always present. Conjunctivitis can occasionally be painful, particularly if there is an associated keratitis (see below) (e.g. adenovirus infection, herpetic infection). The cause can be infective (bacteria, viruses or CHLAMYDIA) chemical (e.g. acids, alkalis) or allergic (e.g. in hay-fever). Conjunctivitis may be caused by contact lenses. Preservatives in eye drops or even the drugs in eye drops may cause conjunctival inflammation. Conjunctivitis may also occur in association with other illnesses, e.g. with upper-respiratory-tract infection, STEVENS–JOHNSON SYNDROME, REITER'S SYNDROME. The treatment depends on the cause. In many patients acute conjunctivitis is self-limiting.

Dacryocystitis Inflammation of the lacrimal sac. This may present acutely as a red, painful swelling between the nose and the lower lid. An abscess may form which points through the skin or may need to be drained by incision. Systemic antibiotics may be necessary. Chronic dacryocystitis may occur with recurrent discharge from the openings of the tear ducts and recurrent swelling of the lacrimal sac. Obstruction of the tear duct is accompanied by watering of the eye. If the symptoms are troublesome, the patient's tear passageways need to be surgically reconstructed.

Ectropion The lid margin is everted, usually the lower lid. Ectropion is most commonly associated with ageing, when the tissues of the lid become lax. It can also be caused by shortening of the skin of the lids such as happens with scarring or mechanical factors – e.g., a tumour pulling the skin of the lower lid downwards. Ectropion tends to cause watering and an unsightly appearance. The treatment is surgical.

Entropion The lid margin is inverted, usually the lower lid. Entropion is most commonly associated with ageing, when the tissues of the lid become lax. It can also be caused by shortening of the inner surfaces of the lids due to scarring – e.g., trachoma or chemical burns. The inwardly directed lashes cause irritation and can abrade the cornea. The treatment is surgical.

Episcleritis Inflammation of the EPISCLERA. There is usually no apparent cause. The inflammation may be diffuse or localized and may affect one or both eyes. It sometimes recurs. The affected area is usually red and moderately painful. Episcleritis is generally not thought to be as painful as scleritis and does not lead to the same complications. Treatment is generally directed at improving the patient's symptoms.

The inflammation may respond to non-steroidal anti-inflammatory drugs or topical corticosteroids.

Keratitis Inflammation of the cornea which is a response to a variety of insults – viral, bacterial, chemical, radiation, or mechanical trauma. Keratitis may be superficial or involve the deeper layers, the latter being generally more serious. The eye is usually red, painful and photophobic. Treatment is directed at the cause.

Nystagmus Involuntary rhythmic oscillation of one or both eyes. There are several causes including nervous disorders, vestibular disorders, eye disorders and certain drugs including alcohol.

Pinguecula A benign degenerative change in the connective tissue at the nasal or temporal limbus. This is visible as a small flattened yellow-white lump adjacent to the cornea.

Pterygium Overgrowth of the conjunctival tissues at the limbus on to the cornea. This usually occurs on the nasal side and is associated with exposure to sunlight. The pterygium is surgically removed for cosmetic reasons or if it is thought to be advancing towards the visual axis.

Ptosis Drooping of the upper lid. May occur because of a defect in the muscles which raise the lid (levator complex), sometimes the result of ageing or trauma. Other causes include HORNER'S SYNDROME, third cranial nerve palsy, MYASTHENIA GRAVIS, and DYSTROPHIA MYOTONICA. The cause needs to be determined and treated if possible. The treatment for a severely drooping lid is surgical, but other measures can be used to prop up the lid with varying success.

Scleritis Inflammation of the sclera. This can be localized or diffuse, can affect the anterior or the posterior sclera and can affect one or both eyes. The affected eye is usually red and painful. Scleritis can lead to thinning and even perforation of the sclera. This can happen sometimes with little sign of inflammation. Posterior scleritis in particular may cause impaired vision and require emergency treatment. There is often no apparent cause, but there are some associated conditions, for example, HERPES ZOSTER OPHTHALMICUS, RHEUMATOID ARTHRITIS, gout , and an autoimmune disease affecting the nasal passages and lungs called Wegener's granulomatosis. Treatment depends on severity but may involve NON-STEROIDAL ANTI-INFLAMMATORY DRUGS, topical CORTICOSTEROIDS or systemic IMMUNOSUPPRESSIVE drugs.

Stye Infection of a lash follicle. This presents as a painful small red lump at the lid margin. It often resolves spontaneously but may require antibiotic treatment if it persists or recurs.

Sub-conjunctival haemorrhage Haemorrhage between the conjunctiva and the underlying episclera. It is painless. There is usually no apparent cause and it resolves spontaneously.

Trichiasis Inward misdirection of lashes. Trichiasis occurs due to inflammation of or trauma to the lid margin. Treatment involves removal of the patient's lashes. Re-growth may be prevented by electrolysis or CRYOTHERAPY to the lid margin or possible surgery.

For the subject of artificial eyes see under PROSTHESES; CATARACT, GLAUCOMA, RETINA, DISORDERS OF, SQUINT, and UVEITIS are dealt with under these headings.

EYE DROPS (AND OINTMENT) are used extensively in the treatment of eye disease. They should be used as instructed by the prescribing physician. Most can be used for one month after the bottle has been opened but should then be discarded and a repeat prescription obtained if necessary. Any eye drops or ointment can have side effects and any difficulty with them should be referred to the prescribing physician.

EYE INJURIES Victims of eye injuries are advised to seek prompt medical advice if the injury is at all serious or does not resolve with simple first-aid measures – for example, by washing out a foreign body using an eye bath.

Blunt injuries These may cause haemorrhage inside the eye, cataract, retinal detachment or even rupture of the eye. Injuries from large blunt objects – for example, a squash ball – may also cause a 'blow-out fracture' of the orbital floor causing double vision. Surgical treatment may be required depnding on the patient's specific problems.

Chemical burns Most chemical splashes cause conjunctivitis and superficial keratitis in the victim; both conditions are self-limiting. Alkalis are, however, more likely to penetrate deeper into the eye and cause permanent damage, particularly to the cornea. Prompt irrigation is important. Further treatment may involve testing the pH of the tears, topical antibiotics and CORTICOSTEROIDS and VITAMIN C (drops or tablets; see APPENDIX 5: VITAMINS), depending on the nature of the injury.

Corneal abrasion Loss of corneal epithelium (outermost layer). Almost any sort of injury to the eye may cause this. The affected eye is usually very painful. In the absence of other problems the epithelium heals very rapidly. Small defects may close within 24 hours. Treatment conventionally consists of antibiotic ointment and sometimes a pad over the injured eye.

Foreign bodies Most foreign bodies which hit the eye are small and are found in the conjunctival sac or on the cornea; most are superficial and can be easily removed. A few foreign bodies penetrate deeper and may cause infection, cataract, retinal detachment or haemorrhage within the eye. The foreign body is usually removed and the damage repaired; nevertheless the victim's sight may have been permanently damaged. Particularly dangerous activities include hammering or chiselling on metal or stone and people carrying out these activities and others such as hedge cutting and grass strimming should wear protective goggles.

F

FACE is that part of the head extending from the forehead to the chin. It is supported by 14 bones: 2 nasal bones. 2 superior maxillae which carry the upper teeth. 2 lacrimal bones, 2 zygomatic bones, 2 palatine bones, 2 nasal bones at the sides of the nose, the vomer, forming a partition between the nostrils, and the mandible carrying the lower teeth. The lower jaw forms a joint of hinge-shape with the temporal bones of the skull, whilst the other bones of the face are firmly fixed together by sutures. The face in man is relatively small, as compared with that in lower animals, on account of the development of the cranium containing the brain. For the same reason, the face has an almost vertical direction instead of being sloped backwards as in animals.

The general character of the features depends chiefly upon the presence of air spaces in the frontal bone, situated immediately behind the eyebrows and in the upper jaw-bones. The varying expressions which are connected with the emotions and the general expression denoting character are chiefly due to the action of numerous thin muscles situated around the openings of the eyes, nose, and mouth. (See MUSCLE.) These are controlled by the 7th cranial nerve, which starts from the back part of the brain, passes through the skull to the ear, and, emerging immediately below the latter, passes forward on to the face round the edge of the lower jaw. In this position it is vulnerable to damage. Injury may result in a flat and expressionless appearance of one side of the face known as BELL'S PALSY (or paralysis) or facial paralysis. The sensory nerve of the face is the 5th cranial nerve, which originates from the neighbouring part of the brain and within the skull divides into three portions called, respectively, ophthalmic, maxillary, and mandibular divisions. Each of these sends branches on to the face through a notch that can be felt near the inner end of the eyebrow, through an opening immediately beneath the eye, and through another opening near the middle of the chin. On their way to the face these nerves supply the parts about the eye, the teeth, and the muscles which move the lower jaw in chewing. The various parts of this nerve are subject to a particularly painful form of neuralgia, known sometimes as tic douloureux. (See NEURALGIA.)

FACE LIFT An operation to reduce wrinkles and lift 'loose' skin on the face of mature persons with the aim of making them look younger. It can be performed under local anaesthetic as an outpatient or with general anaesthesia as an inpatient. The operation is regarded as cosmetic and is usually done privately. The results are not always satisfactory.

FACIAL NERVE is the seventh cranial nerve, and supplies the muscles of expression in the face, being purely a motor nerve. It enters the face immediately below the ear after splitting up into several branches. (See BELL'S PALSY.)

FACIES is a term applied to the expression or appearance of the face.

FACTOR VIII A coagulative blood protein that is a constituent of the COAGULATION cascade, an essential component in the clotting of blood. Those people with the inherited disorder, HAEMOPHILIA, have abnormally low amounts of factor VIII and so bleed more when cut. They are treated with a concentrated version to reduce the tendency to bleed.

FAECES or STOOLS These consist of the remainder of the food after it has passed through the alimentary canal and been subjected to the action of the digestive juices, and after the nutritious parts have been absorbed by the intestinal mucous membrane. The stools also contain various other matters, such as pigment, derived from the BILE, and large quantities of bacteria which are the main component of human stools. The stools are passed once daily by most people, but infants have several evacuations of the bowels in twenty-four hours and many adults may defaecate only two or three times weekly. Sudden changes in bowel habit, persistent diarrhoea or a change from the normal dark brown (caused by the bile pigment stercobilin) to very pale or very dark stools are reasons for seeking medical advice. Blood in the stools may be due to HAEMORRHOIDS or something more serious, and anyone with such symptoms should see a doctor.

Incontinence of the bowels, or inability to retain the stools, is found in certain diseases in which the sphincter muscles, that naturally keep the bowel closed, relax. It is also a symptom of disease in, or injury to, the spinal cord.

Pain on defaecation is a characteristic symptom of a FISSURE at the ANUS or of inflamed haemorrhoids, and is usually sharp. Pain of a duller character associated with the movements of the bowels may be caused by inflammation in the other pelvic organs.

CONSTIPATION and DIARRHOEA are considered under separate headings.

FAINTING, or SYNCOPE, is a temporary loss of consciousness caused by inadequate brain perfusion. It may be preceded by nausea, sweating, loss of vision, and ringing in the ears. It is most often caused by pooling of blood in the extremities, which reduces venous return and thus cardiac output. This may be caused by hot weather or prolonged standing. Occasionally fainting on standing occurs in people with low blood pressure, autonomic neuropathy (in which normal vasomotor reflexes are absent), or those taking antihypertensive drugs. A prolonged rise in intrathoracic pressure caused by coughing, micturition, or the valsalva manoeuvre also impedes venous return and may cause fainting. HYPOVOLAEMIA produced by bleeding, prolonged diarrhoea, or vomiting may also cause fainting. Fainting is also produced by severe pain or emotional upset. Cardiac causes, such as severe stenotic valve disease or rhythm disturbances (particularly complete heart block or very rapid tachycardias), may result in fainting. Treatment must be directed towards the underlying cause, but immediate first aid consists of laying the patient down and elevating the legs.

FAITH HEALING   The facility that some people claim they have to cure disease by a healing force present in their make-up. The healer 'transmits' the force by direct contact with the person seeking treatment. Strong religious beliefs are usually the characteristics of the healer and his or her subject. The force is inexplicable to science but some medically qualified doctors have been convinced of its beneficial effect in some people.

FALLEN ARCHES   Weakness in the muscles that support the bony arches of the FOOT. The result is flat feet, a condition that can adversely affect the person's ability to walk and run normally.

FALLING SICKNESS is an old name for epilepsy. (See EPILEPSY.)

FALLOPIAN TUBES, or UTERINE TUBES, are tubes, one on each side, which are attached at one end to the womb, and have the other unattached but lying close to the ovary. Each is between 10 to 12·5 cm (4 to 5 inches) long, large at the end next the ovary, but communicating with the womb by an opening which admits only a bristle. These tubes conduct the ova from the ovaries to the interior of the womb. Blockage of them by a chronic inflammatory process resulting from infection is a not uncommon cause of infertility in women. (See REPRODUCTIVE SYSTEM.)

FALLOT'S TETRALOGY   A hereditary defect of the heart in which intraventricular septal defect, pulmonary stenosis, right ventricular hypertrophy and a wrongly positioned aorta occur. It is usually treatable by surgery.

FALSE MEMBRANE   The deposit which forms upon the walls of the air passages in cases of diphtheria. It consists partly of fibrin derived

from the blood, partly of the destroyed surface of the mucous membrane upon which it rests, and it contains bacteria in enormous numbers. If it is removed, it leaves a raw and bleeding surface upon which new membrane quickly forms.

FALSE-MEMORY SYNDROME   (see RECOVERED-MEMORY SYNDROME).

FAMILIAL   A description of a disorder, illness or characteristic that runs in families.

FAMOTIDINE   An H$_2$-RECEPTOR-ANTAGONIST drug used to heal gastric and duodenal output by cutting the output of gastric acid by blocking H$_2$ receptors. The drug is taken orally. Side-effects may include dizziness, changed bowel habit, fatigue, rashes, confusion, reversible liver damage and headache.

FANSIDAR   A combination of PYRIMETHAMINE and SULFADOXINE used in conjunction with other antimalarial drugs to treat *falciparum* malaria (see MALARIA).

FARMER'S LUNG   A form of external allergic alveolitis (see ALVEOLITIS) caused by the inhalation of dust from mouldy hay or straw.

FASCIA   Sheets or bands of fibrous tissue which enclose and connect the muscles.

FASCIITIS   Inflammation of FASCIA. The commonest site for it is the sole of the foot where it is known as plantar fasciitis. It is characterized by gnawing pain. There is no specific treatment, but it usually clears up spontaneously though over a considerable time.

FASCIOLIASIS   Disease caused by the liver fluke, *Fasciola hepatica*. This is found in sheep, cattle and other herbivorous animals, in which it is the cause of the condition known as liver rot. It measures about 35 × 13 mm, and is transmitted to man from the infected animals by snails. In Britain it is the commonest disease found in animal slaughterhouses. The danger to man is in eating vegetables, particularly wild watercress, that have been infected by snails. There have been several outbreaks of fascioliasis in Britain due to eating contaminated wild watercress. Much larger outbreaks of fascioliasis due to eating wild watercress have also been reported in France. The disease is characterized by fever, dyspepsia, heavy sweating, loss of appetite, abdominal pain, urticaria, and a troublesome cough. In the more serious cases there may be severe damage to the liver with or without jaundice. The diagnosis is clinched by the finding of the eggs of the fluke in the stools. The two drugs used in treatment are bithionol and chloroquine. Even though many cases are quite mild and recover spontaneously, prevention is particularly important. This consists primarily of never eating wild watercress, as this is the main cause of infestation. Lettuces have also been found to be infested.

FASCIOTOMY An operation to relieve pressure on muscles caused by tight surrounding fascia or fibrous connective tissue. The fascia is slit with an incision.

FASTIGIUM The highest temperature reached in a feverish state or the period when a disease process reaches its peak. It also describes the top of the roof of the fourth ventricle of the brain.

FASTING is the abstention from, or deprivation of, food and drink. It may result from a genuine desire to lose weight – in an attempt to improve one's health or appearance – or may result from a MENTAL ILLNESS. such as depression, or an EATING DISORDER. Certain religious customs and practices may demand periods of fasting. Forced fasting, often extended, has been used for many years as an effective means of torture.

Without food and drink the body rapidly becomes thinner and lighter as it draws upon its stored energy reserves, initially mainly fat. The temperature gradually falls, and muscle is progressively broken down as the body struggles to maintain its vital functions. Dehydration, leading to cardiovascular collapse, inevitably follows unless a basic amount of water is taken, particularly if the body's fluid output is high, such as may occur with excessive sweating.

After prolonged fasting the return to food should be gradual, with careful monitoring of blood-pressure levels and concentrations of serum ELECTROLYTES. Feeding should consist mainly of liquids and light foods at first, with no heavy meals being taken for several days.

FAT A food has more energy-producing power weight for weight than any other food. Animal fat is a mixture in varying proportions of stearic, palmitic, and oleic acids combined with glycerin. Butter contains about 80 per cent of fat, ordinary cream contains 20 per cent fat, and rich cream 40 per cent, whilst olive oil is practically a pure form of fat. Fat requires, when taken to a large extent in the diet, to be combined with a certain proportion of either carbohydrate or protein in order that it may be completely consumed, otherwise harmful products, known as ketones, may form in the blood. Each gram of fat has an energy-producing equivalent of 9·3 Calories.

Fats are divided into saturated fats, that is, animal fats and dairy produce, and unsaturated fats which include vegetable oils from soya bean, maize and sunflower, and marine oils from fish (eg. cod-liver oil). (See ADIPOSE TISSUE; LIPID; OBESITY.)

FATIGUE Tiredness: a physiological state in which muscles become fatigued by the lactic

acid accumulating in them as the result of their activity. For the removal of lactic acid in the recovery phase of muscular contraction oxygen is needed. If the supply of oxygen is not plentiful enough, or cannot keep pace with the work the muscle is doing, then lactic acid accumulates and fatigue results. There is also a nervous element in muscular fatigue: it is diminished by stimulation of the sympathetic nervous system. (See MUSCLE.)

Chronic fatigue is a symptom of some illnesses such as ANAEMIA, HYPOTHYROIDISM, MONONUCLEOSIS, MOTOR NEURONE DISEASE, MYASTHENIA GRAVIS, MYALGIC ENCEPHALITIS (ME) and others. Some drugs may also produce a feeling of fatigue.

FAT NECROSIS In injury to, or inflammation of, the pancreas the fat-splitting enzyme in it may escape into the abdominal cavity, causing death of fat-containing cells.

FATTY DEGENERATION As a result of anaemia, interference with blood or nerve supply, or because of the action of various poisons, body cells may undergo abnormal changes accompanied by the appearance in their substance of fat droplets.

FAUCES The somewhat narrowed opening between the mouth and throat. It is bounded above by the soft palate, below by the tongue, and on either side by the tonsil. In front of, and behind, the tonsil are two ridges of mucous membrane, the anterior and posterior pillars of the fauces.

FAVISM A type of haemolytic ANAEMIA, attacks of which occur within an hour or two of eating broad beans (*Vicia fava*). It is a hereditary disease due to lack of an essential enzyme called glucose-6-phosphate dehydrogenase which plays an important part in the metabolism of glucose and is necessary for the continued integrity of the red cell. This defect is inherited as a sex- linked dominant trait, and the red cells of patients with this abnormality have a normal life span until challenged by certain drugs or fava beans when the older cells are rapidly destroyed, resulting in haemolytic anaemia. Fourteen per cent of American Negroes are affected and 60 per cent of Yemenite Jews in Israel. The perpetuation of the gene is due to the greater resistance against malaria that it carries. Severe and even fatal haemolysis has followed the administration of the antimalarial compounds pamaquine and primaquine in sensitive individuals. These red cells are sensitive not only to fava beans and primaquine but also to sulphonamides, acetanilide, phenacetin, para- aminosalicyclic acid, nitrofurantoin, probenecid and vitamin K analogues.

FAVUS Another name for honeycomb ringworm. (See RINGWORM.)

FEAR An emotional condition provoked by danger and usually characterized by unpleasant subjective feelings accompanied by physiological and behavioural changes. The heart rate increases, sweating occurs and the blood pressure rises. Sometimes fear of certain events or places may develop into a phobia: for example, agoraphobia, a fear of the open.

FEBRILE Having a fever. Describes a patient whose body temperature is greater than normal (36·9–37·8 °C).

FEBRILE CONVULSION Convulsion occurring in a child with a high temperature in which the limbs twitch and he or she may lose consciousness. The condition is common, with 1 child in 20 suffering from it. It is a result of immature HOMEOSTATIC control and is not usually serious, occurring generally as a result of an infection such as measles or tonsillitis. The brain and nervous system are normal in most cases. Treatment is tepid sponging and attention to the underlying cause, with the child placed in the recovery position (see APPENDIX 1: FIRST AID).

FEEDBACK MECHANISM Many glands which produce HORMONES are influenced by other hormones, particularly those secreted by the HYPOTHALAMUS (a controlling centre in the brain) and the PITUITARY GLAND. If the amount of hormone produced by a gland rises, negative feedback mechanisms operate by instructing the pituitary gland, via the hypothalamus, to produce less of the stimulating hormones. This cuts activity in the target gland. Should the amount of hormone produced fall, the feed-

back mechanism weakens with the result that the output of stimulating hormones increases.

FEMINIZATION The development of a feminine appearance in a man, often the result of an imbalance in the sex hormones. Castration, especially before puberty, causes feminization as may the use of hormones to treat an enlarged PROSTATE GLAND.

FEMORAL Adjective relating to the femur or the region of the thigh. For example, the femoral nerve, artery, vein and canal.

FEMUR The thigh bone which is the longest and strongest bone in the body. As the upper end is set at an angle of about 120 degrees to the rest of the bone, and since the weight of the body is entirely borne by the two femora, fracture of one of these bones close to its upper end is a common accident in old people, whose bones are often weakened by OSTEOPOROSIS. The femur fits, at its upper end, into the acetabulum of the pelvis, forming the hip-joint, and, at its lower end, meets the tibia and patella in the knee-joint.

FENESTRATION An operation to make a new opening into the labyrinth of the ear. It has proved most valuable in restoring hearing to patients with OTOSCLEROSIS, particularly in young people with this disease.

FENNEL The seed-like fruit of *Foeniculum vulgare* used as a carminative: i.e. to relieve griping, flatulence, and distension of the stomach. Fennel water used to be a popular remedy for griping.

Feedback mechanism

1 uterus
2 fetal head in position for normal delivery
3 cervix
4 symphysis pubis
5 vagina
6 superior vena cava
7 fetal liver

8 placental vein
9 placenta
10 fetal lungs
11 fetal heart ventricles
12 fetal aorta
13 inferior vena cava
14 placental arteries

(Left) Vertical section of mother's abdomen with fetus in the womb (viewed from the left side). (Right) Diagram of fetal circulation.

FERTILIZATION The process by which male and female gametes (spermatozoa and oöcytes respectively) fuse to form a zygote which develops by a complex process of cell division and differentiation into a new individual of the species. In humans fertilization occurs in the FALLOPIAN TUBES. Sperm deposited in the upper vagina traverse the CERVIX and UTERUS to enter the fallopian tube. Many sperm attempt to penetrate the zona pellucida surrounding the oöcyte, but only one is able to penetrate the oöcyte proper and this prevents any other sperm entering. Once the sperm has entered the oöcyte, their nuclei fuse before the zygote begins to divide.

FESTER A popular term used to mean any collection or formation of pus. It is applied to both abscesses and ulcers. (See ABSCESS; ULCER; WHITLOW.)

FESTINATION The involuntary quickening of gait seen in some nervous diseases, especially in PARKINSONISM.

FETISHISM This is a form of sexual deviation in which the person becomes sexually stimulated by parts of the body, such as the feet, which are not usually regarded as erotogenic.

FETUS The name given to the unborn child after the eight week of development. The human being, like the young of all animals, begins as a single cell, the ovum, in the ovary. After fertilization with a spermatozoon the ovum becomes embedded in the mucous membrane of the uterus, its covering being known as the decidua. Increase in size is rapid, and development of complexity is still more marked. The original cell divides again and again to form new cells, and these become arranged in three layers, known as the ectoderm, mesoderm, and endoderm. From the first are produced the skin, the brain and spinal cord, and the nerves; from the second the bones, muscles, blood-vessels, and connective tissues; while the third develops into the lining of the digestive system and the various glands attached to it.

The ovum produces not only the fetus but several membranes and appendages which serve it till birth, and are then cast away. The embryo develops upon one side of the ovum, its first appearance consisting of a groove, the edges of which grow up and join to form a tube, which in turn develops into the brain and spinal cord. At the same time, a part of the ovum beneath this is becoming pinched off to form the body, and within this the endoderm forms a second tube, which in time is changed in shape and lengthened to form the digestive canal. From the gut there grows out very early a process called the allantois, which attaches itself to the wall of the UTERUS, forming later on the navel-string and afterbirth, by which nourishment is gained for growth. (See PLACENTA.)

The remainder of the ovum, which within two weeks of conception has increased to about 2 mm (1/12 inch) in size, splits into an outer and inner shell, from the outer of which are developed two covering membranes, the chorion and amnion, while the inner constitutes the yolk sac, attached by a pedicle to the developing gut of the embryo. From two weeks after conception onward, the various organs and limbs appear and grow, the name of embryo being applied to the developing being while almost indistinguishable in appearance from the embryo of other animals, till the middle of the second month, when it begins to show a distinctly human form. After this stage it is called the fetus. The property of 'life' is present from the very beginning, although the movements of the fetus are not felt by the mother till the fifth month.

During the first few days after conception the eye begins to be formed, beginning as a cup-shaped outgrowth from the mid-brain, its lens being formed as a thickening in the skin. It is very soon followed by the beginnings of the nose and ear, both of which arise as pits on the surface, which increase in complexity, and are joined by nerves that grow outward from the brain. These three organs of sense have practically their final appearance as early as the beginning of the second month.

As already stated, the body closes in from behind forward, the sides growing forward from the spinal region. In the neck, the growth takes the form of five arches, similar to those which bear gills in fishes. From the first of these the lower jaw is formed, from the second the hyoid bone, all the arches uniting, and the gaps between them closing up by the end of the second month. At this time the head and neck have assumed quite a human appearance.

The digestive canal begins as a simple tube running from end to end of the embryo, but it grows in length and becomes twisted in various directions to form the stomach and bowels. From this tube also the lungs and the liver arise as two little buds, which quickly increase in size and complexity. The kidneys also appear very early, but go through several changes before their final form is reached.

The genital organs appear late. The swellings, which form the ovary in the female and the testicle (or testis) in the male, are produced in the region of the loins, and gradually descend to their final positions. The outward organs are exactly similar in the two sexes till the end of the third month, and the sex is not clearly distinguishable till late in the fourth month.

The blood-vessels appear in the ovum even before the embryo. The heart, originally double, forms as a dilatation upon the arteries which later produce the aorta. These two hearts later fuse into one. (For the circulation in the fetus, see CIRCULATION OF BLOOD.)

The limbs appear about the end of the third week as buds which increase quickly in length and split at their ends into five parts, for fingers or toes. The bones at first are formed of cartilage, in which true bone begins to appear during the third month.

The following table gives the average size and weight of the fetus at different periods:

Age	Length	Weight
4 weeks	5 mm	1·3 grams
3 months	8 to 9 cm	30 to 60 grams
5 months	15 to 25 cm	170 to 340 grams
7 months	32 to 35 cm	1360 to 1820 grams
Birth	45 to 60 cm	3200 grams

Approximate length and weight of the fetus at different periods.

FEVER, or PYREXIA, is the abnormal rise in body temperature that frequently accompanies disease in general.

Causes The cause of fever is the release of an endogenous pyrogen by phagocytic cells called MONOCYTES and MACROPHAGES. The cause of the fever is a small protein which is produced in response to a variety of infectious, immunological and neoplastic stimuli. The LYMPHOCYTES play a part in fever production because they recognize the antigen and release substances called lymphokines and these lymphokines promote the production of endogenous pyrogen. The pyrogen then acts on the thermoregulatory centre in the hypothalamus and this results in an increase in heat generation and a reduction in heat loss, resulting in a rise in body temperature.

This process is usually the result of infection by bacteria or viruses.

The average temperature of the body in health ranges between 36·9 and 37·5 °C (98·4 and 99·5 °F). It is liable to slight variations from such causes as the ingestion of food, the amount of exercise, the menstrual cycle, and the temperature of the surrounding atmosphere. There are, moreover, certain appreciable daily variations, the lowest temperature being between the hours of 01.00 and 07.00 hours, and the highest between 16.00 and 21.00 hours, with trifling fluctuations during these periods. (See TEMPERATURE.)

The development and maintenance of heat within the body depends on the metabolic oxidation consequent on the changes continually taking place in the processes of nutrition. In health this constant tissue disintegration is exactly counterbalanced by the consumption of food, whilst the uniform normal temperature is maintained by the adjustment of the heat developed, and of the processes of exhalation and cooling which take place, especially from the lungs and skin. During a fever this balance breaks down, the tissue waste being greatly in excess of the food supply. The body wastes rapidly, the loss to the system being chiefly in the form of nitrogen compounds (e.g. urea). In the early stage of fever a patient excretes about three times the amount of urea that he would excrete on the same diet if he were in health. Fever is measured by how high the temperature rises above normal. At 41.1°C (106°F) the patient is in a dangerous state of hyperpyrexia and, if above this figure for very long, the patient usually dies.

The body's temperature will also rise if exposed too long to a high ambient temperature. (See HEAT STROKE.)

Symptoms The onset of a fever is usually marked by a rigor or shivering. The skin feels hot and dry, and the raised temperature will often be found to show daily variations – namely, an evening rise and a morning fall. There is a relative increase in the pulse and breathing rates. The tongue is dry and furred; the thirst is intense, while the appetite is gone; the urine is scanty, of high specific gravity, containing a large quantity of solid matter, particularly urea. The patient will have a headache and sometimes nausea, and children may develop convulsions (see FEBRILE CONVULSIONS).

The fever falls by the occurrence of a crisis, i.e. a sudden termination of the symptoms, or by a more gradual subsidence of the temperature, technically termed a lysis. If death ensues, this is due to failure of the vital centres in the brain or of the heart, as a result of either the infection or hyperpyrexia.

Fever may be continuous as in typhoid fever; relapsing as in Borrelia infection; intermittent as in malaria; remittent as in some tropical diseases.

Treatment Fever is a symptom, and the correct treatment is therefore that of the underlying condition. Occasionally, however, it is also necessary to reduce the temperature by more direct methods: physical cooling by, for example, tepid sponging, and the use of antipyretic drugs such as aspirin.

FIBRE, DIETARY (see ROUGHAGE).

FIBREOPTIC ENDOSCOPY has transformed the management of gastro-intestinal disease. In chest disease fibreoptic bronchoscopy has now replaced the rigid wide-bore metal tube which was previously used for examination of the tracheo-bronchial tree. The principle of fibreoptics is that a light from a cold light source passes down a bundle of quartz fibres to illuminate the lumen of the gastro-intestinal tract or the bronchi. The reflected light is returned to the observer's eye via the image bundle which may contain up to 20,000 fibres. The tip of the instrument can be angulated in both directions and finger-tip controls are provided for suction, air insufflation and for water injection to clear the lens or the mucosa. The oesophagus, stomach and duodenum can be visualized. Furthermore, visualization of the pancreatic duct and direct endoscopic cannulation is now possible, as is visualization of the bile duct. Fibreoptic colonoscopy can visualize

the entire length of the colon and it is now possible to biopsy polyps or suspected carcinomas and to perform polypectomy. The flexible smaller fibreoptic bronchoscope has many advantages over the rigid tube and extends the range of view to all segmental bronchi and enables biopsy of pulmonary parenchyma itself. A biopsy forceps can be directed well beyond the tip of the bronchoscope itself and the more flexible fibreoptic instrument causes less discomfort to the patient. (See ENDOSCOPE, BRONCHOSCOPE, LARYNGOSCOPE, LAPAROSCOPE, COLPOSCOPE, COLONOSCOPE.)

Fibreoptic laparoscopy is a valuable technique that allows the direct vizualisation of the female pelvic organs, in order to detect the presence of suspected lesions (and, in certain cases, their subsequent removal), to check on the development and position of the fetus, and to test the patency of the Fallopian tubes.

FIBRILLATION A term applied to rapid contraction or tremor of muscles, especially to a form of abnormal action of the heart muscle in which individual bundles of fibres take up independent action. It is believed to be due to a state of excessive excitability in the muscle associated with the stretching which occurs in dilatation of the heart. The main causes are ATHEROSCLEROSIS, chronic RHEUMATIC heart disease and hypertensive heart disease. Fibrillation is distinguished as atrial or ventricular, depending on whether the muscle of the atria or of the ventricles is affected. In atrial fibrillation the heart beats and the pulse become extremely irregular, both as regards time and force. When the atrium is fibrillating there is no significant contraction of the atrial muscle but the cardiac output is maintained by ventricular contraction. In ventricular fibrillation there is no significant contractile force so that there is no cardiac output. The commonest cause is myocardial infarction. Administration of DIGOXIN may restore normal rhythm and in some patients cardioversion – a controlled direct-current shock given via a modified defibrillator – is effective.

FIBRIN A substance formed in the BLOOD as it clots. Its formation indeed causes clotting. The substance is produced in threads. After the threads have formed a close meshwork through the blood, they contract, and produce a dense felted mass. The substance is formed not only from shed blood but also from LYMPH which exudes from the lymph-vessels. Thus fibrin is found in all inflammatory conditions within serous cavities like the PLEURA, PERITONEUM, and PERICARDIUM, and forms a thick coat upon the surface of the inflamed membranes. It is also found in inflamed joints, and in the lung as a result of pneumonia. (See COAGULATION.)

FIBRINOLYSIS The way in which blood clots are removed from the circulation. The insoluble protein FIBRIN is broken down by the ENZYME plasmin (see PLASMINOGEN) which is activated at the same time as the coagulation process of blood. There is normally a balance between coagulation and fibrinolysis; an abnormal increase in the latter causes excessive bleeding.

FIBRINOGEN The soluble protein in the blood which is the precursor of FIBRIN, the substance in blood-clot.

FIBROADENOMA A benign tumour of glandular epithelium containing fibrous elements. The commonest benign tumour of the breast, often occurring in young women.

FIBROCYSTIC DISEASE OF THE PANCREAS (see CYSTIC FIBROSIS).

FIBROID, or fibromyoma, is the commonest form of tumour of the uterus (see UTERUS, DISEASES OF), and one of the most common tumours of the human body. It is composed of a mixture of muscular and fibrous tissue. The tumour may be small or as large as a grapefruit. Fibroids may cause pain and heavy menstrual bleeding and usually occur in women over 30 years of age. In some women the fibroid may be small enough to remove surgically but, if it is large, a HYSTERECTOMY is often necessary. Small, symptomless fibroids are no danger and can be left untreated.

FIBROMA is a tumour, consisting mainly of fibrous tissue, and most commonly occurring on the skin. In association with the skin disease TUBEROSE SCLEROSIS, two forms of fibromata are seen: periungal – multiple nodules around the nails, and perivascular – raised, red nodules on the face, mainly around the nose. Considerable cosmetic improvement may be achieved by DIATHERMY or surgical removal of the latter.

FIBROMYALGIA SYNDROME Rarely reported in children, most patients are in their 40s or 50s, about 90 per cent being women. It is widely reported in the USA, Canada and Europe, but racial and social predispositions have not been adequately studied.

Symptoms These vary, with pain and fatiguability generally prominent, sometimes causing considerable disability. Patients can usually dress and wash independently but cannot cope with a job or household activities. Pain is mainly axial, but may affect any region. ANALGESICS, NON-STEROIDAL ANTI-INFLAMMATORY DRUGS and local physical treatments are generally ineffective.

Patients often have a poor sleep pattern, often waking exhausted. Unexplained headache, urinary frequency and abdominal symptoms are common, but no cause has been found. Patients generally score highly on measures of anxiety and depression. Fibromyalgia is not an ideal description; idiopathic diffuse-pain syndrome and non-restorative sleep disorder are increasingly preferred terms.

Clinical findings are generally unremarkable; most important is the presence of multiple hyperalgesic tender sites (e.g. low cervical spine, low lumbar spine, suboccipital muscle, mid upper trapezius, tennis-elbow sites, upper outer quadrants of buttocks, medial fat pad of knees). In fibromyalgia, hyperalgesia (excessive discomfort) is widespread and symmetrical, but absent at sites normally non-tender. Claims by patients to be tender all over are more likely to be due to fabrication or psychiatric disturbance. OSTEOARTHRITIS and periarticular syndrome are much more common and should be excluded, together with other conditions, such as HYPOTHYROIDISM, SYSTEMIC LUPUS ERYTHEMATOSUS and inflammatory MYOPATHY, which may present with similar symptoms.

Cause There is no investigational evidence of inflammatory, metabolic or structural abnormality, and the problem seems functional rather than pathological. Serotonin deficiency has a significant role in fibromyalgia syndrome.

Management Controlled trials have confirmed the usefulness of low-dose AMITRIPTYLINE or DOTHIEPIN and a graded exercise programme to increase aerobic fitness. How it works is still unclear; its efficacy may be due to its normalizing effects on the sleep centre or 'pain gating' (reduction of pain sensation) at the spinal-cord level. Prognosis is often poor. Nevertheless suitable advice and training can help most patients to learn to cope better with their condition and avoid unnecessary investigations and drug treatments.

FIBROSARCOMA A cancer of the connective tissue arising in the fibroblasts, stem cells that produce connective tissue cells. The tumours can develop in bone or soft tissue and occur most commonly in the limbs. Treatment is by surgery or radiotherapy.

FIBROSING ALVEOLITIS (See ALVEOLITIS.)

FIBROSIS The formation of fibrous or scar tissue, which is usually due to either infection or injury.

FIBROSITIS, also known as MUSCULAR RHEUMATISM, describes pain and muscular stiffness and inflammation affecting the soft tissues of the arm, legs and trunk. The cause is unknown but may include immunological factors, muscular strain and psychological stress. Treatment is usually palliative.

FIBROUS DYSPLASIA A rare disease in which areas of bone are replaced by FIBROUS TISSUE. This renders the bone fragile and liable to fracture. It may involve only one bone, usually the thigh bone, or FEMUR, or several bones. This latter form of the disease may be accompanied by pigmentation of the skin and the early onset of puberty.

FIBROUS TISSUE One of the most abundant tissues throughout the body. White fibrous tissue consists of fibres of a substance known as collagen, which yields gelatine on being boiled. Between these fibres lie flattened or star-shaped cells, by which the fibres are produced. The fibres, like the cells, are of microscopic size, and are grouped into bundles which are held together by other fibres running round them. Yellow fibrous tissue is a rarer form, and consists of bundles of long yellow fibres, formed from a substance known as elastin. White fibrous tissue is very unyielding and forms sinews, ligaments, the material which binds muscle fibres together, the substance of the true skin. It is also the tissue which is laid down in the repair of wounds, or as a result of inflammation, and so forms the tissue composing a scar. It has the property of contracting and becoming denser as time goes on, and hence the puckering seen in scars, and the contraction resulting from burns and inflammation. Yellow fibrous tissue is highly elastic, and so is found in the walls of arteries, and in ligaments, like that on the back of the neck, which are often stretched. (See also ADHESION; SCAR; WOUNDS.)

FIBULA The slender outer bone of the leg. The head of this bone articualtes with the TIBIA just below the knee, and at the ANKLE it articulates with the TALUS bone.

FILARIASIS The term used to describe several clinical entities caused by one or other of the nematode filariae; these include *Wuchereria bancrofti/Brugia malayi, Onchocerca volvulus, Loa loa, Dracunculus medinensis* (dracontiasis or guinea-worm disease), *Mansonella perstans*, etc. These organisms have widely differing geographical distributions. Whereas lymphatic filariasis is present throughout much of the tropics and subtropics, onchocerciasis (river blindness) is largely confined to west and central Africa and southern America, loaiasis is an infection of west and central Africa, and dracontiasis involves west and central Africa and western India only. Clinically, the lymphatic filariases characteristically cause elephantiasis (lymphoedema); onchocerciasis gives rise to ophthalmic complications (river blindness), rashes and subcutaneous nodules; loaiasis causes subcutaneous 'Calabar swellings' and subconjunctival involvement; and dracontiasis predisposes to secondary bacterial infections (usually involving the lower limbs). Diagnosis is by finding the relevant filarial nematode, either in blood (day and night films should be examined), or one or other of the body fluids. An eosinophilia is often present in peripheral blood. Serological diagnosis is also of value. In onchocerciasis, skin-snips and the Mazotti reaction are valuable adjuncts to diagnosis. The mainstay of chemotherapy consists of diethylcarbamazine (aimed predominantly at the larval stage of the parasite). However, ivermectin (not available in the UK) is effective in onchocerciasis, and metronidazole or one of the benzimidazole compounds have limited value in dracontiasis. Suramin has been used to kill adult filarial worms. Prevention consists of eradication of the relevant insect vector.

FILARISIDE A generic term for drugs used to treat FILARIAL infections.

FILLING The insertion, in denistry, of a specially prepared material into a cavity drilled into a tooth, usually for the treatment of dental caries.

FINASTERIDE is a drug which inhibits the enzyme that metabolizes TESTOSTERONE into the more potent ANDROGEN dihydrotestosterone, This action results in a reduction of prostate tissue. The drug is used to treat enlarged PROSTATE GLANDS, thus improving urinary flow. Its side-effects include reduced libido and impotence. Finasteride offers an alternative to prostatectomy for some men but a significant minority do not improve. Women of childbearing age should not handle broken or crushed tablets.

FINGERS The hand comprises four fingers and a thumb; fingers have the same basic structure, though their size varies from the smallest, fourth or little, to the second which is the largest. Each finger consists of three bones called phalanges united by hinge-joints and strong ligaments. The thumb, like the great toe, differs from the others in having only two bones. These are bent or flexed, and straightened or extended by powerful tendons, two in front and two behind, which are brought into action by the contraction of muscles in the forearm. The sinews are enveloped in complicated synovial sheaths, through which they slide without friction, and are attached to the bases of the middle and end phalanges, back and front.

Running up each side of each finger are two small arteries and two small nerves, which supply the various structures and especially the overlying skin. The skin of the fingers is specially strong and particularly sensitive, and the end of the finger has a highly specialized part, the nail (see SKIN). Each finger articulates with a bone, the metacarpal, which lies in the substance of the hand between the finger and the carpus or wrist.

FINGERPRINT The unique pattern of fine ridges in the outer horny layer of the skin at the front of the tip of each finger and thumb. The ridges are in three type loops (70 per cent), whorls (25 per cent) and arches (5 per cent). Fingerprint patters are used as a routine FORENSIC test by police forces to identify individuals. Some patterns can indicate that the subject has an inherited disorder.

FIRST AID Emergency procedures to help an ill or injured person before he or she receives expert medical attention or is admitted to hospital. Courses of instruction in first aid comprise six to twelve sessions, each of about two hours' duration. Syllabuses of instruction are published by various organizations, the principal ones being the British Red Cross, the St John Ambulance Association, and the St Andrew's Ambulance Association. (See APPENDIX 1: FIRST AID and APPENDIX 2: ADDRESSES.)

FISSURE A term applied both to clefts of normal anatomical structure and also to small narrow ulcers occurring in skin and mucous membrane. The latter type of fissure occurs especially at the corners of the mouth and at the anus. (See LIPS; RECTUM, DISEASES OF.)

FISTULA An unnatural, narrow channel, leading from some natural cavity, such as the duct of a gland, or the interior of the bowels, to the surface. Or it may be a communication between two such cavities, where none should exist, as, for example, a direct communication between the bladder and bowel.

Cause Fistulas may be congenital or develop as a result of injury or infection. A SALIVARY fistula may develop between the gland and outside of the cheek because of a blockage in the duct from the gland to the mouth. A urinary fistula may be one consequence of a fracture of the PELVIS which has damaged the URETHRA. Anal fistulas are one of the commonest forms and are usually the result of infection and abscess formation.

Treatment As a rule, a fistula is extremely difficult to close, especially after it has persisted for some time. The treatment consists in an operation to restore the natural channel, be it salivary duct, or urethra, or bowel. This is effected by appropriate means in each locality, and when it is attained the fistula heals quickly under simple dressings.

FIT A popular name for a sudden convulsive seizure, although the term is also extended to include sudden seizures of every sort. During the occurrence of a fit of any sort the chief object should be to prevent the patient from doing any harm to himself by the convulsive movements. The person should therefore be laid flat, and the head supported on a pillow or other soft material. To prevent the tongue from being bitten, some object of moderate hardness may be placed between the teeth. (See CONVULSIONS; ECLAMPSIA; EPILEPSY; FAINTING; HYSTERIA; STROKE; URAEMIA; APPENDIX 1: FIRST AID.)

FITNESS An ability to perform daily activies without becoming overtired. Fitness is dependent on strength, flexibility and endurance, and the level of individuals' fitness will often depend on their type of employment and the extent to which they indulge in physical exercise, whether training in the local health club or at home or regularly participating in sports. Regular fitness improves people's health and well-being. Fitness exercises should be matched to the subjects' age and abilities and there is a danger if people regularly exercise beyond their capabilities.

FLACCID Relaxed or lacking in stiffness. Used to describe muscles that are not contracting (or following denervation) and organs, e.g. the penis, that are lying loose, empty, or with wrinkles. The opposite of firm or erect.

FLAIL CHEST (see FRACTURES).

FLAP A section of tissue (usually skin) separated from underlying structures but still attached to its distal end by a pedicle through which it receives its blood supply. The free end may then be sutured into a new position to cover a defect caused by trauma or excision of diseased tissue. A free flap involves detachment of a section of tissue, often including bone and muscle, to a distant site where the artery and vein supplying it are anastomosed to adjacent vessels and the tissue is sutured in place.

FLAT-FOOT, or PES PLANUS, is a deformity of the foot in which its arch sinks down so that the inner edge of the foot comes to rest upon the ground.

Causes The disorder may develop in infancy or occur in adult life, usually resulting from a combination of obesity and/or an occupation involving long periods of standing.

Symptoms There is pain along the instep and beneath the outer ankle, the foot is stiff and broad, walking is tiresome, and the toes turn far out.

Treatment Change of occupation to one which allows sitting is sometimes necessary. In early cases the leg muscles may be strengthened by tiptoe exercises performed for ten minutes night and morning. A pad to support the arch may have to be worn inside the shoe. Some children may require surgery.

FLATULENCE A collection of gas in the stomach or bowels. In the former case the gas is expelled from time to time in noisy eructations by the mouth; in the latter case it may produce rumblings in the bowels, or be expelled from the anus.

Causes When gas is found in large amount in the bowels its production is usually due to fermentation set up by bacteria.

Treatment Flatulence in the stomach is treated by relieving the dyspepsia which causes it. It may also be relieved, or eased, by the administration of CARMINATIVES. Flatulence may be aggravated by anxiety. If the flatulence is due to, or aggravated by, the habit of swallowing air, the patient must try and break the habit. To reduce intestinal flatulence may require a change of diet to easily digestible foods.

FLATUS Gas from the intestines that is passed out via the anus. Colloquially called wind, it is formed in the large intestine as a result of bacteria breaking down carbohydrate and aminoacids in digested food.

FLAVINE (see ANTISEPTICS).

FLEAS (see INSECTS IN RELATION TO DISEASE).

FLEXIBILITAS CEREA An abnormal state in which the limbs remain in any position into which they are moved.

FLEXIBLE TRAINING A term applied to the system of postgraduate medical training that allows young doctors to integrate their domestic commitments with the training requirements necessary to become a fully qualified specialist.

FLEXION The bending of a joint in the SAGITTAL plane. Usually an anterior movement, it is occasionally posterior, as in the case of the knee joint. Lateral flexion refers to the bending of the spine in the coronal plane, that is, from side to side.

FLEXOR A muscle that causes bending of a limb or other body part.

FLEXURE A bend in an organ or body part. The term is used, for example, to describe the skin on the inner aspect of the elbow or knee as in the 'hepatic flexure' of the COLON.

FLIES (see INSECTS IN RELATION TO DISEASE).

FLOODING A popular name for an excessive blood-stained discharge from the womb. (See MENSTRUATION; MENORRHAGIA.) In the majority of cases flooding is the sign of a miscarriage. (See ABORTION.)

FLUCLOXACILLIN A PENICILLINASE-resistant penicillin used to treat penicillin-resistant STAPHYLOCOCCI infection. (see PENICILLIN, ANTIBIOTIC).

FLUCONAZOLE An oral triazole antifungal drug used to treat local and systemic CANDIDIASIS and CRYPTOCOCCAL infections.

FLUCTUATION A sign obtained from collections of fluid by laying the fingers of one hand upon one side of the swelling, and, with those of the other, tapping or pressing suddenly on a distant point of the swelling. The thrill communicated from one hand to the other through the fluid is one of the most important signs of the presence of an abscess, or of effusion of fluid into joints or into the peritoneal cavity.

FLUCYTOSINE A synthetic drug used to treat certain fungal infections such as candidiasis (see CANDIDA) and cryptococcosis.

FLUFENAMIC ACID is a drug with analgesic, anti-inflammatory and anti-pyretic actions used in the treatment of OSTEOARTHROSIS and RHEUMATOID ARTHRITIS.

FLUID BALANCE The appropriate balance of fluid input and output (along with dissolved salts essential for life) over 24 hours. During this period about 2,500 millilitres (ml) of fluid should be taken in by a 70-kg man and the same amount excreted. Of this 2,500, 1,500 ml will be drunk, 800 ml will be in the food eaten and 200 ml produced by food metabolism. Excreted water is made up of 1,500 ml of urine, 800 ml insensible loss and 200 ml in the faeces. A 70-kg man's total body fluid is 42 litres (1) (60 per cent of body weight). Intracellular fluid comprises 28 1, extracellular 14 1 and blood 5 1. Water is controlled mainly by the sodium concentration in the body fluids via the release of ANTIDIURETIC HORMONE from the posterior part of the pituitary gland. In seriously ill subjects close monitoring of fluid intake and output, along with measurements of plasma sodium and calcium concentrations, is an essential factor in treatment.

FLUKES are a variety of parasitic worms. (See FASCIOLIASIS.)

FLUOCINOLONE is a corticosteroid for application to the skin as a cream, lotion or ointment. It is more potent than hydrocortisone. It must not be given by mouth.

FLUORESCEIN is a dye which has the special property of absorbing blue-light energy and emitting this energy as green light. This property is made use of in examining the cornea for scratches or ulceration and it is also used to detect abnormally permeable (or leaking) blood vessels in the retina and iris – especially in diabetic retinopathy and diseases of the macula.

FLUORINE, one of the halogen series of elements. In the form of fluoride it is one of the constituents of bone and teeth. Supplementing the daily intake of fluorine diminishes the incidence of dental caries. American and British evidence indicates that people who, throughout their lives, have drunk water with a natural fluorine content of 1 part per million, have less dental caries than those whose drinking water is fluorine free. All the available evidence indicates that this is the most satisfactory way of giving fluorine, and that if the concentration of fluorine in drinking water does not exceed 1 part per million, there are no toxic effects.

FLUOROSCOPE is an apparatus for rendering X-rays visible after they have passed through the body by projecting them on a screen of calcium tungstate. The technique of using it is known as fluoroscopy. It provides a method of being able to watch, for instance, the beating of the heart, or the movements of the intestine after the administration of a barium meal. (See X-RAYS.)

FLUOROURACIL An antimetabolite drug – a group that disrupts normal cell division – used intravenously to treat recurrent and inoperable carcinoma of the colon and rectum, as well as secondaries from cancer of the breast. It can be used topically for some malignant and premalignant skin lesions. (See CYTOTOXIC.)

FLUOXETINE One of a group of antidepressant drugs that produce their effect by inhibiting the reuptake of SEROTONIN. Termed SELECTIVE SEROTONIN-REUPTAKE INHIBITORS (SSRIs), these drugs seem to be effective in alleviating depressive illness. Their sedative effects are less than those of the tricyclic antidepressive drugs and they have few antimuscarinic effects. Withdrawal of fluoxetine and other SSRIs should be done slowly, and they interact with some other antidepressive drugs. A large number of side-effects have been reported with the use of fluoxetine (trade name Prozac®), including allergic reactions, dyspnoea, nausea, anorexia and anxiety.

FLUPENTHIXOL A tranquillizer used in the treatment of schizophrenia (see MENTAL ILLNESS).

FLUPHENAZINE is one of the phenothiazine derivatives of value as an anti-psychotic drug. (See NEUROLEPTICS.)

FLURAZEPAM (see BENZODIAZEPINES).

FLUTTER, or ATRIAL FLUTTER, is the term applied to a form of abnormal cardiac rhythm, in which the atria contract at a rate of between 200 and 400 beats a minute, and the ventricles more slowly. The abnormal rhythm is the result of a diseased heart. (See FIBRILLATION.)

FOETUS (see FETUS)

FOLIC ACID, one of the constituents of the vitamin B complex, derives its name from the fact that it is found in many green leaves, including spinach and grass. It has also been obtained from liver, kidney, and yeasts. In 1945 it was synthesized by American workers, who proposed that the chemical name should be pteroylglutamic acid. It has proved of value in the treatment of macrocytic anaemias, particularly those associated with sprue and nutritional deficiencies.

In order to prevent neural tube defects and cleft lip or palate, all women planning to become pregnant should be advised to have a diet rich in folic acid in the months before conception until 13 weeks' gestation.

Recent research has suggested that adequate levels of folic aid can prevent the build-up of HOMOCYSTEINE, a compound in the blood closely associated with heart attacks and strokes. It has been suggested that the official recommendation of 200 micrograms a day in the diet should be doubled. (See APPENDIX 5: VITAMINS.)

FOLIUM Latin term for leaf: e.g. digitalis folium is digitalis leaf. (Plural: folia.)

FOLLICLE is the term applied to a very small sac or gland: e.g. small collections of adenoid tissue in the throat and the small digestive glands on the mucous membrane of the intestine.

FOLLICLE-STIMULATING HORMONE A hormone produced by the anterior pituitary gland (see PITUITARY BODY) which stimulates the formation of follicles in the ovary each menstrual cycle and of spermatocytes in the testis. It is under hypothalamic control and in the female there is feedback inhibition by oestrogens from the developing follicle.

FOLLICULAR HORMONE (see OESTRADIOL).

FOMENTATION (see also POULTICES) Any warm application to the surface of the body in the form of a cloth. Usually the fomentation cloth is heated by being wrung out of hot water.

FOMITES A traditional term used to include all articles which have been brought into sufficiently close contact with a person sick of some infectious disease to retain the infective material and spread the disease. For example, clothes, bedding, carpets, toys, books, may all be fomites till disinfected.

FONTANELLE Areas on the head on which bone has not yet formed. The chief of these is the anterior fontanelle, situated on the top of the head between the frontal and two parietal bones. In shape it is four-sided, about 25 mm (1 inch) square at the time of birth, gradually diminishing until it is completely covered by bone, which should happen by the age of 18 months. The pulsations of the brain can be readily felt through it. Delay in its closure is particularly found in cases of rickets, as well as in other states of defective development. The fontanelle becomes more tense than usual in acute fevers, WHOOPING-COUGH, and BRONCHITIS, and tends to bulge in cases of HYDROCEPHALUS.

It becomes unusually depressed in all cases of diminished vitality, such as that due to diarrhoea or wasting from any cause.

FOOD INTOLERANCE   Most cases of food intolerance are not due to allergy. The most common cause of an aversion to food is probably psychological. Other cases of food intolerance are due to idiosyncrasy, that is a genetic defect in the patient, such as alactasia, where the intestine lacks the enzyme that digests milk sugar with the result that individuals so affected develop diarrhoea when they drink milk. Intolerance to specific foods, as distinct from allergy, is probably quite common and may be an important factor in the aetiology of the irritable bowel syndrome.

For the diagnosis of true food allergy it is necessary to demonstrate that there is a reproducible intolerance to a specific food and then that there is evidence of an abnormal immunological reaction to it. Occasionally the allergic response may not be to the food itself but to food contaminants such as penicillin, or to food additives such as tartrazine. There may also be reactions to foods which have pharmacological effects, such as caffeine in strong coffee or histamine in fermented cheese, or such reactions may be due to the irritant effect on the intestinal mucosa, especially if it is already diseased, by highly spiced curries.

FOOD POISONING   This illness is characterized by vomiting, diarrhoea, and abdominal pain and results from eating food contaminated with metallic or chemical poisons, certain micro-organisms or microbial products. Alternatively, the foods, such as undercooked red kidney beans or fish of the scombroid family (mackerel and tuna) may contain natural posions. Food poisoning caused by chemical or metallic substances usually occurs rapidly, within minutes or a few hours of eating. Among micro-organisms, bacteria are the leading cause of food poisoning, particularly *Staphylococcus aereus*, *Clostridium perfringens* (formerly *Cl. Welchii*), *salmonella* spp., *Campylobacter jejuni*, and *Escherichia coli* O157.

Staphylococcal food poisoning occurs after food such as meat products, cold meats, milk, custard, and egg products becomes contaminated before or after cooking, usually through incorrect handling by humans who carry *S. aureus*. The bacteria produce an ENTEROTOXIN which causes the symptoms of food poisoning one to eight hours after ingestion. The toxin can withstand heat; thus subsequent cooking of contaminated food will not prevent illness.

Heat-resistant strains of *Cl.perfringens* cause food poisoning associated with meat dishes, soups, or gravy when dishes cooked in bulk are left unrefrigerated for long periods before consumption. The bacteria are ANAEROBES and form spores; the anaerobic conditions in these cooked foods allow the germinated spores to multiply rapidly during cooling, resulting in heavy contamination. Once ingested the bacteria produce enterotoxin in the intestine, causing symptoms within eight to twenty-four hours.

Many different types of Salmonella (about 2,000) cause food poisoning or ENTERITIS, from eight hours to three days after ingestion of food in which they have multiplied. *S. brendeny, S. enteritidis, S. heidelberg, S. newport, S. thompson* are among those commonly causing enteritis. Salmonella infections are common in domesticated animals such as cows, pigs and poultry whose meat and milk may be infected, although the animals may show no symptoms. Duck eggs may harbour Salmonella (usually *S. typhimurium*), arising from surface contamination with the bird's faeces, and foods containing uncooked or lightly cooked hen's eggs, such as mayonnaise, have been associated with enteritis. The incidence of human *S. enteritidis* infection has been increasing (fifteenfold in England and Wales, from 1,101 to 31,000 cases annually between 1982 and 1993), with a sharp rise in phage type-4 isolates. A serious source of infection seems to be poultry meat and hen's eggs.

Although Salmonella are mostly killed by heating at 60 °C for 15 minutes, contaminated food requires considerably longer cooking and, if frozen, must be completely thawed beforehand, to allow even heating at a sufficient temperature.

Enteritis caused by *Campylobacter jejuni* is usually self-limiting, lasting one to three days. Since reporting of the disease began in 1977, in England and Wales its incidence has increased from 1,349 reports initially to 12,822 in 1982 to over 34,000 in the early 1990s. Outbreaks have been associated with unpasteurized milk: the main source seems to be infected poultry.

Escherichia coli O157 was first identified as a cause of food poisoning in the early 1980s, but its incidence has increased sharply since, with over 1,100 cases in the United Kingdom in 1996. The illness can be severe, with bloody diarrhoea and life-threatening renal complications. The reservoir for this pathogen is thought to be cattle, and transmission results from consumption of raw or undercooked meat products and raw dairy products. Cross-infection of cooked meets by raw meat is a common cause of outbreaks of *Escherichia coli* O157 food poisoning. Water and other foods can be contaminated by manure from cattle, and person-to-person spread can occur, especially in children.

Food poisoning associated with fried or boiled rice is caused by *Bacillus cereus*, whose heat-resistant spores survive cooking. An enterotoxin is responsible for the symptoms, which occur two to eight hours after ingestion and resolve after eight to twenty-four hours.

Viruses are emerging as an increasing cause of some outbreaks of food poisoning from shellfish (cockles, mussels, and oysters).

Public-health measures to control the incidence of food poisoning include agricultural aspects of food production, implementing standards of hygiene in abattoirs and regulating the environment and process of industrial food production, handling, transportation, and storage.

FOOD STANDARDS AGENCY An independent agency planned by the UK government. The aim is for the agency to protect consumers' interests in every aspect of food safety and nutrition. Some food policy functions may be transferred from the Ministry of Agriculture, Fisheries and Food to the Department of Health. The agency is likely to advise ministers and the food industry, conduct research and surveillance and monitor enforcement of food safety and hygiene laws.

FOOT That portion of the lower limb situated below the ankle-joint. Its structure is similar to that of the hand. There are seven tarsal bones, of which the talus, supporting the leg bones, and the calcaneus, forming the heel, are the largest. The others are the navicular, three cuneiform, and the cuboid bones. Then comes a row of five metatarsal bones (known together as the metatarsus), and finally fourteen phalanges contained in the toes, the great toe having two only, while each of the others has three. The arrangement of the arteries and nerves is similar to the found in the hand and fingers.

The arch of the foot is a most important structure. The bones are so arranged that the sole is hollow both from before back and from side to side. In walking, the outer edge only, at the middle of the sole, should touch the ground. The arch is further supported by a short plantar ligament situated in the hollow of the arch, running from the calcaneus to the cuboid bone, and by a long plantar ligament situated nearer the surface. It is also slung up by two sinews on either side, coming from muscles in the leg, the two tibial muscles on the inner side, and the two peroneal muscles on the outer side. When this arch gives way, FLAT-FOOT is the result.

For diseases of the foot see BONE, DISEASES OF; CHAFING OF THE SKIN; CHILBLAIN; CLAW-FOOT; CLEFT-FOOT; CLUB-FOOT; CORNS AND BUNIONS; DROP-FOOT; FLAT-FOOT; GOUT; HALLUX RIGIDUS; HALLUX VALGUS; MALLET TOE; METATARSUS for metatarsus varus; METATARSALGIA; NAILS, DISEASES OF.

FORAMEN The Latin term for a hole. It is especially applied to natural openings in bones, such as the foramen magnum, the large opening in the base of the skull through which the brain and spinal cord are continuous.

FORCED DIURESIS A means of encouraging the renal excretion of a compound by altering the pH and increasing the volume of the urine. Occasionally used after drug overdoses, but potentially dangerous, and so only suitable where proper intensive monitoring of the patient is possible. Excretion of acid compounds, such as SALICYLATES, can be encouraged by raising the pH of the urine to $7 \cdot 5 – 8 \cdot 5$

by the administration of an alkali such as bicarbonate (forced alkali diuresis) and that of bases, such as AMPHETAMINES, by lowering the pH of the urine to $5 \cdot 5 – 6 \cdot 5$ by giving an acid such as ammonium chloride (forced acid diuresis).

FORCED FEEDING (see ENTERAL FEEDING).

FORCEPS Surgical instruments with a pincerlike action which are used for grasping objects firmly. There are many different designs for different uses. Obstetric forceps are designed to fit around the infant's head and allow traction to be applied to aid its delivery.

FORENSIC MEDICINE That branch of medicine concerned with matters of law and the solving of crimes, for example, by determining the cause of a death in suspicious circumstances or identifying a criminal by examining tissue found at the scene of a crime. The use of DNA identification to establish who was present at the 'scene of the crime' is now a widely used procedure in forensic medicine.

FORESKIN (see PREPUCE).

FORMALDEHYDE The *British Pharmacopoeia* preparation, Formaldehyde Solution, also known as FORMALIN, contains 34 to 38 per cent formaldehyde in water. It is a powerful antiseptic, and has also the power of hardening the tissues. The vapour is very irritating to the eyes and nose.

Uses For disinfection it is largely used in the form of a spray. It can also be vaporized by heat. One of its advantages is that it does not damage metals or fabrics. In 3 per cent solution in water it is used for the treatment of warts on the palms of the hands and the soles of the feet.

FORMULARY A list of formulae used as drugs and other medical preparations. The *British National Formulary* is an authoritative six-monthly publication containing information and advice on medicines and drugs. Published jointly by the British Medical Association and the Royal Pharmaceutical Society of Great Britain, with input from the Department of Health, it is distributed to all NHS doctors by the government. Many hospitals and general practices produce formularies for use by doctors working in those facilities.

FOSSA A term applied to various depressions or holes, both on the surface of the body and in internal parts, such as the iliac fossa in each lower corner of the abdomen, and the fossae within the skull which lodge the different parts of the brain.

FOVEA A small depression. In the eye this is an area near the fundus which contains predominantly cones and is the area with greatest visual acuity (see EYE; VISION).

FOXGLOVE (see DIGITALIS).

FRACTURES These occur when there is a break in the continuity of the bone. This happens either as a result of violence or because the bone is unhealthy and unable to withstand normal stresses.

Simple fracture Fracture where the skin remains intact or merely grazed.

Compound fractures have at least one wound which is in communication with the fracture which means that bacteria can enter the fracture site and cause infection. A compound fracture is also more serious because there is greater potential for blood loss. Compound fractures usually need hospital admission, antibiotics and careful reduction of the fracture. Debride-ment (cleaning and excising dead tissue) in a sterile theatre may also be necessary.

Examples of fractures: the fibula (thin bone) has a simple fracture of its shaft and a comminuted fracture at its lower end; the tibia has a compound fracture of its shaft.

The type of fracture depends on the force which has caused it. Direct violence occurs when an object hits the bone often causing a transverse break – which means the break runs horizontally across the bone.

Indirect violence occurs when a twisting injury to the ankle, for example, breaks the calf bone (the tibia) higher up. The break may be more oblique. A fall on the outstretched hand may cause a break at the wrist, in the humerus or at the collar-bone depending on the force of impact and age of the person.

Fatigue fractures These occur after the bone has been under recurrent stress. A typical

example is the March fracture of the second toe which army recruits suffer from after long marches.

Pathological fractures These occur in bone which is already diseased, for example, by osteoporosis in post-menopausal women. A woman has a one-in-two chance of suffering from an osteoporotic fracture in her lifetime. These fractures are typically crush fractures of the vertebrae, fractures of the neck of the femur, and COLLES fractures (wrist). Pathological fractures also occur in bone which has secondary-tumour deposits.

Greenstick fractures These occur in young children whose bones are soft and bend in response to stress rather than break. The bone tends to buckle on the side opposite to the force. These fractures heal quickly but still need any deformity corrected and plaster of Paris to maintain the correction.

Complicated fractures These involve damage to important soft tissue such as nerves, blood vessels or internal organs. In these cases the soft-tissue damage needs as much attention as the fracture site.

Comminuted fractures A fracture with more than two fragments. It usually means the injury was more violent and that there is more risk of vessels and nerves' being damaged. These fractures are unstable and take longer to unite. Rehabilitation tends to be protracted.

Depressed fractures Most commonly found in skull fractures. A fragment of bone is forced inwards so that it lies lower than the level of the bone surrounding it. It may damage the brain beneath it.

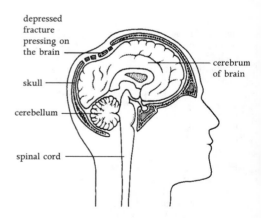

Depressed fracture of the skull (sagittal view).

Hair-line fractures These occur when the bone is broken but the force has not been severe enough to cause visible displacement. These fractures may be easily missed.

Symptoms and signs The fracture site is usually painful, swollen and deformed. There is asymmetry of contour between limbs. The limb is held uselessly. If the fracture is in the upper limb, the arm is usually supported by the patient, if it is in the lower limb the patient is not able to bear weight on it. The limb may appear short because of muscle spasm.

Examination may reveal crepitus – a bony grating – at the fracture site. The diagnosis is confirmed by radiography.

Treatment Healing of fractures (union) begins with the bruise around the fracture's being resorbed and new bone-producing cells and blood vessels migrating into the area. Within a couple of days they form a bridge of primitive bone across the fracture. This is called callus.

The callus is replaced by woven bone which gradually matures as the new bone remodels itself. Treatment of fractures is designed to ensure this process occurs with minimal residual deformity to the bone involved.

Treatment is initially to relieve pain and may involve temporary splinting of the fracture site. Reducing the fracture means restoring the bones to their normal position and this is particularly important at the site of joints where any small displacement may limit movement considerably. A Potts fracture at the ankle joint, for example, may also lead to early osteoarthritis if the congruity of the joint is not fully restored.

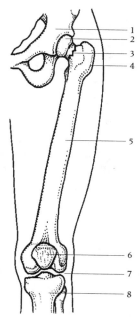

1   pubic bone
2   head of femur (ball and socket joint)
3   fracture of neck of femur
4   greater trochanter of femur
5   shaft of femur
6   patella (knee cap)
7   knee joint (hinge)
8   tibia

Impacted fracture of neck of left femur.

In children it is possible to accept a higher degree of deformity at the fracture site because childrens' bones re-model so well.

Reduction may be done under a general anaesthetic which relaxes muscles and makes manipulation easier. Traction, which means sustained but controlled pulling on the bone, then restores the fragments of the fracture into their normal position. They are then kept in position with plaster of Paris. If closed traction does not work, then open reduction of the fracture may be needed. This may involve fixing the fracture with internal-fixation methods, using metal plates, wires or screws.

This holds the fracture site in a rigid position with the two ends closely opposed. It allows early mobilization after fractures and speeds return to normal use.

External fixators are usually metal devices applied to the outside of the limb to support the fracture site. They are useful in compound fractures where internal fixators are at risk of becoming infected.

Consolidation of a fracture means that repair is complete. The time taken for this depends on the age of the patient, the bone and the type of fracture. A wrist fracture may take six weeks, a femoral fracture three to six months in an adult.

Complications of fractures are fairly common. In non-union the fracture does not unite usually because there has been too much mobility around the fracture site. Treatment may involve internal fixation. Mal-union means that the bone has healed with a persistent deformity and the adjacent joint may then develop early osteoarthritis. Sudeck's atrophy typically occurs after the plaster of Paris cast has been removed from Colles fractures of the wrist. The fingers remain swollen and the wrist is tender. It tends to resolve after six months.

Myositis ossificans commonly occurs at the elbow after a fracture. A big mass of calcified material develops round the fracture site which restricts elbow movements. Late surgical removal (after six to twelve months) is recommended.

Fractured neck of FEMUR typically affects elderly women after a trivial injury. The bone is usually osteoporotic. The leg appears short and is rotated outwards. Usually the patient is unable to put any weight on the affected leg and is in extreme pain. The fractures are classified under Garden's classification which identifies the fractures most likely to result in cutting off the blood supply to the femoral head. Most of these fractures of the neck of femur need fixing by metal plates or hip replacements as immobility in this age group has a mortality of nearly 100 per cent.

In fractures of the SPINAL COLUMN mere damage to the bone, as in the case of the so-called compression fracture, in which there is no damage to the spinal cord, is not necessarily serious. If, however, the spinal cord is damaged, as in the so-called fracture dislocation, the accident may be a very serious one, the usual result being paralysis of the parts of the body below the level

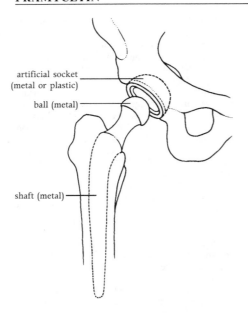

artificial socket
(metal or plastic)

ball (metal)

shaft (metal)

Artificial hip joint showing how the ball of the
prosthesis inserted in the femur fits into the
artificial socket sited in the pubis bone.

T11

T12

L1

L2

T11 Thoracic 11
T12 Thoractic 12
L1 Lumbar 1
L2 Lumbar 2

Injury to the spine: compression fracture of
first lumbar vertebra with no damage to
spinal cord

T11

T12

L1

L2

T11 Thoracic 11
T12 Thoracic 12
L1 Lumbar 1
L2 Lumbar 2

Injury to the spine: fracture/dislocation of
twelfth thoracic vertebra with damage to
spinal cord.

of the injury. Therefore the higher up the spine
is fractured, the more serious the consequences.
The injured person should not be moved till
skilled assistance is at hand, or, if he must be
removed, this should be done on a rigid shutter
or door, not on a canvas stretcher or rug, and
there should be no lifting which necessitates
bending of the back. In such an injury an
operation designed to remove a displaced piece
of bone and free the spinal cord from pressure is
often necessary and successful in relieving the
paralysis. DISLOCATION or SUBLUXATION of the
spine is not uncommon in certain sports, particularly rugby. Anyone who has had such an injury
in the cervical spine (i.e. in the neck) should be
strongly advised not to return to any form of
body-contact sport or vehicular sport.

Simple fissured fractures and depressed fractures of the skull often follow blows or falls on
the head, and may not be serious, though there
is always a risk of damage which is potentially
serious to the brain at the same time.

Compound fractures may result in infection
within the skull, and if the skull is extensively
broken and depressed, surgery is usually required
to check any intercranial bleeding or to relieve
pressure on the brain. Another risk of fracture is
that some of the small arteries on
the inner surface of the skull may be torn and may
bleed, thus causing compression of the brain. For
this reason also the skull is often TREPHINED.

Jaw The lower jaw is often fractured by a
blow on the face. There is generally bleeding
from the mouth, the gum being torn. Also there
are pain and grating sensations on chewing,
and unevenness in the line of the teeth. The
treatment is simple, the line of teeth in the upper
jaw forming a splint, against which the lower
jaw is bound, with the mouth closed.

FRAMYCETIN A broad-spectrum antibiotic
derived from *Streptomyces decaris*. It is active
against a wide range of organisms, and is used
in drops to treat infections of the eyes and ears.

FRECKLES (EPHELIDES) These require no
description. They occur mostly in blond or red-
haired subjects in exposed areas and darken on

sun exposure. MELANOCYTES are not increased in the basal layer of the EPIDERMIS.

FREMITUS Tremors or vibrations in an area of the body, detected by palpating (feeling) with the fingers or the hand or by auscultation (listening). The procedure is most commonly used when examining the chest and assessing what happens when the patient breathes, coughs or speaks. This helps the doctor to diagnose whether disorders such as fluid in the pleural cavity or solidification of a section of the lung have occurred.

Friction fremitus is a grating feeling communicated to the hand by the movements of lungs or heart when the membrane covering them is roughened, as in pleurisy or pericarditis. Vocal fremitus means the sensation felt by the hand when a person speaks; it is increased when the lung is more solid than usual. The 'thrills' felt over a heart affected by valvular disease are also varieties of fremitus.

FREUDIAN THEORY A theory that emotional and allied diseases are due to a psychic injury or trauma, generally of a sexual nature, which did not produce an adequate reaction when it was received and therefore remains as a subconscious or 'affect' memory to trouble the patient's mind. As an extension of this theory Freudian treatment consists in encouraging the patient to tell everything that happens to be associated with trains of thought which lead up to this memory, thus securing a 'purging' of the mind from the original 'affect memory' which is the cause of the symptoms. This form of treatment is also called psychocatharsis or abreaction. The general term, psychoanalysis, is applied, in the first place, to the method of helping the patient to recover buried memories by free association of thoughts. In the second place, the term is applied to the body of psychological knowledge and theory accumulated and devised by Sigmund Freud (1856–1939) and his followers. The term 'psychoanalyst' has traditionally been applied to those who have undergone Freudian training, but Freud's ideas are being increasingly questioned by some modern psychiatrists.

FRICTION The name given either to the fremitus felt, or to the grating noise heard, when two rough surfaces of the body move over one another. It is characteristically obtained over the chest in cases of dry pleurisy.

FRIEDREICH'S ATAXIA A hereditary disease resembling locomotor ataxia, and due to degenerative changes in nerve tracts and nerve cells of the spinal cord and the brain. It occurs usually in children, or at any rate before the twentieth year of life, and affects often several brothers and sisters. Its chief symptoms are unsteadiness of gait, with loss of the knee jerks, followed later by difficulties of speech, tremors of the hands, head, and eyes, deformity of the feet, and curvature of the spine. There is often associated heart disease. The sufferer gets gradually worse, but may live, with increasing disability, for twenty or thirty years.

FRÖHLICH'S SYNDROME A condition in children characterized by obesity, physical sluggishness, and retarded sexual development. It is the result of disturbed pituitary function.

FRONTAL BONE The bone which forms the forehead and protects the frontal lobes of the brain. Before birth, the frontal bone consists of two halves, and this division may persist throughout life, a deep groove remaining down the centre of the forehead. Above each eye is a heavy ridge in the bone, most marked in men, and, behind this, in the substance of the bone, is a cavity on each side, the frontal sinus, which communicates with the nose. Catarrh in these cavities produces the frontal headache characteristic of a 'cold in the head', and sometimes infection develops known as SINUSITIS. (See NOSE, DISEASES OF.)

FRONTAL LOBE The anterior part of the cerebral hemisphere as far back as the central sulcus. It contains the motor cortex and the parts of the brain concerned with personality, behaviour and learning. (See BRAIN.)

FROSTBITE This results from the action of extreme cold (below 0 °C) on the skin. VASOCONSTRICTION results in the reduced blood – and hence, oxygen supply – leading to necrosis of the skin and, in severe cases, the underlying tissues. Chiefly affecting exposed parts of the body, such as the face, and the limbs, it occurs especially in people exercising at high altitudes, or in those at risk of peripheral vascular disease, such as diabetics, who should take particular care of their fingers and toes when in cold situations.

In mild cases, the condition sometimes known as frostnip, the skin on exposed parts of the body, such as the cheeks or nose, becomes white and numb with a sudden and complete cessation of cold and discomfort. In more severe cases blisters develop on the frozen part, and the skin then gradually hardens and turns black until the frozen part, such as a finger, is covered with a black shell of dead tissue. Swelling of the underlying tissue occurs and this is accompanied by throbbing and aching. If, as is often the case, only the skin and the tissues immediately under it are frozen, then in a matter of months the dead tissue peels off. In the most severe cases of all, muscles, bone and tendon are also frozen, and the affected part becomes cold, swollen, mottled and blue or grey. There may be no blistering in these severe cases. At first there is no pain, but in time shooting and throbbing pains usually develop.

Prevention This consists of wearing the right clothing and never venturing on even quite short expeditions in cold weather, particularly on mountains, without taking expert advice as to what should be worn.

Treatment Frostnip is the only form of frostbite that should be treated on the spot. As it usually occurs on exposed parts, such as the face, each member of the party should be on the look out for it in the other. The moment whitening of the skin is seen, the individual should seek shelter and warm the affected part by covering it with his warm hand or a glove until the normal colour and consistency of the affected part are restored. In more severe cases treatment should only be given in hospital or a well-equipped camp. In essentials this consists of warming the affected part, preferably in warm water, against a warm part of the body or warm air. Rewarming should be done for spells of twenty minutes at a time. The affected part should never be placed near an open fire. Generalized warming of the whole body may also be necessary, using hot drinks, and putting the victim in a sleeping bag.

FROZEN SHOULDER A painful condition of the shoulder accompanied by stiffness and considerable limitation of movement. The usual age-incidence is between 50 and 70. The cause is not known. There is no specific treatment, but there is practically always complete recovery, even though this may take twelve to eighteen months.

FRUCTOSE is another name for laevulose, or fruit sugar, which is found along with glucose in most sweet fruits. It is sweeter than sucrose (cane or beet sugar) and this has led to its use as a sweetener.

FRUSEMIDE A potent loop DIURETIC with a rapid onset (30 minutes), and short duration, of action. (See BENZOTHIADIAZINES, DIURETICS.)

FUGUE The term literally means flight and it is used to describe the mental condition in which an individual is suddenly seized with an unconscious motivation to flee from some intolerable reality of everyday existence. This usually involves some agonizing interpersonal relationship. As a rule, it lasts for a matter of hours or days, but may go on for weeks or even months. During the fugue the individual seldom behaves in a particularly odd manner though he may be considered somewhat eccentric. When it is over there is no remembrance of events during the fugue.

Three types of fugue have been identified: (a) hysterical; (b) a manifestation of depression; (c) manifestation of organic mental state such as occurs after an epileptic seizure.

FUMIGATION A means of disinfection by the vapour of powerful antiseptics. (See DISINFECTION).

FUNCTIONAL DISEASES (see PSYCHOSOMATIC DISEASES).

FUNDUS (1) The base of an organ or that part remote from its opening. (2) Point on the retina opposite the pupil through which nerve fibres and blood vessels traverse the retina (see EYE).

FUNGAL INFECTIONS (MYCOSES). The various forms of tinea are caused by multicellular fungi called DERMATOPHYTES which may infect skin, hair or nails (see RINGWORM). PITYRIASIS versicolor and CANDIDOSIS (moniliasis) (see CANDIDA) are caused by unicellular fungi which reproduce by budding (YEASTS). Other fungi, such as ACTINOMYCOSIS, may cause deep systemic infections. Generalized systemic in-fections with candida are rare, and are usually associated with intense IMMUNOSUPPRESSION or antibiotic therapy.

Treatment Confirmation of a suspected diagnosis is obtained by swabbing the lesion. Treatment is usually topical, using nystatin for candida, or miconazole cream or powder for either. Persistent, or severe dermatophyte skin and nail infections require oral anti-fungal therapy with terbinafine (see FUNGUS; MICROBIOLOGY).

FUNGUS A simple plant that is parasitic on other plants and animals. Included in this group are mildews, moulds, mushrooms, toadstools and yeasts. Unlike other plants they do not contain the green pigment chlorophyll. Most of the world's 100,000 different species are harmless or even beneficial to humans. Yeasts are used in the preparation of food and drinks and antibiotics are obtained from some fungi. A few, however, can cause fatal disease and illness in humans.

FUNGUS-POISONING About 2,000 mushrooms (toadstools) grow in England, of which 200 are edible and a dozen are classified as poisonous. Not all the poisonous ones are dangerous. It is obviously better to prevent mushroom poisoning by ensuring correct identification of those that are edible and books and charts are available. If in doubt, do not eat a fungus.

Severe poisoning from ingestion of fungi is very rare, since relatively few species are highly toxic and most species do not contain toxic compounds. The most toxic species are those containing amatoxins such as death cap (*Amanita phalloides*); this species alone is responsible for about 90 per cent of all mushroom-related deaths. There is a latent period of six hours or more between ingestion and the onset of clinical effects with these more toxic species. The small intestine, LIVER and KIDNEYS may be damaged. Therefore any patient with gastrointestinal effects thought to be due to ingestion of a mushroom should be referred immediately to hospital where GASTRIC LAVAGE and treatment with activated charcoal can be carried out, along with parenteral fluids and haemodialysis if the victim is severely ill. In most cases where effects occur, these are early onset gastro-intestinal effects due to ingestion of mush-rooms containing gastrointestinal irritants.

Muscarine is the poisonous constituent of some species. Within two hours of ingesting it, the victim starts salivating and sweating, has visual disturbances, vomiting, stomach cramps, diarrhoea, vertigo, confusion, hallucinations and coma, the severity of symptoms depending on the amount eaten and type of mushroom. Most people recover in 24 hours with treat-ment.

'Magic' mushrooms are a variety that con-tains psilocybin, a hallucinogenic substance. Children who take such mushrooms may de-velop a high fever and need medical care. In adults the symptoms usually disappear within six hours.

Treatment If possible, early GASTRIC LAVAGE should be carried out in all cases of suspected poisoning. Identification of the mushroom spe-cies is a valuable guide to treatment. For muscarine poisoning, ATROPINE is a specific antidote. As stated above, hospital referral is advisable for people who have ingested poison-ous fungi.

FUNNEL CHEST   (see CHEST DEFORMITIES).

FUNNYBONE   Colloquial name for the small area at the back of the elbow where the ULNAR nerve goes over a prominence at the lower end of the HUMERUS bone. If the nerve is hit, acute pain results, accompanied by tingling in the forearm and hand.

FURUNCLE   Another term for a BOIL.

FUSIDIC ACID   A valuable antistaphylo-coccal antibiotic used both orally and topically. It is particularly useful in osteomyelitis (see BONE, DISEASES OF).

G

GABA Gamma aminobutyric acid is an amino acid that occurs in the central nervous system, mainly in the brain tissue. It is a chemical substance that transmits inhibitory impulses from nerve endings across synapses to other nerves or tissues.

GAG A device that when placed between a person's teeth keeps the mouth open.

GAG REFLEX Assessment of victims of major trauma must include maintenance of their airways and breathing. Any false teeth, vomitus and foreign bodies should be removed and the response to digital stimulation of the posterior pharyngeal wall – the 'gag reflex' – assessed. Even with a normal gag reflex, the airway may be seriously threatened if vomiting occurs. During the initial stages of resuscitation, care-ful and constant supervision of the airway is essential, with a high-volume sucker immedi-ately available. If the gag reflex is absent or impaired, an ENDOTRACHEAL tube should be inserted.

GAIT The way in which an individual walks. It may be affected by inherited disorders, by illness – especially neurological disorders – by injury or by drugs and alcohol abuse. Children, as a rule, begin to walk between the ages of twelve and eighteen months, having learned to stand before the end of the first year. If a normal-sized child shows no ability to make movements by this time the possibility of his being mentally retarded must be borne in mind, and if the power of walking is not gained by the time the child is a year and a half old, rickets, cerebral palsy, or a malformation of the hip-joint must be excluded. (See RICKETS; PARALY-SIS.)

In hemiplegia, or paralysis down one side of the body following a STROKE, the person drags the paralysed leg.

Steppage gait occurs in certain cases of alcoholic neuritis, tertiary syphilis (tabes) and other conditions where the muscles that raise the foot are weak and the toes in consequence droop. The person bends the knee and lifts the foot high, so that the toes may clear obstacles on the ground. (See DROP-FOOT.)

In LOCOMOTOR ATAXIA or tabes dorsalis the sensations derived from the lower limbs are blunted, and consequently the movements of the legs are uncertain and the heels planted on the ground with unnecessary force. When the person tries to turn or stands with the eyes shut he may fall over. When he walks he feels for the ground with a stick or keeps his eyes constantly fixed upon it.

In spastic paralysis the limbs are moved with jerks. The foot first of all clings to the ground and then leaves it with a spasmodic movement, being raised much higher than necessary.

In PARKINSONISM the movements are tremu-lous, and as the person takes very short steps, he has the peculiarity of appearing constantly to fall forward, or to be chasing himself.

In CHOREA the walk is bizarre and jerky, the affected child often seeming to leave one leg a step behind him, and then, with a screwing movement on the other heel, go on again.

Hysterical disorders of gait are usually of a striking nature, quite different from those occuring in any neurological conditions. They tend to draw attention to the patient, and are worse when he or she is observed.

GALACTOCELE A cyst-like swelling in the breast which forms as a result of obstruction in the milk-duct draining the swollen area.

GALACTORRHOEA This term may refer to unusually copious secretion of milk from the mamary glands when a mother is feeding her baby. It is also used to describe secretion of milk after the mother has stopped breast feeding.

GALACTOSAEMIA A very rare, recessively inherited disease, with an incidence of around 1 in 75,000 births. Its importance lies in the disastrous consequences of being overlooked. It results from the deficiency of an enzyme, essential for the metabolism of GALACTOSE. Normal at birth, affected infants soon develop jaundice, vomiting, diarrhoea, and fail to thrive on starting milk feeds. If the disorder remains unrecognized, liver disease, cataracts, and mental retardation result. Treatment consists of a lactose-free diet, and special lactose-free milks are now available.

GALACTOSE A constituent of lactose, galactose is a simple sugar that is changed in the liver to glucose. A rare genetic metabolic disease, GALACTOSAEMIA, results in infants' being unable to do this conversion because the enzyme necessary for the reaction is absent.

GALL Another name for bile. (See BILE.)

GALL-BLADDER (see LIVER).

GALL-BLADDER, DISEASES OF The gall-bladder rests on the underside of the liver and joins the common hepatic duct via the cystic duct to form the common bile duct. The gall-bladder acts as a reservoir and concentrator of bile, alterations in the composition of which may result in the formation of gall-stones, the commonest disease of the gall-bladder.

Gall-stones affect 22 per cent of women and 11 per cent of men. The incidence increases with age, but only about 30 per cent of those with gall-stones undergo treatment as the majority of cases are asymptomatic. There are three types of stone: cholesterol, pigment and mixed, depending upon their composition; stones are usually mixed and may contain calcium deposits. The cause of most cases is not clear but sometimes gall-stones will form around a 'foreign body' within the bile ducts or gall-bladder, such as suture material.

BILIARY COLIC Muscle fibres in the biliary system contract around a stone in the cystic duct or common bile duct producing pain in the right upper quarter of the abdomen, with nausea and occasionally vomiting.

JAUNDICE Gall-stones small enough to enter the common bile duct may block the flow of bile and cause jaundice.

ACUTE CHOLECYSTITIS Blockage of the cystic duct may lead to this; the gall-bladder wall becomes inflamed resulting in pain in the right upper quarter of the abdomen, fever and an increase in the white blood cell count. There is characteristically tenderness over the tip of the right ninth rib on deep inhalation (Murphy's sign). Infection of the gall-bladder may accompany the acute inflammation and occasionally an empyema of the gall-bladder may result.

CHRONIC CHOLECYSTITIS A more insidious form of gall-bladder inflammation, producing nonspecific symptoms of abdominal pain, nausea and flatulence which may be worse after a fatty meal.

DIAGNOSIS Stones are usually diagnosed on the basis of the patient's reported symptoms, although asymptomatic gall-stones are often an incidental finding when investigating another complaint. Confirmatory investigations include abdominal radiography – although many gall-stones are not calcified and thus do not show up on these images; ultrasound scanning (see ULTRASOUND), oral cholecystography, which entails a patient's swallowing a substance opaque to X-rays which is concentrated in the gall-bladder, and endoscopic retrograde cholangio-pancreatography (ERCP) – a technique in which an ENDOSCOPE is passed into the duodenum and a contrast medium injected into the biliary duct.

TREATMENT Biliary colic is treated conservatively with bed rest and injection of morphine-like analgesics. Once the pain has subsided, the patient may then be referred for further treatment as outlined below. Acute cholecystitis is treated by surgical removal of the gall-bladder within 2–3 days of admission to hospital. There are two techniques available for this procedure; firstly, conventional cholecystectomy in which the abdomen is opened and the gall-bladder cut out and, secondly, laparoscopic cholecystectomy in which fibreoptic instruments called endoscopes (see FIBREOPTIC ENDOSCOPY) are introduced into the abdominal cavity via several small incisions (see MINIMALLY INVASIVE SURGERY). Laparoscopic surgery has the advantage of reducing the patient's recovery time. Gall-stones may be removed during ERCP, they can be dissolved using ultrasound waves (lithotripsy) or tablet therapy (dissolution chemotherapy), Pigment stones, calcified stones or stones larger than 15 mm in diameter are not suitable for this treatment, which is also less likely to succeed in the overweight patient. Drug treatment is prolonged but stones can disappear completely after two years. Stones may reform on stopping therapy. The drugs used are derivatives of bile salts, particularly chenodeoxycholic acid; side-effects include diarrhoea and liver damage.

Other disorders of the gall-bladder These are rare.

POLYPS may form and, if symptomatic, should be removed. Malignant change is rare.

CARCINOMA of the gall-bladder is a disease of the elderly and is almost exclusively associated with gall-stones. By the time such a cancer has produced symptoms, the prognosis is bleak: 80 per cent of these patients die within one year of diagnosis. If the tumour is discovered early, 60 per cent of patients will survive five years.

GALL-STONES (see GALL-BLADDER, DISEASES OF.)

GAMETE A sexual or germ cell: for example, an OVUM or SPERMATOZOON.

GAMETE INTRAFALLOPIAN TRANSFER (GIFT) A method of helping infertile women to become pregnant. In over half of women diagnosed as infertile their FALLOPIAN TUBES are normal and there are other reasons for failure to conceive. ENDOMETRIOSIS is a common cause. Needle aspiration under laparoscopic or ULTRASONIC control is used remove OVA from the ovary. The ova are mixed with the partner's spermatozoa and introduced into the Fallopian tube so that fertilization can take place, after which the ovum becomes implanted in the wall of the uterus and pregnancy can proceed. Sometimes it is necessary to stimulate the ovary to produce ova by the use of drugs. A variation of GIFT is zygote intrafallopian transfer (ZIFT) in which early development of the fertilized ova is observed in the laboratory before the young embryo is transferred to the Fallopian tubes. About half of women professionally treated for infertility succeed in becoming pregnant.

GAMGEE TISSUE is a surgical dressing composed of a thick layer of cotton-wool between two layers of absorbent gauze, introduced by the Birmingham surgeon, Sampson Gamgee (1828–1886). (Gamgee Tissue has been a registered trade mark since 1911.)

GAMMA AMINOBUTYRIC ACID (GABA) An AMINO-ACID occurring naturally in the central nervous system, mainly in brain tissue where it functions as an inhibitory NEUROTRANSMITTER.

GAMMA BENZENE HEXACHLORIDE A drug that is used in the treatment of PEDICULOSIS and SCABIES.

GAMMA-GLOBULIN describes a group of proteins present in the blood PLASMA. They are characterized by their rate of movement in an electrical field and can be separated by the process of ELECTROPHORESIS. Most gamma-globulins are IMMUNOGLOBULINS. Gamma-globulin injection provides passive or active immunity against HEPATITIS A. (See GLOBULIN, IMMUNITY and IMMUNOLOGY.)

GAMMA RAYS Short-wavelength penetrating electromagnetic rays produced by some radioactive compounds. More powerful than X-rays, they are used in certain RADIOTHERAPY treatments and to sterilize some materials.

GAMMEXANE The proprietary name for a synthetic insecticide which is a formulation of benzene hexachloride. It is active against a large range of insects and pests, including mosquitoes, fleas, lice, cockroaches, house-flies, clothes moths, bed-bugs, ants, and grain pests.

GANGLION This term is used in two senses. In anatomy, it means an aggregation of nerve-cells found in the course of certain nerves (see NERVES). In surgery, it means an enlargement of the sheath of a tendon, containing fluid. The latter occurs particularly in connection with the sinews in front of, and behind, the wrist.

Causes The cause of these dilatations on the tendon-sheaths is either some irregular growth of the synovial membrane which lines them and secretes the fluid that lubricates their movements, or the forcing out of a small pouch of this membrane through the sheath in consequence of a strain. In either case a bag-like swelling forms, whose connection with the synovial sheath becomes cut off, so that synovial fluid collects in it and distends it more and more.

Symptoms A soft, elastic, movable swelling forms, most often on the back of the wrist. It is usually small and gives no problems. Sometimes weakness and discomfort may develop. A ganglion which forms in connection with the flexor tendons in front of the wrist sometimes attains a large size, and extends down to form another swelling in the palm of the hand.

Treatment Sudden pressure with the thumbs may often burst a ganglion and disperse its contents beneath the skin. If this fails, surgical excision is necessary but, as the ganglion may disappear spontaneously, there should be no rush to remove it unless it is causing inconvenience or pain.

GANGRENE The death and decay of body tissues caused by a deficiency or cessation of the blood supply. There are two types, dry and moist. The former is a process of mummification, with the blood supply of the affected area of tissue stopping the tissue withering up. Moist gangrene is characterized by death and putrefactive tissue decay caused by bacterial infection. The dead part, when formed of soft tissues, is called a slough and, when part of a bone, is called a sequestrum.

Causes These include injury – especially injuries caused in war – disease, frostbite, severe burns, ATHEROMA in large blood vessels and diseases, such as DIABETES MELLITUS and RAYNAUD'S DISEASE. Gas gangrene is a form that occurs when injuries are infected with soil contaminated with gas-producing bacilli such as *Clostridium welchii*, which are found in well-cultivated ground.

Treatment Dry gangrene must be kept dry and amputation of the dead tissue done when a clear demarcation line with healthy tissue has formed. Wet gangrene requires urgent surgery and prompt use of appropriate antibiotics.

GARGLES Gargling is a process by which various substances in solution are brought in contact with the throat without being swallowed. The watery solutions used for the purpose are called gargles. Gargles are used in the symptomatic treatment of infections of the throat: i.e. 'sore throat', pharyngitis, and tonsillitis.

GARGOYLISM (also known as HURLER'S SYNDROME) is a rare condition due to lack of a specific ENZYME. It is a progressive disorder usually leading to death before the age of 10 years. The affected child is usually normal during the first few months of life. Mental and physical deterioration then set in. The characteristic features include coarse facial features (hence the name of the condition), retarded growth, chest deformity, stiff joints, clouding of the cornea, enlargement of the liver and spleen, deafness, and heart murmurs, with mental deterioration. It occurs in about 1 in 100,000 births.

GAS (see ANAESTHESIA; CARBON MONOXIDE; NITROUS OXIDE GAS).

GAS GANGRENE (see GANGRENE).

GASTRECTOMY An operation for removal of the whole or part of the stomach. The main indication is in the treatment of peptic ulcers (see STOMACH, DISEASES OF) when complications – especially malignant change – supervene. Total gastrectomy is usually carried out for stomach cancer and the OESOPHAGUS is connected to the DUODENUM. In a partial or subtotal gastrectomy the upper third or half of the stomach is linked to the small intestine. Commonly used to treat severe peptic ulceration before the advent of effective drug treatment in the shape of H_2 receptor antagonists like CIMETIDINE which reduce gastric-acid output, gastrectomy is now used much more selectively. Although most patients are satisfied with the final result, several unpleasant post-gastrectomy syndromes may occur.

GASTRIC Anything connected with the stomach, such as gastric ulcer.

GASTRIC LAVAGE A method of gastric decontamination used in the treatment of POISONING. It is not used routinely. Lavage involves the passage of a lubricated tube via the mouth and oesophagus into the stomach. Patients are positioned on their side with the head lower than the feet. A small quantity of fluid (300 ml) is passed into the stomach and the contents then drained out (by gravity) by lowering the end of the tube. This is repeated until the solution is clear of particulate matter. The procudure should be done only by an experienced health professional.

GASTRIC ULCER (see STOMACH, DISEASES OF).

GASTRIN A hormone produced by the MUCOUS MEMBRANE in the pyloric part of the STOMACH. The arrival of food stimulates production of the hormone which in turn stimulates the production of gastric juice.

GASTRITIS Inflammation of the stomach lining. This may take an acute form when excess alcohol or other irritating substances have been taken, resulting in vomiting. Chronic gastritis may be the result of regular smoking and chronic alcoholism or the condition may be caused by the back flow of BILE from the DUODENUM. The common cause, however, is chronic infection with HELICOBACTER PYLORI. Symptoms are vague but victims are likely to develop gastric ulcers or sometimes cancer. Atrophic gastritis, when the mucosal lining of the stomach withers away, may follow chronic gastritis but sometimes occurs as an AUTOIMMUNE disorder.

GASTROCNEMIUS The large double muscle which forms the chief bulk of the calf, and ends below in the tendo calcaneus.

GASTROENTERITIS Inflammation of the stomach and intestines, usually resulting from an acute bacterial or viral infection. Although generally a mild disease in western countries, it is still reputed to be the fifth commonest cause of death in the UK in children under 1 year, with epidemics of *E. coli* gastroenteritis being particularly serious in neonatal units. The main symptoms are diarrhoea and vomiting, often accompanied by fever and – especially in infants – dehydration. These represent an enormous health problem in developing countries, with over 1·5 million children dying annually from the disease in India – a situation exacerbated by early weaning and malnutrition. Complications may include convulsions, kidney failure, and, in severe cases, brain damage.

Treatment This involves the urgent correction of dehydration, using intravenous saline and dextrose feeds initially, with continuing replacement as required. Antibiotics are not indicated unless systemic spread of bacterial infection is likely. (See FOOD POISONING.)

GASTROENTEROSTOMY An operation performed usually in order to relieve some obstruction to the outlet from the stomach, and consists in making one opening in the lower part of the stomach, another in a neighbouring loop of the small intestine, and stitching the two together.

GASTRO-OESOPHAGEAL REFLUX A disorder in which the contents of the stomach back up into the oesophagus because the usual neuromuscular mechanisms for preventing this are intermittently or permanently failing to work properly. If persistent, the failure may cause OESOPHAGITIS (see OESOPHAGUS, DISEASES OF). If a person develops HEARTBURN, regurgitation, discomfort and OESOPHAGITIS, the condition is called gastro-oesophageal reflux disease and sometimes symptoms are so serious as to warrant surgery. Gastro-oesophageal reflux is sometimes associated with HIATUS HERNIA.

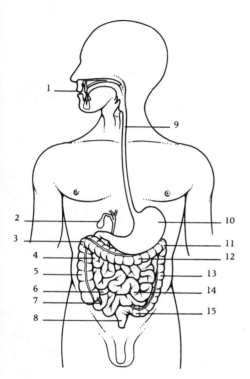

1 mouth	9 oesophagus
2 gall-bladder	10 stomach
3 hepatic flexure	11 splenic flexure
4 duodenum	12 transverse colon
5 ascending colon	13 descending colon
6 ileum	14 jejunum
7 appendix	15 sigmoid flexure
8 rectum	

Gastrointestinal tract.

GASTROINTESTINAL TRACT The passage along which the food passes, in which it is digested (see DIGESTION), and from which it is absorbed by lymphatics and blood-vessels into the circulation. The tract consists of the mouth, pharynx or throat, oesophagus or gullet, stomach, small intestine, and large intestine, in this order. For details see articles under these heads. The total length is about 9 metres in man.

GASTROSCOPE An instrument for viewing the interior of the stomach, by means of a special arrangement of light and mirrors at-

tached to a hollow tube, which is introduced into the stomach via the mouth and gullet. A special camera attachment makes it possible to photograph the interior of the stomach. The modern instruments are fully flexible, transmitting an image through a fibreoptic bundle or by a small videocamera. The operator can see and photograph all areas of the stomach and also take biopsy specimens when required. (See FIBREOPTIC ENDOSCOPY.)

GASTROSTOMY An operation on the stomach by which, when the gullet is blocked by a tumour or other cause, an opening is made from the front of the abdomen into the stomach, so that fluid food can be passed into the organ.

GAUCHER'S DISEASE A disease characterized by abnormal storage of LIPIDS, particularly in the SPLEEN, central nervous system, BONE MARROW, and LIVER. This results in enlargement of the spleen and the liver, particularly the former, and anaemia. It runs a chronic course. Diagnosis is usually by skin fibroblast glucocerebrosidase assay. Death often results from pneumonia or bleeding. Infantile Gaucher's often presents with marked neurological signs of rigid neck DYSPHAGIA, CATATONIA, hyperreflexia and low IQ. The disease can now be treated with enzyme replacement using alglucerase, but the annual cost per patient is substantial.

GEL The term applied to a colloid substance which is firm in consistence although it contains much water: e.g ordinary gelatin.

GELATIN This is derived from COLLAGEN, the chief constituent of connective tissue. It is a colourless transparent substance which dissolves in boiling water, and on cooling sets into a jelly. Such a jelly is a pleasant addition to the invalid diet, especially when suitably flavoured, but it is of relatively little nutritive value as not more than 1 ounce can be taken in the day: i.e. the amount required to make one pint of jelly. Although it is a protein, it is lacking in several of the vital amino-acids. The ordinary household 'stock' made from boiling bones contains gelatin. Mixed with about two and a half times its weight of glycerin, gelatin forms a soft substance used as the basis for many pastilles and suppositories.

GENERAL DENTAL COUNCIL A statutory body set up by the Dentists Act which maintains a register of dentists, promotes high standards of dental education and overseees the professional conduct of dentists. Membership comprises elected and appointed dentists and six appointed lay members.

GENERAL MEDICAL COUNCIL (GMC) A statutory body of elected and appointed medical practitioners and appointed lay members. Its purpose is to protect patients and guide doctors in their professional practice. The council oversees medical education, keeps a register of qualified doctors entitled to practise medicine in the United Kingdom and acts when a doctor's fitness to practise is in doubt. Charges of serious professional misconduct against doctors are heard by the council in public. The GMC is responsible to the Privy Council.

GENERAL OPTICAL COUNCIL The statutory body that regulates the professions of ophthalalmic optician (optometrist) and dispensing optician. It promotes high standards of education and professional conduct and was set up the Opticians Act 1958.

GENERAL PARALYSIS OF THE INSANE An outdated term for the tertiary stage of syphilis (see SYPHILIS)

GENERAL PRACTITIONER is the doctor who provides PRIMARY MEDICAL CARE and is also responsible for community health-care programmes such as VACCINATION. Increasingly called a primary-care physician, he or she is the initial health service contact in the United Kingdom for those seeking medical advice or treatment – or merely reassurance – and so it is vital that the general practitioner establishes a close relationship with his or her patients, with a high degree of trust and confidence. In the National Health Service the general practitioner (GP) or family doctor provides 90 per cent of the medical care for the population. Most illnesses are treated by the GP and, except when emergency patients go direct to hospital, he or she advises whether a patient should see a specialist. This gatekeeper function in the NHS helps to ensure that expensive hospital facilities are used only by those patients who really need them. GPs usually see patients in their surgeries but will also visit them at home when necessary. Around 70 per cent of GPs, of whom there are over 33,000 in the United Kingdom, work in partnerships of two or more, covering each other's work, and on average they each look after 1,900 patients. They are responsible to the health authorities of the National Health Service and are paid in part by capitation fees according to the number of patients registered with them and in part by item of service fees. Almost every person in the country is registered with a GP, who is also allowed to do private practice. General-practitioner training in the UK normally consists of a three-year course, comprising four six-month periods as a junior hospital doctor, working in specialties such as paediatrics, geriatrics, psychiatry and accident and emergency medicine, followed by time spent working under supervision in a general practitioner's surgery.

In the reforms of the NHS that have been a feature of the 1990s, some GPs were given budgets with which they could 'purchase' certain hospital and community services for their patients. Such GPs were known as fundholders. This scheme has recently been modified and the plan is for groups of GPs and health professionals in a locality to decide on the services needed for the patients in the area and to arrange for these to be provided, either by the GPs and other health professionals or the hospital or community health trusts. (The structure and financing of trusts are being reorganized.) (See NATIONAL HEALTH SERVICE.)

GENERIC DRUG A medicinal drug that is sold under its official (generic) name instead of its proprietary (patented brand) name. NHS doctors are advised to prescribe generic drugs where possible as this enables any suitable drug to be dispensed, saving delay to the patient and the sometimes expense to the NHS. (See APPROVED NAMES.)

GENES Humans possess between 50,000 and 100,000 genes which are the biological units of heredity. They are arranged along the length of the 23 pairs of CHROMOSOMES and, like the chromosomes, therefore come in pairs (see GENETIC CODE). Human beings have 46 chromosomes, comprising 2 sex chromosomes and 44 autosomes, but there is also a MITOCHONDRIAL chromosome outside the cell nucleus which is inherited from the mother.

GENE TESTING (see GENETIC SCREENING).

GENE THERAPY Gene therapy is the transfer of a piece of DNA, or gene, into the cell of a person with a disease affecting that gene. The recipient cell then transcribes the gene and translates the resulting messenger RNA to generate protein. First used to treat an American patient in 1990, there are now more than 500 patients receiving gene therapy. In 1988 the European Medical Research Councils of 11 Western European nations, including the UK, produced a joint statement recommending that gene therapy should be limited to interventions aimed at correcting disease or defects and that it should be limited to somatic cells. Intervention on germ-line cells (the sperm and egg), though technically feasible, is not permitted.

GENETIC CODE The message set out sequentially along the human chromosomes. The human gene map is being constructed through the work of the international, collaborative HUMAN GENOME PROJECT. So far only part of the code has been translated and this is the part that occurs in the genes. Genes are responsible for the PROTEIN synthesis of the cell. They instruct the cell how to make a particular polypeptide chain for a particular protein.

Genes carry in coded form the detailed specifications for the thousands of kinds of protein molecules the cell requires for its existence, for its ENZYMES, for its repair work and for its reproduction. These proteins are synthesized from the 20 natural amino-acids, which are uniform throughout nature and which exist in the cell cytoplasm as part of the metabolic pool. The protein molecule consists of AMINO-ACIDS joined end to end to form long polypeptide chains. An average chain contains 100 to 300 amino-acids. The sequence of bases in the nucleic acid chain of the gene corresponds in some fundamental way to the sequence of amino-acids in the protein molecule, and hence it determines the structure of the particular protein. This is the genetic code. DEOXYRIBONU-CLEIC ACID (DNA) is the bearer of this genetic information.

DNA has a long backbone made up of repeating groups of phosphate and sugar deoxyribose. To this backbone four bases are attached as side groups at regular intervals. These four bases are the four letters used to spell out the genetic message. They are adenine, thymine, guanine and cystosine. The molecule of the DNA is made up of two chains coiled round a common axis to form what is called a double helix. The two chains are held together by hydrogen bonds between pairs of bases. Since adenine only pairs with thymine, and guanine only with cystosine, the sequences of bases in one chain fixes the sequence in the other. Several hundred bases would be contained in the length of DNA of a typical gene. If the message of the DNA-based sequences is a continuous succession of thymine, the RIBOS-OME will link together a series of the amino-acid phenylalanine. If the base sequence is a succession of cytosine, the ribosome will link up a series of prolines. Thus each amino-acid has its own particular code of bases. In fact each amino-acid is coded by a word consisting of three adjacent bases. In addition to carrying genetic information, DNA is able to synthesize or replicate itself and so pass its information on to daughter cells.

All DNA is part of the chromosome and so it remains confined to the nucleus of the cell (except in the mitochondrial DNA). Proteins are synthesized by the ribosomes which are in the cytoplasm. DNA achieves control over protein production in the cytoplasm by directing the synthesis of RIBONUCLEIC ACID (RNA). Most of the DNA in a cell is inactive, otherwise the cell would synthesize simultaneously every protein that the individual was capable of forming. When part of the DNA structure becomes 'active', it acts as a template for the ribonucleic acid which itself acts as a template for protein synthesis when it becomes attached to the ribosome. Ribonucleic acid exists in three forms. First 'messenger RNA' carries the necessary 'message' for the synthesis of a specific protein, from the nucleus to the ribosome. Second, 'transfer RNA' collects the individual amino-acids which exist in the cytoplasm as part of the metabolic pool and carries them to the ribosome. Third, there is RNA in the ribosome itself. RNA has a similar structure to DNA but the sugar is ribose instead of deoxyri-

bose and uracil replaces the base thymine. Before the ribosome can produce the proteins, the amino-acids must be lined up in the correct order on the messenger RNA template. This alignment is carried out by transfer RNA, of which there is a specific form for each individual amino-acid. Transfer RNA can not only recognize its specific amino-acid, but also identify the position it is required to occupy on the messenger RNA template. This is because each transfer RNA has its own sequence of bases and recognizes its site on the messenger RNA by pairing bases with it. The ribosome then travels along the chain of messenger RNA and links the amino-acids, which have thus been arranged in the requisite order, by peptide bonds and protein is released. Proteins are important for two main reasons. First, all the enzymes of living cells are made of protein. One gene is responsible for one enzyme. Genes thus control all the biochemical processes of the body and are responsible for the inborn difference between human beings. Second, proteins also fulfil a structural role in the cell so that genes controlling the synthesis of structural proteins are responsible for morphological differences between human beings.

GENETIC COUNSELLING The procedure whereby advice is given about the risks of a genetic disorder and the various options that are open to the individual at risk. This may often involve establishing the diagnosis in the family, as this would be a prerequisite before giving any detailed advice. Risks can be calculated from simple Mendelian inheritance (see MENDELISM) in many genetic disorders. However, in many disorders with a genetic element such as cleft lip or palate, the risk of recurrence is obtained from population studies. Risks include not only the likelihood of having a child who is congenitally affected by a disorder, but also, for adults, that of being vulnerable to an adult-onset disease. The options for individuals would include taking no action, modifying their behaviour, or taking some form of direct action. For those at risk of having an affected child, where prenatal diagnosis is available, this would involve either carrying on with reproduction regardless of risk, deciding not to have children, or deciding to go ahead to have children, but opting for prenatal diagnosis. For an adult-onset disorder such as a predisposition to ovarian cancer, an individual may choose to take no action, to take preventive measures such as use of the oral contraceptive pill, to have screening of the ovaries with measures such as ultrasound, or to take direct action such as removing the ovaries to prevent ovarian cancer occurring.

There are now regional genetics centres throughout the United Kingdom, and patients can be referred through their family doctor or specialists.

GENETIC DISORDERS These are caused when there are mutations or other abnormalities which disrupt the code of a gene or set of genes. These are divided into autosomal dominant, autosomal recessive, sex-linked and polygenic disorders.

Dominant genes A dominant characteristic is an effect which is produced whenever a gene or gene defect is present. If a disease is due to a dominant gene, those affected are heterozygous, that is they only carry a fault in the gene on the one of the pair of chromosomes concerned. Affected people married to normal individuals transmit the gene directly to one half of the children, although this is a random event just like tossing a coin. HUNTINGTON'S CHOREA is due to the inheritance of a dominant gene, as is neurofibromatosis and familial adenomatous polyposis of the colon. Achondroplasia is an example of a disorder in which there is a high frequency of a new dominant mutation, for the majority of affected people have normal parents and siblings. However, the chances of the children of a parent with ACHONDROPLASIA being affected are one in two, as with any other dominant characteristic. Other diseases inherited as dominantcharacteristics include spherocytosis, haemorrhagic telangiectasia and adult polycystic kidney disease.

Recessive genes If a disease is due to a recessive gene, those affected must have the faulty gene on both copies of the chromosome pair (i.e. be homozygous). The possession of a single recessive gene does not result in overt disease, and the bearer usually carries this potentially unfavourable gene without knowing it. If that person marries another carrier of the same recessive gene, there is a one-in-four chance that their children will receive the gene in a double dose, and so have the disease. If an individual sufferer from a recessive disease marries an apparently normal person who is a heterozygous carrier of the same gene, one half of the children will be affected and the other half will be carriers of the disease. The commonest of such recessive conditions in Britain is CYSTIC FIBROSIS, which affects about one child in 2,000. Approximately 5 per cent of the population carry a faulty copy of the gene. Most of the inborn errors of metabolism, such as PHENYLKETONURIA, GALACTOSAEMIA and congenital adrenal hyperplasia (see ADRENOGENITAL SYNDROME), are due to recessive genes.

There are characteristics which may be incompletely recessive, that is, neither completely dominant nor completely recessive and the heterozygotus person, who bears the gene in a single dose, may have a slight defect, whilst the homozygotus, with a double dose of the gene, has a severe illness. The SICKLE-CELL TRAIT is a result of the sickle-cell gene in single dose, and sickle-cell anaemia is the consequence of a double dose.

Sex-linked genes If a condition is sex-linked, affected males are homozygous for the mutated gene as they carry it on their single X chromosome. The X chromosome carries many genes, while the Y chromosome bears few genes, if any, other than those determining masculinity.

The genes on the X chromosome of the male are thus not matched by corresponding genes on the Y chromosome. There is thus no chance of the Y chromosome neutralizing any recessive trait on the X chromosome. A recessive gene can therefore produce disease since it will not be suppressed by the normal gene of the homologous chromosome. The same recessive gene on the X chromosome of the female will be suppressed by the normal gene on the other X chromosome. Such sex-linked conditions include HAEMOPHILIA, CHRISTMAS DISEASE, DUCHENNE type of muscular dystrophy (see MYOPATHY) and nephrogenic DIABETES INSIPIDUS. If the mother of an affected child has another male relative affected, she is a heterozygote carrier; half her sons will have the disease and half her daughters will be carriers. The sister of a haemophiliac thus has a 50-percent chance of being a carrier. An affected male cannot transmit the gene to his son because the X chromosome of the son must come from the mother; all his daughters, however, will be carriers as the X chromosome for the father must be transmitted to all his daughters. Hence sex-linked recessive characteristics cannot be passed from father to son. Sporadic cases may be the result of a new mutation, in which case the mother is not the carrier and is not likely to have further affected children. It is probable that one third of haemophiliacs arise as a result of fresh mutations and these patients will be the first in the families to be affected. Sometimes the carrier of a sex-linked recessive gene can be identified. The sex-linked variety of retinitis pigmentosa (see RETINA, DISORDERS OF) can often be detected by ophthalmoscopic examination.

A few rare disorders are due to dominant genes carried on the X chromosome. An example of such a condition is familial hypophosphataemia with vitamin-D-resistant rickets.

Polygenic inheritance In many inherited conditions the disease is due to the combined action of several genes and the genetic element is then called multi-factorial or polygenic. In this situation there would be an increased incidence of the disease in the families concerned, but it will not follow the Mendelian (see MENDELISM, GENETIC CODE) ratio. The greater the number of independent genes involved in determining a certain disease, the more complicated will be the pattern of inheritance. Furthermore, many inherited disorders are the result of a combination of genetic and environmental influences. Diabetes mellitus is the most familiar of such multi-factorial inheritance. The predisposition to develop diabetes is an inherited characteristic, although the gene is not always able to express itself: this is called incomplete penetrance. Whether or not the individual with a genetic predisposition towards the disease actually develops diabetes will also depend on environmental factors. Diabetes is more common in the relatives of diabetic patients, and even more so amongst identical twins. Non-genetic factors which are important in precipitating overt disease are obesity, excessive intake of carbohydrate foods and pregnancy.

Schizophrenia is another example of the combined effects of genetic and environmental influences in precipitating disease. The risk of schizophrenia in a child, one of whose parents has the disease, is one in ten, but this figure is modified by the early environment of the child.

GENETIC ENGINEERING, or RECOMBINANT DNA TECHNOLOGY, has only developed in the past decade or so; it is the process of changing the genetic material of a cell. Genes from one cell, for example a human cell, can be inserted into another cell, usually a bacterium, and made to function. It is now possible to insert the gene responsible for the production of human insulin, human growth hormone and interferon from a human cell into a bacterium. Segments of DNA for insertion can be prepared by breaking long chains into smaller pieces by the use of restriction enzymes. The segments are then inserted into the affecting organism, usually the bacteria ESCHERICIA COLI by using PLASMIDS and BACTERIOPHAGES. Plasmids are small packets of DNA that are found within bacteria and can be passed from one bacterium to another. Already genetic engineering is contributing to easing the problems of diagnosis. DNA analysis and production of MONOCLONAL ANTIBODIES are other applications of genetic engineering. Genetic engineering has significantly contributed to horticulture and agriculture with certain characteristics of one organism or variant of a species being transfected into another. This has given rise to higher-yield crops and to alteration in colouring and size in produce. Genetic engineering is also contributing to our knowledge of how human genes function as these can be transfected into mice and other animals which can then act as models for genetic therapy. Studying the effects of inherited mutations derived from human DNA in these animal models is thus a very important and much faster way of learning about human disease.

Genetic engineering is a scientific procedure that could have profound implications for the human race. Manipulating heredity would be an unwelcome activity under the control of maverick scientists, politicians or others in positions of power.

GENETIC FINGERPRINTING This technique shows the relationships between individuals. For example, it can be used to prove maternity or paternity of a child. The procedure is also used in FORENSIC MEDICINE whereby any tissue left behind by a criminal at the scene of a crime can be compared genetically with the tissue of a suspect. DNA, the genetic material in living cells, can be extracted from blood, semen, and other body tissues. The technique, pioneered in Britain in 1984, is now widely used.

GENETICS The science which deals with the origin of the characteristics of an individual or the study of heredity.

GENETIC SCREENING A screening procedure that tests whether a person has a genetic make-up that is linked with a particular disease. If so, the person may either develop the disease or pass it on to his or her offspring. When an individual has been found to carry a genetically linked disease, he or she should receive genetic counselling from an expert in inherited diseases.

Genetic screening is proving to be a controversial subject. Arguments are developing over whether the results of such screenings should be made available to employers and insurance companies, a move that could have adverse consequences for some individuals with potentially harmful genetic make-ups. (See GENES; GENETIC DISORDERS.)

GENITAL HERPES (see HERPES).

GENITALIA The external organs of reproduction. The term is usually applied to the external parts of the reproductive system: the VULVA in females and PENIS and SCROTUM in males. Rarely the sex of an individual may not be apparent from the genitalia. Genitals develop from a common embryonic structure and disturbances in the hormone controls of the developing genitalia may produce an individual whose external genitalia are ambiguous. The condition is known as intersex. Some such individuals may be HERMAPHRODITES and some PSEUDOHERMAPHRODITES.

GENITO-URINARY MEDICINE The branch of medicine that deals with sexually transmitted diseases (see VENEREAL DISEASES).

GENITO-URINARY TRACT This consists of the kidneys, ureters, bladder, and urethra and, in the male, the genital organs.

GENOME A complete set of chromosomes derived from one parent, or the total gene complement of a set of chromosomes. An international study is well under way to produce a complete map of the human genome.

GENOTYPE All of an individual's genetic information that is encoded in his or her CHROMOSOMES. It also means the genetic information carried by a pair of alleles which controls a particular characteristic. (See GENES.)

GENTAMICIN An antibiotic derived from a species of micro-organisms, MICROMONOSPORA PURPUREA. Its main value is that it is active against certain micro-organisms such as PSEUDOMONAS PYOCYANEA, E. COLI and AEROBACTER AEROGENES which are not affected by other antibiotics, as well as staphylococci which have become resistant to penicillin.

GENTIAN VIOLET, or CRYSTAL VIOLET, is a dye belonging to the rosaniline group. It is a useful superficial antiseptic for use on unbroken skin.

GENU VALGUM is the medical term for knock-knee, a deformity of the lower limbs in such a direction that when the limbs are straightened the legs diverge from one another. As a result, in walking the knees knock against each other. The amount of knock-knee is measured by the distance between the medial malleoli of the ankles, with the inner surfaces of the knee touching and the knee-caps facing forwards. The condition is so common in children between the ages of 2 to 6 years that it may almost be regarded as a normal phase in childhood. When marked, or persisting into later childhood, it can be corrected by surgery (osteotomy).

GENU VARUM is the medical term for BOW LEG.

GERIATRICS, now increasingly termed MEDICINE OF THE ELDERLY, is a branch of medicine dealing with disorders and diseases associated with old age, particularly their social consequences. (SEE AGEING.)

GERMAN MEASLES (see RUBELLA).

GERM CELL Those embryonic cells with the potential to develop into OVA or SPERMATOZOA.

GERMS (see MICROBIOLOGY).

GERONTOLOGY The study of alterations in the body and mind that occur as a person ages and the problems that result.

GESTALTISM A school of psychology based on the concept that an individual's sense of wholeness is more valuable than a piecemeal approach to perception and behaviour. Founded in Germany early in the 20th century, the school's practitioners regarded the whole as more than a sum of its parts. Aimed at resolving personal problems, the therapy increased subjects' self-awareness of all aspects of themselves in their environment.

GESTATION is another name for pregnancy.

GIARDIASIS A condition caused by a parasitic organism known as *Giardia lamblia*, which is found in the duodenum (see INTESTINE) and the upper part of the small intestine. This organism is usually harmless, but is sometimes responsible for causing diarrhoea. Over 3000 cases of giardiasis, also called lambliasis, a year are reported in Britain. In most of these the infection has been acquired from drinking untreated water in the Middle East or Russia. The illness develops one or two weeks after exposure to infection, and usually starts as an explosive diarrhoea, with the passage of pale fatty stools, abdominal pain and nausea. It responds well to METRONIDAZOLE or MEPACRINE.

GIDDINESS (see VERTIGO).

GIGANTISM Excessive growth (mainly height) caused by overproduction, during childhood or adolescence, of growth hormone by a tumour of the PITUITARY GLAND. Untreated the affected individual may die in early adulthood. Sometimes the tumour appears after the individual has stopped growing and the result then is acromegaly rather than gigantism (see ACROMEGALY).

GILLES DE LA TOURETTE'S SYNDROME Also known as TOURETTE'S SYNDROME, this is a hereditary condition of severe and multiple TICS of motor or vocal origin. It usually starts in childhood and becomes chronic (with remissions). With a prevalance of 1:2,000, a dominant GENE with variable expression may be responsible. The disorder is associated with explosive vocal tics and grunts, occasionally obscene (see COPROLALIA) The patient may also involuntarily repeat the words or imitate the actions of others (see PALILALIAN). HALOPERIDOL, pimozide (an oral antipsychotic drug similar to CHLORPROMAZINE hydrochloride) and CLONIDINE are among drugs that may help to control this distressing, but fortunately rare, disorder.

GINGIVITIS Inflammation of the gums. (See TEETH, DISEASES OF.)

GLANDERS, or EQUINIA, is a specific infectious disease to which certain animals, chiefly those with an undivided hoof – such as horses, asses, and mules – are liable, and communicable by them to man, but this is rare. The cause of glanders is a short rod-shaped organism, known as the *Loefflerella mallei*. It has been eradicated from Britain, but still occurs in Eastern Europe and Asia. Untreated, the acute form of disease may be fatal in humans. About half of those with the chronic form survive without treatment. Antibiotics are the treatment of choice.

GLAND A collection of CELLS or an ORGAN with a specialized ability to make and secrete chemical substances such as enzymes and hormones essential for the normal functioning of the body. Glands are classified into two groups: ENDOCRINE and EXOCRINE. The former secrete their products, hormones, straight into the bloodstream; the latter's secretions are discharged through ducts. (These functional differences are the reason why glands have been

Various types of glands; 1 simple tubular (e.g. intestinal glands); 2 simple coiled tubular (e.g. sweat glands); 3, 4 simple branched tubular (e.g. gastric glands); 5 simple alveolar; 6 simple branched alveolar (e.g. sebaceous glands); 7 compound (e.g. salivary and mammary glands). The secretory part of the gland is black.

defined as ductless and ducted.) Examples of endocrine glands are the adrenals, PITUITARY and THYROID. Exocrine glands include SEBACEOUS glands (in the skin) and the SALIVARY glands in the mouth whose enzymes start the digestion of food. One gland, the PANCREAS, secretes endocrine products (INSULIN) and an exocrine one (CHOLECYSTOKININ). The BREASTS or mammary glands are exocrine glands that secrete milk.

Though strictly speaking not a gland, LYMPH nodes (part of the lymphatic system) are sometimes called that. While they do not produce secretions, lymph glands do release white blood cells, an essential part of the body's defence system.

GLANDULAR FEVER (see MONONUCLEOSIS).

GLANS The term applied to the ends of the PENIS and the CLITORIS. In the penis the glans is the distal helmet-shaped part that is formed by the bulbous corpus spongiosum (erectile tissue). In an uncircumcised man the glans is covered by the foreskin or prepuce when the penis is flaccid.

GLASGOW COMA SCALE A method developed by two doctors in Glasgow that is used to assess the depth of coma or unconsciousness suffered by an individual. The scale is split into three groups: eye opening, motor response, and verbal response, with the level of activity within each group given a score. A person's total score is the sum of the numbers scored in each group and this provides a reasonably objective assessment of the patient's coma state. (see PERSISTENT VEGETATIVE STATE.)

GLAUCOMA A group of disorders characterized by the intraocular pressure being so high as to damage the nerve fibres in the retina and optic nerve as it leaves the eye.

Individuals most at risk have a family history of glaucoma (especially among siblings), are myopic, or have diabetic or thyroid eye disease. People with a strong family history of the disease should have regular eye checks, including tonometry, from the age of 35 years.

Glaucoma is usually classified as being either open-angle glaucoma or narrow-angle glaucoma.

Open-angle glaucoma is a chronic, slowly progressive, usually bilateral disorder. It occurs in 1 in 200 of people over 40 and amounts for 20 per cent of those registered blind in Great Britain. Symptoms are virtually non-existent until well into the disease, when the patient may experience visual problems. It is not painful. The characteristic findings are that the intraocular pressure is raised (normal pressure is up to 21 mm Hg) causing cupping of the optic disc and a glaucomatous visual-field loss. The angle between the iris and the cornea remains open. Treatment is aimed at decreasing the intra-ocular pressure initially by drops, tablets and intravenous drug administration. Surgery may be required later. A trabeculectomy is an operation to create a channel through which fluid can drain from the eye in a controlled fashion in order to bring the pressure down.

Narrow-angle glaucoma affects 1 in 1,000 people over 40 years of age and is more common in women. Symptoms may start with coloured haloes around street lights at night. These may then be followed by rapid onset of severe pain in and around the eye accompanied by a rapid fall in vision. One eye is usually affected first; this alerts the surgeon so that action can be taken to prevent a similar attack in the other eye. Treatment must be started as an emergency with a topical BETA BLOCKER in eye drops with other drugs such as ADRENALINE or pilocarpin added as necessary. Dorzolamide, a topical anhydrase inhibitor, can also be used. ACETA-ZOLAMIDE, also an anhydrase inhibitor, can be given by mouth. In an emergency before surgery mannitol can be given through an intravenous infusion. This is followed by surgery to prevent recurrence. Acute narrow-angle glaucoma occurs because the peripheral iris is pushed against the back of the cornea. This closes off the angle between iris and cornea through which aqueous humour drains out of the eye. Since the aqueous humour cannot drain away, it builds up inside the eye causing a rapid increase in pressure.

GLEET means a chronic form of GONORRHOEA.

GLENOID The term applied to the shallow socket on the shoulder-blade into which the humerus fits, forming the shoulder-joint.

GLIBENCLAMIDE A drug which stimulates the beta cells of the pancreas to liberate insulin, and is used to treat some patients with DIABETES MELLITUS (See SULPHONYLUREAS.)

GLICLAZIDE (see SULPHONYLUREAS).

GLIOMA A tumour in the brain or spinal cord, composed of neuroglia, which is the special connective tissue that supports the nerve-cells and nerve-fibres. Low-grade malignant gliomas cause symptoms by putting pressure on surrounding tissues and organs. Highly malignant gliomas are usually invasive. Gliomas, like other space-occupying tumours in the brain, may present with headaches, seizures, neurological symptoms or symptoms of mental disturbance. Treatment may include surgery, radiotherapy and chemotherapy and should be done in a specialist neurological centre. Gliomas tend to spread within the brain and can be difficult to remove surgically.

GLIPIZIDE (see SULPHONYLUREAS).

GLIQUIDONE (see SULPHONYLUREAS).

GLOBIN A protein which when it combines with haem forms HAEMOGLOBIN, the molecule found in the red blood cell that carries oxygen and carbon dioxide.

GLOBULIN A class of proteins which are insoluble in water and alcohol and soluble in weak salt solution. (See also GAMMA-GLOBULIN.)

GLOBUS A term applied generally to any structures of ball shape, but especially to the sensation of a ball in the throat causing choking, which forms a common symptom of hysteria (globus hystericus).

GLOMERULAR FILTRATION RATE The kidney filters a large volume of blood – 25 per cent of cardiac output or around 1300 ml – through its two million GLOMERULI every minute. The glomeruli filter out cell, protein, and fat-free fluid which, after reabsorption of certain chemicals, is excreted as urine. The rate of this ultrafiltration process, which in health is remarkably constant, is called the glomerular filtration rate (GFR). Each day nearly 180 litres of water plus some small molecular-weight constituents of blood are filtrated. The GFR is thus an indicator of kidney function. The most widely used measurement is CREATININE clearance and this is assessed by measuring the amount of creatinine in a 24-hour sample of urine and the amount of creatinine in the plasma; a formula is applied that gives the GFR.

GLOMERULONEPHRITIS (see KIDNEYS, DISEASES OF)

GLOMERULUS A small knot of blood-vessels about the size of a sand grain, of which around 1,000,000 are found in each kidney, and from which the excretion of fluid out of the blood into the tubules of the kidney takes place.

GLOSSITIS Inflammation of the tongue. Causes include ANAEMIA, CANDIDIASIS and dietary (particularly vitamin) deficiencies. The condition may also occur as a result of friction of the tongue against the sharp edge of a tooth.

GLOSSOPHARYNGEAL nerve is the ninth CRANIAL nerve, which in the main is a SENSORY nerve, being the nerve of taste in the posterior third of the tongue and the nerve of general sensation for the whole upper part of the throat and middle ear. It also supplies the PAROTID GLAND and one of the muscles on the side of the throat.

GLOTTIS The narrow opening at the upper end of the larynx. The glottis is made up of the true vocal cords. (See AIR PASSAGES; CHOKING; LARYNX.)

GLUCAGON A hormone secreted by the alpha cells of the islets of Langerhans in the PANCREAS, which increases the amount of glucose in the blood. This it does by promoting the breakdown of liver GLYCOGEN (glycogenolysis). It is secreted in response to a lowered blood sugar and is used therapeutically to treat HYPOGLYCAEMIA.

GLUCOCORTICOIDS The group of steroid hormones produced by the ADRENAL cortex, which includes cortisol and CORTISONE, and which particularly affect protein, fat and carbohydrate metabolism.

GLUCONEOGENESIS The formation of sugar from amino-acids in the liver.

GLUCOSE (DEXTROSE; GRAPE SUGAR) The form of sugar found in honey and in grapes and some other fruits. It is also the form of sugar circulating in the blood stream and the form into which all sugars and starches are converted in the small intestine before being absorbed. Glucose is a yellowish-white crystalline substance soluble in water and having the property of turning the ray of polarized light to the right. It is often given to patients orally or, sometimes, intravenously as an easily assimilated form of carbohydrate. It has the further practical advantage in this context of not being nearly as sweet-tasting as cane sugar and therefore relatively large amounts can be consumed without sickening the patient. (See SUGAR; URINE.)

GLUCOSE-TOLERANCE TEST A way of assessing the body's efficiency at metabolizing GLUCOSE. The test is used in diagnosing DIABETES MELLITUS. The patient is starved for up to 16 hours after which he is fed glucose by mouth. The concentrations of glucose in the blood and urine are then measured at half-hour intervals over two hours.

GLUCOSIDE A GLYCOSIDE formed from glucose.

GLUE EAR Another name for secretory otitis media. (See EAR, DISEASES OF.)

GLUE SNIFFING (see SOLVENT ABUSE).

GLUTEAL The region of the buttock and the structures situated in it, such as the gluteal muscles, arteries, and nerves.

GLUTEN The constituent of wheat-flour which forms an adhesive substance on addition of water, and allows the 'raising' of bread. It can be separated from the starch of flour, and being of a protein nature is used to make bread for those diabetics who are debarred from starchy and sugary foods.

It is also responsible for certain forms of what is now known as the MALABSORPTION SYNDROME. In these cases an essential part of treatment is a gluten-free diet.

GLUTEUS Three gluteal muscles form each buttock. The gluteus maximus is the large powerful muscle that gives the buttocks their rounded shape. The remaining two muscles are the gluteus medius and gluteus minimus and together the three muscles are responsible for moving the thigh.

GLYCERIN, or GLYCEROL, is an alcohol, $C_3H_8O_3$, which occurs naturally in combination with organic acids in the form of fats or triglycerides. It is a clear, colourless, thick liquid of sweet taste. It dissolves many substances, and absorbs water effectively.

Uses Glycerin has many varied uses. Numerous substances, such as carbolic acid, tannic acid, alum, borax, boric acid, starch, are dissolved in it for application to the body. It is frequently applied along with other remedies to inflamed areas for its action in extracting fluid and thus diminishing inflammation.

GLYCEROL Another name for glycerin.

GLYCERYL TRINITRATE Also known as trinitrin and nitroglycerin, this is a drug used in the treatment of ANGINA PECTORIS and left ventricular failure of the heart. It is normally given as a sublingual tablet or spray, though percutaneous preparations may be useful in the prophylaxis of angina, particularly for patients who suffer attacks at rest, especially at night. Sublingually it provides rapid symptomatic relief of angina, but is only effective for 20–30 minutes. It is a potent vasodilator, and this may lead to unwanted side-effects such as flushing, headache, and POSTURAL HYPOTENSION. Its antispasmodic effects are also valuable in the treatment of ASTHMA, biliary and RENAL COLIC, and certain cases of VOMITING. (See COLIC.)

GLYCO- A prefix meaning of the nature of, or containing, sugar.

GLYCOGEN or ANIMAL STARCH A carbohydrate substance found specially in the liver, as well as in other tissues. It is the form in which carbohydrates taken in the food are stored in the liver and muscles before they are converted into glucose as the needs of the body require.

GLYCOSIDE A compound of a sugar and a non-sugar unit. Glycosides are widespread throughout nature and include many important drugs such as DIGOXIN.

GLYCOSOLATED HAEMOGLOBIN (HbA1) This forms a small proportion of the total HAEMOGLOBIN in the blood. It differs from the major component, HbA, in that it has a glucose group attached. The rate of synthesis of HbA1 is a function of the blood-glucose concentration, and since it accumulates throughout the life span of the red blood cell – normally 120 days – the concentration of HbA1 is related to the mean blood-glucose concentration over the past 3–4 months. It is thus a useful indicator of medium-term diabetic control (see DIABETES MELLITUS) – a good target range would be a concentration of 5 to 8 per cent. When interpreting the HbA1 level, however, it is important to remember that wide fluctuations in blood-glucose concentration, together with ANAEMIA or a reduced erythrocyte life span, may give misleading results.

GLYCOSURIA The presence of sugar in the urine. By far the most common cause of glycosuria is DIABETES MELLITUS, but it may also occur as a result of a lowered renal threshold for sugar when it is called renal glycosuria, and is not indicative of disease. Measurements of the amounts of sugar in the urine is a standard method used by patients (and health professionals) to assess the stability of treatment for diabetes mellitus, indicating whether adjustment is required in the hypoglycaemic agents they are taking.

GOBLET CELL A columnar secretory cell occurring in the epithelium of the respiratory and intestinal tracts. The cells produce the main constituents of MUCUS.

GOITRE is a term applied to a swelling in the front of the neck caused by an enlargement of the THYROID GLAND. The thyroid lies between the skin and the front of the windpipe and in health is not large enough to be seen. The four main varieties of goitre are the simple goitre, the nodular, the lymphadenoid goitre and the toxic goitre.

Simple goitre A benign enlargement of the thyroid gland with normal production of hormone. It is a physiological response to maintain the synthesis of thyroid hormone. It may occur sporadically, but in certain geographical areas of the world it is found more frequently and it is then referred to as 'endemic'. It may be the result of a deficiency of iodine, which is essential for thyroid hormone production. If iodine intake is deficient and the production of thyroid hormone is threatened, the anterior pituitary secretes increased amounts of thyrotrophic hormone with consequent hyperplasia of the thyroid gland. The prevalence of endemic goitre can be, and has been, reduced by the iodinization of domestic salt in many countries. Simple goitres commonly occur at puberty, during pregnancy and at the menopause, which are times of increased demand for thyroid hormone. They may also result from defective utilization of iodine in the synthesis of thyroxine. The immediate cause of simple goitre is increased production of thyrotrophic hormone by the pituitary. The only effective treament is thyroid replacement therapy to suppress the enhanced production of thyrotrophic hormone.

Nodular goitres do not respond as well as the diffuse goitres to thyroxine treatment. They are usually the result of alternating episodes of hyperplasia and involution which lead to permanent thyroid enlargment. The only effective way of curing a nodular goitre is to excise it and thyroidectomy should be recommended if the goitre is causing pressure symptoms or if there is a suspicion of malignancy.

Lymphadenoid goitres are due to the production of antibodies against antigens in the thyroid gland. They are an example of an auto-immune disease. They tend to occur in the 3rd and 4th decade and the gland is much firmer than the softer gland of a simple goitre. Lymphadenoid goitres respond to treatment with thyroxine.

Toxic goitres may occur in GRAVES' DISEASE, though much less frequently autonomous nodules of a nodular goitre may be responsible for the increased production of thyroxine and thus cause THYROTOXICOSIS. Graves' disease is also an auto-immune disease in which an antibody is produced that stimulates the thyroid to produce excessive amounts of hormone, making the patient thyrotoxic.

Rarely, an enlarged gland may be the result of cancer in the thyroid.

TREATMENT A symptomless goitre may gradually disappear or be so small as not to merit treatment. If the goitre is large or is causing the patient difficulty in swallowing or breathing, it may need surgical removal by partial or total thyroidectomy. If the patient is deficient in iodine, fish and iodized salt should be included in the diet.

GOLD SALTS These are used in the treatment of RHEUMATOID ARTHRITIS. Gold may be administered in various forms, such as sodium aurothiomalate. It is injected in very small doses intramuscularly and produces a reaction in the affected tissues which leads to their scarring and healing. If gold is administered in too large quantities skin eruptions, ALBUMINURIA, metallic taste in the mouth, JAUNDICE, and feverishness may be produced, so that it is necessary to prolong a course of this remedy over many months in minute doses. Routine blood and urine tests are also necessary in order to detect any adverse or toxic effect at an early stage.

GOLFER'S ELBOW A term applied to a condition comparable to tennis elbow. It is not uncommon in the left elbow of right-handed golfers who catch the head of their club in the ground when making a duff shot. (See ELBOW.)

GONAD A gland which produces a gamete; an ovary or a testis. There are four stages of sexual development: (1) gonadal differentiation, (2) development of internal genitalia, (3) external genital differentiation, (4) puberty.

The testis and ovary both develop from the undifferentiated gonad which appears in the fourth week of gestation. This indifferent gonad has a cortex and a medulla. In the presence of a Y chromosome the medulla of this structure evolves into a testis and the cortex regresses. In the presence of two X chromosomes the cortex differentiates into an ovary and the medulla regresses. (See GENETIC CODE.)

The internal genitalia also develop from separate primitive structures that transiently co-exist in embryos of both sexes. In the male the Wolffian ducts give rise to the vas deferens, the seminal vesicles and the epididymus, and the Mullerian ducts regress (the prostatic utricle is a remnant). In the female the Mullerian ducts fuse to produce the Fallopian tubes, the uterus and the upper vagina, and the Wolffian ducts regress. The development of the Wolffian ducts and the suppression of the Mullerian ducts requires the presence of a functioning fetal testis from which an 'inducer' diffuses locally to both suppress the Mullerian ducts and stimulate the development of the Wolffian ducts. This inducer is not androgen which is unable to suppress the Wolffian ducts. In the absence of this substance the duct system differentiates along feminine lines irrespective of the genetic sex. Thus if there is no gonad, as in gonadal agenesis, the ducts will develop along female lines. Jost showed in 1947 that surgical castration of the animal fetus before the time of sexual differentiation prevented masculinization and all the litters grew up as apparent females. The developing testis was thus essential for masculinity but the ovary was not essential for feminity. The female form, both internal and external, was that of the neuter sex.

The third stage of sexual development, namely the differentiation of the external genitalia, also involves development from primitive structures common to both sexes. In the female the genital folds become the labia minora, the genital swellings the labia majora and the genital tubercule the clitoris, whilst in the male under the influence of androgens the shaft of the penis, the glans penis and the scrotum are respectively developed. Failure of the genital folds to fuse correctly in the male results in hypospadias. Thus both in the development of the internal genitalia and the external genitalia differentiation to the male form requires a positive influence, otherwise development follows the female pattern.

The final stage of sexual development is puberty when pituitary gonadotrophin production increases to adult levels, and secondary sex characteristics appear.

GONADOTROPHINS, or GONADOTROPHIC HORMONES, are HORMONES that control the activity of the GONADS (i.e. the testes and ovaries). In the male they stimulate the secretion of TESTOSTERONE and the production of SPERMATOZOA. In the female they stimulate the production of ova and the secretion of OESTROGEN and PROGESTERONE. There are two gonadotrophins produced by the pituitary gland. CHORIONIC GONADOTROPHIN is produced in the placenta and excreted in the urine.

GONOCOCCI A bacterium of the species *NEISSERIA GONORRHOEA* responsible for the sexually transmitted disease GONORRHOEA.

GONORRHOEA is an inflammatory disease caused by *NEISSERIA GONOCOCCUS*, affecting especially the mucous membrane of the urethra in the male and that of the vagina in the female, but spreading also to other parts. It is the most common of the VENEREAL DISEASES. According to the WORLD HEALTH ORGANIZATION, 200 million new cases are notified annually in the world. In England the incidence has been falling and in 1996 there were around 12,400 new cases.

Causes The disease is directly contagious from another person already suffering in this manner, usually by sexual intercourse, but occasionally it is conveyed by the discharge on sponges, towels or clothing as well as by actual contact. The gonococcus is found in the discharge expressed from the urethra, which may be spread as a film on a glass slide, suitably stained, and examined under the microscope; or a culture from the discharge may be made on certain bacteriological media and films from this, similarly examined under the microscope. Since discharges resembling that of gonorrhoea accompany other forms of inflammation, the identification of the organism is of great importance.

Symptoms These differ considerably, according to whether the disease is in an acute or a chronic stage.

MEN After an incubation period of between two and ten days, irritation in the URETHRA, scalding pain on passing water, and a viscid yellowish-white discharge appear; the glands in the groin often enlarge and may suppurate. The urine when passed is hazy and is often found to contain yellowish threads of pus visible to the eye. After some weeks, if the condition has become chronic, the discharge is clear and viscid, there may be irritation in passing urine, and various forms of inflammation in neighbouring organs may appear, the TESTICLE, PROSTATE GLAND and BLADDER becoming affected. At a still later stage the inflammation of the urethra is apt to lead to gradual formation of fibrous tissue around this channel. This contracts and produces narrowing, so that the passage of water becomes difficult or may be stopped for a time altogether (the condition known as stricture). Inflammation of some of the joints is a common complication in the early stage, the knee, ankle, wrist, and elbow being the joints most frequently affected, and this form of 'rheumatism' is very intractable and liable to lead to permanent stiffness. The fibrous tissues elsewhere may also develop inflammatory changes, causing lumbago, pain in the foot, etc. In occasional cases, during the acute stage, a general blood-poisoning results, with inflammation of the heart-valves (ENDO-CARDITIS) and abscesses in various parts of the body. The infective matter occasionally is inoculated accidentally into the eye producing a very severe form of conjunctivitis. In the newly born child this is known as ophthalmia neonatorum and until recently was one of the chief causes of blindness. (See EYE DISEASES.)

WOMEN The course and complications of the disease are somewhat different. It begins with a yellow vaginal discharge, pain on passing water, and very often inflammation or abscess of the Bartholin's glands, situated close to the vulva or opening of the vagina. The chief seriousness, however, of the disease is due to the spread of inflammation to neighbouring organs, the uterus, Fallopian tubes, and ovaries, causing permanent destructive changes in these, and leading occasionally to peritonitis through the Fallopian tube, with a fatal result. Many cases of prolonged ill-health and sterility or recurring miscarriages are due to these changes.

Treatment The chances of cure are better the earlier treatment is instituted. The treatment of gonorrhoea was revolutionized by the introduction of the sulphonamides. These, in turn, have now been replaced by the antibiotics. Penicillin is the antibiotic of choice but unfortunately the gonococcus is liable to become resistant to penicillin. In patients who are infected with penicillin-resistant organisms, one of the other antibiotics, such as cefotaxime, ciprofloxacin or spectinomycin, is used. In all cases it is essential that bacteriological investigation should be carried out at weekly intervals for three or four weeks, to make sure that the patient is cured.

GOOD MEDICAL PRACTICE Guidelines for doctors on the provision of good medical care laid down by the GENERAL MEDICAL COUNCIL.

GOUT A term used to describe several disorders associated with a raised concentration of uric acid in the blood, of which various forms of INFLAMMATORY ARTHRITIS and KIDNEY DISEASE are the most important. The condition has an overall prevalence in the UK of around 0·6 per cent.

Causes The cardinal feature of gout is the presence of an excessive amount of uric acid, and its deposition in the joints in the form of sodium monourate. The cause of this excess of uric acid is not known.

Gout has an hereditary element and a family history of the disease is obtained in from 50 to 80 per cent of cases. Inadequate exercise, habitual over-indulgence in animal food and rich dishes, and especially in alcoholic drinks have been indicted as precipitating factors, but the disease can occur in vegetarians and teetotallers.

Gout is infrequent before the age of 40, but it may occasionally affect very young people in whom there is a strong family history. About 95 per cent of patients are males. In women it most often appears during the menopause.

Symptoms An attack of gout may appear without warning, or there may be premonitory symptoms. The affected joint is swollen and the symptoms come and go, usually being worse at night. TOPHI may develop around an affected joint. Urinary calculi (urate based) often occur in patients with gout.

Treatment and prevention NON-STEROIDAL ANTI-INFLAMMATORY DRUGS such as INDOMETHACIN, NAPROXEN, or PHENYLBUTAZONE should be started as soon as possible for an acute attack. After the attack subsides, a lower dose should be continued for at least a week. Salicylates (such as aspirin) and diuretics should be avoided.

In patients prone to recurrent or particularly severe attacks, long-term prophylaxis with AL-LOPURINOL is indicated, especially when associated with kidney disease. This drug, which has few side-effects, lowers the serum urate concentration by preventing the formation of uric acid. A sensible weight-reducing diet is usually helpful.

GRAFT The term applied to a piece of tissue removed from one person or animal and implanted in another, or the same, individual in order to remedy some defect. Skin grafts are commonly used. Bone grafts are also used to replace bone which has been lost by disease: for example, a portion of rib is sometimes removed in order to furnish support for a spine weakened by disease, after the disease has been removed. Also, the bone of young animals is used to afford additional growth and strength to a limb bone which it has been necessary to remove in part on account of disease or injury. Vein grafts are used to replace stretches of arteries which have become blocked, particularly in the heart and lower limbs. The veins most commonly used for this purpose are the saphenous veins of the individual in question provided they are healthy. An alternative is specially treated umbilical vein. (See SKIN-GRAFTING.)

GRAFT VERSUS HOST DISEASE (GVHD) A condition that is a common complication of BONE MARROW transplant. It results from certain LYMPHOCYTES in the transplanted marrow attacking the transplant recipient's tissues, which they identify as 'foreign'. GVHD may appear soon after a transplant or develop several months later. The condition, which is fatal in about a third of victims, may be prevented by immunosuppressant drugs such as cyclosporin (see IMMUNOSUPPRESSION).

GRAM, or GRAMME, is the unit of weight in the metric system and is equal to a little over 15·4 grains. For purposes of weighing food, 30 grams are usually taken as approximately equal to 1 ounce.

GRAM POSITIVE/NEGATIVE   (see GRAM'S STAIN).

GRAM'S STAIN   Bacteria can be stained with an iodine-based chemical dye called Gram's stain (after the scientist who discovered the technique). Different bacteria react differently to exposure to the stain. Broadly, the bacterial specimens are stained first with gentian violet, then with Gram's stain and finally counterstained with a red dye after a decolorizing process. Bacteria that retain the gentian stain are called gram-positive; those that lose it but absorb the red stain are called gram-negative. Some species of staphylococcus, streptococcus and clostridium are gram-positive, whereas some types of salmonella and *Vibrio cholerae* are gram-negative.

GRAND MAL   A convulsive epileptic attack, also known as a tonic-clonic seizure in contrast to petit mal, which includes the milder forms of EPILEPSY.

GRANULATIONS   Small masses of formative cells containing loops of newly formed blood-vessels which spring up over any raw surface, as the first step in the process of healing of wounds. (See ULCER; WOUNDS.)

GRANULOCYTE   White blood cells which, when stained with Romanowsky stains containing thiazine dyes and eosin, are found to contain granules in their cytoplasm. The colour of the granules enables the cells to be further classified as BASOPHILS, EOSINOPHILS, and NEUTROPHILS.

GRANULOMA   A tumour or new growth made up of granulation tissue. This is caused by various forms of chronic inflammation, such as syphilis and tuberculosis.

GRAVEL   The name applied to any sediment which falls down in the urine, but particularly to small masses of uric acid. It produces various unpleasant symptoms. (See URINARY BLADDER, DISEASES OF; GOUT; URINE.)

GRAVES' DISEASE or THYROTOXICOSIS (see HYPERTHYROIDISM).

GRAVID   Pregnant.

GREENSTICK FRACTURE   An incomplete fracture, in which the bone is not completely broken across. It occurs in the long bones of children and is usually due to indirect force. (See FRACTURES.)

GREY MATTER   Those parts of the BRAIN and SPINAL CORD that comprise mainly the interconnected and tightly packed nuclei of nerve cells. The tissue is darker than that of the white matter, which is made of axons from the nerve cells. In the brain grey matter is mainly found in the outer layers of the cerebrum, which is the zone responsible for advanced mental functions. The inner core of the spinal cord is made up of grey matter.

GRIPES   A popular name for the colic of infants, generally due to irregular feeding. (See COLIC.)

GRISEOFULVIN   An antibiotic obtained from *Penicillium griseofulvum Dierckse*, used to treat various forms of ringworm.

GROIN   The region which includes the upper part of the front of the thigh and lower part of the abdomen. A deep groove runs obliquely across it, which corresponds to the inguinal ligament, and divides the thigh from the abdomen. The principal diseased conditions in this region are enlarged glands (see GLANDS), and HERNIA.

GROMMET   A small bobbin-shaped tube used to keep open the incision made in the ear drum in the treatment of secretory otitis media. It acts as a ventilation tube by allowing the Eustachian tube to recover its normal function. (See EAR, DISEASES OF; EUSTACHIAN TUBES.)

GROUP THERAPY   Psychotherapy in which at least two, but more commonly up to ten patients as well as the therapist, take part. The therapist encourages the patients to analyse their own and the others' emotional and psychological difficulties. Group therapy is also used to help patients with the same condition, for instance, alcoholism or compulsive gambling. They discuss their problems for perhaps an hour twice a week and explore ways of resolving them.

GROWING PAINS   Ill-defined discomfort and pains that occur in the limbs of some children. They occur mainly at night between ages of 6 and 12 years. The cause is unknown but the condition is not significant and does not require treatment.

GROWTH   A popular term applied to any new formation in any part of the body. (See CANCER; CYSTS; GANGLION; TUMOUR.) For growth of children, see WEIGHT AND HEIGHT.

GROWTH HORMONE   A product of the anterior part of the pituitary gland that promotes normal growth and development in the body by changing the chemical activity in the cells. The hormone activates protein production in the muscle cells as well as the release of energy from the metabolism of fats. Its release is controlled by the contrasting actions of growth-hormone releasing factor and somatostatin. If the body produces too much growth hormone before puberty GIGANTISM results; in adulthood the result is ACROMEGALY. Lack of growth hormone in children retards growth.

For many years growth hormone was extracted from human corpses and very rarely this caused CREUTZFELDT-JAKOB DISEASE (CJD) in the recipients. The hormone is now genetically engineered.

GUILLAN-BARRÉ SYNDROME A disease of the peripheral nerves causing weakness and numbness in the limbs that customarily occurs up to three weeks after CAMPYLOBACTER infection of the gastrointestinal tract, provoking an allergic response in the nerves. Recovery is usually good.

GUINEA-WORM (see DRACONTIASIS).

GULF WAR SYNDROME A collection of varying symptoms, mainly neurological such as persistent tiredness, amnesia, dizziness, muscle wasting and digestive disturbances that have been attributed to the exposure of soldiers, serving in the 1991 Gulf War, to insecticides and possibly other chemicals. Protective vaccinations against the effects of threatened biological and chemical warfare were also indicted as a cause. Research in the USA and UK into the disorder is still being carried out.

GULLET, or OESOPHAGUS, is the tube down which food passes from the throat to the stomach. (See OESOPHAGUS.)

GUM (a) The soft tissue surrounding the TEETH. Also called the gingiva, this tissue protects underlying structures and helps to keep the teeth tightly in the jaw bones. Inflammation of the gum is called gingivitis and may be due to dental PLAQUE or to systemic disorders such as LEUKAEMIA and SCURVY.

(b) A complex viscid substance which exudes from the stems and branches of various trees, and consists principally of arabin or bassorin. The two best-known gums are gum acacia and gum tragacanth. Gum-resins such as asafoetida, galbanum, and myrrh also contain resin.

GUMBOIL A painful condition of inflammation, ending sometimes as an abscess, situated in the gum about the root of a carious tooth.

GUMMA A hard swelling, or GRANULOMA, characteristic of tertiary SYPHILIS. It normally develops in the skin or subcutaneous tissue, mucous membranes or sub-mucosa, and the long bones. Although often painless, it may produce marked symptoms by interfering with the brain or other internal organs in which it may be located. Treatment with penicillin (or tetracycline if the patient is allergic) usually ensures a rapid disappearance of the gumma.

GUMS, DISEASES OF (see MOUTH, DISEASES OF; TEETH, DISEASES OF).

GYNAECOLOGY The branch of medicine dealing with the female pelvic and urogenital organs, in both the normal and diseased states. It encompasses aspects of CONTRACEPTION, ABORTION, and IN-VITRO FERTILIZATION. Covering the full age range, it is closely related to obstetrics, while involving aspects of both surgery and psychiatry.

GYNAECOMASTIA An abnormal increase in size of the male breast.

GYPSUM Plaster of Paris used to stabilize and externally splint fractured bones.

GYRUS is the term applied to a convolution of the b rain.

H

H₂ RECEPTOR ANTAGONISTS are drugs that block the action of HISTAMINE at the H_2 receptor (which mediates the gastric and some of the cardiovascular effects of histamine). By reducing the production of acid by the stomach, these drugs – chiefly cimetidine, ranitidine, and the newer ones, famotidine and nizatidine – are valuable in the treatment of peptic ulcers (healing when used in high dose, preventing relapse when used as maintenance therapy in reduced dose), reflux oesophagitis (see OESOPHAGUS, DISEASES OF), and the ZOLLINGER-ELLISON SYNDROME. These drugs are now being supplanted by PROTON PUMP INHIBITORS and HELICOBACTER PYLORI eradication therapy. (See DUODENAL ULCER.)

HAEM An iron-containing PORPHYRIN compound that combines with the protein GLOBULIN to make HAEMOGLOBIN, a constituent of erythrocytes (red blood cells).

HAEMANGIOMA Also known as a pyogenic granuloma, this is an acquired lesion that presents as a red papule which bleeds easily. Treatment is normally by cautery. A 'strawberry NAEVUS' is a haemangioma appearing around the time of birth, which may grow to a large size. Treatment is not required, however, as they normally fade.

HAEMARTHROSIS is the process of bleeding into, or the presence of blood in, a joint. It may occur as a result of major trauma (for example, fracture of the patella may lead to bleeding into the knee joint), or, more commonly, following minor trauma, or even spontaneously, in cases of HAEMOPHILIA or other disorders of blood clotting. If repeated several times it may lead to fibrosis of the joint lining and inflammation of the cartilage, causing marked stiffness and deformity.

HAEMATEMESIS means vomiting of blood. Blood brought up from the stomach is generally dark in colour, and is often so far digested as to form small brown granules resembling coffee grounds. Vomiting of blood is one of the chief symptoms of peptic ulcer, but it may also occur in gastritis, especially when this is due to the action of irritant poisons or alcohol, and cancer of the stomach. It should always be remembered that the blood may come from the nose or throat, and, after being swallowed, provoke vomiting. (See HAEMORRHAGE.)

HAEMATIN An organic growth factor. As an intravenous infusion it is increasingly being used as an effective treatment for acute attacks of PORPHYRIA; early use may prevent the chronic neuropathy sometimes associated with this condition.

HAEMATINIC A drug that raises the quantity of HAEMOGLOBIN in the blood. Ferrous sulphate is a common example of iron-containing compounds given to anaemic patients whose condition is due to iron deficiency. Traditionally haematinics have been used to prevent anaemia in pregnant women.

HAEMATOCOELE A cavity containing blood. Generally as the result of an injury which ruptures blood-vessels, blood is effused into one of the natural cavities of the body, or among loose cellular tissue, producing a haematocoele.

HAEMATOCOLPOS The condition in which MENSTRUAL blood is held up in the VAGINA as a result of an imperforate HYMEN.

HAEMATOCRIT Also known as packed cell volume, this is an expression of the fraction of blood volume occupied by the red cells. It is determined by centrifuging a sample of blood in a capillary tube and measuring the height of the resulting packed cells as a percentage of the total sample height.

Normal values: males 42–53%
or 0.42–0.53 mL/dL
females 32–48%
or 0.36–0.48 mL/dL

HAEMATOGENOUS An adjective applied to a biological process which produces blood or to an agent produced in or coming from blood. For example, a haematogenous infection is one resulting from contact with blood that contains a virus or bacterium responsible for the infection.

HAEMATOLOGIST A doctor or scientist who specializes in the study and treatment of blood and blood disorders.

HAEMATOLOGY The study of diseases of the blood.

HAEMATOMA means a collection of blood forming a definite swelling. It is found often upon the head of new-born children after a protracted and difficult labour. It may occur as the result of any injury or operation.

HAEMATOXYLON, or LOGWOOD, is the wood of Haematoxylon campechianum, which is used as a dye in staining tissues in histology. As it has a mildly astringent action, it is used for checking diarrhoea.

HAEMATURIA Blood in the urine. (See URINE.) The blood may come from any part of the urinary tract. When the blood comes from the kidney or upper part of the urinary tract, it is usually mixed throughout the urine, giving the latter a brownish or smoky tinge. This condition is usually the result of glomerulonephritis, or it may be present in persons suffering from high blood-pressure or PYELITIS. Blood may also appear in the urine when a stone or gravel is present in the pelvis of the kidney setting up irritation, especially after exercise. The blood may also originate from a bladder that is inflamed or infected or which contains benign (papilloma) or malignant growths. Inflammation or injury to the urethra can also cause haematuria. Someone with haematuria should seek medical advice. (See KIDNEYS, DISEASES OF.)

HAEMIC MURMUR Unusual sounds heard over the heart and large blood-vessels in severe cases of ANAEMIA. They disappear as the condition is recovered from.

HAEMOCHROMATOSIS, or BRONZED DIABETES, is a disease in which cirrhosis of the liver, enlargement of the spleen, pigmentation of the skin, and diabetes mellitus are associated with the abnormal and excessive deposit in the organs of the body of the iron-containing pigment, haemosiderin.

HAEMODIALYSIS A method of removing waste products or poisons from the circulating blood using the principle of DIALYSIS. The procedure is used on patients with malfunctioning or non-functioning kidneys. It is done using an artificial kidney or dialyser which restores blood to its normal state. The process has to be repeated, sometimes for many months, until a donor kidney is available for transplantation to replace the patient's failing kidneys.

HAEMOFILTRATION A technique similar to haemodialysis. Blood is dialysed using ultra-filtration through a membrane permeable to water and small molecules (molecular weight <12,000). Physiological saline solution is simultaneously reinfused.

HAEMOGLOBIN The colouring compound which produces the red colour of blood. It is a chromoprotein, made up of a protein called globin and the iron-containing pigment, haemin. When separated from the red blood corpuscles, each of which contains about 600 million haemoglobin molecules, it is crystalline in form. It exists in two forms: simple haemoglobin, found in venous blood, and oxyhaemoglobin, which is a loose compound with oxygen, found in arterial blood after the blood has come in contact with the air in the lungs. This oxyhaemoglobin is again broken down as the blood passes through the tissues, which take up the oxygen for their own use. This is the main function of haemoglobin: to act as a carrier of oxygen from the lungs to all the tissues of the body. When the haemoglobin leaves the lungs it is 97 per cent saturated with oxygen. When it comes back to the lungs in the venous blood it is 70 per cent saturated. The oxygen content of 100 millilitres of blood leaving the lungs is 19·5 millilitres, and that of venous blood returning to the lungs is 14·5 millilitres. Thus each 100 millilitres of blood delivers 5 millilitres of oxygen to the tissues of the body. Human male blood contains 13 to 18 grams of haemoglobin per 100 millilitres. In women, there are 12 to 16 grams per 100 millilitres. A man weighing 70 kilograms (154 pounds) has around 770 grams of haemoglobin circulating in his red blood corpuscles.

HAEMOGLOBINOPATHIES Impairment of adult HAEMOGLOBIN formation is the characteristic abnormality of the haemoglobinopathies, which are hereditary haemolytic ANAEMIAS, genetically determined and related to race. The haemoglobin may be abnormal because: (1) there is a defect in the synthesis of normal adult haemoglobin and this occurs in THALASSAEMIA when there may be an absence of one or both of the polypeptide chains characteristic of normal adult haemoglobin, or (2) an abnormal form of haemoglobin such as haemoglobin S, that of SICKLE-CELL DISEASE, is formed instead of adult haemoglobin. This abnormality may involve as little as one amino acid of the 300 in the haemoglobin molecule. In sickle-cell haemoglobin one single amino acid molecule, that of glutamic acid, is replaced by another, that of valine, and this results in such a deficient end product that the ensuing disease is frequently rapidly fatal.

HAEMOGLOBINURIA The presence of blood pigment in the urine caused by the destruction of blood corpuscles in the blood-vessels or in the urinary passages. It turns urine a dark red or brown colour. In some people this condition, known as intermittent haemoglobinuria, occurs from time to time, especially on exposure to cold. It is also produced by various poisonous substances taken in the food. It occurs in malarious districts in the form of one of the most fatal forms of malaria: BLACKWATER FEVER. (See also MARCH HAEMOGLOBINURIA.)

HAEMOLYSIS Destruction of blood corpuscles by the action of poisonous substances, usually of a protein nature, circulating in the blood, or by certain chemicals. It occurs, for example, gradually in some forms of anaemia and rapidly in poisoning by snake venom.

HAEMOLYTIC DISEASE OF THE NEW-BORN A potentially serious disease of the new-born characterized by haemolytic ANAEMIA (excessive destruction of red blood cells) and JAUNDICE. It may be associated with oedema, and if there is a great deal of fluid in the pericardial, pleural, and peritoneal cavities the condition is known as Hydrops fetalis. If jaundice appears within 24 hours of birth it is likely to be due to blood-group incompatibility between the mother and baby. The commonest cause of haemolytic disease of the new-born is rhesus incompatibility (see BLOOD GROUPS) – a previously sensitized rhesus-negative mother produces antibodies which cause haemolysis (destruction of the blood cells) in her rhesus-positive baby.

In mild cases the new-born infant becomes slightly jaundiced with only mild anaemia and no treatment is necessary. If tests during pregnancy suggests that the condition may be severe, delivery of the baby may be induced from 35 weeks onwards. In severely affected fetuses a fetal blood transfusion may be required.

The infant's SERUM BILIRUBIN –the bilirubin present in the blood – concentration should be plotted regularly so that treatment can be given before levels likely to cause brain damage occur. Safe bilirubin concentrations depend on the age of the child, and reference charts should always be used.

High bilirubin concentrations may be treated with PHOTOTHERAPY (treatment with light, involving the use of sunlight, non-visible ULTRA-VIOLET light, visible blue light or LASERS). Extra fluid is given to prevent dehydration and to improve bilirubin excretion by shortening the gut transit time. Severe jaundice and anaemia may require exchange transfusion (see TRANS-FUSION OF BLOOD). Haemolytic disease of the new-born secondary to rhesus incompatibility has become less common since the introduction of anti-D (Rho) immunoglobulin. This anti-body should be given to all rhesus-negative women at any risk of a fetomaternal transfu-sion, to prevent them from mounting an anti-body response. Anti-D is given routinely to rhesus-negative mothers after the birth of a rhesus-positive baby, but doctors should also remember to give it after threatened abortions, antepartum haemorrhages, miscarriages, and terminations of pregnancy.

HAEMOLYTIC URAEMIC SYNDROME

A disease of children resulting in acute OLIGURIC renal failure. A febrile illness of the gastrointestinal or respiratory tracts is followed by intravascular coagulation of blood which results in HAEMOLYSIS, ANAEMIA, THROMBO-CYTOPAENIA and renal failure (resulting from fibrin deposition in renal arterioles and glomerular capillaries).

The death rate is 2–10 per cent and the majority of patients survive without renal fail-ure. The longer the period of oliguria the greater the risk of chronic renal failure.

Treatment is supportive with replacement of blood and clotting factors, control of HYPER-TENSION and careful observance of fluid bal-ance.

HAEMOPERICARDIUM

The presence of blood in the PERICARDIUM, the membranous sac which surrounds the heart. The condition may result from a MYOCARDIAL INFARCTION, leaking ANEURYSM, injury or tumour. Because the peri-cardial blood compresses the heart, the latter's pumping action is impeded, reducing the blood pressure and causing cardiac failure. Urgent surgical drainage of the blood may be required.

HAEMOPHILIA

An inherited disorder of blood COAGULATION which results in prolonged bleeding even after minor injury. There is a deficiency of factor VIII, an essential clotting factor in the coagulation cascade – the complex series of biochemical events that lead from injury of the wall of a blood vessel to the formation of a blood clot that checks bleeding. It is a sex- linked recessive disorder (though a small number of cases arise by spontaneous mutation) so that females carry the disease, half their sons will be affected and half their daugh-ters will be carriers. The sons of haemophiliacs are unaffected but half their daughters will be carriers. Haemophilia affects approximately 1:4,000 of the UK population but only 1:20,000 is severely affected. Severity of the disease depends upon the percentage, compared with normal, of factor VIII activity present. Less than 1 per cent and there will be spontaneous bleeding into joints and muscles; 1–5 per cent and there will be occasional spontaneous bleed-ing and severe bleeding after minor injury; 5–

25 per cent and there will only be severe bleeding after major injury. Before treatment was available, severe haemophiliacs suffered from severe pain and deformity from bleeds into joints and muscles. Bleeding also occurred into the gut, kidney and brain and few survived past adolescence.

Freeze-dried factor VIII may be kept in domestic refrigerators. Haemophiliacs can use it to abort minor bleeds by reconstituting it and injecting it intravenously. More major bleeding or preparation for surgery involves raising factor VIII levels to 30–100 per cent by giving cryoprecipitate.

With treatment most haemophiliacs lead normal lives, though obviously dangerous or contact sports should be avoided. Before do-nors of blood were screened for hepatitis B and C or for HIV infection, some individuals with haemophilia receiving factor VIII were unwit-tingly infected with those diseases. Today's screening procedures make such infections very unlikely.

There is a National Haemophilia Register and each registered sufferer carries a card with details about his condition. Information may also be obtained from NHS haemophilia cen-tres and the Haemophilia Society (see APPENDIX 2: ADDRESSES).

HAEMOPHILUS

A genus of the hetero-geneous group of Parvobacteria, which con-tains several important human (and animal) pathogens. They are gram-negative (see GRAM'S STAIN), rod-like, aerobic, non-sporing and non-motile, parasitic bacteria. Mostly found in the respiratory tract, they may be part of the normal flora, but may also be responsible for several diseases. The main pathogenic species of haemophilus is *H. influenzae*, which may cause severe exacerbations of chronic BRONCHI-TIS, as well as MENINGITIS, EPIGLOTTITIS, SINUSI-TIS, and OTITIS MEDIA. Other species may cause conjunctivitis (see EYE DISEASES) or CHANCROID. *Haemophilus* species are sensitive to a wide range of antibiotics, though generally resistant to penicillin.

HAEMOPOIESIS

The formation of blood cells and platelets, a continuous process through-out life. As ageing cells are removed from the circulation the new ones, generated in the BONE MARROW, replace them.

HAEMOPOEITIC STEM CELL

This is the basic cell from which all types of blood cells originate. Its appearance is believed to be similar to that of a LYMPHOCYTE.

HAEMOPTYSIS

The coughing up of blood from the lungs. The blood is usually bright red and frothy, thus distinguishing it from blood brought up from the stomach. It is a potentially serious sign of lung disease, though in elderly people haemoptysis may be due to a varicose condition of the small veins in the throat, not to haemorrhage in the lungs; while in young people this condition is often due to bleeding from the nose, in which, owing to the position of the head, the blood happens to run backwards instead of forwards through the nostrils. (See HAEMORRHAGE; TUBERCULOSIS.)

HAEMORRHAGE The escape of blood from any of the blood vessels, normally in response to some trauma, or as a result of a clotting disorder such as HAEMOPHILIA. The bleeding may be external, for example, following a skin laceration, or internal, for example, haematemesis (bleeding into the stomach), haemoptysis (bleeding from the lungs), haematuria (bleeding from the kidneys or urinary tract). Bleeding into or around the brain is a major concern following serious head injuries, or in newborn infants following a difficult labour. Haemorrhage is classified as arterial – the most serious type, in which the blood is bright red and appears in spurts (in severe cases the patient may bleed to death in a few minutes); venous, less serious (unless from torn varicose veins) and easily checked, in which the blood is dark and wells up gradually into the wound; and capillary, in which the blood slowly oozes out of the surface of the wound, and soon stops spontaneously. Haemorrhage is also classified as primary, reactionary, and secondary (see WOUNDS). Severe haemorrhage causes SHOCK and ANAEMIA, and blood transfusion is often required.

When a small artery is cut across, the bleeding stops in consequence of changes in the wall of the artery on the one hand, and in the constitution of the blood on the other. Every artery is surrounded by a fibrous sheath, and when cut, the vessel retracts some little distance within this sheath and a blood clot forms blocking the open end (see COAGULATION). When a major blood vessel is torn, such spontaneous closure may be impossible and surgery is required to stop the bleeding.

Three main principles are applicable in the control of a severe external haemorrhage: (*a*) direct pressure on the bleeding point or points; (*b*) elevation of the wounded part; (*c*) pressure on the main artery of supply to the part.

Control of internal haemorrhage is more difficult than for external bleeding. First-aid measures should be taken while professional help is sought. The patient should be laid down with legs raised. He or she should be reassured and kept warm. The mouth may be kept moist but no fluids should be given. (See APPENDIX 1: FIRST AID.)

HAEMORRHOIDS or PILES Varicose (swollen) veins in the lining of the anus. They are very common affecting nearly half of the UK population at some time in their lives, with men having them more often and for a longer time.

Varieties Haemorrhoids are classified into first, second and third degree depending on how far they prolapse through the anal canal. First-degree ones do not protrude; second-degree piles protrude during defaecation; third-degree ones are trapped outside the anal margin, though they can be pushed back. Most haemorrhoids can be described as internal, since they are covered with glandular mucosa, but some large, long-term ones develop a covering of skin. Piles are usually found at the three, seven and eleven o'clock sites when viewed with the patient on his or her back.

Causes The veins in the anus tend to become distended because they have no valves and because they form the lowest part of the PORTAL SYSTEM and are apt to become overfilled when there is the least interference with the circulation through the portal vein, and partly because the muscular arrangements for keeping the rectum closed interfere with the circulation through the haemorrhoidal veins. An absence of fibre from Western diets is probably the most important cause. The result is that people often strain to defaecate hard stools, thus raising intra-abdominal pressure which slows the rate of venous return and engorges the network of veins in the anal mucosa. Pregnancy is an important contributory factor in women developing haemorrhoids. In some people haemorrhoids are a symptom of disease higher up in the portal system, causing interference with the circulation. They are common in heart disease, liver complaints, such as cirrhosis or congestion, and any disease affecting the bowels.

Symptoms Piles cause itching, pain and often bleeding, which may occur whenever the patient defaecates or only sometimes. The piles may prolapse permanently or intermittently. The patient may complain of aching discomfort which, with the pain, may be worsened.

Treatment Prevention is important and a high fibre diet will help to do this and is also necessary after piles have developed. A bulking agent will help and patients should not spend a long time straining on the lavatory. Itching can be lessened if the PERINEUM is properly washed, dried and powdered. Prolapsed piles can be replaced with the finger. Local anaesthetic and steroid ointments can help to relieve symptoms but do not remedy the underlying disorder. If conservative measures fail, then surgery may be required. Piles may be injected, stretched or excised according to the patient's particular circumstances.

Where haemorrhoids are secondary to another disorder such as cancer of the rectum or colon, the underlying condition must be treated, hence the importance of medical advice if piles persist.

HAEMOSIDEROSIS An increase in the amount of iron stored in the body. Rarely, it may be due to ingestion of too much iron. A more likely cause is repeated blood transfusions. The extra iron may affect the function of the heart and liver.

HAEMOSTASIS The process by which bleeding stops. It involves constriction of blood vessels, the formation of a platelet plug, and blood clotting. The term is also used for surgical interventions to stop bleeding, e.g. the use of diathermy. (See COAGULATION and HAEMORRHAGE.)

HAEMOSTATICS A group of drugs used to treat bleeding disorders such as HAEMOPHILIA. Factor VIII is one of the clotting factors available for treatment: preparations of it are injected after abnormal bleeding or before surgery. Vitamin-K preparations are another haemostatic group used to treat an overdose of anticoagulant drugs.

Haemostatic preparations of gelatine and cellulose are used to stem bleeding from the skin, gums or tooth extractions.

HAEMOTHORAX An effusion of blood into the PLEURAL CAVITY.

HAIR (see SKIN; WHITE HAIR).

HAIR, REMOVAL OF (see DEPILATION).

HALF LIFE: The time taken for the plasma concentration of an administered drug to decline by half as a result of redistribution, metabolism and excretion.

HALIBUT-LIVER OIL The oil expressed from fresh, or suitably preserved, halibut liver. It is a particularly rich source of vitamin A (30,000 international units per gram), and also contains vitamin D (2300 to 2500 units per gram). It is available in capsules as a means of providing the two vitamins. (See APPENDIX 5: VITAMINS.)

HALITOSIS Another term for bad breath. This may be a sign of illness – for example, lung disease or SINUSITIS, and a person with diabetes may have breath tainted with acetone if his sugar metabolism is poorly controlled. Usually, however, halitosis is caused by smoking, drinking alcohol, eating certain foods (garlic or onions) or inadequate oral and dental hygiene.

HALLUCINATIONS False perceptions arising without an adequate external stimulus, as opposed to illusions, which are misinterpretations of stimuli arising from an external object. Hallucinations come from 'within', although the affected individual may see them as coming from 'without'. Nevertheless, they may occur at the same time as real perceptions, and may affect any sense (vision, hearing, smell, taste, touch, etc.).

Causes They may be the result of intense emotion or suggestion, sensory deprivation (for example, overwork or lack of sleep), disorders of sense organs, or disorders of the central nervous system. Although hallucinations may occur in perfectly sane people, they are more commonly an indication of a MENTAL ILLNESS. They may be deliberately induced by the use of HALLUCINOGENS.

HALLUCINOGENS Compounds characterized by their ability to produce distortions of perception, emotional changes, depersonalization, and a variety of effects on memory and learned behaviour. They include LYSERGIC ACID DIETHYLAMIDE and MESCALINE. (See also DRUG ADDICTION.)

HALLUX The anatomical name of the great toe.

HALLUX RIGIDUS Stiffness of the joint between the great toe and the foot which induces pain on walking. It is usually due to a crush injury or stubbing of the toe. Such stubbing is liable to occur in adolescents with a congenitally long toe. If troublesome it is treated by an operation to create a false joint.

HALLUX VALGUS Outward displacement of the great toe and is always associated with a bunion. It is due to the pressure of footwear on an unduly broad foot. In adolescents this broad foot is inherited; in adults it is due to splaying of the foot as a result of loss of muscle tone. The bunion is produced by pressure of the footwear on the protruding base of the toe. In mild cases the wearing of comfortable shoes may be all that is needed. In more severe cases the bunion may need to be removed, while in the most severe the operation of ARTHROPLASTY may be needed. (See also CORNS AND BUNIONS.)

HALO A coloured circle seen round a bright light in some eye conditions. When accompanied by headache it is specially likely to be caused by GLAUCOMA.

HALOPERIDOL One of the butyrophenone group of drugs used to treat patients with psychoses. Its action is similar to that of the PHENOTHIAZINE group of drugs. It is also used in depot form, being administered by deep intramuscular injection for maintenance control of SCHIZOPHRENIA and other psychoses. The drug may help to control tics and intractable hiccups.

HALOTHANE A volatile liquid anaesthetic used for many years as a potent inhalant anaesthetic. It provides smooth induction of anaesthesia and is non-irritant and pleasant to inhale. A major drawback, however, is that it can cause severe damage to the liver, especially after repeated anaesthetic exposures, so a careful history is essential before a patient is given halothane. (see HALOTHANE HEPATITIS.)

HALOTHANE HEPATITIS   A very rare form of hepatitis following exposure to halothane during anaesthesia (1:35,000 halothane anaesthetics). Jaundice develops three to four days after exposure and will occasionally develop into a fatal massive hepatic necrosis. It is of unknown aetiology but probably has an immunological basis. It is more common following multiple exposures in a short time (less than 28 days), and in obesity, middle age and females. It is rare in children.

HAMARTOMA   These are benign tumours, usually in the lung, containing normal components of pulmonary tissue such as smooth muscle and connective tissue.

HAMMER-TOE   The deformity in which there is permanent flexion, or bending of the middle joint of the toe. The condition may affect all the toes as in CLAW-FOOT. More commonly it affects one toe, usually the second. It is due to a relatively long toe and the pressure on it of the footwear. A painful bunion usually develops on it. In mild cases relief is obtained by protecting the toe with adhesive pads. If this does not suffice operation is necessary. (See CORNS AND BUNIONS.)

HAMSTRINGS   The name given the tendons at the back of the knee, two on the inner side and one on the outer side, which bend this joint. They are attached to the tibia below. Strains, or 'pulls' and tears, of the hamstring are common in people taking part in strenuous sports such as athletics, football, rugby and tennis (see SPORTS INJURIES).

HAND   The section of the upper limb below the wrist. The hand of man is more highly developed in its structure and in its nervous connections than the corresponding part in any other animal. Indeed the possession of a thumb which can be 'opposed' to the other fingers for grasping objects is one of the distinguishing features of the human race that has contributed to its evolutionary success. Of all the parts of the body, the hand, which is connected with a large area on the surface of the brain, is capable of the highest degree of education.

In structure, the hand has a bony basis of eight small carpal bones in the wrist, five metacarpal bones in the fleshy part of the hand, and three phalanges in each finger, two only in the thumb. From the muscles of the forearm twelve strong tendons or sinews run in front of the wrist. Of these, nine go to the fingers and thumb and are bound down by a strong band, the flexor retinaculum, in front of the wrist. They are enclosed in a complicated synovial sheath, and pass through the palm and down the fingers. (See FINGERS.) Behind the wrist twelve tendons likewise cross from forearm to hand.

Forming the ball of the thumb and that of the little finger, and filling up the gaps between the

1   metatarsal bones of the finger
2   hamate (c)
3   pisiform (c)
4   triquetrum (c)
5   lunate (c)
6   ulna
7   radius
8   capitate (c)
9   scaphoid (c)
10 trapezium (c)
11 trapezoid (c)
12 metatarsal bone of the thumb
13 phalanges of the thumb
14 phalanges of index finger

The bones of the right hand and wrist (anterior view). Bones marked '(c)' form the carpal group of bones.

metacarpal bones, are other muscles, which act to separate and bring together the fingers, and to bend them at their first joints (knuckles).

Deep in the palm the ulnar artery makes an arch across the hand, giving off branches which run down the sides of the fingers; while the radial artery makes an arch across at a still deeper level, lying in close contact with the bones.

The skin of the hand is richly supplied with nerve filaments, in accordance with its highly specialized sense of touch, the outer three and a half digits being supplied in front by the median, behind by the radial nerve, whilst the inner one and a half fingers have their nerve supply both back and front from the ulnar nerve.

HAND, FOOT AND MOUTH DISEASE   A contagious disease due to infection with COXSACKIE A16 virus. Most common in children, the incubation period is three to five days. It is characterized by an eruption of blisters on the palms, the feet (often the toes) and in the mouth.

HANGING is a form of death due to suspension of the body from the neck, either suddenly, as in judicial hanging – not in the United Kingdom as the death penalty is not used in the justice system – so as to damage the spinal column and cord, or in such a way as to constrict the air passages and the blood-vessels to the brain. Death is, in any case, speedy, resulting in two or three minutes, if not instantaneous. Apart from judicial hanging, and in the absence of any signs of a struggle, hanging is usually due to suicide. The resuscitation of people found hanging is similar to that for drowning. (See APPENDIX 1: BASIC FIRST AID, cardiac/respiratory arrest.)

HANG-NAIL A splitting of the skin (cuticle) at the side of a finger nail. It is usually caused by trauma in manual workers, but ISCHAEMIA of the fingers (see RAYNAUD'S DISEASE) may predispose to the condition. Secondary infection and inflammation may make hang-nail a very tender condition; treatment consists of reducing TRAUMA, use of EMOLLIENTS and ANTIBIOTICS if necessary.

HARDNESS is a term applied to water that contains a large amount of calcium and magnesium salts (lime salts) which form an insoluble curd with soap and thus interfere with the use of the water for purposes of washing. Hard water is especially found in districts where the soil is chalky. Temporary hardness, which is due mainly to the presence of bicarbonates of lime, can be remedied by boiling, when the lime is precipitated as carbonate of lime. Permanent hardness is not remedied by boiling, and is due to the presence of a large amount of sulphate of lime. It may be removed by the addition of sodium carbonate (washing soda) or by the Permutit process which involves the use of various combinations of silicate of alumina and soda. In the past hard water was often blamed for many ills – without any convincing evidence. Today epidemiologists are suggesting that the drinking of soft water may lead to heart disease.

HARE-LIP (see PALATE, MALFORMATIONS OF).

HARTMANN'S SOLUTION A solution commonly used as a means of fluid replacement in dehydrated patients. Each litre contains 3·1 grams of sodium lactate, 6 grams of sodium chloride, 0·4 gram of potassium chloride, and 0·7 gram of calcium chloride.

HASHIMOTO'S DISEASE A condition in which the whole of the THYROID GLAND is diffusely enlarged and firm. It is one of the diseases produced by AUTOIMMUNITY. The enlargement is due, not to increase of colloid, but to diffuse infiltration of LYMPHOCYTES and increase of fibrous tissue. This form of goitre appears in middle-aged women, does not give rise to symptoms of THYROTOXICOSIS, and tends to produce MYXOEDEMA (see HYPOTHYROIDISM).

HAVERSIAN CANALS The fine canals in bone which carry the blood-vessels, lymphatics, and nerves necessary for the maintenance and repair of bone. (See BONE.)

HAY FEVER or ALLERGIC RHINITIS This is caused by an ALLERGY to the pollen of grasses, trees and other plants. Contact with the particular pollen that the sufferer is allergic to causes HISTAMINE release resulting in a blocked, runny nose and itchy watering eyes. It affects approximately 3 million people each year in the UK.

The mainstays of treatment are ANTIHISTAMINES and the use of steroid nasal spray and eyedrops. Occasionally desensitization may work if the particular allergen is known.

HEAD (see BRAIN; FACE; SCALP; SKULL).

HEADACHE A very common condition which may vary considerably in severity and type. Its significance and cause may vary tremendously, at one extreme indicating the presence of a tumour or meningitis, while at the other extreme it may merely indicate a common cold or tiredness. Even so, persistent or recurrent headaches should always be taken seriously. Although the brain itself is insensitive to pain, the surrounding membranes – meninges – are very sensitive, and changes in intracranial arteries, or spasm of the neck or scalp muscles, which may occur for various reasons, may cause considerable pain. In most cases a clinical diagnosis should be possible; further investigations should only be necessary following head injury, if headaches recur or if neurological signs such as drowsiness, vomiting, confusion, seizures, or focal signs, develop.

Some of the more common causes of headaches are as follows. Anxiety is probably the most common cause of headache and, where possible, the reason for the anxiety – overwork, family problems, unemployment, financial difficulties, etc. – should be tackled. Some people are more prone to anxiety than others. An unpleasant environment such as traffic pollution, badly ventilated or overcrowded working conditions, excessive smoking, etc., may provoke headaches in some people. MIGRAINE is a characteristic and often disabling type of headache. High blood pressure may cause headaches. Occasionally refractive errors of the eyes are associated with headaches. SINUS infections are often characterized by frontal headaches. Rheumatism in the muscles of the neck and scalp produce headaches. Fever is commonly accompanied by a headache, and SUNSTROKE and HEATSTROKE customarily result in headaches. Finally, as already stated, diseases in the brain such as MENINGITIS, tumours and haemorrhage may first manifest themselves as persistent or recurrent headaches.

Treatment Obtaining a reliable diagnosis – with the help of further investigations when indicated – should always be the initial aim;

treatment in most cases should then be aimed at the underlying condition. This same principle applies whether the cause is physical or stress induced. Used sensibly, a low dose of aspirin or paracetamol, for a limited period, may be helpful. In many cases of stress-induced headache, however, the most effective treatment is relaxation, possibly aided initially with a little alcohol or a mild sedative.

HEAD INJURY Any injury to the head, whether associated with a skull fracture or not. Patients with head injuries should be assessed for signs of neurological damage, which may not develop at once. Patients with drowsiness, vomiting, confusion, or any focal neurological signs after a head injury should be seen by a doctor. Particular care should be taken with individuals who have consumed alcohol and sustained a head injury in a fight, fall or vehicle accident. Symptoms indicative of a severe head injury may be attributed (wrongly) to the effects of alcohol and crucial time lost in treating the injury.

People suffering the results of such injuries and their relatives can obtain help and advice from Headway (National Head Injuries Association) (see APPENDIX 2: ADDRESSES).

HEAF TEST A skin test to find out if a person is immune to TUBERCULOSIS. TUBERCULIN (a preparation derived from the TUBERCLE bacillus) is injected via punctures in the skin of the forearm, using a spring-loaded gunlike instrument with six very short needles set in circular form. A positive test is indicated by a red raised reaction of the skin: this means the subject is immune. If the result is negative, the subject can be given BCG VACCINE.

HEALING (see WOUNDS).

HEALTH The state of health implies much more than freedom from disease, and good health may be defined as the attainment and maintenance of the highest state of mental and bodily vigour of which any given individual is capable. Environment, including living and working conditions, plays an important part in determining a person's health. The UK government is now placing much greater emphasis on health promotion and the prevention of disease and has published national targets for reducing the incidence of some major diseases. The 1978 World Health Organization statement declares that primary care should 'be made universally accessible to individuals and families in the community, by means acceptable to them, through their full participation, and at the cost that the community and country can afford to maintain in the spirit of self-reliance . . . [and] addresses the main health problems in the community, providing promotive, preventative, curative and rehabilitative services accordingly'. Factors affecting access to health include finance, ideology, and education.

HEALTH AND SAFETY EXECUTIVE The statutory body in Britain responsible for the health and safety of workers. The address of the HSE can be found in APPENDIX 2: ADDRESSES.

HEALTH CARE PRIORITIES As the needs and demands of patients and the costs of health care of populations have risen sharply in recent years, governments and health-care providers – whether tax funded, insurance based, employer provided or a mix of these – have increasingly had to face the dilemma of what services a country or a community can afford to provide. As a result, various techniques for deciding priorities of care and treatment are evolving. In the United Kingdom priorities were for many years based on the decisions of individual clinicians who had wide freedom to prescribe the most appropriate care. This clinical freedom is increasingly being circumscribed by managerial, community and political decisions driven in part by the availability of resources and increasingly by what people want. Rationing services, however, is not popular and as yet no broadly agreed consensus has emerged, either in Western Europe or North America, as to how priorities can be decided that have broad community support and which can be afforded.

HEALTH CENTRE An imprecise term that may refer to a group of doctors and supporting staff operating from one building owned or leased by the doctors, or a building owned or leased by a district health authority that contains staff or services from one or more sections of the National Health Service.

HEALTH EDUCATION The process of educating the public to adopt a healthy lifestyle and abandon dangerous or unhealthy behaviour. With the rising cost of health care and the increasing amount of illness and injury resulting from preventable causes, health professionals, governments and the World Health Organization are strongly supporting more and better health education for everyone from schoolchildren to the elderly. Information on all aspects of health education in the United Kingdom can be obtained from the Health Education Authority (see APPENDIX 2: ADDRESSES).

HEALTH PROMOTION A surveillance plan based on a community and aimed at maintaining an optimum state of health and quality of life for those who make up the community – both as individuals and as a group. Programmes would include immunization targets, health education, screening tests, as well as environmental procedures such as monitoring atmosphere, improving housing, water and food supplies, and encouraging safe and healthy working practices.

HEALTH SERVICE COMMISSIONER An official, responsible to the United Kingdom's parliament, appointed to protect the interests of National Health Service patients in matters concerning the administration of the health service. Known colloquially as the health ombudsman, the commissioner presents regular reports on the complaints dealt with.

HEALTH-SERVICE MANAGEMENT The administrative machinery for planning, delivering and monitoring health care provided by health professionals and their supporting staff. This may range from running a small primary-care centre to organizing a large hospital or being responsible for meeting the health needs of a region or a nation. Whether the overall structure for proving care is state funded, insurance based, private practice or a mixture of these, health-service management is essential in an era of rapidly evolving and expensive scientific medicine. Health-service managers are administrators with special training and skills in managing health care; sometimes they are doctors, nurses or other health professionals but many have been trained in management in commercial, civil service or industrial environments.

HEALTH VISITORS are nurses with a special training who form an important part of the primary health care team. Working in close conjunction with GENERAL PRACTITIONERS, they are primarily responsible for the health care of children and elderly people in the community. Health education and general promotion of health are an important part of their role. Contact the Health Visitors' Association (see APPENDIX 2: ADDRESSES).

HEARING (see DEAFNESS; EAR).

HEARING AIDS Nearly two-thirds of people aged over 70 have some degree of hearing impairment (see DEAFNESS). Hearing aids are no substitute for definitive treatment of the underlying cause of poor hearing, so examination by an ear, nose and throat surgeon is sensible before a hearing aid is issued (and is essential before one can be given through the NHS). The choice of aid depends on the age, manipulative skills, and degree of hearing impairment of the patient and the underlying cause of the deafness. The choice of hearing aid for a deaf child is particularly important as impaired hearing can hinder speech development.

Ear trumpets, although old fashioned, may occasionally help an elderly person who is unable to manage an electronic aid.

Electronic aids consist, essentially, of a microphone, an amplifier, and an earphone. In postaural aids the microphone and amplifier are contained in a small box worn behind the ear or attached to spectacles. The earphone is on a specially moulded earpiece. Some patients find it difficult to manipulate the controls of an aid worn behind the ear, and they may be better off with a device worn on the body. Some hearing aids are worn entirely within the ear and are very discreet. They are particularly useful for people who have to wear protective headgear such as helmets.

All types have a volume control and a special setting for use with telephone and in rooms fitted with an inductive coupler that screens out background noise.

In making a choice therefore from the large range of effective hearing aids now available, the expert advice of an ear specialist must be obtained. The RNID (Royal National Institute for Deaf People) (see APPENDIX 2: ADDRESSES), provides a list of clinics where such a specialist can be consulted. It also gives reliable advice concerning the purchase and use of hearing aids.

HEART A hollow muscular pump with four cavities, each provided at its outlet with a valve, whose function is to maintain the circulation of the blood. The two upper cavities are known as atria, the two lower ones as ventricles. The term auricle is applied to the ear-shaped tip of the atrium on each side.

Position The heart lies in the chest between the two lungs, but projecting more to the left side than to the right. On the left side its apex reaches out in the adult between 8 and 9 cm (3½ and 4 inches), almost to the nipple, and lies beneath the fifth rib, while its right border extends only a short distance, at most 2·4 cm, beyond the margin of the breast-bone. Its lower border rests upon the diaphragm, by which it is separated from the liver and stomach, and this close connection has an important influence upon the heart in several disorders of the stomach. Above, the heart extends to the level of the second rib, where the great vessels, the aorta on the right side and the pulmonary artery on the left, lie behind the breast-bone.

1	superior vena cava	6	pulmonary artery
2	right lung	7	left lung
3	right atrium	8	left ventricle
4	right ventricle	9a	liver (left lobe)
5	aorta	9b	liver (right lobe)

Diagram of the heart as seen on X-ray film.

superior vena cava

right lung

inferior vena cava

aorta

pulmonary artery

pulmonary veins

left lung

heart

aorta

Diagram of blood vessels linking heart and lungs.

Shape and size   The heart of any individual is about the size and shape of the clenched fist. Its weight in the male varies from 280 to 340 grams, and in the female from 230 to 280 grams. It continues to increase in weight and size up to a ripe old age, more so in men than in women. One end of the heart is pointed (apex), the other is broad (base), and is deeply cleft at the division between the two atria. One groove running down the front and up the back shows the division between the two ventricles; a circular, deeper groove marks off the atria above from the ventricles below. The capacity of each cavity is somewhere between 90 and 180 ml.

Structure   The heart lies within a strong fibrous bag, known as the pericardium, and since the inner surface of this bag and the outer surface of the heart are both covered with a smooth, glistening membrane faced with flat cells and lubricated by a little serous fluid (around 20 millilitres), the movements of the heart are accomplished almost without friction. The main thickness of the heart wall consists of bundles of muscle fibres, which run, some in circles right round the heart, others in loops, first round one cavity, then round the corresponding cavity of the other side. Within all the cavities is a smooth lining membrane, continuous with that lining the vessels which open into the heart. The investing smooth membrane is known as epicardium, the muscular substance as myocardium, and the smooth lining membrane as endocardium.

Important nerves regulate the heart's action, especially via the vagus nerve and with the sympathetic system. In the near part of the atria lies a collection of nerve cells and connecting fibres, known as the sinuatrial node, which forms the starting-point for the impulses that initiate the beats of the heart. Hence its alternative name of the pacemaker of the heart. In the groove between the ventricles and the atria lies another collection of similar nerve tissue, known as the atrioventricular node. Running

down from there into the septum between the two ventricles is a band of special muscle fibres, known as the atrioventricular bundle, or the bundle of His. This splits up into a right and a left branch for the two ventricles, and the fibres of these distribute themselves throughout the muscular wall of the ventricles and control their contraction. (For illustrations of the heart and its blood vessels see CIRCULATION OF THE BLOOD.)

Openings   There is no direct communication between the cavities on the right side and those on the left; but the right atrium opens into the right ventricle by a large circular opening, and similarly the left atrium into the left ventricle. Into the right atrium open two large veins, the superior and inferior venae cavae, with some smaller veins from the wall of the heart itself, and into the left atrium open two pulmonary veins from each lung. One opening leads out of each ventricle, to the aorta in the case of the left ventricle, to the pulmonary artery from the right.

Before birth the fetus's heart has an opening (foramen ovale) from the right into the left atrium through which the blood passes; but when the child first draws air into his lungs this opening closes and is represented in the adult only by a depression (fossa ovalis). (For illustration of internal anatomy of heart see CIRCULATION OF THE BLOOD.)

Valves   The heart contains four valves. The mitral valve consists of two triangular cusps, the tricuspid valve of three smaller cusps. The aortic and pulmonary valves each consist of three semilunar-shaped segments. The structure of a valve is a double layer of the lining membrane of the heart (endocardium) strengthened by fibrous tissue between. Two valves are placed at the openings leading from atrium into ventricle, the tricuspid valve on the right side, the mitral valve on the left, so as completely to prevent blood from running back into the atrium when the ventricle contracts. Two more, the pulmonary valve and the aortic valve, are at

1 aortic valve
2 mitral valve

Interior of the left ventricle, showing structure
of mitral and aortic valves.

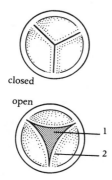

closed

open

1 cavity of left ventricle
2 valve cusp

Aortic valve, a semilunar-type valve. The
pulmonary valve is also of this type.

the entrance to these arteries, and prevent regurgitation into the ventricles of blood which has been driven from them into the arteries. The noises made by these valves in closing constitute the greater part of what are known as the heart sounds, and can be heard by anyone who applies his ear to the front of a person's chest. Murmurs heard accompanying these sounds indicate defects in the valves, and form one of the chief signs of heart disease.

Action At each heart-beat the two atria contract and expel their contents into the ventricles, which at the same time they stimulate to contract together, so that the blood is driven into the arteries, to be returned again to the atria after having completed a circuit in about

fifteen seconds through the body or lungs as the case may be. The heart beats from sixty to ninety times a minute, the rate in any given healthy person being about four times that of the respirations. The heart is to some extent regulated by a nerve centre in the MEDULLA, closely connected with those centres which govern the lungs and stomach, and nerve fibres pass to it in the vagus nerve. By some of these fibres its rate and force can be diminished, by others increased, according to the needs of the various organs of the body. If this nerve centre is injured or poisoned, for example, by lack of oxygen, the heart stops beating in human beings, although in some of the lower animals – e.g. frogs, fishes, and reptiles – the heart may under favourable conditions go on beating for hours even after its entire removal from the body.

HEARTBURN A burning sensation experienced in the region of the heart and up the back to the throat. It is caused by an excessive acidity of the gastric juice – often aggravated by dietary indiscretions – and is relieved temporarily by taking alkaline substances, such as 1·2 grams of bicarbonate of soda or commercial preparations such as aluminium-containing antacid tablets such as Aluminium Hydroxide Tablets, BP. The frequency of heartburn attacks can be lessened by eating a sensible diet, avoiding fatty or indigestible foods and restricting alcohol consumption.

HEART DISEASES: The heart is essentially a muscle pump which receives its own nutrient supply through the coronary arteries. It contains four valves which are designed to direct blood flow and the heart itself sits in a silky sac known as the pericardium. The action of the heart is determined by a sophisticated electric circuit known as the conducting system (see HEART).

Heart disease can affect any of the structures and more than one at a time.

Congenital heart disease accounts for 1–2 per cent of all cases of organic heart disease. It may be inherited, present at birth for no obvious reason or in rare cases related to RUBELLA in the mother or to drugs taken in pregnancy. The commonest forms are holes in the heart (atrial septal defect, ventricular septal defect (see SEPTAL DEFECT), a patent DUCTUS ARTERIOSUS and COARCTATION OF THE AORTA. Many complex forms also exist and can be diagnosed in the womb by fetal echocardiography which can lead to elective termination of pregnancy. Surgery to correct many of these abnormalities is feasible, even for the most severe abnormalities, but may only be palliative giving rise to major difficulties of management as the children become older. Heart transplantation is now increasingly employed for the uncorrectable lesions.

Coronary artery disease, also known as ischaemic heart disease, is the most important cause of symptoms and death in the adult population. It may present for the first time as sudden death but more usually it causes ANGINA PECTORIS, myocardial infarction (heart attack) or heart failure. It can also lead to a disturbance of heart rhythm. Its cause is not fully known but factors associated with an increased risk of developing coronary artery disease include male sex, increasing age, diabetes, cigarette smoking, high blood pressure and a raised concentration of cholesterol in the blood. Around 133,000 people died of coronary-artery disease in England and Wales in 1995; it was the biggest single cause of death.

Heart muscle disease or cardiomyopathy usually indicates a weakness of the left ventricle which secondarily affects the right ventricle. The efficiency of the pump deteriorates, the heart attempts to compensate by increasing muscle thickness (hypertrophy) and by dilating (enlarged heart), but after a variable time it fails, leading to the symptoms of breathlessness due to fluid accumulation in the lungs (pulmonary oedema). With a failure to pump efficiently the output falls and fatigue becomes a problem. When more advanced, fluid distends the liver and the ankles may become swollen.

Cardiomyopathy may be secondary to coronary artery disease, present in the absence of coronary artery disease and of no obvious cause, due to an inflammation of the heart muscle (myocarditis) most commonly caused by a virus infection or due to excessive consumption of alcohol. Myocarditis may resolve, as may cardiomyopathy due to excessive alcohol consumption if drinking is stopped, but most forms of cardiomyopathy are progressive, needing regular medication to maintain quality and quantity of life.

Valvular heart disease primarily affects the mitral and aortic valves which can become narrowed (stenosis) or leaking (incompetence). Pulmonary valve problems are usually congenital (stenosis) and the tricuspid valve is sometimes involved when rheumatic heart disease primarily affects the mitral or aortic valves RHEUMATIC FEVER, usually in childhood, remains a common cause of chronic valvular heart disease causing stenosis, incompetence or both of the aortic and mitral valves, but each valve has other separate causes for malfunction.

Aortic valve disease is more common with increasing age. When narrowed the heart hypertrophies and may later fail. Symptoms of angina or breathlessness are common and dizziness or blackouts (syncope) also occur. Replacing the valve is a very effective treatment, even with advancing age. Aortic stenosis may be caused by degeneration (senile calcific), inheriting two leaflets instead of the usual three (bicuspid valve) or rheumatic fever. Aortic incompetence again leads to hypertrophy, but dilatation is more common as blood leaks back into the ventricle. Breathlessness is the more common complaint. The causes are the same as stenosis but also include inflammatory conditions such as SYPHILIS or ANKYLOSING SPONDYLITIS and other disorders of connective tissue. The valve may also leak if the aorta dilates stretching the valve ring as with HYPERTENSION, aortic ANEURYSM and MARFAN'S SYNDROME – an inherited disorder of connective tissue that causes heart defects. Infection (endocarditis) can worsen acutely or chronically destroy the valve and sometimes lead to abnormal outgrowths on the valve (vegetations) which may break free and cause devastating damage such as a stroke or blocked circulation to the bowel or leg.

Mitral valve disease leading to stenosis is rheumatic in origin. Mitral incompetence may be rheumatic but in the absence of stenosis can be due to ISCHAEMIA, INFARCTION, inflammation, infection and a congenital weakness (prolapse). The valve may also leak if stretched by a dilating ventricle (functional incompetence). Infection (endocarditis) may affect the valve in a similar way to aortic disease. Mitral symptoms are predominantly breathlessness which may lead to wheezing or waking at night breathless and needing to sit up or stand for relief. They are made worse when the heart rhythm changes (atrial fibrillation) which is frequent as the disease becomes more severe. This leads to a loss of efficiency of up to 25 per cent and a predisposition to clot formation as blood stagnates rather than leaves the heart efficiently. Mitral incompetence may remain mild and be of no trouble for many years but infection must be guarded against (endocarditis prophylaxis).

Endocarditis is an infection of the heart which may acutely destroy a valve or lead to chronic destruction. Bacteria settle usually on a mild lesion. Antibiotics taken at vulnerable times can prevent this happening (antibiotic prophylaxis); one of the most common occasions is before dental treatment. If established, vigorous intravenous antibiotic therapy is needed and surgery is often necessary. The mortality is 30 per cent but may be higher if the infection settles on a replaced valve (prosthetic endocarditis). Complications include heart failure, shock, embolization (generation of small clots in the blood) and cerebral (mental) confusion. PERICARDITIS is an inflammation of the sac covering the outside of the heart. The sac becomes roughened and pain occurs as the heart and sac rub together. This is heard by stethoscope as a scratching noise (pericardial rub). Fever is often present and a virus the main cause. It may also occur with rheumatic fever, kidney failure, tuberculosis or from an adjacent lung problem such as pneumonia or cancer. The inflammation may cause fluid to accumulate between the sac and the heart (effusion) which may compress the heart causing a fall in blood pressure, a weak pulse and circulatory failure (tamponade). This can be relieved by aspirating the fluid. The treatment is then directed at the underlying cause.

Disturbances of rhythm are common and of several types. Many do not reflect underlying disease. Usually the patient becomes aware of his heart beat (palpitations) which may be fast or appear to miss a beat or kick. Stress or stimulants such as caffeine or alcohol are a frequent cause. Occasionally the disturbance can be troublesome, even though not dangerous, and merit treatment, but drugs should be avoided if no obvious disease exists.

Disturbances reflecting disease may lead to the heart's going fast or slow or both intermittently.

Atrial fibrillation may occur without obvious disease but usually presents when there is coronary artery disease, cardiomyopathy, high blood pressure or mitral valve disease. The rhythm is very irregular and may lead to rapid poorly co-ordinated contractions of the ventricle leading to heart failure. It predisposes to clots' forming in the heart. Treatment may be directed to converting the heart back to normal (sinus) rhythm by drugs or electric shock treatment or to controlling the speed with drugs such as DIGOXIN. It is a serious irregularity. Blood-thinning medication such as WARFARIN is often prescribed.

Extrasystoles are very common and usually perceived as missed beats or extra beats (a kick or thump). They are not usually serious but they may, however, complicate coronary artery disease or heart muscle disease when certain forms need specialized therapy.

Heart block refers to a failure to conduct normally through the electric circuit of the heart. There are three types; 1st degree which can be a normal variation and does not cause slowing; 2nd degree which causes intermittent slowing and 3rd degree or complete block where there is no electrical connection and heart beats are slow and unpredictable leading to blackouts (Stokes-Adams attacks) and/or heart failure. For most 2nd degree and all complete cases a pacemaker relieves symptoms and improves life expectancy.

Sinus node disease The main electrical control of the heart is the sinus node. If this is diseased or inherits a malfunction, the heart may develop rapid, slow or both rapid and slow rhythms. Often a tape recording for 24 hours (Holter) is used to document the irregularities. The heart itself may well be normal but these electrical disturbances can be very symptomatic. Treatment may include drugs, a CARDIAC PACEMAKER or both.

Miscellaneous There are many infrequent causes of heart problems which for the affected individual are a cause of debility. These include a problem of heart muscle thickening (hypertrophic cardiomyopathy), which can cause angina, irregular heart beats and sudden death, and Wolf Parkinson White Syndrome which causes the heart to race due to an extra fast conducting section in the circuit. This may induce pain, dizziness and blackouts. Some electrical conditions of the heart merit specific study known as electrophysiology (EPS) which allows the abnormality to be mapped out, thus facilitating drug or intervention treatment (ablation) to stop abnormal conduction.

Some disorders of the heart can be remedied with HEART SURGERY or for a few diseases heart transplants (see also TRANSPLANTATION)

HEART LUNG MACHINE A device that temporarily takes over the function of the heart and lungs. It is used in certain operations in the chest, giving the surgeon more time for operations such as open-heart surgery, heart transplants and heart-lung transplants. The machine also ensures an operating area largely free of blood which helps the surgeon to work more quickly. A pump replaces the heart and an oxygenator replaces the lungs. When connected up, the machine in effect bypasses normal cardiopulmonary activity. It also contains a heat exchanger to warm or cool the patient's blood according to the requirements of the operation. The patient is given an anticoagulant (HEPARIN) to counteract clotting which may occur when blood cells get damaged during the machine's use. Patients are on the machine only for a few hours because blood supply to vital organs begins to be reduced.

HEART SURGERY Open-heart surgery permits the treatment of many previously inoperable conditions that were potentially fatal or made the patient chronically disabled. CORONARY-ARTERY BYPASS, used to remedy obstruction of the arteries supplying the heart muscle, was first done in the mid 1960s and is now widely practised. About the same time the first heart transplant was performed (in South Africa) and the use of this operation is now limited only by the availability of suitable heart donors. Constricted heart valves are now routinely dilated by MINIMALLY INVASIVE techniques such as ANGIOPLASTY and laser treatment and faulty valves can be replaced with mechanical alternatives (see VALVULOPLASTY).

Heart transplants Replacement of a person's unhealthy heart with a normal heart from a healthy donor. The donor's heart needs to be removed immediately after death and kept chilled in saline before rapid transport to the recipient. These are technically demanding operations used to treat patients with progressive untreatable heart disease but whose other body systems are in good shape. They usually have advanced coronary-artery disease and damaged heart muscle (CARDIOMYOPATHY). Apart from the technical difficulties of the operation, preventing rejection of the transplanted heart by the recipient's immune system requires complex drug treatment. But once the patient has passed the immediate postoperative phase, the chances of five-year survival is as high as 80 per cent in some cardiac centres.

HEAT-CRAMPS Painful cramps in the muscles occurring in workers, such as stokers, who labour in hot conditions. The cramps are the result of loss of salt in the sweat, and can be cured by giving salty water to drink. (See HEAT-STROKE.)

HEAT SPOTS A vague term applied to small inflamed and congested areas which appear especially upon the skin of the face, neck, and chest or other parts of the body in warm weather.

HEAT STROKE A condition resulting from environmental temperatures which are too high for compensation by the body's thermo-regulatory mechanism(s). It is characterized by hyperpyrexia, nausea, headache, thirst, confusion, and dry skin. If untreated, coma and death ensue. Its occurence is sporadic; whereas a single individual may be affected (occasionally with fatal consequences), his or her colleagues may remain unaffected. Predisposing factors include unsatisfactory living or working conditions, inadequate acclimatization to tropical conditions, unsuitable clothing, underlying poor health, and possibly dietetic or alcoholic indiscretions. It can be a major problem during pilgrimages, e.g., the Hadj. Four clinical syndromes are recognized:

Heat collapse is characterized by fatigue, giddiness, and temporary loss of consciousness. It is accompanied by hypotension and bradycardia; there may be vomiting and muscular cramps. Urinary volume is diminished. Recovery is usual.

Heat exhaustion is characterized by increasing weakness, dizziness, and insomnia; in the majority, sweating is defective; there are few, if any, signs of dehydration. Pulse rate is normal, and urinary output good. Body temperature is usually 37·8–38·3 °C.

Heat cramps (usually in the legs, arms, or back and occasionally involving the abdominal muscles) are associated with hard physical work at a high temperature. Sweating, pallor, headache, giddiness, and intense anxiety are present. Body temperature is only mildly raised.

Heat hyperpyrexia is heralded by energy loss and irritability; this is followed by mental confusion and diminution of sweating. The individual rapidly becomes restless, comatose, and body temperature rises to 41–42 °C or even higher. The condition is fatal unless expertly treated as a matter of urgency.

Treatment With the first two syndromes, the affected individual must be removed immediately to a cool place, and isotonic saline administered, intravenously in a severe case. The fourth syndrome is a medical emergency. The patient should be placed in the shade, stripped, and drenched with water; fanning should be instigated. He or she should be wrapped in a sheet soaked in cool water and fanning continued. When rectal temperature has fallen to 39 °C the patient is wrapped in a dry blanket. Immediately after consciousness returns, normal saline should be given orally; this usually provokes sweating. The risk of circulatory collapse exists. Convalescence may be protracted and the patient should be repatriated to a cool climate. Prophylactically, personnel intended for work in a tropical climate must be very carefully selected. Adequate acclimatization is also essential; severe physical exertion must be avoided for several weeks. Light clothes should be worn. The diet should be light but nourishing, and fluid intake adequate. Those performing hard physical work at a very high ambient temperature should receive sodium chloride supplements. Attention to ventilation and air-conditioning is essential; fans are also of value.

HEBEPHRENIA A form of mental disorder coming on in youth and marked by depression and gradual failure of mental faculties with egotistic and self-centred delusions. It is one of the forms of schizophrenia.

HEBERDEN'S NODES Small hard knobs which appear at the sides of the last phalanges of the fingers in people who have osteoarthrosis.

HEEL is the hinder part of the foot formed by the calcaneus and the specially thick skin covering it. It is not subject to many diseases. Severe pain in the heel is sometimes a sign of gout or rheumatism.

HEIGHT (see WEIGHT AND HEIGHT).

HELICOBACTER PYLORI A genus of flagellated gram-negative bacterium. It colonizes the mucosal layer of the stomach and duodenum causing inflammation – gastritis and duodenitis respectively. In England and Wales 60 per cent of the annual 4,000 or so people who die from PEPTIC ULCERATION have *H. pylori* infection. The bacterium, which usually becomes apparent in middle age, is linked with 75 per cent of deaths from gastric cancer. In the developed world most people are infected by the age of 10. *H. pylori* gastroduodenitis is now a disease in its own right. It can be diagnosed on a blood test but a biopsy of the stomach lining is a more accurate method. The latest development in treatment is the use of PROTON PUMP INHIBITOR triple therapy – a proton pump inhibitor plus two antibiotics, usually clarithromycin and amoxicillin or metronidazole. Success rates are around 90 per cent and the infection rarely recurs. *H. pylori* used to be classified as *CAMPYLOBACTER PYLORI*.

HELIUM This is the lightest gas known, with the exception of hydrogen. This property renders it of value in ANAESTHESIA, as its addition to the anaesthetic means that it can be inhaled with less effort by the patient. Thus it can be used in the presence of any obstruction to the entry of air to the lungs.

HELMINTHS Another name for parasitic worms such as FLUKES, tapeworms (TAENIASIS) and nematodes (ASCARIASIS).

HEMIANAESTHESIA Loss of touch-sense down one side of the body.

HEMIANOPIA, HEMIANOPSIA, and HEMIOPIA are terms meaning loss of half the usual area of vision. The affected person may see everything clearly to the left or to the right, the field of vision stopping abruptly at the middle line, or he may see things only when straight in front of him, or thirdly, he may see objects far out on both sides, although there is a wide area straight in front for which he is quite blind. The position of the blind area is important in localizing the position in the brain of the disease responsible for the condition.

HEMIATROPHY Atrophy of one side of the body, or of part of the body on one side: for example, facial hemiatrophy, in which one-half of the face is smaller than the other either in the course of development or as a result of some nervous disorder.

HEMIBALLISMUS Involuntary movements similar to choreiform movements but of much greater amplitude and force. They are violent throwing movements of the limbs which are usually unilateral. They tend to occur acutely as a result of vascular damage to the mid-brain.

HEMICOLECTOMY An operation to remove the right or left half of the colon, usually with end-to-end anastomosis of the remaining portion of the intestine. This is often used for the treatment of malignant or inflammatory diseases of the colon.

HEMICRANIA A headache limited to one side of the head. (See MIGRAINE.)

HEMIMELIA This consists of defects in the distal part of the extremities such as the absence of a forearm or hands. This is a congenital defect and large numbers of cases resulted from the administration of Thalidomide during pregnancy.

HEMIPARESIS Paralysis affecting the muscles of one side of the body. This most commonly follows a stroke and occurs when parts of the brain serving motor function on the opposite side of the body are damaged.

HEMIPLEGIA Paralysis limited to one side of the body. (See PARALYSIS.)

HEMP (see CANNABIS).

HENLE, LOOP OF That part of the nephron (see KIDNEYS) between the proximal and distal convoluted tubules. It extends into the renal medulla as a hairpin-shaped loop. The ascending link of the loop actively transports sodium from the lumen of the tube to the interstitium, and this, combined with the 'counter-current' flow of fluid through the two limbs of the loop, plays a part in concentrating the urine.

HENOCH-SCHÖNLEIN PURPURA This is an inflammatory condition of the small blood vessels, the cause of which is not known but may be an allergic response to food or drugs. Commonest among young children, especially boys, the inflammation causes blood to leak into joints, kidneys, intestine and skin. Symptomatic treatment is usually sufficient but severely ill patients may need corticosteroid drugs.

HEPARIN is a naturally produced ANTICOAGULANT) with a rapid effect which is thought to act by neutralizing thrombin (see COAGULATION). Inactive when taken orally, it is normally given intravenously – it may be given for a few days, combined with an oral anticoagulant such as warfarin, to initiate anticoagulation. Low-dose heparin may be given by subcutaneous injection for longer periods, for the prophylaxis of deep-vein thrombosis or pulmonary embolism in 'high-risk' patients, such as those with obesity or a history of thrombosis, or post-operatively. If haemorrhage occurs, withdrawal of heparin is usually sufficient, but protamine sulphate is a rapidly active and specific antidote. Prolonged treatment with heparin may cause osteoporosis.

HEPATECTOMY The operation for removal of the liver, or part of it.

HEPATITIS Hepatitis, or inflammation of liver cells (see LIVER), may be acute or chronic and symptoms may be absent or non-specific. Acute hepatitis causes JAUNDICE, itching, abdominal pain and liver tenderness, malaise, ANOREXIA, fever and nausea. Treatment consists of bed-rest and relief of symptoms. All unnecessary drugs must be stopped and alcohol should be avoided. Chronic hepatitis can cause any of the symptoms above, but they tend to be more insidious in onset.

Diagnostic investigations include blood tests to assess liver function, liver biopsy to classify the type and cause of hepatitis and ultrasound scanning (see ULTRASOUND).

There are many causes; some agents can produce both acute and chronic hepatitis. Alcohol abuse is the commonest cause in Great Britain.

Viral hepatitis classically refers to infection with one of the so-called hepatitis viruses, of which there are at least five: A, B, C, D and E. Many other virus infections produce liver inflammation and these include glandular fever and HIV, but these five viruses specifically target liver cells. Treatment with many drugs causes hepatitis as a side-effect; HALOTHANE general anaesthesia, methyl dopa and paracetamol in overdose are examples. Autoimmune diseases such as RHEUMATOID ARTHRITIS may exhibit associated chronic hepatitis.

Fulminant hepatitis is the severest form of liver inflammation; there is massive destruction of liver cells resulting in liver failure with severe jaundice, impaired consciousness, fluid retention and a bleeding tendency. Kidney failure may follow. Causes include alcohol abuse, acute viral hepatitis and paracetamol overdose. Liver transplantation has dramatically improved the outlook of this condition.

Infectious hepatitis is caused by hepatitis A and E viruses. These varieties are transmitted primarily by faeces-contaminated drinking water: A is common throughout the globe but E is found mainly in developing countries. They may also be transmitted by eating food contaminated with faecal material from an infected individual, particularly seafood, and it is common in areas where standards of hygiene are poor. In temperate climates it tends to occur in late summer; in the tropics there is no seasonal variation. Incubation period is 15 to 45 days. Patients should not return to work until at least 7 days after complete clinical recovery, when the prognosis is good and there is no risk of chronic infection. Hepatitis E virus is similar to Hepatitis A, except that in pregnancy the mortality rate of the former may be as high as 20 per cent.

Serum hepatitis is due to infection with viruses B, C or D. They share the same routes of infection – through transfusion of infected blood, sharing needles for injection of drugs, tattooing or through sexual intercourse with an infected individual – and tend to have a longer incubation period, up to 180 days in the case of virus B. These virus infections carry a much higher mortality rate (1–3 per cent in hepatitis B and C, up to 20 per cent in virus D) and the viruses may remain in the blood for many years, causing chronic carrier status (such individuals remain an infectious risk to others) and chronic hepatitis. Diagnosis of these various types of viral infection is by the demonstration of specific ANTIBODIES and ANTIGENS in the blood. Following the discovery of the responsible virus, non-A non-B hepatitis is now known as hepatitis C.

Persistence of hepatitis B virus in the blood with hepatic inflammation lasting more than 6 months after hepatitis B infection is defined as chronic type-B hepatitis. Hepatocellular carcinoma is common in areas of the world where hepatitis-B carrier status is frequent and chronic hepatitis – of any cause – may result in cirrhosis. Therefore much effort has gone into finding treatments for chronic type-B hepatitis, the most successful of which has been antiviral chemotherapy with INTERFERON. The response

to this treatment may be disappointing with a high rate of relapse.

A vaccine to prevent hepatitis B is available but is usually given only to people at high risk such as health-care workers or those travelling frequently to high-risk areas. Protection against hepatitis A and B can be given by passive immunization using IMMUNOGLOBULIN injections. The UK government is planning to immunize infants against hepatitis C. People in high-risk areas should observe good standards of personal and food hygiene. Infection with hepatitis B can be reduced by using CONDOMS during sexual intercourse.

HEPATOLENTICULAR DEGENERATION
(see WILSON'S DISEASE).

HEPATOMA   A primary malignant tumour of liver cells. It has marked geographical variation, being most common in parts of Africa and the Far East. It is more common in men and with those who have pre-existing CIRRHOSIS.

HEPATOMEGALY   Enlargement of the liver. This may be caused by congestion (e.g. in heart failure), infection (e.g. hepatitis), malignancy, inflammation, or early CIRRHOSIS.

HERBAL MEDICINE   Varieties of medical treatment using different plants. For many centuries herbal medicine was the most commonly used medical treatment in cultures throughout the world.

HEREDITY   The principle on which various peculiarities of bodily form or structure, or of physical or mental activity are transmitted from parents to offspring. (See GENES.)

HERMAPHRODITE   An individual in whom both ovarian and testicular tissue is present. Hermaphrodites may have a testis on one side and an ovary on the other, or an ovotestis on one side and an ovary or testis on the other, or there may be an ovotestis on both sides. Both gonads are usually intra-abdominal. The true hermaphrodite usually has a uterus and at least one fallopian tube on the side of the ovary. On the side of the testis there is usually a vas deferens. Most true hermaphrodites are raised as males but external virilization is not usually complete. Even when significant phallic development is present hypospadias and cryptorchism are common. At puberty gynaecomastia develops and menstruation is common, as ovarian function is usually more nearly normal than testicular function. The condition is rare. A more common condition is pseudohermaphroditism: these are individuals who possess the gonads of only one sex but their external genitalia may be ambiguous. The cause is a hormonal imbalance and can usually be corrected by hormone treatment.

HERNIA The protrusion of an organ, or part of an organ through the wall of the cavity that normally contains it. The most common types of hernia involve the organs of the abdomen which can herniate externally through the abdominal wall, or internally usually through a defect in the diaphragm. External hernias appear as a swelling, covered with skin, which bulge out on coughing or straining but which can normally be made to disappear with gentle pressure.

Types The commonest hernia is the inguinal hernia, which appears in the groin at the site of inguinal canal, which contains the spermatic chord in males. Less common is the femoral hernia which appears just below the groin, passing through a defect close to the main blood vessels of the leg. The inguinal hernia is commoner in males and the femoral hernia in

1 transverse abdominis muscle
2 external oblique muscle
3 internal oblique muscle
4 spermatic cord
5 epidydimis
6 testis
7 scrotum
8 abdominal contents
9 abdominal peritoneum
10 rectus femoris
11 internal spermatic fascia
12 tunica vaginalis

Anatomy of indirect inguinal hernia: arrow shows direction of displaced loop of intestine moving into scrotum.

Site of inguinal hernia (shaded).

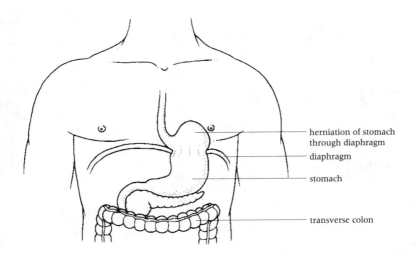

herniation of stomach through diaphragm

diaphragm

stomach

transverse colon

Diaphragmatic or hiatus hernia showing the stomach pushing through the diaphragm into the chest cavity.

females. Other common types of abdominal hernia include an incisional hernia, through a defect in any abdominal surgical scar, a paraumbilical hernia arising just to the side of the umbilicus and an epigastric hernia in the mid line above the umbilicus. In children, herniation may occur through the umbilicus itself, which is a natural weak spot. The commonest internal hernia is a hiatus hernia, when part of the stomach slips upwards into the chest through the DIAPHRAGM.

Causes Hernias may be due to a defect present at birth (congenital), or may develop later in life (acquired). Acquired hernias arise due to the development of a defect or injury of the abdominal wall or due to increased pressure within the abdominal cavity, which forces the organ through a potential weakness. Such causes include chronic coughing or excessive straining due to constipation.

Complications Small hernias may cause no problems at all. However, some may be large and cumbersome, or may give rise to a dragging sensation or even pain.

Although most hernias will reduce spontaneously under the effects of gravity or gentle pressure, any organs that may have been displaced inside some hernias may become stuck, when they are said to be irreducible. If the contents become so trapped that their blood supply is cut off, then strangulation occurs. This is a surgical emergency because the strangulated organs will soon die or rupture. When strangulation does occur, the hernia becomes irreducible, red, and very painful. If the hernia contains bowel, then the bowel may also become obstructed.

Treatment Conservative treatment with a compression belt, or truss, is now less popular than in previous eras. Surgical repair is the preferred option whenever possible, and consists of returning the herniated organs to their proper place, and then repairing the defect through which the hernia occurred. This may be done safely under local or general anaesthetic, often as a day-case procedure, and most operative repairs result in a permanent cure.

HERNIOPLASTY A surgical technique for repair of a HERNIA. The abnormal opening is sewn up or the weakness is strengthened with sutures or the insertion of a polypropylene mesh.

HERNIORRAPHY Surgical repair of a hernia. This may be done as an open operation or as MINIMALLY INVASIVE SURGERY using a LAPAROSCOPE.

HEROIN Also known as diacetyl morphine, this drug is an opiate, a group which includes morphine, codeine, pethidine, and methadone. It is a powerful analgesic and cough suppressant, but its capacity to produce euphoria rapidly induces dependence. Popular with addicts, its mostly pleasant effects soon produce tolerance, and the need to inject the drug, with associated risks of HIV infection, has affected its use by addicts (see DRUG ADDICTION). Withdrawal symptoms include restlessness, insomnia, muscle cramps, vomiting, and diarrhoea; signs include dilated pupils, raised pulse rate, and disturbed temperature control. Although rarely life threatening, they may cause great distress; for this reason methadone, which has a slower and less severe withdrawal syndrome, is commonly used when weaning addicts off heroin. Legally still available to doctors in the UK, heroin is normally only used in patients with severe pain, or to comfort the dying.

HERPANGINA is a short febrile illness in which minute vesicles or punched-out ulcers develop in the posterior parts of the mouth. It is due to infection with the group A COXSACKIE VIRUSES.

HERPES GENITALIS or genital herpes A sexually transmitted HERPES SIMPLEX infection of the GENITALS in either sex.

HERPES SIMPLEX An acute infectious disease, characterized by the development of groups of superficial vesicles, or blebs, in the skin and mucous membrane. It is due to a virus, and infection can occur at any time from birth onwards, but the usual time for primary infection is between the second and fifteenth year. Once an individual is infected, the virus persists in the body for the rest of the individual's life. It is one of the causes of scrum-pox.

Symptoms The symptoms vary with the age of infection. In young infants it may cause a generalized infection which may prove fatal. In young children the infection is usually in the mouth, and this may be associated with enlargement of the glands in the neck, general irritability and fever. The condition usually settles in seven to ten days. In adults the vesicles may occur anywhere in the skin or mucous membranes. The more common sites are the lips, mouth and face where they are known as cold sores. The vesicles may also appear on the genitalia, when it is known as Herpes genitalis, or in the conjunctiva or cornea and the brain may be infected, causing encephalitis or meningitis. The first sign is the appearance of small painful swellings. These quickly develop into vesicles, containing clear fluid, and surrounded by a reddened area of skin. Some people are particularly liable to recurrent attacks, and these often tend to be associated with some debilitating condition or infection, such as pneumonia.

Except in the case of herpes of the cornea, the eruption clears completely unless it becomes contaminated with some other organism. In the case of the cornea, there may be residual scarring, which may impair vision.

Treatment Aciclovir is effective both topically as cream or eye drops or orally. In severe systemic infections it can be given intra-venously.

HERPES VIRUSES   One member of a group of viruses containing DNA which cause latent infections in animal and man. Viruses from this group cause HERPES SIMPLEX, HERPES ZOSTER (shingles) and CHICKENPOX and include CYTOME-GALOVIRUS and EPSTEIN-BARR VIRUS.

HERPES ZOSTER, or SHINGLES, is a skin eruption of acute nature, closely related to chickenpox, consisting in the appearance of small yellow VESICLES, which spread over an area, dry up, and heal by scabbing. It receives its name from the Greek word, for a 'circingle' or girdle, because it spreads in a zone-like manner round half the chest. Herpes of the face also occurs, particularly on the brow and round the eye.

Causes   It is due to a virus identical with that of chickenpox. This invades the ganglia of the nerves, particularly the spinal nerves of the chest and the fifth cranial nerve which supplies the face. In spite of its being due to the same virus as chickenpox, it is rare for herpes zoster to occur as a result of contact with a case of chickenpox. On the other hand, it is not unusual for a patient with herpes zoster to infect a child with chickenpox. It is a disease of adults rather than children, and the older the person the more likely is he to develop the disease. Thus in adults under 50 the incidence is around 2·5 per 1000 people a year. Between 50 and 60 it is around 5 per 1000, whilst in octo-genarians it is 10 per 1000. Most adults who acquire the disease have had chickenpox in child-hood. Occasionally it may be associated with some serious underlying disease such as leukaemia, lymphadenoma, or multiple my-eloma.

Symptoms   The first symptoms of herpes are much like those of any feverish attack. The person feels unwell for some days, has a slight rise of temperature, and vague pain in the side or in various other parts. The pain finally settles at a point in the side, and, two or three days after the first symptoms, the rash appears. Minute yellow blebs or vesicles as they are known are seen on the skin of the back, of the side, or of the front of the chest, or simultane-ously on all three, the points corresponding to the space between one pair of ribs right round. These blebs increase in number for some days, and spread till there is often a complete half girdle round one side of the chest. The pain in this stage is severe, but it appears to vary a good deal with age, being slight in children and very severe in old people, in whom indeed herpes sometimes forms a serious illness. After one or two weeks, most of the vesicles have dried up and formed scabs. The pain may not pass off when the eruption disappears, but may remain for weeks or even months: a condition known as post-herpetic neuralgia. Old people are prone to develop this condition.

Treatment   ACICLOVIR or famciclovir can be given orally, and are effective if started in large doses early in the attack. Later topical antibi-otics may be required. Analgesics may be necessary if neuralgia is severe.

HERTZ   The SI (International System of Units) unit of frequency. It indicates the number of cycles per second (c/s). The abbreviation for hertz is Hz.

HETEROGRAFT   A transplant from one animal to another of a different species. It is also known as a xenograft.

HETEROSEXUAL   Sexual attraction to in-dividuals of the opposite sex. (See HOMOSEXUAL-ITY.)

HETEROZYGOUS   An individual having dis-similar members of the pair of genes coding for a given characteristic (see GENES).

HEXACHLOROPHANE   A widely used an-tiseptic which is active against a range of micro-organisms, including gram-positive and gram-negative organisms, *Shigella dysenteriae*, and *Salmonella typhi*. One of its advantages is that it retains its activity in the presence of soap, and it is therefore often used in soaps and creams in a concentration of 1 to 2 per cent. It must be used with caution in babies as it can be absorbed through the skin and prove harmful.

HEXAMINE   A substance which, when ex-creted by the kidneys, releases formaldehyde, that has an antiseptic action. It is given to patients with recurrent cystitis. It acts only in urine with an acid reaction, and, if the urine is alkaline, ascorbic acid may acidify it. Hexam-ine is used prophylactically and for long-term treatment of recurrent urinary-tract infections.

Hg   The chemical symbol for mercury. BLOOD PRESSURE is traditionally measured in milli-metres (mm) of mercury using a SPHYGMO-MANOMETER consisting of an inflatable cuff (usually wrapped round the upper arm) con-nected by a rubber tube to a column of mercury calibrated in mm of mercury.

HIATUS HERNIA   A displacement of a por-tion of the stomach through the opening in the diaphragm through which the oesophagus passes from the chest to the abdominal cavity. (see HERNIA.)

HICCUP   An involuntary spasmodic contrac-tion of the DIAPHRAGM which produces an indrawing of breath during which there is a sudden closure of the vocal cords. This results in the well-known sound and sensation.
   It is usually of benign cause (e.g. indigestion)

but may be a symptom of medullary brain damage, uraemia, typhoid fever or encephalitis lethargica.

There are many folk remedies for hiccups but most subside spontaneously. Prolonged hiccups due to disease may respond to treatment with chlorpromazine.

HIGH-DEPENDENCY UNIT A hospital unit equipped and staffed to nurse patients who require a high level of technically supported care. Patients are usually moved to such units when they have made satisfactory progress in an intensive-care unit (ICU) and do not require the one-to-one nursing necessary in ICUs. Patients who have undergone major surgery are often transferred from the recovery ward to a high-dependency unit until they are well enough to be cared for in a standard ward.

HILUM A term applied to the depression on organs such as the lung, kidney, and spleen, at which the vessels and nerves enter it and round which the lymphatic glands cluster. The hilum of the lung is also known as its root.

HIP That part of the body on each side of the pelvis where it articulates with the head of the femur (thigh bone).

HIP-JOINT The joint formed by the head of the thigh-bone and the deep cup-shaped hollow on the side of the pelvis which receives it (acetabulum). The joint is of the ball-and-socket variety, is dislocated only by very great violence, and is correspondingly difficult to reduce to its natural state after dislocation. The joint is enclosed by a capsule of fibrous tissue, strengthened by several bands, of which the principal is the ilio-femoral or Y-shaped ligament placed in front of the joint. A round ligament also unites the head of the thigh-bone to the margin of the acetabulum.

For hip-joint disease see under JOINTS, DISEASES OF.

HIPPOCRATIC OATH An oath traditionally taken by doctors on qualification that sets out the moral precepts of their profession and binds them to a code of behaviour and practice. It is named after Hippocrates (460–370 BC), the Greek 'father of medicine'.

HIPPUS is a tremor of the iris which produces alternating contraction and dilatation of the pupil.

HIRSCHSPRUNG'S DISEASE, or MEGA COLON, is a congenital condition in childhood which is characterized by great hypertrophy and dilatation of the colon. The RECTUM and lower COLON have failed to develop a normal nerve network, thus disturbing normal contraction and expansion of these structures. Treat-

ment is surgical removal of the affected sections with the remaining colon being joined to the anus.

HIRSUTISM, or HYPERTRICHOSIS, is the growth of hair of the male type and distribution in women. It is either due to the excess production of androgens or to undue sensitivity of the hair follicle to normal female levels of circulating androgens. The latter is called idiopathic because the cause is unknown. The increased production of androgens in the female may come from the ovary and be due to the polycystic ovary syndrome or an ovarian tumour, or the excess androgen may come from the adrenal cortex and be the result of congenital adrenal hyperplasia, an adrenal tumour or Cushing's syndrome. However there is a wide range of normality in the distribution of female body hair. It varies with different racial groups. The Mediterranean races have more body hair than Nordic women and the Chinese and Japanese have little body hair. Many normal women, especially those with dark hair, have hair apparent on the upper lip and a few coarse hairs on the chin and around the nipples are not uncommon. Extension of the pubic hair towards the umbilicus is frequently found in normal women. Dark hair is much more apparent than fair hair and this is why bleaching is of considerable benefit in the management of hirsutism.

The treatment of hirsutism is that of the primary cause. When it is idiopathic hirsutism it must be managed by simple measures such as bleaching the hair and the use of depilatory waxes and creams. Coarse facial hairs can be removed by electrolysis, although this is time consuming. Shaving is often the most effective remedy and neither increases the rate of hair growth nor causes the hairs to become coarser.

HISTAMINE An AMINE derived from HISTIDINE. It is widely distributed in the tissues of plants and animals, including man. It is a powerful stimulant of gastric juice, a constrictor of smooth muscle including that of the bronchi, and a dilator of arterioles and capillaries. It is this last action which is responsible for the eruption of URTICARIA.

HISTIDINE An amino-acid from which histamine is derived.

HISTOLOGY The study of the minute structure of the tissues using special staining processes which are combined with electron and light microscopy. The specialty is staffed by medically qualified pathologists (histologists) and scientifically qualified technicians.

HISTOPLASMOSIS A disease due to a yeast-like fungus known as *Histoplasma capsulatum*. Most cases have been reported from USA. In infants it is characterized by fever, anaemia, enlargement of the liver and spleen, and involvement of the lungs and gastro-intestinal tract. In older children it may resemble pulmonary tuberculosis, whilst in adults it may be confined to involvement of the skin.

HIV Human immunodeficiency virus: the virus that is responsible for AIDS. It is one of the family of human T-cell lymphocytotrophic viruses, others of which may cause lymphomas in man. (See AIDS/HIV.)

HIVES A popular term applied to eruptions of the nature of URTICARIA.

HLA SYSTEM The major histocompatibility complex, or human leucocyte antigen (HLA) region, consists of genetically determined antigens, situated on chromosome 6. Found in most tissues, though to a differing extent, the four gene loci are known as A, B, C, D, while the individual alleles at each locus are numbered 1, 2, 3, etc. The number of possible combinations is thus enormous, and the chance of two unrelated people being identical for HLA is very low. HLA incompatibility causes the immune response, or rejection reaction, that occurs with unmatched tissue grafts. Strong associations between HLA and susceptibility to certain diseases – notably the autoimmune diseases such as rheumatoid arthritis, insulin-dependent diabetes, and thyrotoxicosis – have been described. Certain HLA antigens occur together more frequently than would be expected by chance (linkage disequilibrium), and may have a protective effect, conferring resistance to a disease.

HODGKIN'S DISEASE, so called after Thomas Hodgkin (1798–1866), the Guy's Hospital pathologist who first described it, or LYMPHADENOMA, is an uncommon malignant form of LYMPHOMA in which the lymphatic glands all over the body undergo progressive enlargement. The spleen is also affected. The cause is not known. The glands affected may reach a great size. The male:female ratio is 1·4:1 and the disease is rare before 10, peaking in the twenties and late middle age. The patient often runs a characteristic form of fever (Pel-Ebstein fever), in which bouts of fever alternate with several days of normal body temperature. The patient becomes progressively weaker and develops anaemia and impairment of the immune system. There is a serious risk of life-threatening infections. Diagnosis is by biopsy of affected gland or organs. Treatment consists of radiotherapy when the disease is relatively localized. When it is more widespread, however, chemotherapy is the treatment of choice. This is now given in the form of a combination of drugs, rather than one single drug. CYTOTOXIC drugs used include doxorubicin, lomustine, mustine, vinblastine, vincristine and procarbazine. Prednisolone is also given. The results of treatment are now such that over 80 per cent treated by radiotherapy, and 78 per cent of those treated by combined chemotherapy, are still alive after five years.

HOLISTIC A method of medical care in which patients are treated as a whole and which takes into account their physical and mental state as well as social background rather than just treating the disease alone.

HOMATROPINE is an alkaloid derived from atropine, which is used to produce dilatation of the pupil and to paralyse accommodation temporarily for the purpose of examining the interior of the eye. It is used in 1 per cent solution, and its effects pass away in the course of a few hours.

HOMEOSTASIS The normal physiological process that ensures that the body's internal systems, such as its metabolism, blood pressure and body temperature, maintain an equilibrium whatever the conditions of the outside environment. For example, the body temperature remains at around 37 °C (98.4 °F) in a cold or a hot climate.

HOMOCYSTEINE An intermediate product in the body's synthesis of the amino-acid CYSTEINE.

HOMOCYSTINURIA is a congenital disease due to the inability of the affected individual to metabolize, or utilize properly one of the essential AMINO-ACIDS known as methionine. The main features of the condition are abnormality of the lens of the eye, mental retardation, fair complexion and fair hair and a high cheek colour.

HOMOEOPATHY A system of medicine founded by Hahnemann at the end of the eighteenth century. It is based upon the theory that diseases are curable by those drugs which produce effects on the body similar to symptoms caused by the disease (similia similibus curantur). In administering drugs, the theory is also held that their effect is increased by giving them in minute doses obtained by substantially diluting them. (see APPENDIX 13: COMPLEMENTARY MEDICINE.)

HOMOGRAFT A piece of tissue or an organ, such as a kidney, transplanted from one animal to another of the same species: e.g. from man to man. It is also known as an allograft.

HOMOSEXUALITY Sexual activity with a member of the same sex. There has been considerable debate among psychiatrists as to whether homosexuality should be regarded as a normal sexual variant or as a psycho-pathological development or deviation. Although homosexuality is found in virtually every society and culture there is no society in which it is the predominant or preferred mode of sexual activity. Various attempts have been made to link homosexuality to hormonal factors, particularly lowered testosterone levels, or to find a genetic explanation, but there is no evidence for either. Psycho-analytic theories link homosexuality to early child-rearing influences, in particular the close binding and intimate mother.

The number of homosexual men and women in the UK is unknown. There has never been a representative population survey. Re-analysis of the Kinsey report suggests that only 3 per cent of adult men have exclusively homosexual leanings and a further 3 per cent have extensive homosexual and heterosexual experience. Homosexuality among women (lesbianism) seems to be less common. Some homosexual men have high rates of sexual activity and multiple partners and, as with heterosexual men and women, this increases the risk of acquiring sexually transmitted diseases, unless they take appropriate precautionary measures, for example, the use of condoms for penetrative sex, whether vaginal or anal. It was in homosexual males that the virus responsible for AIDS was first identified, but the infection now occurs in both sexes.

There are still differences in the way homosexuals and heterosexuals are treated in British law. The age of consent for homosexuals is 18, while for heterosexuals it is 16.

HOMOZYGOUS An individual having identical members of the pair of genes coding for a given characteristic, (see GENES).

HOOKWORM (see ANCYLOSTOMIASIS).

HORMONE REPLACEMENT THERAPY (see MENOPAUSE).

HORMONES These are 'chemical messengers' that are dispersed by the blood and act on target organs to produce effects distant from their point of release. The main organs involved in hormone production are the PITUITARY, PANCREAS, OVARY, TESTIS, THYROID, and ADRENAL. The release of many hormones is, ultimately, under the control of the central nervous system via a series of inhibiting and releasing factors from the HYPOTHALAMUS. Hormones are involved in maintaining homeostasis: e.g. insulin regulates the concentration of glucose in the blood. They also participate in growth and maturation: e.g. growth hormone promotes growth and helps to regulate fat, carbohydrate, and protein metabolism; and the sex hormones promote sexual maturation and reproduction. (See ENDOCRINE GLANDS.)

HORNER'S SYNDROME This is the description given to a combination of changes resulting from paralysis of the sympathetic nerve in the neck. They are: small pupil, a drooping upper lid and an apparently (though not actually) sunken eye.

HORRIPILATION Another term for gooseflesh, due to contraction of the small muscles in the skin which make the hairs erect.

HORSESHOE KIDNEY (see KIDNEYS, DISEASES OF).

HOSPICE A hospital that cares only for the terminally ill and dying. The emphasis is on providing quality of life and special care is taken in providing pain relief by whichever methods are deemed best suited to the person's needs. In the United Kingdom hospice care has been greatly developed, in particular with the leadership of Dr (Dame) Cicely Saunders. Many hospices are funded by charitable funds and their activities supported by voluntary workers.

HOSPITAL An institution providing treatment for sick and injured persons. This may be done on an inpatient or outpatient basis. It provides investigative and therapeutic services which are not available on a domiciliary basis. Hospitals are broadly divided into general hospitals (available in each district in the United Kingdom) and hospitals specializing in particular ailments (e.g. ophthalmology, ear, nose and throat, neurology, etc.). In addition there are teaching hospitals which have the dual function of patient care and the education of medical staff. (See NATIONAL HEALTH SERVICE.)

In the UK all patients are entitled to hospital care provided by their NHS trust (see NATIONAL HEALTH SERVICE) when referred by their GENERAL PRACTITIONER or admitted via the accident and emergency department. (In exceptional cases patients with severe mental illness can be compulsorily admitted by the authorities.) Admission will depend on clinical priority as demand commonly exceeds supply of beds in some localities. Private hospital care is available under the care of a consultant of choice, provided that the patient is covered by appropriate private medical insurance or can pay direct the substantial hospital and medical fees.

HOSPITAL-ACQUIRED INFECTION Infections acquired by patients while they are in hospital. Because of the high level of antibiotic use in hospital some bacteria become resistant to them – for example, METHICILLIN-RESISTANT *STAPHYLOCOCCUS AUREUS* (*MRSA*). This makes hospital-acquired infections potentially dangerous and sometimes life-threatening. It is one of the developments that is prompting calls for greater care in the prescribing of antibiotics.

HOSPITAL CHAPLAINCY A service provided by a religious denomination primarily aimed at meeting the spiritual and religious needs of patients in hospitals. In the UK NHS hospital trusts employ both full-time and part-time chaplains, usually representing the mainline Christian churches (Anglican, Free and Roman

Catholic). Their duties vary but always at least involve meeting the specifically religious needs of patients as well as of relatives and staff who may ask for help. Public services in chapels, the bedside administration of the Word and Sacraments, prayers and radio services are among chaplains' duties. When requested by patients, chaplains also liaise with representatives of other world faiths.

Chaplains have a broad responsibility for the spiritual health care of all in hospital. They share this with other staff members, particularly the nursing staff, to whom the chaplains can be a resource. Chaplains also train and use volunteers from local churches to help with ward visiting and other chaplaincy duties. Much of the time spent with patients takes the form of a listening ministry, helping patients to find their own answers to what is happening to them in hospital and in life generally. Spiritual health can be seen as a quest for right relationships in four areas – to other people, oneself, the world around and 'Life' itself. The religious person subsumes all that in his/her relationship to God. The link between spiritual dis-ease and physical ill-health is well established. The chaplain therefore helps a hospital to provide a holistic approach to health care. Chaplains also give time to the care of staff who increasingly face stress at work. They make use of support groups, counselling, meditation, etc. Chaplains support patients' relatives facing a crisis, e.g. by being with them over the period of a death, and by providing regular bereavement services for those who have lost babies. Some chaplains have a particular expertise in ethics and are members of the various hospital ethics committees. A chaplain may have a 'non-management' view of the health of the hospital itself, which can be of use to hospital management. (See SPIRITUAL PAIN.)

HOST   An organism on which a parasite lives.

HOUR-GLASS STOMACH   The term given to the X-ray appearance of a stomach which is constricted in its middle part because of either spasm of the stomach muscle or contraction of scar tissue from a gastric ulcer.

HOUSEMAID'S KNEE   An inflammation of the bursa in front of the knee-cap, often mistaken for some disease in the joint itself (see BURSITIS).

HUMAN CHORIONIC GONADOTRO-PHIN   A glycoprotein hormone secreted by the placenta (see PLACENTA) in early pregnancy which stimulates the CORPUS LUTEUM within the OVARY to secrete OESTROGEN, PROGESTERONE, and relaxin. It is essential for the maintenance of pregnancy up to about 6–8 weeks of gestation. A RADIO-IMMUNO ASSAY can be used to detect it and pregnancy can be diagnosed as early as six days after conception by testing for

it in the urine. Some tumours also secrete human chorionic gonadotrophin, particularly HYDATIDIFORM MOLES, which produce large amounts.

HUMAN FERTILIZATION AND EMBRY-OLOGY ACT   An Act of the United Kingdom's Parliament (passed in 1990) that legislates for the procedures involved in the production of EMBRYOS and children conceived by ARTIFICIAL INSEMINATION, in vitro fertilization or any other means of assisted conception. A person must give written informed consent before tissue is removed for use in assisted conception. The Act sets out definitions of the legal parents in the varying circustances of fertilization techniques. It also set up the Human Fertilization and Embryology Authority: this body controls and reviews research using embryos and issues licences for such research and for treatment in assisted conception.

HUMAN GENOME PROJECT   The human genome project is a global initiative which will locate and determine the DNA (deoxyribonucleic acid) sequence of all our genes. DNA is the genetic material of nearly all living organisms which controls heredity. This project will provide a major contribution to our understanding of the genetic basis of human diseases and their treatment. There are more than 90,000 human genes (see GENES and GENETIC CODE) and the 15-year project aims to be completed by 2004. The first phase, virtually complete, has been to form a map detailing the position of all the genes on the CHROMOSOMES. The second phase is to define the DNA sequence of each gene. Stringent ethical guidelines are being developed in tandem with the work. The initiative will cost $3 billion and is supported in Britain by the Medical Research Council, the Wellcome Trust and industry. Commercial companies have also been investing heavily in gene mapping and major controversy has been prompted by attempts to patent genes identified by commercial interests. This could stifle medical research in this field.

HUMAN IMMUNODEFICIENCY VIRUS (see AIDS/HIV).

HUMAN LEUCOCYTE ANTIGEN (see HLA SYSTEM).

HUMERUS   The bone of the upper arm. It has a rounded head, which helps to form the shoulder joint, and at its lower end presents a wide pulley-like surface for union with the radius and ulna. Its epicondyles form the prominences at the sides of the elbow.

HUMIDIFICATION   The air we breathe must be moist for the efficient working of the lungs. (See RESPIRATION.) Humidification, or moistening the air, is achieved largely by the NOSE which acts as an air-conditioner, warming, moistening, and filtering the 10,000 litres of air which we inhale daily, in the process of which, incidentally, it produces around 1·5 litres of secretion daily. Humidity is expressed as relative humidity (RH). This is the amount of moisture in the air expressed as a percentage of the maximum possible at that temperature. If the temperature of a room is raised without increasing the moisture content, the RH falls. The average outdoor RH in Britain is around 70 to 80 per cent. With central heating it may drop to 25 per cent or lower.

This is why humidification, as it is known, of the air is essential in buildings heated by modern heating systems. The aim should be to keep the RH around 30 to 50 per cent. In houses this may be achieved quite satisfactorily by having a jug or basin of water in the room, or some receptacle that can be attached to the heater. In offices some more elaborate form of humidifier is necessary. Those suffering from chronic bronchitis are particularly susceptible to dry air, as are those individuals with disorders of the eye because the secretions that bathe the eyes and keep them moist are unnaturally dried out. (See also VENTILATION.)

HUMIDIFIER FEVER   A form of ALVEOLITIS caused by contamination of the water used to humidify, or moisten, the air in air-conditioning plants. The breathing of the contaminated air results in infection of the lung, which is characterized by fever, cough, shortness of breath and malaise, worse on Monday and tending to improve during the course of the week. (See also LEGIONNAIRE'S DISEASE.)

HUMOUR   A traditional term applied to any fluid or semi-fluid tissue of the body: e.g. the aqueous and vitreous humours in the eye. The term, humour, is also associated with a theory regarding the causation of disease, which originated with Pythagoras and lasted in a modified form until the early part of the nineteenth century. According to this theory diseases are due to an improper mixture in the body of blood, bile, phlegm and black bile.

HUNGER   A craving for food or other substance necessary to bodily activity. Hunger for food is supposed to be directly produced by strong contractions of the stomach which occur when it is empty or nearly so. (See also THIRST.) AIR HUNGER is an instinctive craving for oxygen resulting in breathlessness, either when a person ascends to great heights where the pressure of air is low, or in some diseases such as pneumonia and diabetes mellitus which affects the body's METABOLISM and therefore its need for oxygen, an essential constituent in this process.

HUNTINGTON'S CHOREA   A hereditary disease characterized by involuntary movements and dementia. Each child of a parent with the disease has a 50:50 chance of developing it. The usual time of onset is between 35 and 45, but 10 per cent of cases occur under the age of 20. Some patients show more severe mental disturbance, others more severe disturbances of movement, but in all it pursues an inexorable downward course over a period of ten to twenty years to a terminal state of physical and mental helplessness. It is estimated that there are around 6,000 cases in Britain. The defective gene (located on chromosome no. 4) has now been identified and GENETIC SCREENING is possible for those at risk. Genetic therapy may one day be possible, meanwhile genetic counselling of affected families is very important. People with Huntington's chorea and their relatives can obtain help and guidance from Huntington's Disease Association (see APPENDIX 2: ADDRESSES).

HURLER'S SYNDROME (see GARGOYLISM).

HUTCHINSON'S TEETH   The term applied to the narrowed and notched permanent incisor teeth which occur in congenital syphilis. They are so named after Sir Jonathan Hutchinson (1828–1913), the London physician who first described them.

HYALINE   Tissue material that has a glass-like appearance when stained and viewed under the microscope. It occurs in a variety of tissues and diseases, particularly Respiratory Distress Syndrome (see ADULT RESPIRATORY DISTRESS SYNDROME), hyaline degeneration of arterioles and alcoholic liver disease.

HYALINE MEMBRANE DISEASE   A condition found in premature infants and infants born by CAESAREAN SECTION, characterized by the onset of difficulty in breathing a few hours after birth. About half the affected babies die, death usually occurring before the third day. At post-mortem examination the alveoli and the finer bronchioles of the lungs are found to be lined with a dense membrane. The cause of the condition is obscure. (See ADULT RESPIRATORY DISTRESS SYNDROME.)

HYALURONIDASE is an ENZYME which hydrolyses hyaluronic acid. The latter is a gel-like substance which is widely distributed throughout the body and which helps to bind together the tissue cells and also acts as a lubricant in joints. By virtue of its action in hydrolysing hyaluronic acid, hyaluronidase is now used in subcutaneous injections of fluid as it facilitates the spread of the injected fluid and therefore its absorption.

HYCOSY   The acronym of hysterosalpingo-contrast sonography which is an outpatient procedure for testing whether a woman's FALLOPIAN TUBES are blocked. The flow along the tubes can be identified using ultrasonography (via the vagina) and an echo contrast medium. (See ULTRASOUND).

HYDATID A cyst produced by the growth of immature forms of a tapeworm. (See TAENIASIS.)

HYDATIDIFORM MOLE, or VESICULAR MOLE as it is sometimes known, is a rare complication of pregnancy, in which there is tremendous proliferation of the epithelium of the chorion (the outer of the two fetal membranes). It seldom occurs during a first pregnancy. Treatment consists of immediate evacuation of the womb.

HYDRADENITIS SUPPURATIVA A chronic inflammatory disease of the apocrine sweat glands (see PERSPIRATION). It is more common in women, in whom it usually occurs in the armpit, than in men in whom it is most common in the perineum of the drivers of lorries and taxis. It occurs in the form of painful, tender lumps underneath the skin, which burst often in a week or so. Treatment consists of removal by operation.

HYDRALAZINE A vasodilator hypotensive drug, useful as an adjunct to other treatment for HYPERTENSION.

HYDRAMNIOS A condition characterized by excess of fluid in the amniotic cavity. (See AMNION.)

HYDROCEPHALUS An abnormal accumulation of cerebrospinal fluid within the skull. It is due to one or more of three main causes: (i) excessive production of spinal fluid (see CEREBROSPINAL FLUID); (ii) defective absorption of cerebrospinal fluid; (iii) blockage to the circulation of cerebrospinal fluid. The causes of these disturbances of circulation of cerebrospinal fluid may be congenital (most commonly associated with SPINA BIFIDA, meningitis, or a tumour).

Symptoms In children the chief symptoms observed are the gradual increase in size of the upper part of the head, out of all proportion to the face or the rest of the body. The head is globular, with a wide anterior fontanelle and separation of the bones at the sutures. The veins in the scalp are prominent, and there is a 'crackpot' note on percussion. The normal infant's head should not grow more than 2·5 cm (1 inch) in each of the first two months of life and much more slowly subsequently. Growth beyond this rate should arouse suspicions of hydrocephalus. Another useful rule is that the circumference of the head should not exceed that of the chest. In chronic hydrocephalus, the head of an infant 3 months old has been known to measure 72·5 cm (29 inches); and in the case of the man, Cardinal, who died in Guy's Hospital, the head measured 82·5 cm (33 inches). The cerebral ventricles are widely distended, and the convolutions of the brain flattened, while occasionally the fluid escapes into the cavity of the cranium, which it fills, pressing down the brain to the base of the skull. As a consequence of such changes, the functions of the brain are interfered with, and in general the mental condition of the patient is impaired. The child is dull and listless, irritable and sometimes suffers from severe mental subnormality. The special senses become affected as the disease advances, especially vision, and sight is often lost, as is also hearing. Towards the end paralysis is apt to occur.

The outlook for children with hydrocephalus is not as gloomy as was at one time thought to be the case. Such a child has a 50 per cent chance of survival with the disease arrested. He then has a 75 per cent chance of being educable. Almost one-third of arrested cases can be expected to enjoy normal intelligence with little or no physical disability.

Treatment Numerous ingenious operations have been devised for the treatment of hydrocephalus. The most satisfactory of these utilize the Holter or Pudenz unidirectional valves and shunts (tubes), whereby the cerebrospinal fluid is by-passed into the right atrium of the heart or the peritoneal cavity, but it is only in a proportion of affected children that these operations produce a satisfactory result. The shunt may have to be left in position indefinitely.

HYDROCHLORIC ACID A colourless, pungent, fuming liquid. Secreted by the parietal cells in the lining of the stomach, it aids in the digestion of the food.

HYDROCHLOROTHIAZIDE (see BENZOTHIADIAZINES).

HYDROCOELE A collection of fluid connected with the testis or spermatic cord. When there is no obvious cause, it is classified as primary. Such hydrocoeles are usually large and tense, and are commonly found in middle-aged and younger men, presenting as a large, painless scrotal swelling. Congenital hydrocoeles may occur in infants, when they are often associated with a hernial sac. Hydrocoele of the cord is rare. Secondary hydrocoele is generally smaller and lax; it is usually secondary to a tumour or inflammation of the underlying testis or epididymis.

Treatment Congenital hydrocoeles usually disappear spontaneously and may be safely watched; surgery is only indicated when there is a hernia, or if it persists after the first year. Hydrocoeles in adults should be tapped and the testis palpated to exclude primary lesions. Primary hydrocoeles may be managed by intermittent tapping, or preferably, by surgical removal. Secondary hydrocoeles require treatment of the underlying condition.

HYDROCORTISONE has the chemical formula, 17-hydroxycorticosterone. It is closely allied to CORTISONE both in its structure (cortisone is an oxidation product of hydrocortisone) and in its action. Available in tablet, topical or injection form, hydrocortisone is used in adrenocortical insufficiency, for the suppression of local and systemic inflammatory and allergic disorders and in the treatment of shock. Its mineralocorticoid effects – control of salt and water balance – mean that the drug should not be used long term except as replacement therapy in the treatment of ADDISON'S DISEASE or following adrenalectomy when hydrocortisone should be given with the mineral corticoid fludrocortisone (see ADRENAL GLANDS and CORTICOSTEROIDS).

HYDROGEN PEROXIDE A thick colourless liquid with the formula H_2O_2 (water is H_2O), possessing only one oxygen atom in its molecule). Available in solution with water and as a cream, It is readily reduced to water giving up oxygen in the process, which causes the characteristic frothing seen when used. H_2O_2 has antiseptic and deodorizing properties. Thus it is used as a mouthwash, to clean wounds and ulcers and occasionally to disinfect body cavities at operation. It is also a bleach.

HYDROMORPHONE HYDROCHLORIDE A recently introduced opioid ANALGESIC drug used to relieve severe pain in cancer. It is taken in capsule form or the powder may be sprinkled over soft food.

HYDRONEPHROSIS A chronic disease in which the kidney becomes greatly distended with fluid. It is caused by obstruction to the flow of urine at the pelvi-ureteric junction. If the ureter is obstructed the ureter proximal to the obstruction will dilate and pressure will be transmitted back to the kidney to cause hydronephrosis. Obstruction may occur at the bladder neck or in the urethra itself. Enlargement of the prostate is a common cause of bladder-neck obstruction. This would give rise to hypertrophy of the bladder muscle and both dilatation of the ureter and hydronephrosis. If the obstruction is not relieved progressive destruction of renal tissue will occur. As a result of the stagnation of the urine infection is probable and cystitis and pyelonephritis may occur.

HYDROPHOBIA Another name for RABIES.

HYDROPS FETALIS (see HAEMOLYTIC DISEASE OF THE NEW-BORN).

HYDROSTATIC ACCOUCHEMENT The management of normal childbirth with the mother partly immersed in a water bath.

HYDROTHERAPY Treatment using water in the form of baths, douches, etc.

HYDROTHORAX A collection of fluid in the pleural cavities.

HYDROXOCOBALAMIN, or vitamin B_{12}, has now replaced CYANOCOBALAMIN in the treatment of pernicious anaemia. (See ANAEMIA.) It has the practical advantage that fewer injections are required than in the case of cyanocobalamin. Like cyanocobalamin it belongs to the group of substances known as cobalamins which have an ENZYME action in practically every metabolic system in the body and are essential for normal growth and nutrition.

HYDROXYUREA A drug that is proving of value in the treatment of chronic myeloid leukaemia.

HYDROXYZINE HYDROCHLORIDE One of the many ANTIHISTAMINE DRUGS that can be taken orally, it is used to treat itching and for short-term treatment of anxiety states (see BENZODIAZEPINES). The drug is particularly useful in such conditions as parasitophobia (fear of parasites) where patients have both itch and mental disorder.

HYGIENE The science of health and the study of ways of its preservation, particularly by widespread education and promotion of cleanliness. Especially valuable in developing countries, where it plays a vital role in helping to spread the limitation of infectious diseases.

HYMEN The thin membranous fold partially closing the lower end of the virginal vagina. If the opening is small, the hymen will tear at the time of first intercourse, usually with a little bleeding. In a few women the hymen is abnormally tough and surgical cutting may be necessary for the women to have normal intercourse.

HYOID is a U-shaped bone at the root of the tongue. It can be felt from the front of the neck, lying about 2·5 cm above the prominence of the thyroid cartilage.

HYOSCINE Also called scopalamine, this is an ALKALOID obtained from the plant henbane (hyoscyamus). It is an ANTICHOLINERGIC DRUG sometimes used as a premedicant in patients undergoing anaesthesia for its sedative and antiemetic effects and its ability to reduce saliva production. It may cause confusion in the elderly.

HYPER- Prefix denoting abnormally increased or excessive.

HYPERACTIVITY A pattern of behaviour in children who have problems concentrating and who are always overactive. The condition is also known as attention deficit disorder. Medical opinion differs over its incidence: doctors in the UK believe it is an uncommon disorder. The cause is unclear: but there may be a familial element and minor brain damage might be a factor. Treatment is difficult. Stimulant drugs like amphetamine may help and behaviour therapy and family counselling can benefit the child. Psychological and educational support are advisable.

HYPERACUSIS means an abnormally acute sense of hearing.

HYPERAEMIA means congestion or presence of an excessive amount of blood in a part.

HYPERAESTHESIA Over-sensitiveness of a part of the body, as found, for example, in certain nervous diseases. (See TOUCH.)

HYPERALGESIA Excessive sensitiveness to pain. (See PAIN; TOUCH.)

HYPERBARIC A pressure that is greater than that of the atmosphere. Hyperbaric oxygenation is a procedure in which the patient is exposed to high-pressure oxygen. The technique is used for the treatment of people suffering from CARBON MONOXIDE poisoning, compressed-air illness, gas GANGRENE and serious breathing disorders. Occasionally it is used for patients undergoing cardiac surgery.

HYPERCALCAEMIA A state in which the plasma calcium concentration is significantly raised. The most important causes are HYPERPARATHYROIDISM, malignant bone disease and other (non-metastatic) cancers, and chronic renal failure. Less common causes include SARCOIDOSIS, MYELOMATOSIS, VITAMIN D overdosage (see APPENDIX 5: VITAMINS), HYPERTHYROIDISM, and immobilization.

Signs and symptoms A general malaise and depression are common, with generalized muscular weakness, anorexia and vomiting. Disturbed renal function causes increased urine output and thirst, with calcium deposits eventually leading to renal stones. Primary bone disease may cause pain and weakness, with an increased incidence of fractures, and there may be gritty deposits of calcium in the eyes. Severe hypercalcaemia produces anuria, with confusion and coma leading to death.

Treatment The patient should be rehydrated and a diuretic given. Attention should then be focused on the underlying cause – usually a parathyroid adenoma or bone tumour – and surgical removal should produce complete clinical cure, provided advanced renal disease is not already present.

HYPERCALCIURIA An abnormally large amount of calcium in the urine. It is the most common single cause of stones in the KIDNEYS in Britain.

HYPERCAPNIA An abnormal increase in the amount of carbon dioxide in the blood or in the lungs (see BLOOD GASES). It may be caused by a reduced respiratory rate or effort, diseases of the chest wall and lung (affecting breathing) and cyanotic heart disease.

HYPERCHLORHYDRIA Excessive production of hydrochloric acid in the stomach. It is a characteristic finding in certain forms of DYSPEPSIA, particularly that associated with a duodenal ulcer. It causes HEARTBURN and WATERBRASH. (See DUODENAL ULCER; DYSPEPSIA; STOMACH, DISEASES OF.)

HYPERCHOLESTEROLAEMIA (see CHOLESTEROL and HYPERLIPIDAEMIA).

HYPEREMESIS GRAVIDARUM A rare condition (less than 0·2 per cent) of pregnancies in which there is severe vomiting. If untreated it can result in severe dehydration, ketoacidosis (an excess of KETONE acids) and liver damage. More common in multiple pregnancy it may recur in subsequent pregnancies.

HYPERGLYCAEMIA An excess of sugar in the blood that may occur in various diseases, typically in DIABETES MELLITUS. The normal blood glucose level in the fasting state is between 3.5–5.5 mmol/1 blood (see APPENDIX 6: MEASUREMENTS IN MEDICINE); four or five times that amount in diabetes, owing to insufficient insulin in the blood, possibly accompanied by an excessive carbohydrate intake. Untreated, it may lead to diabetic coma.

HYPERIDROSIS, or HYPERHIDROSIS, means excessive sweating. (See PERSPIRATION.)

HYPERKALAEMIA A plasma POTASSIUM concentration above the normal range. Often caused by renal failure or excessive intake of potassium, perhaps in a drug. It may be complicated by cardiac dysrhythmias (abnormal rhythm of the heart).

HYPERKERATOSIS Thickening of the horny (outer) layer of skin, this disorder may be inherited, affecting the palms and soles.

HYPERKINETIC SYNDROME (see HYPERACTIVITY).

HYPERLIPIDAEMIA An excess of fat in the blood characterizing a group of metabolic disorders. The two most important fats circulating in the blood are CHOLESTEROL and TRIGLYCERIDES. Raised blood levels of cholesterol predispose to ATHEROMA and CORONARY

ARTERY DISEASE and raised triglycerides predispose to pancreatitis. Six types of hyperlipidaemia have been identified; they are differentiated by the amount that their blood concentrations are higher than normal. Some of the hyperlipidaemias are familial and some are secondary to other diseases such as HYPOTHYROIDISM, DIABETES MELLITUS, nephrotic syndrome and alcoholism. Hyperlipidaemias are associated with serious disorders such as ATHEROSCLEROSIS and coronary artery disease. Diagnosis of the different types depends on blood tests to discover lipid levels. There is evidence that therapy which lowers the lipid concentration reduces the progression of premature atheroma, particularly in those who suffer from the familial disorder. Treatment should include appropriate diets, usually food low in cholesterol and saturated fats. There are a number of drugs available for lowering the lipid content of the plasma but these should be reserved for patients in whom severe hyper-lipidaemia is inadequately controlled by weight reduction. Anion-exchange resins – clofibrate, bezafibrate and gemfibrozil, for example – and statins such as atorvastatin and simvastatin, as well as nicotinic acid, all lower plasma cholesterol and plasma triglyceride concentration through their effect on reducing the hepatic production of lipoproteins. Cholestyramine and colestipol, both of which are anion-exchange resins, bind bile salts in the gut and so decrease the absorption of the cholesterol that these bile salts contain and hence lower plasma cholesterol concentrations. Probucol lowers plasma cholesterol concentrations by increasing the metabolism of low-density lipoproteins.

The statins (atorvastatin, cerivastatin, fluvastatin, pravastatin and simvastatin) inhibit an enzyme involved in synthesizing cholesterol, especially in the liver. They are more effective than anion-exchange resins in lowering LDL (low-density lipoprotein) cholesterol – a form of low-density cholesterol carried in the blood stream, high levels of which are believed to be the main cause of ATHEROMA. Statins are, however, less effective than the clofibrate group in reducing TRIGLYCERIDES and raising HDL (high-density lipoprotein) cholesterol (high-density cholesterol).

HYPERMETROPIA or HYPEROPIA, is a term applied to long- sightedness, in which the eye is too flat from front to back and rays of light are brought to a focus behind the retina. (See VISION.)

HYPERNATRAEMIA   A serum sodium concentration above normal. It is usually caused by dehydration (either from inadequate intake or excessive loss of water). Occasionally it may be caused by excessive sodium intake and rarely by a raised level of aldosterone hormone.

HYPERNEPHROMA   Now named renal cell carcinoma, this is a malignant tumour resembling the tissue of the suprarenal gland and occurring in the kidney. The tumour may be symptomless for many years. Fever, loin pain, HAEMATURIA, and swelling are among the presenting symptoms. Surgical removal is the initial treatment, and the tumours are fairly insensitive to cytotoxic drugs and radiotherapy. Hormone treatment may help. The tumours are prone to spread via the bloodstream, for example, to the lungs.

HYPERPARATHYROIDISM   Increased activity of the parathyroid gland. Parathyroid hormone increases serum calcium. Hyperparathyroidism may be primary (due to an adenoma or hyperplasia of the gland), secondary (in response to hypocalcaemia) or tertiary (when secondary hyperparathyroidism causes the development of an autonomous adenoma).

HYPERPITUITARISM   Overactivity of the anterior lobe of the PITUITARY causing ACROMEGALY (GIGANTISM).

HYPERPLASIA means an abnormal increase in the number of cells in a tissue.

HYPERPROLACTINAEMIA   Overproduction of the hormone prolactin, usually as a result of a tumour of the putuitary gland (prolactinoma). (see PROLACTIN.)

HYPERPYREXIA   High fever. (See FEVER; TEMPERATURE.)

HYPERSENSITIVITY   The abnormal immunological reaction produced in certain individuals when re-exposed to antigens that are innocuous to normal individuals. An antigen or allergen stimulates an allergic response. This produces a state of altered re-activity or an allergic state. Such a state of altered re-activity may be beneficial to the host, as in establishing a state of immunity, or it may be harmful to the host and produce a state of disease. Hypersensitivity is thus an allergic reaction in an individual sensitized by previous exposure to the antigen and in whom the allergic process constitutes the disease.

HYPERTENSION   This may be defined as a blood pressure above 160/90 mm Hg. Some people's blood pressure, particularly the systolic measurement, may vary with daily activity, rising with exercise or anxiety. Circadian variations also occur. Systolic blood pressure also rises with age in people living in the developed world. In more than 90 per cent of people with high blood pressure the cause is not identified and this 'variety' is often described as essential hypertension. Some individuals, especially the elderly, seem to adjust to being hypertensive and the condition is discovered by chance.

Hypertension can be divided into primary and secondary types.

Primary hypertension can be characterized as: labile (as in opening paragraph); isolated systolic due to arteriosclerotic changes in the elderly; essential or BENIGN; malignant or accelerated phase due to breakdown in the tissues and nervous control of the blood vessels; and hypertension in pregnancy, which may lead to PRE-ECLAMPSIA and ECLAMPSIA.

Secondary hypertension is a consequence of disease elsewhere in the body, for example, chronic renal failure, endocrine disorders, such as PHAEOCHROMOCYTOMAS, congenital defects, and rare disorders such as PORPHYRIA, and lead poisoning. Drugs given for other disorders – for example, arthritis – can also cause a rise in blood pressure.

Treatment This varies according to the type of hypertension and careful investigation is often needed to decide the correct diagnosis and treatment. Attention to risk factors is important. Those affected should not smoke and should control their alcohol intake. A low-fat and low-salt diet is advisable, and obese patients should lose weight. Moderate exercise and avoidance of stress may help to reduce blood pressure, as may relaxation therapy. Such changes should be done after medical advice. Drugs being given for other conditions – for example, arthritis – may have to be stopped.

If these measures fail then drug treatment will probably be necessary. Drug regimens will depend on the type and severity of hypertension and they need careful monitoring. Among the commonly used drugs, sometimes given in combination, are: DIURETICS; CALCIUM-CHANNEL BLOCKERS; BETA-ADRENORECEPTOR BLOCKERS and ANGIOTENSIN-CONVERTING ENZYME (ACE) INHIBITORS. Treatments are now very effective in controlling blood pressure and thus reducing markedly the incidence of complications such as STROKE, CORONARY THROMBOSIS and RENAL FAILURE.

Hypertension in pregnancy requires skilled treatment, often in hospital. Malignant hypertension, a potentially fatal condition, may require urgent hospital admission with bed rest and a combination of drug regimens prescribed. Surgery may be necessary to treat hypertension due to a PHAEOCHROMOCYTOMA, the abnormal ADRENAL GLAND being removed.

HYPERTHERMIA means abnormally high body temperature. A rapid rise of temperature to dangerous levels – called malignant hyperthermia – may be precipitated by general anaesthesia but the condition is rare (1:50,000 operations) and is usually inherited. The anaesthetic is stopped and icepacks are used to cool the patient. Pure oxygen and intravenous sodium choride are also administered.

It is also the name given to the treatment of disease by the artificial production of fever. This can be achieved by various methods, such as radiation heat cabinets boosted with radio frequency (RF); immersion in a hot wax bath; heated suits or blankets; techniques using electromagnetic waves (e.g. RF, MICROWAVES); ULTRASOUND of appropriate frequencies. It is sometimes of help as an adjunct to surgery, chemotherapy, or radiotherapy in the treatment of cancer.

HYPERTHYROIDISM Excessive activity of the thyroid gland. It is a common disorder affecting between 2 and 5 per cent of all females at some time in their lives. Most cases are the result of disease of the thyroid gland. The commonest cause is GRAVES' DISEASE, also called thyrotoxicosis. Single or multiple ADENOMAS or nodules in the thyroid also cause hyperthyroidism. There are several other rare causes, including inflammation caused by a virus, autoimmune reactions and cancer. The symptoms of hyperthyroidism affect many of the body's system as a consequence of the much increased metabolic rate: these include the cardiovascular, nervous, alimentary and musculoskeletal systems.

Graves' disease is a syndrome consisting of diffuse GOITRE, overactivity of the thyroid gland and EXOPHTHALMOS (protruding eyes). Patients lose weight and develop an increased appetite, heat intolerance and sweating. They are anxious, irritable, hyperactive, suffer from tachycardia, breathlessness and muscle weakness and are sometimes depressed. The hyperthyroidism is due to the production of antibodies to the TSH receptor which stimulate the receptor with resultant production of excess thyroid hormones. The goitre is due to antibodies that stimulate the growth of the thyroid gland. The exophthalmos is due to another immunoglobulin called the ophthalmopathic immunoglobulin which is an antibody to a retro-orbital antigen on the surface of the retro-orbital eye muscles. This provokes inflammation in the retro-orbital tissues which is associated with the accumulation of water and mucopolysaccharide which fills the orbit and causes the eye to protrude forwards.

Although Graves' disease may affect any age group the peak incidence is in the 3rd decade. Females are affected ten times as often as males. The prevalence in females is one in 500. As with many other auto-immune diseases, there is an increased prevalence of auto-immune thyroid disease in the relatives of patients with Graves' disease. Some of these patients may have hypothyroidism and others thyrotoxicosis. Patients with Graves' disease may present with a goitre or with the eye signs or, most commonly, with the symptoms of excess thyroid hormone production. Thyroid hormone controls the metabolic rate of the body so that the symptoms of hyperthyroidism are those of excess metabolism.

The diagnosis of Graves' disease is confirmed by the measurement of the circulating levels of the two thyroid hormones, thyroxine and tri-iodothyronine.

Treatment There are several effective treatments for Graves' disease.

ANTITHYROID DRUGS: these drugs inhibit the iodination of tyrosine and hence the formation of the thyroid hormones. The most commonly used drugs are the thiourea compounds carbimazole and propylthiouricil. They will control the excess production of thyroid hormones in virtually all cases. Once the patient has been rendered euthyroid the dose can be reduced to a maintenance dose and is usually continued for two years. The disadvantage of antithyroid drugs is that even after two years' treatment nearly half the patients will relapse and will then require more definitive therapy.

PARTIAL THYROIDECTOMY: removal of three-quarters of the thyroid gland is effective treatment of the hyperthyroidism of Graves' disease. It is the treatment of choice in those patients with large goitres. The patient must however be rendered euthyroid (normally functioning thyroid) before surgery is undertaken, or thyroid crisis and arrhythmias may complicate the operation.

RADIOACTIVE IODINE THERAPY: this has been in use for many years. It is an effective means of controlling hyperthyroidism. One of the disadvantages of radioactive iodine is that the incidence of hypothyroidism is much greater than with other forms of treatment. However the management of hypothyroidism is simple and requires thyroxine tablets and regular monitoring for hypothyroidism. There is no evidence of any increased incidence of cancer of the thyroid or LEUKAEMIA following radio-iodine therapy. It has been the pattern in Britain to reserve radio-iodine treatment to those over the age of 35 or those whose prognosis is unlikely to be more than 30 years as a result of cardiac or respiratory disease. Radioactive iodine treatment should not be given to a seriously thyrotoxic patient.

BETA-ADRENOCEPTOR-BLOCKING DRUGS, usually PROPRANOLOL, are useful for symptomatic treatment during the first 4 to 8 weeks until the longer-term drugs have reduced thyroid activity.

HYPERTONIC (1) Referring to one solution which has a greater osmotic pressure than another. Physiologically it is used to describe solutions which have a greater osmotic pressure than body fluids. (2) Muscles with abnormally increased tone (e.g. following a stroke).

HYPERTROPHY The increase in size which takes place in an organ as the result of an increased amount of work demanded of it by the bodily economy. For example, when valvular disease of the heart is present, compensation occurs by an increase in thickness of the heart-muscle, and the organ, by beating more powerfully, is able to overtake the strain thrown upon it. Similarly, if one kidney is removed, the other hypertrophies or grows larger to overtake the double work.

HYPERVENTILATION An abnormally rapid resting respiratory rate. If voluntary it causes lightheadedness and then unconsciousness by lowering the blood tension of carbon dioxide. It is a manifestation of chest and heart diseases which raise carbon dioxide tension or cause HYPOXIA (e.g. severe chronic obstructive pulmonary disease or pulmonary oedema). Mechanically ventilated patients may be hyperventilated to lower carbon dioxide tension in order to reduce INTRACRANIAL PRESSURE.

HYPERVOLAEMIA An increase in the volume of circulating blood above the normal range.

HYPNOTICS These are drugs that induce SLEEP. Before a hypnotic is prescribed, it is important to establish – and, where possible, treat – the cause of the insomnia. They are most often needed to help an acutely distressed patient, for example, following bereavement, or in cases of jet lag, or in shift workers. They may be required in states of chronic distress, whether induced by disease or environment; in these cases it is especially important to limit their use in order to prevent undue reliance on the drugs, and not to allow the use of hypnotics and sedatives to become a means of evading the patient's real problem. In many cases, such as chronic depression, overwork, and alcohol abuse, hypnotics are quite inappropriate; some form of counselling and relaxation therapy is often preferable.

Hypnotics should always be chosen and prescribed with care, bearing in mind the patient's full circumstances. They are generally best avoided in the elderly (confusion is a common problem), and in children – apart from special cases. The most commonly used hypnotics are the BENZODIAZEPINES) such as nitrazepam and temazepam; chloral derivatives, while useful in children, are generally second choice. They should be used in the lowest possible dose for the minimum period. Side-effects include daytime drowsiness – which may interfere with driving and other skilled tasks – and insomnia following withdrawal, especially after prolonged use, is a hazard. Zolpidem and zopiclone are two drugs similar to the benzodiazepines, indicated for short-term treatment of insomnia in the elderly. Adverse effects include confusion, incoordination and unsteadiness, and falls have been reported.

HYPNOTISM The process of producing a state of mind known as hypnosis. Although a process which has been known for hundreds of years, its precise nature is still ill understood. One modern writer has defined hypnosis as 'a temporary condition of altered attention, the most striking feature of which is greatly increased suggestibility'. There is no evidence, as has been claimed, that women can be more easily hypnotized than men. Children and young adults are the more easily hypnotized, middle-aged people being more resistant. There are various methods of induction of hypnosis, but the basis of them is some rhythmic stimulus accompanied by the repetition of carefully worded suggestions. The most commonly used method is to ask the patient to fix his eye on a given spot, or light, and then keep on repeating to him, in a quiet soothing voice, that his eyes will gradually become tired and that he will want to close them. There are various levels of hypnosis, usually classified as light, medium, and deep, and it has been estimated that 10 per cent of people cannot be hypnotized, 35 per cent can be taken into light hypnosis, 35 per cent into medium hypnosis, and 20 per cent into deep hypnosis.

Hypnosis can be used as a treatment for some psychiatric patients and in some people with psychosomatic conditions in which emotional or psychological disturbances precipitate physical disorders such as skin lesions or headaches. Hypnosis may help to relieve pain in childbirth; asthma may also respond to it. Some people may find hypnosis of help 'in overcoming addictions to smoking, alcohol or gambling. Hypnosis has risks and its use in treatment should be by doctors trained in the technique.

HYPO A prefix meaning below, under less than normal: for example, hypotension (low blood pressure) and hypodermic (under the skin).

HYPOCALCAEMIA A serum concentration of calcium below the normal range (9–11 mg of calcium per 100 ml of serum). This may cause TETANY, acutely, and chronically may give rise to rickets, OSTEOMALACIA or OSTEOPOROSIS. It may be caused by HYPOPARATHYROIDISM, VITAMIN D DEFICIENCY (see APPENDIX 5: VITAMINS), malabsorption, renal failure or acute pancreatitis (see PANCREAS, DISEASES OF).

HYPOCAPNIA A blood tension of carbon dioxide below normal. It is produced by hyperventilation which may be voluntary, mechanical (if the patient is on a ventilator) or in response to a physiological insult such as metabolic acidosis or brain injury.

HYPOCHLORHYDRIA An insufficient secretion of hydrochloric acid from the digestive cells of the stomach lining.

HYPOCHONDRIASIS A DELUSION of ill health, often severe, such that patients may believe they have a brain tumour or incurable insanity. Furthermore, patients may believe that they have infected others, or that their children have inherited the condition. It is a characteristic feature of depression, but may also occur in SCHIZOPHRENIA, when the delusions may be secondary to bodily HALLUCINATIONS, and a sense of subjective change. Chronic hypochondriasis may be the result of an abnormal personality development, for example, the insecure, bodily conscious person. Delusional preoccupations with

the body – usually the face – may occur, such that the patient is convinced that his or her face is twisted, or disfigured with acne.

Treatment Hypochondriacal patients may also develop physical illness, and any new symptoms must always be carefully evaluated. In most patients the condition is secondary, and treatment should be directed to the underlying depression or schizophrenia. In the rare cases of primary hypochondriasis, supportive measures are the mainstay of treatment.

HYPODERMIC A term pertaining to, the region immediately under the skin. Thus, a hypodermic injection means an injection given underneath the skin. A hypodermic syringe is a small syringe which, fitted with a fine needle, is used to give such injections.

HYPOGASTRIC A term means pertaining to the lower middle part of the abdomen just above the pubis.

HYPOGLOSSAL NERVE The twelfth cranial nerve, which supplies the muscles of the tongue, together with some others lying near it.

HYPOGLYCAEMIA A deficiency of glucose in the blood – the normal range being 3·5–7·5 mmol/l (see DIABETES MELLITUS). It most commonly occurs in diabetic patients, for example, after an excessive dose of insulin, heavy exercise, particularly with inadequate or delayed meals. It may also occur in non-diabetic people, however, for example, in very cold situations or after periods of starvation. Hypoglycaemia is normally indicated by characteristic warning signs and symptoms – particularly if the blood-glucose concentration is falling rapidly. These include anxiety, tremor, sweating, breathlessness, raised pulse rate, blurred vision, often with reduced concentration, leading – in severe cases – to unconsciousness. These may be relieved by taking some sugar, some sweet biscuits or drink. In emergencies, such as when the patient is comatose, an intramuscular injection of GLUCAGON, or intravenous glucose should be given. Early treatment is vital, since prolonged hypoglycaemia, by starving the brain cells of glucose, may lead to irreversible brain damage.

HYPOGLYCAEMIC AGENTS or ORAL ANTIDIABETIC DRUGS include three groups: sulphonylureas, biguanides and other antidiabetics. They are used in the treatment of non-insulin dependent (type 2) diabetes, when they should be used in addition to the diet, and not as a replacement. They should not be prescribed until patients have been shown not to respond adequately to at least three months' restriction of energy and carbohydrate intake.

Sulphonylureas, the main group, act on the beta cells to stimulate insulin release; consequently they are effective only when there is some residual pancreatic beta-cell activity (see INSULIN). They also act on peripheral tissues to increase sensitivity, although this is less important. All sulphonylureas may lead to HYPOGLYCAEMIA four hours or more after food, but this is relatively uncommon, and usually an indication of overdose. There are several different sulphonylureas; apart from some differences in their duration or action (and hence in their suitability for individual patients) there is little difference in their effectiveness. Only chlorpropamide has appreciably more side-effects – mainly because of its prolonged duration of action and consequent risk of hypoglycaemia. There is also the common and unpleasant chlorpropamide/alcohol-flush phenomenon when the patient takes alcohol. Selection of an individual sulphonylurea depends on the patient's age and renal function, and often just on personal preference. Elderly patients are particularly prone to the risks of hypoglycaemia when long-acting drugs are used. In these patients chlorpropamide, and preferably glibenclamide, should be avoided and replaced by others such as gliclazide or tolbutamide.

These drugs may cause weight gain and are indicated only if poor control persists despite adequate attempts at dieting. They should not be used during breast feeding, and caution is necessary in the elderly and those with renal or hepatic insufficiency. They should be avoided in PORPHYRIA. During surgery and intercurrent illness (such as myocardial infarction, coma, infection and trauma), insulin therapy should be temporarily substituted. Insulin is generally used during pregnancy and should be used in the presence of ketoacidosis.

SIDE-EFFECTS Chiefly gastrointestinal disturbances and headache; these are generally mild and infrequent. After drinking alcohol, chlorpropamide may cause facial flushing. It also may enhance the action of ANTIDIURETIC HORMONE, very rarely causing HYPONATRAEMIA.

Sensitivity reactions are very rare, usually occurring in the first six to eight weeks of therapy. They include transient rashes which rarely progress to ERYTHEMA MULTIFORME and exfoliate dermatitis, fever and jaundice; chlorpropamide may also occasionally result in photosensitivity. Rare blood disorders include THROMBOCYTOPENIA, AGRANULOCYTOSIS and aplastic anaemia.

Biguanides Metformin, the only available member of this group, acts by reducing GLUCONEOGENESIS and by increasing peripheral utilization of glucose. It can act only if there is some residual insulin activity, hence it is only of value in the treatment of non-insulin dependent (type 2) diabetics. It may be used alone or with a sulphonylurea, and is indicated when strict dieting and sulphonylurea treatment have failed to control the diabetes. It is particularly valuable in overweight patients, in whom it may be used first. Metformin has several advantages: hypoglycaemia is not usually a problem, weight gain is uncommon, and lower plasma insulin

levels. Gastrointestinal side-effects are initially common and persistent in some patients, especially when high doses are being taken. Lactic acidosis is a rarely seen hazard occurring in patients with renal impairment, in whom metformin should not be used.

Other antidiabetics Acarbose is an inhibitor of intestinal alpha glucosidases (enzymes that process GLUCOSIDES), delaying the digestion of starch and sucrose, and hence the increase in blood glucose concentrations after a meal containing carbohydrate. It has been recently introduced for the treatment of type 2 patients inadequately controlled by diet or diet with oral hypoglycaemics.

Guar gum, if taken in adequate doses, acts by delaying carbohydrate absorption, and therefore reducing the postprandial blood glucose levels. It is also used to relieve symptoms of the DUMPING SYNDROME.

HYPOGONADISM is the condition characterized by deficient production of the hormones secreted by the gonads: that is, the OVARIES and TESTES.

HYPOKALAEMIA The abnormal low concentration of potassium in the blood.

HYPOMANIA is a slight degree of mania. The individual is elated to an extent that he or she may make unwise decisions and social behaviour may become animated and uninhibited. To the casual observer individuals may, however, seem normal. Treatment is advisable to prevent them from harming their own or their family's interests. Treatment is for mania (see MENTAL ILLNESS).

HYPONATRAEMIA A serum concentration of sodium below the normal range. It may be produced by dilution of blood (giving large volumes of salt-poor solutions intravenously), excessive water retention (inappropriate secretion of antidiuretic hormone), excessive sodium loss, and, rarely, by inadequate salt intake.

HYPOPARATHYROIDISM Underactivity of the PARATHYROID GLANDS. Thus there is a lack of parathyroid hormone resulting in HYPOCALCAEMIA. It may be caused by inadvertent removal of the glands when the thyroid gland is surgically removed or by failure of the glands because of autoimmune disease.

HYPOPHYSECTOMY Surgical excision of the PITUITARY GLAND.

HYPOPHYSIS Another name for the PITUITARY GLAND.

HYPOPIESIS The condition, or state, characterized by abnormally low blood-pressure.

HYPOPITUITARISM Underactivity of the PITUITARY GLAND. It can cause dwarfism (see DWARF), delayed puberty, impotence, infertility, AMENORRHOEA, HYPOTHYROIDISM, and hypoadrenalism. Causes include tumours, irradiation of the gland, SARCOIDOSIS, and necrosis associated with postpartum haemorrhage (Sheehan's syndrome).

HYPOPLASIA Excessive smallness of an organ or part, arising from imperfect development.

HYPOSPADIAS A developmental abnormality in the male, in which the urethra opens on the under-surface of the penis or in the PERINEUM. The condition is treatable with surgery, but several operations over a period of years may be required to ensure normal urinary and sexual functions.

HYPOSTASIS The term applied to the condition in which blood accumulates in a dependent part of the body as a result of poor circulation. Congestion of the base of the lungs in old people from this cause, and infection, is called hypostatic PNEUMONIA.

HYPOTENSION The term to describe normally low blood-pressure. Postural hypotension is the abnormal fall in blood-pressure which may occur on suddenly standing up. It is more liable to occur in the elderly.

HYPOTHALAMUS That part of the forebrain situated beneath and linked with the THALAMUS on each side and forming the floor of the third ventricle. Also linked to the PITUITARY GLAND beneath it, the HYPOTHALAMUS contains collections of nerve cells believed to form the controlling centres of (1) the SYMPATHETIC and (2) the PARASYMPATHETIC nervous systems. The hypothalamus is the nervous centre for primitive physical and emotional behaviour. It contains nerve centres for the regulation of certain vital processes: the metabolism of fat, carbohydrate and water; sleep; body temperature and sexual functions.

HYPOTHERMIA A core body temperature of less than 35 °C. As the temperature of the body falls, there is increasing dysfunction of all the organs, particularly the central nervous and cardiovascular systems. The patient becomes listless and confused, with onset of unconsciousness between 33–28 °C. Cardiac output at first rises with shivering but then falls progressively, as do the oxygen requirements of the tissues. Below 17–26 °C cardiac output is insufficient even to supply this reduced demand for oxygen by the tissues. The heart is susceptible to spontaneous ventricular fibrillation below 28 °C. Metabolism is disturbed and the concentration of blood GLUCOSE and POTASSIUM rises as the temperature falls. Cooling of the kidneys produces a diuresis and further fluid loss from the circulation to the tissues causes HYPOVOLAEMIA.

Severe hypothermia is sometimes complicated by gastric erosions and haemorrhage and pancreatitis. Infants and the elderly are less efficient at regulating temperature and conserving heat than other age groups and are therefore more at risk from accidental hypothermia during cold weather, if their accommodation is not warm enough. Approximately half a million elderly people are at risk in Britain each winter from hypothermia. The other major cause of accidental hypothermia is near drowning in icy water. Deliberate hypothermia is sometimes used to reduce metabolic rate so that prolonged periods of cardiac arrest may occur without tissue hypoxia developing. This technique is used for some cardiac and neurosurgical operations and is produced by immersion of the anaesthetized patient in iced water or by cooling an extracorporeal circulation.

Treatment of hypothermia is by warming the patient and treating any complications that arise. Passive warming is usual with conservation of the patient's own body heat with insulating blankets. If the core temperature is below 28 °C, then active rewarming should be instituted by means of warm peritoneal, gastric or bladder lavage or using an extracorporeal circulation. Care must be taken in moving hypothermic patients as a sudden rush of cold peripheral blood to the heart can precipitate ventricular fibrillation. Prevention of hypothermia in the elderly is important. Special attention must be paid to diet, heating the home and adequate clothing in several layers to limit heat loss.

HYPOTHYROIDISM A condition characterized by thickening and coarsening of the skin. Other body tissues can be affected, particularly the nose and lips. It is most commonly caused by underactivity of the THYROID GLAND. The thyroid gland secretes two hormones – thyroxine and triodothyronine – and these hormones are responsible for the metabolic activity of the body. Hypothyroidism may result from developmental abnormalities of the gland or a deficiency of the enzymes necessary for the synthesis of the hormones. It may be a feature of endemic goitre and retarded development, but the most common cause of hypothyroidism is the auto-immune destruction of the thyroid known as chronic thyroiditis. It may also occur as a result of radio-iodine treatment of thyroid overactivity and is occasionally secondary to pituitary disease in which inadequate THYROID-STIMULATING-HORMONE (TSH) production occurs. It is a common disorder, occurring in fourteen per one thousand females and one per one thousand males. Most patients present between the age of thirty and sixty years. The term myxoedema was introduced in 1878 to describe the swelling of the skin and sub-cutaneous tissues that characterized severe forms of hypothyroidism.

Symptoms As thyroid hormones are responsible for the metabolic rate of the body, hypothyroidism usually presents with a general slowing-up. This affects both physical and mental activities. The intellectual functions become slow, the speech deliberate and the formation of ideas and the answers to questions take longer than in healthy people. Physical energy is reduced and patients frequently complain of lethargy and generalized muscle aches and pains. Patients become intolerant of the cold and the skin becomes dry and swollen. The larynx also becomes swollen and gives rise to a hoarseness of the voice. Most patients gain weight and develop constipation. The skin becomes dry and yellow due to the presence of increased carotine. Hair becomes thinned and brittle and even baldness may develop. Swelling of the soft tissues may give rise to a carpal tunnel syndrome and middle-ear deafness. The diagnosis is confirmed by measuring the levels of thyroid hormones in the blood which are low and of the pituitary TSH which is raised in primary hypothyroidism.

Treatment consists of the administration of THYROXINE. Although triodothyronine is the metabolically active hormone, thyroxine is converted to triodothyronine by the tissues of the body. Treatment should be started cautiously with a small dose of not more than 0·05 mg of thyroxine and this can be slowly increased to 0·2 mg daily, the equivalent of the maximum output of the thyroid gland. If too large a dose is given initially palpitations and tachycardia are likely to result and in the elderly heart failure may be precipitated.

HYPOTONIC (1) Referring to a solution which has a lower osmotic pressure (see OSMOSIS) than another. Physiologically it describes a solution with a lower osmotic pressure than body fluids. (2) Muscles with abnormally reduced tone.

HYPOVENTILATION Shallow and/or slow breathing, often caused by the effects of injury or drugs on the respiratory centre. It causes HYPERCAPNIA and HYPOXIA

HYPOVOLAEMIA A reduced circulating blood volume. Acutely it is caused by unreplaced losses from bleeding, sweating, diarrhoea, vomiting or diuresis. Chronically it may be caused by inadequate fluid intake.

HYPOXIA A low blood tension of oxygen. It may be caused by low inspired concentration of oxygen, an abnormal breathing pattern, lung disease or heart disease. If severe and prolonged it will cause organ damage and death as cellular function is dependent on oxygen.

HYSTERECTOMY Surgical removal of the uterus. Hystero-oophorectomy is the term applied to removal of the uterus and ovaries.

HYSTERIA A traditional description for a symptom (or symptoms) with no obvious organic cause, which is an unconscious reaction and from which the person may benefit. It is now recognized as a dissociative disorder. Such disorders – AMNESIA, FUGUES, multiple personality states and trancelike conditions – are powerful defence mechanisms against severe stress of someone's inability to cope with life. Mass hysteria is a phenomenon characterized by extreme suggestibility in a group of often emotionally charged people.

The name originates from the idea that hysteria – a Greek-based word for 'uterus' – was in some way associated with the womb. Hence the old-fashioned association of hysteria with women and supposed sexual disturbances. Doctors should eliminate a diagnosis of physical disease before diagnosing a dissociative disorder. Most hysterical conversion reactions subside spontaneously. If not, the individual needs psychiatric advice. Treatment is difficult. Reasons for stress should be explored and, if possible, resolved. Hypnosis to help the person to relive stressful episodes – known as ABREACTION – may be of value.

HYSTEROSCOPY is the direct visualization of the interior of the uterus using FIBREOPTIC ENDOSCOPY. The technique, which allows minor surgical procedures to be carried out at the same time, has transformed the management of uterine disorders.

HYSTEROTOMY An operation in which the UTERUS is opened to remove a FETUS before 28 weeks' gestation. After 28 weeks it would be called a CAESAREAN SECTION. It is now seldom used as a means of abortion.

I

IATRIC Anything pertaining to a physician.

IATROGENIC DISEASE Disease induced by a physician: commonly a drug-induced disease.

IBUPROFEN An anti-inflammatory drug with analgesic properties used to treat rheumatoid arthritis and other forms of rheumatism as well as headaches and muscular pains. (See NON-STEROIDAL ANTI-INFLAMMATORY DRUGS.)

ICD See INTERNATIONAL CLASSIFICATION OF DISEASE.

ICHTHAMMOL, ICHTHYOL, is ammonium ichthosulphonate, an almost black, thick liquid of fishy smell, prepared from a bituminous shale. It is used in chronic ECZEMA.

ICHTHYOSIS A disorder in which the skin is permanently dry and scaly. It is usually genetically determined and several different forms are recognized:

Ichthyosis vulgaris Common and inherited as a dominant trait. Beginning in early childhood, it is often associated with atopic eczema. The limb flexures and face are spared.

X-linked ichthyosis is much less common, more severe and appears earlier than ichthyosis vulgaris. The fish-like scales are larger and darker and do not spare the flexures and face.

Ichthyosiform erythroderma Of two types and very rare: in the recessive form the appearance at birth is of the so-called 'collodion baby'; in the dominant form the baby is born with universally red, moist and eroded skin with an unpleasant smell. Gradually over several months, thick scales replace the erythema.

Treatment Minor forms are helped by constant use of EMOLLIENTS and moisturizing applications. Cream containing urea can be valuable. The rare erythrodermic patterns in the NEONATE require skilled intensive care as thermo-regulation is disturbed and massive fluid loss occurs through the skin. Later in childhood, oral RETINOIDS are useful.

ICTERUS is another name for jaundice.

ICTUS is another term for a stroke.

IDIOPATHIC is a term applied to diseases to indicate that their cause is unknown.

IDIOPATHIC THROMBOCYTOPENIC PURPURA This is an AUTOIMMUNE disorder in which blood PLATELETS are destroyed. This disturbs the blood's coagulative properties and spontaneous bleeding (purpura) occurs into the skin. The disease may be acute in children but they usually recover without treatment. Adults may develop a more serious, chronic variety which requires treatment with CORTICOSTEROIDS and sometimes SPLENECTOMY. Should the disease persist despite these treatments, IMMUNOSUPPRESSIVE drugs are worth trying. Should the bleeding threaten life, concentrates of PLATELETS should be administered.

IDIOSYNCRASY An inherent abnormal qualitative reaction to a drug that is primarily the result of a constitutional defect in the patient. The abnormal sensitivity of patients with PORPHYRIA to BARBITURATES and SULPHONAMIDES is an example. Hereditary biochemical defects of red blood cells are responsible for many drug-induced haemolytic anaemias and for FAVISM. Drug-sensitive red cells are deficient

in the enzyme glucose phosphate dehydrogenase which plays an important part in the metabolism of glucose and is necessary for the continued integrity of the cell. When patients with porphyria are given certain drugs, particularly barbiturates and sulphonamides, they are liable to develop acute neurological episodes with peripheral and respiratory paralysis which may result in death. Porphyria variegata, the South African variety of porphyria, is an example of an inborn error of metabolism which was without serious symptoms until the advent of barbiturate drugs. Taking these drugs can precipitate total paralysis and death.

IDOXURIDINE An iodine containing antiviral agent still widely used in the treatment of cases of herpes simplex involvement of the cornea of the eye (see EYE DISEASES).

IFOSFAMIDE (see CYTOTOXIC).

ILEITIS Inflammation of the ileum. It may be caused by CROHN'S DISEASE, TYPHOID, TUBERCULOSIS or the bacterium *Yersinia enterocolitica*. Ileitis may also accompany ulcerative colitis (see COLITIS).

Patients and their relatives can obtain help and guidance from the National Association for Colitis and Crohn's Disease (see APPENDIX 2: ADDRESSES).

ILEO-CAECAL The term applied to the region of the junction between the small and large intestines in the right lower corner of the abdomen. The ileo-caecal valve is a structure which allows the contents of the intestine to pass onwards from the small to the large intestine, but, in the great majority of cases, prevents their passage in the opposite direction.

ILEOSTOMY The operation by which an artificial opening is made into the ileum and brought through the abdominal wall to create an artificial opening or stoma. It is most often performed as part of the operation for cancer of the rectum, in which the rectum has usually to be removed. An ileostomy is then performed which acts as an artificial anus, to which a bag is attached to collect the waste matter. Distressing though this may at first be, the vast majority of people with an ileostomy learn to lead a fully active and normal life. Help and advice in adjusting to what can be described as an 'ileostomy life' can be obtained from the Ileostomy Association of Great Britain and Ireland (see APPENDIX 2: ADDRESSES). (See STOMA.)

ILEUM The lower part of the small intestine. (See INTESTINE.)

ILEUS Paralysis of the bowel muscle. (See INTESTINE, DISEASES OF.)

ILIUM The uppermost of the three bones forming each side of the pelvis. (See BONE; PELVIS.)

ILLUSIONS (see HALLUCINATIONS).

IMIDAZOLE A group of antifungal drugs active against a wide range of FUNGI and YEASTS. Some are also effective against bacteria and HELMINTH infections. Econazole, clotrimazole, ketoconazole, fluconazole and itraconazole are examples: the drugs are given by mouth or externally as creams.

IMIPRAMINE One of the tricyclic anti-depressants used to treat depression. (See ANTI-DEPRESSANTS.)

IMMERSION FOOT The term applied to a condition which develops as a result of prolonged immersion of the feet in cold or cool water. It was a condition commonly seen during the 1939–45 War in shipwrecked sailors and airmen who had crashed in the sea and spent long periods before being rescued. Such prolonged exposure results in vasoconstriction of the smaller arteries in the feet, leading to coldness and blueness of the feet, and finally, in severe cases, to ulceration and gangrene.

IMMUNE SYSTEM (see IMMUNITY).

IMMUNITY The body's defence against foreign substances. Its major function is to combat infectious micro-organisms (bacteria, viruses and parasites) but it also protects against drugs, toxins, and cancer cells. Immunity is partly non-specific since it does not depend on previous exposure to the foreign substance. For example, micro-organisms are engulfed and inactivated by polymorphonuclear leucocytes as a first line of defence before specific immunity has developed. Acquired immunity depends on specific recognition of the foreign substance and is the usual outcome of natural infection or prophylactic immunization. Foreign substances which provoke an immune response are termed 'antigens'. These are usually proteins but smaller molecules such as drugs and chemicals can also induce an immune response. Proteins are taken up and processed by specialized cells called 'antigen presenting cells', strategically sited where microbial infection may enter the body. The complex protein molecules are broken down into short amino-acid chains (peptides) and transported to the cell surface where they are presented by structures called HLA antigens. These antigens are the human form of histocompatibility antigens which confer individuality on the cells of most mammalian species.

Foreign peptides presented by HUMAN LEUCO-CYTE ANTIGEN (HLA) molecules are recognized by cells called T lymphocytes. These originate in the bone marrow and migrate to the thymus where they are educated to distinguish between foreign PEPTIDES which elicit a primary immune response and self-antigens which do not. Non-responsiveness to self-antigens is termed 'tolerance' (see AUTO-IMMUNITY). Each population or clone of T cells is uniquely responsive to a single peptide sequence because it expresses a surface molecule ('receptor') which fits only that peptide. The responsive T cell clone induces a specific response in other T and B lymphocyte populations. Cytotoxic T cells penetrate infected tissues and kill cells which express peptides derived from invading micro-organisms, thereby helping to eliminate the infection.

B lymphocytes secrete ANTIBODIES which are collectively termed GAMMA-GLOBULINS or IMMUNOGLOBULINS (Ig). Each B cell population (clone) secretes antibody uniquely specific for antigens encountered in the blood, extracellular space, and the lumen of organs such as the respiratory passages and gastrointestinal tract. Antibodies belong to different Ig classes; IgM antibodies are initially synthesized followed by smaller and therefore more penetrative IgG molecules. IgA antibodies are adapted to cross the surfaces of mucosal tissues so that they can adhere to organisms in the gut, upper and lower respiratory passages, thereby preventing their attachment to the mucosal surface. IgE antibodies also contribute to mucosal defence but are implicated in many allergic reactions (see ALLERGY).

Antibodies are composed of constant portions, which distinguish antibodies of different class, and variable portions, which confer unique antigen-binding properties on the product of each B cell clone. In order to match the vast range of antigens the immune system has to combat, the variable portions are synthesized under the instructions of a large number of encoding genes whose products are assembled to make the final antibody. The antibody produced by a single B cell clone is called a MONOCLONAL ANTIBODY; monoclonal antibodies are synthesized in vivo and in vitro for diagnostic and therapeutic purposes. Primary immune responses induce memory for the initiating antigen which persists in selected lymphocytes. Further challenge with the same antigen stimulates an accelerated, more vigorous secondary response by both T and B lymphocytes. Priming the immune system in this manner forms the physiological basis for immunization programmes.

Populations of LYMPHOCYTES with different functions and other cells engaged in immune responses carry distinctive protein markers. By convention these are classified and enumerated by their 'CD' markers, using monoclonal antibodies specific for each marker.

Immune responses are influenced by cytokines which function as hormones acting over a short range to accelerate the activation and proliferation of other cell populations contributing to the immune response. Specific immune responses collaborate with non-specific defence mechanisms. These include the COMPLEMENT SYSTEM, a protein cascade reaction designed to

Age	Disease and mode of administration
3 days	BCG (Bacille Calmette-Guerin) by injection if tuberculosis in family in past 6 months.
2 months	Poliomyelitis (oral); adsorbed diphtheria, whooping-cough (pertussis)[1] and tetanus[2] (triple vaccine given by injection); HIb injection[3]
3 months	Poliomyelitis (oral); diphtheria, whooping-cough (pertussis)[1] and tetanus[2] (triple vaccine given by injection); HIb injection[3]
4 months	Poliomyelitis (oral); diphtheria, whooping-cough (pertussis)[1] and tetanus[2] (triple vaccine given by injection); HIb injection[3]
12–18 months	Measles, mumps, and rubella (German measles)[4] (given together live by injection)

SCHOOL ENTRY

4–5 years	Poliomyelitis (oral); adsorbed diphtheria and tetanus (given together by injection); give MMR vaccine if not already given at 12–18 months
10–14 females	Rubella (by injection) if they have missed MMR
10–14	BCG (Bacille Calmette-Guerin) by injection to tuberculin-negative children to prevent tuberculosis
15–18	Poliomyelitis single booster dose (oral); tetanus (by injection)

1 Pertussis may be excluded in certain susceptible individuals.
2 Known as DPT or triple vaccine.
3 *Haemophilus influenzae* immunization (type B) is being introduced to be given at same time, but different limb.
4 Known as MMR vaccine.

Recommended immunization schedules in the United Kingdom

eliminate antigens neutralized by antibodies and to recruit cell populations which kill microorganisms.

IMMUNIZATION is the introduction of antigens into a body (by injection, orally or via a nasal spray) to provoke immunity usually against infectious diseases such as whooping-cough, measles and poliomyelitis.

IMMUNIZATION The introduction of ANTIGENS into a body to produce IMMUNITY The table above gives the immunization programme recommended by the UK government.

IMMUNO-ASSAY Procedures which measure the concentration of any antigenic material to which an antibody can be created. The amount of antigen bound to this antibody is proportional to the parent substance. Enzymes (ELISA) or radioactive labels (RADIO-IMMUNO ASSAY) are used to measure the concentration of antigenic material.

IMMUNODEFICIENCY Impaired immunity resulting from inherited or acquired abnormalities of the immune system. This leads to increased vulnerability to infection (see IMMUNITY). Important inherited examples of immunodeficiency are defects in function of GRANULOCYTES and the COMPLEMENT SYSTEM. Common acquired forms of immunodeficiency are defective function of B-type LYMPHOCYTES and hence antibody deficiency in 'common variable hypogammaglobulinaemia' and grossly deficient CD4 T-cell function – malfunctioning

T-type LYMPHOCYTES – in AIDS, secondary to HIV infection.

IMMUNOGENICITY The characteristic of a substance that can provoke an immune response (see IMMUNITY). This includes how 'foreign' a substance entering or contacting the body is, route of entry, dose, number and period of exposure to antigen and the genetic make-up of the host.

IMMUNOGLOBULINS are a group of naturally occurring proteins that act as ANTIBODIES. They are structurally related, their differences determining their biological behaviour. Man has 5 types of immunoglobulin with different protective functions: IgA, IgD, IgE, IgG and IgM. In the laboratory they are separated and identified by a chemical process called electrophoresis. Most antibodies have a molecular weight of 160,000.

Certain immunoglobulins can be used in the active or passive immunity of people against infectious diseases such as rabies and viral hepatitis (see IMMUNITY and GAMMA-GLOBULIN).

IMMUNOLOGIST A specialist (medically or scientifically qualified) who practises or researches immunology.

IMMUNOLOGY The study of immune responses to the environment. Its main clinical applications include improving resistance to microbial infections (see IMMUNITY), combating the effects of impaired immunity (see IMMUNO-DEFICIENCY), controlling harmful immune reactions (see ALLERGY), and manipulating immune responses (see IMMUNOSUPPRESSION and IMMUNOTHERAPY) to prevent harmful immunological responses such as graft rejection and autoimmune diseases (see AUTOIMMUNITY). The clinical study of disordered immunity now forms the allied discipline of clinical immunology, which is closely linked to the laboratory-based discipline of immunopathology.

IMMUNOSUPPRESSANT A drug that reduces the body's resistance to infection and other foreign agents. It does so by suppressing the activity of the immune system (see IMMUNITY). Examples of such drugs are AZATHIOPRINE, CYCLOPHOSPHAMIDE and CYCLOSPORIN A. Immunosuppressants are used to help transplanted organs and tissues to survive the potential immune reaction from the host. They are also used to treat AUTOIMMUNE disorders such as RHEUMATOID ARTHRITIS.

IMMUNOSUPPRESSION The suppression of harmful immune responses. The prevention of organ rejection by recipients of kidney, heart, and bone-marrow transplants is the most clear-cut application. Immunosuppression is also necessary in many diseases mediated in whole or in part by abnormal immune reactions (see ALLERGY and AUTOIMMUNITY). Most immunosuppressive drugs in current clinical practice are non-specific since they inhibit protective immunity and not just the harmful immune reaction. CORTICOSTEROIDS are most commonly used. The anti-proliferative drugs AZATHIOPRINE and METHOTREXATE are also widely employed. The introduction of more selective drugs such as CYCLOSPORIN and biological agents (see IMMUNOTHERAPY) promises to improve the situation. Tacrolimus is a recently introduced MACROLIDE IMMUNOSUPPRESSANT. It is indicated for primary immunosuppression in liver and kidney allograft recipients and also for allograft rejection resistant to conventional immunosuppressive regimens. Although chemically unrelated to cyclosporin, it seems to act in a similar way with similar side-effects; the incidence of neurotoxity and nephrotoxicity appears to be greater, CARDIOMYOPATHY has been reported, as have disturbances of GLUCOSE METABOLISM.

IMMUNOSUPPRESSIVE A drug that lowers the body's resistance to infection and other 'foreign' bodies by suppressing the IMMUNE system. These drugs are essential to the success of transplant surgery as they help the transplanted organ to survive. They are also valuable in treating AUTOIMMUNE diseases such as RHEUMATOID ARTHRITIS. The immunosuppressive drug normally used in transplant surgery is cyclosporin.

IMMUNOTHERAPY The manipulation of immunity by immunological means to reduce

harmful reactions or to boost beneficial responses. Severe allergy to wasp or bee stings is often treated by a course of injections with allergen purified from insect venom. There are current attempts to treat autoimmune diseases with monoclonal antibodies to the T-cell populations or cytokines implicated in the immunopathogenesis of the disorder (see AUTOIMMUNITY and IMMUNITY).

Strategies are also being evaluated for treating cancer by boosting the patient's own immunity to cancer cells. One approach is immunization with cancer cells manipulated *in vivo* to increase a T-lymphocyte attack on antigens expressed by tumour cells. Another method is to manipulate the cytokine network into encouraging an immune attack on or self-destruction ('apoptosis') of malignant cells.

However immunotherapy is a developing science and its place in the routine treatment of immunological and malignant diseases still evolving.

IMPACTION A term applied to a condition in which two things are firmly lodged together. For example, when after a fracture one piece of bone is driven within the other, this is known as an impacted fracture; when a tooth is firmly lodged in its socket so that its eruption is prevented, this is known as dental impaction.

IMPETIGO An infectious skin disease caused usually by *Staphylococcus aureus* and less often by *Streptococcus pyogenes*. The itching rash is particularly seen on the face but may spread widely. Vesicles and pustules erupt and dry to form yellow-brown scabs. Untreated it may last for weeks. In very young infants large blisters may form (bullous impetigo).

Treatment Crusts should be gently removed with saline. Mild cases respond to frequent aplication of mupiricin or NEOMYCIN/BACITRACIN ointment. More severe cases should be treated orally with FLUCLOXACILLIN or CEPHALOSPORIN. If the patient is allergic to penicillin, erythromycin can be used.

For severe intractable acne an oral retinoid drug called isotretinoin (commercially produced as Roaccutane®) can be used. It is given systemically but treatment must be supervised by a consultant dermatologist as serious side-effects, including possible psychiatric disturbance, can occur. The drug is also teratogenic so women who are, or who may become, pregnant must not take isotretinoin. It acts mainly by suppressing sebum production in the sebaceous glands and can be very effective. Recurrent bouts of impetigo should raise suspicion of underlying scabies or head lice.

IMPOTENCE The inability to perform the sexual act. It may be partial or complete, temporary or permanent. Of the many classifications of this quite common condition, the most satisfactory is probably that which divides it into two main groups: organic and psychological. Among organic causes are lesions of the external genitalia, e.g. a tight foreskin; disturbances of the endocrine glands, such as diminished activity of the gonads, thyroid gland or pituitary gland; diseases of the central nervous system, e.g. tabes dorsalis; any severe disturbance of health, such as diabetes mellitus, addiction to alcohol and the like. Psychological factors are the commonest cause and these are anxiety, ignorance, fear, guilt, weakness of sexual desire or abnormality of such desire. Counselling or sex therapy, preferably with the partner, has a 50-per-cent chance of helping to cure long-term impotence of psychological origin.

An oral drug for treating erectile function has recently been approved by the USA's Food and Drug Administration. Sildenafil citrate (tradename (Viagra®) is the first in a new class of drugs called phosphodiesterase type 5 inhibitors. They work by improving blood flow to the penis. The pill can be taken an hour before intercourse. The drug is not an aphrodisiac, and side-effects include headache, facial flushing and indigestion. There are some suggestions that it may, however, affect retinal function.

IMPRINTING   In the context of animal behaviour this is a quick and irreversible type of learning in which patterns are imprinted on the animal's mind during the first few hours of life. The smell and feel of its mother are one such imprint.

INANITION   Exhaustion in an individual caused by lack of appropriate nutrients in the circulating blood. Starvation, malnutrition or intestinal disorders are among the causes.

INBREEDING   The birth of offspring to parents who are closely related. In traditional rural communities marriage between cousins was common and this could lead to a higher than average number of children with congenital anomalies or learning difficulties

INCIDENCE   One of the main ways to measure the frequency of a disease in a particular population; the incidence of a disease is the number of new cases that occur during a particular time. Prevalence, the other measure, is the total number of cases of disease present at any one time and covers both old and new cases.

INCISION   A cut or wound and is a term specially applied to surgical openings.

INCISOR   The term for the four front teeth of each jaw. (See TEETH.)

INCOMPATIBILITY   (1) In the pharmacological context, the use of two or more drugs in treatment which together produce adverse consequences for the patient. The *British National*

Formulary carries an appendix devoted to drug interactions. (2) In the haematological context, an adverse reaction in a patient given a blood transfusion in which the donor blood is incompatible with that of the recipient. (See TRANSFUSION OF BLOOD.)

INCOMPETENCE is a term applied to the valves of the heart when, as a result of disease in the valves or alterations in size of the chambers of the heart, the valves become unable to close the orifices which they should protect. (See HEART DISEASES.)

INCONTINENCE

Urinary incontinence is the involuntary loss of urine. This distressing condition affects 5 per cent of the population, 8 per cent of women and 3 per cent of men. The two main groups of urinary incontinence are urge and stress incontinence.

Urge incontinence   This is the involuntary loss of urine associated with the strong desire to void, and is the result of bladder dysfunction. Urge incontinence may be the result of overactive motor nerves to the bladder, which may be due to spinal problems such as MULTIPLE SCLEROSIS, nerve problems such as DIABETES or secondary to bladder outflow obstruction as a result of PROSTATE DISEASE, or IDIOPATHIC causes. Similarly urge incontinence may be the result of overactive sensory nerves, which is associated with cystitis, bladder stones, or bladder tumours.

Stress incontinence   This is the involuntary loss of urine during activities, such as coughing, exercise, or lifting. Caused by weakness in the urethral muscle which holds the urine in the bladder, stress incontinence is usually the result of obesity, childbirth or, in men, a broken pelvis, or an operation on the prostate gland.

Investigations   These would include, in women, a vaginal examination to look for PROLAPSE, a urine test to exclude any infections, and specific tests to assess the function of the bladder known as urodynamics.

Treatment   Urge incontinence can be treated by bladder-training measures, by the use of drugs to calm the bladder, or by distending the bladder under an anaesthetic. Stress incontinence is treated by the individual's performing pelvic-floor exercises, which can be supplemented by stimulation of the pelvic floor. An operation designed to raise and support the bladder and urethra may also be effective.

Faecal incontinence is the inability to control bowel movements and may be due to severe constipation, especially in the elderly, local disease or to injury or disease of the spinal cord or nervous supply to rectum and anal muscles. Those with the symptom need investigation.

INCOORDINATION   A term applied to irregularity of movements produced either by loss of the sensations by which they are governed or by defects in the muscles themselves or their nerves.

INCUBATION means the period elapsing between the time when a person becomes infected by some agent and the first appearance of the symptoms of the disease. Most acute infectious diseases have fairly definite periods of incubation, and it is of great importance that people who have run the risk of infection should know the length of time which must elapse before they can be sure whether or not they are to contract the disease in question. A person who has been exposed to infection is, during the incubation period, technically known as a contact. By isolating and watching contact cases medical officers can often successfully check a threatened epidemic. It must be noted that diseases are not communicated to others by a person while passing through the stage of incubation. Some diseases, however, such as measles, become infectious as soon as the first symptoms set in after the incubation period is over; others, like scarlet fever and smallpox, are not so infectious then as in their later stages. The incubation period for any given disease is remarkably constant, although in the case of a severe attack the incubation is usually slightly shortened, and if the oncoming attack be a mild one, the period may be lengthened. All of these may, however, take a few days longer than the time stated to show themselves. (See INFECTION.) Several also, and especially whooping-cough, may be difficult to recognize in their early stages.

	days
Chickenpox	14–21
Diphtheria	2–5
German measles	14–21
Measles	10–15
Mumps	18–21
Poliomyelitis	3–21
Smallpox	10–16
Typhoid fever	7–21
Whooping-cough	7–10

Incubation periods of the commoner infectious diseases.

INDEX FINGER   The forefinger or second digit of the hand (see FINGERS).

INDEX MEDICUS   A monthly publication produced by the National Library of Medicine in the USA. The publication indexes leading biomedical literature from throughout the world. Indexing is by author and subject.

INDIAN HEMP (see *CANNABIS INDICA*).

INDIGESTION (see DYSPEPSIA).

INDOMETHACIN   One of many NON-STEROIDAL INFLAMMATORY DRUGS used in the treatment of gout and rheumatoid arthritis. A proprionic-acid derivative, it may help to relieve night pain and morning stiffness. It is also used to treat the congenital abnormality of the heart known as DUCTUS ARTERIOSUS.)

The drug is graded as being associated with 'intermediate risks' in the *British National Formulary*. It causes headaches, dizziness and gastrointestinal disturbances.

INDORAMIN   An alpha-adreno-receptor-blocking drug used in the treatment of high blood-pressure. It has several side-effects including sleepiness, dizziness, depression and failure to ejaculate. (See ADRENERGIC RECEPTORS.)

INDUCTION   Bringing about a particular event, for example, the induction or starting of labour; the induction of anaesthesia.

INDURATION   The pathological hardening of a tissue or organ. This may occur when a tissue is infected or when it is invaded by cancer.

INDUSTRIAL DISEASES (see OCCUPATIONAL DISEASES).

INFANT   A baby who is under 1 year old.

INFANT FEEDING   The new-born infant may be fed naturally from the breast or artificially from a bottle.

Breast-feeding   Unless there is a genuine contra-indication, every baby should be breast-fed. The nutritional components of human milk are in the ideal proportions to promote the healthy growth of the human new-born. The mother's milk, especially colostrum (the fluid secreted before full lactation is established) contains immune cells and antibodies that increase the baby's resistance to infection. In addition, breast milk does not require elaborate and expensive preparation rituals. From the mother's point of view, breast-feeding helps the womb to return to its normal size and helps her to lose excess body fat gained during pregnancy. Most importantly, breast-feeding promotes intimate contact between mother and baby. A final point to be borne in mind, however, is that drugs taken by a mother can be excreted in her milk. These include antibiotics, sedatives, tranquillizers, alcohol, nicotine and high-dose steroids or vitamins.

Artificial feeding   Unmodified cows' milk is not a satisfactory food for the human new-born and may cause dangerous metabolic imbalance. If breast-feeding is not feasible, one of the many commerciallly available formula milks should be used. Most of these are made from cows' milk which has been modified to reflect the composition of human milk as nearly as possible. For the rare infant who develops cows'-milk-protein intolerance, a milk based on soya-bean protein is indicated.

Feeding and weight gain The main guide as to whether an infant is being adequately fed is the weight. During the first days of life a healthy infant loses weight, but, however, by the end of the second week, should return to birth weight. From then on, weight gain should be approximately 6oz. (170g) each week.

The timing of feeds reflects social convention rather than natural feeding patterns. Among the most primitive hunter-gatherer tribes of South America, babies are carried next to the breast and allowed to suckle at will. Fortunately for developed society, however, babies can be conditioned to intermittent feedings.

As the timing of breast-feeding is more flexible, little or no preparation time being required, mothers can feed their babies on demand. Far from spoiling the baby, demand feeding is likely to lead to a contented infant. The only necessary caution being that a crying baby is not always a hungry baby.

In general, a new-born will require feeding every two to four hours and, if well, is unlikely to sleep for more than six hours. After the first months, a few lucky parents will find their infant sleeping through the night.

Weaning Weaning on to solid foods is again a matter of some individuality. Most babies will become dissatisfied with a milk-only diet round about six months and develop enthusiasm for cereal-based weaning foods. Introduction of solids before the age of four months is unusual and, unless really necessary to quell an apparently insatiable appetite, should be avoided. Similarly, delaying the commencement of weaning beyond nine months is nutritionally undesirable. As weaning progresses, the infant's diet requires less milk. Once established on a varied solid diet, breast and formula milks can be safely replaced with cows' milk. There is, however, no nutritional contra-indication to continued breast-feeding until the mother wishes to stop.

It is during weaning that infants realize that they can arouse extreme maternal anxiety by refusing to eat. This can lead to force-feeding and battles of will which may culminate in a breakdown of the mother–child relationship. To avoid this, parents must resist the temptation to coax the child to eat. If the child refuses solid food, the meal should be taken away with a minimum of fuss. Children's appetites reflect their individual genetic structure and a well child will eat enough to grow and maintain satisfactory weight gain. If a child is not eating properly, weight gain will be inadequate over a prolonged period and an underlying illness is the most likely cause. Indeed, failure to thrive is the paediatrician's best clue to chronic illness.

Advice on feeding Many sources of conflicting advice are available to new parents. It is impossible to satisfy everyone and ultimately it is the well-being of the mother and infant and the closeness of their relationship that matter. In general, mothers should be wary of rigid advice. An experienced midwife, health visitor or well-baby-clinic nursing sister are among the most reliable sources of information.

	Protein per cent	Fat per cent	Sugar per cent	Calories per cent
Human milk	1·1	4·2	7·0	70
Cow's milk	3·5	3·9	4·6	66

Composition of human and cow's milk

INFANTILE PARALYSIS An old name for POLIOMYELITIS.

INFANTILISM The condition characterized by imperfect sexual development at puberty. It may or may not be associated with small stature. It may be due to lack of development of certain of the endocrine glands: i.e. the GONADS, pituitary gland or the adrenal glands. In other cases it may be associated with a generalized disease such as diabetes mellitus, asthma, ulcerative colitis and rheumatoid arthritis.

INFANT MORTALITY is the number of deaths of infants under one year of age. The infant mortality rate in any given year is calculated as the number of deaths in the first year of life in proportion to every 1000 registered live births in that year. Along with PERINATAL MORTALITY, it is accepted as one of the most important criteria for assessing the health of the community and the standard of the social conditions of a country.

The improvement in the infant mortality rate has occurred mainly in the period from the second month of life. There has been much less improvement in the neonatal mortality rate: i.e. the number of infants dying during the first four weeks of life, expressed as a proportion of every 1000 live births. During the first week of life the main causes of death are asphyxia, prematurity, birth injuries and congenital abnormalities. After the first week the main cause of death is infection.

Social conditions also play an important rôle in infant mortality. In England and Wales the infant mortality rate in 1930–32 was: Social Class I (professional), 32·7; Social Class III (skilled workers), 57·6; Social Class V (unskilled workers), 77·1. The comparable figures for Scotland for 1939–45 were: Class I, 30·9; Class III, 53·4; Class V, 78·6. Many factors come into play in producing these social variations, but overcrowding is undoubtedly one of the most important. For instance, in 1936 the infant mortality rate in Bournemouth, where only 0·3 per cent of working-class families were overcrowded, was 78 per cent of that for the entire country, compared with 145 per cent in Newcastle-upon-Tyne where 10·7 per cent of working-class families were overcrowded. The same discrepancy persists to the present day.

1838–9	146	1950–52	30
1851–60	154	1960–62	22
1900–02	142	1970–72	18
1910–12	110	1980–82	12
1920–22	82	1990–82	7
1930–32	67	1996 (prov.)	6·2
1940–42	59		

Infant mortality rate in the United Kingdom 1838–1996. Deaths of infants under 1 year of age per thousand live births.

It is thus evident that for a reduction of the infant mortality rate to the minimum figure the following conditions must be met. Mothers and potential mothers must be housed adequately in healthy surroundings. The pregnant and nursing mother must be ensured an adequate diet. Effective antenatal supervision must be available to every mother, as well as skilled supervision during labour. The new-born infant must be adequately nursed and adequately fed and mothers encouraged to breast feed. Environmental and public-health measures must be taken to ensure adequate housing, a clean milk supply and full availability of such protective measures as immunization against diphtheria, measles, poliomyelitis and whooping-cough. (See also PERINATAL MORTALITY.)

INFARCTION   The changes in an organ when an artery is suddenly blocked, leading to the formation of a dense, wedge-shaped mass in the part of the organ supplied by the artery. It occurs as the result of embolism or of thrombosis. (See EMBOLISM.)

INFECTION   The process by which a disease is communicated via micro-organisms from one person to another. All diseases so communicable are called infectious. This micro-organism may be a BACTERIUM, a RICKETTSIA, a VIRUS, a PROTOZOON, or a METAZOON. Invasion of the body by a metazoon (e.g. by an intestinal worm) is more often known as an infestation.

The skin is an important protection against micro-organisms entering the body tissues. A large measure of protection is afforded by the factors which ensure immunity against diseases. (See IMMUNITY.)

Modes of infection   The infective material may be transmitted to the person by direct contact with a sick person, when the disease is said to be contagious, although such a distinction is purely artificial. Different diseases are specially infectious at different periods of their course. Protecting people can be difficult since some diseases are infectious before the patient shows any symptoms.

Infection may be conveyed on dust, in drinking-water, food, particularly milk, the body's waste products and secretions, or even clothes and linen which have been in contact with the infected individual.

Some people who have suffered from a disease, or who have simply been in contact with an infectious case, harbour the infectious agent. This is particularly the case in typhoid fever, the bacillus continuing to develop in the gall-bladder of some people, who have had the disease, maybe for years after the symptoms have disappeared. In the case of cholera, which is endemic in some developing countries with hot climates, 80 per cent or more of the population may harbour the bacillus and spread infection when other circumstances favour this. Similarly in the case of DYSENTERY, people who have completely recovered may still be capable of infecting dust and drinking-water by their stools. DIPHTHERIA and cerebrospinal MENINGITIS, which is particularly liable to infect children, are other examples.

Flies can infect milk and other food with the organisms causing TYPHOID FEVER and food poisoning. Mosquitoes carry the infective agents of MALARIA, DENGUE FEVER and YELLOW FEVER, these undergoing part of their development in the body of the mosquito. Fleas convey the germ of plague from rat to man, lice are responsible for inoculating TYPHUS fever and one form of RELAPSING FEVER by their bite. A tick is responsible for spreading another form of relapsing fever, and kala-azar (or LEISHMANIASIS) is spread by the bites of sandflies.

Notifiable diseases   Certain of the common and most serious infectious diseases are notifiable in the United Kingdom. A doctor diagnosing someone infected by a notifiable disease must inform the authorities. For the current list of notifiable infectious diseases in the UK see NOTIFIABLE DISEASES.

Prevention is an important aspect of the control of infectious diseases and various steps can be taken to check the spread of such infections as dysentery, tuberculosis, malaria and others. (See also IMMUNITY; INCUBATION.)

INFECTIOUS MONONUCLEOSIS (see MONONUCLEOSIS).

INFERTILITY   This is diagnosed when a couple have not achieved a pregnancy after one year of regular unprotected sexual intercourse. Between 15–20 per cent of couples have difficulties in conceiving. The 'deficiency' lies with the male partner in about a third of cases, with the female partner in about a third and with both partners in about a third. Couples should be investigated together efficiently and as quickly as possible to decrease the distress which is invariably associated with the diagnosis of infertility. In about 10–15 per cent of women suffering from infertility ovulation is disturbed. Mostly they will have either irregular periods or no periods at all.

Checking a hormone profile in the woman's blood will help in the diagnosis of ovulatory disorders like polycystic ovaries, an early menopause, anorexia or other endocrine illnesses. Ovulation itself is best assessed by ultrasound scan at mid-cycle or by a blood hormone progesterone level in the second half of the cycle.

The FALLOPIAN TUBES may be damaged or blocked in 20–30 per cent of infertile women. This is usually caused by previous pelvic infection or ENDOMETRIOSIS, where menstrual blood is thought to flow backwards through the fallopian tubes into the pelvis and seed with cells from the lining of the uterus in the pelvis. This process often leads to scarring of the pelvic tissues; 5–10 per cent of infertility is associated with endometriosis.

To assess the Fallopian tubes adequately a procedure called LAPAROSCOPY is performed. A telescope is inserted through the umbilicus and at the same time a dye is pushed through the tubes to assess their patency. The procedure is performed under a general anaesthetic.

In a few cases the mucus around the cervix may be hostile to the partner's sperm and therefore prevents fertilization.

Defective SPERM production is responsible for up to a quarter of infertility. It may result from the failure of the TESTES to descend in early life, from infections of the testes or previous surgery for testicular torsion. The semen is analysed to assess the numbers of sperm and their motility and to check for abnormal forms.

In a few cases the genetic make-up of one partner does not allow the couple ever to achieve a pregnancy naturally.

In about 25 per cent of couples no obvious cause can be found for their infertility.

Ovulation may be induced with drugs.

In some cases damaged fallopian tubes may be repaired by tubal surgery. If the tubes are destroyed beyond repair a pregnancy may be achieved with IN VITRO FERTILIZATION.

Endometriosis may be treated either with drugs or laser therapy and pregnancy rates after both forms of treatment are between 40–50 per cent, depending on the severity of the disease.

Few options exist for treating male-factor infertility. These are artificial insemination by husband or donor and more recently in vitro fertilization. Drug treatment and surgical repair of VARICOCELES have disappointing results.

Following investigations between 30 and 40 per cent of infertile couples will achieve a pregnancy usually within two years. (see ARTIFICIAL INSEMINATION; ASSISTED CONCEPTION.)

INFESTATION A term applied to the occurrence of animal parasites in the intestine, hair or clothing. (See INSECTS IN RELATION TO DISEASE.)

INFILTRATION The invasion of tissues or organs by cells or fluid that are not normally present. Local anaesthetic is infiltrated into an area of tissue to produce ANALGESIA in a defined area.

INFLAMMATION The reaction of the tissues to any injury, which may be the result of trauma, infection or chemicals. The victim feels pain and the affected tissue becomes hot, red and swollen. Inflammation also interferes with function. Local blood vessels dilate, thus increasing blood flow to the injured site. White blood cells invade the affected tissue engulfing bacteria or other foreign bodies; related cells consume any dead cells, thus producing pus after which the site starts to heal. If the infection is severe it may persist locally – chronic inflammation – or spread elsewhere in the body – systemic infection.

INFLUENZA is an acute infectious disease, characterized by a sudden onset, fever and generalized aches and pains, which usually occurs in epidemics and pandemics.

Cause The disease is caused by a virus of the influenza group. There are at least three types of influenza virus, known respectively as A, B and C. One of their most characteristic features is that infection with one type provides no protection against another type. Equally important is the ease with which the influenza virus can change its character. It is these two characteristics which explain why one attack of influenza provides little, if any, protection against a subsequent attack, and why it is so difficult to prepare an effective vaccine against the disease.

Epidemics of influenza due to virus A occur in Britain at two- to four-year intervals, and outbreaks of virus B influenza in less frequent cycles. Virus A influenza, for instance, was the prevalent infection in 1949, 1951, 1955 and 1956, whilst virus B influenza was epidemic in 1946, 1950, 1954 and, along with virus A, in 1958–59. The pandemic of 1957, which swept most of the world, though fortunately not in a severe form, was due to a new variant of virus A – the so-called Asian virus – and it has been suggested that it was this variant that was responsible for the pandemics of 1889 and 1918. Since 1957, variants of virus A have been the predominating causes of influenza accompanied on occasions by virus B. In 1997 an outbreak of Chinese avian influenza caused alarm. The influenza virus had apparently jumped species to infect some people in Hong Kong and, because no vaccine was available, some experts feared it might start an epidemic. In the event, it did not.

Symptoms The incubation period of influenza A and B is two to three days and the disease is characterized by a sudden onset. In most cases this is followed by a short, sharp febrile illness of two to four days' duration, associated with headache, prostration, generalized aching and respiratory symptoms. In many cases the respiratory symptoms are restricted to the upper respiratory tract, and consist of signs of irritation of the nose, pharynx and larynx. There may be nose-bleeds, and a dry hacking cough is often a prominent and troublesome symptom. The fever is usually remittent and the temperature seldom exceeds 39·4 °C (103 °F), tending to fluctuate between 38·3 and 39·4 °C (101 and 103 °F).

The most serious complication is infection of the lungs. This infection is usually due to organisms other than the influenza virus. It is a complication which can have serious results in elderly people.

The very severe form which tends to occur during pandemics – and which was so common during the 1918–19 pandemic – is characterized by the rapid onset of broncho-pneumonia and severe prostration. Because of the toxic effect on the heart there is a particularly marked form of cyanosis, known as heliotrope cyanosis.

Convalescence following influenza tends to be prolonged. Even after an attack of average severity there tends to be a period of weakness and depression.

Treatment Expert opinion is still divided as to the real value of influenza vaccine in preventing the disease. Part of the trouble is that, as already pointed out, there is no value in giving any vaccine until it is known which particular virus is causing the infection. As this varies from winter to winter, and as the protection given by vaccine does not exceed one year, it is obviously not worth while attempting to vaccinate the whole community. The general rule therefore is that, unless there is any evidence that a particularly virulent type of virus is responsible, only those should be vaccinated who are particularly vulnerable, such as children in boarding schools, elderly people, pregnant women, and people who suffer from chronic bronchitis. In the face of an epidemic, people in key positions, such as doctors, nurses and those concerned with public safety, transport and other public utilities should be vaccinated.

For an uncomplicated attack of influenza, treatment is symptomatic: that is, rest in bed, analgesics to relieve the pain, sedatives, and a light diet. A linctus is useful to sooth a troublesome cough. The best analgesic is ASPIRIN – either alone, or combined with PARACETAMOL and CODEINE. None of the sulphonamides or the known antibiotics has any effect on the influenza virus. On the other hand, should the lungs become infected, antibiotics should be given immediately, because, as has already been pointed out, such an infection is usually due to other organisms. If possible, a sample of sputum should be examined to determine which organisms are responsible for the lung infection. The choice of antibiotic then depends upon which antibiotic the organism is most sensitive to.

INFORMATION TECHNOLOGY IN MEDICINE

The advent of computing has had widespread effects in all areas of society with medicine no exception. Computer systems are vital, as they are in any modern enterprise, for the administration of hospitals, general practices and health authorities, supporting payroll, finance, stock ordering and billing, resource and bed management, word-processing correspondence, laboratory-result reporting, appointment and record systems, and management audit.

The imaging systems of COMPUTED TOMOGRAPHY (CT) and MAGNETIC RESONANCE IMAGING (MRI) have powerful computer techniques underlying them.

Computerized statistical analysis of study data, population databases and disease registries is now routine, leading to enhanced understanding of the interplay between diseases and the population. And the results of research, available on computerized indexes such as MEDLINE, can be obtained in searches that take only seconds, compared with the hours or days necessary to accomplish the same task with its paper incarnation, *Index Medicus*.

Medical informatics The direct computerization of those activities which are uniquely medical – history taking, examination, diagnosis and treatment – has proved an elusive goal, though it is hotly pursued by doctors, engineers and scientists working in the discipline of medical informatics. Computer techniques have scored some successes: patients are, for example, more willing to be honest about taboo areas, such as their drug or alcohol consumption, or their sexual proclivities with a computer than face to face with a clinician, but the practice of taking a history remains the cornerstone of clinical practice. The examination of the patient is unlikely to be supplanted by technological means in the foreseeable future; visual and tactile recognition systems are still in their infancy. Skilled interpretation of the result by machine rather than the human mind seems equally as remote. Working its way slowly outward from its starting point in mathematical logic, ARTIFICIAL INTELLIGENCE that in any way mimics its natural counterpart seems a distant prospect. Though there have been successes in computer-supported diagnosis in some specialized areas, such as the diagnosis of abdominal pain, workable systems that could supplant the mind of the generalist are still the dream of the many developers pursuing this goal, rather than a reality available to doctors in their consulting rooms now.

In therapeutics, computerized prescribing systems still require the doctor to make the decision about treatment, but facilitate the process of writing, issuing, and recording the prescription. In so doing, the system can provide automated checks, warning if necessary about allergies, potential drug interactions, or dosing errors. The built-in safety that this process offers is enhanced by the superior legibility of the script that ensues, reducing the potential for error when the medicine is dispensed by the nurse or the pharmacist.

Success in these individual applications continues to drive development, though the process has its critics, who are not slow to point to the lengthier consultations that arise when a computer is present in the consulting room and its distracting effect on communication with the patient.

Underlying these many software applications lies the ubiquitous personal computer – more powerful today than its mainframe predecessor of only twenty years ago – combined with networking technology that enables interconnection and the sharing of data. As in essence the doctor's role involved the acquisition, manipulation and application of information – from the individual patient, and from the body of medical knowledge – great excitement surrounds the development of open systems that allow different software and hardware platforms to interact. Many problems remain to be solved, not least the fact that for such systems to work, the whole organization, and not just a few specialized individuals, must become computer literate. It must be easy to learn to use, which requires an intuitive interface between the user and the computer system that is predictable and logical in its ordering and presentation of information.

Many other issues stand in the way of the development towards computerization: standard systems of nomenclature for medical concepts have proved surprisingly difficult to develop, but are crucial for successful information sharing between users. Sharing information between existing legacy systems is a major challenge, often requiring customized software and extensive human intervention to enable the previous investments that an organization has made in individual systems (e.g. laboratory-result reporting) to be integrated with newer technology. The beginnings of a global solution to this substantial obstacle to networking progress is in sight: the technology that enables the Internet – an international network of telephonically linked personal computers – also enables the establishment of intranets, in which individual servers (computers dedicated to serving information to other computers) act as repositories of 'published' data, which other users on the network may 'browse' as necessary in a client–server environment.

Systems that support this process are still in early stages of development but the key conceptualizations are in place. Developments over the next five to ten years will centre on the electronic patient record available to the clinician on an integrated clinical workstation. The clinical workstation – in essence a personal computer networked to the hospital or practice system – will enable the clinician to record clinical data and diagnoses, automate the ordering of investigations and the collection of the results, and facilitate referral and communication between the many professionals and departments involved in any individual patient's care.

Once data is digitized, it may be as freely networked globally as locally. Consultations in which live video and sound transmissions are the bonds of the doctor–patient relationship (the techniques of telemedicine) are already reality, and have proved particularly convenient and cost effective in linking the patient and the generalist to specialists in remote areas with low population density.

As these problems are solved, concerns about privacy and confidentiality arise. While paper records were often only confidential by default, the potential for breaches of security in computerized networks is much graver. External breaches of the system by hackers are one serious concern, but internal breaches by authorized users making unauthorized use of the data are a much greater risk in practice. Governing network security so that clinical users have access on a need-to-know basis is a difficult business: the software tools to enable this – encryption, anonymization (ensuring that clinical information about patients is anonymous to prevent confidential information about them leaking out) of data collected for management and research processes, and KEY ESCROW exist in the technical domain but remain a complex conundrum for solution in the real world.

INFORMED CONSENT   Patients' rights are a growing concern for doctors and patients. A controversial aspect of their clinical relationship is consent: doctors need signed agreement from patients before carrying out operations or procedures, before entering patients in clinical trials, and, increasingly, before publishing photographs of patients for medical education in print or electronic media. Consent is informed when patients are fully aware of the consequences and risks of signing a consent for any purpose. For example, doctors and other health professionals should tell patients of the complications of a treatment and the likelihood of its success. They should make sure that the patients understand the information given and patients should be given the opportunity to ask questions and, where appropriate, immediate relatives should be involved in the process. Doctors are often inclined to highlight the benefits of a treatment, while downplaying the risks, but the General Medical Council in the United Kingdom has shown its willingness to discipline doctors who go beyond the consent that they were given by patients. Some doctors, however feel that, especially in relation to research and medical education, consent need not be fully informed as the overall benefit to patients outweighs the risk to an individual. Others, both doctors and patients, argue that overlooking the autonomy of competent individuals is against the spirit of the Helsinki Declaration (see ETHICS COMMITTEES), which states that the 'interests of the subject must always prevail over the interest of science or society.' Although the exact limits will remain difficult to define in some settings, informed consent should be obtained from patients in accordance with guidelines from professional medical organizations. Patients or close relatives could consult the local NHS authorities or help groups (see APPENDIX 2: ADDRESSES) if they are dissatisfied with their doctors' explanations.

INFUNDIBULUM   A funnel-shaped passage. The word is used specifically to describe the hollow conical stalk that links the HYPOTHALMUS to the posterior lobe of the PITUITARY GLAND.

INFUSION The intravenous or subcutaneous injection of one of a variety of therapeutic solutions, such as saline, glucose, or gum acacia, in the treatment of severe dehydration, hypoglycaemia, or other plasma electrolyte imbalance. Blood infusions may be given in cases of severe anaemia, for example, after heavy bleeding. Infusions may be given in intermittent amounts of around 570 ml (1 pint) at a time, or alternatively by continuous drip-feed over several hours.

INGESTION The act of taking fluid, food, or medicine into the stomach. The way in which a phagocytic cell surrounds and absorbs foreign substances such as bacteria in the blood.

INGUINAL HERNIA An extrusion of the abdominal PERITONEUM, sometimes containing a loop of bowel, through natural openings in the region of either groin (see HERNIA).

INGUINAL REGION The groin, the area of the body where the lower part of the abdomen meets the upper thigh. The inguinal ligaments extend on each side from the superior spines of the iliac bones to the pubic bone. It is also called Poupart's ligament (see diagram of ABDOMEN).

INHALANTS Substances that can be inhaled into the body through the lungs. They may be delivered in traditional form dissolved in hot water and inhaled in the steam or as an aerosol, a suspension of very small liquid or solid particles in the air. The latter are now usually delivered by devices in which the aerosol is kept under pressure in a small hand-held cylinder and delivered in required doses by a release mechanism.

Aerosols Asthmatic patients find aerosol devices of value in controlling their attacks. They provide an effective and convenient way of applying drugs directly to the bronchi, thus reducing the risks of unwanted effects accompanying systemic therapy. They are of particular use in asthma. Broncho-dilator aerosols contain either a beta-sympathomimetic agent or ipratropium bromide which is an anti-cholinergic drug. Of the BETA-ADRENOCEPTOR AGONISTS ISOPRENALINE was the first compound to be widely used as an aerosol. It did however stimulate beta$_1$ receptors in the heart as well as beta$_2$ receptors in the bronchi and so produced palpitations and even dangerous cardiac arrhythmias. Newer beta-adrenoceptor agonists are specific for the beta$_2$ receptors and thus have a greater safety margin. They include SALBUTAMOL, TERBUTALINE, rimiterol, fenoterol and reproterol. Unwanted effects such as palpitations, tremor and restlessness are uncommon with these more specific preparations. In patients who get insufficient relief from the beta- adrenoreceptor agonist the drug ipratropium bromide is worth adding. Salmeterol is a longer-acting BETA-2 ADRENOCEPTOR STIMU-LANT for twice daily administration. It is not intended for the relief of acute attacks, for which shorter acting beta-2 stimulants such as SALBUTAMOL should be used. Salmeterol should be added to existing corticosteroid therapy, rather than replacing it. (See ASTHMA.)

Patients must be taught carefully and observed while using their inhalers. It is important that patients should realize that if the aerosol no longer gives more than slight transient relief they should not increase the dose but seek medical help.

INHALATION A method of applying drugs in a finely divided or gaseous state, so that, when breathed in, they may come in contact with the nose, throat and lungs. There are two chief means by which drugs are mingled with the air and so taken in by breathing. These are traditional steam inhalations and modern aerosol devices which deliver a fine spray direct into the mouth.

INHALER A device for administering a drug in the form of a powder or vapour. This method of delivery is particularly valuable in the treatment of respiratory disorders such as ASTHMA or BRONCHITIS (see INHALANTS).

INHERITANCE The transfer of characteristics, traits and disorders from parents to children by means of GENES carried in the CHROMOSOMES of the GERM CELLS. (see GENETIC CODE; GENETIC DISORDERS.)

INHIBITION means arrest or restraint of some process effected by nervous influence. The term is applied to the action of certain inhibitory nerves: e.g. the vagus nerve which contains fibres that inhibit or control the action of the heart. The term is also applied generally to the mental processes by which instinctive but undesirable actions are checked by a process of self-control.

INJECTIONS The introduction of a substance into the body using a syringe and an attached needle. Injections may be given under the skin (subcutaneous), via a vein (intravenous), deep into a muscle (intramuscular) or into the fluid surrounding the spinal cord (intrathecal).

INNER EAR This comprises three fluid-filled chambers or labyrinths situated in the bony temporal area that are concerned with identifying a person's position in space. Each chamber lies in a different plane and movement of fluid in it is picked up by sensory cells that transmit the information to the brain. Disease or damage to the inner ear upsets the sense of balance and causes vertigo. MOTION SICKNESS is caused by the inner ear's being unable to accommodate to the changes in position resulting from motion. (see EAR.)

INNERVATION The nerve supply to a tissue, organ or part of the body. It carries motor impulses to and sensory impulses away from the part.

INOCULATION The process by which infective material is brought into the system through a small wound in the skin or in a mucous membrane. Many infectious diseases and blood-poisoning are contracted by accidental inoculation of microbes. Inoculation is now used as a preventive measure against many infectious diseases. (See VACCINE.)

INOSITOL A sugar compound that is one constituent of some phospholipids (see LIPIDS) found in cells. It is found in many foods but, though sometimes classified as a vitamin, it is not a vital part of the human diet.

INOTROPIC Adjective describing anything that affects the force of muscle contraction. It is usually applied to the heart muscle and an inotrope such as DIGOXIN is a drug that improves its contraction. Beta blocker drugs such as PROPRANOLOL have negative inotropic properties.

INPATIENT A person who requires a hospital bed for investigation or treatment. (See HOSPITAL.)

INQUEST An official inquiry conducted by a coroner into the cause of an individual's death. The coroner is a judicial officer who, when a death is sudden, unexpected or occurs in suspicious circumstances, considers the results of medical and legal investigation and, sitting with a jury or on his own, makes the conclusions public. He has wide powers and in deaths of uncertain cause no official death certificate can be issued without his or her approval. A coroner may be legally or medically qualified (or both). In Scotland the comparable officer is the procurator fiscal.

INSANITY (see MENTAL ILLNESS).

INSECT REPELLENTS (See DIBUTYL PHTHALATE; DIMETHYL PHTHALATE.)

INSECTICIDES Substances which kill insects. Since the discovery of the insecticidal properties of DDT in 1940, a steady stream of new ones has been introduced, and their combined use has played an outstanding part in international public health campaigns, such as that of the World Health Organization for the eradication of malaria.

Unfortunately, insects are liable to become resistant to insecticides, just as bacteria are liable to become resistant to antibiotics, and it is for this reason that so much research work is being devoted to the discovery of new ones.

The useful effects of insecticide must be set against the increasing evidence that the indiscriminate use of some of these potent preparations is having an adverse effect, not only upon human beings, but also upon the ecosystems.

Some such as DDT, the use of which is now banned in the UK, are very stable compounds that enter the food chain and may ultimately be lethal to many animals, including birds and fishes.

There have been suggestions that some of the illnesses reported by combatants in the 1991 Gulf War may have been caused by the insecticides used to reduce the risks of catching diseases caused by insect vectors.

INSECTS IN RELATION TO DISEASE
Many insects play an important part in the transmission of infectious diseases. Thus, flies by their feet and their feeding habits carry the organisms which cause typhoid fever, the tsetse fly spreads sleeping sickness, mosquitoes transmit the germs of malaria and yellow fever, fleas convey plague germs and lice convey typhus fever and one form of relapsing fever. In addition, these creatures are nuisances as well as dangers. (see also BITES AND STINGS.)

House-fly (*Musca domestica*) This fly lays its eggs in manure, or in moist, fermenting vegetable matter. The maggot is hatched in eight hours to two days, feeds on the manure, passes through the pupa stage in anything from a few days to four weeks, and, becoming a fly, is capable of egg-laying about three weeks from its own appearance as an egg. As 120 to 150 eggs are laid in a batch by each female fly, this fly is capable, under the most favourable conditions, of producing over half-a-million progeny within her life of three months. The fly gorges on fluid food which it sucks up by means of its proboscis, and it has the habit of repeatedly vomiting and re-swallowing the contents of its crop as it feeds, thus distributing bacteria over uncovered food.

Blow-fly, or **blue-bottle** (*Calliphora erythrocephala*), lays its eggs (450 to 600 in number) on meat, fish or decaying animal matter. The maggot hatches out within a day, passes through the pupa stage and becomes a full-grown fly in about three weeks. Its habits are similar to those of the house-fly, though in numbers it is much less plentiful.

TREATMENT OF FLIES The most important measure is to destroy their breeding grounds near human dwellings. Food should be adequately protected and stored. An insecticide may be used as a powder, a spray or a paint, but care must be exercised that it does not come in contact with food or with surfaces on which food is prepared.

Mites and lice The commonest infestation encountered is SCABIES which is caused by a small mite, *Sarcoptes scabei*.

There are three lice which infest man: the body louse (*Pediculus corporis*), the head louse (*Pediculus capitis*) and the crab louse (*Pediculus pubis*). The head louse is by far the most common in Britain. Infestation is most common in children under school age, but it is not unusual in adults. Head lice spread by close human contact. (See also PEDICULOSIS.)

Lice convey the causative micro-organisms of typhus fever, one form of relapsing fever, and trench fever. The louse is probably responsible for more human deaths than any other insect barring the malaria mosquito (see RELAPSING FEVER; TRENCH FEVER; TYPHUS FEVER).

TREATMENT OF SCABIES AND LICE   Malathion, an organophosphorus insecticide, is used as a lotion or cream to treat scabies, head lice and crab lice. It must be used strictly according to medical and manufacturer's instructions as malathion is potentially harmful if wrongly applied, especially in young children.

The same advice applies to the pyrethroid agents permethrin and phenothrin, as well as to carbaryl (restricted to prescription use only) and benzyl benzoate.

Fleas   *Pulex irritans* is the common flea that afflicts humans. *Xenopsylla cheopis* is the rat flea that conveys *Pasteurella pestis*, the causative organism of plague, from rat to man. The flea lays its eggs singly. They take two to four days in summer, two weeks in winter, to hatch into larvae which are fully grown in a fortnight. The larva then becomes a pupa from which the adult emerges two weeks later. The flea can survive for a long time without food.

TREATMENT OF FLEAS   Human beings vary tremendously in their susceptibility to flea bites. For those who are susceptible the best preventive is dimethyl phthallate sprayed on the trousers or socks where it is effective for several days. In the absence of dimethyl phthallate, alternative methods of prevention are the smearing of the skin with oil of pennyroyal, oil of lavender, or 10 per cent crotamiton cream or lotion, or dusting the socks and underclothing with pyrethrum powder, menthol or camphor. For disinfestation of buildings, a solution of insecticide in kerosene is effective. Other anti-flea agents are pyrethrum, flaked naphthalene, or parachlorbenzene.

Bed bugs (*Cimex lectularius*) are best got rid of by a solution of insecticide in kerosene, with or without the addition of pyrethrum. (See BED BUG.)

Mosquitoes   One of these (*Anopheles gambiae*) is responsible for conveying the parasite of malaria, another (*Aedes aegypti*) for distributing the infection of yellow fever.

TREATMENT OF MOSQUITOES   See under MALARIA; YELLOW FEVER.

INSEMINATION   The ejaculation of semen in the vagina in the act of sexual intercourse. In artificial insemination the semen is placed there by the use of an instrument. (See ASSISTED CONCEPTION.)

INSIGHT   A person's knowledge of him or herself. The description is especially relevant to

a person's realization that he or she has psychological difficulties. Thus someone with a psychosis (see MENTAL ILLNESS) lacks insight. Insight also refers to an individual's concept of his or her personality and problems.

INSOLATION   A term applied both to treatment by exposure to the sun's rays and to fever caused by excessive heat (see HEAT-STROKE).

INSOMNIA   (see SLEEP, DISORDERS OF; HYPNOTICS).

INSPISSATION   The process of the drying or thickening of fluids or excretions by evaporation.

INSTITUTIONALIZATION   A condition brought about by a prolonged stay in an impersonal institution. The individual becomes apathetic and listless as a result of inadequate stimulation in an uninteresting environment. The condition can occur in mental institutions or long-stay nursing homes; the affected person loses the ability to make any decisions.

INSUFFLATION   means the blowing of powder or vapour into a cavity, especially through the air passages, for the treatment of disease.

INSULIN   A POLYPEPTIDE HORMONE produced in the PANCREAS by the beta cells of the ISLETS OF LANGERHANS. It plays a key role in the body's regulation of CARBOHYDRATE, FAT, and PROTEIN METABOLISM, and its deficiency leads to DIABETES MELLITUS. Diabetic patients are described as type 1 (insulin dependent), or type 2 (non-insulin dependent), though many of the latter may need insulin later on, in order to maintain good control.

Insulin is extracted mainly from pork pancreas and purified by crystallization or made biosynthetically by recombinant DNA technology using *Escherichia coli* or semisynthetically by enzymatic modification of porcine insulin to produce human insulin – the form now generally used, though some patients find it unsuitable and have to return to porcine insulin.

First isolated in a pure form by McLeod, Banting and Best in 1921, the hormone acts by enabling the muscles and other tissues requiring sugar for their activity to take up this substance from the blood. All insulin preparations are to a greater or lesser extent IMMUNOGENIC in man, but immunological resistance to insulin action is uncommon.

Previously available in three strengths, of 20, 40, and 80 units per millilitre (U/ml), these have now largely been replaced by a standard strength of 100 U/ml (U100). Numerous different insulin preparations are listed; these differ in their speed of onset and duration of action, and hence vary in their suitability for individual patients.

Insulin is inactivated by GASTROINTESTINAL ENZYMES and is therefore generally given by subcutaneous injection, usually into the upper arms, thighs, buttocks, or abdomen. Some insulins are also available in cartridge form, which may be administered by injection devices ('pens'). The absorption may vary from different sites and with strenuous activity. About 25 per cent of diabetics require insulin treatment: most children from the onset, and all patients presenting with ketoacidosis. Insulin is also often needed by those with a rapid onset of symptoms, such as weight loss, weakness, sometimes vomiting, often associated with ketonuria.

The aim of treatment is to maintain good control of blood glucose concentration, while avoiding severe HYPOGLYCAEMIA; this is usually achieved by a regimen of PREPRANDIAL injections of short-acting insulin (often with a bedtime injection of long-acting insulin). Insulin may also be given by continuous subcutaneous infusion with an infusion pump. This technique has many disadvantages; patients must be well motivated and able to monitor their own blood glucose, with access to expert advice both day and night; it is therefore rarely used.

HYPOGLYCAEMIA is a potential hazard for many patients converting from porcine to human insulin, because human insulin may result in subjects' being unaware of classical hypoglycaemic warning symptoms.

Drivers must be particularly careful, and individuals may be forbidden to drive if they have frequent or severe hypoglycaemic attacks. For this reason, insurance companies should be warned, and diabetics should – after taking appropriate medical advice – either return to porcine insulin or consider stopping driving.

INSULINOMA A tumour in the beta cells in the Islets of Langerhans in the PANCREAS that produces insulin.

INSULIN SHOCK A disorder in which the body produces excess insulin which then reduces the amount of glucose in the blood (HYPOGLYCAEMIA). Treatment is with glucose or GLUCAGEN. Untreated the patient goes into a coma and dies.

INTEGUMENT Another name for skin. The term is also used for a layer or membrane surrounding any of the body's organs.

INTELLIGENCE QUOTIENT Usually known as IQ, this is the ratio between the mental age and chronological age multiplied by 100. Thus, if a boy of 10 years of age is found to have a mental age of 12 years, his IQ will be: 120.

On the other hand, if he is found to have a mental age of 8 years his IQ will be: 80.

The mental age is established by various tests, the most widely used of which are the Stanford-Binet Scale, the Wechsler Adult Intelligence Scale, and the Mill Hill Vocabulary Test.

Average intelligence is represented by an IQ of 100, with a range of 85 to 115. For practical purposes it is taken that the intellectual level reached by the average 15-year-old is indistinguishable from that of an adult.

INTELLIGENCE TEST A standardized procedure of mental assessment to determine an individual's intellectual ability. The result is produced as a score termed the INTELLIGENCE QUOTIENT. The Wechsler Adult intelligence Scale (WAIS) and one for children, the Wechsler Intelligence Scale for Children (WICS), are commonly used, as is the Stanford-Binet Scale. Assessments are made for educational purposes and to help in the diagnoses of people with possible mental retardation or intellectual deterioration.

INTENSIVE THERAPY UNIT (ITU) A hospital unit in which patients undergo specialized resuscitation, monitoring and treatment procedures. People who have had severe injuries, heart attacks, or major operations – for example, cardiac surgery – are admitted to ITUs, which are staffed 24 hours a day with highly trained nurses, technicians and doctors and equipped with electronic monitoring devices that allow continuous assessment of vital body functions such as heart rate, blood pressure and blood chemistry. (see HIGH-DEPENDENCY UNIT.)

INTERCOSTAL The term applied to the nerves, vessels and muscles that lie between the ribs, as well as to diseases affecting these structures.

INTERFERON It has been known for many years that one virus will interfere with the growth of another. In 1957, UK research workers isolated the factor that was responsible for the phenomenon. They gave it the name of interferon. There are now known to be three human interferons. They are glycoproteins and are released from cells infected with virus or exposed to stimuli which mimic virus infection. They not only inhibit the growth of viruses. They also inhibit the growth and reduplication of cells. This is the basis for their investigation as a means of treating cancer. Hitherto the major difficulty has been obtaining sufficient supplies, but methods have now been evolved which promise to provide adequate amounts of it. The most promising of these is by means of what is known as genetic engineering, or manipulation, whereby a portion of DNA from interferon is inserted into the micro-organism known as *Escherichia coli* (see ESCHERICHIA) which thus becomes a source of almost unlimited amounts of interferon as it can be grown so easily. The evidence to date indicates that interferon is of value in treating certain virus infections, particularly different forms of herpes and viral hepatitis (see HEPATITIS). Interferon is also now used in the treatment of hairy cell leukaemia (see LEUKAEMIA) and MULTIPLE SCLEROSIS.

INTERLEUKINS   Interleukins are lymphokines, that is POLYPEPTIDES produced by activated LYMPHOCYTES. They are involved in signalling between cells of the IMMUNE SYSTEM and are released by several cell types, including lymphocytes. They interact to control the immune response of cells and also participate in haemopoiesis. There are seven varieties, interleukins 1 to 7. For example, interleukin 1 is produced as a result of inflammation and it stimulates the proliferation of T and B lymphocytes. They enhance the immune response by stimulating other lymphocytes and activating dormant T cells. Interleukin 2 has anti-cancer effects as it is able to activate T lymphocytes to become killer cells which destroy foreign ANTIGENS such as cancer cells, and this anti-cancer effect is being developed for clinical use. The remaining interleukins have a range of properties in cell growth and differentiation.

INTERMITTENT   A term applied to fevers which continue for a time, subside completely and then return again. The name is also used in connection with a pulse in which occasional heart-beats are not felt, in consequence of irregular action of the heart.

INTERMITTENT CLAUDICATION   A condition occurring in middle-aged and elderly people, which is characterized by pain in the legs after walking a certain distance. The pain is relieved by resting for a short time. It is due to arteriosclerosis (see ARTERIES, DISEASES OF) of the arteries to the leg, which results in inadequate blood supply to the muscles. Drugs usually have little effect in easing the pain, but useful preventive measures are to stop smoking, reduce weight (if overweight) and to take as much exercise as possible within the limits imposed by the pain.

INTERMITTENT SELF CATHETERIZATION   A technique in which a patient (of either sex) inserts a disposable CATHETER through the URETHRA into the BLADDER to empty it of urine. Increasingly used to manage patients with chronic retention of urine or whose bladders do not empty properly – usually the result of neurological disorder affecting the bladder (neuropathic bladder). (See BLADDER, DISEASES OF.)

INTERN   A doctor in training who carries out his duties and training in hospital and usually spends some of his time living in the hospital. The description is used mainly in North America. Alternative terms are house officer or resident which are used in the United Kingdom.

INTERNATIONAL CLASSIFICATION OF DISEASE   A World Health Organization classification of all known diseases and syndromes. The diseases are divided according to system (respiratory, renal, cardiac, etc.) or type (accidents, malignant growth, etc.). Each of them is given a three-digit number to facilitate computerization. This classification allows mortality and morbidity rates to be compared nationally and regionally.

INTERNET   Access to medical information via the internet is now widespread in some populations, often serving more patients than doctors. In addition to the huge variety of information available, patients can share experiences via electronic discussion groups, or obtain e-mail advice on a fee-for-service basis. Some professional organizations and journals provide free access to information, and the internet can be a useful resource for medical practitioners and researchers. Concerns have arisen about the growth in electronic medical information. Some believe that patients who have unlimited access to information via the internet will be less likely to tolerate health-care rationing or will demand treatments that may be inappropriate in their individual circumstances. Other criticisms relate to the quality and accuracy of the information provided, potential breaches of patient confidentiality and also the risk of unwarranted accusations of medical negligence.

INTERNODE   The length of the AXON (of a nerve cell) that is covered with a MYELIN sheath. The nodes of Ranvier, which have no myelin sheath, separate the internodes. (See NERVES.)

INTERSEXUALITY is a state of indeterminate sexuality of an individual, and may present in many different forms. A characteristic is that only one type of gonad – testis or ovary – is present; in HERMAPHRODITES both types are present. Intersexuality may be due to a fault in the genetic mechanism of sex determination as early as conception, or to later errors in sexual differentiation of the embryo and fetus, or after birth. Some cases may result from abnormal metabolism of the sex hormones, or may be drug-induced (for example, women given ANDROGENS or PROGESTERONE for repeated miscarriages may give birth to girls with some genital virilization). Abnormalities of the sex chromosomes may be associated with delayed (or failure of) sexual development, so that the individual shows some of the characteristics (often underdeveloped) of both sexes. Some of the more common presentations of the condition include HYPOGONADISM, CRYPTORCHIDISM, and primary AMENORRHOEA.

Intersexuality inevitably leads to considerable psychological disturbance as the child grows up. It is therefore important to reach an early decision as to the child's sex – or at least, the sex that he (or she) is to be brought up as. Surgical or hormonal means should then be employed, when appropriate, to develop the attributes of that sex and diminish those of the other, together with psychological counselling.

INTERSTITIAL is a term applied to indifferent tissue set among the proper active tissue of an organ. It is generally of a supporting character and formed of fibrous tissue. The term is also applied to the fluid always present in this in a small amount, and to diseases which specially affect this tissue, such as interstitial keratitis. (See EYE DISEASES.)

INTERTRIGO Inflammation between two skin surfaces in contact, typically in the toe clefts, axillae, under the breasts or in the anogenital folds. Heat, friction and obesity are aggravating factors. Secondary fungal or bacterial infection with candida or bacteria is common.

INTERVENTION STUDY Comparison of outcomes between two or more groups of patients who have been intentionally given different treatments or preventative measures, for example, diets. The subjects in the trial should be randomly allocated to the various groups with one group – called the control group – receiving no active treatment. If possible, neither patients nor doctors participating in a study should know which patients are receiving what treatment (double blind study/ trial). Furthermore groups should exchange treatments after a prearranged time (crossover study/trial).

INTERVERTEBRAL DISC The fibrous disc that acts as a cushion between the bony vertebrae, enabling them to rotate and bend one on another. The disc tends to degenerate with age and may get ruptured and displaced – prolapsed or slipped disc – as a result of sudden strenuous action. Prolapsed disc occurs mainly in the lower back and is more common in men than women and in the 30–40 age group.

INTESTINE All the alimentary canal situated below the stomach. In it most digestion is carried on, and through its walls all the food material is absorbed into the blood and lymph streams. (See DIGESTION.) The length of the intestine in man is about 8·5 to 9 metres (28 to 30 feet), and it takes the form of one continuous tube suspended in loops in the abdominal cavity.

Divisions The intestine is divided into small intestine and large intestine. The former comprises that part of the tube which extends from the stomach onwards for 6·5 metres (22 feet) or thereabout, and at its broadest point is about 35 mm (1½ inches) in width. The large intestine is the second part of the tube, and though shorter (about 1·8 metres (6 feet) long) is much wider than the small intestine, reaching in places a width of 65 mm (2½ inches). The small intestine

1 anulus fibrosus
2 nucleus pulposus

Cross-section of intervertebral disc.

1 intervertebral disc
2 vertebral body
3 anulus fibrosus
4 spinal cord
5 vertebral spine
6 nucleus pulposus (protruding into spinal cord)

Lateral view of prolapsed intervertebral disc.

is divided rather arbitrarily into three parts: the duodenum, consisting of the first 25 or 30 cm (10 or 12 inches), into which the ducts of the liver and pancreas open; the jejunum, which is generally found empty after death, and comprises the next 2·4 or 2·7 metres (8 or 9 feet); and finally the ileum, which at its lower end opens into the large intestine.

The large intestine begins in the lower part of the abdomen on the right side. The first part is known as the caecum, and into this opens the appendix vermiformis. The appendix is a small tube, about the thickness of a quill, from 2 to 20 cm (average 9 cm) in length, which has much the same structure as the rest of the intestine. At one end it is closed, at the other it opens into the caecum, and although it appears to play little or no part in digestion, it is important because of the frequency with which it becomes inflamed. (See APPENDICITIS.) The caecum is continued into the colon. This is subdivided into: the ascending colon which ascends through the right flank to beneath the liver; the transverse colon which crosses the upper part of the abdomen transversely to the left side; the descending colon which bends downwards and descends through the left flank into the pelvis where it becomes the sigmoid colon. The last part of the large intestine is known as the rectum, which passes straight down through the back part of the pelvis, to open to the exterior through the anus.

Structure The intestine, both small and large, consists of four coats, which vary slightly in structure and arrangement at different points, but are broadly the same throughout the entire length of the bowel. On the inner surface there is a mucous membrane; outside this is a loose submucous coat, in which blood-vessels run; next comes a muscular coat in two layers; and finally a tough, thin peritoneal membrane. The total thickness of all four coats amounts to about 3 mm.

MUCOUS COAT The interior of the bowel is completely lined by a single layer of pillar-like cells placed side by side. These rest upon a smooth, fine membrane, beneath which is a loose network of connective tissue and muscular fibres, richly supplied with blood-vessels and lymphatic-vessels. The surface in the small intestine is much increased by countless ridges with deep furrows between them that run across the upper part, and the whole surface is thickly studded with short hair-like processes called villi. As blood- and lymph-vessels run up to the end of these villi, the digested food passing slowly down the intestine is brought into close relation with the circulation. Between the bases of the villi are set little openings, each of which leads into a simple, tubular gland lined by cells, which are similar to those covering the surface, and which produce a digestive fluid. In the small and large intestines, many cells are devoted to the production of mucus for lubricating the passage of the food through the bowel. A large number of minute masses, called lymph follicles, similar in structure to the tonsils and lymphatic glands, are scattered over the inner surface of the intestine. In the lower part of the small intestine these are grouped into patches of 2·5 square centimetres in size, known as Peyer's patches, which are of special interest, because the inflammation and ulceration of the bowels that occur in typhoid fever are limited to them and to the scattered follicles. The large intestine is bare both of ridges and of villi, and, as already stated, its mucous membrane produces mucus in large amount.

SUBMUCOUS COAT This consists of a loose connective tissue which allows the mucous membrane to play freely over the muscular coat. The blood-vessels and lymphatic-vessels which absorb the food in the villi pour their contents into a network of large vessels lying in this coat.

MUSCULAR COAT The muscle in the small intestine is arranged in two definite layers, in the outer of which all the fibres run lengthwise with the bowel, whilst in the inner they pass circularly round it.

PERITONEAL COAT forms the outer covering for almost the whole intestine except parts of the duodenum and of the large intestine. It is a tough, fibrous membrane, covered upon its outer surface with a smooth layer of cells.

1 villi	6 circular muscles
2 lymph follicle	7 longitudinal muscles
3 intestinal gland	8 peritoneum
4 muscularis mucosae	9 duodenal gland
5 submucous coat	

Longitudinal section of intestinal wall. (Left section) Duodenum;
(right section) small intestine.

Support The duodenum and greater part of the large intestine are covered only in front by the peritoneum which lines the abdominal cavity, and this tough membrane serves to bind these parts of the intestine firmly against the back wall of the abdomen. The jejunum and ileum, the transverse colon, and the first part of the rectum are not only completely surrounded by peritoneum, but a double layer of this membrane suspends these parts of the bowel at a distance of several inches from the lines on the back of the abdomen, where the two layers become continuous with the rest of the peritoneum. In this way freedom is given to the movements of these parts of the bowels. These suspending structures are known as mesenteries. That of the small intestine is the largest, being shaped like a fan, 200 mm (8 inches) long at its attached margin, and spreading out to 6·5 metres (22 feet) at its frilled border, where it meets the intestine. The vessels and nerves which supply the intestine run between the two layers of the mesentery.

INTESTINE, DISEASES OF The principal signs of trouble which has its origin in the intestines consist of pain somewhere about the abdomen, sometimes vomiting, and irregular bowel movements: constipation, diarrhoea or alternating bouts of these.

Several diseases are treated under separate headings. (See APPENDICITIS; CHOLERA; COLITIS; CONSTIPATION; DIARRHOEA; DYSENTERY; ENTERIC FEVERS; HERNIA; ILEITIS; INTUSSUSCEPTION; IRRITABLE BOWEL SYNDROME; PERITONITIS; PILES; RECTUM, DISEASES OF.)

Inflammation of the bowel may affect either its outer or its inner surface. The outer surface is covered by peritoneum, and peritonitis is a serious disease. (See PERITONITIS.) Inflammation of the inner surface is known generally as enteritis, inflammation of special parts receiving the names of colitis, appendicitis, and the like. Enteritis may form the chief symptom of certain infective diseases due to special organisms: for example in TYPHOID FEVER, CHOLERA, DYSENTERY. Again, it may be acute, though not connected with any definite organism, when, if severe, it is a very serious condition, particularly in young children. Or it may be chronic, especially as the result of dysentery, and then constitutes a less serious though very troublesome complaint.

Perforation of the bowel may take place as the result either of injury or of disease. Stabs and other wounds which penetrate the abdomen may damage the bowel, and severe blows or crushes may tear it without any external wound. Ulceration, as in typhoid fever, or, more rarely, in TUBERCULOSIS, may cause an opening in the bowel-wall also. Again, when the bowel is greatly distended above an obstruction, faecal material may accumulate and produce ulcers, which rupture with the ordinary movements of the bowels. Whatever the cause, the symptoms are much the same.

SYMPTOMS The contents of the bowel pass out through the perforation into the peritoneal cavity, and, making their way between the coils of intestine, set up a general peritonitis. In consequence, the abdomen is painful, and after a few hours becomes extremely tender to the touch, as a result of the peritonitis. The abdomen swells, particularly in its upper part, owing to gas having passed also into the cavity. Vomiting is a symptom, and the person passes into a state of collapse. Such a condition is almost invariably fatal in two, or at most three, days, if not promptly treated.

TREATMENT All food should be withheld, because whatever is taken into the stomach is either vomited or is liable to pass out of the perforation into the peritoneal cavity. An operation is urgently necessary, the abdomen being opened in the middle line, the perforated portion of bowel found, and the perforation stitched up.

Obstruction of the bowels means a stoppage to the passage down the intestine of the partially digested food. Obstruction may be due either to some cause within the abdomen or to the thrusting of a loop of bowel through an opening in the wall of this cavity. The latter class of cases has been referred to under HERNIA. Obstruction may be acute when it comes on suddenly with intense symptoms, or it may be chronic, when the obstructing cause gradually increases and the bowel becomes slowly more narrow till it closes altogether, or when slight obstruction comes and goes till it ends in an acute attack. In chronic cases the symptoms are much the same as those of the acute variety, although they are milder in degree and more prolonged.

CAUSES Obstruction may be due to causes outside the bowel altogether, for example, the pressure of tumours in neighbouring organs, the twisting round the bowel of bands produced by former peritonitis, or even the twisting of a coil of intestine round itself so as to cause a kink in its wall. Chronic and partial forms of obstruction are sometimes due to such kinks near the end of the small intestine, sometimes to the pressure of the mesentery on the upper end of the small intestine. Chronic causes of the obstruction may exist in the wall of the bowel itself: for example, a tumour, or the contracting scar of an old ulcer. The condition of INTUSSUSCEPTION, where part of the bowel passes inside of the part beneath it, in the same way as one turns the finger of a glove outside in, causes obstruction and other symptoms. Finally some body, such as a concretion, or the stone of some large fruit, or even a mass of hardened faeces, may become jammed within the bowel and stop up its passage.

SYMPTOMS There are four chief symptoms of this condition, and any case in which these are combined demands immediate treatment. These are pain, vomiting, constipation and swelling of the abdomen.

TREATMENT As a rule the surgeon opens the abdomen, finds the obstruction and relieves it or if possible removes it altogether.

Tumours are relatively uncommon in the small intestine and, when they do occur, they are usually benign. Conversely, they are relatively common in the large intestine where they are usually cancerous. The most common site for cancer of the large intestine is the rectum, with the sigmoid, caecum and ascending colon next in order of frequency. It is a disease of the older age-groups, occurs with equal frequency in men and women and is the second commonest cancer (after lung cancer) in the United Kingdom. Nearly 28,000 cases a year occur in England and Wales. A history of altered bowel habit, in the form of increasing constipation or diarrhoea, or an alternation of these, or of bleeding from the anus, in a middle-aged person is an indication for taking medical advice. If the condition is cancer, then the sooner it is operated on, the better the result.

INTIMA The innermost coat lining the arteries and the veins.

INTOLERANCE An adverse reaction of a patient to a drug or treatment. (See ADVERSE REACTIONS TO DRUGS.)

INTOXICATION A term applied to states of poisoning. The poison may be some chemical substance introduced from outside, e.g. alcohol (see ALCOHOL), or it may be due to the products of bacterial action, the bacteria either being introduced from outside or developing within the body. The term auto-intoxication is applied in the latter case.

INTRA- Prefix indicating inside or within. For example, intracellular: within a cell; intra-articular: within a joint.

INTRACORONARY ARTERY STENTING A narrowed or blocked CORONARY ARTERY can compromise the blood supply to the HEART MUSCLE (see HEART DISEASES). A supportive tube or stent passed into each affected artery can restore the blood supply. The stent has a HEPARIN coating to stop blood clots from forming. Since it was first performed in 1987 intracoronary stents have cut the reblockage rate from one in three patients who have had coronary ANGIOPLASTY only to fewer than one in ten in cases where a stent was used with angioplasty.

INTRACRANIAL is the term applied to structures, diseases, and the like, contained in or rising within the head.

INTRACRANIAL PRESSURE This is the pressure that is maintained by the brain tissue,

intracellular and extracellular fluid, cerebrospinal fluid and blood. An increase in intracranial pressure may occur as a result of inflammation, injury, haemorrhage, or tumour in the brain tissue as well as of some congenital conditions. The pressure is measured by lumbar puncture in which a syringe attached to a mamometer (pressure-measuring device) is inserted into the cerebrospinal fluid surrounding the lower part of the spinal cord.

INTRACYTOPLASMIC SPERM INJECTION Intracytoplasmic sperm injection (ICSI) is the most significant therapeutic advance in male infertility treatment in the past 30 years. The technique is used when IN VITRO FERTILIZATION (IVF) is not possible because the man has very few, motile, normal SPERM, or when previous attempts at IVF have not produced a fertilized EMBRYO. ICSI requires a single sperm which is injected directly into the cytoplasm of an egg previously retrieved from the woman. Once fertilized the embryo is transferred to her uterus. For men with no sperm in the semen, it may be possible to retrieve sperm by needle aspiration of the EPIDIDYMIS under LOCAL ANAESTHETIC. Other techniques involve microsurgical retrieval from the epididymis or TESTICLE under a general anaesthetic. Potential complications include scrotal pain, bruising, HAEMATOMA formation and infection. ICSI and surgical sperm retrieval require extensive training and expertise and is currently available in only a few selected infertility units. Safety concerns relate to a higher than expected rate of sex CHROMOSOME abnormalities after ICSI and also the potential risk of transmitting paternal genetic defects in the Y chromosome to sons born after ICSI.

INTRATHECAL means within the membranes or meninges which envelop the spinal cord. The intrathecal space, between the arachnoid and the pia mater, contains the cerebrospinal fluid.

INTRAUTERINE CONTRACEPTIVE DEVICE (IUCD) A mechanical device, commonly a coil, inserted into the uterus to prevent conception, probably by interfering with the implantation of the embryo. For many, though not all, women IUDs are an effective and acceptable form of contraception, though only about 10 per cent of women in the UK use them. The devices are of various shapes and made of plastic or copper; most have a string that passes through the cervix and rests in the vagina.

About one-third of women have adverse effects as the result of IUCDs: common ones are backache and heavy menstrual bleeding. The frequency of unwanted pregnancies is about 2 per 100 women years of use. (See CONTRACEPTION.)

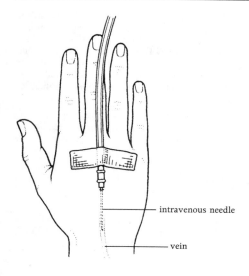

Position of intravenous needle inserted into vein
on back of hand for administration of
intravenous fluid or blood transfusion.

INTRAVENOUS   A term which means inside a vein. An intravenous injection is one that is given into a vein. Blood transfusions are given intravenously, as are other infusions of fluid.

INTRAVENOUS UROGRAM   A procedure for getting X-ray pictures of the urinary tract. A radio-opaque medium is injected into a vein and, when it is excreted by the kidneys, the substance can be identified on X-rays. Any abnormalities in structure or foreign bodies such as calculi are outlined by the dye.

INTROSPECTION   The observation of one's own thoughts or feelings. It is generally applied to this process when it occurs to an abnormal extent in association with melancholia.

INTROVERT   Physically it means turning inside out: for example, a uterus (rarely) inverts after a very difficult delivery. Psychologically the term refers to an individual whose character looks inward on him or herself and who may also be obsessive and have few friends.

INTUBATION   A simple operation consisting in the introduction, through the mouth into the larynx, of a tube designed to keep the air passage open at this point.

INTUITION   The immediate understanding of a situation by someone without the customary mental process of reasoning.

INTUSSUSCEPTION   A form of obstruction of the bowels in which part of the intestine enters within that part immediately beneath it. This can best be understood by observing what takes place in the fingers of a tightly fitting glove as they turn outside in when the glove is pulled off the hand. The people affected are almost always infants. The cause is not known. The point at which it most often occurs is the junction between the small and the large intestines, the former passing within the latter. The symptoms are those of intestinal obstruction in general, and in addition there is often a discharge of blood-stained mucus from the bowel. The treatment consists – unless the symptoms rapidly subside, when it may be assumed that the bowel has righted itself – of either hydrostatic reduction by means of a barium enema, or an operation. At operation the intussusception is either reduced or, if this not possible, the obstructed part is cut out and the ends of the intestine then stitched together. If treated adequately and in time, the mortality is now reduced to around 1 per cent.

INVASION   The entry of bacteria into the body. The spread of cancer into normal, nearby tissues or organs.

IN VITRO   A term commonly used in medical research and experimental biology. Literally 'in a glass', it refers to observations made outside the body: e.g. on the action of drugs on bacteria. The opposite term is IN VIVO, which refers to observations of processes in the body.

IN VITRO FERTILIZATION (IVF)   Fertilization of the egg outside the body. The fertilized ovum is then incubated until the blastocyst stage develops when it is implanted into the uterus. The procedure was developed in Britain and the first successful in vitro baby, a girl, was born in 1978. IVF is used when a woman has blocked FALLOPIAN TUBES or when the sperm and ovum are unable to fuse in the reproductive tract. Hormone treatment results in the potential mother's producing several mature ova, some of which are removed from the ovary using a LAPAROSCOPE and fertilized with her partner's semen. (See ASSISTED CONCEPTION.)

IN VIVO   A Latin term to describe biological events that take place inside the bodies of living organisms.

INVOLUCRUM   The sheath of new bone which is formed round a piece of dead bone in, for example, osteomyelitis.

INVOLUNTARY MUSCLE   Muscle that does not operate under a person's conscious control. Involuntary muscle, also called smooth muscle because the cells do not contain the striations that occur in VOLUNTARY MUSCLE, is found in blood vessels, the heart, stomach, and intestines.

INVOLUTION The process of change whereby the uterus returns to its resting size after parturition. The term is also applied to any retrograde biological change, as in senility.

IODIDES Salts of iodine, those which are especially used in medicine being the iodide of potassium and iodide of sodium. Iodides are excreted in the mucus secretions, as well as in the urine, saliva and sweat, and have an action in liquefying the mucus secretion of the bronchial tree. They are therefore used in expectorant mixtures. They are also used to assist in providing a supply of iodine in patients with goitre, or in individuals who live in an area where goitre is liable to occur because of a deficiency of iodine in the drinking water. They may be given in the form of iodized salt. (See GOITRE.)

Over-dosage of iodides results in IODISM.

IODINE A non-metallic element which is found largely in seaweed. The body contains about 30 mg, largely concentrated in the thryoid gland where it is used to synthesize thyroid hormones. Iodine has a highly irritating action and when applied to the skin, stains the latter dark brown and causes it to peel off in flakes, while internally it is a violent irritant poison in large doses.

Externally iodine is used as an antiseptic. Its drawback is that it is fixed by protein, which reduces its antiseptic efficiency in open wounds. Its main use in this sphere therefore is for sterilizing the unbroken skin, as before an operation. Radioactive iodine is used for diagnosing and treating disease of the thyroid gland.

IODISM A condition resulting from an over-dose of iodides, but in some susceptible individuals iodism may be produced by very small amounts of iodides. It is characterized by running of the eyes and nose, sore throat, a heavy, dull feeling over the eyes, increased secretion of saliva and a typical skin eruption. These manifestations usually disappear rapidly upon the drugs being withdrawn.

ION EXCHANGE RESINS Synthetic organic substances, capable of exchanging ions – cationic or anionic – from the contents of the intestine. Originally used in the prevention of OEDEMA, they have been superseded in this role by the modern DIURETICS, and are now used chiefly in the treatment of HYPERKALAEMIA. They are usually taken by mouth or as an enema.

IONIZATION means the breaking up of a substance in solution into its constituent ions.

IPECACUANHA, IPECAC, or HIPPO, is the root of Cephaëlis ipecacuanha, a Brazilian shrub. It contains an alkaloid, emetine, which acts as an irritant when brought in contact with the interior of the stomach, producing vomiting. Formerly used to induce vomiting among young children after poisoning and if still alert, but now of uncertain value after intense debate among clinical toxicologists. Activated charcoal, however, does reduce absorption. (See POISONS.)

Uses Ipecacuanha was a constituent of many traditional expectorant mixtures given in the treatment of bronchitis.

IPRATROPIUM An anticholinergic, bronchodilator drug of value in the treatment of asthma, bronchitis and rhinitis.

IRIDECTOMY The operation by which a hole is made in the iris, as, for example, in the treatment of GLAUCOMA or as part of CATARACT SURGERY.

IRIDENCLEISIS An operation formerly used in the treatment of glaucoma. It has now been replaced by trabeculectomy (see GLAUCOMA).

IRIDOLOGY The study of the iris (see EYE). It is an old practice dating back to the days of Aristotle, which has been revived as a non-conventional treatment (see NON-CONVENTIONAL MEDICINE).

IRIS (see EYE).

IRITIS (see UVEITIS).

IRON A metal which is an essential constituent of the red blood corpuscles, where it is present in the form of haemoglobin. It is also present in muscle, myoglobin, and in certain respiratory pigments which are essential to the life of many tissues in the body. Iron is absorbed principally in the upper part of the small intestine. It is then stored: mainly in the liver; to a lesser extent in the spleen and kidneys, where it is available, when required, for use in the bone marrow to form the haemoglobin in red blood corpuscles. The daily iron requirement of an adult is 15 to 20 milligrams. This requirement is increased during pregnancy.

Uses The main use of iron is in the treatment of iron-deficiency anaemias, usually in the form of a ferrous sulphate but many formulations are available. (See ANAEMIA.) Iron preparations sometimes cause irritation of the gastro-intestinal tract, and should therefore always be taken after meals. They sometimes produce a tendency towards constipation. Whenever possible, iron preparations should be given by mouth. If parenteral administration is clinically necessary because of malabsorption of or side-effects from oral preparation, a suitable preparation is iron sorbitol injection given intramuscularly. Most patients respond successfully to oral iron preparations.

IRRADIATION The use of naturally occurring isotopes, or artificially produced X-rays, in the killing of tumour cells. The amount of radiation is the adsorbed dose; the SI unit is the gray (Gy). Different tumours seem to be particularly sensitive to radiation; radiotherapy plays an important role in the management of germ-cell tumours (SEMINOMA, TERATOMA) and LYMPHOMAS. Many head and neck tumours, gynaecological cancers, and localized prostate and bladder cancers are curable with radiotherapy. It may be used to reduce the pain – for example, from bone metastases.

Unwanted effects of radiation Generalized: lethargy, loss of appetite. Skin: erythema, dry desquamation with itching, moist desquamation. Patients should keep treated area dry and clean and avoid soap, antiseptic mouth washes, smoking and spicy food if possible. (see ISOTOPE; RADIATION SICKNESS; RADIOTHERAPY).

IRRIGATION is the method of washing out wounds, or cavities of the body, like the bladder and bowels. (See DOUCHE; ENEMA.)

IRRITABLE BOWEL SYNDROME A motility disorder of the intestinal tract. Sometimes, inaccurately, called spastic colon or irritable colon. Some of the symptoms of the irritable bowel syndrome affect more than 10 per cent of the normal adult population, but most people accept these symptoms as a minor nuisance. The cause is not fully understood but the main abnormality seems to be a disturbance of involuntary muscle movement in the large intestine. The structure of the intestines are, however, normal and the victims do not usually lose weight. The disease affects up to 20 per cent of adults and accounts for half of the patients seen by gastroenterologists. The disease may well be stress related. Only those with severe symptoms or those who worry about their symptoms should consult a doctor.

Symptoms Abdominal pain is the commonest symptom and it frequently moves from one area of the abdomen into another. A disturbed bowel habit is also common and this may alternate between diarrhoea and constipation. A feeling of abdominal distension is common, as is heartburn. Some patients suffer from painless, watery diarrhoea. The symptoms are either due to abnormal motility of the gut or to increased intestinal sensitivity to distension. The pain can, in fact, often be produced in patients by balloon inflation within the colon or other parts of the gut. The symptoms frequently start after an acute intestinal infection, and acute psychological stresses can also influence the activity of the bowel.

Treatment is largely symptomatic. Patients require reassurance and explanation of the functional nature of the disorder. Anticholinergic drugs inhibit colonic motor activity and the antispasmodic drug mebeverine has a direct relaxant effect on intestinal smooth muscle.

Anti-diarrhoeal drugs such as codeine phosphate reduce the frequency and urgency of defaecation. Bulking agents speed colonic transit and allow the passage of softer, bulkier motions. High-fibre diets are beneficial. Cophenotrope (a mixture of diphenoxylate and ATROPINE) is indicated as an adjunct to rehydration in acute DIARRHOEA, and in the treatment of chronic mild ULCERATIVE COLITIS. (Young children are particularly susceptible to overdosage and should be carefully observed for at least 48 hours after ingestion.) Loperamide sometimes helps.

ISCHAEMIA Bloodlessness of a part of the body, due to contraction, spasm, constriction or blocking (by embolus or by thrombus) of the arteries: for example, of the heart.

ISCHAEMIC HEART DISEASE (see CORONARY THROMBOSIS).

ISCHIO-RECTAL ABSCESS An abscess arising in the space between the rectum and ischial bone and often resulting in a fistula. It may occur spontaneously or be secondary to an anal fissure, thrombosed haemorrhoids or other anal disease. The disorder is painful and usually accompanied by fever. Treatment is by a combination of antibiotics and surgery.

ISCHIUM is the bone which forms the lower and hinder part of the pelvis. It bears the weight of the body in sitting.

ISHIHARA'S TEST A test for colour vision, introduced by a Japanese doctor, comprising several plates with round dots of different colours and sizes. It is also the name of a type of blood test for syphilis.

ISLETS OF LANGERHANS: Groups of specialized cells distributed throughout the PANCREAS, that produce three hormones, INSULIN, GLUCAGON, and SOMATOSTASIN.

ISOCARBOXAZID is a monoamine-oxidase inhibitor antidepressive drug. (See ANTIDEPRESSANTS).

ISO-IMMUNIZATION is the IMMUNIZATION of one member of a species by an antigen lacking in it but present naturally in other members of the species, as, for example, the immunization of an Rh-negative mother by an Rh-positive fetus, the mother as a result producing anti-Rh agglutinins which injure the fetus. (See also HAEMOLYTIC DISEASE OF THE NEWBORN; BLOOD GROUPS.)

ISOLATION This is important when treating patients with serious infection or whose immune systems are severely compromised by illness or radio- or chemotherapy. The procedure also protects staff caring for infectious patients. (See INCUBATION; INFECTION; QUARANTINE.)

ISOLEUCINE   One of the essential aminoacids, which are fundamental components of all proteins. It cannot be synthesized by the body and so must be obtained from the diet.

ISOMETRIC   Of similar measurement. Isometric exercises are based on the isometric contraction of the muscles. Fibres are provoked into working by pushing or pulling an immovable object but this technique prevents them from shortening in length. These exercises improve a person's fitness and builds up his or her muscle strength.

ISONIAZID   One of the anti-tuberculous drugs. It has the advantages of being relatively non-toxic and of being active when taken by mouth. Unfortunately, like streptomycin, it may render the *Mycobacterium tuberculosis* resistant to its action. This tendency to produce resistance is considerably reduced if it is given in conjunction with RIFAMPICIN and PYRAZINAMIDE.

ISOPRENALINE   An INOTROPIC SYMPATHOMIMETIC drug which is used as a short-term emergency treatment of HEART BLOCK or severe BRADYCARDIA. (See HEART DISEASES.)

ISOTONIC   A term applied to solutions which have the same power of diffusion as one another. An isotonic solution used in medicine is one which can be mixed with body fluids without causing any disturbance. An isotonic saline solution for injection into the blood, so that it may possess the same osmotic pressure as the blood serum, is one of 0·9-per-cent strength or containing 9 grams of sodium chloride to 1 litre of water. This is also known as normal or physiological salt solution. An isotonic solution of bicarbonate of soda for injection into the blood is one of 1·35-per-cent strength in water. An isotonic solution of glucose for injection into the blood is one of 5-per-cent strength in water.

Solutions which are weaker, or stronger than, the fluids of the body with which they are intended to be mixed are known as hypotonic and hypertonic, respectively.

ISOTOPE   This is a form of a chemical element with the same chemical properties as other forms but which has a different atomic mass. It contains an identical number of positively charged particles called protons, in the nucleus, giving it the same atomic number, but the numbers of neutrons differ. A radioactive isotope, or radionuclide, is one that decays into other isotopes, and in doing so emits alpha, beta or gamma radiation.

Applications of radionuclides to diagnosis   The use of radionuclides in diagnosis is based on the fact that it is possible to tag many of the substances normally present in the body with a radioactive label. Certain synthetic radioactive elements such as technetium can also be used. Because it is possible to detect minute quantities of radioactive material, only very small doses are needed, making the procedure a safe one. Furthermore the body pool of the material is therefore not appreciably altered, and metabolism is not disturbed. Thus in studies of iodine metabolism the ratio of radioactive atoms administered to stable atoms in the body pool is of the order of 1 to 1,000 million. By measuring radioactivity in the body, in blood samples, or in the excreta it is possible to gain information about the fate of the labelled substance, and hence of the chemically identical inactive material. Hence it is theoretically possible to trace the absorption, distribution and the excretion of any substance normally present in the body, provided that it can be tagged with a suitable radioactive label.

If the investigation necessitates tracing the path of the material through the body by means of external counting over the body surface it is obviously essential to use an isotope that emits gamma radiation or positrons. If, however, only measurements on blood sample or excreta are required it is possible to use pure beta emitters. Whole-body counters measure the total radioactivity in the body, and these are of great value in absorption studies.

Moving images can provide information on body functions such as the movements of the heart, blood flow, bile flow in the liver and urine in the kidneys. The development of COMPUTED TOMOGRAPHY or CT SCANNING has replaced radionuclide scanning for some imaging procedures.

Five main groups of diagnostic uses may be defined:

(1) METABOLIC STUDIES   The use of radioactive materials in metabolic studies is based on the fundamental property that all isotopes of an element are chemically identical. The radioactive isotope is used as a true isotope tracer – that is, when introduced into the body (in whatever form) it behaves in the same way as the inactive element. For example, isotopes of iodine are used to measure thyroid function, and isotopes of calcium enable kinetic studies of bone formation and destruction to be performed.

(2) ABSORPTION AND DISTRIBUTION STUDIES   The fate of labelled substances given by mouth can be followed to assess their absorption, utilization and excretion. In most of these studies the isotope is a true isotope tracer. For example, iron absorption can be measured with radioactive iron; vitamin-B_{12} absorption may be investigated with vitamin B_{12} tagged with radioactive cobalt.

(3) BODY COMPOSITION BY DILUTION STUDIES   By introducing an isotope into a compartment, such as the blood or extracellular space, it is possible to measure the volume of that compartment by determining the dilution of radioactivity when equilibrium has been reached.

(4) PHYSICAL TRACING STUDIES In this type of study the isotope is not necessarily used as a true isotopic tracer. In other words, it does not trace the path of the corresponding inactive isotope. For example, xenon-133 is used in measurements of blood flow in muscles, and in lung-function studies; krypton-85 is used to detect intracardiac shunts (abnormal blood flows in the heart). Neither of these elements is normally present in the body. The survival of ERYTHROCYTES may be followed and the organ of sequestration revealed by labelling them with radioactive chromium.

(5) SCANNING OF ORGANS AND TISSUES Scanning is a technique which is used to determine the distribution of radioactive isotopes within the body or within one particular organ. In the conventional scanner the radiation detector, which is a scintillation counter, 'sees' only a small cross-sectional area of the body at a time. The activity 'seen' at each point is registered, and a 'map' of the activity seen over the scanned area is recorded. Various methods of presentation have been used, and the recently improved display systems present the information gathered by the scanner more effectively. More recent developments are stationary detectors such as the gamma camera, auto-fluoroscope, and other devices which can view the whole of the area simultaneously. Thus when selective concentration of an isotope in a tissue occurs it is possible to examine the distribution of that isotope by means of scanning. A toxic nodule in the thyroid may be identified by its selective concentration of iodine-131. Areas of absent function on the radioactive scan ('cold' areas) suggest the presence of tumours, abscesses, and similar lesions. Iodine-131 may be used to localize tumours of the thyroid, and chlormerodrin labelled with mercury-197 to delineate tumours of the kidneys. Of even greater practical application is the localizing of brain tumours with human serum albumin labelled with iodine-131 or with radioactive technetium.

Treatment Radioactive isotopes are also used in medical treatment. The overactivity of the thyroid gland in thyrotoxicosis can be treated by the ingestion of radioactive iodine. The ingested iodine is taken up by the thyroid gland where local irradiation of the gland takes place, reducing its activity. Radioactive phosphorus is used in the treatment of polycythemia rubra vera. It is largely taken up in bone as this is the main source of body phosphate and irradiation of the bone marrow results, controlling the overactivity that is characteristic of POLYCYTHEMIA rubra vera. In cobalt teletherapy the isotope cobalt 60 is used to deliver 1·2–1·3-million-volt radiation which is equivalent to X-rays generated at a peak voltage of 3–4-million-volts. (See RADIOTHERAPY.)

ISSUE is an old term for a suppurating sore.

ITCH is a popular name for SCABIES.

ITCHING (see PRURITUS).

-ITIS A suffix added to the name of an organ to signify any diseased condition of that organ.

ITRACONAZOLE A triazole antifungal drug taken orally for oropharyngeal and vulvovaginal CANDIDIASIS, PITYRIASIS versicolor and tinea corporis and pedis (RINGWORM). It is also used for systemic fungal infections such as ASPERGILLOSIS, candidiasis and cryptococcosis where other fungicidal drugs have not worked. Itraconazole is metabolized in the liver so should not be given to patients who have or have had liver disease. The drug can be given as maintenance treatment of AIDS patients to prevent resurgence of underlying fungal disease to which they are vulnerable.

IUCD/IUD An abbreviation for an intrauterine contraceptive device (coil). It acts mechanically to prevent conception but the coil is not suitable for all women and has a failure rate of 2·3 per cent

IUS (intrauterine system) A hormonal contraceptive device that is placed in the UTERUS. It is a long-term reversible method of contraception.

IVF or IN VITRO FERTILIZATION (see ASSISTED CONCEPTION).

IVORY, or DENTINE, is the hard material which forms the chief bulk of the teeth. (See TEETH.)

J

JACKSONIAN EPILEPSY (see EPILEPSY).

JAUNDICE is a yellow discoloration of the skin due to the deposition of bile pigment in its deeper layers. It is the main sign of several disorders of the liver and biliary system. Many babies develop jaundice soon after birth because of the accumulation of bilirubin (yellow bile pigment) in the blood. This is unusually due to liver immaturity and soon disappears, but a serious disorder, HAEMOLYTIC DISEASE OF THE NEW-BORN, is a potentially dangerous type of neonatal jaundice that requires treatment.

Types In adults three types of jaundice occur. They are all the result of disturbance in the mechanism by which HAEMOGLOBIN from the breakdown of ageing red blood cells (erythrocytes) is not properly processed in the liver. Normally the breakdown product of this haemoglobin – bilirubin – is made water soluble in the liver and excreted via the bile ducts into the small intestine, where it colours the stools dark brown.

HAEMOLYTIC JAUNDICE   In this type the amount of bilirubin produced is too much for the liver to deal with, the excess usually being the result of an abnormal level of haemoglobin. This haemolytic anaemia, as it is known, has several causes (see ANAEMIA).

HEPATOCELLULAR JAUNDICE   In this disorder bilirubin builds up in the blood because liver cells have been damaged or have died – usually as a result of a viral infection (there are four types) causing hepatitis, or by liver failure (see HEPATITIS).

OBSTRUCTIVE JAUNDICE   Also called cholestatic jaundice, this type is characterized by the inability of bile to be discharged from the liver because the BILE DUCTS are blocked as a result of GALLSTONES or a growth. Sometimes the ducts are absent (atresia) or have been destroyed in the liver as a result of cirrhosis. (See also BILIRUBIN; HAEMOLYTIC DISEASE OF THE NEW-BORN; KERNICTERUS.)

Symptoms   Yellowness, appearing first in the whites of the eyes and later over the whole skin, is the symptom that attracts notice. Indigestion, nausea, poor appetite and general malaise are other symptoms. The skin may itch, the whites of the eyes are yellow and the faeces are grey or white because of the absence of bile.

Treatment   The essential step is to treat the underlying cause if possible: for instance, gallstones, if these be the cause of the jaundice. Comprehensive laboratory investigations are usually required. Supportive measures are needed. (See LIVER DISEASES.).

JAW   The name applied to the bones that carry the teeth. The two upper jaw-bones, the maxillae, are firmly fixed to the other bones of the face. The lower jaw, the mandible, is shaped somewhat like a horseshoe, and, after the first year of life, consists of a single bone. It forms a hinge-joint with the squamous part of the temporal bone, immediately in front of the ear. Both upper and lower jaw-bones possess deep sockets, known as alveoli, which contain the roots of the teeth. (See DISLOCATIONS; FRACTURES; GUMBOIL; MOUTH; TEETH.)

JEJUNUM   Part of the small intestine. (See INTESTINE.)

JELLY (see GELATIN).

JENNER   Edward Jenner was an English country practitioner (1749–1823). He had noticed that cowpox, which milkmaids caught from cattle, gave these women immunity from the scourge of smallpox. In 1796 he transformed this observation into the medical technique of vaccination, innoculating a country boy with matter from the arm of a milkmaid infected with cowpox. Despite hostility from some doctors, Parliament voted him a grant of £10,000 for a society to promote vaccination and the technique spread world-wide, giving benefit to an immense number of people. (See VACCINATION; SMALLPOX.)

JERK   A sudden involuntary movement. The term is often used to describe the tendon reflexes.

JOINT-MOUSE is a popular term for a loose body in a joint. It is found especially in the knee. (See JOINTS, DISEASES OF.)

JOINTS   A joint is the articulation point between different parts of the skeleton, whether bone or cartilage. They are divided into those which are fixed or relatively fixed (fibrous and cartilaginous joints), and those which allow free movement (synovial joints). In the former, exemplified by the sutures between the bones of the skull, a layer of cartilage or fibrous tissue lies between the bones, binding them firmly together. Amphiarthrodial joints, exemplified by the joints between the vertebral bodies, have a thick disc of fibro-cartilage between the bones. Although the individual joint is capable of very little movement, a series of these gives to the spinal column, as a whole, a flexible character.

All movable joints involve four structures: the bones whose junction forms the joint; a layer of cartilage covering the ends of these, making them smooth; a fibrous sheath, the capsule, thickened at various points into bands or ligaments, which hold the bones together; and, finally, the synovial membrane, which lines the capsule and produces a synovial fluid, lubricating the movements of the joint. In addition, the bones are kept in position at the joints by the various muscles passing over them and atmospheric pressure. Where the ends of the bones do not quite correspond, a subsidiary disc of fibro-cartilage may help to adapt the ends of the bones more perfectly to each other. Larger cavities may be filled by movable pads of fat under the synovial membrane, giving additional protection to the joint.

Varieties   After this main division of joints into those which are fixed and those movable, the movable joints may be further subdivided. In gliding joints, such as the wrist and ankle, the bones have flat surfaces capable of only a limited amount of movement. In hinge joints, such as the elbow and knee, movement takes place around one axis. Ball-and-socket joints, exemplified by the shoulder and hip, allow free movement in any direction. Subsidiary varieties are named according to the shape of the bones which enter the joint.

JOINTS, DISEASES OF   'Rheumatism' is the colloquial term for non-specific musculo-skeletal symptoms arising in the joints, ligaments, tendons and muscles. 'Arthritis' describes a pathological musculoskeletal disorder. Most

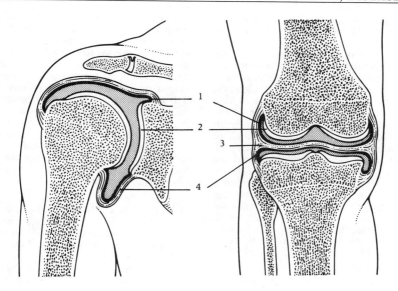

1 synovial membrane
2 articular cartilage
3 articular disc
4 capsule

Diagram of synovial joints. (Left) A right shoulder joint (simple synovial) from the front. (Right) Right knee joint (synovial with articular disc) from the front.

common are sprains of ligaments, strains of tendons and muscles, BURSITIS, TENDINITIS and non-specific back pain. At any one time about 20 per cent of people will have back pain; 80 per cent will have it some time in their lives. Rheumatic symptoms may arise from over-use of healthy tissues (sports injuries) or from unusual strain on normal tissue: the 'weekend professional' problem.

Back disorders are particularly poorly understood and chronic back pain is linked to emotional problems such as stress and depression. The nucleus pulposus – the soft centre of the intervertebral disc – is at risk of prolapse under the age of 40 through an acquired defect in the fibrous cartilage ring surrounding it. Over 40 this nucleus is firmer and 'slipped disc' is less likely to occur. Once prolapse has taken place, however, that segment of the back is never quite the same again, as OSTEOARTHRITIS develops in the adjacent facet joints. Stiffness and pain may develop, sometimes many years later. There may be accompanying pain in the legs: 'Sciatica' is pain in the line of the sciatic nerve, while its rarer analogue at the front of the leg is cruralgia, following the femoral nerve. Leg pain of this sort may not be true nerve pain but referred from arthritis in the spinal facet joints. Only about 5 per cent of patients with back pain have true sciatica, and spinal surgery is most successful (about 85 per cent) in this group.

When the complaint is of pain alone, surgery is much less successful. Manipulation by prop-erly trained physiotherapists, doctors, osteopaths or chiropractors can relieve symptoms temporarily, but seems to make little difference to the ultimate outcome

Osteoarthritis (OA) rarely starts before 40, but by 80 affects 80 per cent of the population. There are structural and functional changes in the articular cartilage, as well as changes in the collagenous matrix of tendons and ligaments. OA is not purely 'wear and tear'. Various subgroups have a genetic component. Early OA may be precipitated by localized alteration in anatomy, such as a fracture or infection of a joint. Reactive new bone growth typically occurs, causing sclerosis beneath the joint, and osteophytes – outgrowths of bone – are characteristic at the margins of the joint. The commonest sites are the first metatarsal (great toe), spinal facet joints, the knee, the base of the thumb and the terminal finger joints (Heberden's nodes).

OA has a slow but variable course, with periods of pain and low-grade inflammation. Acute inflammation, common in the knee, may result from release of pyrophosphate crystals, causing pseudo-gout.

Urate gout results from crystallization of URIC ACID in joints, against a background of hyperuricaemia. This high concentration of uric acid in the blood may result from genetic and environmental factors, such as excess dietary purines, alcohol or diuretic drugs.

Inflammatory arthritis is less common, but potentially much more serious. Several types exist:

SPONDYLARTHRITIS affects younger men, chiefly involving spinal and leg joints. This may lead to inflammation and eventual ossification of the enthesis, where the ligaments and tendons are inserted into the bone around joints. This may be associated with other parts of the body: skin (psoriasis), bowel and genito-urinary inflammation, sometimes resulting in infection of the organs (such as dysentery). The syndromes most clearly delineated are ankylosing (see SPINE AND SPINAL CORD, DISEASES AND INJURIES OF), psoriatic or colitic spondylitis and REITER'S SYNDROME. The diagnosis is made clinically and radiologically; no association has been found with AUTOANTIBODIES. A particularly clear gene locus, HLA B27, has been identified in ankylosing spondylitis. Psoriasis can be associated with a characteristic peripheral arthritis.

Systemic autoimmune rheumatic diseases (see AUTOIMMUNE DISORDERS).

RHEUMATOID ARTHRITIS (RA) The commonest of these diseases. Acute inflammation causes lymphoid synovitis, leading to erosion of the cartilage, and associated joints and soft tissues. Fibrosis follows, causing deformity. Auto-antibodies are common, particularly Rheumatoid Factor. A common complication of RA is Sjögren's syndrome, when inflammation of the mucosal glands may result in a dry mouth and eyes.

SYSTEMIC LUPUS ERYTHEMATOSUS (SLE) and various overlap syndromes occur, such as systemic sclerosis and dermatomyositis. Autoantibodies against nuclear proteins such as DNA lead to deposits of immune complexes and VASCULITIS in various tissues, such as kidney, brain, skin and lungs. This may lead to various symptoms, sometimes even organ failure.

Infective arthritis includes:

SEPTIC ARTHRITIS, an uncommon but potentially fatal disease if not diagnosed and treated early with approriate antibiotics. Common causes are TUBERCLE bacilli and STAPHYLOCOCCI. Particularly at risk are the elderly and the immunologically vulnerable, such as those under treatment for cancer, or on CORTICOSTEROIDS or IMMUNOSUPPRESSANTS.

RHEUMATIC FEVER is the most common of these, but is now rare in Western countries. Resulting from a reaction to a streptococcal infection, it is characterized by a migratory arthritis, rash and cardiac involvement.

Other infections which may be associated with arthritis include RUBELLA, PARVOVIRUS and LYME DISEASE.

Treatment Septic arthritis is the only type that can be cured, while the principles of treatment for the others are similar: to reduce risk factors (such as hyperuricaemia); to suppress inflammation; to improve function with physiotherapy and, in the event of joint failure, to perform surgical arthroplasty. NON-STEROIDAL ANTI-INFLAMMATORY drugs (NSAIDs) include aspirin, paracetamol and many recently developed ones, such as the proprionic acid derivatives IBUPROFEN and NAPROXEN, along with other drugs that have similar properties such as PIROXICAM. They all carry a risk of toxicity, such as renal dysfunction, or gastro-intestinal irritation with haemorrhage. Stronger suppression of inflammation requires corticosteroids and CYTOTOXIC DRUGS such as azathioprine or cyclophosphamide. Recent research promises more specific and less toxic anti-inflammatory drugs, such as the cytokines. An important treatment for some osteoarthritic joints is surgical replacement of the joints.

JOINT REPLACEMENT Also known as arthroplasty, this is the surgical replacement of a joint or part of a joint. Hip replacements were the first type to be introduced and many types of artificial joint are successful, installed with generally excellent results. As many knee joints as hips are now replaced, with finger, shoulder and elbow joints now commonly given artificial articular surfaces. The co-operation between engineers and surgeons (bioengineering) will undoubtedly widen the scope of successful joint replacements, with plastic and metal the prime surface materials. The artificial part may be 'cemented' in place or the bone encouraged to 'fuse' with the plastic or metal.

JOULE is the unit of energy in the International System of Units. The official abbreviation is J. 4186·8 J = 1 Calorie (or kilocalorie). (See also CALORIE; APPENDIX 6: WEIGHTS AND MEASURES.)

JUGULAR is a general name for any structure in the neck, but is especially applied to three large veins, the anterior, external and internal jugular veins, which convey blood from the head and neck regions to the interior of the chest.

JUNG, KARL GUSTAV (1875–1961) was a Swiss psychiatrist. Born in Basel, he studied medicine there, working under Eugen Bleuler at the Burgholzli mental clinic in Zurich (1900–9). His early works *Studies in Word Association* (1904–9). in which he coined the term 'complex', and *The Psychology of Dementia Praecox* (1906–7) led to his meeting Sigmund Freud in Vienna in 1907. Initially Freud's collaborator, his independent researches, which he published in *The Psychology of the Unconscious* (1911–12), made him increasingly critical of Freud's insistence on the psychosexual origins of the neuroses. This led to a break in 1913. From then he went on to develop his own school of 'analytical psychology', introducing the concepts of 'introvert' and 'extrovert' personalities, and developing the theory of the 'collective unconscious' with its archetypes of man's basic psychic nature. In contrast with Freudian analysis, in Jungian analysis the relationship between therapist and patient is less one-sided because the therapist is more willing to be active and to reveal information about himself. (See FREUD'S THEORY; PSYCHO-ANALYSIS.)

K

KALA-AZAR   Another name for visceral leishmaniasis. (See LEISHMANIASIS.)

KANAMYCIN is an antibiotic derived from *Streptomyces kanamyceticus*. It is active against a wide range of organisms, including *Staphylococcus aureus* and *Mycobacterium tuberculosis*.

KAOLIN (china clay), is a smooth white powder consisting of natural white aluminium silicate resulting from the decomposition of minerals containing felspar. It is used as a dusting powder for eczema and other forms of irritation in the skin. It is also used internally in cases of diarrhoea. Talc, French chalk and Fuller's earth are similar silicates.

Kaolin poultice contains kaolin, boric acid, glycerin and various aromatic substances.

KAOLINOSIS is a form of PNEUMOCONIOSIS caused by the inhaling of clay dust.

KAPOSI'S SARCOMA   Once a very rare disease in Western countries, though more common in Africa, it is now a feature of AIDS. Its increasing occurrence was one of the first pointers to the development of AIDS. It is a condition in which malignant skin tumours develop, originating from the blood vessels. The tumours form purple lumps which customarily start on the feet and ankles, then spread up the legs and develop on the arm and hands. In AIDS the sarcoma appears in the respiratory tract and gut and it causes serious bleeding. Radiotherapy normally cures mild cases of Kaposi's sarcoma but severely affected patients will need anti-cancer drugs to check the tumour's growth. (See AIDS.)

KAWASAKI DISEASE   Also called mucocutaneous lymph node syndrome, this disorder of unknown origin occurs mainly in children under five. It was first described in Japan but has now spread to Europe. It is characterized by high fever, conjunctivitis (see EYE DISEASES), skin rashes and swelling of the neck glands. It is possible that the disease is caused by an infection. Most patients recover spontaneously.

Arteritis is a common complication and results in the development of coronary artery aneurysms in up to 60 per cent of those affected.

These aneurysms and myocardial infarction are often detected after the second week of illness. The disease can be hard to diagnose. Six deaths occurred in the UK in one year recently but only one was diagnosed during life. The incidence in the UK is over 3 per 100,000 children under five years of age. Most cases occur in Japan but a third of incidents were reported in the USA.

KELOID   Hard lumpy nodule of the skin due to overgrowth of fibrous tissue in the dermis. It usually follows surgical or accidental trauma or burns, but, rarely, may complicate acne on the upper trunk. Most commonly seen in the skin over the sternum, shoulders and upper back; coloured people are particularly prone. Injection of corticosteroid into the keloid may cause partial resolution. Excision should be avoided.

KERATIN   The substance of which horn and the surface layer of the skin are composed. (See SKIN.)

KERATITIS (see EYE DISEASES).

KERATOMALACIA   Softening of the cornea due to a severe vitamin A deficiency (see EYE DISEASES).

KERATOPLASTY   Technical term for a corneal graft.

KERATOSIS (ACTINIC KERATOSIS)   Rough scaly area on exposed skin caused by chronic solar damage from exposure to sun. The face and backs of the hands are most commonly affected. (See also MELANOMA; SUNBURN.) CRYOTHERAPY is effective, but prevention by appropriate clothing and sun-blocking creams is a better strategy.

KERION   A suppurating form of RINGWORM.

KERNICTERUS   The staining with bile of the basal nuclei of the brain, with toxic degeneration of the nerve cells, which sometimes occurs in HAEMOLYTIC DISEASE OF THE NEW-BORN.

KERNIG'S SIGN   This is found in MENINGITIS. A healthy person's thigh can be bent to a right angle with the body when the knee is straight; in cases of meningitis the knee cannot be straightened when the knee is bent this way or, if so, the patient suffers intense pain.

KETOCONAZOLE   An imidazole antifungal drug available for both oral and topical use. Better absorbed orally than other imidazoles, it also has an anti-androgen effect which may give rise to GYNAECOMASTIA and IMPOTENCE in men. In view of its potential hepatotoxicity it should not be given orally for trivial infections but reserved for systemic fungal infections.

KETOGENESIS The production of KETONES in the body. Abnormal ketogenesis may result in KETOSIS.

KETOGENIC DIET This contains such an excess of fats that acetone and other ketone bodies appear in the urine. It is sometimes used in the treatment of epilepsy and chronic infections of the urinary tract by *Escherichia coli*. In this diet, butter, cream, eggs and fat meat are allowed, whilst sugar, bread and other carbohydrates are cut out as far as possible.

KETONE Another name for acetone or dimethyl ketone. The term, ketone bodies, is applied to a group of substances closely allied to acetone, especially beta-hydroxybutyric acid and acetoacetic acid. These are produced in the body from imperfect oxidation of fats and protein foods, and are found in specially large amount in severe cases of diabetes mellitus. Ketonuria is the term applied to the presence of these bodies in the urine.

KETOPROFEN (see NON-STEROIDAL ANTI-IN-FLAMMATORY DRUGS).

KETOSIS A condition in which an excessive amount of KETONES are produced by the body and these accumulate in the blood stream. The affected person becomes drowsy, suffers a headache, breathes deeply, and may lapse into a coma. The condition results from an unbalanced metabolism of fat, which may occur in DIABETES MELLITUS or starvation.

KEY ESCROW A secure encryption system in which the key to the code for obtaining access to computerized confidential information (on patients) is stored for use by a third party who can use it only under clearly defined circumstances. Examples might be a medical practitioner treating the patient or a law enforcement agency. (See INFORMATION TECHNOLOGY.)

KEYHOLE SURGERY (see MINIMALLY INVASIVE SURGERY).

KIDNEY, ARTIFICIAL (see DIALYSIS).

KIDNEYS These are a pair of glands located in the upper abdomen close to the spine. Level with the last dorsal and upper two lumbar vertebrae, each is covered behind by the twelfth rib of its own side. They are kept in this position by the fat and loose connective tissue in which they are embedded, by the large vessels which supply them with blood, and by the peritoneal membrane stretched over their front surface.

Structure Each is about 10 cm long, 6.5 cm wide, 5 cm thick, and weighs around 140 grams. The size of kidneys found in individuals, how-

1 calyx minor	7 ureter
2 hilum	8 fibrous capsule
3 renal artery	9 cortex
4 pelvis	10 pyramid
5 renal vein	11 papilla
6 calyx major	12 medulla

Vertical section through the kidney

1a afferent arteriole
1b efferent arteriole
2 glomerulus
3 interlobular artery
4 arcuate artery
5 arcuate vein
6 descending limb of Henle's loop
7 proximal convoluted tubule
8 distal convoluted tubule
9 collecting tubule
10 urineferous interlobular vein
11 ascending limb of Henle's loop

Diagram of renal tubules and blood supply of the kidney positioned in the cortex and medulla (see vertical-section diagram).

1 afferent vessel	4 efferent blood vessel
2 capillary tuft	5 glomerular capsule
3 tubule	6 capsule

Diagram of glomerulus (Malphigian corpuscle).

ever, varies considerably with the development, and probably habits, of the individual, maintaining a remarkably constant ratio to body weight. The left kidney is slightly longer and narrower than the right, and lies a little higher in the abdomen.

Adult kidneys have a smooth exterior, although in early life (as in many animals) the organ is divided up into distinct lobes, corresponding to the pyramids found in the interior. It is enveloped by a tough fibrous coat, bound to the kidney only by loose fibrous tissue and by a few blood vessels that pass between it and the kidney. The outer margin of the kidney is convex, while the inner is concave, with a deep depression, known as the hilum, where the vessels enter. At this point the renal vein lies in front of the renal artery, the former joining the inferior vena cava, while the latter arises from the aorta almost at right-angles. The URETER, which conveys URINE down to the bladder, is also joined at this point. The ureter is spread out into an expanded, funnel-like end, known as the pelvis, to which the capsule of the kidney is firmly attached, and which further divides up into little funnels known as the calyces. A vertical section through a kidney (see diagram) shows two distinct layers: an outer one, about 4 mm thick, known as the cortex, and an inner, the medulla, lying closer to the hilum. The medulla consists of around a dozen pyramids arranged side by side, with their base on the cortex and their apex projecting into the calyces of the ureter. The apex of each pyramid is studded with tiny holes, which are the openings of the microscopic uriniferous tubes.

In effect, each pyramid, taken together with the portion of cortex lying along its base, is an independent mini-kidney. About twenty small

tubes are on the surface of each pyramid; these, if traced up into its substance, repeatedly subdivide so as to form bundles of convoluted tubules, known as medullary rays, passing up towards the cortex (see diagram). One of these may be traced further back; ending, after a tortuous course, in a small rounded body: the Malpighian corpuscle or glomerulus (see diagram). Each glomerulus and its convoluted tubule is known as a nephron, which constitutes the functional unit of the kidney. Each kidney contains around one million nephrons.

After entering the kidney, the renal artery divides into branches, forming arches where the cortex and medulla join. Small vessels come off these arches and run up through the cortex, giving off small branches in each direction. These end in a tuft of capillaries, enclosed in Bowman's capsule, which forms the end of the uriniferous tubules just described; capillaries with capsule constitute a glomerulus. After circulating in the glomerulus, the blood leaves by a small vein, which again divides into capillaries on the walls of the uriniferous tubules. From these it is finally collected into the renal veins and then leaves the kidney. This double circulation (first through the glomerulus and then around the tubule) allows a large volume of fluid to be removed from the blood in the glomerulus, the concentrated blood passing on to the uriniferous tubule for removal of parts of its solid contents. Other arteries come straight from the arches and supply the medulla direct; the blood from these passes through another set of capillaries and finally into the renal veins. This circulation is confined purely to the kidney, although small connections by both arteries and veins exist which pass through the capsule and, joining the lumbar vessels, communicate direct with the aorta.

Function The kidneys work to separate fluid and certain solids from the blood. The glomeruli filter from the blood the non-protein portion of the plasma – around 150–200 litres in 24 hours, 99 per cent of which is reabsorbed on passing through the convoluted tubules.

Three main groups of substances are classified according to their extent of uptake by the tubules:

(1) SUBSTANCES ACTIVELY REABSORBED, such as amino-acids, glucose, sodium, potassium, calcium, magnesium and chlorine.

(2) SUBSTANCES DIFFUSING THROUGH THE TUBULAR EPITHELIUM when their concentration in the filtrate exceeds that in the plasma, such as urea, uric acid and phosphates.

(3) SUBSTANCES NOT RETURNED TO THE BLOOD from the tubular fluid, such as creatine.

In diseased kidneys the number of glomeruli and tubules decline, leading to a gradual loss of efficiency. Partial closure of the kidney vessels by disease – for example, arteriosclerosis – leads to a rise in blood pressure, aimed at forcing more blood through the kidneys. In consequence, this type of renal disease causes marked changes in the cardiovascular system.

Total failure of the kidneys leads to accumulation of these solid waste substances in the blood. The resulting general 'poisoning' is known as URAEMIA.

KIDNEYS, DISEASES OF The complex nature of the kidney's structure and functions means that any disorders of it can have a serious systemic effect. Traditionally kidney diseases were divided into medical and surgical. As understanding has grown about how the kidney works and how various disorders affect it, clinical boundaries have blurred and its diseases are now the province of specialist nephrologists who call on surgical skills when these are needed.

The disease affecting the kidneys can be broadly classified into congenital and genetic disorders; autoimmune disorders; malfunctions caused by impaired blood supply; infections; metabolic disorders and tumours of the kidney. Outside factors may cause functional disturbances – for example, obstruction in the urinary tract preventing normal urinary flow may result in hydronephrosis, and the CRUSH SYNDROME, which releases proteins into the blood as a result of seriously damaged muscles (rhabdomyolosis), can result in impaired kidney function. Another outside factor, medicinal drugs, can also be hazardous to the kidney. Large quantities of ANALGESICS taken over a long time damage the kidneys and acute tubular NECROSIS can result from certain antibiotics.

Fortunately the body has two kidneys and as most people can survive on one, there is a good 'functional reserve' of kidney tissue.

Symptoms suggestive of kidney problems include loin pain associated with obstruction (renal colic) or due to infection, fevers, swelling (oedema), usually of the legs but occasionally including the face and arms, blood in the urine (haematuria), excess quantities of urine (polyuria), including at night (nocturia) due to failure of normal mechanisms in the kidney for concentrating urine. Patients with chronic renal failure often have very diffuse symptoms including nausea and vomiting, tiredness due to anaemia, shortness of breath, skin irritation, pins and needles (paraesthesia) due to damage of the peripheral nerves (peripheral neuropathy) and eventually (rarely seen nowadays) clouding of consciousness and death. Many patients with kidney disorders do not have any symptoms, even when the condition is quite advanced.

Signs of kidney disease include loin tenderness, enlarged kidneys, signs of fluid retention, high blood pressure and, in patients with end-stage renal failure, pallor, pigmentation and a variety of neurological signs including absent reflexes, reduced sensation, and a coarse flapping tremor (asterixis) due to severe disturbance of the body's normal metabolism.

Renal failure Serious kidney disease may lead to impairment or failure of the kidney's ability to filter waste products from the blood and excrete them in the urine, a process that controls the body's water and salt balance and helps to maintain a stable blood pressure. Failure of this process causes URAEMIA – an increase in urea and other metabolic waste products – as well as other metabolic upsets in the blood and tissues, all of which produce varying symptoms. Failure can be sudden or develop more slowly (chronic). In the former function usually returns to normal once the underlying cause has been treated. Chronic failure, however, usually irreparably reduces or stops normal function.

Acute failure commonly results from physiological shock following a bad injury or major illness. Serious bleeding or burns can reduce blood volume and pressure to the point where blood supply to the kidney is greatly reduced. Acute myocardial infarction or pancreatitis may produce a similar result. A mismatched blood transfusion can produce acute failure. Obstruction to the urine flow by a stone (calculus) in the urinary tract, a bladder tumour or an enlarged prostate can also cause acute renal failure, as can glomerulonephritis (see below) and the haemolytic-uraemia syndrome.

HYPERTENSION, DIABETES MELLITUS, polycystic kidney disease (see below) or amyloidosis are among conditions that cause chronic renal failure. Others include stone, tumour, prostatic enlargement and overuse of analgesic drugs. Chronic failure may eventually lead to end-stage renal failure, a life-threatening situation that will need DIALYSIS or a renal transplant (see TRANSPLANTATION).

Familial renal disorders include autosomal dominant inherited polycystic kidney disease and sex-linked familial nephropathy. Polycystic kidney disease is an important cause of renal failure in the UK. Patients, usually aged 30 to 50, present with haematuria, hypertension, loin or abdominal discomfort or, rarely, urinary-tract infection, hypertension and enlarged kidneys. Diagnosis is based on ultrasound examination of the abdomen. Complications include renal failure, hepatic cysts and, rarely, SUBARACHNOID HAEMORRHAGE. No specific treatment is available. Familial nephropathy occurs more often in boys than girls and commonly presents as Alport's syndrome (familial nephritis with nerve deafness) with PROTEINURIA, HAEMATURIA, progressing to renal failure and DEAFNESS. The cause of the disease lies in an absence of a specific ANTIGEN in a part of the glomerulus. The treatment is conservative, with most patients eventually requiring dialysis or transplantation.

Acute glomerulonephritis is an immune-complex disorder due to entrapment within glomerular capillaries of ANTIGEN (usually derived from B haemolytic STREPTOCOCCI) antibody complexes initiating an acute inflammatory response (see IMMUNITY). The disease affects children and young adults, classically presents with a sore throat followed two weeks later by a fall in urine output (oliguria), haematuria, hypertension and mildly abnormal renal function. The disease is self limiting with 90 per cent of patients spontaneously recovering. Treatment consists of control of blood pressure, reduced fluid and salt intake, occasional DIURETICS and ANTIBIOTICS.

Chronic glomerulonephritis is also due to immunological renal problems and is also classified by taking a renal biopsy. It may be subdivided into various histological varieties as determined by renal biospy. Proteinuria of various degrees is present in all these conditions but the clinical presentations vary as do their treatments. Some resolve spontaneously. Others are treated with steroids or even the cytotoxic drug CYCLOPHOSPHOMIDE or the immunosuppressant cyclosporin. Prognoses are generally satisfactory but some patients may require renal dialysis or kidney transplantation, an operation with a good success rate.

Impaired blood supply may be the outcome of diabetes mellitus and physiological shock, which lowers the blood pressure, also affects the blood supply. The result can be acute tubular necrosis. POLYARTERIS NODOSA and SYSTEMIC LUPUS ERYTHEMATOSUS (SLE) may damage the large blood vessels in the kidney. Treatment is of the underlying condition.

Infection of the kidney is called pyelonephritis, a key predisposing factor being obstruction of urine flow through the urinary tract. This causes stagnation and provides a fertile ground of bacterial growth. Acute pyelonephritis is more common in women, especially during pregnancy when bladder infection (CYSTITIS) spreads up the URETERS to the kidney. Symptoms are fever, malaise and backache. Antibiotics and high fluid intake are the most effective treatment. Chronic pyelonephritis may start in childhood as a result of congenital deformities that permit urine to flow up from the bladder to the kidney (reflux). Persistent reflux leads to recurrent infections causing permanent damage to the kidney. Specialist investigations are usually required as possible complications include hypertension and kidney failure.

Tumours of the kidney are fortunately rare. Non-malignant ones commonly do not cause symptoms. Even malignant tumours (renal cell carcinoma) may be asymptomatic for many years. As soon as symptoms appear – haematuria, back pain, nausea, malaise, sometimes secondary growths in the lungs, bones or liver, and weight loss – urgent treatment including surgery, radiotherapy and chemotherapy is necessary. This cancer occurs mostly in adults over 40 and has a hereditary element. The prognosis is not good unless diagnosed early. In young children a rare cancer called nephroblastoma (Wilm's tumour) can occur; treatment is with surgery, radiotherapy and chemotherapy. It may grow to a substantial size before being diagnosed.

Cystinuria is an inherited metabolic defect in the renal tubular reabsorption of cystine, ornithine, lysine and arginine. Cystine precipitates in an alkaline urine to form cystine stones.

Triple phosphate stones are associated with infection and may develop into a very large branching calculi (staghorn calculi). Stones present as renal or ureteric pain, or as an infection. Treatment has undergone considerable change with the introduction of MINIMALLY INVASIVE SURGERY and the destruction of stone by sound waves (LITHOTRIPSY).

KIDNEY (RENAL) FAILURE (see KIDNEY, DISEASES OF).

KINAESTHETIC SENSATIONS A term used to describe those sensations which underlie muscle tension and position of joint and muscle. These sensations send impulses along nerves to the brain, and thus inform it of the position of the limb in space and of the relative position to each other of individual muscles and muscle-groups and of joints.

KININS Substances present in the body which are powerful VASODILATORS. They also induce pain and are probably involved in the production of the headache of MIGRAINE. In addition, they play a part in the production of ALLERGY and ANAPHYLAXIS.

KISS OF LIFE Emergency mouth-to-mouth resuscitation of an unconscious person (see APPENDIX 1: BASIC FIRST AID).

KLEBSIELLA A GRAM-NEGATIVE bacteria found in the intestinal, respiratory, and urogenital tracts of man and animals. Varieties of the bacteria, which are rod shaped and nonmotile, can cause PNEUMONIA and URINARY INFECTIONS.

KLEPTOMANIA A psychological disorder in which the person afflicted has an irresistible compulsion to steal things, without necessarily having any need for the object stolen.

KLINEFELTER'S SYNDROME The original syndrome described by Klinefelter consisted of GYNAECOMASTIA, testicular atrophy and INFERTILITY. Intelligence was unimpaired. Patients have been described who have associated mental defects and striking tallness of stature but the only constant feature of the syndrome is testicular atrophy with resulting azoospermia and infertility. The atrophy of the TESTIS is the result of a peritubular fibrosis which begins to appear in childhood and progresses until all the seminiferous tubules are replaced by fibrous tissue. Gynaecomastia, mental retardation and EUNUCHOIDISM (loss of male secondary sexual characteristics – small penis, loss of body hair and a high pitched voice) – may be associated but the first is inconstant and the two last are infrequent. Most patients with Klinefelter's syndrome have 47 chromosomes instead of the normal 46. The extra chromosome is an X chromosome so that the sex chromosome constitution is XXY instead of XY. Klinefelter's syndrome is one of the most common chromosome abnormalities and occurs in 1 in 300 of the male population. Patients with this syndrome show that the Y chromosome is strongly sex determining. Thus a patient who has an XXY chromosome constitution may have the appearance of a normal male and the only incapacity is infertility. However the loss of a Y chromosome leads to the development of a bodily form which is essentially feminine (see TURNER'S SYNDROME).

KLUMPKE'S PARALYSIS Injury as a result of the stretching of a baby's brachial plexus during its birth may cause partial paralysis of the arm with atrophy of the muscles of the forearm and hand.

KNEE The joint formed by the femur, tibia and patella (knee-cap). It belongs to the class of hinge-joints, although movements are much more complex than the simple motion of a hinge, the condyles of the femur partly rolling, partly sliding over the flat surfaces on the upper end of the tibia, and the acts of straightening and of bending the limb being finished and begun, respectively, by a certain amount of rotation. The cavity of the joint is very intricate: it consists really of three joints fused into one, but separated in part by ligaments and folds of the synovial membrane. The ligaments which bind the bones together are extremely strong, and include the popliteal and the collateral ligaments, a very strong patellar ligament uniting the patella to the front of the tibia, two cruciate ligaments in the interior of the joint, and two fibro-cartilages which are interposed between the surfaces of tibia and femur at their edge. All these structures give to the knee-joint great strength, so that it is seldom dislocated.

A troublesome condition often found in the knee – and common among athletes, footballers and other energetic sports people – consists of the loosening of one of the fibro-cartilages lying at the head of the tibia, especially of that on the inner side of the joint. The cartilage may either be loosened from its attachment and tend to slip beyond the edges of the bones, or it may become folded on itself. In either case, it tends to cause locking of the joint when sudden movements are made. This causes temporary inability to use the joint until the cartilage is replaced by forcible straightening, and the accident is apt to be followed by an attack of synovitis, which may last some weeks, causing lameness with pain and tenderness especially felt at a point on the inner side of the knee. This condition can be relieved by an operation – sometimes by keyhole surgery (see MINIMALLY INVASIVE SURGERY) – to remove the loose portion of the cartilage. Patients whose knees are severely affected by osteoarthritis or rheumatoid arthritis which cause pain and stiffness can now have the joint replaced with an artificial one. (See also JOINTS, DISEASES OF.)

KNEE JERK (See REFLEX ACTION).

KNEE-JOINT REPLACEMENT A surgical operation to replace a diseased – usually osteoarthritic – knee with an artificial (metal or plastic) implant which covers the worn cartilage. As much of the original joint as possible is retained. The operations, like hip replacements, are usually done on older people (there is some restriction of movement) and about 90 per cent are successful.

KNOCK-KNEE (GENU VALGUM) This is a deformity of the lower limbs in such a direction that when the limbs are straightened the legs diverge from one another. As a result, in walking the knees knock against each other. The amount of knock-knee is measured by the distance between the medial malleoli of the ankles, with the inner surfaces of the knee touching and the knee-caps facing forwards. The condition is so common in children between the ages of 2 to 6 years that it may almost be regarded as a normal phase in childhood. When marked, or persisting into later childhood, it can be corrected by surgery (osteotomy).

KOCH'S BACILLUS The original name for *Mycobacterium tuberculosis*, which causes TUBERCULOSIS. It stems from the name of the German doctor who first identified the bacillus.

KOILONYCHIA The term applied to nails that are hollow and depressed like a spoon, a condition sometimes associated with chronic iron deficiency.

KOPLIK SPOTS Bluish-white spots appearing on the mucous membrane of the mouth in cases of MEASLES about the third day, and forming the first part of the rash in this disease.

KORSAKOFF'S SYNDROME A form of mental disturbance occurring in chronic alcoholism and other toxic states, such as URAEMIA, LEAD poisoning and cerebral SYPHILIS. Its special features are talkativeness with delusions in regard to time and place, the patient, although clear in other matters, imagining that he has recently made journeys.

KREBS CYCLE A series of cellular chemical reactions starting and ending with oxaloacetic acid. Also called the citric acid or tricarboxylic acid cycle, it produces energy in the form of adenosine triphosphate and is the last stage in the biological oxidation of fats, proteins, and carbohydrates. Named after Sir Hans Kreb, a German biochemist working in England in 1900, who won the Nobel Prize for his discovery.

KUPFFER CELLS Star-shaped cells present in the blood-sinuses of the LIVER. They form part of the RETICULO-ENDOTHELIAL system and are to a large extent responsible for the breakdown of HAEMOGLOBIN into the BILE pigments.

KURU   A slowly progressive fatal disease due to spongiform degeneration in the central nervous system, particularly the cerebellum (see BRAIN). It is confined to the Fore people in the Eastern Highlands of New Guinea. It is believed to be due to an infection with a PRION, similar to that causing CREUTZFELDT-JAKOB DISEASE (CJD), acquired from the cannibalistic rite of eating the organs, particularly the brains, of deceased relatives (out of respect). This origin of the disease was suggested by the fact that originally it was a disease of women and children, and it was they who practised this rite. Since the rite was given up, the disease has largely disappeared in children, but still occurs in women as it has an incubation period of up to 20 years.

KVEIM TEST is the characteristic histological test used for the diagnosis of SARCOIDOSIS. The test involves an intradermal injection of sarcoid SPLEEN tissue. If positive, non-caseating GRANULOMATA are seen at the injection site in 4–6 weeks. A positive test is highly specific for sarcoid, but if negative, this would not be excluded.

KWASHIORKOR   One of the most important causes of ill health and death among children in the tropics. It is predominantly a deficiency disease due to a diet short of protein. There is also some evidence of a lack of the so-called essential fatty acids. It affects typically the small child weaned from the breast and not yet able to cope with an adult diet, or for whom an adequate amount of first-class protein is not available, and it is mainly found in the less well-developed countries.
    The onset of the disease is characterized by loss of appetite, often with diarrhoea and loss of weight. The child is flabby, the skin is dry, and the hair is depigmented, dry, sparse and brittle. At a later stage oedema develops and the liver is often enlarged. In the early stages the condition responds rapidly to a diet containing adequate first-class protein, but in the later stages this must be supplemented by careful nursing, especially as the child is very liable to infection.

KYPHOSCOLIOSIS: A combination of SCOLIOSIS and KYPHOSIS in which the spine (see SPINAL COLUMN) is abnormally curved sideways and forwards. The condition may be the result of several diseases affecting the spinal muscles and vertebrae or it may happen during development for no obvious reason. Although braces may reduce the deformity, an operation may be necessary to correct it.

KYPHOSIS   The term applied to curvature of the spine in which the concavity of the curve is directed forwards. (See SPINE AND SPINAL CORD, DISEASES AND INJURIES OF.)

L

LABETALOL is an alpha- and beta-adrenoceptor blocker (see ADRENERGIC RECEPTORS) used to treat hypertension. Beta blockers block the beta-adrenoceptors in the HEART, peripheral blood vessels and bronchi. Many of this group of drugs are now available and are all equally effective but with differences that may make them suitable for a particular patient. Labetalol has the added property of dilating ARTERIOLES, thus lowering resistance in the small peripheral blood vessels and helping to reduce blood pressure.

LABIA   Lips. The labia majora and labia minora are the outer and inner lip-like folds of skin surrounding the entrance to the vagina (see diagrams in REPRODUCTIVE SYSTEM).

LABIUM is the Latin word for a lip or lip-shaped organ.

LABOUR   Also known by the traditional term PARTURITION, this is the process by which the products of conception, normally a fully developed baby, are expelled from the mother's body by regular contractions of the UTERUS. The onset of labour is difficult to pinpoint accurately, but any one of the following suggests that labour may start soon: the protective mucus plug comes away from the CERVIX and the mother passes a small amount of blood-stained mucus vaginally – a 'show'. The membranes around the fetus rupture and the mother loses amniotic fluid vaginally. The mother becomes aware of painful contractions of the uterus. When these become regular, labour is said to be 'established'.
    Labour is divided into three stages: the first stage is from the onset of labour to full (10 cm) dilation of the opening of the neck of the womb (cervical os). The duration of the first stage is very variable. During the first stage the strength and frequency of the uterine contractions are often measured and the fetal heart rate is monitored frequently. Abnormal responses of the fetal heart during labour can indicate that the baby is suffering from the effects of labour and may need expert assistance to be delivered safely.
    The second stage is from full cervical dilation to delivery of the baby. At the onset of this stage the mother usually experiences an irresistible urge to push and a combination of strong co-ordinated uterine contractions and maternal effort gradually moves the baby down the birth canal. The duration of the second stage is variable. The mother can become exhausted by the effort of pushing and, if the second stage is very long, she may need expert assistance from the doctor or midwife. This may mean enlarging the vaginal opening with an episiotomy (cutting the outlet) or applying special obstetric FORCEPS to the baby's head to allow the baby to be pulled out. Sometimes, if no progress is being made in the second stage because the baby's position is unsatisfactory or because the

baby is becoming distressed, a CAESAREAN SECTION may be necessary.

The third stage of labour is from delivery of the baby to delivery of the placenta. This usually occurs within a few contractions. The birth attendant must check that the placenta and membranes are complete as any retained products of conception can lead to serious bleeding or infection later.

Ventouse (see VACUUM EXTRACTOR).

LABYRINTH A convoluted system of structures forming the inner ear and involved in hearing and balance. (See EAR.)

LACERATION A wound to the skin or surface of an organ which results in a cut with irregular edges (cf. an incision produced with a knife which has smooth, regular edges).

LACRIMAL Gland, duct, apparatus (see EYE DISEASES).

LACTASE An enzyme produced by glands in the small INTESTINE which changes LACTOSE (milk sugar) into glucose and galactose during the process of digestion.

LACTATION The period during which an infant is suckled on the mother's breast. (See BREASTS, DISEASES OF; INFANT FEEDING.)

LACTEAL A lymphatic vessel that transmits CHYLE from the intestine. (See LYMPH.)

LACTIC ACID A colourless, syrupy, sour liquid, which is produced by the action of a bacterium upon LACTOSE, the sugar found in milk. The growth of this organism and consequent formation of lactic acid cause the souring of milk, and the same change takes place to a limited extent when food is long retained in the stomach.

Lactic acid ($CH_3.CHOH.COOH$) is produced in the body during muscular activity, the lactic acid being derived from the breakdown of glycogen. Muscle fatigue is associated with an accumulation of lactic acid in the muscle. Recovery follows when enough oxygen gets to the muscle, part of the lactic acid being oxidized and most of it then being built up once more into glycogen.

LACTIC ACID BACILLI These were introduced by Metchnikoff to prepare milk as a special article of diet. The bacilli, which are issued in various forms, are added to fresh milk, allowed to act on it in a warm place for several hours (according to the degree of sourness desired), and the milk is then consumed with the active bacilli. These, after a course of such treatment, come to replace the bacteria naturally found in the intestines, and are supposed to be less injurious to the system. The bacilli, which are harmless, have, in some cases of intestinal

disease or of rheumatism, a beneficial action. Buttermilk has a similar effect. (See YOGHURT.)

LACTOSE The official name for sugar of milk. (See SUGAR.)

LACTOSE INTOLERANCE A form of allergic indigestion which is much more common in certain non-Caucasian races than in Caucasian. It is due to lack in the intestine of the ENZYME known as LACTASE which is responsible for the digestion of lactose, the sugar in milk. In individuals the taking of milk is followed by nausea, a sensation of bloating, or distension, in the gut, abdominal pain and diarrhoea. Such disturbances after taking milk may also be due to the individual's being allergic to milk. Treatment is by means of a low-lactose diet. Foodstuffs high in lactose, such as fresh or powdered milk, and milk puddings should be avoided. Most people subject to it can tolerate fermented milk products and the small amounts of milk used in baking and added to margarine and sausages. In Britain it is said to occur in up to 80 per cent of non-Caucasian adults but only 5 per cent of Caucasian adults.

LACUNA A small pit or depression.

LAMBLIA (see GIARDIASIS).

LAMELLA A small disc of glycerin jelly, 3 mm (⅛ inch) in diameter, containing an active drug for application to the eye. It is applied by insertion behind the lower lid.

LAMINECTOMY An operation in which the arches of one or more vertebrae in the spinal column are removed so as to expose a portion of the spinal cord for removal of a tumour, relief of pressure due to a fracture, or disc protrusion.

LANGERHANS CELLS Clear, dendritic cells found in the granular layer of the EPIDERMIS that are thought to participate in ANTIGEN activity (see SKIN).

LANOLIN Derived from wool fat, it has properties valuable in ointments and creams but may cause allergic contact dermatitis.

LANUGO Soft fine hair covering the fetus. It disappears by the ninth month of gestation and is therefore only seen on premature babies.

LAPAROSCOPE An instrument, consisting, essentially, of a rigid or flexible cylinder, an eyepiece and a light source, which is inserted through a small incision into the abdominal cavity (which has already been distended with carbon dioxode gas). The laparoscope allows the contents of the abdominal cavity to be examined without performing a LAPAROTOMY. Some operations may be performed using the laparoscope to guide the manipulation of instruments inserted through another small incision (e.g. STERILIZATION, CHOLECYSTECTOMY). (See ENDOSCOPE.)

LAPAROSCOPY A technique by which the contents of the abdomen may be examined, biopsies taken, and minor surgical procedures carried out, by the insertion of a tube through a small hole made in the abdominal wall (see LAPAROSCOPE; ENDOSCOPE). The advances of FIBREOPTIC ENDOSCOPY have transformed the management of abdominal disease, particularly gastrointestinal problems.

LAPAROTOMY A general term applied to any operation in which the abdominal cavity is opened.

LARVA The pre-adult stage in insects and nematodes occurring between the egg and the sexually mature adult.

Larva migrans is a self-limiting, intensely itching skin eruption caused by NEMATODE larvae, usually of the dog and cat HOOKWORM. The migrating larvae leave red raised irregular tracks in the skin, often on the foot and less frequently elsewhere. The disease is usually acquired by people who take their holidays on tropical beaches. It can be cured by a three-day course of oral ALBENDAZOLE.

LARYNGECTOMY Operation for removal of the larynx. (See APPENDIX 2: ADDRESSES.)

LARYNGITIS Inflammation of the mucous membrane of the larynx and vocal chords and may be acute or chronic. The cause is usually an infection, most commonly viral, although it may be the result of secondary bacterial infection, voice abuse or irritation by gases or chemicals.

Acute laryngitis may accompany any form of upper-respiratory-tract infection. The main symptom is of hoarseness and often pain in the throat. Swelling of the cords may occur, the voice becomes husky or it may be lost. Cough, breathing difficulties and sometimes STRIDOR may occur. Acute airway obstruction is unusual following laryngitis but may occasionally be serious in children (see CROUP), when immediate specialist referral is needed.
TREATMENT Steam inhalations and symptomatic treatments are often soothing and reduce swelling. Antibiotics are seldom necessary. Rarely airway intervention, either ENDOTRACHEAL INTUBATION or tracheostomy may be necessary if severe airway obstruction develops (see APPENDIX 1: FIRST AID). Affected patients should rest their voice and avoid smoking.

Chronic laryngitis can result from repeated attacks of acute laryngitis; excessive use of the voice – loud and prolonged, singing or shouting; tumours, which may be benign or malignant; or secondary to diseases such as tuberculosis and syphilis.

Benign tumours or small nodules, such as singer's nodules, may be surgically removed by direct LARYNGOSCOPY under general ANAESTHETIC; while cancer of the larynx may be treated either by RADIOTHERAPY or by SURGERY, depending on the extent of the disease. Hoarseness may be the only symptom of vocal-chord disturbance or of laryngeal cancer, and any case which has lasted for six weeks should be referred for a specialist opinion. Laryngectomy clubs are being established throughout the country (see APPENDIX 2: ADDRESSES) to support patients following laryngectomy. Speech therapists provide speech rehabilitation.

Functional disorders They usually occur in young women at times of emotional stress, producing hysterical paralysis of the adductors of both vocal chords or phonation. The voice may be lost completely (aphomia) or reduced to a whisper. Although patients may not speak, they often cough. This is usually psychological in origin; after excluding any local pathology, speech therapy is again invaluable.

LARYNGOLOGY That branch of medical science concerned with disorders and diseases of the larynx.

LARYNGOSCOPE Examination of the larynx may be performed indirectly with use of a laryngeal mirror, or directly by use of a laryngoscope. The direct examination is usually performed under general anaesthetic.

LARYNGO-TRACHEO-BRONCHITIS (CROUP) An acute infection of the respiratory tract in infants and young children. It is usually a virus infection or may be caused by *Haemophilus influenzae*. The onset is variable but the croupy cough and stridulous breathing usually occur a few days after the onset of a viral upper-respiratory-tract infection. The harsh barking cough is typical of the condition. The majority of children with this condition can be treated with humidification and antibiotics if necessary, but they should always be referred for specialist assessment and hospitalization is preferable in all cases. Rarely, some form of intervention is necessary and this will either be in the form of endotracheal intubation or of a tracheostomy.

LARYNX The organ of voice which also forms one of the higher parts of the air passages. It is placed high up in the front of the neck and there forms a considerable prominence on the surface. It is covered in front by the skin, a layer of fibrous tissue and a thin layer of muscles, whilst its sides are protected by the lateral lobes of the thyroid gland and by the large sterno-cleidomastoid muscles.
The larynx is almost 5 cm or 2 inches in height and forms a sort of box, well protected in front by cartilages, rather more open behind and communicating above with the pharynx at the root of the tongue and below the windpipe or trachea. The larynx is enclosed by five large

1 thyroid cartilage
2 arytenoid cartilage
3 upper border of cricoid cartilage
4 posterior cricoarytenoid muscles
5 muscular processes
6 vocal processes

Diagram of the opening of the larynx to show the action of the muscles. A horizontal section has been made at the level of the true vocal cords. The two cords are widely separated by the action of 4.

cartilages: the thyroid cartilage, whose prominent pointed front forms the Adam's apple; the cricoid cartilage, a ring placed below it; the epiglottis, a leaf-like cartilage projecting above the thyroid cartilage into the interior of the throat at the root of the tongue; and a pair of arytenoid cartilages jointed to the top edge of the cricoid cartilage behind, where the thyroid cartilage is deficient. There are also four small nodules of cartilage above the arytenoids. The edges of the laryngeal cartilages do not fit closely together, and the spaces between are filled up by membranes. Certain of the ligaments which bind the cartilages together are of great importance. These pass along each side of

1 thyroid cartilage   5 muscular processes
2 arytenoid cartilage   6 vocal processes
3 lateral arytenoid   7 thyroarytenoid
4 arytenoid muscles

Diagram of the opening of the larynx to show the action of the muscles. The cords are now held together by the action of 3, 4 and 7.

the larynx, from the arytenoid cartilage behind to the thyroid cartilage in front, two bands of elastic fibres covered by the mucous membrane which lines the whole larynx. One pair of these bands lies directly above the other, the upper pair being known as the false vocal cords; the lower pair are the true vocal cords. The latter are capable of various degrees of tenseness and slackness and of approximation and separation, these results being achieved by several small muscles, which are attached to the arytenoid cartilages and governed in their movements through branches of the vagus nerves. Between the true and false cord is a deep depression on each side known as the ventricle of the larynx. The larynx is lined throughout by mucous membrane, which generally is covered by ciliated cells; but over the true cords, which are subject to much friction in the production of the voice, the surface consists of flattened cells similar to those of the skin.

The vocal cords vibrating in different notes, according to their tenseness and the like, produce the sounds of VOICE AND SPEECH.

LASER stands for Light Amplification by Stimulated Emission of Radiation. The light produced by a laser is of a single wavelength and all the waves are in phase with each other, allowing a very high level of energy to be projected as a parallel beam or focused on to a small spot. Various gases, liquids and solids will emit light when they are suitably stimulated. A gassed laser is pumped by the ionizing effect of a high voltage current. This is the same process as that used in a fluorescent tube. Each type of laser has a different effect on biological tissues and this is related to the wavelength of the light produced. The wavelength determines the degree of energy absorption by different tissues and because of this different lasers are needed for different tasks. The argon laser produces light in the visible green wavelength which is selectively absorbed by haemoglobin. It heats and coagulates tissues and it is thus possible to seal bleeding blood vessels and to selectively destroy pigmented lesions. The carbon-dioxide laser is the standard laser for cutting tissue. The infra-red beam it produces is strongly absorbed by water and so vaporizes cells. Thus by moving a finely focused beam across the tissue it is possible to make an incision.

The two main uses of the laser in surgery are the endoscopic photocoagulation of bleeding vessels and the incision of tissue. Lasers have important applications in ophthalmology in the treatment of such disorders of detachment of the retina and the diabetic complication of proliferative retinopathy. The destruction of abnormal cells – a sign of premalignancy – in the cervix is done using lasers. The beams may be used to remove scar tissue from the FALLOPIAN TUBES resulting from infection, thus unblocking the tubes and improving the chances of conception. Lasers also have several important applications in dermatology. They are used in the treatment of pigmented lesions such as lentigo,

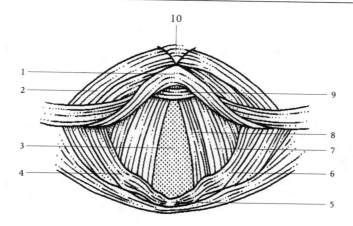

1 epiglottis	6 aryepiglottic fold
2 vallecula	7 vestibular fold
3 trachea	8 vocal fold
4 ventricular fold	9 tubercle of epiglottis
5 cornic cartilage	10 glossoepiglottic fold

A laryngoscopic view of the interior of the larynx.

larynx from behind

larynx from left side

1 epiglottis	12 ventricle
2 aryepiglottic fold	13 thyroid cartilage
3 tubercle	14 cricothyroid membrane
4 ventricular fold	15 cricoid cartilage
5 vocal fold	16 vocal cord
6 interior thyroarytenoid muscle	17 respiratory glottis
7 cricothyroid membrane	18 false vocal cord
8 cricothyroid membrane	19 arytenoideus muscle
9 ventricle of larynx	20 corniculate cartilage
10 thyroid cartilage	21 cuneiform cartilage
11 adipose tissue	22 epiglottis

Anatomy of the larynx.

in the obliteration of port-wine stains, in the removal of small, benign tumours such as verrucas, and finally in the removal of tattoos.

Low-intensity laser beams promote tissue healing and reduce inflammation, pain and swelling. Their effect is achieved by stimulating blood and lymph flow and by cutting the production of PROSTAGLANDINS, which provoke inflammation and pain. The beams are used to treat ligament sprains, muscle tears and inflamed joints and tendons.

The three great advantages of lasers are their potency, their speed of action, and the ability to focus on an extremely small area. For these reasons they are being used increasingly, and have allowed great advances to be made in microsurgery, and particularly FIBREOPTIC ENDOSCOPY.

LASSA FEVER, which derives its name from the fact that it was first reported in Lassa in Nigeria. The cause is an arenavirus. This may be transmitted by rodents or direct from an infected person to those around him. The incubation period is three to twenty-one days. It is characterized by headache, lethargy and severe muscular pains, and there is often a rash due to bleeding into the skin and mucous membranes. Sore throat is often present. It may carry a high mortality rate, particularly in pregnant women. As it is a virus infection, there is no specific treatment, and all that can be done is supportive nursing.

LASSAR'S PASTE   Officially known as Zinc and Salicylic Acid Paste, BP, this preparation is used as a remedy for ECZEMA.

LATERAL Referring to the sides of an organ or the body or that part furthest from the midline or median plane.

LATISSIMUS DORSI   A large flat triangular muscle in the back (see MUSCLE).

LAUDANUM   The traditional name for tincture of OPIUM.

LAUGHING-GAS   A popular name for NITROUS OXIDE GAS.

LAVAGE   The name applied to the washing out of the stomach. (See GASTRIC LAVAGE.)

LAXATIVES (see PURGATIVES).

LEAD A metallic element that has no action itself upon the body, but its salts, when absorbed in any quantity, or for any length of time, have very important effects. When a lead salt comes in contact with a wound or with any mucous surface, it combines with the albuminous material of the discharge or secretion to form a whitish glaze, which affords protection to the surface. It also has an astringent action upon the blood-vessels, helping to stop bleeding or relieve the congestion of inflammation. If one of the soluble lead salts is taken internally, in large amount, it has an irritant action. (See LEAD POISONING.)

LEAD POISONING   Lead and lead compounds are used in a variety of products including petrol additives, piping – lead water pipes were once a common source of poisoning – weights, professional paints, dyes, ceramics, ammunition, homeopathic remedies and ethnic cosmetic preparations. Lead compounds are toxic by ingestion, inhalation and, rarely, by skin exposures. Metallic lead, if ingested, is absorbed if it remains in the gut. The absorption is greater in children. Toxicity of lead salts is dependent on solubility. Fumes from molten lead or petrol can cause serious toxicity.

Acute poisonings are rare. Clinical features include metallic taste, abdominal pain, vomiting, diarrhoea, anorexia, fatigue, muscle weakness and shock. Neurological effects may include headache, drowsiness, convulsions and coma. Inhalation results in severe respiratory-tract irritation and systemic symptoms as above.

Chronic poisonings cause gastrointestinal disturbances and constipation. Other effects are anaemia, weakness, pallor, anorexia, insomnia, renal hypertension and mental fatigue. There may be a bluish 'lead line' on the gums, although this is rarely seen. Neuromuscular dysfunction may result in motor weakness and paralysis of the extensor muscles of the wrist and ankles. Encephalopathy and nephropathy are severe effects. Chronic low-level exposures in children are linked with reduced intelligence and behavioural and learning disorders.

Management of patients who have been poisoned is supportive with removal from source, gastric decontamination if required, and X-RAYS to monitor passage of metallic lead through gut if ingested. It is essential to ensure adequate hydration and renal function. Concentrations of lead in the blood should be monitored. Where these are found to be toxic, chelation therapy should be started. Several chelators are now available such as DMSA (Meso-2,3-dimercaptosuccinic acid), sodium calcium edetate (see EDTA) and PENICILLAMINE. (See POISONS and APPENDIX 2: ADDRESSES.)

LEARNING DISABILITY (MENTAL HANDICAP)   Learning disability, previously called mental handicap is a problem of markedly low intellectual functioning, usually caused by a genetic abnormality. People with learning disability were, until about 20 years ago, usually cared for in large long-stay hospitals. But this proved unnecessary, and often detrimental. People with learning disability want to be seen as themselves, to learn new skills, to choose where to live, to have good health care, to have girlfriends or boyfriends, to make decisions about their lives, and to have enough money to live on. Many now live at home with their families, or in small residential units with access to work and leisure and to other people in ordinary communities. Some people with learning disabilities, however, also have MENTAL ILLNESSES. Most can be treated as outpatients, but a few need more intensive inpatient treatment, and a very small minority with disturbed behaviour need secure (i.e. locked) settings.

In the United Kingdom the 1993 Education Act uses 'learning difficulties': generalized (severe or moderate), or specific (e.g. DYSLEXIA, dyspraxia (or APRAXIA), language disorder). The 1991 Social Security (Disability Living Allowance) Regulations use the term 'severely mentally impaired' if a person suffers from a state of arrested development or incomplete physical development of the brain which results in severe impairment of intelligence and social functioning. This is distinct from the consequences of dementia. Though 'mental handicap' is widely used, 'learning disability' is preferred by the Department of Health.

Originally 'handicap' referred to weights in horse racing. Now distinction is drawn between impairment (a biological deficit), disability (the functional consequence) and handicap (the social consequence).

People with profound learning disability are unable to walk or talk, have multiple disabilities and are dependent on others for care and mobility. Children with severe learning disability develop at up to half the rate of normal children of the same age and, as adults, reach the average level of a child of 3–8 years. Some achieve basic functional literacy (recognition of name, common signs) and numeracy (some understanding of money) but most have a life-long dependency for aspects of self-care (some fastenings for clothes, preparation of meals, menstrual hygiene, shaving) and need supervision for outdoor mobility.

Children with moderate learning disability develop at between half and three-quarters of the normal rate and reach the standard of an average child of 8–11 years. They become independent for self-care and public transport unless they have associated disabilities. Most are capable of supervised or sheltered employment. Living independently and raising a family may be possible.

Occurrence   Profound learning disability affects about 1 person per thousand, severe learning disability 3 per thousand and moderate learning disability requiring special service 1 per cent. With improved health care, survival of people with profound or severe learning disability is increasing.

Causation   Most children with profound or severe learning disability have a diagnosable biological brain disorder. Forty per cent have a chromosome disorder (three quarters of whom have DOWN'S SYNDROME). A further 15 per cent have other genetic causes, brain malformations or recognizable syndromes. About 10 per cent suffered brain damage during pregnancy (e.g. from CYTOMEGALOVIRUS INFECTION). A similar proportion suffer post-natal brain damage from

head injury, accidental or not, near-miss cot death or drowning, cardiac arrest, brain infection (ENCEPHALITIS or MENINGITIS) or in association with severe seizure disorders.

Explanations for moderate learning disability include Fragile X or other CHROMOSOME abnormalities in a tenth, NEUROFIBROMATOSIS, fetal alcohol syndrome and other causes of intra-uterine growth retardation. Genetic counselling should be considered for children with learning disability. Prenatal diagnosis is sometimes possible.

Medical complications   EPILEPSY affects 1 in 20 with moderate, 1 in 3 with severe and 2 in 3 with profound learning disability, though only 1 in 50 with Down's syndrome is affected. One in 5 with severe or profound learning disability has CEREBRAL PALSY, many being difficult to feed in early years. Dental treatment is difficult also. Impairments of vision and/or hearing are common. Those with Down's syndrome are prone to heart and bowel malformations, thyroid insufficiency, GLUE EAR, MYELOID LEUKAEMIA and ALZHEIMER'S DISEASE.

Psychological and psychiatric needs   Over half of the people with profound or severe and many with moderate learning disability show psychiatric or behavioural problems, especially in early years or adolescence. Symptoms may be atypical and hard to assess. Psychiatric disorders include AUTISTIC BEHAVIOUR and schizophrenia (see MENTAL ILLNESS). Emotional problems include anxiety, dependence and depression. Behavioural problems include tantrums, hyperactivity, self-injury, passivity, masturbation in public and resistance to being shaved or helped with menstrual hygiene. There is greater vulnerability to abuse with its behavioural consequences.

Respite and care needs   Respite care is arranged with link families for children or staffed family homes for adults where possible. Responsibility for care lies with social services departments which can advise also about benefits.

Education   Special educational needs should be met in the least restrictive environment available to allow access to the national curriculum with appropriate modification and support. For older children with learning disability and for young children with severe or profound learning disability this may be in a special day or boarding school. Some children can be provided for in mainstream schools with extra classroom support. The 1993 Education Act lays down stages of assessment and support up to a written statement of special educational needs with annual reviews.

Pupils with learning disability are entitled to remain at school till aged 19 and most with severe or profound learning disability do so. Usually those with moderate learning disability move to further education after the age of 16.

Advice is available from the Mental Health Foundation, the British Institute of Learning Disabilities, Mencap (Royal Society for Mentally Handicapped Children and Adults), and the Scottish Society for the Mentally Handicapped (see APPENDIX 2: ADDRESSES).

LEBER'S DISEASE, or HEREDITARY OPTIC ATROPHY, is a hereditary disease in which blindness comes on at about the age of twenty.

LECITHIN A very complex fat found in various tissues of the body, but particularly in the brain and nerves, of which it forms a large part. It is also found in large quantities in the yolk of an egg.

LEECHES Animals belonging to the class Vermes, provided with suckers and living a semi-parasitic life, their food being mainly derived from the blood of other animals. They abstract blood by means of a sucker surrounding the mouth, which is provided with several large sharp teeth. Land leeches live in tropical forests and can attach themselves to a person's ankles and lower legs. Aquatic leeches are found in warm water and may attach themselves to swimmers. Their bites are painless, their saliva reducing the clotting properties of blood with hirundin. The result is that the wound continues to bleed after the leech has detached itself or been gently removed (lighted match, alcohol, salt and vinegar are effective removal agents). The medicinal leech, *Hirudo medicinalis*, was formerly employed for the abstraction of small quantities of blood in inflammatory and other conditions. Nowadays it is occasionally used to drain haematomas.

LEG This term is generally applied to the whole lower extremity but, properly speaking, includes that part between the knee and ankle joints. The lower limb is attached to the pelvic bones by strong muscles, especially the gluteal and hamstring muscles behind and the abductor muscles on the inner side of the thigh. The head of the femur, or thigh bone, lies in a deep cup-shaped hollow, the acetabulum, on the outer side of the pelvis. The femur, which is the longest and strongest bone in the body, forms at its lower end the joint of the knee with the tibia. The knee-joint is protected in front by the patella or knee-cap. Along the outer side of the tibia lies the smaller fibula, which does not extend up to the knee but which, along with the tibia, forms the ankle joint. The two prominences on the ankle (malleoli) are formed by the tibia on the inner side and the fibula on the outer side. Seven tarsal bones comprise the hinder part of the foot, of which the talus takes the weight of the body from the tibia and fibula. There are five metatarsal bones in the front portion of the foot and each toe has three phalangeal bones, excepting the great toe which has two. The powerful quadriceps extensor muscle in front of the thigh is attached to the knee-cap, which in turn is attached to the front of the tibia by the patellar ligament. This muscle straightens the knee and keeps the body in an erect posture. Below the knee the muscles of the calf, attached to the heel through the tendo calcaneus, or tendon of Achilles, raise the heel off the ground in walking. In front of and to the outside of the leg lie the tibial and peroneal muscles, which bend the ankle upwards and raise the toes. In the sole of the foot are a number of small muscles which bend the toes downwards. The arch of the foot is an important structure. (See FOOT.)

Most of the blood supply to the lower limb is carried by the femoral artery which, below the knee, divides into anterior and posterior tibial vessels. The blood returns from the leg partly by deep veins lying alongside the arteries, but to a large extent by the great saphenous vein which joins the FEMORAL vein in the GROIN.

The chief nerve in the lower limb is the sciatic nerve which runs down the middle of the back of the thigh deeply embedded in muscles. Above the knee it divides into two parts: the tibial and common peroneal nerves. (See also FOOT; FRACTURES; JOINTS; KNEE; LIMBS; VEINS.)

LEGIONNAIRE'S DISEASE A form of pneumonia due to a bacterium known as *Legionella pneumophila*. The bacterium is widely distributed in nature and is commonly found in surface water and soil. Legionellae are ubiquitous in water. Stationary water and sludge in water tanks provide favourable conditions for primary multiplication. Inhalation of water aerosols seems the most likely way that people acquire the disease. The organism is able to multiply at water outlets. Some rubber outlets in showers and taps are able to support the growth of legionellae so that high concentrations of the organism are released when the tap is first used in the morning. In the presence of the disease the treatment of infected water systems is essential by cleaning, chlorination or heating or a combination of all three.

The PNEUMONIA caused by legionnellae has no distinctive clinical or radiological features, so that the diagnosis is based on laboratory findings. This depends on the detection of antibodies by the indirect fluorescent antibody test. There is no evidence that the disease is transmitted directly from person to person. The predominant root of infection is by inhalation. The incubation period is two to ten days. The disease starts with aches and pains followed rapidly by a rise in temperature, shivering attacks, cough and shortness of breath. The X-ray tends to show patchy areas of consolidation in the lungs. The assessment of treatment is still hampered by the lack of proper clinical trials but it does seem that erythromycin and rifampicin are the most useful antibiotics. Rifampicin, however, should never be given alone because of the rapid development of drug resistance. In England in 1984 there were 151 cases reported and between 1985 and 1987 200 cases were reported each year. By the late 90s the number of cases reported had dropped to double figures.

LEG ULCER (see VENOUS ULCER).

LEIOMYOMA A benign tumour made up of unstriped or involuntary muscle fibres.

LEISHMANIASIS A group of infections caused by flagellate protozoan parasites of the genus Leishmania spp., transmitted to man by sandfly species of the genera Phlebotomus (Old World leishmaniasis) and Lutzomiya (New World leishmaniasis). The causative organism(s) was first visualized by Leishman and Donovan in 1903 and 1904 respectively.

Visceral leishmaniasis (kala-azar) A systemic infection caused by *Leishmania donovani* which occurs in tropical and subtropical Africa, Asia, the Mediterranean littoral (and some islands), and in tropical South America. Several mammals, including dogs, can act as zoonotic reservoirs of infection. In the Mediterranean region it is predominantly a disease of infants; in Africa, it occurs more commonly in adolescents and young adults. It constitutes an opportunistic infection in the presence of HIV (AIDS) infection. Onset is frequently insidious; incubation period is 2–6 months. Enlargement of spleen and liver may be gross; fever, anaemia, and generalized lymphadenopathy are usually present. Diagnosis is usually made from a bone-marrow specimen, splenic-aspirate, or liver-biopsy specimen; amastigotes (Leishman-Donovan bodies) of *L. donovani* can be visualized. Several serological tests are of value in diagnosis. Untreated, the infection is fatal within two years, in approximately 70 per cent of patients. Treatment traditionally involved sodium stibogluconate (a pentavalent antimonial compound). Other chemotherapeutic agents (including allupurinol, ketoconazole, and immunotherapy) are now in use, the most recently used being liposomal amphotericin B. Although immunointact persons usually respond satisfactorily, they usually relapse if they have HIV infection. Response to chemotherapy varies geographically, longer courses being required in India compared with the Mediterranean area.

Cutaneous leishmaniasis This form is caused by infection with *L. tropica, L. major, L. aethiopica*, and other species. The disease is widely distributed in the Mediterranean region, Middle East, Asia, Africa, Central and South America, and the former Soviet Union; it is less common than formerly in northern Australia. It is characterized by localized cutaneous ulcers – usually situated on exposed areas of the body. There is no visceral involvement. Diagnosis is by demonstration of the causative organism in a skin biopsy-specimen; the leishmanin skin test is of value. Most patients respond to sodium stibogluconate (see above); local heat therapy is also used. Recently, paromomycin cream has been successfully applied locally.

Mucocutaneous leishmaniasis This form is caused by *L. braziliensis* and rarely *L. mexicana*.

It is present in Central and South America, particularly the Amazon basin. It is characterized by highly destructive, ulcerative, granulomatous lesions of the skin and mucus membranes, especially involving the mucocutaneous junctions of the mouth, nasopharynx, genitalia, and rectum. Infection is usually via a superficial skin lesion at the site of a sandfly bite. However, spread is by haematogenous routes (usually after several years) to a mucocutaneous location. Diagnosis and treatment are the same as for cutaneous leishmaniasis.

LENS OF THE EYE (see EYE).

LENTIGO Lentigines are brown MACULES varying in diameter from 1 mm to 10mm or more. Simple lentigines arise in childhood, not necessarily on exposed areas. They may also occur on the lips and are harmless and usually very small. Solar or actinic lentigines are common on the face, neck and backs of the hands in older people and reflect the total cumulative lifetimes exposure to sunlight.

LEPROSY A chronic bacterial infection caused by *Mycobacterium leprae* affecting the skin, mucous membranes, and nerves. *M. leprae* (demonstrated by Hansen in Norway in 1873) is taxonomically related to *M. tuberculosis*; it also possesses an acid-fast staining reaction. Although widespread in northern Europe and other temperature areas in the past (in medieval times it was a major problem in England and Scandinavia), infection is now almost confined to tropical and subtropical countries, mostly in Africa and India. A suggestion is that underlying tuberculosis protects against leprosy, but the reverse is clearly supported in the published literature. There is no clear evidence that underlying HIV infection predisposes to the disease. There are two distinct (polarized) clinical forms: tuberculoid and lepromatous. The former usually takes a benign course and is frequently self-limiting, whereas the latter is relentlessly progressive; between these two polar forms lies an intermediate/dimorphous group. It is very unusual in childhood. Susceptibility may be increased by malnutrition. Nasal secretions (especially in lepromatous disease) are teeming with *M. leprae* and constitute the main source of infection; however, living in close proximity to an infected individual seems necessary for someone to contract the disease. *M. leprae* can also be transmitted in breast milk from an infected mother. Only a small minority of those exposed to *M. leprae* develop the disease; those in contact with a lepromatous case are far more likely to contract it than is the case with the tuberculoid form. The incubation period is three to five years or longer. The major clinical manifestations involve skin and nerves. The former range from depigmented, often anaesthetic areas, to massive nodules. Nerve involvement ranges from localized nerve swelling(s) to extensive areas of anaesthesia.

Advanced nerve destruction gives rise to severe deformities: foot-drop, wrist-drop, claw-foot, extensive ulceration of the extremities with loss of fingers and toes, and bone changes. Eye involvement can produce blindness. Laryngeal lesions produce hoarseness and more serious sequelae. Clinical manifestations vary in different ethnic groups; whereas European and Mongoloid groups frequently acquire the lepromatous form, this is less often so in Indian and African groups. The diagnosis is essentially a clinical one; however, skin-smears, histological features and the lepromin skin-test help to confirm the diagnosis and to enable the form of disease to be graded. Introduction of the sulphone compound, dapsone, revolutionized management of the disease. More recently, rifampicin and clofazimine, have been added as first-line drugs for treatment. Second-line drugs include minocycline, ofloxacin and clarithromycin; a number of regimens incorporating several of these compounds (multi-drug regimens – introduced in 1982) are now widely used. A three-drug regime is recommended for multibacillary leprosy and a two-drug one for parcibacillary leprosy. Dapsone resistance is a major problem worldwide, but occurs less commonly when multi-drug regimens are used. Older compounds – ethionamide and prothionamide – are no longer used because they are severely toxic to the liver. Corticosteroids are sometimes required in patients with 'reversal reaction'. Supportive therapy includes physiotherapy; both plastic and orthopaedic surgery may be necessary in advanced stages of the disease. Improvement in socio-economic conditions, and widespread use of BCG vaccination are of value as preventive strategies. Early diagnosis and prompt institution of chemotherapy should prevent long-term complications. The WHO objective is to eliminate the infection as a public health problem by the year 2000, a challenging target. Attempts are being made to produce a vaccine against leprosy.

LEPTOMENINGITIS Inflammation of the inner and more delicate membranes of the brain or spinal cord.

LEPTOSPIRA A group, or genus, of spiral micro-organisms, normally found in rodents and other small mammals in which they cause no harm. When transmitted to man by these animals, either directly or indirectly as through cows, they give rise to various forms of illness.

LEPTOSPIROSIS The disease caused by infection with Leptospira. The three most common members of this group in the United Kingdom are *L. icterohaemorrhagiae*, *L. canicola*, and *L. hebiomadis*. It is an occupational hazard of farmers, sewage and abattoir workers, fish cutters and veterinary surgeons, but the infection can also be acquired from bathing in contaminated water. The disease varies in intensity from a mild influenza-like illness to a fatal form of jaundice due to severe liver disease. The kidneys are often involved and there may be meningitis. Penicillin or tetracycline are the usual treatment but unless they are given early in the disease their effect is limited.

Spirochaetosis icterohaemorrhagica, or Weil's disease, is the term applied to infection with the *Leptospira icterohaemorrhagiae* which is transmitted to man by rats, these animals excreting the organism in their urine; hence the liability of sewer workers to the disease. The condition is characterized by fever, jaundice, enlarged liver, nephritis, and bleeding from mucous membranes.

LESBIAN A female HOMOSEXUAL; lesbianism is a condition in which a woman is sexually attracted to another woman. Lesbians form about 2 per cent of the female population in the UK. Some engage in active sexual behaviour with another woman, with MASTURBATION, mutual stimulation of the clitoris and oral sex being the usual techniques for achieving ORGASM.

LESION meant originally an injury, but is now applied generally to all disease changes in organs and tissues.

LETHARGY or LASSITUDE means a loss of energy. It is a common presenting complaint to both the general practitioner and hospital consultant. It may have a physical cause or a psychological cause. It may be the result of inadequate rest, environmental noise, boredom, insomnia or recent illness. It may be the result of medicinal drugs, the most common of which are beta-blockers and diuretics. Drugs of abuse may also be a cause (see ADDICTION). The common psycho-social problems producing lethargy are depression and anxiety. If the patient with lethargy runs a fever the differential diagnosis is that of a PUO (Pyrexia of unknown origin). Many patients with fatigue can establish the onset of the symptom to a febrile illness even though they no longer run a fever. The lethargy that follows glandular fever and other viral infections is well recognized. Some of these patients have a true depressive illness and their presentation and response to treatment is little different to sufferers from any other depressive illness. MYALGIC ENCEPHALOMYELITIS (ME) or chronic fatigue syndrome is another disorder associated with lethargy and tiredness. Organic causes of lethargy include anaemia, malnutrition, hypothyroidism, uraemia, alcoholism and diabetes mellitus.

LEUCINE One of the essential, or indispensable, AMINO-ACIDS. They are so called because they cannot be synthesized, or manufactured, in the body, and are therefore essential constituents of the diet.

LEUCO- (or LEUKO-) A prefix meaning white.

LEUCOCYTE The scientific name for white blood cells. Leucocytes differ from ERYTHRO-CYTES (red blood cells) in that they contain no haemoglobin and are therefore colourless, and contain a well- formed nucleus. Most of them are larger than erythrocytes, being 8 to 15 micrometres in diameter, and there are many fewer in the blood – usually about 8000 per cubic millimetre of blood. There are three main classes of white cells: granulocytes, lymphocytes, and monocytes.

Granulocytes, or polymorphonuclear leucocytes as they are sometimes termed, which normally constitute 70 per cent of the white blood cells, have a lobed nucleus and a granular cytoplasm. They are divided into three groups according to the staining reactions of these granules: neutrophils, which stain with neutral dyes and constitute 65 to 70 per cent of all the white blood cells; eosinophils, which stain with acid dyes (e.g. eosin) and constitute 3 to 4 per cent of the total white blood cells; and basophils, which stain with basic dyes (e.g. methylene blue) and constitute about 0·5 per cent of the total white blood cells.

Lymphocytes, which constitute 25 to 30 per cent of the white blood cells, have a clear non-granular cytoplasm and a relatively large nucleus which is only slightly indented. They are divided into two groups: small lymphocytes which are slightly larger than erythrocytes (about 8 micrometres in diameter); large lymphocytes, which are about 12 micrometres in diameter.

Monocytes, which constitute about 5 per cent of the white blood cells, are 10 to 15 micrometres in diameter and differ from lymphocytes in having a rather smaller nucleus which tends to be more indented and to be placed more eccentrically. Monocytes are motile phagocytic cells that circulate in the blood and migrate into the tissues where they develop into various forms of macrophages such as tissue MACROPHAGES and KUPFFER CELLS. They remove micro-organisms from the body and identify and present antigenic material to lymphocytes. The cytoplasm is non-granular. (See illustration, BLOOD.)

SITE OF ORIGIN The granulocytes are formed in the red bone marrow. The lymphocytes are formed predominantly in lymphoid tissue. There is some controversy as to the site of origin of monocytes: some say they arise from lymphocytes, whilst others contend that they are derived from histiocytes: i.e. the RETICULO-ENDOTHELIAL SYSTEM.

FUNCTION The leucocytes constitute one of the most important of the defence mechanisms against infection. This applies particularly to the neutrophil leucocytes. (See LEUCOCYTOSIS.) (See also ABSCESS; BLOOD; INFLAMMATION; PHAGO-CYTOSIS; WOUNDS.)

LEUCOCYTOSIS A temporary condition in which the polymorphonuclear LEUCOCYTES in the blood are increased in number. It occurs in many different circumstances, and forms a valuable means of diagnosis in certain diseases. It may occur, however, as a normal reaction in certain conditions: e.g. pregnancy, menstruation, and during muscular exercise. Apart from these conditions, leucocytosis is usually due to the presence of inflammatory processes. It is part of the body's defence mechanism against infection with micro-organisms, the purpose of the increase in the number of leucocytes being to help to destroy the invading bacteria. Thus, during many acute infective diseases, such as pneumonia, the number is greatly increased. In all suppurative conditions there is also a leucocytosis, and if it seems that an abscess is forming deep in the abdomen, or in some other site where it cannot be readily examined, as, for example, an abscess resulting from appendicitis, the examination of a drop of blood gives a valuable aid in the diagnosis, and may be sufficient, in the absence of other signs, to point out the urgent need of an operation. TYPHOID FEVER constitutes the major exception to the statement that acute infective diseases show this increase of white cells in the blood, and, accordingly, in the case of this disease, the presence of an increase is a specially reliable sign of abscess formation, or other severe complication.

Other infective conditions in which a leucocytosis does not occur include measles and influenza.

LEUCODERMA, or LEUCODERMIA, is a condition of the skin in which areas of it become white, as the result of various skin diseases.

LEUCOPENIA A condition in which the white corpuscles of the blood are greatly reduced in numbers.

LEUCOPLAKIA (see LEUKOPLAKIA).

LEUCORRHOEA Discharge of mucus from the VAGINA. It may be whitish or yellowish and is normal in some women, usually increasing before and after menstruation. Oral contraceptives may increase or diminish the amount of discharge, as does sexual stimulation. Abnormal discharges are excessive in amount with an offensive smell and yellow or green colouring. They may be caused by micro-organisms or by fungal infection such as *Candida albicans*. Another causative agent is the protozoan parasite, *Trichomonas vaginalis* (see TRICHOMONIASIS). A pessary or tampon that a woman has forgotten to remove will cause a substantial and offensive discharge. Treatment depends on the cause, with an antibiotic or antifungal drug used as required. Children rarely have vaginal discharge; if they do, it is usually due to an infection or foreign body in the vagina. (See also UTERUS, DISEASES OF.)

LEUCOTOMY (see PSYCHOSURGERY).

LEUKAEMIA, or LEUCOCYTHAEMIA, is a malignant disorder of white blood cells which proliferate in a disorganized manner. The disease is also characterized by great enlargement of the SPLEEN, changes in the marrow of the bones, and by enlargement of the LYMPH glands all over the body. The condition may be either acute or chronic. According to the type of corpuscles chiefly present the acute form is called acute lymphoblastic leukaemia, or acute myeloid leukaemia. The names for the corresponding chronic forms of the disease are chronic lymphatic leukaemia, and chronic myeloid leukaemia. Acute lymphoblastic leukaemia is most common in the first five years of life, and rare after the age of 25. Acute myeloid leukaemia is most common in children and young adults, but may occur at any age. Chronic lymphatic leukaemia occurs at any age between 35 and 80, most commonly in the 60s, and is twice as common in men as in women. Chronic myeloid leukaemia is rare before the age of 25, and most common between 30 and 65. Men and women are equally affected. About 2,500 patients with acute leukaemia are diagnosed in the United Kingdom, with a similar number annually diagnosed with chronic leukaemia; around 3,500 die from two varieties.

Cause Both types of acute leukaemia seem to arise from a MUTATION in a single white cell. The genetically changed cell then goes through an uncontrolled succession of divisions resulting in many millions of abnormal white cells in the blood, bone marrow and other tissues. Possible causes are virus infection, chemical exposure, radiation and genetic background. The cause of chronic lymphocytic leukaemia is not known; the chronic myeloid version may have a genetic background.

Symptoms In the acute cases the patient shows pallor, occasional purpuric rash, and enlargement of the lymphatic glands and spleen. The temperature is raised, and the condition may be mistaken for an acute infection. Such cases usually run a rapid course, lasting a few weeks or months. In the chronic type of the disease the onset is gradual, and the first symptoms which occasion discomfort are either swelling of the abdomen and shortness of breath, due to painless enlargement of the spleen, or the enlargement of glands in the neck, armpits and elsewhere, or the pallor, palpitation, and other symptoms of anaemia which often accompany leukaemia. Occasional bleeding from the nose, stomach, gums, or bowels may occur, and may be severe. Generally, there is a slight fever. When the blood is examined microscopically, not only is there an enormous increase of the white cells, which may be multiplied thirty- or sixty-fold, but various immature forms are found. In the lymphatic form of the disease most white cells resemble lymphocytes, which, in healthy blood, are present only in small numbers. In the myeloid form, myelocytes, or large immature cells from the bone-marrow, which are never present in healthy blood, appear in large numbers, and there may also be large numbers of immature, nucleated erythrocytes.

Although there is still no guaranteed cure, the outlook in both acute and chronic leukaemia has greatly improved, particularly for the acute form of the disease. Thus, in those with acute lymphoblastic leukaemia, which accounts for around 85 per cent of all childhood leukaemias, the overall survival rate may be as high as 60 per cent, with the chance of inducing a remission reaching 90 per cent. The results in acute myeloid leukaemia are not as good. In the case of chronic lymphatic leukaemia the average period from the time of diagnosis to death is around six years, although quite a number of patients, particularly the elderly, survive for ten years or more. In chronic myeloid leukaemia the average survival time is around three to four years, with 20 per cent surviving for more than five years.

Treatment Promising results are being obtained in the control of the disease using blood transfusions, CHEMOTHERAPY, RADIOTHERAPY and bone-marrow TRANSPLANTATION. In the case of acute leukaemia the drugs now being used include MERCAPTOPURINE, METHOTREXATE, CYCLOPHOSPHAMIDE, and VINCRISTINE. But CORTISONE and its derivatives sometimes produce dramatic temporary improvement. Blood transfusion plays an important part in controlling the condition during the period before the response to chemotherapy or hormone therapy can be expected. Chemotherapy has almost completely replaced radiotherapy in the treatment of chronic leukaemia. For the myeloid form BUSULPHAN is the most widely used drug, replaced by hydroxyurea, mercaptopurine, or one of the NITROGEN MUSTARD DERIVATIVES in the later stages of the disease. For the lymphatic form the drugs used are CHLORAMBUCIL, CYCLOPHOSPHAMIDE, and the nitrogen mustard derivatives.

Prognosis Between 50 and 60 per cent of patients with acute lymphoblastic leukaemia may be cured; between 20 and 50 per cent of those with acute myeloid leukaemia have much improved survival rates. Prognosis of patients with chronic lymphocytic leukaemia is often good, depending on early diagnosis.

LEUKO- (see LEUCO-).

LEUKOPLAKIA A white plaque on mucous membranes caused by overgrowth of the tissues. It is occasionally a precancerous condition.

LEUKOTRIENES A group of naturally occurring slow-reacting substances (SRSS) which have powerful smooth-muscle stimulating properties, particularly on bronchial smooth muscle. Leukotrienes are a metabolic derivative of PROSTAGLANDINS.

LEVALLORPHAN TARTRATE is an antidote to morphine. It is usually given intravenously.

LEVAMISOLE is a drug that is used to treat ASCARIASIS. Its main advantage seems to be in mass treatment as one dose may prove effective. It is also being used in the treatment of a group of diseases of obscure origin including CROHN'S DISEASE and rheumatoid arthritis. The drug is unavailable in the UK.

LEVATOR (1) Any muscle that raises the organ or structure into which it is inserted. (2) A surgical instrument for raising depressed fragments of bone in a fracture, particularly a fracture of the skull.

LEVODOPA A drug used in the treatment of PARKINSON'S DISEASE. It is converted to dopamine in the brain, correcting the deficiency which causes the disorder. Levodopa is often given with carbidopa or benserazide, both dopamine decarboxylase inhibitors, to prevent its conversion to DOPAMINE in the body before it reaches the brain. It may cause nausea, HYPOTENSION or cardiac dysrhythmias.

LEVORPHANOL A synthetic derivative of morphine. It is an effective analgesic but, like morphine, is a drug of addiction.

LIBIDO The natural desire for sexual intercourse. Lack of desire or diminished libido may occur in any general medical illness as well as in endocrine diseases when there is a lack of production of the sex hormones. The strength or weakness of the sexual drive may be associated with psychiatric diseases; it may also be the result of certain drugs. It must be distinguished from impotence, where the desire for intercourse is normal but the performance is defective due to the inability to achieve or maintain an erection.

LIBRIUM (see CHLORDIAZEPOXIDE).

LICE (see INSECTS IN RELATION TO DISEASE; PEDICULOSIS).

LICHEN (LICHENIFICATION) is a term used to describe a thickening of chronically inflamed skin to give a bark-like appearance.

Lichen simplex (neurodermatitis) is a form of eczema perpetuated by constant rubbing of the affected skin. Typically, well-defined plaques occur on one or both sides of the nape of the neck, on the ulnar forearm near the elbow, or on the sides of the calves. It is often associated with emotional stress.

Lichen planus is a less common inflammation of the skin characterized by small shiny flat-topped violaceous PAPULES which may coalesce to form large PLAQUES. Itching can be intense. Typically seen on the flexor aspects of the wrists, the lower back and on the legs below the knees, it may also affect the mucous mem-

branes of the mouth and lips. The cause is unknown. While in some patients the disorder appears to be nervous or emotional in origin, it can be caused by certain drugs such as gold a CHLOROQUINE. Severe cases may require oral CORTICOSTEROIDS to control the eruption.

LIFE EXPECTANCY The number of years an individual can expect to live. Life expectancy at birth in most Western countries is around 75 years for women and 70 for men, a figure that has been steadily rising as living standards have improved. The longer a person lives, the greater is his or her life expectancy. A 70-year-old may live a further 15 years.

LIGAMENTS Strong bands of fibrous tissue which serve to bind together the bones entering into a joint. They are, in some cases, cord-like, in others flattened bands, whilst most joints are surrounded by a fibrous capsule or capsular ligament. (See JOINTS.)

LIGATION Tying off – for example, a blood vessel – by completely encircling it with a tight band usually of catgut or some other suture material.

LIGATURE A cord or thread used to tie round arteries in order to stop the circulation through them, or to prevent escape of blood from their cut ends. Ligatures are generally made of catgut or silk, and are tied with a reef-knot.

LIGHT REFLEX Pupillary constriction in the eye in response to light. The direct light reflex involves pupillary constriction in the eye into which a light is shone; the consensual light reflex is the pupillary constriction that occurs in the other eye. The afferent or inward pathway of the reflex is via the optic nerve (see EYE) and the efferent or outward pathway is via the occulomotor nerve.

LIGHTNING INJURIES These are not uncommon – it is estimated that lightning strikes somewhere on the earth an average of 100 times a second, but the majority of those struck by lightning recover. A direct hit, however, means instantaneous death, with the clothes torn off, and the victim may be hurled quite a long distance. Even the individual who recovers has usually fallen unconscious the moment he is struck. Those who are a little farther away experience tingling of the skin and their hair may stand on end.

Preventive measures indoors during a lightning storm consist of keeping away from the fireplace, the main electrical switch, the bathroom, the kitchen sink and the television aerial. It is perfectly safe to use the telephone. Out of doors, solitary trees, walls, wire fences and other metallic structures, ponds and river banks should be avoided. So also should flat open spaces, such as golf courses, where an individual may form the highest point. To use a metal-tipped umbrella or a golf club is potentially dangerous. There is no risk inside a vehicle. In a severe storm the safest thing is to lie down in a ditch. In Britain, there are around 10 deaths a year from lightning strikes.

Treatment of an individual struck by lightning consists of artificial respiration, which may need to be prolonged for several hours. (See APPENDIX 1: BASIC FIRST AID.)

LIGNOCAINE A local anaesthetic. It is also used in the treatment of certain disorders of cardiac rhythm known as ventricular arrhythmias which may be particularly dangerous following a CORONARY THROMBOSIS.

LIMBS, ARTIFICIAL (see PROSTHESES).

LIMBIC SYSTEM A circular complex system of nerve pathways in the middle of the brain. This connected cluster of neuronal nuclei is involved in the working of the AUTONOMIC system, helping to control the expression of instinct and mood in activities of the motor systems and the endocrine glands of the body. The brain regions involved include the amygdala (an almond-shaped basal ganglion deep in each cerebral hemisphere (see BRAIN)) and the HYPOTHALAMUS. If the limbic system is impaired by injury or disease, the person may suffer abnormal emotional responses such as unprovoked rage, unreasonable fear and anxiety, depression, greater than normal sexual interest and crying or laughing for no good reason.

LIMB LENGTHENING An orthopaedic procedure in which the length of a limb, usually a leg, is increased. The bone is surgically divided and slowly stretched in a special frame. The operation is usually done on people with unequal leg lengths as a result of injury or from PARALYSIS in childhood. Exceptionally, it may be done in both legs to help people of short stature.

LIMBS Outgrowths from the sides of the body, which, in man as in all the higher animals, number four. The limbs of all the higher animals, though differing much in outward appearance, are constructed on a similar plan, modified to suit the requirements of the owner, the fore-limb, for example, developing in birds into a wing, in seals into a flipper. In all, however, the various muscles, bones, and blood-vessels, though differing in size and shape, correspond in arrangement. The bones, muscles, and main arteries of the arm, forearm, and hand have all representatives in the thigh, leg, and foot. (See ARM; LEG.)

In structure, each limb consists of four segments, the shoulder, arm, forearm, and hand in the case of the upper limb, corresponding to the haunch, thigh, leg and foot in the lower limb.

The diseases affecting the limbs are those of the skin, muscles, bones, etc., forming them. (For injuries of the limbs see FRACTURES; HAEMORRHAGE; JOINTS, DISEASES AND INJURIES OF; WOUNDS.)

LIME-JUICE A yellow liquid obtained by squeezing lime-fruit, *Citrus limetta*. In common with lemon-juice, it is a rich source of vitamin C (16·8 to 62·5 mg per 100 ml) and contains a large quantity of citric acid. It is used as a refreshing drink and as a preventive of, and remedy for, SCURVY. Lime-juice which has been boiled, or preserved for a prolonged period, loses its anti-scorbutic properties.

LINCTUS A term applied to any thick syrupy medicine. Most of these are remedies for excessive coughing.

LINDANE An insecticide effective in scabies and lice infestations; however, head lice are now often resistant (see INSECTS IN RELATION TO DISEASE). Used excessively, it may be neurotoxic.

LINEA ALBA is the line of fibrous tissue stretching down the mid-line of the belly from the lower end of the sternum to the pubic bone (see PUBIS). The linea alba gives attachment to the muscles of the belly wall.

LINEA NIGRA During pregnancy the LINEA ALBA becomes pigmented and appears as a dark line down the middle of the belly, and is called the linea nigra.

LINEAR ACCELERATOR (see RADIOTHERAPY).

LINGUAL Referring or related to the tongue: e.g. the lingual nerve supplied sensation to the tongue.

LINIMENTS, or EMBROCATIONS, are oily mixtures intended for external application by rubbing. Their chief use is in the production of pain relief, particularly in rheumatic conditions. They may be highly toxic if taken orally – a particular danger with children.

LINT This was originally made of teased-out linen; now it consists of a loose cotton fabric, one side of which is fluffy, the other being smooth and applied next to the skin when the surface is broken. Marine lint consists of tow impregnated with tar, and is used where large quantities of some absorbent and deodorizing dressing are required. Cotton lint is impregnated with various substances, the most common being boracic lint. Lint containing perchloride of iron (15 per cent) is valuable as a styptic.

LIPAEMIA The presence of an excessive amount of fat in the blood.

LIPASE An enzyme widely distributed in plants, and present also in the liver and gastric and pancreatic juices, which breaks down fats to the constituent fatty acids and glycerol.

LIPID A substance which is insoluble in water, but soluble in fat solvents such as alcohol and ether. The main lipid groups are the triglycerides, phospholipids, and glycolipids. They play an important role in nutrition, health (particularly in the functioning of the cell membranes, and the immune response), and disease (notably cardiovascular disease). There is a strong correlation between the concentration of CHOLESTEROL in the blood (transported as lipoproteins) and the risk of developing ATHEROMA and coronary heart disease (see HEART DISEASES). Lipoproteins are classified by their density and mobility, the chief groups being low-density (LDL) and high-density (HDL). High serum concentrations of LDL increase the risk of cardiovascular disease, while HDL is though to protect the vessel wall by removing cholesterol, and has an inverse relationship to risk. The various serum lipid abnormalities have been classified into five groups, according to the cause and particular lipoprotein raised. Most important are type II (increased LDL, genetically determined) and type IV (increased VLDL, associated with obesity, diabetes, and excess alcohol). Various lipid-lowering drugs are available, such as CHOLESTYRAMINE and CLOFIBRATE, but any drug treatment must be combined with a strict diet, reduction of blood pressure, and cessation of smoking.

LIPIDOSIS Any disorder of lipid metabolism in body cells. Some hereditary disorders cause deposition of lipids within the brain.

LIPODYSTROPHY A congenital mal-Edistribution of fat tissue. Subcutaneous fat is totally absent from a portion of the body and hypertrophied in the remainder. Another form of lipodystrophy occurs at the site of INSULIN injections. These are much less frequently seen nowadays as the new synthetic preparations of insulin are pure and unlikely to cause this reaction which was not uncommon with the older preparations. Occasionally the converse occurs at the site of insulin injections where the lipogenic action of insulin stimulates the fat cells to hypertrophy. This can also be disfiguring and usually results from using the same site for injections too frequently.

LIPOLYSIS The enzymatic breaking down of fat.

LIPOMA A tumour mainly composed of fat. Such tumours arise in almost any part of the body, developing in fibrous tissues, particularly in that beneath the skin. They are simple in nature, and seldom give any trouble beyond that connected with their size and position. (See TUMOUR.)

LIPOSARCOMA A malignant tumour of adipose or fatty tissue. It occurs most frequently in the thighs, buttocks or retroperitoneum. The four main types are: well differentiated, myxoid, round cell and pleomorphic (variety of forms).

LIPOSOMES These are essentially tiny oil droplets consisting of layers of fatty material known as phospholipid separated by aqueous compartments. Drugs can be incorporated into the liposomes, which are then injected into the bloodstream or into the muscles, or given by mouth. Using this method of giving drugs, it is possible to protect them from being broken down in the body before they reach the part of the body where their curative effect is required: for example, in the liver or in a tumour.

LIPS These form a pair of curtains before the mouth, each composed of a layer of skin and of mucous membrane, between which lies a considerable amount of fat and of muscle fibres.

The diseases to which the lips are liable are not numerous.

Fissures, coming on in cold weather, form a troublesome condition often difficult to get rid of. Such peeling and cracking of the vermilion of the lips is common in those exposed for long periods to wind and sunlight. Treatment consists of the application of aqueous cream. If the main cause is excessive exposure to sunlight, in which case the lower lip is mainly affected, the best application is mexenone cream.

Herpes, in the form of what are known as 'cold sores', often develops on the lip as a result of a cold or other feverish condition, but quickly passes off. (See HERPES.)

Ulcers may form on the inner surface of the lip, usually in consequence of bad teeth or of dyspepsia.

Small cysts sometimes form on the inner surface of the lip, and are seen as little bluish swellings filled with mucus; they are of no importance.

Hare-lip is a deformity sometimes present at birth. (See PALATE, MALFORMATIONS OF.)

Cancer of the lip sometimes occurs, almost always in men, and usually on the lower lip. (See also MOUTH, DISEASES OF.)

LIQUOR (see SOLUTION).

LIQUORICE The root of *Glycyrrhiza glabra*, a plant of southern Europe and Asia. It is a mild expectorant, but is mainly used to cover the taste of disagreeable and more powerful drugs. Solid and liquid extracts are made from it, but the most commonly used preparation is compound liquorice powder, which contains also senna and sulphur.

LISTERIOSIS A rare disease, although the causal organism, *Listeria monocytogenes*, is widely distributed in soil, silage, water, and various animals, with consequent risk of food contamination. Neonates are the main age group affected – often as a result of a mild or inapparent infection in the pregnant mother. The disease presents in two main forms: MENINGO-ENCEPHALITIS, or SEPTICAEMIA with enlarged lymph glands. Elderly adults occasionally develop the first form, while younger adults are more likely to develop a mild or even inapparent form. The disease generally responds well to antibiotics such as AMPICILLIN or CHLORAMPHENICOL; nevertheless, the incidence rose over the past decade but seems to have levelled out at around 100 a year.

LITHIASIS A general name applied to the formation of calculi and concretions in tissues or organs: e.g. cholelithiasis means the formation of calculi in the gall-bladder.

LITHIUM CARBONATE A drug widely used in the prophylaxis treatment of certain forms of mental illness. The drug should be given only on specialist advice. The major indication for its use is acute mania. It induces improvement or remission in over 70 per cent of such patients. In addition, it is effective in the treatment of manic-depressive patients, preventing both the manic and the depressive episodes. There is also evidence that it lessens aggression in prisoners who behave antisocially and in patients with learning difficulties who mutilate themselves and have temper tantrums. It is not recommended for children. Because of its possible toxic effects – including kidney damage –it is a drug that must only be administered under medical supervision and with monitoring of the blood levels as the gap between therapeutic and toxic concentrations is narrow. Because of the risk of its damaging the unborn child, it should not be prescribed, unless absolutely necessary, during pregnancy, particularly in the first three months. Mothers should not take it while breast feeding as it is excreted in the milk in high concentrations. The drug should not be taken with diuretics.

LITHOLAPAXY is the term applied to the operation in which a stone in the bladder is crushed by an instrument introduced along the urethra, and the fragments washed out through a catheter.

LITHOTOMY The operation of cutting for stone in the bladder. The operation is of great historic interest, because more has probably been written about it in early times than about any other type of surgery, and because, for long, it formed almost the only operation in which the surgeon dared to attack diseases of the internal organs.

LITHOTRIPSY Extracorporeal shock-wave lithotripsy (ESWL) causes disintegration of renal and biliary stones (see CALCULI) without physical without contact and is therefore an attractive procedure for patients and surgeons. Stones in the upper urinary tract are a common condition in the United Kingdom causing considerable morbidity and requiring large and lengthy operations with an extensive convalescent period. Percutaneous renal surgery has changed this picture but it requires at least puncture of the kidney and possibly open nephrolithotomy for large branched calculi. Extracorporeal shock-wave lithotripsy causes disintegration of the stone without contact and is therefore a far more attractive procedure.

The generation of shock waves as a form of treatment for urinary calculi was first described in 1955 by the Russian engineer Yutkin. Shock waves generated outside the body can be accurately focused with a reflector whilst the patient is suspended in water to facilitate transmission of the waves. These are focused on the calculus. The resultant fine fragments are passed spontaneously in the urine with minimal, if any, discomfort. The procedure has been shown to be safe, short and effective and is most acceptable to patients.

LITMUS, which is prepared from several lichens, is a vegetable dye-substance, which on contact with alkaline fluids becomes blue, and on contact with acid fluids, red. Slips of paper, impregnated with litmus, form a valuable test for the acidity of the secretions and discharges.

LITTLE'S DISEASE is a form of cerebral palsy. (See CEREBRAL PALSY.)

LIVER The liver is the largest gland in the body, serving numerous functions, chiefly involving various aspects of metabolism.

Form The liver is divided into four lobes, the greatest part being the right lobe, with a small left lobe, while the quadrate and caudate lobes are two small divisions on the back and under surface. Around the middle of the under surface, towards the back, a transverse fissure, the porta hepatis, is placed, by which the hepatic artery and portal vein carry blood into the liver, and the right and left hepatic ducts emerge, carrying off the bile formed in the liver to the gall-bladder attached under the right lobe, where it is stored.

Position Occupying the right hand upper part of the abdominal cavity four-fifths of the organ lie to the right of the midline of the body. Above, it is separated from the right lung by just the DIAPHRAGM and PLEURAL membrane,

1 liver
2 gall-bladder
3 ampulla of Vater (leading into duodenum)
4 hepatic ducts
5 bile duct
6 common bile duct

Positions of liver, gall-bladder and connecting
bile-ducts.

while the liver rests on various abdominal organs: chiefly the right KIDNEY and SUPRA-RENAL GLAND, the large INTESTINE, DUODENUM, and STOMACH.

Size The adult liver weighs more than 1.5 kg, varying with the size of the individual. It is relatively larger in young children, making up about one-eighteenth of the total body weight and contributing to their protuberant abdomen.

Vessels The blood supply differs from that of the rest of the body, in that the blood collected from the stomach and bowels into the PORTAL VEIN does not pass directly to the heart, but is first distributed to the liver, where it breaks up into capillary vessels. As a result, some harmful substances are filtered from the blood stream and destroyed, while various constituents of the food are stored in the liver for use in the body's metabolic processes. The liver also receives the large HEPATIC artery from the coeliac axis. After circulating through capillaries, the blood from both sources is collected into the hepatic veins, which pass directly from the back surface of the liver into the inferior vena cava.

Minute structure The liver is enveloped in a capsule of fibrous tissue – Glisson's capsule – from which strands run along the vessels and penetrate deep into the organ, binding it together. Subdivisions of the hepatic artery, portal vein, and bile duct lie alongside each other, finally forming the interlobular vessels, which lie between the lobules of which the whole gland is built up. Each is about the size of a pin's head and forms a complete secreting unit; the liver is built up of hundreds of

thousands of such lobules. These contain small vessels, capillaries, or sinusoids, lined with stellate KUPFFER CELLS, which run into the centre of the lobule, where they empty into a small central vein. These lobular veins ultimately empty into the hepatic veins. Between these capillaries lie rows of large liver cells in which metabolic activity occurs. Fine bile capillaries collect the bile from the cells and discharge it into the bile ducts lying along the margins of the lobules. Liver cells are among the largest in the body, each containing one or two large round nuclei. The cells frequently contain droplets of fat or granules of GLYCO-GEN, that is animal starch.

Functions The liver is, in effect, a large chemical factory and the heat this produces contributes to the general warming of the body. The liver secretes BILE, chief constituents of which are the bile salts (sodium glycocholate and taurocholate), the bile pigments (BILIRUBIN and BILIVER-DIN), CHOLESTEROL, and LECITHIN. These bile salts are collected and formed in the liver and are eventually converted into the bile acids. The bile pigments are the iron-free and globin-free remnant of haemoglobin, formed in the Kupffer cells of the liver. (They can also be formed in the spleen, lymph glands, bone marrow and connective tissues.) Bile therefore serves several purposes. It excretes pigment, the breakdown products of old red blood cells. The bile salts by increasing fat absorption and activating pancreatic lipase thus aid the digestion of fat. Bile is necessary for the absorption of vitamins D and E.

The other important functions of the liver are as follows:
- In the embryo it forms red blood cells, while the adult liver stores vitamin B₁₂, necessary for the proper functioning of the bone marrow in the manufacture of red cells.
- It manufactures FIBRINOGEN, ALBUMIN, and GLOBULIN from the blood.
- It stores IRON and copper, necessary for the manufacture of red cells.
- It produces HEPARIN, and with the aid of VITAMIN K, PROTHROMBIN.
- Its Kupffer cells form an important part of the RETICULO-ENDOTHELIAL system, which breaks down red cells, and probably manufactures ANTIBODIES.
- Noxious products made in the intestine and absorbed into the blood are detoxicated in the liver.
- It stores carbohydrate in the form of glycogen, maintaining a two-way process: glucose ⇆ glycogen.
- CAROTENE forms vitamin A, and B vitamins are stored.
- It splits up aminoacids and manufactures urea and uric acids.
- It plays an essential role in the storage and metabolism of fat.

LIVER DISEASES The liver may be extensively diseased without any obviously serious symptoms, unless the circulation through it is impeded, the outflow of bile checked, or neighbouring organs implicated. JAUNDICE, which is a symptom of several liver disorders, is dealt with elsewhere. ASCITES, which may be caused by interference with the circulation through the portal vein of the liver, as well as by other causes, is also considered separately. The presence of gall-stones is a complication of some diseases connected with the liver, and is treated under GALL-BLADDER, DISEASES OF. For hydatid cyst of the liver see TAENIASIS. Liver diseases in a tropical environment are dealt with later in this section.

Inflammation of the liver, or HEPATITIS, may occur as part of a generalized infection or may be a localized condition. Infectious hepatitis, which is the result of infection with a virus, is one of the most common forms of hepatitis. (See HEPATITIS.) There are many other viruses that can cause hepatitis, including that responsible for GLANDULAR FEVER. Certain spirochaetes may also be the cause, particularly that responsible for LEPTOSPIROSIS, as can many drugs. Hepatitis may also occur if there is obstruction of the bile duct, as by a gall-stone.

Cirrhosis of the liver A disorder caused by chronic damage to liver cells. The mechanism is still unclear. The liver develops areas of fibrosis or scarring and in response the remaining normal liver cells increase and form regeneration nodules. Those islands of normality, however, suffer from inadequate blood supply, thus adversely affecting liver function. Experimentally it has been shown that the condition can be produced by a deficiency of certain of the amino-acids found in protein, but this only explains a small proportion of the cases found in man. It is probable that three factors are involved: a nutritional deficiency, a toxic factor, and an infective factor. More than one factor may be at work in an individual with cirrhosis. Alcohol is the most common cause of cirrhosis in the United Kingdom and the USA. In Africa and many parts of Asia, infection with hepatitis B virus is a common cause. Certain drugs, for example, paracetamol, may damage the liver if taken in excess. Unusual causes of cirrhosis include defects of the BILE DUCTS, HAEMOCHROMATOSIS (raised iron absorption from the gut), CYSTIC FIBROSIS, cardiac cirrhosis (the result of heart failure causing circulatory congestion in the liver), and WILSON'S DISEASE (raised copper absorption).

SYMPTOMS Some people with cirrhosis exhibit no signs or symptoms and the disease may be diagnosed at a routine medical examination. Others may develop JAUNDICE, OEDEMA (including ascites, fluid in the abdomen), fever, confusion, HAEMATEMESIS (vomiting blood), loss of appetite and lethargy. On examination cirrhotic patients often have an enlarged liver and/or spleen and HYPERTENSION. Liver function tests, cholangiography (X-ray examination of the bile ducts) and biopsy of liver tissue will help to reach a diagnosis.

TREATMENT Nothing can be done to repair a cirrhosed organ, but the cause, if known, must be removed and further advance of the process thus prevented. In the case of the liver a high-protein, high-carbohydrate, low-fat diet is given, supplemented by liver extract and vitamins B and K. The consumption of alcohol should be banned. In patients with liver failure and a poor prognosis, liver transplantation is worthwhile but only after careful consideration. (See TRANSPLANTATION.)

Abcess of the liver When an abscess develops in the liver, it is usually a result of amoebic DYSENTERY, appearing sometimes late in the disease, even after the diarrhoea is cured (see below). It may also follow upon inflammation of the liver due to other causes. In the case of an amoebic abscess treatment consists of oral metronidazole.

Acute hepatic necrosis is a destructive and often fatal disease of the liver which is very rare. It may be due to chemical poisons, such as carbtetrachloride, chloroform, phosphorus and industrial solvents derived from benzene. It may also be the cause of death in cases of poisoning with fungi. Very occasionally it may be a complication of acute infectious hepatitis.

Cancer of the liver is not uncommon, although it is rare for the disease to begin in the liver, the involvement of this organ being usually secondary to disease situated somewhere in the stomach or bowels. Cancer originating in the liver is more common in Asia and Africa. It usually arises in a fibrotic (or cirrhotic) liver and in carriers of the hepatitis B virus. There is great emaciation, which increases as the disease progresses. The liver is much enlarged, and its margin and surface are rough, being studded with hard cancer masses of varying size, which can often be felt through the abdominal wall. Pain may be present. Jaundice and oedema often appear.

LIVER DISEASE IN THE TROPICS

Acute liver disease Many viruses can be responsible for acute hepatocellular jaundice. The hepatitis viruses (A–F) are of paramount importance. Hepatitis E (HEV), which causes a disease overall very similar to HAV infection, often produces acute hepatic failure in pregnant women; extensive epidemics – transmitted by contaminated drinking-water supplies – have been documented at Delhi and Kashmir. HBV, especially in association with HDV, also causes acute liver failure in infected patients in several tropical countries; however, the major importance of HBV is that the infection leads to chronic liver disease (see below). Other hepatotoxic viruses include the Epstein-Barr virus, cytomegalovirus, yellow fever, Marburg/ Ebola viruses, etc. Acute liver disease also occurs in the presence of several acute bacterial infections, including *Salmonella typhi*, brucellosis, leptospirosis, syphilis, etc. Also, the complex type of jaundice associated with acute systemic bacterial infection – especially pneumococcal pneumonia and pyomiositis – assumes a major importance in many tropical countries, especially those in Africa and Papua New Guinea. Of protozoan infections, PLASMO-DIUM falciparum malaria, leishmaniasis, and toxoplasmosis should be considered. Ascaris lumbricoides (the roundworm) can produce obstruction to the biliary system.

Chronic liver disease   Long-term disease is dominated by sequelae of HBV and HCV infections (often acquired during the neonatal period), both of which can cause chronic active hepatitis, cirrhosis, and hepatocellular carcinoma ('hepatoma'), one of the world's most common malignancies. Chronic liver disease is also caused by schistosomiasis (usually Schistosoma mansoni and S. japonicum), and acute and chronic alcohol ingestion. Furthermore, many local herbal remedies and also orthodox chemotherapeutic compounds (e.g. those used in tuberculosis and leprosy) can result in chronic liver disease. Haemosiderosis ('Bantu siderosis') is a major problem in southern Africa. Hepatocytes contain excessive iron – derived primarily from an excessive intake, often present in locally brewed beer; however, a genetic predisposition seems likely. Indian childhood cirrhosis – associated with an excess of copper – is a major problem in India and surrounding countries. Epidemiological evidence shows that much of the copper is derived from copper vessels used to store milk used after weaning. Veno-occlusive disease was first described in Jamaica. However, this disease, which can present acutely, subacutely, chronically and is caused by pyrrolyzidine alkaloids (present in bush-tea), including heliotropium, is now known to occur far more widely. The previously held view that severe malnutrition predisposes to cirrhosis and other forms of chronic liver disease can no longer be upheld. Several HIV-associated 'opportunistic' infections can give rise to hepatic disease.

A localized (focal) form of liver disease in all tropical/subtropical countries results from invasive Entamoeba histolytica infection (amoebic liver 'abscess'); serology and imaging techniques assist in diagnosis. This should be differentiated form pyogenic liver abscess, which usually occurs secondarily to another intra-abdominal infection. Hydatidosis also causes localized liver disease; one or more cysts usually involve the right lobe of the liver. Serological tests and imaging techniques are of value in diagnosis. Whilst surgery formerly constituted the sole method of management, prolonged courses of albendazole and/or praziquantel have now been shown to be effective; however, surgical intervention is still required in some cases.

Hepato-biliary disease is also a problem in many tropical/subtropical countries. In southeast Asia, Clonorchis sinensis and Opisthorchis viverini infections cause chronic biliary-tract infection, complicated by adenocarcinoma of the biliary system. Praziquantel is effective chemotherapy before advanced disease ensues.

Fasciola hepatica (the liver fluke) is a further hepato-biliary helminthic infection; treatment is with bithionol or triclabendazole, praziquantel being relatively ineffective.

LIVER-FLUKE is the popular name of Fasciola hepatica, a parasite which infests sheep, and which is occasionally found in the bile-passages and liver of man. (See FASCIOLIASIS.)

LIVER PILLS (see CHOLAGOGUES).

LIVER SPOTS   A misnomer applied to the brown MACULES often seen on the backs of the hands of those chronically exposed to sunlight. (See LENTIGO.) They have no connection with any liver disorder.

LIVING WILL   Known formally as an advance statement about medical treatment, this is a written statement, agreed and signed by an adult individual who is of sound mind, requesting his or her doctors to withhold or withdraw treatment to sustain his or her life if the person suffers from an incurable and fatal condition and a loss of mental capacity. An advance statement can be of various types, ranging from a reflection of the individual's aspirations and preferences to a clear instruction refusing some or all medical procedures.

Though some countries have legislation recognizing living wills, the United Kingdom does not, but the existence of such a will would guide doctors in their decisions. In 1995 the British Medical Association issued a code of practice on the subject.

LOBE   The term applied to the larger divisions of various organs, such as to the four lobes of the liver, the three lobes of the right and the two lobes of the left lung, which are separated by fissures from one another, and to the lobes or superficial areas into which the brain is divided. The term lobar is applied to structures which are connected with lobes of organs, or to diseases which have a tendency to be limited by the boundaries of lobes, such as lobar pneumonia.

LOBECTOMY   The operation of cutting out a lobe of the lung in such diseases as abscess of the lung and bronchiectasis and carcinoma.

LOBOTOMY is the cutting of a lobe. (See PSYCHOSURGERY).

LOBULE   The term applied to a division of an organ smaller than a lobe: for example, the lobules of the lung are of the size of millet seeds, those of the liver slightly larger. Lobules form the smallest subdivisions or units of an organ, each lobule being similar to the others, of which there may be perhaps several hundred thousand in the organ.

LOCAL ANAESTHESIA Loss of sensation produced in a part of the body to stop pain while a person is examined, investigated or treated. The anaesthesia is effected by giving drugs in a local area temporarily to stop the action of pain-carrying nerve fibres. To anaesthetize a large area, a nerve block is done. Various drugs are used, depending on the depth and length of local anaesthesia required (see ANAESTHESIA).

LOCHIA is the discharge which takes place during the first week or two after child-birth. During the first four days it consists chiefly of blood; after the fifth day the colour should become paler, and after the first week the quantity should diminish. If the discharge becomes smelly, it may indicate an infection and immediate investigation and treament necessary. (SEE PUERPERIUM).

LOCKED-IN SYNDROME This describes a condition in which a patient is awake and retains the power of sense perception but is unable to communicate except by limited eye movements because the motor nervous system is paralysed. Several diseases can cause this syndrome which results from interruption of some of the nerve tracts between the mid brain and the pons (see BRAIN). Sometimes the syndrome is caused by severe damage to muscles or the nerves enervating them. Locked-in syndrome may sometimes be confused with a PERSISTENT VEGETATIVE STATE

LOCKJAW A painful spasm of the jaw muscles making it hard to open the mouth. It is a prominent symptom of tetanus and was once the popular name for this condition.

LOCOMOTOR ATAXIA The uncoordinated movements and unsteady lurching gait that occurs in the tertiary stage of untreated SYPHILIS.

LOCUM TENENS A doctor who stands in for another.

LOGORRHOEA is the technical term for garrulousness, a feature which may be exaggerated in certain states of mental instability.

LOIASIS is the disease caused by the filarial worm *Loa loa*, a thread-like worm which differs from *W. bancrofti* in that it is shorter and thicker, and it is found in the blood-stream during the day, not at night. It is transmitted by the mango fly, *Chrysops dimidiata*, but other flies of this genus can also transmit it. It is confined to West and Central Africa. The characteristic feature of the disease is the appearance of fugitive swellings which may arise anywhere in the body in the course of the worm's migration through the body. These are

known as Calabar swellings. The worm is often found in the eye, hence the old name of the worm in Africa – the eye worm. Satisfactory results are being reported from the use of diethylcarbamazine in the treatment of this form of FILARIASIS.

LOIN is the name applied to the part of the back between the lower ribs and the pelvis. (For pain in the loins see BACKACHE; LUMBAGO.)

LONG-SIGHT (see REFRACTION).

LOOP DIURETICS Drugs used in pulmonary oedema (excess fluid in the lungs) caused by failure of the left VENTRICLE of the HEART. DIURETICS cause an increase in excretion of URINE, thus reducing the amount of fluid in the body. Intravenous administration of loop diuretics relieves patients' breathlessness. They work by inhibiting resorption of fluid in the renal tubule loops of the KIDNEY. Frusemide and bumetanide are commonly used loop diuretic drugs.

LOPERAMIDE A drug that reduces the motility of the gastrointestinal tract and is of limited use as an adjunct to fluid replacement in acute diarrhoea in adults and older children.

LORAZEPAM is a benzodiazepine tranquillizer shown to be of limited use in the short-term treatment of anxiety or insomnia, in status epilepticus, or for perioperative use. Its use is not recommended for children. As with other benzodiazepines, the smallest possible dose should be given for the shortest possible time, as dependence is a well-recognized danger.

LORDOSIS An unnatural curvature of the spine forwards. It occurs chiefly in the lumbar region, where the natural curve is forwards, as the result of muscular weakness, spinal disease, etc. (See SPINAL COLUMN.)

LOTIONS Fluid preparations intended for bringing in contact with, or for washing, the external surface of the body. Lotions are generally of a watery or alcoholic composition, and many of them are known as 'liquors'. Those external applications which are of an oily nature, and intended to be rubbed into the surface, are known as liniments.

LOUSE (see INSECTS IN RELATION TO DISEASE).

LOZENGES These are small tablets containing drugs mixed with sugar, gum, glycerin-jelly, or fruit-paste. They are used in various affections of the mouth and throat, being sucked and slowly dissolved by the saliva, which brings the drugs they contain in contact with the affected surface. Some of the substances used in lozenges are benzalkonium (disinfectant), benzocaine (analgesic), betamethasone (corticosteroid), bismuth (disinfectant), formaldehyde (disinfectant), hydrocortisone (corticosteroid), liquorice, penicillin (antibiotic).

LSD (see LYSERGIC ACID DIETHYLAMIDE).

LUDWIG'S ANGINA An uncommon bacterial infection affecting the floor of the mouth. It can spread to the throat and become life threatening. Usually caused by infected gums or teeth, it causes pain, fever and swelling, resulting in difficulty in opening the mouth or swallowing. Urgent ANTIBIOTIC treatment is called for, otherwise the patient may need a tracheostomy to relieve breathing problems.

LUGOL'S SOLUTION is a compound solution of iodine and potassium iodide used in the preoperative preparation of patients with THYROTOXICOSIS. The solution is taken orally.

LUMBAGO Pain in the lower (lumbar) region of the back. It may be muscular, skeletal or neurological in origin. A severe form associated with SCIATICA may be due to a prolapsed INTERVERTEBRAL DISC. Less severe forms may be caused by OSTEOARTHRITIS of the spine, a trapped nerve, inflammation of connective tissue or may follow an old injury.

   The treatment will depend on the cause but mild lumbago will usually respond to NONSTEROIDAL ANTI-INFLAMMATORY DRUGS and the application of warmth. Victims should remember to bend their knees rather than their backs when lifting objects.

LUMBAR A term used to denote structures in, or diseases affecting, the region of the loins, as, for example, the lumbar vertebrae, lumbar abscess.

LUMBAR PUNCTURE A procedure for removing cerebrospinal fluid from the spinal canal in the lumbar region in order: (1) to diagnose disease of the nervous system; (2) to introduce medicaments: spinal anaesthetics, or drugs, or serum.

LUMBAR SYMPATHECTOMY Destruction of the lumbar chain of SYMPATHETIC nerves by means of surgery, DIATHERMY or injection of chemicals (phenol or alcohol). The technique is used to improve the blood flow to the leg in patients with peripheral vascular disease and to treat some types of chronic leg pain. The technique has only limited success.

LUMBAR VERTEBRA There are five lumbar vertabrae in the lower spinal column between the thoracic vertebrae and the sacrum (see SPINAL COLUMN).

Site of lumbar puncture: between third and fourth lumbar vertebrae.

1 dura mater
2 filum terminale
3 cauda equina

Cross-section of lumbar vertebra to show needle in position in the cerebrospinal fluid.

LUMBRICUS is a name sometimes applied to the roundworm or *Ascaris lumbricoides*. (See ASCARIASIS.)

LUMEN   (1) The space enclosed by a tubular structure or hollow organ (e.g. the gastro-intestinal tract or bladder). (2) The SI unit of luminous flux (1 lumen (1m) = the amount of light emitted per second in a unit solid angle of 1 steradian by a 1-candela point source).

LUMPECTOMY An operation for breast cancer in which the tumour is removed from the breast rather than with it (see MASTECTOMY).

LUNATIC A general and traditional term applied to people of disordered mind, because lunacy was supposed at one time to be largely influenced by the moon. It should no longer be used in medicine. (See MENTAL ILLNESS.)

LUNGS Positioned in the chest, the lungs serve primarily as respiratory organs (see RESPIRATION), also acting as a filter for the blood.

Form and position Each lung is a spongelike cone, pink in children and grey in adults. Its apex projects into the neck, with the base resting on the diaphragm. The rounded outer surface is in contact with the ribs and the heart lies between the lungs. The right lung has three lobes, the left lung two, and their combined weight, generally heavier in men, is about 1.1 kg. Each lung is enveloped by a closed cavity, the pleural cavity, consisting of two layers of pleural membrane separated by a thin layer of fluid. In healthy states this allows expansion and retraction as breathing occurs. In some diseases air escapes into the pleural cavity, causing the lung temporarily to collapse; in other disorders, large amounts of fluid collect there, compressing the lung.

Changes at birth The inrush of blood at birth as the infant starts breathing doubles the weight of the lungs; their colour changes from yellowish to rose red; they become spongy as air is inhaled. These changes are important from the medicolegal point of view, in determining whether a dead infant was born alive or not.

Heart/lung connections The heart lies in contact with the two lungs, so changes in lung volume inevitably affect the pumping action of the heart. Furthermore, both lungs are connected by blood vessels to the heart (see diagram on page 244). The PULMONARY ARTERY passes from the right ventricle and divides into two branches, one of which runs straight outwards to each lung, entering its substance along with the bronchial tube at the hilum or root of the lung. From this point also emerge the pulmonary veins, which carry the blood oxygenated in the lungs back to the left atrium.

Fine structure of lungs Each main bronchial tube, entering the lung at the root, divides into branches, which subdivide again and again, to be distributed all through the substance of the lung, till the finest tubes, known as respiratory bronchioles, have a width of only 0·25 mm ($^1/_{100}$ inch). All these tubes consist of a mucous membrane surrounded by a fibrous sheath. The surface of the mucous membrane comprises columnar cells provided with cilia (hairlike structures) which sweep mucous and unwanted matter such as bacteria to the exterior.

The smallest divisions of the bronchial tubes, or bronchioles, divide into a number of tortuous tubes known as alveolar ducts terminating eventually in minute sacs, known as alveoli, of which there are around 300 million.

The branches of the pulmonary artery accompany the bronchial tubes to the furthest recesses of the lung, dividing like the latter into finer and finer branches, and ending in a dense network of capillaries. The air in the air-vesicles is separated therefore from the blood only by two delicate membranes: the wall of the air-vesicle and the capillary wall, through which exchange of gases (oxygen and carbon dioxide) readily takes place. The essential oxygenated blood from the capillaries is collected by the pulmonary veins, which also accompany the bronchi to the root of the lung.

The lungs also contain an important system of lymph vessels, which start in spaces situated between the air-vesicles and eventually leave the lung along with the blood-vessels, and are connected with a chain of bronchial glands lying near the end of the trachea.

LUNGS, DISEASES OF The general symptoms and signs of chest diseases are mentioned under CHEST DISEASES and the chief affections to which these organs are liable are also treated under special headings. (See ASTHMA; BRONCHIECTASIS; CHEST, DEFORMITIES OF; CHRONIC OBSTRUCTIVE PULMONARY DISEASE (CPOD); CHILLS AND COLDS; EMPHYSEMA; EXPECTORATION; HAEMOPTYSIS; HAEMORRHAGE; OCCUPATIONAL DISEASES; PLEURISY; PNEUMONIA; PULMONARY EMBOLISM; TUBERCULOSIS.)

Inflammation of the lungs is generally known as pneumonia when it is due to infection, as alveolitis when the inflammation is immunological and as pneumonitis when it is due to physical or chemical agents. (See PNEUMONIA.) ABSCESS OF THE LUNG consists of a collection of pus within the lung tissue. Causes include inadequate treatment of pneumonia, inhalation of vomit, obstruction of the bronchial tubes by tumours and foreign bodies, pulmonary EMBOLI and septic emboli. The patient becomes generally unwell with cough and fever. BRONCHOSCOPY is frequently performed to detect any obstruction to the bronchi. Treatment is with a prolonged course of antibiotics. Rarely, surgery is necessary.

Pulmonary oedema (CONGESTION OF THE LUNGS) is the accumulation of fluid in the pulmonary tissues and air spaces. This may be caused by cardiac disease (heart failure or disease of heart valves) or by an increase in the permeability of the pulmonary capillaries allowing leakage of fluid into the lung tissue (see ADULT RESPIRATORY DISTRESS SYNDROME).

Heart failure (left ventricular failure) can be caused by a weakness in the pumping action of the heart leading to an increase in back pressure which forces fluid out of the blood vessels into the lung tissue. Causes include heart attacks and HYPERTENSION (high blood pressure). Narrowed or leaking heart valves hinder the flow of blood through the heart; again, this produces an increase in back pressure which raises the capillary pressure in the pulmonary vessels and causes flooding of fluid into the interstitial spaces and alveoli. Accumulation of fluid in lung tissue produces breathlessness. Treatments

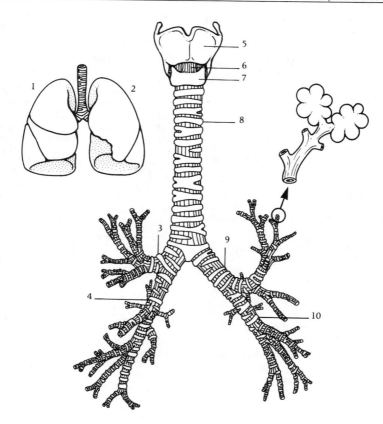

1 right lobes
2 left lobes
3 right bronchus
4 right hyparterial bronchus
5 thyroid cartilage

6 cricothyroid ligament
7 cricoid cartilage
8 trachea
9 left bronchus
10 left hyparterial bronchus

Lower air passages (centre) and their position relative to the lungs (left).
Respiratory bronchiole and alveolus (right).

include DIURETICS and other drugs to aid the pumping action of the heart. Surgical valve replacement may help when heart failure is due to valvular heart disease.

ADULT RESPIRATORY DISTRESS SYNDROME (ARDS) produces pulmonary congestion because of leakage of fluid through pulmonary capillaries. It complicates a variety of illnesses such as sepsis, trauma, aspiration of gastric contents and diffuse pneumonia. Treatment involves treating the cause and supporting the patient by providing oxygen.

Collapse of the lung may occur due to blockage of a bronchial tube by tumour, foreign body or a plug of mucus which may occur in bronchitis or pneumonia. Air beyond the blockage is absorbed into the circulation causing the affected area of lung to collapse. Collapse may also occur when air is allowed into the pleural space – the space between the lining of the lung and the lining of the inside of the chest wall.

This is called a pneumothorax and may occur following trauma, or spontaneously, for example when there is a rupture of a subpleural air pocket (such as a cyst) allowing a communication between the airways and the pleural space. Lung collapse by compression may occur when fluid collects in the pleural space (pleural effusion). When this fluid is blood it is known as a haemothorax. If it is due to pus it is known as an empyema. Collections of air, blood, pus or other fluid can be removed from the pleural space by insertion of a chest drain, thus allowing the lung to re-expand.

Tumours of the lung are the most common cause of cancer in men and along with breast cancer are a major cause of cancer in women. Several types of lung cancer occur, the most common being squamous cell carcinoma, small (or oat cell) carcinoma, adenocarcinoma and large cell carcinoma. All but the adenocarcinoma have a strong link with smoking. Each type has a different pattern of growth and responds differently to treatment. Over 36,000 men and women died of cancer of the trachea, bronchus and lung in 1995.

The commonest presenting symptom is cough; others include haemoptisis (coughing up blood), breathlessness, chest pain, wheezing and weight loss. As well as spreading locally in the lung – the rate of spread varies – lung cancer commonly spawns secondary growths in the liver, bones or brain. Diagnosis is confirmed by X-rays and bronchoscopy with biopsy.

If diagnosed early, lung cancer can be treated surgically either by pneumonectomy (removal of a lung) or lobectomy (removal of part of a lung). Anti-cancer drugs and chemotherapy are used to restrict the spread of cancer. Fewer than 20 per cent of lung cancer patients survive five years after diagnosis. Early diagnosis is the key to effective treatment.

Wounds of the lung may cause damage to the lung and by admitting air into the pleural cavity cause the lung to collapse with air in the pleural space (pneumothorax). This may require the insertion of a chest drain to remove the air from the pleural space and allow the lung to re-expand. The lung may be wounded by the end of a fractured rib or by some sharp body pushed between the ribs.

LUNG VOLUMES The volume of air within the lungs changes with the respiratory cycle. The volumes defined below can be measured and may be useful indicators of some pulmonary diseases.

Total lung capacity (TLC) The volume of air that can be held in the lungs at maximum inspiration.

Tidal volume (TV) The volume of air taken into and out of the lungs with each breath.

Inspiratory reserve volume (IRV) The volume of air that can still be inspired at the end of a normal quiet inspiration.

Expiratory reserve volume (ERV) The volume of air that can still be expired at the end of a normal quiet expiration.

Residual volume (RV) The volume of air remaining in the lungs after a maximal expiration.

Vital capacity (VC) The maximum amount of air that can be expired after a maximal inspiration.

Functional residual capacity (FRC) The volume of air left in the lungs at the end of a normal quiet expiration.

Normal values for a 60-kg man are:	
	ml
TLC	5000–6000
TV	400–600
IRV	3300–3750
ERV	950–1200
RV	1200–1700
VC	3400–4800
FRC	2300–2600

LUPUS This is the Latin word for wolf, a term applied to certain chronic skin diseases which can destroy skin, underlying cartilage and even bone to cause serious deformity if uncontrolled.

Lupus vulgaris is a form of TUBERCULOSIS of the skin. It typically begins in childhood and may spread slowly for decades if untreated. The face and neck are the usual sites. In untreated disease, large well-demarcated areas may be affected with redness, scaling and thickening. If the affected skin is blanched by pressure, yellow-brown foci may be observed – the so-called apple-jelly nodules. The disease causes extensive scarring as it spreads and may destroy cartilage in its path, e.g. on the nose or ear, causing gross deformity. The disease was common in the UK up to 50 years ago, but is now rare. It is treated with a combination of tuberculostatic drugs.

Lupus erythematosus is an autoimmune disease which can affect skin or internal organs. In discoid lupus erythematosus only the skin is affected. Sharply defined red, scaly and eventually atrophic patches appear on the face, especially on the nose and cheeks. ALOPECIA with scarring is seen if the scalp is affected. It is aggravated by sunlight. Topical CORTICOSTEROIDS are helpful.

Systemic lupus erythematosus (SLE) is a less common disease, usually occurring in women. Typically, a bright erythema in a 'butterfly' distribution on the nose and cheeks is later associated with arthritis and involvement of internal organs, especially the kidneys, heart and central nervous system, which may be fatal if untreated. A characteristic pattern of autoantibodies is found in the blood. The disorder is hard to diagnose in its early stages but with early diagnosis and treatment the long-term outlook is good. Large doses of oral corcicosteroid and other immunosuppressive drugs may be needed to suppress the disease. The cause of lupus erythematosus is unknown but rarely certain drugs can cause a similar syndrome. (See APPENDIX 2: ADDRESSES.)

LUTEINIZING HORMONE A hormone secreted by the anterior pituitary which stimulates ovulation, maturation of the corpus luteum and the synthesis of progesterone by the ovary and testosterone by the testis.

LUX The unit of illumination. The abbreviation is lx.

LUXATION Another word for dislocation. (See DISLOCATIONS.)

LYCANTHROPY Morbid delusion that one is a wolf.

LYING-IN (see LABOUR).

LYME DISEASE This comprises arthritis associated with skin rashes, fever and sometimes ENCEPHALITIS or carditis (inflammation of the heart). It is caused by a SPIROCHAETE which is transmitted by tick bite. Treatment is with antibiotics.

LYMPH is the fluid which circulates in the lymphatic vessels of the body. It is a colourless fluid, like blood plasma in composition, only rather more watery. It contains salts similar to those of blood plasma, and the same proteins, though in smaller amount: FIBRINOGEN, SERUM ALBUMIN, and serum GLOBULIN. It also contains LYMPHOCYTES (white blood cells), derived from the glands. In some lymphatic vessels, the lymph contains, after meals, a great amount of fat in the form of a fine milky emulsion. These are the vessels which absorb fat from the food passing down the intestine, and convey it to the thoracic duct; they are called lacteals because their contents look milky (See CHYLE.)

The lymph is derived, initially, from the blood, the watery constituents of which exude through the walls of the CAPILLARIES into the tissues, conveying material for the nourishment of the tissues and absorbing waste products.

The spaces in the tissues communicate with lymph capillaries, which have a structure similar to that of the CAPILLARIES of the blood-vessel system, being composed of delicate flat cells joined edge to edge. These unite to form fine vessels, resembling minute veins in structure, called lymphatics. These ramify throughout the body, passing through lymphatic glands, and ultimately discharge their contents into the jugular veins in the root of the neck. Other lymph vessels commence in great numbers as minute openings on the surface of the PLEURA and PERITONEUM, and act as drains for these otherwise closed cavities. When fluid is effused into these cavities, as in a pleural effusion, for example, its absorption takes place through the lymphatic vessels. The course of these vessels is described under the entry on GLANDS.

Lymph circulates partly by reason of the pressure at which it is driven through the walls of the blood capillaries, but mainly in consequence of incidental forces. The lymph capillaries and vessels are copiously provided with valves, which prevent any back flow of lymph, and every time these vessels are squeezed, as by the contraction of a muscle, or movement of a limb, the lymph is pumped along.

The term lymph is also applied to the serous fluid contained in the vesicles which develop as the result of vaccination, and used for the purpose of vaccinating other individuals. (See VACCINATION.)

LYMPHADENITIS Inflammation of lymphatic glands.

LYMPHADENOMA Another name for HODGKIN'S DISEASE.

LYMPHADENOPATHY Medical description of swollen lymph glands. One cause is HIV infection (see AIDS).

LYMPHANGIECTASIS means an abnormal dilatation of the lymph vessels, as in FILARIASIS.

LYMPHANGIOGRAPHY, or LYMPHOGRAPHY, is the procedure whereby the LYMPHATICS and lymphatic glands can be rendered visible on X-ray films by means of the injection of radio-opaque substances.

LYPHANGIOMA An uncommon non-malignant tumour occurring in the skin or the tongue. It comprises an abnormal collection of lymph vessels and tends to be present from birth. Sometimes it disappears spontaneously but it may need surgical removal.

LYMPHANGITIS Inflammation situated in the lymphatic vessels.

LYMPHATICS Vessels which convey the LYMPH. (For an account of their arrangement, see GLANDS.)

LYMPH NODE Swellings which occur at various points in the lymphatic system through which lymph drains. They consist of a cortex, medulla and lymph sinuses and have two main functions: (1) The interception and removal of abnormal or foreign material from the lymph.

1 hilum: (a) efferent lymph vessel
             (b) venuole
             (c) arteriole
2 afferent lymph vessel
3 lymph valve
4 capsule
5 reticulin matrix
6 follicle: (a) lymphatic follicular node
             (b) medulla
7 trabecula
8 subscapula sinus

Structure of lymph node.

1 submandibular lymph node
2 right bronchomediastinal trunk
3 right lumbar trunk
4 occipital lymph node
5 parotid lymph nodes
6 cervical lymph node
7 jugular trunk
8 subclavian trunk.
9 axillary lymph node.
10 thoracic lymph node
11 thoracic duct
12 cisterna chyli
13 intestinal trunk
14 left lumbar trunk
15 iliac lymph node
16 inguinal lymph node
17 popliteal lymph node

Lymphatic system of body.

(2) The production of immune responses. The lymph nodes become enlarged when the area of the body which they drain is the site of infection or as a manifestation of some systemic diseases. Occasionally they are the site of primary or metastatic malignant disease.

LYMPHOCYTE A variety of white blood cell produced in the lymphoid tissues and lymphatic glands of the body. It contains a simple rounded nucleus surrounded by proto-plasm generally described as non-granular. Two varieties of lymphocyte are described, small and large, and together they form over 20 per cent of the white cells of the blood. They play an important part in the production of ANTIBODIES, and in the rejection of transplanted organs such as the heart. (See TRANSPLANTA-TION.) This they do in two different ways. What are known as B lymphocytes produce ANTIBOD-IES, while T lymphocytes attack and destroy ANTIGENS directly. They are known as T lymphocytes because they are produced by the THYMUS GLAND. Their numbers are increased in TUBERCULOSIS and certain other diseases. Such an increase is known as lymphocytosis.

LYMPHOCYTOSIS An increase in the number of lymphocytes in the blood, e.g. in response to infection or in chronic LYMPHOCYTIC LEUKAEMIA.

LYMPHOEDEMA Swelling of a part or organ due to obstruction to the lymph-vessels draining it.

LYMPHOGRANULOMA INGUINALE, LYM-PHOGRANULOMA VENEREUM; PORADENITIS VENEREA; LYMPHOPATHIA VENEREUM, is a vene-real disease in which the chief characteristic is enlargement of glands in the groin, the infecting agent being a virus.

LYMPHOID TISSUE Tissue involved in the formation of lymph, lymphocytes, and anti-bodies. It consists of the lymph nodes, thymus, tonsils and spleen.

LYMPHOKINES Lymphokines are poly-peptides that are produced by lymphocytes as part of their immune response to an antigen and their function is to communicate with other cells of the immune system. Some lymphokines stimulate B cells to differentiate into ANTIBODY-producing plasma cells; others stimulate T lymphocytes to proliferate and other lympho-kines become INTERFERONS.

LYMPHOMA is a malignant proliferation of lymphoid tissue classified into two main types: HODGKIN'S and non-Hodgkin's. Another vari-ety is found in children in Africa; sometimes called BURKITT'S LYMPHOMA after the surgeon who first described it. Because of its geographi-cal distribution it is thought to be due to a virus which is transmitted by mosquitoes, but no virus has yet been definitely isolated from the tumour. Hodgkin's and non-Hodgkin's lym-phomas present as enlarged lymph glands, mainly in the neck and axillae in the former and more generally in the latter variety. The differ-ence rests in the histology of the enlarged glands. Radiotherapy and chemotherapy can be used for both types with more aggressive treatment needed for Hodgkin's lymphoma. Both types are graded according to severity and the grade is a guide to survival rates which are much improved with modern treatments.

LYMPHOSARCOMA A malignant growth of the lymphoid elements of the body, and is characterized by generalized enlargement of the lymphatic glands, spleen, and liver. The majority of cases – about 55 per cent – occur in the 60 to 70 age-group, but it may occur at any age. The prognosis is poor, 80 per cent of cases dying within six years. Treatment is by means of irradiation or chemotherapy.

LYSERGIC ACID DIETHYLAMIDE (LSD) belongs to the ergot group of ALKALOIDS. It has various effects on the brain, notably analgesic and hallucinogenic, thought to be due to its antagonism of 5-hydroxytry tryptamine (5-HT). In small doses it induces psychic states, in which the individual may become aware of repressed memories. For this reason it may help in the treatment of certain anxiety states, if used under skilled supervision. LSD rapidly induces tolerance, however, and psychological depend-ence may occur, though not physical depend-ence. Serious side-effects include psychotic reactions, with an increased risk of suicide (see DRUG ADDICITION).

LYSINE An essential AMINO-ACID, lysine was first isolated in 1889 from casein, the principal protein of milk. Like other essential amino-acids it ensures optimum growth in infants and balanced nitrogen metabolism in adults.

LYSIS The gradual ending of a fever, and the opposite of crisis, which signifies the sudden ending of a fever. (See CRISIS.) It is also used to describe the process of dissolution of a blood-clot, or the destruction of CELLS as a result of damage to or rupture of the plasma membrane, thus allowing the cell contents to escape.

LYSOL A brown, clear, oily fluid with anti-septic properties, made from coal-tar and con-taining 50 per cent cresol. When mixed with water it forms a clear soapy fluid. (See CRESOL.)

LYSOL POISONING When lysol is swal-lowed there is a sense of burning about the mouth and throat. There are signs of corrosion around and in the mouth, with brown discol-oration, and the characteristic smell of lysol is very evident in the breath. If the lysol is not speedily removed, unconsciousness and stupor gradually come on and death may occur within 24 hours. Septic pneumonia is also liable to supervene, and may produce death at a later period.

Treatment If the skin has been contaminated with the lysol, it must be washed with water, and any lysol-contaminated clothing must be taken off. Large quantities of tepid water and salt may be given at once to dilute the lysol if it has been swallowed, and produce vomiting.

LYSOZYME An enzyme present in tears and eggwhite which catalyses the destruction of some bacteria by damaging their walls.

LYSSA is another term for RABIES.

M

McBURNEY'S POINT (see APPENDICITIS).

MACERATION is the softening of a solid by soaking in fluid.

MACR- (MACRO- Prefix denoting large-size cell – for example, MACROPHAGE, a large PHAGOCYTE.

MACROCYTE is an unusually large red blood cell (ERYTHROCYTE) especially characteristic of the blood in pernicious anaemia.

MACROCYTOSIS This condition is particularly associated with PERNICIOUS ANAEMIA but can also be caused by a number of other things, such as alcohol, pregnancy, MYXOEDEMA and MYELOMA, and also by vitamin B_{12} deficiency: this occurs sometimes in vegans and also in patients with CROHN'S DISEASE.

MACROGLOSSIA An abnormally large tongue.

MACROLIDES A group of antibiotics. The original macrolide, ERYTHROMYCIN, was discovered in the early 1950s and used successfully as an alternative to PENICILLIN. The name derives from the molecular structure of this group, two new drugs of which are clarithromycin and azithromycin. Macrolides check PROTEIN synthesis in BACTERIA and the latest ones are, like erythromycin, active against several bacterial species including GRAM-POSITIVE COCCI and rods. In addition they act against *Haemophilus influenzae*. Clarithromycin is potent against

CHLAMYDIA TRACHOMITIS and *Helicobacter pylori*. Azithromycin is efective against infections caused by *Legionella* spp. (see LEGIONNAIRE'S DISEASE), GONOCOCCI and *MYCOPLASMA PNEUMONIAE*.

MACROPHAGE A large PHAGOCYTE that forms part of the RETICULO-ENDOTHELIAL system. It is found in many organs and tissues, including connective tissues, bone marrow, lymph nodes, spleen, liver and central nervous system. Free macrophages move between cells and, using their scavenger properties, collect at infection sites to remove foreign bodies, including bacteria. Fixed macrophages are found in connective tissue.

MACROPSIA Condition in which objects appear larger than normal. It can be due to disease of the MACULA of the eye.

MACULA A spot or area of tissue that is different from surrounding tissue. An example is the macula letea, the yellow spot in the retina of the eye (see EYE).

MACULES Areas of skin discoloration which may be seen but not felt. They may occur in a wide range of conditions such as ECZEMA, PSORIASIS, SYPHILIS and after burns, as well as in pregnancy.

MACULOPAPULAR A skin rash that is made up of macules (discoloration of the skin) and papules (raised abnormality of the skin).

MADURA FOOT Tropical infection of the foot by deeply invasive fungi which cause chronic swelling and suppuration with multiple discharging sinuses. Antibiotics are of limited value and advanced disease may require amputation.

MAGNESIUM is a light metallic element. Magnesium is one of the essential mineral elements of the body, without which it cannot function properly. The adult body contains around 25 grams, the greater part of which is in the bones. More than two-thirds of our daily supply come from cereals and vegetables. As most other foods also contain useful amounts, there is thus seldom any difficulty in maintaining an adequate amount in the body. It is an essential constituent of several vital enzymes. Deficiency leads to muscular weakness and interferes with the efficient working of the heart. The salts of magnesium used as drugs are the hydroxide of magnesium, the oxide of magnesium, generally known as 'magnesia', and the carbonate of magnesium, all of which have an antacid action; also the sulphate of magnesium generally known as 'Epsom salts', which acts as a purgative.
Uses Compounds of magnesia are used to correct hyperacidity of the stomach and as a laxative.

MAGNESIUM TRISILICATE A white powder with antacid properties. A mild antacid with prolonged action, it is used for treating peptic ulceration, commonly combined with quickly acting antacids. It has no side-effects so can be used in large doses.

MAGNETIC RESONANCE IMAGING (MRI) (see MRI).

MALABSORPTION SYNDROME This term includes a multiplicity of diseases, all of which are characterized by faulty absorption from the intestine of essential foodstuffs, such as fat, vitamins and mineral salts. Among the conditions in this syndrome are COELIAC DISEASE, SPRUE, CYSTIC FIBROSIS and PANCREATITIS. Surgical removal of the small intestine also causes the syndrome. Symptoms include ANAEMIA, diarrhoea, OEDEMA, vitamin deficiencies, weight loss and, in severe cases, MALNUTRITION.

MALACIA is a term applied to softening of a part or tissue in disease: e.g. OSTEOMALACIA or softening of the bones.

MALAISE A vague feeling of feverishness, listlessness, and languor, which often precedes the onset of serious acute diseases, or accompanies passing illnesses, such as dyspepsia, chills, and colds.

MALAR Anything relating to the cheek. For example, the malar (zygomatic) bone is also known as the cheek bone, and a malar flush is reddening of the cheeks.

MALARIA The term is derived from the Italian *mal aria*. Disease is caused by four species of Plasmodium: *P. falciparum*, *P. vivax*, *P. ovale*, and *P. malariae*. Clinically, malaria is characterized by recurrent febrile episodes, sometimes associated with rigors; enlargement of the spleen is common. *P. falciparum* infection can also be associated with several serious – often fatal – complications (see below); although other species cause chronic disease, acute mortality is unusual.

Malaria is a disease of great antiquity; one suggestion is that it contributed significantly to the fall of the Roman Empire. An association with marshes was recognized in ancient times, and an association with mosquitoes had been suggested on many occasions historically. However, it was not until 1897–8, that Ronald Ross working in India was able to establish clearly a host–mosquito–host cycle in avian malaria. Shortly afterwards the human–mosquito–human cycle was established beyond doubt; groups of British (led by Patrick Manson) and Italian (A. Bignami and others) researchers helped in this discovery.

The infection(s) is very widely distributed in tropical and subtropical countries; *P. falciparum* is, however, confined very largely to Africa, Asia, and South America. Not only are areas of transmission increasing, but *Plasmodium* spp. parasites are also increasingly developing resistance to various chemoprophylactic and chemotherapeutic agents. Malaria also constitutes a significant problem in travellers; so it is essential that travellers obtain sound advice on chemoprophylaxis before embarking on tropical trips (see APPENDIX 3: TRAVEL AND HEALTH), especially to a rural area where intense transmission can occur. Transmission has also been recorded at airports, and following blood transfusion.

During a bite by the female mosquito, one or more sporozoites are injected into the human circulation; these are taken up by the hepatocytes (liver cells). Following division, merozoites (minute particles resulting from the division) are liberated into the bloodstream where they invade the erythrocytes. These in turn divide, releasing further merozoites. Merozoites are periodically liberated into the bloodstream, causing characteristic fevers, rigors, etc. To complete the life-cycle, sexual forms (gametocytes) are taken up during a further mosquito bite.

Diagnosis is by demonstration of trophozoites – a stage in the parasite's life-cycle that takes place in red blood cells – in thick/thin blood-films of peripheral blood. Serological tests are of value in deciding whether an individual has had a past infection, but are of no value in acute disease.

Prophylaxis United Kingdom malaria specialists have produced guidance for residents travelling to ENDEMIC areas for short stays. Drug choice takes account of:

- risk of exposure to malaria;
- extent of drug resistance;
- efficacy of recommended drugs and their side-effects;
- criteria relevant to the individual (e.g. age, pregnancy, kidney or liver impairment).

Personal protection against being bitten by mosquitoes is essential. Permethrin-impregnated nets are an effective barrier while skin barrier protection and vaporized insecticides are helpful. Lotions, sprays or roll-on applicators all containing diethyltoluamide (DEET) are safe and work when put on the skin. Their effect, however, lasts only for a few hours. Long sleeves and trousers should be worn after dark.

Drug prophylaxis should be started at least a week before travelling into countries where malaria is endemic (two or three weeks in the case of mefloquine). Drug treatment should be continued for at least four weeks after leaving endemic areas. Even if all recommended anti-malarial programmes are followed, it is possible that malaria may occur any time up to three months afterwards. Medical advice should be sought if any illness develops. Chloroquine can be used as a prophylactic drug where the risk of resistant falciparum malaria is low. Otherwise mefloquine or proguanil hydrochloride should be used. Travellers to malaria-infested areas should seek expert advice on appropriate prophylactic treatment well before departing.

Various chemoprophylactic regimes are widely used. Those commmonly prescribed include: chloroquine + paludrine, mefloquine, and Maloprim (trimethoprim + dapsone); Fansidar (trimethoprim + sulphamethoxazole) has been shown to have significant side-effects, especially when used in conjunction with chloroquine, and is now rarely used. No chemotherapeutic regimen is totally effective so other preventive measures are again being used. These include people avoiding mosquito bites, covering exposed areas of the body between dusk and dawn, and using mosquito repellents.

Chemotherapy was for many years dominated by the synthetic agent chloroquine. However, with the widespread emergence of chloroquine-resistance, quinine is again being widely used. First introduced into Europe from South America as the 'bark' in the 17th century, it was first included in the *London Pharmacopoeia* (3rd edition) in 1677 as *Cortex Peruanus*. Quinine should be administered intravenously in a severe infection; the oral route is used subsequently and in minor cases. Other agents currently in use include mefloquine, halofantrine, doxycycline, and the artemesinin alkaloids ('qinghaosu').

Complications of *P. falciparum* infection include cerebral involvement, due to adhesion of immature trophozoites on to the cerebral vascular endothelium; these lead to a high death rate when inadequately treated. Renal involvement (frequently resulting from haemoglobinuria), pulmonary oedema, hypotension, hypoglycaemia, and complications in pregnancy are also important. In complicated disease, haemodialysis and exchange transfusion have been used. No adequate controlled trial using the latter regimen has been carried out, however, and possible benefits must be weighed against numerous potential side-effects – for instance, the introduction of a wide range of infections, overloading the circulatory system with infused fluids and other complications.

P. vivax and *P. ovale* infections cause less severe disease, although overall there are many clinical similarities with *P. falciparum* infection; acute complications are unusual, but chronic anaemia is often present. Primaquine is necessary to eliminate the exoerythrocytic cycle in the hepatocyte (liver cell).

P. malariae usually produces a chronic infection, and chronic renal disease (nephrotic syndrome) is an occasional sequel, especially in tropical Africa.

Gross splenomegaly (hyperreactive malarious splenomegaly, or tropical splenomegaly syndrome) can complicate all four human *Plasmodium* spp. infections. The syndrome responds to long-term malarial chemoprophylaxis. BURKITT'S LYMPHOMA is found in geographical areas where malaria infection is endemic; the Epstein-Barr virus is aetiologically involved.

The World Health Organization reported that in 1997 malaria was one of Europe's top ten infectious diseases. In 1992 20,000 cases were reported: this had risen to 200,000 in 1995. The resurgence of malaria has been worldwide, in part the result of resistant strains of the disease developing and in part because many countries have failed (or been unable) to implement environmental measures to eliminate mosquitoes. Near 40 years ago the WHO forecast that by 1980 only four million people would be affected worldwide. In the late 1990s around 500 million people a year get malaria and 1.5 million (possibly more) die from the disease.

MALATHION Organo-phosphorus insecticide which is a preferred scabicide and pediculocide; applied externally; resistance rare (see INSECTS AND DISEASE).

MALFORMATION (see DEFORMITIES).

MALIGNANT A term applied in several ways to serious disorders. Tumours are called malignant when they grow rapidly, tend to infiltrate surrounding healthy tissues, and to spread to distant parts of the body, leading eventually to death. (See CANCER.) The term is also applied to types of disease which are much more serious than the usual form, such as malignant HYPERTENSION and malignant SMALLPOX. Malignant pustule is another name for ANTHRAX

MALIGNANT HYPERPYREXIA (see MALIGNANT HYPERTHERMIA).

MALIGNANT HYPERTENSION has nothing to do with cancer. It derives its name from the fact that, if untreated, it runs a rapidly fatal course. (See HYPERTENSION.)

MALIGNANT HYPERTHERMIA This disorder is a rare complication of general ANAESTHESIA caused, it is believed, by a combination of an inhalation anaesthetic (usually HALOTHANE) and a muscle-relaxant drug (usually succinycholine). A life-endangering rise in temperature occurs, with muscular rigidity the first sign. TACHYCARDIA, ARRYTHMIA, ACIDOSIS and SHOCK usually occur. About 1:20,000 patients having general anaesthesia suffer from this disorder, which progresses rapidly and is often fatal. Surgery and anaesthesia must be stopped immediately and appropriate corrective measures taken, including the administration of DANTROLENE intravenously. It is a dominantly inherited genetic condition; therefore when a case is identified it is most important that relatives are screened.

MALIGNANT LYMPHOMA or LYMPHOMA A malignant tumour of the lymph nodes. It includes HODGKIN's disease and non-Hodgkin's lymphomas. The malignancy varies and the outlook varies from death after a few months to many years. The disease presents as multiple enlarged lymph nodes accompanied by systemic symptoms such as fever, sweating and loss of weight. It may be widespread or occur in just a single area – for instance, a tonsil. Drugs such as CHLORAMBUCIL or combinations of CYCLOPHOSPHAMIDE, VINCRISTINE and PREDNISONE. DOXORUBICIN and/or BLEOMYCIN may also be used. The results from these anticancer drugs may be dramatic. Local disease may require radiotherapy before chemotherapy. A bone-marrow transplant is sometimes necessary for patients with non-Hodgkin's lymphoma who fail to respond to chemotherapy.

MALIGNANT MELANOMA (see MELANOMA.)

MALINGERING is a term applied to the feigning of illness. In the great majority of cases a person who feigns illness has a certain amount of disability, but exaggerates the illness or discomfort for some ulterior motive – for example, to take time off work or to obtain compensation.

MALLEOLUS Name of either of the two bony prominences at the ankle. (See LEG.)

MALLET FINGER Deformation of a finger due to sudden forced flexion of the terminal joint of a finger, resulting in rupture of the tendon. As a result the individual is unable to extend the terminal part of the finger which remains bent forward. The middle, ring and little fingers are most commonly involved. Treatment is by splinting the finger. The end result is satisfactory provided the victim has sufficient patience.

MALLET TOE The condition in which it is not possible to extend the terminal part of the toe. It is usually due to muscular imbalance but may be due to congenital absence of the extensor muscle. A CALLOSITY often forms on it which may be painful. Should this be troublesome, treatment consists of removal of the terminal phalanx.

MALLEUS The hammer-shaped lateral bone of the group of three that form the sound-transmitting ossicles in the middle ear. (See EAR.)

MALNUTRITION The condition arising from an inadequate or unbalanced diet. The causes may be a lack of one or more essential nutrients or inadequate absorption from the intestinal tracts. A diet that is deficient in CARBOHYDRATE usually contains inadequate protein, and this type of malnutrition occurs in Africa and Asia as a result of poverty, famine or war. (See DIET.)

MALOPRIM A combination of PYRIMETHAMINE and DAPSONE which is used for the prevention of MALARIA in limited circumstances.

It has the advantage of only needing to be taken once weekly. It should not be taken by anyone hypersensitive to sulphonamides, and should not be used for the treatment of an acute attack.

MALPRACTICE Improper or inadequate medical treatment that fails to match the standards of skill and care that is reasonably expected from a qualified health care practitioner – usually a doctor or dentist. Litigation against health professionals for malpractice has been running at substantial levels in the USA for some years. During the past decade the number of cases has been rising sharply in the United Kingdom, in part because of failings in the NHS and in part because the population has more understanding of health care and people are more aware when possible malpractice has occurred. In the UK the GENERAL MEDICAL COUNCIL, GENERAL DENTAL COUNCIL and THE UNITED KINGDOM CENTRAL COUNCIL FOR NURSING (see NURSING), MIDWIFERY AND HEALTH VISITING are responsible for professional standards among, respectively, doctors, dentists and nurses.

MALPRESENTATION A situation during childbirth in which a baby is not in the customary head-first position before delivery. The result is usually a complicated labour in which a caesarean operation may be necessary to effect the birth. (See LABOUR.)

MALTA FEVER (see BRUCELLOSIS).

MAMMARY GLAND (see BREASTS).

MAMMOGRAPHY The special technique whereby X-rays are used to show the structure of the breast or any abnormalities in it. It is an effective way of distinguishing benign from malignant tumours. It can detect tumours that are not palpable. In a multi-centre study in the USA, called The Breast Cancer Detection Demonstration Project, which involved nearly 300,000 women in the 40–49 age group, 35 per cent of the tumours were found by mammography alone, 13 per cent by physical examination and 50 per cent by both methods. The optimum frequency of screening is debatable. The American College of Radiologists recommends a baseline mammogram at the age of 40 years with subsequent mammography at one to two year intervals up to the age of 50. Thereafter, annual mammography is recommended. In the United Kingdom a less intensive screening programme is in place with women over 50 being screened every three years. As breast cancer is the commonest malignancy in Western women and is increasing in frequency, the importance of screening for this form of cancer is obvious.

MAMMOPLASTY A surgical operation to reconstruct a breast after part or all of it has been removed to treat breast cancer, to enlarge small breasts or to reduce the size of overlarge breasts. The routine method for breast enlargement used to be the insertion of SILICONE implants under the skin. Controversy about the long-term safety of silicone, however, has restricted their use, mainly to women needing reconstruction of their breasts after cancer surgery. Side-effects have included hardening of breast tissue, leaking of implants and development of scar tissue.

MANAGED HEALTH CARE This process aims to reduce the costs of health care while maintaining the quality of care. The concept originated in the United States but has attracted interest in the United Kingdom and Europe where the spiralling costs of health care have been causing widespread concern. Managed care works through changing clinical practice but it is not a discrete entity. The American I. J. Iglehart has defined it as 'a variety of methods of financing and organizing the delivery of comprehensive health care in which an attempt is made to control costs by controlling the provision of services.' Managed care has three facets: health policy, how that policy is managed and how individuals needing health care are dealt with. The process and its applications are still evolving and it is likely that different health-care systems will adapt it to suit their own particular circumstances.

MANDELIC ACID A non-toxic keto-acid used in the treatment of infections of the urinary tract, especially those due to the *Escherichia coli* and the *Streptococcus faecalis* or *Enterococcus*. It is administered in doses of 3 grams several times daily. As it is only effective in an acid urine, ammonium chloride must be taken at the same time.

MANDIBLE The bone of the lower jaw.

MANGANESE A metal, oxides of which are found abundantly in nature. Permanganate of potassium is a well-known disinfectant.

MANIA A form of mental disorder characterized by great excitement. (See MENTAL ILLNESS.)

MANIC-DEPRESSION, or CYCLOTHYMIA, is a form of mental illness characterized by alternate attacks of mania and depression. (See MENTAL ILLNESS.)

MANIPULATION The passive movement – often forceful – of bones, joints, or soft tissues, carried out by orthopaedic surgeons, PHYSIOTHERAPISTS, OSTEOPATHS and CHIROPRACTORS as an important part of treatment, often highly effective. It may be used for three chief reasons: correction of deformity (mainly the reduction of fractures and dislocations, or to overcome deformities such as congenital CLUB FOOT); treatment of joint stiff-ness (particularly after an acute limb injury, or FROZEN SHOULDER); and relief of chronic pain (particularly when due to chronic strain, notably the spinal joints (see PROLAPSED INTERVERTEBRAL DISC)). Depending on the particular injury or deformity being treated, and the estimated force required, manipulation may be used with or without anaesthesia. Careful clinical and radiological examination, together with other appropriate investigations, should always be carried out before starting treatment, to reduce the risk of harm, or disasters such as fractures or the massive displacement of an intervertebral disc.

MANNITOL An osmotic DIURETIC given intravenously. (See DIURETICS.)

MANOMETER An instrument for measuring the pressure or tension of liquids or gases. (See BLOOD-PRESSURE.)

MANTOUX TEST, also known as MENDEL'S TEST, is a test for TUBERCULOSIS. It consists in injecting into the superficial layers of the skin (i.e. intradermally) a very small quantity of old tuberculin. A positive reaction of the skin – swelling and redness – shows that the person so reacting has been infected with the *Mycobacterium tuberculosis*. But it does not mean that such a person is suffering from active tuberculosis. (See TUBERCULIN.)

MANUBRIUM The uppermost part of the STERNUM or breast-bone.

MARASMUS Progressive wasting, especially in young children, when there is no ascertainable cause. It is generally associated with defective feeding. (See ATROPHY; INFANT FEEDING.)

MARBURG DISEASE This is also known as GREEN MONKEY DISEASE and VERVET MONKEY DISEASE because the first recorded cases acquired their infection from monkeys of this genus. It is a highly dangerous viral infection with a high mortality rate. The incubation period is 4 to 9 days. The onset is sudden with marked nausea and severe headache. This is followed by rising temperature, diarrhoea, and vomiting. Towards the end of the first week a rash appears which persists for a week and is accompanied by internal bleeding. In those who recover convalescence is slow and prolonged. The world distribution of the causative virus is unknown, but apart from laboratory infections acquired through working with vervet monkeys, all the cases so far reported have occurred in Africa.

MARCH FRACTURE A curious condition in which a fracture occurs of the second (rarely the third) metatarsal bone in the foot without any obvious cause. The usual story is that a pain suddenly developed in the foot while walking or marching, (hence the name) and that it has persisted ever since. The only treatment needed is immobilization of the foot and rest, and the fracture heals satisfactorily.

MARCH HAEMOGLOBINURIA A complication of walking and running over long distances. It is due to damage to red blood cells in the blood-vessels of the sole of the feet. This results in HAEMOGLOBIN being released into the bloodstream, which is then voided in the urine, the condition known as HAEMO-GLOBINURIA. No treatment is required.

MARFAN'S SYNDROME An inherited disorder affecting about one person in 50,000 in which the connective tissue is abnormal. The result is defects of the heart, skeleton and eyes. The victims are unusually tall and thin with deformities of the chest and spine. They have spider-like hands and their joints and ligaments are weak. Orthopaedic intervention may help, as will drugs to control the heart problems. As affected individuals have a 50-per-cent chance of passing on the disease to their children, they should receive genetic counselling.

MARIJUANA Another term for CANNABIS INDICA, or hemp, or hashish. (See DRUG ADDICTION.)

MARRIAGE GUIDANCE (see RELATE MARRIAGE GUIDANCE).

MARROW (see BONE MARROW).

MARSH FEVER (see MALARIA).

MASK A device that covers the nose and mouth to enable inhalation ANAESTHETICS or other gases such as oxygen to be administered. It is also a covering for the nose and mouth to ensure antiseptic conditions are maintained during surgery, when dressing a wound or nursing a patient in conditions of isolation. The term mask is also applied to the expressionless appearance that occurs in certain disorders – for example, PARKINSON'S DISEASE.

MASOCHISM A condition in which a person gets pleasure from physical or emotional pain inflicted by others. The term is often used in the context of achieving sexual excitement through inflicted pain. Masochism may be a conscious or subconscious activity.

MASSAGE, or RUBBING A method of treatment in which the operator uses his hands, or occasionally other appliances, to rub the skin and deeper tissues of the person under treatment. It is often combined with (a) passive movements, in which the masseur moves the limbs in various ways, the person treated making no effort; or (b) active movements, which are performed with the combined assistance of masseur and patient. Massage is also often combined with baths and gymnastics in order to strengthen various muscles. Massage helps to improve circulation, prevent adhesions in injured tissues, relax muscular spasm, improve muscle tone and reduce any oedema. (See also CARDIAC MASSAGE.)

Massage for medical conditions is best done by trained practitioners. A complete list of members of the Chartered Society of Physiotherapy can be obtained on application to the Secretary of the Society (see APPENDIX 2: ADDRESSES).

MASSETER An important muscle of mastication that extends from the zygomatic arch in the cheek to the mandible or jaw bone. It acts by closing the jaw.

MASS HYSTERIA (see HYSTERIA).

MASS MINIATURE RADIOGRAPHY is a method of obtaining X-ray photographs of the chests of large numbers of people. It has been used on a large scale as a means of screening the population for pulmonary TUBERCULOSIS. It is no longer used in the United Kingdom.

MASTALGIA The term applied to pain in the breast.

MAST CELLS Round or oval cells found predominantly in the loose CONNECTIVE TISSUES. They contain HISTAMINE and HEPARIN, and carry immunoglobulin E, the ANTIBODY which plays a predominant part in allergic reactions. Although known to play a part in inflammatory reactions, allergy, and hyper-sensitivity, their precise function in health and disease is still not quite clear.

MASTECTOMY The operation for removal of a breast usually because of cancer. When the diagnosis of a breast lump is uncertain the surgeon may perform a lumpectomy (removal of the lump) and have this tissue assessed in the laboratory. If cancer cells are found, it may be necessary to proceed to a full mastectomy. In the United Kingdom a national protocol for the treatment of breast cancer has been recommended. Patients who have had a mastectomy will usually need a prosthesis to ensure a balanced figure. It is an operation that can cause considerable psychological disturbance. Those who find it difficult to adjust to the situation after the operation will obtain helpful advice from Breast Cancer Care (see APPENDIX 2: ADDRESSES).

MASTICATION The act whereby, as a result of movements of the lower jaw, lips, tongue, and cheek, food is reduced to a condition in which it is ready to be acted on by the gastric juices in the process of digestion. Adequate mastication is an essential part of the digestive process. (See DIGESTION.)

MASTITIS The term applied to inflammation of the breast. (See BREASTS, DISEASES OF.)

MASTOID PROCESS The large process of the temporal bone of the skull which can be felt immediately behind the ear. It contains numerous cavities, one of which, the mastoid antrum, communicates with the middle ear, and is liable to suppurate when the middle ear is diseased. (See EAR, DISEASES OF.)

MASTURBATION The production of an orgasm by self-manipulation of the PENIS or CLITORIS.

MAT BURN A combination of a burn and an abrasion which occurs in wrestlers when the skin over the bony points is rubbed against the unyielding canvas mat.

MATCH-WORKERS' DISEASE (see PHOSPHORUS POISONING).

MATERIA MEDICA The branch of medical study which deals with the sources, preparations, and uses of drugs. (See MEDICINES.)

MATERNITY AND CHILD WELFARE In the United Kingdom the proper care of pregnant women, mothers, infants and young children started largely on a voluntary basis early in the 20th century. With official backing it has now developed into an extensive network of clinics in NHS general practices, hospitals and local-authority premises, where skilled antenatal, postnatal and paediatric care is provided by consultants, general practitioners, midwives, health visitors and nurses. Local authorities also have certain responsibilities for the provision of appropriate accommodation for mothers with young children on low incomes. Various welfare benefits are available to young families, provided they meet official criteria. Day nurseries, some run by local authorities, others on a voluntary or privately funded basis are available in some areas to young mothers, especially those who are working. Efforts are being made to increase the numbers of such nurseries.

A recent official review of maternity and child health services called for substantial changes in professional practice to secure a 'woman-centred service'. The aim was greater acceptability and accessibility of maternity care founded on 'clinical practices of known effectiveness'.

MAXILLA The name applied to the upper jaw-bones, which bear the teeth.

ME (see MYALGIC ENCEPHALOMYELITIS).

MEASLES, also known as MORBILLI, is an acute infectious disease occurring mostly in children and caused by an RNA paramyxovirus. The name, measles, comes from the teutonic root, *maes*, meaning a spot. Morbilli is a diminutive of morbus, a disease. It appears to have been known from an early period in the history of medicine, mention being made of it in the writings of Rhazes and others of the Arabian physicians in the tenth century. For long, however, its specific nature was not recognized, and it was held to be a variety of smallpox. Measles and SCARLET FEVER were long confused with each other; and in the account given by Sydenham of epidemics of measles in London in 1670 and 1674, it is evident that even that accurate observer had not as yet clearly perceived their pathological distinction, although it would seem to have been made a century earlier by Ingrassia, a physician of Palermo. The disease known as German measles, or RUBELLA, is a much milder disease than measles. Measles is compulsorily notifiable in Britain.

Causes Measles is a virus disease of the earlier years of childhood. Like most other infectious maladies, it is rare in infants under 6 months old on account of the antibodies that they have acquired from their mothers before birth. It is rare in adults because most have undergone an attack in early life, although second attacks can occur. The incubation period is 7 to 21 days.

There has been a dramatic fall in numbers from 1986 when over 80,000 cases were reported. This is due to the introduction in 1988 of the measles, mumps and rubella vaccine (MMR) (see IMMUNIZATION); 1990 was the first year in which no deaths from measles were reported. Even so, fears of side-effects of the vaccine against measles meant that some children in the UK were not immunized. Side-effects are, however, rare and the government is campaigning to raise the rate of immunization, with GPs being set targets for their practices.

There are few diseases so infectious as measles, and its rapid spread in epidemics is no doubt due to the fact that this viral infection is most potent in the earlier stages. Hence the difficulty of timely isolation and the readiness with which the disease is spread, which is mostly by infected droplets.

Symptoms Prodromal symptoms are catarrh, conjunctivitis (see EYE DISEASES), fever and a feeling of wretchedness. Then Koplik spots – a classic sign of measles – appear on the roof of the mouth and lining of the cheeks. The macular body rash, typical of measles, appears three to five days later.

Treatment Isolation of the patient and treatment of any secondary bacterial infection.

Children usually run a high temperature which can be relieved with cool sponging and antipyretic drugs. Calamine lotion may alleviate any itching.

MEASURES (see APPENDIX 6: MEASUREMENTS IN MEDICINE).

MEAT (see PROTEIN).

MEATUS A term applied to any passage or opening: e.g. external auditory meatus, the passage from the surface to the drum of the EAR.

MECKEL'S DIVERTICULUM A hollow process sometimes found attached to the small intestine. It is placed on the small intestine about 90 to 120 cm (3 or 4 feet) from its junction with the large intestine, is several cms long, and ends blindly.

MECONIUM The brown, semi-fluid material which collects in the bowels of a fetus before birth, and which should be discharged either at the time of birth or shortly afterwards. It consists partly of bile secreted by the liver before birth, partly of debris from the mucous membrane of the intestines.

MEDIA The middle layer of an organ or tissue, but more usually applied to the wall of an artery or vein, where the media comprises layers of elastic and smooth muscle fibres.

MEDIAL Near the middle of tissue, organ or body.

MEDIAL TIBIAL SYNDROME is the term applied by athletes to a condition characterized by pain over the inner border of the shin, which occurs in most runners and sometimes in joggers. The syndrome, also known as shin splints, is due to muscular swelling resulting in inadequate blood supply in the muscle: hence the pain. The disorder may be the result of compartment syndrome (build-up of pressure in the muscles), TENDINITIS, muscle or bone inflammation or damage to the muscle. It usually disappears within a few weeks, responding to rest and PHYSIOTHERAPY, with or without injections. In some cases, however, it becomes chronic and so severe that it occurs even at rest. If the cause is the compartment syndrome, relief is usually obtained by a simple operation to relieve the pressure in the affected muscles.

MEDIASTINUM is the space in the chest which lies between the two lungs. It contains the heart and great vessels, the gullet, the lower part of the windpipe, the thoracic duct, the phrenic nerves, as well as numerous structures of less importance

MEDICAID A joint state and federal health insurance scheme in the United States that provides cover for poorer people in the population.

MEDICAL DEFENCE SOCIETIES These are UK organizations that provide doctors with insurance cover against claims for medical negligence in their clinical practice. The societies advise doctors on all legal aspects of their work, including patients' complaints. The sharp rise in claims for medical negligence in the NHS in the 1980s persuaded the UK Health Departments to introduce a system in which the government would accept liability for negligence by NHS hospital doctors. The defence societies also provide cover for doctors in some other countries.

MEDICAL DEVICES AGENCY An executive agency of the Department of Health in the UK. Set up in 1994, it is responsible for regulating and advising on sale or use of any product, other than a medicine, used in the health-care environment for the diagnosis, prevention, monitoring or treatment of illness or disease. Equipment ranges from CARDIAC PACEMAKERS to PROSTHESES and from SYRINGES to MRI.

MEDICAL EDUCATION This term is used to define the process of learning and knowledge acquisition in the study of medicine. It also encompasses the expertise required to develop education and training for students and learners in all aspects of medical health care. Studies for undergraduate students, postgraduate students and individual health-care practitioners from the initial stages to the ongoing development of a career in medicine or associated health fields are also included in medical education. The word 'pedagogy' is sometimes applied to this process.

A range of research investigations has developed within medical education. These apply to course monitoring, audit, development and validation, assessment methodologies and the application of educationally appropriate principles at undergraduate and postgraduate levels. Research is undertaken by medical educationalists whose backgrounds include teaching, social sciences and medicine and related health-care specialties and who will hold a medical or general educational diploma, degree or other appropriate postgraduate qualification.

Development and validation for all courses are an important part of continuing accreditation processes. The relatively conservative courses at both undergraduate and postgraduate levels, including diplomas and postgraduate qualifications awarded by the specialist medical royal colleges (responsible for standards of specialist education) and universities, have undergone a range of reassessment and redefinition driven by the changing needs of the individual practitioner in the last decade. The stimuli to change aspects of medical training have come from the government through the then Chief Medical Officer, Sir Kenneth Calman, and the introduction of new approaches to specialist training (The Calman programme), from the GENERAL MEDICAL COUNCIL and its document 'Tomorrow's Doctors' and from the profession itself through the activities of the British Medical Association and the medical royal colleges. The evolving expectations of the public in their perception of the requirements of a doctor into the next century and changes in education of other groups of health professionals have also led to pressures for changes.

Consequently, many new departments and units devoted to medical education within university medical schools, royal colleges and elsewhere within higher education have been established. These developments have built upon practice developed elsewhere in the world, particularly in North America, Australia and some European countries. Undergraduate education has seen application of new educational methods, including problem-based learning (PBL) in Liverpool, Glasgow and Manchester, clinical and communication skill teaching, early patient contact and the extensive adoption of Internet (World Wide Web) support and Computer Aided Learning (CAL). In postgraduate education, driven by European directives and practices, changes in specialist training and the needs of community medicine, new courses have developed around the membership and fellowship examinations for the royal colleges. Examples of these changes driven by medical education expertise include the STEP course for the Royal College of Surgeons of England and distance-learning courses for diplomas in primary care and rheumatology as well as examples of good practice as adopted by the Royal College of General Practitioners.

Continuing Professional Development (CPD) and Continuing Medical Education (CME) are also important aspects of medical education now being developed in the United Kingdom, and are evolving to meet the needs of individuals at all stages of their careers.

Bodies closely involved in medical educational developments and their review include the General Medical Council, SCOPME (The Standing Committee on Postgraduate Medical Education), all the medical royal colleges and medical schools and the British Medical Association through its Board of Medical Education. The National Health Service (NHS) is also involved in education and is a key to facilitation of CPD/CME as the major employer of doctors within the United Kingdom.

Several learned societies embrace medical education at all levels. These include ASME (The Association for the Study of Medical Education), MADEN (The Medical and Dental Education Network) and AMEE (The Association for Medical Education in Europe). Specialist journals are devoted to research reports relating to medical educational developments (e.g. *Academic Medicine, Health Care Education, Medical Education*). The more general medical journals (e.g. *British Medical Journal, New England Journal of Medicine, The Lancet, Annals of the Royal College of Surgeons*) also carry articles on educational matters. Finally, the World Wide Web (WWW) is a valuable source of information relating to courses and course development and other aspects of modern medical education.

MEDICAL INFORMATICS (see INFORMATION TECHNOLOGY IN MEDICINE).

MEDICAL RECORD The information recorded and kept by health professionals about an individual's illness(es). The information is normally confidential to those responsible for caring for the patient and to the patient, if he or she should wish to see it.

MEDICAL RESEARCH COUNCIL A statutory body in the United Kingdom that promotes the balanced development of medical and related biological research and aims to advance knowledge that will lead to improved health care. It employs its own research staff in more than 40 research establishments. These include the National Institute for Medical Research, the Laboratory of Molecular Biology and the Clinical Sciences Centre. Grants are provided so that individual scientists can do research which complements the research activities of hospitals and universities. There are several medical charities and foundations – for example, the Imperial Cancer Research Fund, the British Heart Foundation, the Nuffield Laboratories and the Wellcome Trust foster medical which fund and foster research.

MEDICARE A health insurance scheme in the United States, managed by the federal government, that provides cover for Americans over the age of 65 who have certain disabilities.

MEDICATED Description of a substance that contains a medicinal drug, commonly applied to items such as sweets and soaps.

MEDICINE (1) The skills and science used by trained practitioners to prevent, diagnose, treat and research disease and its related factors.
(2) A drug used to treat an individual with an illness or injury.
(3) The diagnosis and treatment of those diseases not normally requiring surgical intervention.

Defensive medicine Diagnostic or treatment procedures undertaken by practitioners with the aim of reducing the likelihood of legal action by patients.

MEDICINE OF AGEING Diseases developing during a person's lifetime may be the result of his or her lifestyle, environment, genetic factors and natural ageing factors.

Lifestyle While this may change as people grow older – for instance, physical activity is commonly reduced – some lifestyle factors are unchanged: for example, cigarette smoking, commonly started in adolescence, may be continued as an adult and result in smoker's cough and eventually chronic BRONCHITIS and EMPHYSEMA, widespread ATHEROSCLEROSIS causing heart attacks and STROKES, OSTEOPOROSIS producing bony fractures and cancer affecting the lungs and bladder.

Environmental factors These may result in illnesses which include ASTHMA and BRONCHITIS from dusts and pollen, skin cancer after chronic exposure to the sun and intellectual impairment that may be attributed by those with ageist attitudes merely to 'old age' but, in fact, may be caused by organic solvents.

Genetic factors can cause SICKLE CELL DISEASE, HUNTINGTON'S CHOREA and POLYCYSTIC KIDNEYS.

Ageing process This is associated with the menopause in women and, in both sexes, with a reduction in the body's tissue elasticity and often a deterioration in mental and physical capabilities. When compared with illnesses described in much younger people, similar illnesses in old age present in an atypical manner – for example, confusion and changed behaviour due to otherwise asymptomatic heart failure causing a reduced supply of oxygen to the brain. Social adversity in old age may result from the combined effects of reduced body reserve, atypical presentation of illness, multiple disorders and POLYPHARMACY.

Age-related change in the presentation of illnesses This was first recognized by the specialty of geriatric medicine which is concerned with the medical and social management of advanced age. Before the 1960s sick elderly people were usually looked after in NHS institutions, many of them old poor-law hospitals, with variable standards of medical input and often unsatisfactory nursing care. This led some health professionals to argue that with proper diagnosis and treatment many of these seemingly chronic inpatients could be mobilized and thus return to their own homes or to residential or day-status care.

This change in approach was largely a consequence of the development of the specialty of geriatrics whose practitioners took a positive, dynamic approach and transformed the care of ill or disabled elderly people. Now the aim is to assess, treat and rehabilitate such patients. The number of institutional beds has been steadily cut, while availability of day-treatment centres and respite facilities have been boosted – though still inadequate to cope with the growing number of people over 65.

These developments, along with day social centres, provide relatives and carers with a break from the often demanding task of look-ing after the frail or ill elderly. As the proportion of elderly in the population rises, along with the cost of hospital inpatient care, close co-operation between hospitals, COMMUNITY CARE services and PRIMARY CARE teams becomes increasingly important if senior citizens are not to suffer from the consequences of the tight operating budgets of the various medical and social agencies with responsibilities for the care of the elderly. Private or voluntary nursing and residential homes have expanded in the past 15 years and now care for many elderly people who previously would have been ocupying NHS facilities. This trend has been accelerated by a tightening of the benefit rules for funding such care. Local authorities are now responsible for assessing the needs of elderly people in the community and deciding whether they are eligible for financial support (in full or in part) for nursing-home care.

With a substantial proportion of hospital inpatients in the United Kingdom being over 60 it is sometimes argued that all health professionals should be skilled in the care of the elderly and thus the need for doctors and nurses trained in the specialty of geriatrics is diminishing. Even so, as more people are reaching their 80s, there seems to be a reasonable case for training staff in the type of care these individuals need and to facilitate research into illness at this stage of life.

MEDICINES are drugs made stable, palatable and acceptable for administration. In Britain the Medicines Act 1968 controls the making, advertising, and selling of substances used for 'medicinal purposes', which means diagnosing, preventing, or treating disease, or altering a function of the body. Permission to market a medicine has to be obtained from the government through the Medicines Control Agency, or from the European Commission through the European Medicines Evaluation Agency. It takes the form of a Marketing Authorization (formerly called a Product Licence), and the uses to which the medicine can be put are laid out in the Summary of Product Characteristics (which used to be called the Product Data Sheet).

There are three main categories of licensed medicinal product. Drugs in small quantities can, if they are perceived to be safe, be licensed for general sale (GSL – general sales list), and may then be sold in any retail shop. P (pharmacy-only) medicines can be sold from a registered pharmacy by or under the supervision of a PHARMACIST; no prescription is needed. P and GSL medicines are together known as OTCs, that is, 'over-the-counter medicines'. POM (prescription-only medicines) can only be obtained from a registered pharmacy on the prescription of a doctor or dentist. As more information is gathered on the safety of drugs, and more emphasis is put on individual responsibility for health, there is a trend towards allowing drugs that were once POM to be more widely available as P medicines. Examples include HYDROCORTISONE 1-per-cent cream for skin rashes, CIMETIDINE for indigestion, and ACICLOVIR for cold sores. Care is needed to avoid taking a P medicine that might alter the actions of another medicine taken with it, or that might be unsuitable for other reasons. Patients should read the patient-information leaflet, and seek the pharmacist's advice if they have any doubt about the information. They should tell their pharmacist or doctor if the medicine results in any unexpected effects.

Methods of administration The ways in which drugs are given are increasingly ingenious. Most are still given by mouth. Some oral preparations ('slow release' or 'controlled release' preparations) are designed to release their contents slowly into the gut, to maintain the action of the drug. We may see a revolution in ways of giving medicines, such as insulin, which have at present to be injected, if they can be 'packaged' in minute protective spheres of fat that pass through the gut wall before releasing their contents.

Buccal preparations are allowed to dissolve in the mouth, and sublingual ones are dissolved under the tongue. The other end of the gastrointestinal tract can also absorb drugs: suppositories inserted in the rectum can be used for their local actions, for example, as laxatives; or to allow absorption when taking the drug by mouth is difficult or impossible, for example, during a convulsion, or when vomiting.

Small amounts of drug can be absorbed through the intact skin, and for very potent drugs like OESTROGENS (female sex hormones) or the anti-anginal drug GLYCERYL TRINITRATE, a drug-releasing 'patch' can be used. Drugs can be inhaled into the lungs as a fine powder to treat or prevent ASTHMA attacks. They can also be dispersed ('nebulized') as a fine mist which can be administered with compressed air or oxygen. Spraying a drug into the nostril, so that it can be absorbed through the lining of the nose into the bloodstream, can avoid destruction of the drug in the stomach. This route is used for a small number of drugs like antidiuretic hormone.

Injection remains an important route of administering drugs both locally (for example, into joints or into the eyeball), and into the bloodstream. For this latter purpose, drugs can be given under the skin, that is, subcutaneously (s.c. – also called hypodermic injection); into muscle – intramuscularly (i.m.), or into a vein – intravenously (i.v.). The ultra-fine disposable needles now available make subcutaneous injection much less painful than it once was. Oily or crystalline preparations of drugs injected subcutaneously form a 'depot' from which they are absorbed only slowly into the blood. The action of drugs such as TESTOSTERONE and INSULIN can be prolonged by using such preparations, which also allow contraceptive 'implants' that work for some months.

Safe disposal of unwanted medicines Unwanted medicines are a form of 'controlled waste' under the Environmental Protection Act 1990 and must be disposed of in an appropriate way.

The best thing is to take any extra or unwanted medicines to a registered pharmacy. Syringes and needles, used by diabetic patients, for example, pose problems. Devices exist to cut off and retain the needle; and some local authorities in the United Kingdom arrange for collection and safe disposal. There are also local 'needle exchange' schemes for intravenous drug abusers.

Safe use of medicines All medicines can have unwanted effects ('side-effects' or, more strictly adverse effects) that are unpleasant and sometimes harmful. It is best not to take any medicine, prescribed or othewise, unless there is a clear reason for doing so; the possible adverse effects of treatment, and the risk of their occurring, have to be set against any likely benefit. Remember too that one treatment can affect another already being taken. For example, some over-the-counter (OTC) medicines, and many prescription-only medicines (POMs), interfere with treatment with the ANTICOAGULANT WARFARIN. Many adverse effects depend on the dosage, so the recommended dosage should not be exceeded. Some people, for example, those with ALLERGIES to a particular group of drugs, or those with kidney or liver disease, are more likely to suffer adverse effects than otherwise healthy people.

When an individual begins a course of treatment he or she should take it as instructed. With ANTIBIOTIC treatments especially, it is important to take the whole course of tablets prescribed, because brief exposure of bacteria to an antibiotic can make them resistant to treatment. Increasing bacterial resistance to antibiotics is a serious world-wide problem. The UK government has urged its doctors to prescribe antibiotics only when such treatment is necessary and likely to be effective. Most drugs can be stopped at once, but some treatments can cause unpleasant, and occasionally dangerous, symptoms if stopped abruptly. Sleeping tablets, anti-EPILEPSY treatment, and medicines used to treat ANGINA are among the agents which can cause such 'withdrawal symptoms'. CORTICOSTEROIDS are a particularly important group of medicines in this respect, because prolonged courses of treatment with high doses can suppress the ability of the body to respond to severe stresses (such as surgical operations) for many months or even years.

MEDICOLEGAL A term that relates to the practice of medicine and law (see FORENSIC MEDICINE).

MEDLARS Medical Literature Analysis and Retrieval System, a computerized index system produced by the US National Library of Medicine.

MEDLINE A computer-based telephone line linkage to MEDLARS for rapid transmission of medical information held by that library. Information can be accessed worldwide.

MEDULLA The inside part of an organ or tissue that is distinct from the outer part – for example, the marrow in the centre of a long bone or the inner portion of the kidneys or adrenal glands.

MEDULLA OBLONGATA is the hindmost part of the brain and is continued into the spinal cord. In it are situated several of the nerve-centres which are most essential to life, such as those governing breathing, the action of the heart, swallowing. (See BRAIN.)

MEFENAMIC ACID A non-steroidal anti-inflammatory drug that is an analgesic for mild to moderate pain in RHEUMATOID and OSTEOARTHRITIS and other musculoskeletal disorders. Also used for DYSMENNORRHOEA and MENORRHAGIA. It must be used with care as it has several side-effects, in particular DIARRHOEA and occasional HAEMOLYTIC ANAEMIA. It must not be used in patients with inflammatory bowel disease.

MEGA- and MEGALO- are prefixes denoting largeness.

MEGACOLON A greatly enlarged colon that may be present at birth or develop later. It can occur in all age groups and the condition is typified by severe chronic constipation. Megacolon is caused by obstruction of the colon which may be due to faulty innervation, or to psychological factors. Other causes are HIRSCHSPRUNG'S DISEASE or ULCERATIVE COLITIS. In old people the persistent use of powerful laxative drugs may cause the condition.

MEGALOMANIA A delusion of grandeur or an insane belief in a person's own extreme greatness, goodness, or power.

MEIBOMIAN GLANDS Numerous glands within the tarsal plates of the eyelids. Their secretions form part of the tears. (See EYE.)

MEIOSIS or REDUCTION DIVISION is the form of cell division that only occurs in the gonads, that is the testis and the ovary, giving rise to the germ cells of the sperms and the ova. Two types of sperm cells are produced. One contains 22 autosomes and a Y sex chromosome and the other contains 22 autosomes and an X sex

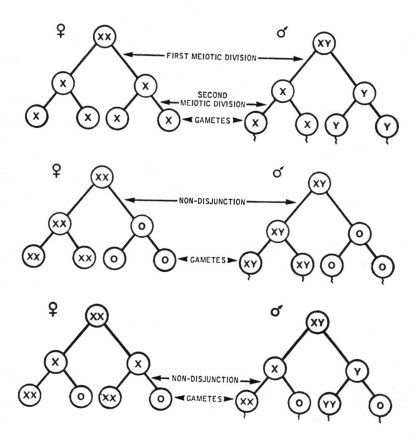

The formation of gametes. Top, normal meiosis. Centre, non-disjunction at first meiotic division. Bottom, non-disjunction at second meiotic division.

chromosome. All the ova, however, produced by normal meiosis have 22 autosomes and an X sex chromosome. Two divisions of the nucleus occur and only one division of the chromosomes, so that the number of chromosomes in the ova and sperms is half that of the somatic cells. Each chromosome pair divides so that the gametes receives only one member of each pair. The number of chromosomes is restored to full complement at fertilization so the the zygote has a complete set, each chromosome from the nucleus of the sperm pairing up with its corresponding partner from the ovum.

The first stage of meiosis involves the pairing of homologous chromosomes which join together and synapse lengthwise. The chromosomes then become doubled by splitting along their length and the chromatids so formed are held together by centromeres. As the homologous chromosomes, one of which has come from the mother and the other from the father, are lying together genetic interchange can take place between the chromatids and in this way new combinations of genes arise. All four chromatids are closely interwoven and recombination may take place between any maternal or any paternal chromatids. This process is known as crossing over or recombination. After this period of interchange homologous chromosomes move apart, one to each pole of the nucleus. The cell then divides and the nucleus of each new cell now contains 23 and not 46 chromosomes. The second meiotic division then occurs, the centromeres divide and the chromatids move apart to opposite poles of the nucleus so there are still 23 chromosomes in each of the daughter nuclei so formed. The cell divides again so that there are four gametes, each containing a half number (haploid) set of chromosomes. However, owing to the recombination or crossing over the genetic material is not identical with either parent or with other spermatozoa.

MELAENA Blood in the faeces in which dark, tarry masses are passed from the bowel. It is due to bleeding from the stomach or from the higher part of the bowel, the blood undergoing chemical changes under the action of the secretions, and being finally converted in large part into sulphide of iron. It is a serious symptom meriting medical investigation. It can indicate peptic ulcer or carcinoma of the stomach.

MELANCHOLIA A form of mental illness characterized by great mental and physical depression. (See MENTAL ILLNESS.)

MELANIN Pigment which confers colour on the SKIN, HAIR and EYE. It is produced by cells called MELANOCYTES interspersed along the basal layer of the epidermis. The maturation of the epidermis into stratum corneum cells packed with melanin granules confers an ultraviolet light barrier which protects the skin against the harmful effects resulting from continued solar exposure. The races do not differ in the number of melanocytes in their skin, only in the rate and quantity of melanin production. Exposure to bright sunlight stimulates melanin production and distribution causing 'suntan'. A hormone from the PITUITARY GLAND may stimulate melanin production on the face in pregnancy. (See CHLOASMA.)

MELANOCYTE Clear branching cell in the epidermis that produces tyrosinase (an enzyme) and MELANIN.

MELANOMA Malignant tumour arising from MELANOCYTES. It may start in an existing MOLE or arise *de novo*. Increasing exposure to sunlight of white populations in the last half century has resulted in an alarming increase in the incidence of this cancer. It is mainly seen in those over 40 years, especially on the legs in women and on the back in men. An enlarging pigmented macule or nodule with irregular contuour, profile or colour distribution is always suspect.

Treatment is excision with a margin of normal tissue. The prognosis depends on the depth of invasion. Very superficial melanomas carry an excellent outlook once removed, but deeper tumours may spread to regional lymph glands and beyond with fatal results. Public awareness campaigns have led to the earlier presentation of melanomas in recent years, with corresponding benefit. (See SUNBURN.)

MELATONIN A hormone that plays a key role in the body's diurnal (night and day) rhythms. Produced by the PINEAL GLAND and derived from SEROTONIN, it acts on receptors in an area of the brain above the OPTIC CHIASMA, synchronizing them to the diurnal rhythm. Melatonin is under investigation as a possible agent to treat insomnia in the elderly and in shift workers. It may also help people with SEASONAL AFFECTIVE DISORDER SYNDROME (SAD) and those who suffer from jet lag.

MELPHALAN An ALKYLATING AGENT used to treat certain forms of malignant disease including BREAST tumours, OVARIAN cancer, MELANOMA and HODGKIN'S LYMPHOMA. It can be given orally or by injection. (See CYTOTOXIC.)

MEMBRANES (see BRAIN; CROUP; DIPHTHERIA; LABOUR).

MEMORY The capacity to remember. It is complex and probably occurs in many areas of the brain including the LIMBIC system and the TEMPORAL LOBES. Despite such poor knowledge of the anatomy of memory, research has revealed much about how the process works. There are three main steps: registration, storage, and recall.

During registration information from the sense organs and the cerebral cortex is put into codes for storage in the short-term memory system. The codes are usually acoustic (based on the sounds and words that would be used to describe the information) but may use any of the five senses. This system can take only a few chunks of information at a time. Research shows, for example, that only about seven longish numbers can be retained and recalled at once – the next new number displaces an earlier one that is then forgotten. And if a subject is asked to describe a person he has just met, he will recall only seven or so facts about that person. This depends on attention span and can be improved by concentration and rehearsal, for example, by reciting the list of things that must be remembered.

Material needing storage for several minutes stays in the short-term memory. More valuable information goes to the long-term memory where it can be kept for any period from a few minutes to a lifetime. Storage is more reliable if the information is in meaningful codes – it is much easier to remember people's names if their faces and personalities are memorable too. Using techniques such as mnemonics takes this into account.

The final stage is retrieval. Recognizing and recalling the required information involves searching the memory. In the short-term memory this takes about 40 thousandths of a second per item, a rate that is surprisingly consistent, even in people with disorders such as SCHIZOPHRENIA.

Most kinds of forgetting or amnesia occur during retrieval. Benign forgetfulness is usually caused by interference from similar items because the required information was not clearly coded and well organized. Retrieval can be improved by recreating the context in which the information was registered. This is why the police reconstruct scenes of crimes, and why revision for exams is more effective if facts are learnt in the form of answers to mock questions.

Loss of memory or amnesia mainly affects long-term memory (information which is stored indefinitely) rather than short-term memory which is measured in minutes. Short-term memory may, however, be affected by unconsciousness caused by trauma. Drivers involved in an accident may be unable to recall the event or the period leading up to it. The cause of amnesia is disease of or damage to the parts of the brain responsible for memory. Degenerative disorders such as ALZHEIMER'S DISEASE, brain tumours, infections (for example, ENCEPHALITIS), STROKES, SUBARACHNOID HAEMORRHAGE and alcoholism all cause memory loss. Some psychiatric illnesses feature loss of memory and ageing is is usually accompanied by some memory loss, though the age of onset and severity vary greatly.

MENARCHE The start of MENSTRUATION. The average age at which it occurs in British girls is 12·5 years, a year or two after the first physical indications of PUBERTY start. In London girls it is 13·1 years. There is considerable racial and geographical variation.

MENDELISM The term applied to a law enunciated by G. J. Mendel that the offspring is not intermediate in type between its parents, but that the type of one or other parent is predominant. Characteristics are classed as either dominant or recessive. The offspring of the first generation tend to inherit the dominant characteristics, whilst the recessive characteristics remain latent and appear in some of the offspring of the second generation. If individuals possessing recessive characters unite, recessive characters then become dominant characters in succeeding generations. The law may be expressed by the following formula:

$$n(DD+2DR+RR)$$

in which DD represents dominant offspring, RR recessive offspring, and DR offspring with mixed characters. (See GENETICS).

MENDELSON SYNDROME Inhalation of regurgitated stomach contents, usually as a complication of general ANAESTHESIA. It may cause death from ANOXIA or result in extensive lung damage.

MENIÈRE'S DISEASE So called after the Frenchman, Prosper Menière, who first described it in 1861, the disease is characterized by TINNITUS, deafness and intermittent attacks of VERTIGO. It usually occurs in middle age, and is slightly more common in men than in women. The first manifestation is usually deafness on one side. Then, as a rule many months later, there is a sudden attack, without any warning, of intense vertigo. The acute giddiness usually lasts for two to three hours with some unsteadiness persisting for a few days. The time interval between attacks varies from a week to a few months. When they do recur, they tend to occur in clusters. The tinnitus, which tends to be high-pitched, comes on about the same time as the deafness. It is often described as being like rushing water or escaping steam. The deafness becomes gradually worse until it is complete. The condition is due to excessive fluid in the labyrinth of the ears (see EAR). The cause of this accumulation is not known, though it has been suggested that it might be a form of allergy, or might be due to spasm of the small blood-vessels. The disorder is diagnosed from AUDIOMETRY, the CALORIC test and other investig-ations.

Treatment Acute vertigo symptoms can sometimes be alleviated with drugs such as CYCLIZINE and NICOTINIC ACID, but the disorder is notoriously difficult to treat and no certain cure is available. Surgical decompression of the fluid in the ear's balancing mechanism may relieve vertigo and prevent the disease worsening. The vestibular nerve to the ear can also be cut to relieve vertigo while preserving hearing. (See TINNITUS.)

MENINGES The membranes surrounding the brain and spinal cord. (See BRAIN.) The membranes include the DURA MATER, a tough, fibrous membrane closely applied to the inside of the skull; the ARACHNOID, a more delicate membrane, enveloping the brain but separated from its irregular surface by spaces containing fluid; and the pia mater, a delicate network of fibres containing blood-vessels and uniting the arachnoid to the brain. The two last are sometimes referred to as the pia-arachnoid. These membranes bear the blood-vessels which nourish the surface of the brain and the interior of the skull. Meningeal haemorrhage from these vessels forms one of the chief dangers arising from fracture of the skull.

MENINGISM A condition with symptoms closely resembling those of MENINGITIS. Most commonly occurring in children, it is usually a symptom of chest infection or of inflammation in the upper respiratory tract. Given the serious implications of meningitis, medical advice should be sought. Examination of the CEREBROSPINAL FLUID may be necessary: in meningism the fluid is normal.

MENINGITIS Inflammation affecting the membranes of the brain or spinal cord or usually both. Meningitis may be caused by bacteria, viruses, fungi, malignant cells or blood (after SUBARACHNOID HAEMORRHAGE). The term is, however, usually restricted to inflammation due to a BACTERIUM or VIRUS. Viral meningitis is normally a mild, self-limiting infection of a few days' duration. Bacterial meningitis is life threatening, and 70 per cent of cases of acute bacterial meningitis in the UK are caused by three bacteria: *Neisseria meningitidis* (meningococcus), *Haemophilus influenzae* and *Streptococcus pneumoniae* (pneumococcus). Other bacteria include *Escherichia coli*, *Mycobacterium tuberculosis* (see TUBERCULOSIS), *Treponema pallidum* (see SYPHILIS) and *STAPHYLOCOCCI* spp. Bacterial meningitis may occur by spread from nearby infected foci such as the nasopharynx, middle ear, mastoid and sinuses. Direct infection may be the result of penetrating injuries of the skull from accidents or gunshot wounds. Meningitis may also be a complication of neurosurgery despite careful aseptic precautions. Immunocompromised patients – those with AIDS or on cytoxic drugs – are vulnerable to infections. Bacterial meningitis is an emergency: the infection has a high mortality, even in the developed world. Untreated, it is fatal: the death rate among treated patients may be as high as 15 per cent.

First recognized in France in 1837, when there was an epidemic, bacterial meningitis has occurred in occasional epidemics in Europe and America since then. Spread is particularly likely in schools and similar communities. Many people harbour the meningococcus without developing meningitis. In recent years small clusters of cases, mainly in schoolchildren and young people at college, have occurred in Britain. In 1996 the steady rise in meningococcal meningitis occurring over the previous decade continued, reaching the highest total for 50 years: 1,136 cases out of a total of 2,313 for all types of meningitis. The (estimated) number of deaths from meningitis in 1996 was 234, higher than in 1989, the last peak year.

Symptoms of meningitis are severe with rapidly developing malaise accompanied by fever, severe headache, PHOTOPHOBIA, vomiting, irritability, rigors, drowsiness and neurological disturbances. Neck stiffness and a positive KERNIG'S SIGN appearing within a few hours of infection are key diagnostic signs.

Diagnosis and treatment are urgent and, if bacterial meningitis is suspected, antibiotic treatment should be started even before laboratory confirmation of the infection. Analysis of the CEREBROSPINAL FLUID (CSF) by means of a LUMBAR PUNCTURE is an essential step in diagnosis. The CSF is clear or turbid in viral meningitis, turbid or viscous in tuberculous infection and turbulent or purulent when meningococci or staphylococci are the infective agents. Cell counts and biochemical make-up of the CSF are other diagnostic pointers. Serological tests are done to identify possible syphilitic infection, which is now rare in Britain.

Patients with suspected meningitis should be admitted to hospital quickly. Meningococcal and pneumococcal infections are treated with large doses of intravenous PENICILLIN; meningitis due to *H. influenzae* is treated with intravenous CHLORAMPHENICOL. Local infections such as SINUSITIS or middle-ear infection require treatment, and appropriate surgery for skull fractures or meningeal tears should be carried out as necessary. Tuberculous meningitis is treated for at least nine months with antituberculous drugs (see TUBERCULOSIS). If bacterial meningitis causes convulsions, these can be controlled with DIAZEPAM and analgesics will be required for the severe headache.

Treatment of close contacts such as family, school friends, medical and nursing staff is recommended if the patient has *H. influenzae* or *N. meningitidis*: RIFAMPICIN provides effective prophylaxis. Contacts of patients with pneumococcal infection do not need preventive treatment. Vaccines for meningococcal meningitis may be given to family members in small epidemics and to any contacts who are especially at risk such as infants, the elderly and immunocompromised individuals.

The outlook for a patient with bacterial meningitis depends on age – the young and old are vulnerable, speed of onset – sudden onset worsens the prognosis – and how quickly treatment is started, hence the urgency of diagnosis and admission to hospital.

Prevention One type of bacterial meningitis, haemophilus, has been largely controlled by vaccination. For most varieties, however, the best protection is to give antibiotic drugs to people who have been in contact with sufferers. Research continues on trying to find more effective vaccines. (See APPENDIX 2: ADDRESSES.)

MENINGOCELE is a protusion of the meninges of the brain through a defect in the skull. (See SPINA BIFIDA.)

MENINGOCOCCUS (see NEISSERIA).

MENINGOENCEPHALITIS is the term applied to infection of the membranes, or meninges, of the brain and the underlying brain matter. In practically all cases of MENINGITIS there is some involvement of the underlying brain. It is when this involvement is considerable that the term, meningoencephalitis, is used. One form that has attracted attention in recent years is that caused by AMOEBAE, particularly that known as *Naegleria fowleri*, in which the infection is acquired through bathing in contaminated water. Effective chlorination of swimming baths kills this micro-organism.

MENINGOMYELOCELE A protrusion of the meninges of the spinal cord through a defect in the spine. (See SPINA BIFIDA.)

MENISCUS A crescentic fibro-cartilage in a joint, such as the cartilages in the knee-joint.

MENOPAUSE This is the term applied to the cessation of menstruation at the end of reproductive life. Usually it occurs between the ages of 45 and 50, although it may occur before the age of 30 or after the age of 50. It can be a psychologically disturbing experience which is quite often accompanied by physical manifestations. These include hot flushes, tiredness, irritability, lack of concentration, palpitations, aching joints and vaginal irritation. There may also be loss of *libido*. Most women can and do live happy, active lives through the menopause, the length of which varies considerably. The loss of OESTROGEN which occurs at the menopause causes atrophy of the genital tract. VASOMOTOR instability in the form of hot flushes, sweats and palpitations occur and can be very debilitating. Urinary urgency, loss of libido and depression are not uncommon manifestations and are remediable with treatment.

One of the major problems of the menopause which does not give rise to symptoms until many years later is OSTEOPOROSIS. After the menopause 1 per cent of the bone is lost per annum to the end of life. This is a factor in the frequency of fractures of the femur in elderly women as a result of osetoporosis but it can be prevented by hormone-replacement therapy.

Hormone replacement therapy (HRT) This term has become synonymous with the scientifically correct term 'OESTROGEN replacement therapy' to signify the treatment of menopausal symptoms and signs with oestrogens, now usually combined with PROGESTOGEN. Oestrogen relieves the short-term symptoms such as hot flushes, sweats and vaginal dryness. Atrophic VAGINITIS and VULVITIS also usually respond to treatment with oestrogens. Oestro-

gen therapy reduces the demineralization of bone which normally occurs after the menopause and, if it is started early and continued for years, it may prevent the development of osteoporosis. Oestrogen is far more effective than calcium supplements and has been shown greatly to reduce fractures affecting the spine, wrists and legs after the age of 50. Cyclical therapy is necessary to avoid abnormal bleeding in women who have reached the menopause. If oestrogens are given alone there is a slightly increased risk of endometrial hyperplasia which may proceed to endometrial cancer. This can be prevented by the administration of oestrogen-progestogen combinations. There is good evidence that a combination of oestrogen and a progestogen avoids the endometrial hyperstimulation produced by the oestrogen alone and relieves most of the symptoms of vasomotor instability of the menopause and prevents the bone loss associated with the menopause. HRT is indicated for menopausal women whose lives are inconvenienced by vasomotor instability or vaginal atrophy. (The latter may respond to local oestrogen treatment.) For vasomotor symptoms systemic treatment should be given for at least a year. In terms of oestrogenic activity natural oestrogen such as oestradiol, oestrone and oestriol are more appropriate for HRT than synthetic oestrogens like ethinyloestradiol, mestranol and diethylstilboestrol.

It has been suggested there was a relationship between oestrogen treatment and breast tumours. However a study by the Boston Collaborative Drug Surveillance Program showed that there was no evidence of any association between oestrogen therapy and either benign or malignant breast tumours. HRT produces minor adverse effects which include breast tenderness, fluid retention, leg cramps and nausea. A few women may face a greater risk of abnormal blood clotting, so HRT is not normally recommended for women who smoke heavily or have had THROMBOSIS, severe HYPERTENSION, STROKE or liver disease.

HRT has, however, brought great benefits to menopausal women, but careful consideration of the woman's medical history and menopausal symptoms is necessary in deciding what combination of drugs should be given and for how long. Long-term treatment is usually favourable in risk-benefit terms for menopausal women without a UTERUS, and they do not require progestogen: treatment may be given for ten years. The position of women with a uterus is less clear because the progestogen they need to take may reduce the protective effect of low-dose oestrogen against MYOCARDIAL INFARCTION and STROKE.

A recently introduced non-hormonal drug, raloxifene hydrochloride, is being used in postmenopausal women to prevent bone loss and reduce the risk of non-traumatic fractures of vertebrae bones.

MENORRHAGIA means an over-abundance of the menstrual discharge.

MENSTRUATION A periodic change occurring in human beings and the higher apes, and consists chiefly in a flow of blood from the cavity of the womb, and associated with various slight constitutional disturbances. It begins between the ages of 12 and 15, as a rule, although its onset may be delayed till as late as 20, or it may begin as early as 10 or 11. Along with its first appearance the body develops the secondary sex characteristics of the sex: e.g. enlargement of the breasts, characteristic hair distribution. The duration of each menstrual period varies in different persons from two to eight days. It recurs in the great majority of cases with regularity, most commonly at intervals of twenty-eight days or thirty days, less often with intervals of twenty-one or twenty-seven days, ceasing only during pregnancy and lactation, till the age of 45 or 50 arrives, when it stops altogether, as a rule ceasing early if it has begun early, and vice versa. The final stoppage is known as the MENOPAUSE or the CLIMACTERIC.

Menstruation depends upon a functioning ovary and this upon a healthy PITUITARY GLAND. The regular rhythm may depend upon a centre in the HYPOTHALAMUS, which is in close connection with the pituitary. After menstruation the denuded uterine endometrium is regenerated under the influence of the follicular hormone, oestradiol. The epithelium of the endometrium proliferates, and about a fortnight after the beginning of menstruation great development of the endometrial glands takes place under the influence of progesterone, the hormone secreted by the corpus luteum. These changes are made for the reception of the fertilized OVUM. In the absence of fertilization the uterine endometrium breaks down in the subsequent menstrual discharge.

Disorders of menstruation In most healthy women, menstruation proceeds regularly for thirty years or more, with the exceptions connected with childbirth. In many women, however, menstruation may be absent, excessive or painful. The term amenorrhoea is applied to the condition of absent menstruation. The terms menorrhagia and metrorrhagia describe excessive menstrual loss, the former if the excess occurs at the regular periods, the latter if it is irregular. Dysmenorrhoea is the name given to painful menstruation.

AMENORRHOEA If menstruation has never occurred the amenorrhoea is termed primary. If it ceases after having once become established it is known as secondary amenorrhoea. The only value of these terms is that some patients with either chromosome abnormalities or malformations of the genital tract fall into the primary category. Otherwise the age of onset of symptoms is more important.

The causes of amenorrhoea are numerous and treatment requires dealing with the primary cause. The commonest cause is pregnancy. Psychological stress or eating disorders can cause amenorrhoea. Poor nutrition or loss of weight by dieting may do so and any serious underlying disease such as TUBERCULOSIS or MALARIA may also result in the cessation of periods. The excess secretion of PROLACTIN, whether this is the result of a micro-adenoma of the PITUITARY GLAND or whether it is drug induced, will cause amenorrhoea and possibly GALACTORRHOEA as well. Malfunction of the pituitary gland will result in a failure to produce the gonadotrophic hormones with consequent amenorrhoea. Excessive production of cortisol, as in CUSHING'S SYNDROME, or of ANDROGENS, as in the adrenogenital syndrome or the polycystic ovary syndrome, will result in amenorrhoea. Amenorrhoea occasionally follows use of the oral contraceptive pill and may be associated with both hypothyroidism and obesity.

Patients should be reassured that amenorrhoea can often be successfully treated and does not necessarily affect their ability to have normal sexual relations and to conceive. When weight loss is the cause of amenorrhoea, restoration of body weight alone can result in spontaneous menstruation. Patients with raised concentration of serum gonadotrophin hormones have primary ovarian failure. It is not amenable to treatment. Cyclical oestrogen/progestogen therapy will usually establish withdrawal bleeding. If the amenorrhoea is due to mild pituitary failure menstruation may return after treatment with clomiphene, a non-steroidal agent which competes for oestrogen receptors in the HYPOTHALAMUS. The patients who are most likely to respond to clomiphene are those who have some evidence of endogenous oestrogen and gonadotrophin production.

IRREGULAR MENSTRUATION This is a change from the normal monthly cycle of menstruation, the duration of bleeding or the amount of blood lost (see MENORRHAGIA). Such changes may be the result of an upset in the balance of OESTROGEN hormones and PROGESTERONE hormones which between them control the cycle. Cycles may be irregular after the MENARCHE and before the MENOPAUSE. Unsuspected pregnancy may manifest itself as an 'irregularity' as can an early miscarriage. Disorders of the UTERUS, OVARIES or organs in the pelvic cavity can also cause irregular menstruation. Women with the condition should seek medical advice.

MENORRHAGIA Excessive menstruation may be due to the same systemic conditions which produce amenorrhoea. The underlying disorder should be treated and this will usually result in restoration of a normal cycle. Menorrhagia may occur when menstruation first starts and during the months leading up to the menopause, when periods also tend to become irregular. Local conditions in the reproductive tract are the commonest cause of menorrhagia, often accompanied by an irregular cycle (metrorrhagia). Polypus, FIBROID, and other tumours, displacements of the uterus and inflammation following childbirth or miscarriage are the most common causes of this type. Treatment involves remedying the local cause. (See UTERUS, DISEASES OF.)

DYSMENORRHOEA This varies from discomfort to serious pain and sometimes vomiting and general malaise. ANAEMIA is sometimes a cause of painful menstruation as well as of stoppage of this function.

Inflammation of the uterus, OVARIES or the FALLOPIAN TUBES is a common cause of dysmenorrhoea which comes on for the first time late in life, especially when the trouble follows the birth of a child. In this case the pain exists more or less at all times, but is aggravated at the periods. Treatment with analgesics and remedying the underlying cause is called for.

Many cases of dysmenorrhoea appear with the beginning of menstrual life, and accompany every period. It has been estimated that 5 to 10 per cent of girls in their late teens or early twenties are severely incapacitated by dysmenorrhoea for several hours each month. Various causes have been suggested for the pain, one being an excessive production of PROSTAGLANDINS. There may be a psychological factor in some sufferers and, whether this is the result of inadequate sex instruction, fear, family, school or work problems, it is important to offer advice and support, which in itself may resolve the dysmenorrhoea. Symptomatic relief is of value.

MENTAL HANDICAP (See LEARNING DISABILITY.)

MENTAL ILLNESS Defined simply, this is a disorder of the brain's processes that makes the sufferer feel or seem ill and may prevent that person from coping with daily life. Psychiatrists – doctors specializing in diagnosing and treating mental illness – have, however, come up with a range of much more complicated definitions over the years.

Psychiatrists like to categorize mental illnesses because mental signs and symptoms do occur together in clusters or syndromes, each tending to respond to certain treatments. The idea that illnesses can be diagnosed simply by recognizing their symptom patterns may not seem very scientific in these days of high technology. For most common mental illnesses, however, this is the only method of diagnosis; whatever is going wrong in the brain is usually too poorly understood and too subtle to show up in laboratory tests or computed tomography scans of the brain. And symptom-based definitions of mental illnesses are, generally, a lot more meaningful than the vague lay term 'nervous breakdown', which is used to cover an attack of anything from AGORAPHOBIA to total inability to function normally.

There is still a lot to learn about the workings of the brain, but psychiatry has developed plenty of practical knowledge about the probable causes of mental illness, ways of relieving symptoms, and aiding recovery. Most experts now believe that mental illnesses generally arise from different combinations of inherited risk and psychological STRESS, sometimes with additional environmental exposure, e.g. to VIRUSES, DRUGS or ALCOHOL.

The range of common mental illnesses includes anxiety states, PHOBIAS, DEPRESSION, alcohol and drug problems, the EATING DISORDERS ANOREXIA and BULIMIA NERVOSA, manic depression, SCHIZOPHRENIA, DEMENTIA, and a group of problems related to coping with life that psychiatrists call personality disorders.

Of these mental illnesses, dementia is the best understood. It is an irreversible and fatal form of mental deterioration (starting with forgetfulness and eventually leading to severe failure of all the brain's functions), caused by rapid death of brain cells and consequent brain shrinkage. Schizophrenia is another serious mental illness which disrupts thought processes, speech, emotions and perception (how the brain handles signals from the five senses). Manic depression, in which prolonged 'highs' of extremely elevated mood and overexcitement alternate with abject misery, has similar effects on the mental processes. In both schizophrenia and manic depression the sufferer loses touch with reality, develops unshakeable but completely unrealistic ideas (delusions), and hallucinates (vividly experiences sensations that are not real, e.g. hears voices when there is nobody there). This triad of symptoms is called psychosis and it is what lay people, through fear and lack of understanding, sometimes call lunacy, madness or insanity.

The other mental illnesses mentioned above are sometimes called neuroses. But the term has become derogatory in ordinary lay language. Indeed, many people assume that neuroses are mild disorders that only affect weak people who cannot pull themselves together, while psychoses are always severe. In reality, psychoses can be brief and reversible and neuroses can cause lifelong disability.

However defined and categorized, mental illness is a big public-health problem. A national survey in England in 1995 suggested that one in five women and around one in seven men had mental illness. About half a million people in Britain suffer from schizophrenia: it is three times commoner than cancer. And at any one time up to a tenth of the adult population is ill with depression.

Treatment settings Most people with mental health problems get the help they need from their own family doctors, without ever seeing psychiatrists. General practictitioners in Britain treat 9 out of 10 recognized mental-health problems and see around 12 million adults with mental illness each year. Even for the 1 in 10 of these patients referred to psychiatrists, general practitioners usually handle those problems that continue or recur

Psychiatrists, psychiatric nurses, social workers, psychologists, counsellors and therapists often see patients at local doctors' surgeries and will do home visits if necessary. Community mental-health centres – like general-practice health centres but catering solely for mental-health problems – offer another short cut to psychiatric help. The more traditional, and still more common, route to a psychiatrist for many people, however, is from the general practititioner to a hospital outpatient department.

Specialist psychiatric help In many ways a visit to a psychiatrist is much like any trip to a hospital doctor and, indeed, psychiatric clinics are often based in the outpatient departments of general hospitals. First appointments with psychiatrists can last an hour or more because the psychiatrist – and sometimes other members of the team such as nurses, doctors in training, and social workers – need to ask lots of questions and record the whole consultation in a set of confidential casenotes.

Psychiatric assessment usually includes an interview and an examination and is sometimes backed up by a range of tests. The interview begins with the patient's history, the personal story that explains how and, to some extent, why help is needed now. Mental-health problems almost invariably develop from a mixture of causes – emotional, social, physical, and familial – and it helps psychiatrists to know what the people they see are normally like and what kind of lives they have led. These questions may seem unnecessarily intrusive, but they allow psychiatrists to understand patients' problems and decide on the best way to help them.

The next stage in assessment is the mental-state examination. This is how psychiatrists examine minds, or at least their current state. Mental-state examination entails asking more questions and using careful observation to assess feelings, thoughts, and mental symptoms and the way the mind is working (for example, in terms of memory and concentration). During first consultations psychiatrists usually make diagnoses and explain them. The boundary between a life problem that will clear up spontaneously and a mental illness that needs treatment is sometimes quite blurred; one consultation may be enough to put the problem in perspective and help to solve it.

Further assessment in the clinic may be needed, or some additional tests. Simple blood tests can be done in outpatient clinics but other investigations will mean referral to another department, usually on another day.

Further assessment and tests

PSYCHOLOGICAL TESTS Psychologists work in or alongside the psychiatric team, helping in both assessment and treatment. The range of psychological tests studies memory, intelligence, personality, perception and capability for abstract thinking.

PHYSICAL TESTS Blood tests and brain scans may be useful to rule out a physical illness causing psychological symptoms.

SOCIAL ASSESSMENT Many patients have social difficulties that can be teased out and helped by a psychiatric social worker. 'Approved social workers' have special training in the use of the Mental Health Act, the law that authorizes compulsory admissions to psychiatric hospitals and compulsory psychiatric treatments. These social workers also know about all the mental-health services offered by local councils and voluntary organizations and can refer clients to them. The role of some social workers has been widened greatly in recent years by the expansion of community care.

OCCUPATIONAL THERAPY ASSESSMENT Mental-health problems causing practical disabilities – for instance, inability to work, cook or look after oneself – can be assessed and helped by occupational therapists.

Treatment The aims of psychiatric treatment are to help sufferers shake off, or at least cope with, symptoms and to gain or regain an acceptable quality of life.

PSYCHOLOGICAL TREATMENTS

Counselling This is a widely used 'talking cure', particularly in general practice. Counsellors listen to their clients, help them to explore feelings, and help them to find personal and practical solutions to their problems. Counsellors do not probe into clients' pasts or analyse them.

Psychotherapy This is the best known 'talking cure'. The term psychotherapy is a generalization covering many different concepts. They all started, however, with Sigmund FREUD, the father of modern psychotherapy. Freud was a doctor who discovered that, as well as the conscious thoughts that guide our feelings and actions, there are powerful psychological forces of which we are not usually aware. Applying his theories to his patients' freely expressed thoughts, Freud was able to cure many illnesses, some of which had been presumed completely physical. This was the beginning of individual analytical psychotherapy, or PSYCHOANALYSIS. Although Freud's principles underpin all subsequent theories about the psyche, many different schools of thought (sometimes contradicting each other) have emerged and influenced psychotherapists (see ADLER; JUNG; PSYCHOTHERAPY).

Behaviour therapy This springs from theories of human behaviour, many of which are based on studies of animals. The therapists, mostly psychologists, help people to look at problematic patterns of behaviour and thought and change them. Cognitive therapy is very effective, particularly in depression and eating disorders.

PHYSICAL TREATMENTS The most widely used physical treatments in psychiatry are drugs. Tranquillizing and anxiety-reducing BENZODIAZEPINE drugs like diazepam, well known by its trade name of Valium, were prescribed widely in the 1960s and 70s because they seemed an effective and safe substitute for barbiturates. Benzodiazepines are, however, addictive and are now recommended only for short-term relief of anxiety that is severe, disabling, or unacceptably distressing. They are also used for short-term treatment of patients drying out from alcohol.

ANTIDEPRESSANTS like amitriptyline and fluoxetine, well known by its commercial name Prozac, are given to lift depressed mood and to relieve the physical symptoms that sometimes occur in depression, such as insomnia and poor appetite. Antidepressants' side effects are mostly relatively mild, although one group, the monoamine oxidase inhibitors can lead to sudden and dangerous high blood-pressure if taken with certain foods.

Manic depression virtually always has to be treated with mood-stabilizing drugs. Lithium carbonate is used in acute mania to lower mood and stop psychotic symptoms. It can also be used in severe depression. However lithium's main use is to prevent relapse in manic depression. Long-term unwanted effects may include kidney and thyroid problems. Short-term problems in the nervous system and kidney may occur if the blood concentration of lithium is too high – therefore it must be monitored by regular blood tests. Carbamazepine, a treatment for epilepsy, has also been found to stabilize mood, and also necessitates blood tests.

Antipsychotic drugs, also called neuroleptics and major tranquillizers, are the only effective treatments for relieving serious mental illnesses with hallucinations and delusions. They are used mainly in schizophrenia and they include the short-acting drugs chlorpromazine and clozapine and the long-lasting injections given once every few weeks like fluphenazine decanoate. In the long term, however, some of the older antipsychotic drugs can cause a brain problem called TARDIVE DYSKINESIA that affects control of movement and is not always reversible. And the antipsychotic drugs' short-term side-effects such as shaking and stiffness sometimes have to be counteracted by other drugs called anticholinergic drugs such as procyclidine and benzhexol. Newer antipsychotic drugs such as clozapine do not cause tardive dyskinesia. But clozapine cannot be given as a long-lasting injection and its concentration in the body has to be monitored by regular blood tests to avoid toxicity.

OTHER PHYSICAL TREATMENTS The other two physical treatments used in psychiatry are particularly controversial: electroconvulsive therapy (ECT) and psychosurgery. In ECT, which can be life-saving for patients who have severe life-threatening depression, a small electric current is passed through the brain to induce a fit or seizure. Before the treatment the patient is anaesthetized and given a muscle-relaxing injection that reduces the magnitude of the fit to a slight twitching or shaking. Scientists do not really understand how ECT works, but it does, for carefully selected patients. Psychosurgery – operating on the brain to alleviate psychiatric illness or difficult personality traits – is extremely uncommon these days. Stereotactic surgery, in which small cuts are made in specific brain fibres under X-ray guidance, has superseded the more generalized lobotomies of old. The Mental Health Act 1983 ensures that psychosurgery is performed only when the patient has given fully informed consent and a second opinion has agreed that it is necessary. For all other psychiatric treatments (except another rare treatment, hormone implantation for reducing the sex drive of sex offenders)

either consent or a second opinion is needed, not both.

Treating patients with acute psychiatric illness Psychiatric emergencies – patients with acute psychiatric illness – may develop from psychological, physical, or practical crises. Any of these crises may need quick professional intervention. Relatives and friends often have to get this urgent help because the sufferer is not fit enough to do it or, if psychotic, does not recognize the need. First, they should ring the person's general practitioner. If the general practitioner is not available and help is needed very urgently, relatives or friends should phone the local social services department and ask for the duty social worker (on 24-hour call). In a dire emergency, the police will know what to do.

Any disturbed adult who threatens his or her own or others' health and safety and refuses psychiatric help may be moved and detained by law. The Mental Health Act of 1983 authorizes emergency assessment and treatment of any person with apparent psychiatric problems that fulfil these criteria.

Although admission to hospital may be the best solution, there are other ways that psychiatric services can respond to emergencies. In some districts there are 'crisis intervention' teams of psychiatrists, nurses, and social workers who can visit patients urgently at home (at a GP's request) and, sometimes, avert unnecessary admission. And research has shown that home treatment for a range of acute psychiatric problems can be effective.

Treatment in hospital Psychiatric wards do not look like medical or surgical wards and staff may not wear uniforms. Patients do not need to be in their beds during the day, so the beds are in separate dormitories. The main part of most wards is a living space with a day room, an activity and television room, quiet rooms, a dining room, and a kitchen. Ward life usually has a certain routine. The day often starts with a community meeting at which patients and nurses discuss issues that affect the whole ward. Patients may go to the occupational therapy department during the day, but there may also be some therapy groups on the ward, such as relaxation training. Patients' symptoms and problems are assessed continuously during a stay in hospital. When patients seem well enough they are allowed home for trial periods; then discharge can be arranged. Patients are usually followed up in the outpatient clinic at least once.

Long-term treatment and community care Long-term treatment is often provided by GPs with support and guidance from psychiatric teams. That is fine for people whose problems allow them to look after themselves and for those with plenty of support from family and friends. But some people need much more intensive long-term treatment and many need help with running their daily lives.

Since the 1950s successive governments have

closed the old psychiatric hospitals and have tried to provide as much care as possible outside hospital – in 'the community'. Community care is effective as long as everyone who needs inpatient care, or residential care, can have it. But demand exceeds supply. Research has shown that some homeless people have long-term mental illnesses and have somehow lost touch with psychiatric services. Many more have developed more general long-term health problems, particularly related to alcohol, without ever getting help.

The NHS and Community Care Act 1990, in force since 1993, established a new breed of professionals called care managers to assess people whose long-term illnesses and disabilities make them unable to cope completely independently with life. Care managers are given budgets by local councils to assess people's needs and arrange for them tailor-made packages of care, including services like home helps and day centres. But co-ordination between health and social services has sometimes failed – and resources are limited – and the government decided in 1997 to tighten up arrangements and pool community-care budgets.

Since 1992 psychiatrists have had to ensure that people with severe mental illnesses have full programmes of care set up before discharge from hospital, to be overseen by named key workers. And since 1996 psychiatrists have used a new power called Supervised Discharge to ensure that the most vulnerable patients cannot lose touch with mental-health services. There is not, however, any law that allows compulsory treatment in the community.

There is ample evidence that community-care can work and that it need not cost more than hospital care. Critics argue, however, that even one tragedy resulting from inadequate care, perhaps a suicide or even a homicide, should reverse the march to community care. And, according to the National Schizophrenia Fellowship, many of the 10–15 homicides a year carried out by people with severe mental illnesses result from inadequate community care.

Further information can be obtained from the Mental Health Act Commission, and from MIND, The National Association for Mental Health. MIND also acts as a campaigning and advice organization on all aspects of mental health. (See APPENDIX 2: ADDRESSES.)

MEPACRINE HYDROCHLORIDE A synthetic acridine product used in the treatment of MALARIA. It came to the fore during the 1939–45 War, when supplies of quinine were short, and proved of great value both as a prophylactic and in the treatment of malaria. It is now used only to treat infestation with tapeworms. (See TAENIASIS.)

MERALGIA PARAESTHETICA A condition characterized by pain and PARAESTHESIA on the front and outer aspect of the thigh. It is more common in men than in women, and the victims are usually middle-aged, overweight and out of condition. It is due to compression of the lateral cutaneous nerve of the thigh. It is exacerbated by an uncomfortable driving position when motoring long distances. Reduction in weight, improvement in general fitness and correction of faulty posture usually bring relief. If these fail, surgical decompression of the nerve may bring relief.

MERCAPTOPURINE One of the ANTI-METABOLITE group of drugs, which includes methotrexate, fluorouracil and thioguanine. These drugs are incorporated into new nuclear material in the cell or combine irreversibly with vital cellular enzymes, preventing normal cellular metabolism and division. Mercaptopurine is used mainly for the maintenance treatment of acute LEUKAEMIAS, though it is increasingly proving valuable in the treatment of CROHN'S DISEASE. As with all CYTOTOXIC DRUGS, dosage must be carefully controlled; in particular it must be reduced if used concurrently with allopurinol. Side-effects include gastrointestinal upsets, including ulceration, and bone-marrow depression.

MERCURY, also known as QUICKSILVER or HYDRARGYRUM, is a heavy fluid metal which, with its salts, has been used in medicine for many centuries.

Action The salts of mercury fall into two groups: the mercuric salts, which are very soluble and powerful in action; and the mercurous salts, which are less soluble and act more slowly and mildly. The mercuric salts are all highly poisonous both to man and to bacterial life, so that they are strongly antiseptic.

Uses Externally the mercuric salts are used as antiseptics, anti-parasitic agents and fungicides. Mercury has been widely used in dental amalgams for filling teeth, though doubts have recently been raised whether the metal can be absorbed into the body tissue, with unwanted results.

MESCALINE Derived from the Mexican peyote cactus, *Anhalonium lewinii*, it is a hallucinogen used for many centuries by Indian tribes in Mexico as an intoxicant to produce ecstatic states for religious celebrations. In recent times its ability to produce temporary psychotic symptoms has beeen used to investigate the mechanism of PSYCHOSIS. Mescaline has similar effects to those of LSD: changes in mood and thought, illusions, self-absorption, an altered perception of time and illusions. Experience of the drug may subsequently provoke panic attacks, deliberate self-injury, real psychosis and sometimes addiction. (See DRUG ADDICTION.)

MESENCEPHALON is the mid-brain connecting the cerebral hemispheres with the pons and cerebellum.

MESENTERY is the double layer of peritoneal membrane which supports the small intestine. It is of a fan shape, and its shorter edge is attached to the back wall of the abdomen for a distance of about 15 cm (6 inches), while the small intestine lies within its longer edge, for a length of over 6 metres (20 feet). The terms mesocolon, mesorectum, etc., are applied to similar folds of peritoneum that support parts of the colon, rectum, etc.

MESMERISM (see HYPNOTISM).

MESOCOLON The double fold of peritoneum by which the large intestine is suspended from the back wall of the abdomen.

MESOTHELIOMA A malignant tumour of the pleura, the membrane lining the chest cavity. The condition is commoner in people exposed to asbestos dust. It may be asymptomatic or cause pain, cough, and breathing troubles. Surgery or radiotherapy may be effective but often the disease has spread too far before it is discovered.

METABOLIC DISORDERS A collection of disorders in which some part of the body's internal chemistry (see METABOLISM) is disrupted. Some of these disorders arise from inherited deficiencies in which a specific enzyme is absent or abnormal or does not function properly. Other metabolic disorders occur because of malfunctions in the ENDOCRINE system. There may be over- or underproduction of a hormone involved in the control of metabolic activities. A prime example is DIABETES MELLITUS – a disorder of sugar metabolism; others include CUSHING'S SYNDROME, HYPOTHYROIDISM, HYPERTHYROIDISM and insulinoma (an insulin-producing tumour of the PANCREAS). The bones can be affected by metabolic disorders such as OSTEOPOROSIS, OSTEOMALACIA, RICKETS and PAGET'S DISEASE. PORPHYRIA, HYPERLIPIDAEMIA, HYPERCALCAEMIA and gout are other examples of disordered metabolism.

There are also over 200 identified disorders described as inborn errors of metabolism. Some cause few problems, others are serious threats to an individual's life. Individual disorders are, fortunately, rare – probably one child in 10,000 or 100,000; overall these inborn errors affect around one child in 1,000. Examples include GALACTOSAEMIA, PHENYLKETONURIA, PORPHYRIAS, TAY SACHS DISEASE and varieties of mucopolysaccharidosis, HOMOCYSTINURIA and hereditary fructose (a type of sugar) intolerance.

METABOLISM This means tissue change and includes all the physical and chemical processes by which the living body is maintained, and also those by which the energy is made available for various forms of work. The constructive, chemical and physical, processes by which food materials are adapted for the use of the body are collectively known as anabolism. The destructive processes by which energy is produced with the breaking down of tissues into waste products is known as catabolism. *Basal metabolism* is the term applied to the energy changes necessary for essential processes such as the beating of the heart, respiration, and maintenance of body warmth. This can be estimated, when a person is placed in a state of complete rest, by measuring the amounts of oxygen and carbon dioxide exchanged during breathing under certain standard conditions. (See CALORIE.)

METACARPAL BONES The five long bones which occupy the hand between the carpal bones at the wrist and the phalanges of the fingers. The large rounded 'knuckles' at the root of the fingers are formed by the heads of these bones. (See HAND.)

METAPHYSIS The extremity of a long bone where it joins the EPIPHYSIS.

METAPLASIA The term applied to a change of one kind of tissue into another. Though not usually harmful,it may be precancerous if occurring in the CERVIX, BLADDER or lining of the airways (BRONCHI).

METASTASIS and **METASTATIC** are terms applied to the process by which malignant disease spreads to distant parts of the body, and also to the secondary tumours resulting from this process. For example, a cancer of the breast may produce metastatic growths in the glands of the armpit, cancer of the stomach may be followed by metastases in the liver.

METATARSAL BONES The five bones in the foot which correspond to the metacarpal bones in the hand, lying between the tarsal bones, at the ankle, and the toes. (See FOOT.)

METATARSALGIA Pain affecting the metatarsal region of the foot. It is common in adolescents associated with FLAT-FOOT. In adults it may be a manifestation of rheumatoid arthritis. Morton's metatarsalgia is a form associated usually with the nerve to the second toe cleft often induced by the compression of tight shoes.

METATARSUS is the group name of the five metatarsal bones in the FOOT. Metatarsus varus is the condition characterized by deviation of the forefoot towards the other foot. It is a common condition in new-born babes and almost always corrects itself spontaneously. Only in the rare cases in which it is due to some deformity of the bones or muscles of the foot is any treatment required.

METEORISM The distension of the abdomen by gas produced in the intestines. (See FLATULENCE.)

METFORMIN is a BIGUANIDE which lowers the blood sugar – HYPOGLYCAEMIA. This it does by increasing cellular uptake of glucose. It is active when taken by mouth and is used to treat some patients with DIABETES MELLITUS, usually in addition to another hypoglycaemic drug.

METHADONE HYDROCHLORIDE Also known as physeptone, this is a synthetic drug structurally similar to morphine, one of many OPIOID drugs used to treat severe pain. Methadone is, however, less sedating and has a longer half-life. Furthermore, it is more reliable when taken orally, and although vomiting is common, it is generally less severe than with morphine.

Methadone is valuable as a cough suppressant for non-productive cough, acting on the medullary 'cough centre' in the central nervous system. It is also helpful in weaning addicts off morphine and heroin, having a slower onset of dependence and a less severe withdrawal syndrome. When used for prolonged periods, methadone should not be given more often than twice daily, to avoid the risks of accumulation and opioid overdosage. (See DRUG ADDICTION.)

METHAEMOGLOBIN A derivative of haemoglobin in which the iron has been oxidized from ferrous to ferric form. It does not combine with oxygen and therefore plays no part in oxygen transport. Normal concentration of methaemoglobin in red blood cells is less than one per cent of the total haemoglobin. When a large concentration of the haemoglobin is in the form of methaemoglobin the patient will suffer from hypoxia and will be cyanosed. Most cases of methaemoglobinaemia are due to chemical agents.

METHAEMOGLOBINAEMIA is a condition due to the presence in the blood of METHAEMO-GLOBIN. It is characterized by CYANOSIS which turns the skin and lips a blue colour, shortness of breath, headache, fatigue and sickness. There are two main forms: a hereditary form and a toxic form. The latter is caused by certain drugs, including acetanilide, phenacetin, the sulphonamides and benzocaine. The treatment of the toxic form is the withdrawal of the causative drug. In the more severe cases the administration of methylene blue or ascorbic acid may also be needed, and these are the drugs used in the hereditary form.

In recent years attention has been drawn to a form known as infantile methaemoglobinaemia in bottle-fed babies under the age of 6 months. This is due to the presence of excess nitrate in the drinking water. Nitrate pollution of water has been increasing due to the purification of sewage effluent to a high standard before its discharge to water-courses, and to changes in agricultural policy leading to better drainage of land and increased use of artificial fertilizers. As a result, especially where rainfall is low and the land low-lying, as in eastern and south-east England, underground supplies of water contain more than 50 mg of nitrate per litre, which is the level recommended by the World Health Organization, and may even exceed the maximum acceptable level of 100 mg per litre. High nitrate concentrations may also occur in surface waters after heavy rain. The cause of the methaemoglobinaemia is nitrite into which the nitrate is converted either in the baby's bottle or in his gut. Few serious cases have been recorded in Britain, and most of those which have occurred have been due to water from private sources.

Arrangements are now in force whereby water authorities inform the appropriate health authority if water with a nitrate content of 50 mg per litre has to be supplied, and alternative low-nitrate water is made available, sometimes in the form of bottled water, by local authorities for infants below the age of 6 months. The EEC has recommended an even more stringent criterion: that water used for baby feeds should not contain more than 25 mg of nitrate per litre.

METHANE An odourless, colourless highly flammable gas. It occurs naturally in gas from coal mines and oil wells, where it is a hazard because of its explosive properties. 'Natural' gas supplied to homes and industries is almost 100 per cent methane. Unlike coal gas, it is not poisonous unless present in large amounts, when it may displace oxygen and thus asphyxiate anyone exposed to it. Decomposition of organic matter produces methane.

METHANOL A variety of alcohol used as a solvent to remove paint or a constituent of some antifreeze fluids. It is poisonous: sometimes people drink it as a substitute for ethyl (ordinary) alcohol. Symptoms appear up to 24 hours after imbibing methanol and include nausea, vomiting, dizziness, headache and sometimes unconsciousness. Treatment is to induce vomiting (in conscious victims) and to do a stomach washout (see GASTRIC LAVAGE) but such steps must be taken within two hours of ingestion. Hospital treatment is usually required, when intravenous infusion of sodium bicarbonate (and sometimes ethanol which slows up breakdown of methanol by the liver) is administered.

METHICILLIN-RESISTANT *STAPHYLO-COCCUS AUREUS* (MRSA) Most STAPHY-LOCOCCI have now evolved resistance to benylpenicillin (see PENICILLIN) because of their ability to produce PENICILLINASES. Cloxacillin and flucloxacillin (see PENICILLIN) are antibiotics still effective against most staphylococci. At one time methicillin was used to combat resistant strains but in hospital environments bacteria acquired immunity to this powerful drug (now withdrawn from use) and to cloxacillin. RIFAMPICIN, VANCOMYCIN, TEICOPLANIN and TEMOCILLIN, are still active against most PENICIL-

LINASE-producing GRAM-negative bacteria. There is, however, a growing threat to health because of the rise in the number of antibiotic-resistant bacteria.

METHIONINE is an essential AMINO-ACID that contains sulphur and is necessary for normal growth in infants and to maintain nitrogen balance in adults.

METHOHEXITONE A quick-acting, short-term intravenous barbiturate ANAESTHETIC. It produces anaesthesia in one arm-brain circulation time and, as it may cause APNOEA and low blood pressure, the anaesthetist must have adequate resuscitative facilities on hand. Particular care is called for if the patient is having surgery of the mouth, pharynx or larynx or if he or she is in shock or has cardiovascular problems (see ANAESTHESIA).

METHOTREXATE One of the ANTIMETABOLITES used to treat certain forms of malignant disease. Acting to inhibit the enzyme dihydrofolate reductase, which is essential for purine and pyrimidine synthesis, it is given orally, intravenously, intramuscularly or intrathecally. Methotrexate is used as maintenance therapy for childhood acute LYMPHOBLASTIC LEUKAEMIA, while other uses include CHORIOCARCINOMA, non-Hodgkin LYMPHOMAS, and various solid tumours. Intrathecally, it is used in the prophylaxis of childhood acute lymphoblastic leukaemia, and as treatment for established meningeal cancer or lymphoma.

Side-effects include suppression of myelocytes in bone marrow, inflammation of mucous membranes, and, rarely, PNEUMONITIS. It should be avoided whenever significant renal impairment is present, while significant pleural effusion or ascites is also a contraindication. Blood counts should be carefully monitored whenever intrathecal methotrexate is given. Oral or parenteral folinic acid helps prevent or speed recovery from myelosuppression or mucositis.

Methotrexate is used in dermatology, where it may be indicated for cases of severe uncontrolled PSORIASIS unresponsive to conventional therapy; it may also be indicated for severe active RHEUMATOID ARTHRITIS. Because of its potentially severe haematological, pulmonary, gastrointestinal, and other toxicities it should be used only by specialists and appropriate renal and liver function tests carried out before and during treatment. It should be avoided in pregnancy, and conception should be avoided for at least six months after stopping, as should breast feeding. Concurrent administration of aspirin or other NSAIDS (NON-STEROIDAL ANTI-INFLAMMATORY DRUGS) reduce methotrexate excretion, increasing its toxicity, and should therefore be avoided whenever possible.

METHYL is an organic radical whose chemical formula is CH_3, and which forms the centre of a wide group of substances known as the methyl group. For example, methyl alcohol is obtained as a by-product in the manufacture of beet-sugar, or by distillation of wood; methyl salicylate is the active constituent in oil of wintergreen; methyl hydride is better known as marsh gas.

Methyl alcohol, or wood spirit (see METHANOL), is distilled from wood and is thus a cheap form of alcohol. It has actions similar to, but much more toxic than, those of ethyl alcohol. It has a specially pronounced action on the nervous system, and in large doses is apt to cause neuritis, especially of the optic nerves, leading to blindness, partial or complete.

METHYLCELLULOSE A COLLOID which absorbs water to swell to about 25 times its original volume. It is used in the treatment of constipation and also in the management of obesity. The rationale for its use in obesity is that by swelling up in the stomach it reduces the appetite.

METHYLDOPA A centrally acting anti-hypertensive drug often used in conjunction with a DIURETIC. It can be effective in controlling high blood-pressure in pregnancy. The drug is also safe to use in patients with ASTHMA or heart failure.

METHYLENE BLUE, or methylthionin chloride, is valuable in a dose of 75–100 mg, as a 1-per-cent intravenous injection, in the treatment of methaemoglobinaemia, which may occur following high doses of local anaesthetics such as prilocaine.

METHYLPREDNISOLONE A MINERALCORTICOID drug with an action comparable to that of prednisolone, but effective at a somewhat lower dose.

METHYLTESTOSTERONE A synthetic male sex hormone given by mouth to treat men who are sexually underdeveloped. It can be used to treat menstrual and menopausal disorders and breast cancer. The drug will will also suppress lactation.

METHYSERGIDE A drug used to prevent attacks of MIGRAINE. The drug requires hospital supervision as it has to be used with care because of the toxic effects it sometimes produces, such as nausea, drowsiness and retroperitoneal fibrosis.

METOCLOPRAMIDE This drug antagonizes the actions of dopamine. Given orally, intramuscularly, or intravenously, it is used to treat nausea and vomiting, particularly in gastrointestinal disorders, or when associated with cytotoxics or radiotherapy. It is useful in the early treatment of MIGRAINE.

Caution is indicated in prescribing metoclopramide for elderly and young patients, and whenever hepatic or renal impairment is present, and it should be avoided in pregnancy or cases of PORPHYRIA. Adverse effects include EXTRAPY-RAMIDAL effects, HYPERPROLACTINAEMIA with occasional TARDIVE DYSKINESIA or prolonged administration. There have also been occasional reports of drowsiness, restlessness, diarrhoea, depression, NEUROLEPTIC malignant syndrome, with rare cardiac conduction abnormalities following intravenous administration.

METOLAZONE A thiazide-type DIURETIC particularly effective when combined with a LOOP DIURETIC when it produces profound diuresis. The drug is also useful for treating kidney stones. (See BENZOTHIADIAZINES.)

METOPROLOL A beta-adrenergic receptor blocking agent. (See ADRENERGIC RECEPTORS.)

METRE The basic unit of length in the modern version of the metric system, known as the International System of Units (SI). (See APPENDIX 6: MEASUREMENTS IN MEDICINE.) It is equivalent to 39·37 inches.

METRITIS Inflammation of the uterus (see UTERUS, DISEASES OF).

METRONIDAZOLE An antimicrobial drug particularly active against ANAEROBIC bacteria and PROTOZOA. Given by mouth, by rectum or intravenously, it is used to treat infections of the urinary, genital, and digestive systems, such as TRICHOMONIASIS, AMOEBIASIS, GIARDIASIS, and acute ulcerative GINGIVITIS, and is a useful treatment for dental abscesses. Topically, it is used in the management of ROSACEA and it reduces the odour produced by anaerobic bacteria in fungating tumours.

It may cause a DISULFIRAM-like reaction with alcohol; caution is similarly indicated in patients with impaired liver function, hepatic encephalopathy, pregnancy or breast feeding. Rare side-effects include nausea, vomiting, unpleasant taste, furred tongue and gastrointestinal disturbances; rashes, URTICARIA, and ANGIOEDEMA; drowsiness, headache, dizziness, ATAXIA and ANAPHYLAXIS.

METROPATHIA HAEMORRHAGICA A disorder characterized by irregular bouts of uterine bleeding – without previous ovulation – due to excessive oestrogenic activity. It is associated with endometrial hyperplasia and cysts of the ovary.

METRORRHAGIA Uterine bleeding otherwise than at the proper period. It is usually due to a uterine lesion. (See MENSTRUATION.)

METYRAPONE is a drug that inhibits the production of CORTISOL in the adrenal cortex which results in an increase in ACTH production and (completing the feedback control cycle) thus greater synthesis of the chemical precursors of cortisol. Metyrapone is used to treat patients with CUSHING'S SYNDROME (a condition caused by excess amounts of CORTICOSTEROID hormones in the body) where surgery is not possible.

MICONAZOLE One of the IMIDAZOLE group of antifungals which includes clotrimazole and ketoconazole. Active against a wide range of fungi and yeasts, their main indications are vaginal candidiasis and dermatophyte skin infections. Miconazole is used as a cream or ointment; it may also be given orally (for oral or gastrointestinal infections), or parenterally (for systemic infections such as aspergillosis or candidiasis). (See MYCOSIS.)

MICROANGIOPATHY Disease of the CAPILLARIES.

MICROBE (see BACTERIA).

MICROBIOLOGY The study of all aspects of micro-organisms (microbes) – that is, organisms which individually are generally too small to be visible other than by microscopy. Few ecological habitats are devoid of micro-organisms – even extreme environments such as salt pans and thermal springs support microbial life – and the range of habitats the microbes can colonize is reflected in their extraordinary diversity in terms of morphology and development; metabolic abilities; and behaviour in response to stimuli in their immediate environment, adverse conditions, and other organisms.

The term micro-organism is applicable to VIRUSES; BACTERIA; and microscopic forms of FUNGI, algae, and protozoa. Some micro-organisms have affinities with both plants and animals, and it is preferable to consider micro-organisms as belonging to a separate kingdom, the protista, rather than attempting to categorize them according to the conventional dichotomy of the plant and animal kingdoms.

Among the smallest and simplest micro-organisms are the viruses. First described as filterable agents, and ranging in size from 20–30 nm to 300 nm, they may be directly visualized only by electron microscopy. They consist of a core of DEOXYRIBONUCLEIC or RIBONUCLEIC acid (DNA or RNA) within a protective protein coat, or capsid, whose subunits confer a geometric symmetry. Thus viruses are usually cubical (icosahedral) or helical; the larger viruses (pox-, herpes-, myxo-viruses) may also have an outer envelope. Their minimal structure dictates that viruses are all obligate parasites, relying on living cells to provide essential components for their replication. Apart from animal and plant cells, viruses may infect and replicate in bacteria (bacteriophages) or fungi (mycophages), which are damaged in the process.

Bacteria are larger (0·01–5000µm) and more complex. They are prokaryotes, with a subcellular organization which generally includes DNA and RNA, a cell membrane, organelles such as ribosomes, and a complex and chemically variable cell envelope. Rickettsiae, chlamydia, and mycoplasmas, once thought of as viruses because of their small size and absence of a cell wall (mycoplasma) or major wall component (chlamydia), are now acknowledged as bacteria. Rickettsiae and chlamydia are obligate intracellular parasites of medical importance. Bacteria may also possess additional surface structures, such as capsules and organs of locomotion (flagella) and attachment (fimbriae and stalks). Individual bacterial cells may be spheres (cocci); straight (bacilli), curved (vibrio), or flexuous (spirilla) rods; or oval cells (coccobacilli). On examination by light microscopy bacteria may be visible in characteristic configurations (as pairs of cocci (diplococci), or chains (streptococci), or clusters); actinomycete bacteria grow as filaments with externally produced spores. Bacteria grow essentially by increasing in cell size and dividing by fission, a process which in ideal laboratory conditions some bacteria may achieve about once every 20 minutes. Under natural conditions growth is usually much slower.

As a group bacteria have a wide repertoire of metabolic and physiological capabilities. Some can synthesize their complex organic cellular components and biochemical intermediates if provided with light or chemical energy; others require sources of existing organic molecules from other micro-organisms, plants, or animals.

Eukaryotic micro-organisms comprise fungi, algae, and protozoa. These organisms are larger, and they have in common a well-developed internal compartmentation into subcellular organelles. Algae additionally have chloroplasts, which contain photosynthetic pigments; fungi lack chloroplasts; and protozoa lack both a cell wall and choroplasts but may have a contractile vacuole to regulate water uptake and, in some, structures for capturing and ingesting food. Fungi grow either as discrete cells (yeasts), multiplying by budding, fission, or conjugation, or as thin filaments (hyphae) which bear spores, though some may show both morphological forms during their life cycle. Algae and protozoa generally grow as individual cells or colonies of individuals and multiply by fission.

Micro-organisms of medical importance include representatives of the five major microbial groups that obtain their essential nutrients at the expense of their hosts. Many bacteria and most fungi, however, are SAPROPHYTES, being major contributors to the natural cycling of carbon in the environment and to biodeterioration; others are of ecological and economic importance because of the diseases they cause in agricultural or horticultural crops or because of their beneficial relationships with higher organisms. Additionally, they may be of industrial or biotechnological importance. Fungal diseases of humans tend to be most important in tropical environments and in immuno-compromised subjects.

For the micro-organism to be considered pathogenic and therefore capable of causing disease, it should fulfil a classic set of criteria termed Koch's postulates, which are designed to establish pathogenicity unequivocally. Some pathogens, for example, those that are not cultivable *in vitro* or in an alternative animal host, cannot fulfil all of the criteria and their status as true pathogens may have to rely on indirect methods.

Pathogenic micro-organisms display to a varying extent special characteristics, or virulence factors, that enable them to colonize their hosts and overcome or evade physical, biochemical, and immunological host defences. For bacteria, whose pathogenic properties have been intensively researched, the role of specific virulence factors and their relation to disease is better understood. Thus the presence of capsules, as in the bacteria that cause anthrax (*Bacillus anthracis*), one form of pneumonia (*Streptococcus preumoniae*), scarlet fever (*S. pyogenes*), bacterial meningitis (*Neisseria meningitidis, Haemophilus influenzae*) is directly related to the ability to cause disease because of their antiphagocytic properties. Fimbriae are related to virulence, enabling tissue attachment – for example, in gonorrhoea (*N. gonorrhoeae*) and cholera (*Vibrio cholerae*). Many bacteria excrete extracellular virulence factors; these include enzymes and other agents that impair the host's physiological and immunological functions. Some bacteria produce powerful toxins (excreted exotoxins or endogenous endotoxin), which may cause local tissue destruction and allow colonization by the pathoGEN OR WHOSE SPECIFIC ACTION MAY EXPLAIN THE DISEASE MECHANISM. In *Staphylococcus aureus* exfoliative toxin produces the staphylococcal scalded-skin syndrome, TSS toxin-1 toxic-shock syndrome, and enterotoxin food poisoning. The pertussis exotoxin of *Bordetella pertussis*, the cause of whooping cough, blocks immunological defences and mediates attachment to tracheal cells, and the exotoxin produced by *Corynebacterium diphtheriae* causes local damage resulting in a pronounced exudate in the trachea.

Viruses cause disease by cellular destruction arising from their intracellular parasitic existence. Attachment to particular cells is often mediated by specific viral surface proteins; mechanisms for evading immunological defences include latency, change in viral antigenic structure, or incapacitation of the immune system – for example, destruction of CD 4 lymphocytes by the human immunodeficiency virus.

Mechanisms of pathogenicity are generally less well understood for fungi and protozoa; further discussion of these topics is to be found in major textbooks on medical micro-biology.

Recently microbiology has contributed to significant advances in genetics by pioneering techniques of genetic engineering (see GENETICS).

MICROCEPHALY Abnormal smallness of the head, usually associated with learning disability. It may occur as a result of infection of the fetus by, for example, RUBELLA (German measles) or from the consequences of X-ray examinations of the mother early in pregnancy. Damage to the brain during birth may also cause microcephaly.

MICROCYTE A small red blood cell.

MICROFILARIA The mobile embryo of certain parasitic nematode worms which are found in the blood or lymph of patients infected with filarial worms. The microfilariae develop into larva in the body of a blood-sucking insect, for example, a mosquito.

MICROGRAM is the 1/1000th part of a milligram. The abreviation for it is µg. (See APPENDIX 6: MEASUREMENTS IN MEDICINE.)

MICROMETRE, or MICRON, is the 1/1000th part of a millimetre. The abbreviation for it is µm. (See APPENDIX 6: MEASUREMENTS IN MEDICINE.)

MICRO-ORGANISM A very small, single-celled living organism that cannot usually be seen by the naked eye. The most important micro-organisms in medicine are those that cause disease. This 'pathogenic' group, however, forms only a small proportion of the enormous number of known micro-organisms. The main pathogenic ones are BACTERIA. Others are FUNGI and RICKETTSIA. Though not true cells, VIRUSES are usually classified as micro-organisms. (see BACTERIA).

MICROPSIA Condition in which objects appear smaller than normal. It can be due to disease of the macula.

MICROSCOPE An optical instrument – first developed by Antony van Leeuwenhoek in the seventeenth century – comprising adjustable magnifying lenses that greatly enlarge a small object under study – for example, an insect, blood cells, or bacteria. Some microscopes use electron beams to magnify minute objects such as chromosomes, crystals, or even large molecules. Optical microscopes are also used for microsurgery when the area being operated on is otherwise inaccessible, for example, in eye and inner ear surgery, for the removal of tumours from the brain or spinal cord and for resuturing damaged blood vessels and nerves.

MICROSPORUM One of the three genera of dermatophytes (fungi) which cause tinea. Microsporum of human or animal origin is an important cause of tinea capitis, or ringworm of the scalp. (See RINGWORM.)

MICROSURGERY Surgery performed with the use of an operating microscope. It is used routinely in certain operations on the eye, the ear and the larynx. In recent years it has been used, with increasing success, in attempts to reunite severed legs and arms. Under the operating microscope, surgical sutures invisible to the naked eye are used to reunite blood vessels 0·5 millimetre in diameter. The severed limb will survive for up to eight hours at room temperature, longer if cooled – as by ice in the ambulance taking the patient to hospital. Success depends primarily on restoration of the circulation to the limb. Once this has been achieved, attention is later turned to restoring the continuity of the nerves.

MICROWAVES Non-ionizing electro-magnetic radiations in the frequency range of 30–300,000 megahertz. They are emitted from electronic devices, such as heaters, some domestic ovens, television receivers, radar units and diathermy units. There is no scientific evidence to justify the claims that they are harmful to man or produce any harmful effect in the GENES. The only known necessary precaution is the protection of the eyes in those using them in industry, as there is some evidence that prolonged exposure to them in this may induce cataract. (See also DIATHERMY.)

MICTURITION The act of urination.

MIDDLE EAR That portion of the ear lying between the TYMPANIC MEMBRANE and the INNER EAR. It contains the ossicles, the three small bones that transmit sound. (See EAR.)

MIDGES (see BITES AND STINGS).

MID-LIFE CRISIS A colloquial description of the feelings of anxiety and distress experienced by some individuals in early middle age. They realize that by 45 years of age they are no longer young and men in particular try to turn the clock back by changing jobs, dressing trendily, taking up energetic or unusual sports or engaging in extramarital liaisons. Sometimes those in mid-life crises develop mild or even serious depression. The feelings of anxiety and insecurity usually disappear with time but some people may benefit from counselling.

MIDWIFE A member of the profession which provides care and advice during pregnancy, supervises the mother's labour and delivery and looks after her and the baby after birth. Should a pregnancy or labour develop complications, the midwife will seek medical advice. Most midwives are registered general nurses who have also done an 18-month course in midwifery. Trained midwives are registered with the UK Central Council for Nursing Midwifery and Health visiting and work in hospitals or a domiciliary setting. Midwives practise in hospitals, health units or in a domiciliary (home) setting (see APPENDIX 9: STATUTORY ORGANIZATIONS and APPENDIX 10: PROFESSIONAL ORGANIZATIONS (Royal College of Midwives).

MIDWIFERY (see LABOUR; MIDWIFE).

MIGRAINE, or HEMICRANIA as it was sometimes known from the Greek word for half a skull, is a common condition characterized by recurring intense headaches. It is much commoner in women than men and affects around 10 per cent of the population. It has been defined as 'episodic headache accompanied by visual or gastro-intestinal disturbances, or both, attacks lasting hours with total freedom between episodes'.

It usually begins at puberty – though young children can be affected – and often tends to stop in middle age: e.g. in women attacks often cease after menopause. It often disappears during pregnancy. The disorder tends to run in families, though how is not clearly understood. In susceptible individuals attacks may be provoked by a wide variety of causes including: anxiety, emotion, depression, shock, and excitement; physical and mental fatigue; prolonged focusing on television or cinema screen; noise, especially loud and high-pitched sounds; certain foods: e.g. chocolate, cheese, citrus fruits, pastry; alcohol; prolonged lack of food; irregular meals; menstruation and the premenstrual period.

Anything that can provoke a headache in the ordinary individual can probably precipitate an attack in a migrainous subject. It seems as if there is an inherited predispostion that triggers a mechanism whereby in the migrainous subject the headache and the associated sickness persist for hours, a whole day or even longer.

The precise cause is not known, but the generally accepted view is that in susceptible individuals one or other of these causes produces spasm or constriction of the blood-vessels of the brain. This in turn is followed by dilatation of these blood-vessels which also become more permeable and so allow fluid to pass out into the surrounding tissues. This combination of dilatation and outpouring of fluid is held to be responsible for the headache.

Two types of migraine have been recognized: classical and common. The former is relatively rare and the headache is preceded by a slowly extending area of blindness in one or both eyes, usually accompanied by intermittent 'lights'. The phenomenon lasts up to 30 minutes and is followed by a bad, often unilateral headache with nausea, sometimes vomiting and sensitivity to light. Occasionally, passing neurological symptoms such as weakness in a limb may accompany the attack. The common variety has similar but less severe symptoms. It consists of an intense headache, usually situated over one or other eye. The headache is usually preceded by a feeling of sickness and blurring of sight. In 15 to 20 per cent of cases this disturbance of sight takes the form of bright lights: the so-called aura of migraine. The majority of attacks are accompanied by vomiting. The duration of the headache varies, but in the more severe cases the victim is usually confined to bed for twenty-four hours.

Treatment consists, in the first place, of trying to avoid any precipitating factor. Patients must find out which drug, or drugs, give them most relief, and they must always carry these about with them wherever they go. This is because it is a not uncommon experience to be aware of an attack coming on and to find that there is a critical quarter of an hour or so during which the tablets are effective. If not taken within this period, they may be ineffective and the unfortunate victim finds himself prostrate with headache and vomiting. In addition he should immediately lie down, and at this stage a few hours' rest may prevent the development of a full attack. When an attack is fully developed, rest in bed in a quiet, darkened room is essential; any loud noise or bright light intensifies the headache or sickness. The less food that is taken during an attack the better, provided the individual drinks as much fluid as he wants. Group therapy, in which groups of around ten migrainous subjects learn how to relax, is often of help in more severe cases, whilst in others the injection of a local anaesthetic into tender spots in the scalp reduces the number of attacks. Drug treatment is not very satisfactory. Analgesics such as PARACETAMOL, aspirin and CODEINE phosphate sometimes help. A combination of buclizine hydrochloride and analgesics, taken when the visual aura occurs, prevents or diminishes the severity of an attack in some people. Perhaps the most effective remedy for the condition is ERGOTAMINE TARTRATE which causes the dilated blood vessels to contract, but this must only be taken under medical supervision. In many cases METOCLOPRAMIDE, followed ten minutes later by three tablets of either aspirin or paracetamol, provides a most effective form of treatment if taken early in an attack. In milder attacks, aspirin, with or without codeine and paracetamol, may be of value. Sumatriptan (5-hydroxytryptamine ($5HT_1$) AGONIST – also known as a SEROTONIN agonist) is of value for acute attacks. It is used orally or by subcutaneous injection but should not be used for patients with ischaemic heart disease. Naratriptan is another (recently introduced) $5HT_1$ agonist that is an effective treatment for acute attacks.

People with migraine and their relatives can obtain help and guidance from the British Migraine Association (see APPENDIX 2: ADDRESSES).

MILIA These are small keratin cysts appearing as white papules on the cheek and eyelids.

MILIARIA (PRICKLY HEAT) An intensely itchy vesicular and erythematous rash induced by intense heat and humidity. It is caused by a disturbance of sweat gland function.

MILIARY A term, expressing size, applied to various disease products which are about the size of millet seeds: e.g. miliary aneurysms, miliary tuberculosis.

MILIUM is a pinhead white cyst of the skin of the face containing corneal cells. They can be removed on the point of a sterile needle.

MILK The natural food of all animals belonging to the class of mammalia for a considerable period following their birth. It is practically the only form of animal food in which protein, fat, carbohydrate, and salt are all represented in sufficient amount, and it therefore contains all the constituents of a standard diet. Milk is important in human nutrition because it contains first-class animal protein of high biological value, because it is exceptionally rich in calcium, and because it is a good source of vitamin A, thiamine and riboflavine. It also contains a variable amount of ascorbic acid (vitamin C) and of vitamin D, the amount of the latter being higher during the summer months than during the winter months. Raw milk yields 67 Calories per 100 millilitres, in which are present (in grams) 87·6 of water, 3·3 of protein, 3·6 of fat, 4·7 of carbohydrate, and 0·12 of calcium. Heat has no effect on the vitamin A or D content of milk, or on the riboflavine content, but it causes a considerable reduction in the vitamin C and thiamine content.

The ready digestibility of milk, especially when mixed with lime water, or when 125 to 200 mg of citrate of soda have been added for 30 ml of milk in order to soften the curd, makes it a specially suitable food for children or people whose illness affects their normal appetite. Some children lose the enzyme that breaks down LACTOSE to simpler sugars making the milk more difficult to digest. Milk allergy occurs in some infants because they are allergic to the proteins in animal milk.

Preparation of milk Milk may be prepared for food in various ways. Boiling destroys the bacteria, especially any *Mycobacteria tuberculosis* which the milk may contain. It also partly destroys vitamin C and thiamine, as does pasteurization. Curdling of milk is effected by adding rennet, which carries out the initial stage of digestion and thus renders milk more suitable for people who could not otherwise tolerate it. Souring of milk is practised in many countries before milk is considered suitable for food; it is carried out by adding certain organisms such as the lactic acid bacillus, the Bulgarian bacillus, and setting the milk in a warm place for several hours. (See LACTIC ACID BACILLI.) Sterilization, which prevents fermentation and decomposition, is usually carried out by raising the milk to boiling temperature (100 °C) for fifteen minutes and then hermetically sealing it. Condensed, unsweetened milk – usually known as evaporated milk – is concentrated in vacuo at low temperature; the milk is then placed in tins, which are sealed, and is sterilized by heat at a temperature of 105 °C. This destroys 60 per cent of the vitamin C and 30 to 50 per cent of the thiamine. Sweetened condensed milk is not exposed to such a high temperature. The sugar, which prevents the growth of micro-organisms, is added before the condensing, and finally reaches a concentration of about 40 per cent. Dried milk is prepared by evaporating all the fluid so that the milk is reduced to the form of powder. Humanized milk is cow's milk treated to render it closely similar to human milk.

MILK TEETH are the temporary teeth of children. (For the time of their appearance, see TEETH.)

MILLILITRE is the 1000th part of 1 litre. It is practically the equivalent of a cubic centimetre ($1 \text{ cm}^3 = 0.999973 \text{ ml}$); ml is the usual abbreviation.

MINERALCORTICOID (see CORTICO-STEROIDS).

MINIMALLY INVASIVE SURGERY (MIS) Also called MINIMAL-ACCESS SURGERY or, more popularly, 'keyhole surgery', MIS is surgical intervention, whether diagnostic or curative, that causes patients the least possible physical trauma. This branch of surgery has grown speedily from a technique used by gynaecologists, urologists and innovative general surgeons to one regularly used in general surgery, GYNAECOLOGY, UROLOGY, thoracic surgery, ORTHOPAEDIC surgery and OTORHINOLARYNGOLOGY. MIS is commonly carried out by means of an operating laparoscope (a type of ENDOSCOPE) that is slipped through a small incision in the skin. The technique became feasible in the early 1980s, when the silicon-chip television camera was invented. A small attachment on the end of the laparoscope (an instrument first used in humans in 1910 by a German surgeon) provided an image that could be magnified on a screen, leaving the surgeon's hands free to operate while his assistant operated the laparoscope. Halogen bulbs, fibreoptic cables and rod lenses have all contributed to the technical advancement of laparoscopes. Operations done in this manner include extracorporeal shock-wave LITHOTRIPSY for stones in the gall bladder and biliary ducts and in the urinary system and removal of the gall bladder. MIS is also used to remove cartilage or loose pieces of bone in the knee joint. This method of surgery usually means that patients can be treated on a day or overnight basis allowing them to resume normal activities more quickly than with conventional surgery. It is also more cost effective, allowing hospitals to treat

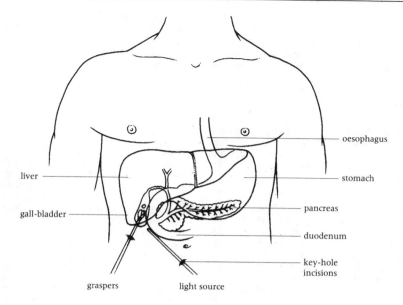

Removal of stones from gall-bladder using the technique of minimally invasive surgery.

more patients in a year. Surgeons undertake special training in the use of MIS, a highly skilled technique, before they are permitted to use the procedures on patients.

MINOCYCLINE A form of TETRACYCLINE mainly used in the long-term suppression of acne vulgaris (see ACNE). Overusage in high dosage may lead to a characteristic pattern of skin pigmentation.

MIOSIS Condition of constriction (reduction in size) of the pupil. It may be the result of disease affecting the AUTONOMIC NERVOUS SYSTEM. Bright light causes miosis and some drugs – for example, PILOCARPINE or OPIUM – have the same effect.

MISCARRIAGE (see ABORTION).

MITHRIDATISM A term applied to immunity against the effects of poisons produced by administration of gradually increasing doses of the poison itself. The process is named after Mithridates, King of Pontus, who rendered himself immune against poisoning by this means.

MITOCHONDRIA The rod-like bodies in the cells of the body which contain the enzymes necessary for the activity of the cell. They have been described as the 'power plant of the cell'. (See CELLS.)

MITOSIS The process of cell division for somatic cells and for the ovum after fertilization.

Each chromosome becomes doubled by splitting lengthwise and forming two chromatids which remain held together by the centromere. These chromatids are exact copies of the original chromosomes and contain duplicates of all the genes they bear. When cell division takes place the pull of the spindle splits the centromere and each double chromatid separates, one passing to one pole of the nucleus and the other to the opposite pole. The nucleus and the cell itself then also divide, forming two new daughter cells containing precisely the same 23 pairs of chromosomes and carrying exactly the same complement of genes as did the mother cell. (See CHROMOSOMES, FERTILIZATION, GENES, HEREDITY.)

MITRAL INCOMPETENCE A defect in the MITRAL VALVE or the HEART allows blood to leak from the left VENTRICLE into the left ATRIUM. It is also known as mitral regurgitation; incompetence may occur along with MITRAL STENOSIS. The left ventricle has to work harder to compensate for the faulty valve, so it enlarges, but eventually the ventricle cannot cope with the extra load and left-sided heart failure may develop. A common cause of mitral incompetence is RHEUMATIC FEVER or damage following a heart attack. The condition is treated with drugs to help the heart but in severe cases heart surgery may be required.

MITRAL STENOSIS Narrowing of the opening between the left ATRIUM and left VENTRICLE of the heart as a result of rigidity of, and adhesion between, the cusps of the mitral valve. It is due, almost invariably, to the infection of RHEUMATIC FEVER. The atrium has to work harder to force blood through the narrowed channel. The effects are similar to those of mitral incompetence. Shortness of breath and palpitations and irregular beating (fibrillation) of the atrium are common consequences in adults. Drug treatment with DIGOXIN and DIURETIC drugs helps but surgery to dilate or replace the faulty valve may be necessary.

MITRAL VALVE, so called from its resemblance to a bishop's mitre, is the valve which guards the opening between the atrium and ventricle on the left side of the heart. (See HEART.)

MMR VACCINE A combined vaccine offering protection against MEASLES, MUMPS, and RUBELLA (German measles), it was introduced in the UK in 1988 and has now replaced the measles vaccine. The combined vaccine is offered to all infants in their second year, and the present rate of uptake is around 90 per cent. Health authorities have an obligation to ensure that all children have received the vaccine by school entry – it should be given with the pre-school booster doses against diphtheria, tetanus, and polio, if not earlier – unless there is a valid contra-indication (such as partial immunosuppression, parental refusal, or evidence of previous infection. MMR vaccine may also be used in the control of measles outbreaks, if offered to susceptible children within three days of exposure to infection. The vaccine is effective and generally safe, though minor symptoms such as malaise, fever and rash may occur 5–10 days after immunization. Very rarely a child may suffer brain damage from the measles component of MMR but the potential benefits greatly outweigh the small risk. The incidence of all three diseases has dropped substantially since MMR was introduced in the UK and USA (see IMMUNIZATION).

MOCLOBEMIDE A reversible MONOAMINE OXIDASE INHIBITOR (MAOI), this drug is used for patients with severe depression. As with all MAOIs those taking moclobemide should avoid taking too much tyramine-rich food – mature cheese, yeast extracts, fermented soya-bean products – and they should not take the drug with another antidepressant.

MOLAR TEETH The last three teeth on each side of the jaw. (See TEETH.)

MOLE A term used to describe the common pigmented spots which occur on human skin. It arises from a collection of abnormal melanocytes in the dermis adjacent to the epidermodermal junction. Moles are usually not present at birth and appear in childhood or adolescence. Most moles are less than 5 mm in diameter and are macular at first, becoming raised later. Rarely, moles are present at birth and may occasionally be massive. There is a substantial risk of future malignancy in massive congenital moles and prophylactic surgical removal is advised if feasible. All humans have moles but their number varies from 10 or less to 100 or more. The members of some families are genetically predisposed to large numbers of moles, some of which may be large and irregular in shape and colour. This 'atypical mole syndrome' is associated with an increased risk of future malignant melanoma. (See MELANOMA; SKIN.)

MOLLUSCUM CONTAGIOSUM Common papular eruption of the skin caused by a VIRUS. Most common in children, it is highly contagious and often transmitted in swimming pools and sauna baths. Mollusca are often multiple and persistent in children with atopic ECZEMA, and epidemics may occur in boarding schools. The typical molluscum is 2–3 mm in diameter, skin coloured and translucent, with a dimpled centre. The armpits and adjacent chest, upper inner thighs and genital areas are common sites in young children. In adults the infection is usually transmitted sexually and affects the pubic area and lower belly. Mollusca eventually disappear spontaneously, but cure can be expedited by curettage under surface anaesthesia.

MONGOLIAN BLUE SPOTS Irregularly shaped areas of bluish-black pigmentation found occasionally on the buttocks, lower back or upper arms in new-born infants of African, Chinese and Japanese parentage and sometimes in the babies of black-haired Europeans. They measure from one to several centimetres in diameter, and usually disappear in a few months. They are commonly mistaken for bruises.

MONGOLISM (see DOWN'S SYNDROME).

MONILIASIS The infection caused by monilia, the genus of fungi now known as Candida albicans. The infection may occur in the mouth, where it is known as THRUSH, lungs, intestine, vagina, skin, or nails.

MONKEYPOX A smallpox-like disease, due to a virus which occurs in monkeys kept in captivity. Since 1970, when first reported, fewer than 100 human cases have been recorded. Most of these have been in Zaïre, and all have been in the equatorial rain-forest of West and Central Africa (Zaïre, Liberia, Sierra Leone, Nigeria, Ivory Coast and Cameroon). The case-fatality rate to date has been 17 per cent. It does not appear to be highly infectious and it is not at the moment considered to be a great risk to human beings.

MONOAMINE OXIDASE INHIBITORS (MAOIs) are drugs that destroy, or prevent the action of, monoamine oxidase (MAO). Monoamines, which include NORADRENALINE and tyramine, play an important part in the metabolism of the brain, and there is some evidence that excitement is due to an accumulation of monoamines in the brain. MAO is a naturally occurring ENZYME which is concerned in the breakdown of monoamines. MAOIs were among the earliest antidepressants used but they are now used much less than TRICYCLIC and related antidepressants or SELECTIVE SEROTONIN-REUPTAKE INHIBITORS (SSRIS) and related antidepressants because of the dangers of dietary or drug interactions and because MAOIs are less effective than these two groups.

An excessive accumulation of monoamines can induce a dangerous reaction characterized by high blood-pressure, palpitations, sweating and a feeling of suffocation. Hence the care with which MAOI drugs are administered. What is equally important, however, is that in no circumstances should a patient receiving any MAOI drug eat cheese, yeast preparations such as Marmite, tinned fish, or high game. The reason for this ban is that all these foodstuffs contain large amounts of tyramine which increases the amount of certain monoamines such as noradrenaline in the body. (See MENTAL ILLNESS.)

There are also certain drugs, such as AMPHETAMINE and PETHIDINE, which must not be taken by a patient who is receiving an MAOI drug. The MAOIs of choice are phenelzine or isocarboxazid because their stimulant effects are less than those of other MAOIs, making them safer.

MONOCLONAL ANTIBODIES An artificially prepared ANTIBODY obtained from cell clones – a genetically identical group of cells – and comprising a single type of immunoglobulin. It neutralizes only one specific ANTIGEN. The antibodies are prepared by linking antibody-forming LYMPHOCYTES from the spleen of mice with MYELOMA CELLS from mice. Monoclonal antibodies are used in the development of new vaccines and in the study of human cells, hormones, and micro-organisms. Research is under way for their use in the treatment of some forms of cancer. (See IMMUNOLOGY.)

MONOCYTE A type of white blood cell which has a single kidney-shaped nucleus. Present in the tissues and lymphatic system as well as the circulation, it ingests foreign particles such as tissue debris and bacteria. Monocytes are about 20μm in diameter and 1 mm³ of blood contains around 7500 of them, many times fewer than the five million erythrocytes (red blood cells).

MONOMANIA is a form of mental illness, in which the affected person has a delusion upon one subject, though he or she can converse rationally and is a responsible individual upon other matters.

MONONUCLEOSIS An acute viral infection in which the patient developes a sore throat, swollen lymph glands and fever. Also known as glandular fever, infectious mononucleosis is caused by members of the HERPES group of viruses – EPSTEIN BARR and CYTOMEGALOVIRUS. The disease is more common among adolescents aged 15 to 17, an age when their immune defence machanisms are not fully developed. In the UK many thousands of teenagers catch the disease every year, and kissing is believed to be the method of transmission among many of them. The blood contains many atypical LYMPHOCYTES and the diagnosis is confirmed with the heterophil antibodies test. Patients normally recover within six weeks without treatment, but they may feel tired and depressed for several months afterwards. There is debate as to whether mononucleosis is related to myalgic encephalomyelitis (ME) and other chronic fatigue syndromes related to viral infections.

MONOPLEGIA Paralysis of a single limb or part. (See PARALYSIS.)

MONOSACCHARIDE A sugar having six carbon atoms in the molecule, such as glucose, galactose, and laevulose.

MONOZYGOTIC TWINS Twins who develop from a single ovum fertilized by a single spermatozoa. Also known as identical or uniovular twins (see MULTIPLE BIRTHS).

MORBID ANATOMY The study of the structural changes that diseases cause in the body, in particular those that can be seen with the naked eye at POST-MORTEM EXAMINATIONS.

MORBIDITY The condition of being diseased. The morbidity rate is the number of cases of disease occurring within a particular number of the population.

MORBILLI Another name for measles.

MORBILLIVIRUSES are the group of viruses which include those responsible for measles, canine distemper and rinderpest (a plague affecting cattle).

MORBUS, the Latin word for disease, is used in such terms as morbus cordis (heart disease), morbus coxae (hip-joint disease).

MORIBUND In a state of dying.

MORON A traditional term used to describe individuals with mild learning difficulties. It should no longer be used.

MORPHINE, or MORPHIA, is the name of the chief alkaloid upon which the action of opium depends. (See OPIUM; DRUG ADDICTION.)

MORPHOEA A form of circumscribed scleroderma. (See SCLERODERMA.)

MORTALITY (see DEATH, CAUSES OF; DEATH RATE; INFANT MORTALITY).

MORTIFICATION is another name for gangrene. (See GANGRENE.)

MOSAICISM If non-dysjunction occurs after the formation of a ZYGOTE, that is during a mitotic cell division and not a meiotic cell division, some of the cells will have one chromosome constitution and others another. The term mosaicism describes a condition in which a substantial minority of cells in an individual's body differ from the majority in their chromosome content. How substantial this minority will depend on how early during cleavage the zygote undergoes non-dysjunction. Mosaicism can cause disorders such as DOWN's and TURNER's syndrome. The proportion and type of abnormal cells affect the physical appearance of the affected individual. This may range from normal to the features typical of people with a chromosomal-abnormality syndrome. (See MEIOSIS.)

MOSQUITOES. (See ANOPHELES; BITES AND STINGS; MALARIA.)

MOTILIN is a HORMONE formed in the DUODENUM and the JEJUNUM which plays a part in controlling the movements of the stomach and the gut.

MOTION Waste products evacuated in a bowel movement, also called faeces or stool.

MOTION (TRAVEL) SICKNESS A characteristic set of symptoms experienced by many people when subjected to the constant changes of position caused, for example, by the pitching and rolling motion of a vessel at sea. Depression, giddiness, nausea and vomiting are the most prominent.

Causes Although the vast majority of people appear to be liable to this ailment at sea, they do not all suffer alike. Many endure acute distress, whilst others are simply conscious of transient feelings of nausea and discomfort. A smaller proportion of people suffer from air and car sickness. The symptoms are a result of overstimulation of the organs of balance in the inner ear by continuous changes in the body's position. The movements of the horizon worsen this situation.

Symptoms The symptoms generally show themselves soon after the journey has started, by the onset of giddiness and discomfort in the head, together with a sense of nausea and sinking at the stomach, which soon develops into intense sickness and vomiting. Most people recover quickly when the motion stops.

Treatment Innumerable preventives and remedies have been proposed. Cinnarizine 30 mg orally is useful 2 hours before travel, then 15 mg every 8 hours during journey if necessary. Dimenhydrinate and promethazine are also commonly taken for motion sickness.

MOTOR A term usually applied to nerves, used to describe anything that results in movement. Motor nerves stimulate muscles to contract, producing movement. (See SENSORY.)

MOTOR NEURONE DISEASE (MND) A group of disorders of unknown origin. Certain cells in the neurological system's motor nerves degenerate and die. Upper and lower motor neurones may be affected but sensory cells retain their normal functions. Three types of MND are identified: amyotrophic lateral sclerosis (50 per cent of patients); progressive muscular atrophy (25 per cent) in which the prognosis is better than for AML; bulbar palsy (25 per cent). Men are affected more than women and the disorder affects about seven people in every 100,000. Those affected develop weakness and wasting of their muscles and usually die within three to five years and the average age of death is 60 years. The diagnosis is confirmed with various tests including the measurement of electrical activity in muscles, electromyography, muscle BIOPSY, blood tests and X-ray examination of the spine. There is no medical treatment: patients need physical and psychological support with aids to help them overcome disabilities. The Motor Neurone Disease Association provides excellent advice and help for sufferers and their relatives. (See APPENDIX 2: ADDRESSES).

MOUNTAIN SICKNESS (see ALTITUDE SICKNESS).

MOUTH The start of the alimentary canal. It is bounded anteriorly by the lips and posteriorly by the fauces which is the narrow passage between the tonsils. Immediately behind the lips are the teeth, embedded in the jaw, and behind the lower teeth is the tongue. The upper part of the mouth is the palate. The anterior or hard palate is firm and immovable as it consists of bone covered by mucosa, while the posterior part is soft and mobile. The soft palate moves during swallowing and speech. The salivary glands discharge their saliva into the mouth through small ducts. Two of these ducts are large and can be easily seen; the parotid duct opens into the cheek opposite the upper second molar tooth and the submandibular gland duct can be seen under the tongue in the midline.

Food in the mouth is prepared for digestion by being broken up by the teeth and mixed with saliva prior to being projected into the stomach via the oesophagus.

MOUTH, DISEASES OF The mucous membrane of the mouth can indicate the health of the individual and internal organs, e.g. pallor or pigmentation may indicate anaemia, jaundice or Addison's disease.

Conditions of the tongue At rest the tongue touches all the lower teeth and is slightly arched from side to side. It has a smooth surface with a groove in the middle and an even but definite edge. It is under voluntary control and the tip can be moved in all directions.

Ankyloglossia or tongue-tie is found when the frenum or band connecting the lower surface of the tongue to the floor of the mouth is so short or tight that the tongue cannot be protruded. Surgery can remedy the defect.

Gross enlargement of the tongue can make speech indistinct or make swallowing and even breathing difficult. This is known as macroglossia and may be such that the tongue is constantly protruded from the mouth. The cause may be congenital as in severe cases of DOWN'S SYNDROME or it may occur as a result of ACROMEGALY or be due to abnormal deposits as in amyloid disease.

A marked tremor of the tongue when protruded may be seen in various neurological diseases but may be caused by alcoholism.

After a STROKE involving the motor nerve centre the control of one side of the tongue musculature will be lost. This will result in the protruded tongue pointing to the side of the body which is paralysed. The sense of taste on one side of the tongue may also be lost in some diseases of the brain and facial nerve.

The presence of fur on the tongue may be obvious and distressing. This is due to thickening of the superficial layers of the tongue which may appear like hairs which trap food debris and become discoloured. Furring is common during fever and as a result of mouth breathing and smoking.

In some conditions the tongue may appear dry, red and raw (GLOSSITIS). An inflamed beefy tongue is characteristic of pellagra, a disease caused by deficiency of NICOTINIC ACID in the diet. A magenta-coloured tongue may be seen when there is a lack of RIBOFLAVIN.

Thrush is characterized by the presence of white patches on the mucous membrane which bleeds if the patch is gently removed. It is caused by the growth of a parasitic mould known as *Candida albicans*. Antifungal agents usually suppress the growth of Candida. Candidal infiltration of the mucosa is often found in cancerous lesions.

Leukoplakia literally means a white patch. In the mouth it is often due to an area of thickened cells from the horny layer of the epithelium. It appears as a white patch of varying density and is often grooved by dense fissures. There are many causes, most of them of minor importance. It may be associated with smoking, syphilis, chronic sepsis or trauma from a sharp tooth. Cancer must be excluded.

Ulcers of the tongue are similar to those elsewhere in the mouth. The most common are aphthous ulcers which are small red and painful

and last for about ten days. They are associated with stress, mild trauma, and occasionally with folic acid and vitamin B_{12} deficiency. Ulcers of the tongue are sometimes found in patients with chronic bowel disease.

Stomatitis (inflammation of the mouth) arises from the same causes as inflammation elsewhere, but among the main causes are the cutting of teeth in children, sharp or broken teeth, excess alcohol, tobacco smoking and general ill-health. The mucous membrane becomes red, swollen and tender and ulcers may appear. Treatment consists mainly of preventing secondary infection supervening before the stomatitis has resolved. Antiseptic mouthwashes are usually sufficient.

Gingivitis (see TEETH, DISEASES OF) is inflammation of the gum where it touches the tooth. It is caused by poor oral hygiene and is often associated with the production of calculus or tartar on the teeth. If it is neglected it will proceed to periodontal disease.

Ulcers of the mouth These are usually small and arise from a variety of causes. Aphthous ulcers are the most common. They last about ten days and usually heal without scarring. They may be associated with stress or dyspepsia. There is no ideal treatment.

Herpetic ulcers are similar but usually there are many ulcers and the patient appears feverish and unwell. It is more common in children.

Alveolar abscess, dental abscess or gumboil This is an abscess caused by an infected tooth. It may present as a large swelling or cause trismus (inability to open the mouth). Treatment is drainage of the pus, extraction of the tooth or antibiotics.

Calculus   (a) Salivary; a calculus or stone may develop in one of the major salivary gland ducts. This may result in a blockage which will cause the gland to swell and be painful. It usually swells before a meal and then slowly subsides. The stone may be passed but often has to be removed in a minor operation. If the gland behind the calculus becomes infected, then an abscess forms and, if this persists, the removal of the gland may be indicated. (b) Dental, also called TARTAR: This is a calcified material which adheres to the teeth and it often starts as the soft debris found on teeth which have not been well cleaned and is called plaque. If not removed, it will gradually destroy the periodontal membrane and result in the loss of the tooth.

Ranula   This is a cystlike swelling found in the floor of the mouth. It is often caused by mild trauma to the salivary glands with the result that saliva collects in the cyst instead of discharging into the mouth. Surgery may be required.

Mumps is an acute infective disorder of the major salivary glands. It causes painful enlargement of the glands which lasts for about two weeks (see MUMPS).

Tumours occur in all parts of the mouth. They may be benign or malignant. Benign tumours are common and may follow mild trauma or are an exaggerated response to irritation. Polyps are found in the cheeks and on the tongue and become a nuisance as they may be bitten frequently. They are easily excised.

A mucocoele is found mainly in the lower lip.

An exostosis or bone outgrowth is often found in the mid-line of the palate and on the inside of the MANDIBLE. This only requires removal if it becomes unduly large or pointed and easily ulcerated.

Malignant tumours within the mouth are often large before they are noticed, whereas those on the lips are usually seen early and are more easily treated. The cancer may arise from any of the tissues found in the mouth including epithelium, bone, salivary tissue and tooth-forming tissue remnants. Oral cancers represent about 5 per cent of all reported malignancies, and in England and Wales around 3,300 people are diagnosed annually as having cancer of the mouth and pharynx.

Cancer of the mouth is less common below the age of 40 years and more common in men. It is often associated with chronic irritation from a broken tooth or ill-fitting denture. It is also more common in those who smoke and those who chew betel leaves. LEUKOPLAKIA may be a precursor of cancer. Spread of the cancer is by way of the lymph nodes in the neck. Early treatment by surgery, radiotherapy or chemotherapy, will often be effective, except for the posterior of the tongue where the prognosis is very poor. Although surgery may be extensive and potentially mutilating, recent advances in repairing defects and grafting tissues from elsewhere have made treatment more acceptable to the patient.

MOUTH-TO-MOUTH RESPIRATION (see APPENDIX 1: BASIC FIRST AID).

MRI or MAGNETIC RESONANCE IMAGING   A non-invasive method of imaging the body and its organs. It may also be used to study tissue metabolism. The body is placed in a magnetic field which causes certain atomic nuclei to align in the direction of the field. Pulses of radio-frequency radiation are then applied and interpretation of the frequencies absorbed and re-emitted allows an image in any body plane to be built up. (See diagram.)

MRSA (see METHICILLIN-RESISTANT STAPHYLOCOCCUS AUREUS).

MUCILAGE   This is prepared from acacia or tragacanth gum, and is used as an ingredient of mixtures containing solid particles in order to keep the latter from settling, and also as a demulcent.

MUCOCOELE   An abnormally dilated cavity in the body due to the accumulation of mucus; such a 'cyst' may therefore form wherever there is mucous membrane.

MUCOCUTANEOUS LYMPH NODE SYNDROME   (see KAWASAKI DISEASE).

MRI scanner

Nuclear magnetic resonance imaging (MRI) scanner. The MRI scanner comprises a strong electromagnet, a radio-wave emitter and a radio-wave detector. The subject is rotated through different planes to obtain a series of images which are viewed on a computer-controlled monitor screen.

MUCOLYTIC The term used to describe the property of destroying, or lessening the tenacity of, mucus. It is most commonly used to describe drugs which have this property and are therefore used in the treatment of bronchitis. The inhalation of steam, for example, has a mucolytic action.

MUCOPOLYSACCARIDOSIS A collection of familial metabolic disorders, the best known of which is Hurler's syndrome. Others include Hunter's, Maroteaux-Lamy and Scheie's syndromes. The disorders, which result from a faulty gene-producing abnormality in a specific ENZYME, affect one child in 10,000. Those affected usually die before reaching adulthood.

MUCOSA A term for mucous membrane.

MUCOUS MEMBRANE The general name given to the membrane which lines many of the hollow organs of the body. These membranes vary widely in structure in different sites, but all have the common character of being lubricated by mucus, derived in some cases from isolated cells on the surface of the membrane, but more generally from definite glands placed beneath the membrane, and opening here and there through it by ducts. The air passages, the gastrointestinal tract and the ducts of glands which open into it, and also the urinary passages, are all lined by mucous membrane.

In structure a mucous membrane consists of a basis of fibrous tissue resembling the true skin, though looser and lighter in texture, in which the blood-vessels, nerves, and mucous glands lie. This is covered on its surface by a layer of epithelium resembling the epithelium covering the SKIN, although the cells are in all cases of a more soft and succulent nature than those on the outer surface of the body.

It is in the character and properties of these cells that the various mucous membranes chiefly differ. In the air passages they are – almost everywhere except over the VOCAL CORDS – of a pillar-like shape and provided with thread-like processes, being known as ciliated cells. On the vocal cords the cells, which are exposed to constant friction, resemble those of the skin. In the alimentary system generally they are of a simple pillar-like or columnar type placed side by side, though in the mouth and gullet, where the food causes much friction, the surface, like that of the vocal cords, closely resembles the epidermis of the skin.

Lying close beneath the epithelium there is, in most mucous membranes, a thin layer of involuntary muscle fibres, and to this, coupled with the extremely loose attachment of mucous membranes to the organs which they line, is due the great pliability and elasticity of these membranes.

MUCOVISCIDOSIS (see CYSTIC FIBROSIS).

MUCUS The general name for the slimy secretion derived from mucous membranes. It is mainly composed of a substance called mucin, which varies according to the particular mucous membrane from which it is derived, and it contains other substances, such as cells cast off from the surface of the membrane, enzymes, and dust particles. Mucin has the following characteristics: it is viscid, clear, and tenacious; when dissolved in water it can be precipitated by addition of acetic acid; and when not in solution already, it is dissolved by weak alkalis, such as lime-water.

Under normal conditions the surface of a mucous membrane is lubricated by only a small quantity of mucus; the appearance of large quantities is a sign of inflammation.

MULLERIAN DUCTS The Mullerian and the Wolffian ducts are separate sets of primordia that transiently co-exist in embryos of both sexes. In female embryos the Mullerian ducts grow and fuse in the midline producing the FALLOPIAN TUBES, the uterus and the upper third of the vagina whereas the Wolffian ducts regress. In the male the Wolffian ducts give rise to the vas deferens, the seminal vesicles and the epididymis and the Mullerian ducts disappear. This phase of development requires a functioning testis from which an inducer substance diffuses locally over the primordia to bring about the suppression of the Mullerian duct and the development of the Wolffian duct. In the absence of this substance development proceeds along female lines regardless of the genetic sex.

MULTIGRAVIDA A pregnant woman who has had more than one pregnancy.

MULTIPARA A woman who has borne several children.

MULTIPLE BIRTHS Twins occur about once in eighty pregnancies, triplets once in 6000, quadruplets about once in 500,000. Quintuplets are exceedingly rare. Such is the natural state of affairs. In recent years, however, the position has been altered by the introduction of the so-called fertility drugs, such as CLOMIPHENE, and human menopausal gonadotrophin which, through the medium of the pituitary gland, stimulate the production of ova. Their wide use in the treatment of infertility has resulted in an increase in the number of multiple births, a recognized hazard of giving too large a dose. So far as fraternal, or binovular, twins are concerned, multiple pregnancy may be an inherited tendency; it certainly occurs more often in certain families, but this may be partly due to chance. A woman who has already given birth to twins is ten times more likely to have another multiple pregnancy than one who has not previously had twins. The statistical chance of a third pair of twins is 1 in 512,000. Identical twins do not run in families.

Twins may be binovular or uniovular. Binovular, or fraternal, twins are the result of the mother's releasing two ova within a few days of each other and both being fertilized by separate spermatozoa. They both develop separately in the mother's womb and are no more alike than is usual with members of the same family. They are three times as common as uniovular, or identical, twins, who are developed from a single ovum fertilized by a single spermatozoon, but which has split early in development. This is why they are usually so remarkably alike in looks and mental characteristics. Unlike binovular twins, who may be of the same or different sex, they are always of the same sex.

The relative proportion of twins of each type varies in different races. Identical twins have much the same frequency all over the world: around 3 per 1000 maternities. Fraternal twins are rare in Mongolian races: less than 3 per 1000 maternities. In Caucasians they occur two or three times as often as identical twins: between 7 (Spain and Portugal) and 10 (Czech and Slovak Republics and Greece) per 1000 maternities. They are more common in Africocaribbeans, reaching 30 per 1000 maternities in certain West African populations. (See also SIAMESE TWINS.)

'False twins' are not uncommon, when 'twin' children have been fathered by different men.

Parents of twins, triplets or more can obtain advice and help from the Twins and Multiple Births Association (TAMBA) (see APPENDIX 2: ADDRESSES).

MULTIPLE PERSONALITY DISORDER

The individual with this psychiatric disorder has two or more different personalities, often contrasting. The dominant personality at the time determines the behaviour and attitude of the individual, who customarily seems not to know about the other personality – or personalities. The switch from one personality to another is abrupt and the mental condition of the differing personalities is usually normal. It is possible that child abuse is a factor in the disorder, which is treated by psychotherapy. The classic multiple personality was the fictional form of Dr Jekyll and Mr Hyde.

MULTIPLE SCLEROSIS (MS) is a progressive disease of the brain and spinal cord, which, though slow in its onset, in time may produce marked symptoms, such as paralysis and tremors, and may ultimately result in a severely disabled invalid. Formerly known as disseminated sclerosis, the disorder consists of hardened patches, from the size of a pin-head to that of a pea or larger, scattered here and there irregularly through the brain and spinal cord. Each patch is made up of a mass of the connective tissue (neuroglia), which should be present only in sufficient amount to bind the nerve-cells and fibres together. In the earliest stage, the insulating sheaths (MYELIN) of the nerve-fibres in the hardened patches break up, are absorbed, and leave the nerve-fibres bare, the connective tissue being later formed between these.

Cause Although this is one of the most common diseases of the central nervous system in Europe – there are around 50,000 affected individuals in Britain alone – the cause is still not known. The disease comes on in young people (onset being rare after the age of 40), apparently without previous illness. The rate of women to men victims is three to two. It is more common in first and second children than in those later in birth order, and in small rather than big families. There may be a hereditary factor, for MS, which could be an autoimmune disorder: the body's defence system attacks the myelin in the central nervous system as if it were a 'foreign' tissue.

Symptoms These depend greatly upon the part of the brain and cord affected by the sclerotic patches. Temporary paralysis of a limb, or of an eye muscle, causing double vision, and tremors upon exertion, first in the affected parts, and later in all parts of the body, are early symptoms. Stiffness of the lower limbs causing the toes to catch on small irregularities in the ground and trip the person in walking, is often an annoying symptom and one of the first to be noticed. Great activity is shown in the reflex movements obtained by striking the tendons and by stroking the soles of the feet. The latter reflex shows a characteristic sign (Babinski sign) in which the great toe bends upwards and the other toes spread apart as the sole is stroked, instead of the toes collectively bending downwards as in the normal person. Tremor of the eye movements (nystagmus) is usually found. Trembling handwriting, interference with the functions of the bladder, giddiness, and a peculiar 'staccato' or 'scanning' speech are common symptoms at a later stage. Numbness and tingling in the extremities occur commonly, particularly in the early stages of the disease. As the disease progresses, the paralyses, which were transitory at first, now become confirmed, often with great rigidity in the limbs. In many cases patients the disease progresses very slowly.

People with multiple sclerosis, and their relatives, can obtain help and guidance from the Multiple Sclerosis Society of Great Britain and Northern Ireland. Another helpful organization is the Multiple Sclerosis Resource Centre. Those with sexual or marital problems arising out of the illness can obtain information from SPOD (Association to Aid the Sexual and Personal Relationships of People with a Disability). See APPENDIX 2: ADDRESSES.

Treatment is unsatisfactory, because the most that can be done is to lead a life as free from strain as possible, to check the progress of the disease. The use of INTERFERON seems to slow the progress of MS and clinical trials are in progress in various countries to assess the effectiveness of this costly drug. Corticosteroids may be of help to some patients. It is important to keep the nerves and muscles functioning, and therefore the patient should remain at work as long as he or she is capable of doing it, and in any case should regularly exercise.

MUMPS, also known as EPIDEMIC PAROTITIS, is an infectious disease characterized by inflammatory swelling of the parotid and other SALIVARY GLANDS, often occurring as an epidemic, and affecting mostly young people. Its name comes from the old verb, 'mump', meaning to mope or assume a disconsolate appearance – an apt description of the victim of the disease at its height.

Causes Mumps is due to infection with a virus and is highly infectious from person to person. It is predominantly a disease of childhood and early adult life, but it can occur at any age. Epidemics usually occur in the winter and spring. It is infectious for two or three days before the swelling of the glands appears. A vaccine is now available that gives a high degree of protection against the disease, the incidence of which is falling sharply. The vaccine is combined with those for MEASLES and RUBELLA (MMR). (See IMMUNIZATION.)

Symptoms There is an incubation period of two to three weeks after infection before the glands begin to swell. The gland first affected is generally the parotid, situated in front of and below the ear. The swelling usually spreads to the submaxillary and sublingual glands lying beneath the jaw. The patient is feverish and the gland is tender. The swelling disappears after about five days. In 15 to 30 per cent of males, inflammation of the testicles (orchitis) develops. This usually occurs during the second week of the illness, but may not occur until two or three weeks later. It may result in partial atrophy of the TESTICLES, but practically never in infertility. In a much smaller proportion of females with mumps, inflammation of the OVARIES or breasts may occur. Inflammation of the pancreas, accompanied by tenderness in the upper part of the abdomen and digestive disturbances, sometimes occurs. MENINGITIS is also an occasional complication. The various complications are found much more often when the disease affects adults than when it occurs in childhood.

Treatment There is no specific treatment but ANALGESICS and plenty of fluid are available. The child may need to be in bed for a few days and should not return to school until the symptoms have settled. Adults with orchitis may need strong painkillers, and CORTICOSTEROID drugs may be required to reduce the painful swelling.

MUNCHAUSEN'S SYNDROME, also known as 'hospital addiction' syndrome, is a type of factitious disorder (one in which the patient's symptoms mimic those of a genuine illness) in which patients may present repeatedly to hospitals with symptoms and signs (often simulated) suggestive of serious physical illness. More common among men than women, it differs from malingering in that no obvious reward results from the imagined or simulated symptoms. Patients may simulate signs and symptoms in a bizarre way, for instance, by swallowing blood or inserting needles into the chest. Abdominal symptoms are particularly common. They have a history of multiple hospital admissions and operations, and show extensive pathological lying and lack of personal rapport. Although the cause is unclear, it is thought to be a form of hysterical behaviour in a severely disordered personality. Patients are often masochistic, attention seeking, and constantly trying to obtain ANALGESIC drugs. Occasionally there may be a degree of treatable DEPRESSION, but on the whole management is very difficult, as patients often abscond from psychiatric treatment.

A variation of the syndrome – Munchausen by proxy – has recently been identified. The persons affected inflict damage on others, usually children, in their care – thus drawing attention to themselves.

MURMUR The uneven, rustling sound heard by auscultation over the heart and various blood-vessels in abnormal conditons. For example, murmurs heard when the stethoscope is applied over the heart are highly characteristic of valvular disease of this organ.

MUSCAE VOLITANTES ('FLYING FLIES') Spots before the eyes due to small opacities in the vitreous humour casting shadows on the retina. In themselves vitreous floaters are harmless but anyone with 'spots before the eyes' of sudden onset should seek specialist advice.

MUSCARINE The poisonous principle found in some toadstools. (See FUNGUS-POISONING.) It is a cholinergic substance with pharmacological properties resembling those of ACETYLCHOLINE, a chemical neurotransmitter released at the junctions (synapses) of PARASYMPATHETIC nerves and at the junctions where nerves enter muscles.

MUSCLE Muscular tissue is divided, according to its function, into three main groups, voluntary muscle, involuntary muscle or skeletal, of which the former is under control of the will, whilst the latter discharge their functions independently. The term striped muscle is often given to voluntary muscle, because under the microscope all the voluntary muscles show a striped appearance, whilst involuntary muscle is, in the main, unstriped or plain. Heart muscle, is partially striped, while certain muscles of the throat, and two small muscles inside the ear, not controllable by will-power, are also striped.

Structure of muscle Skeletal or voluntary muscle forms the bulk of the body's musculature and contains over 600 such muscles. They are classified according to their methods of action. A flexor muscle closes a joint, an extensor opens it; an abductor moves a body part outwards, an adductor moves it in; a depressor lowers a body part and a levator raises it; while a constrictor (sphincter) muscle

1 frontalis
2 greater zygomatic
3 masseter
4 sternohyoid
5 trapezius
6 deltoid
7 serratus anterior
8 biceps
9 triceps
10 brachialis
11 pronator teres
12 palmaris longus
13 flexorcarpus radialis
14 ileopsoas
15 pectineus
16 adductor longus
17 gracilis
18 vastus lateralis
19 anterior tibial
20 peroneus brevis
21 extensor hallucis longus
22 orbicularis oculi
23 orbicularis oris
24 depressor anguli oris
25 sternocleidomastoid
26 pectoralis major
27 latissimus dorsi
28 pectoralis minor
29 linea alba
30 external oblique
31 brachioradialis
32 flexor carpi ulnaris
33 inguinal ligament
34 iliacus
35 palmar carpal ligament
36 sartorius
37 rectus
38 vastus medialis
39 peroneus longus
40 gastrocnemius
41 soleus
42 superior extensor retinaculum

Muscles of the body: front view.

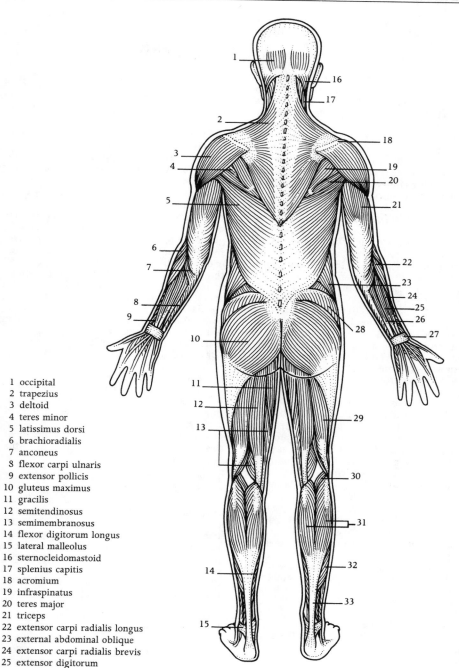

1 occipital
2 trapezius
3 deltoid
4 teres minor
5 latissimus dorsi
6 brachioradialis
7 anconeus
8 flexor carpi ulnaris
9 extensor pollicis
10 gluteus maximus
11 gracilis
12 semitendinosus
13 semimembranosus
14 flexor digitorum longus
15 lateral malleolus
16 sternocleidomastoid
17 splenius capitis
18 acromium
19 infraspinatus
20 teres major
21 triceps
22 extensor carpi radialis longus
23 external abdominal oblique
24 extensor carpi radialis brevis
25 extensor digitorum
26 extensor carpi ulnaris
27 extensor retinaculum
28 gluteus medius
29 vastus externus
30 plantaris
31 gastrocnemius
32 soleus
33 calcaneal tendon (Achilles)

Muscles of the body: back view.

surrounds an orifice, closing and opening it. Each muscle is enclosed in a sheath of fibrous tissue, known as fascia or epimysium, and, from this, partitions of fibrous tissue, known as perimysium, run into the substance of the muscle, dividing it up into small bundles. Each of these bundles consists in turn of a collection of fibres, which form the units of the muscle. Each fibre is about 50 micrometres in thickness and ranges in length from a few millimetres to 300 millimetres. If the fibre is cut across and examined under a high-powered microscope, it is seen to be further divided into fibrils. Each fibre is enclosed in an elastic sheath of its own, which allows it to lengthen and shorten, and is known as the sarcolemma. Within the sarcolemma lie numerous nuclei belonging to the muscle fibre, which was originally developed from a simple cell. To the sarcolemma, at either end, is attached a minute bundle of connective-tissue fibres which unites the muscle fibre to its neighbours, or to one of the connective tissue partitions in the muscle, and by means of these connections the fibre affects muscle contraction. Between the muscle fibres, and enveloped in a sheath of connective tissue, lie here and there special structures known as muscle-spindles. Each of these contains thin muscle fibres, numerous nuclei, and the endings of sensory nerves. (See TOUCH.) The heart muscle comprises short fibres which communicate with their neighbours via short branches and have no sarcolemma.

Plain or unstriped muscle is found in the following positions: the inner and middle coats of the STOMACH and INTESTINES; the URETERS and urinary BLADDER; the TRACHEA and bronchial tubes; the ducts of glands; the GALL-BLADDER; the UTERUS and FALLOPIAN TUBES; the middle coat of the blood- and lymph-vessels; the iris and ciliary muscle of the eye; the dartos muscle of the SCROTUM; and in association with the various glands and hairs in the skin. The fibres are very much smaller than those of striped muscle, although they vary greatly in size. Each has one or more oval nuclei and a delicate sheath of sarcolemma enveloping it. The fibres are grouped in bundles, much as are the striped fibres, but they adhere to one another by cement material, not by the tendon bundles found in voluntary muscle.

Development of muscle All the muscles of the developing individual arise from the central layer (mesoderm) of the embryo, each fibre taking origin from a single cell. Later on in life, muscles have the power both of increasing in size, as the result of use, for example, in athletes, and also of healing, after parts of them have been destroyed by injury. An example of the great extent to which unstriped muscle can develop to meet the demands made on it is the uterus whose muscular wall develops so much during pregnancy that the organ increases from the weight of 30 to 40 g (1 to 1½ oz.) to a weight of around 1 kg (2 lb.), decreasing again to its former small size in the course of a month after child-birth.

Physiology of contraction A muscle is an elaborate chemico-physical system for producing heat and mechanical work. The total energy liberated by a contracting muscle can be exactly measured. From 25 to 30 per cent of the total energy expended is used in mechanical work. The heat of contracting muscle makes an important contribution to the maintenance of the heat of the body. (See also MYOGLOBIN.)

The energy of muscular contraction is derived from a complicated series of chemical reactions. Complex substances are broken down and built up again, supplying each other with energy for this purpose. The first reaction is the breakdown of adenyl-pyrophosphate into phosphoric acid and adenylic acid (derived from nucleic acid); this supplies the immediate energy for contraction. Next phosphocreatine breaks down into creatine and phosphoric acid, giving energy for the resynthesis of adenyl-pyrophosphate. Creatine is a normal nitrogenous constituent of muscle. Then glycogen through the intermediary stage of sugar bound to phosphate breaks down into lactic acid to supply energy for the resynthesis of phospho-creatine. Finally part of the lactic acid is oxidized to supply energy for building up the rest of the lactic acid into glycogen again. If there is not enough oxygen, lactic acid accumulates and fatigue results.

All of the chemical changes are mediated by the action of several enzymes.

Involuntary muscle has several peculiarities of contraction. In the heart rhythmicality is an important feature, one beat appearing to be, in a sense, the cause of the next beat. Tonus is a character of all muscle, but particularly of unstriped muscle in some localities, as in the walls of arteries.

Fatigue occurs when a muscle is made to act for some time and is due to the accumulation of waste products, especially sarcolactic acid. These substances affect the end plates of the nerve controlling the muscle, and so prevent destructive over-action of the muscle. As they are rapidly swept away by the blood, the muscle, after a rest, particularly if the rest is accompanied by massage or by gentle contractions to quicken the circulation, recovers rapidly from the fatigue. Muscular activity over the whole body causes prolonged fatigue which is remedied by rest to allow for metabolic balance to be re-established.

The distribution of the skeletal muscles is shown in the diagrams on pages 368 and 369.

MUSCLE CRAMP A sudden painful involuntary maximal contraction of a muscle or muscle group. It may last up to 10 minutes and occurs in normal individuals. Cramps usually occur in bed at night when the individual is at rest. Night cramps are especially common in the elderly, during pregnancy and in patients with DIABETES or peripheral vascular disease. They can be caused by sodium loss from excessive sweating, vomiting or diarrhoea. It may also be due to HYPOKALAEMIA as a result of treatment with DIURETICS. Drugs such as the BETA-ADRENERGIC stimulants may be responsible. Sometimes an attack can be thwarted by actively contracting the opposing muscle. The most common cramp is in the calf or foot, so the foot should be dorsiflexed at the ankle and the leg straightened. When the cramp is in the calf muscles, getting out of bed and standing up will stretch the calf muscles and ease the attack. When attacks of cramp occur frequently at night, treatment with quinine bisulphate may help.

MUSCLE RELAXANTS These drugs produce partial or complete paralysis of skeletal muscle. Drugs in clinical use are all reversible and are used to help insert a breathing tube into the trachea (endotracheal tube) during general anaesthesia and artificial ventilation. (see ANAESTHESIA.) They may be broadly divided into depolarizing and non-depolarizing muscle relaxants. Depolarizing muscle relaxants act by binding to acetylcholine receptors at the motor end plate where nerves are attached to muscle cells and producing a more prolonged depolarization than acetylcholine which results in initial muscle fasciculation (overactivity) and then flaccid paralysis of the muscle. The only commonly used depolarizing drug is succinylcholine which has a rapid onset of action and lasts approximately three minutes. Non-depolarizing muscle relaxants bind to the acetylcholine receptors, preventing acetylcholine from gaining access to them. They have a slower onset time and longer duration than depolarizers, though this varies widely between different drugs. They are competitive antagonists and they may be reversed by increasing the concentration of acetylcholine at the motor end plate using an anticholinesterase agent such as neostigmine. These drugs are broken down in the liver and excreted through the kidney and their action will be prolonged in liver and renal failure. Other uses include the relief of skeletal muscle spasms in TETANUS, PARKINSON'S DISEASE and spastic disorders. The drugs dantrolene and diazepam are used in these circumstances.

MUSCLES, DISEASES OF

Inflammation (myositis) of various types may occur. As the result of injury, an abscess may develop (see ABSCESS), although wounds affecting muscle generally heal well. A growth due to SYPHILIS, known as a gumma, sometimes forms a hard, almost painless swelling in a muscle. Rheumatism is a vague term traditionally used to define intermittent and often migratory discomfort, stiffness or pain in muscles and joints with no obvious cause. The most common form of myositis is the result of immunological damage as a result of auto-immune disease. Because it affects many muscles it is called polymyositis.

Myositis ossificans, or deposition of bone in muscles, may be congenital or acquired. The congenital form, which is rare, first manifests

itself as painful swellings in the muscles. These gradually harden and extend until the child is encased in a rigid sheet. There is no effective treatment and the outcome is fatal.

The acquired form is a result of a direct blow on muscle, most commonly on the front of the thigh. The condition should be suspected whenever there is severe pain and swelling following a direct blow over muscle. The diagnosis is confirmed by hardening of the swelling. Treatment consists of short-wave diathermy (see DIATHERMY) with gentle active movements. Recovery is usually complete.

Rupture of a muscle may occur, without any external wound, as the result of a spasmodic effort. It may tear the muscle right across, as sometimes happens to the feeble plantaris muscle in running and leaping, or part of the muscle may be driven through its fibrous envelope, forming a hernia of the muscle. The severe pain experienced in many cases of lumbago is due to tearing of one of the muscles in the back. These conditions are usually relieved by rest and massage. Partial muscle tears, such as occur in sport, require energetic treatment. In the early stages this consists of the application of cold (see COLD, USES OF), firm compression, elevation of the affected limb, rest for a day or so and then gradual mobilization (see SPORTS MEDICINE).

Compression syndrome is the tense painful state of muscles induced by excessive accumulation of INTERSTITIAL fluid in them, following unusual exercise. This condition is more liable to occur in the muscles at the front of the shin because they lie within a tight fascial membrane. Here the syndrome is known as the anterior tibial syndrome. Prevention consists of always keeping fit and in training for the amount of exercise to be undertaken. Equally important is what is known in sporting circles as 'warming down': i.e., at the end of training or a game, exercise should be gradually tailed off. Treatment consists of elevation of the affected limb, compression of it by compression bandages, with ample exercise of the limb within the bandage, and massage. In more severe cases DIURETICS may be given. Occasionally surgical decompression may be necessary.

Myasthenia (see MYASTHENIA GRAVIS) is muscle weakness due to a defect of neuro-muscular conduction.

Pain, quite apart from any inflammation or injury, may be experienced on exertion. This type of pain, known as myalgia, tends to occur in unfit individuals and is relieved by rest and physiotherapy.

Parasites sometimes lodge in the muscles, the most common being *Trichinella spiralis*, producing the disease known as TRICHINOSIS.

Tumours occur occasionally, the most common being fibroid, fatty, and sarcomatous growths.

Myopathy is a term applied to an acquired or developmental defect in certain muscles. (See MYOPATHY.)

Wasting of muscles sometimes occurs as a symptom of disease in other organs: for example, damage to the nervous system, as in poliomyelitis or in the disease known as progressive muscular atrophy. (See PARALYSIS.)

MUSCULAR DYSTROPHY (see MYOPATHY).

MUSCULOSKELETAL An adjective that relates to muscle and/or bone. The musculoskeletal system comprises the bones of the skeleton and all the muscles attached to them.

MUSHROOM POISONING (see FUNGUS-POISONING).

MUSHROOM-WORKER'S LUNG A form of lung disease that occurs in mushroomworkers as a result of their being hypersensitive to mushrooms. (See ALVEOLITIS.)

MUSTINE An alkylating drug – one that acts (like ionizing radiation) by damaging DNA – used to treat HODGKIN'S DISEASE. A toxic compound, it is now much less commonly used than a few years ago. (See CYTOTOXIC.)

MUTAGEN A chemical or physical agent that has the property of increasing the rate of MUTATION among cells. A mutagen does not usually increase the range of mutations. Chemicals, ionizing radiation, and viruses may act as mutagens.

MUTATION A change occurring in the genetic material (DNA) in the CHROMOSOMES of a cell. It is caused by a fault in the replication of a cell's genetic material when it divides to form two daughter cells. Mutations may occur in somatic cells which may result in a local growth of the new type of cells. These may be destroyed by the body's defence mechanism or they may develop into a tumour. If mutation occurs in a germ cell or gamete – the organism's sex cells – the outcome may be a changed inherited characteristic in succeeding generations. Mutations occur rarely but a small steady number are caused by background radiation in the environment. They are also caused by MUTAGENS. (See CHROMOSOME; GENETIC DISORDERS.)

MUTISM (see VOICE AND SPEECH).

MYALGIA Pain in a muscle. (See MUSCLES, DISEASES OF; BORNHOLM DISEASE; LUMBAGO.)

MYALGIC ENCEPHALOMYELITIS (ME) A syndrome in which tiredness, muscle pain, lack of concentration, panic attacks, memory loss and depression occur. Its existence and causes have been the subject of controversy reflected in the variety of names given to the syndrome: post-viral fatigue syndrome, Royal Free disease, epidemic neuromyasthenia and Icelandic disese. ME often follows virus infections of the upper respiratory tract or gut. It may occur in epidemics or as individual cases. Physical examination shows no evidence of disease and there is no diagnostic test – diagnosis usually being made by excluding other possible disorders. The sufferer usually recovers in time, though sometimes recovery may take many months. There is no specific curative treatment, but symptomatic treatment such as resting in the early stages, may help. Sufferers may find it helpful to consult the ME Association (see APPENDIX 2: ADDRESSES).

MYASTHENIA GRAVIS A serious disorder in which the chief symptoms are muscular weakness and a special tendency for fatigue to come on rapidly when efforts are made. The prevalence is around 1 in 30,000. Two-thirds of the patients are women, in whom it develops in early adult life. In men it tends to develop later in life.

It is a classical example of an auto-immune disease (see AUTO-IMMUNITY). The body develops antibodies which interfere with the working of the nerve endings in muscle that are acted on by ACETYLCHOLINE. It is acetylcholine that transmits the nerve impulses to muscles. If this transmission cannot be effected, as in myasthenia gravis, then the muscles are unable to contract. Not only the voluntary muscles, but those connected with the acts of swallowing, breathing, and the like, become progressively weaker, though there is no very marked wasting. Rest and avoidance of undue exertion are necessary, and regular doses of neostigmine bromide, or pyridostigmine at intervals enable the muscles to be used and in some cases have a curative effect. These drugs act by inhibiting the action of cholinesterase. This is an ENZYME produced in the body which destroys any excess of acetylcholine. In this way they increase the amount of available acetylcholine which compensates for the deleterious effect of antibodies on the nerve endings.

The THYMUS GLAND plays the major part in the cause of myasthenia gravis, possibly by being the source of the original acetylcholine receptors to which the antibodies are being formed. At all events, thymectomy, or removal of the thymus, is increasingly important in the management of patients with myathenia gravis. The incidence of remission following thymectomy increases with the number of years after the operation. Complete remission or substantial improvement can be expected in 80 per cent of patients.

The other important aspect in the management of patients with myasthenia gravis is IMMUNOSUPPRESSION. Drugs are now available that suppress ANTIBODY production and so reduce the concentration of antibodies to the acetylcholine receptor. The problem is that they not only suppress abnormal antibody production, but also suppress normal antibody production. The main groups of immunosuppressive drugs used in myasthenia gravis are the CORTICOSTEROIDS and AZATHIOPRINE. Improvement following steroids may take several weeks to become manifest and an initial deterioration is often found during the first week or ten days of treatment. Azathioprine is also effective in producing clinical improvement and reducing the antibodies to acetylcholine receptors. These affects occur more slowly than with steroids and the mean time for an azathioprine remission is nine months.

The Myasthenia Gravis Association, which provides advice and help to sufferers, was created and is supported by myasthenics, their families and friends (see APPENDIX 2: ADDRESSES).

MYCOBACTERIUM   A GRAM-POSITIVE rod-like genus of aerobic BACTERIA, some species of which are harmful to man and animals. For example, *M. tuberculosis* (Koch's bacillus) and *M. leprae* cause, respectively, tuberculosis and leprosy.

MYCOPLASMA   A genus of micro-organisms which differ from bacteria in that they lack a rigid cell wall. They are responsible for widespread epidemics in cattle and poultry. For a long time the only member of the genus known to cause disease in man was *Mycoplasma pneumoniae* which is responsible for the form of pneumonia known as primary atypical pneumonia (see PNEUMONIA). Another, *Mycoplasma genitalium*, has now been isolated which is responsible for certain cases of non-gonococcal urethritis. Mycoplasma infections respond to TETRACYCLINE drugs. (See NON-SPECIFIC GENITAL INFECTION.)

MYCOSIS   The general term applied to diseases due to the growth of fungi in the body. Among some of the simplest and commonest mycoses are RINGWORM, FAVUS, and THRUSH. The MADURA FOOT of India, ACTINOMYCOSIS, and occasional cases of PNEUMONIA and suppurative ear disease are also due to the growth of moulds in the bodily tissues. Other forms of mycosis include ASPERGILLOSIS, CANDIDIASIS, CRYPTOCOCCOSIS and HISTOPLASMOSIS.

MYCOSIS FUNGOIDES   An old term for a chronic eruption of the skin characterized by ERYTHEMATOUS itching PLAQUES (raised patches on the skin resulting from the merging or enlargement of papules), which, if left untreated, eventually form tumours and ulcers. The disease is now known to be a form of cancer of LYMPHOCYTES called T-cell LYMPHOMA. It may be responsive to PHOTOCHEMOTHERAPY in its early stages and to RADIOTHERAPY when more advanced.

MYDRIASIS   Dilation or widening of the pupil of the eye. Occurring naturally when it is dark or when someone is emotionally aroused; mydriasis can also result from the administration of ATROPINE eye drops. Alcohol consumption also has a mydriatic effect.

MYECTOMY   Removal of all or part of a muscle by surgery. It may be used to correct a squint (caused by unbalanced eye muscles) or to remove a FIBROID from the muscular wall of the UTERUS.

MYELIN   A substance made up of protein and phospholipid that forms the sheath surrounding the axons of some neurons. These are described as myelinated or medullated nerve fibres (see NERVES), and electric impulses pass along them faster than along non-myelinated nerves. Myelin is produced by Schwann cells which occur at intervals along the nerve fibre. (See MULTIPLE SCLEROSIS.)

MYELITIS is inflammation of the spinal cord.

MYELOCYTE   The name given to one of the cells of bone-marrow from which the granular white cells of the blood are produced. They are found in the blood in certain forms of leukaemia.

MYELOGRAPHY   The injection of a radio-opaque substance into the central canal of the spinal cord in order to assist in the diagnosis of diseases of the spinal cord or spine using X-ray examination.

MYELOID   An adjective that relates to the granulocyte precursor cell in the bone marrow. For example, myeloid leukaemia, which arises from abnormal growth in the blood-forming tissue of the marrow.

MYELOMA (see MYELOMATOSIS).

MYELOMATOSIS, or MULTIPLE MYELOMA.   A malignant disorder of plasma cells, derived from B LYMPHOCYTES. In most patients the bone marrow is heavily infiltrated with atypical, monoclonal plasma cells, which gradually replace the normal cell lines, inducing ANAEMIA, leucopenia, and thrombocytopenia. Bone absorption occurs, producing diffuse OSTEOPOROSIS. In some cases only part of the immunoglobulin molecule is produced by the tumour cells, appearing in the urine as Bence Jones proteinuria. The disease is rare under the age of 30, frequency increasing with age to peak between 60 and 70 years. It is more common in men than women, and in black people than white. There may be a long pre-clinical phase, sometimes as long as 25 years. When symptoms do occur, they tend to reflect bone involvement, reduced immune function, renal failure, anaemia or hyperviscosity of the blood. Vertebral collapse is common, with nerve root pressure and reduced stature. The disease is usually fatal, infection being a common cause of death. Local skeletal problems should be treated with radiotherapy, and the general disease with chemotherapy, chiefly melphalan or cyclophosphamide. Red-blood-cell transfusion is usually required, together with plasmapheresis (see PLASMA EXCHANGE), and orthopaedic surgery may be necessary following fractures. With sensitive counselling to increase the patient's morale, the prognosis may be significantly improved.

MYELOSUPPRESSION A fall in the production of blood cells in the bone marrow. This fall often occurs after chemotherapy for cancer. ANAEMIA, infection and abnormal bleeding are symptomatic of myelosuppression.

MYIASIS Infestation of the skin, deeper tissues or the intestine by larvae of the tropical tumbu fly.

MYOCARDIAL INFARCTION (see CORONARY THROMBOSIS).

MYOCARDITIS Inflammation of the muscular wall of the HEART.

MYOCARDIUM is the muscular substance of the heart. (See MUSCLES.)

MYOCLONUS A brief, twitching muscular contraction which may involve only a single muscle or many muscles. It may be too slight to cause movement of the affected limb, or so violent as to throw the victim to the floor. The cause is not known, but in some cases may be a form of epilepsy. A single myoclonic jerk in the upper limbs occasionally occurs in petit mal. (See EPILEPSY.) The myoclonic jerks which many people experience in falling asleep are a perfectly normal phenomenon.

MYOGLOBIN The protein which gives MUSCLE its red colour. It has the property of combining loosely and reversibly with oxygen. This means that it is the vehicle whereby muscle extracts OXYGEN from the HAEMOGLOBIN in the blood circulating through it, and then releases the oxygen for use by the muscle.

MYOGLOBINURIA The occurrence of MYOGLOBIN in the URINE. This is the oxygen binding pigment in muscle and mild myoglobinuria may occur during exercise. Severe myoglobinuria will result from severe injuries, particularly crushing injuries, to muscles.

MYOMA The term applied to a tumour, almost invariably of a simple nature, which consists mainly of muscle fibres. These muscle tumours often occur in the UTERUS.

MYOMECTOMY Removal by surgery of FIBROIDS from the muscular wall of the UTERUS.

MYOMETRIUM The muscular coat of the UTERUS.

MYOPATHY A generic term covering all primary muscle disease. It is not a neurological disease, and should be distinguished from neuropathic conditions (see NEUROPATHY) such as MOTOR NEURONE DISEASE, which tend to affect the distal limb muscles. The main subdivisions are genetically determined, congenital, metabolic, drug induced, and myopathy (often inflammatory) secondary to a distant carcinoma. Progressive muscular dystrophy is characterized by symmetrical wasting and weakness, the muscle fibres being largely replaced by fatty and fibrous tissue, with no sensory loss. Inheritance may take several forms, thus affecting the sex and age of victims.

The commonest type is Duchenne's muscular dystrophy which is inherited as a sex-linked disorder. It nearly always occurs in boys.

Symptoms There are three chief types of myopathy. The commonest, known as pseudo-hypertrophic muscular dystrophy, affects particularly the upper part of the lower limbs of children. The muscles of the buttocks, thighs and calves seem excessively well developed, but nevertheless the child is clumsy, weak on his legs, and has difficulty in picking himself up when he falls. In another form of the disease, which begins a little later, as a rule about the age of 14, the muscles of the upper arm are first affected, and those of the spine and lower limbs become weak later on. In a third type, which begins about this age, the muscles of the face, along with certain of the shoulder and upper arm muscles, show the first signs of wasting. All the forms have this in common: that the affected muscles grow weaker till their power to contract is quite lost. In the first form, the patients seldom reach the age of 20, falling victims to some disease which, to ordinary people, would not be serious. In the other forms the wasting, after progressing to a certain extent, often remains stationary for the rest of life. Myopathy may also be acquired when it is the result of disease such as THYROTOXICOSIS, OSTEOMALACIA or CUSHING'S DISEASE, and the myopathy resolves when the primary disease is treated.

Treatment Some myopathies may be the result of inflammation or arise from an endocrine or metabolic abnormality. Treatment of these is the treatment of the cause with supportive physiotherapy and any necessary physical aids while the patient is recovering. Treatment for the hereditary myopathies is supportive since, at present, there is no cure, though developments in gene research raise the possibility of future treatment. Physiotherapy, physical aids, counselling and support groups may all be helpful in caring for these patients.

The education and management of these unfortunate children raise many difficulties. Much help in dealing with these problems can be obtained from the Muscular Dystrophy Group of Great Britain (see APPENDIX 2: ADDRESSES).

MYOPIA (see REFRACTION).

MYOSITIS Inflammation of a muscle. (See MUSCLES, DISEASES OF.)

MYOSITIS OSSIFICANS (see MUSCLE).

MYOTONIA A condition in which the muscles, though possessed of normal power, contract only very slowly. The stiffness disappears as the muscles are used.

MYRINGOPLASTY The sealing by a surgical tissue graft of a hole or perforation in the eardrum, which separates the middle and outer sections of the EAR. It is aimed at improving the subject's hearing. Sometimes the operation is done to stop persistent discharge.

MYRINGOTOMY is the operation of cutting the drum of the ear in cases of acute inflammation of the middle ear.

MYRRH is a gum-resin obtained from *Commiphora molmol*, an Arabian myrtle tree. It stimulates the function of mucous membranes with which it is brought in contact or by which it is excreted. Tincture of myrrh is used for a gargle in sore throat, as a tooth-wash when the gums are inflamed, and as an ingredient of cough mixtures.

MYXOEDEMA (see HYPOTHYROIDISM).

MYXOMA A tumour consisting of very imperfect connective tissue, and containing a peculiar mucus-like juice.

MYXOVIRUSES These include the influenza viruses A, B and C; the para-influenza viruses, types 1 to 3. Respiratory syncytial virus, which is an important cause of respiratory disease in the early years of life, is caused by the related paramyxoviruses. Myxoviruses have an affinity for protein receptors in red blood cells.

N

NAEVUS A congenitally determined tissue abnormality. In the skin, naevi of blood vessels are best known, but a MOLE is a MELANOCYTE naevus and warty streaked and linear naevi of the epidermis occasionally occur. There are several patterns of vascular naevi:

Naevus simplex ('salmon patch') About a third of white children are born with macular pink areas of erythema on the nape, brow or eyelids which usually disappear after a few months, but patches on the nape may persist.

Naevus flammeus (port-wine stain) is present at birth. It is unilateral, usually on the face and may be extensive. It tends to darken with age and is permanent. Laser treatment is effective.

Strawberry naevus (cavernous haemangioma) is usually not present at birth but appears within a few weeks and grows rapidly, reaching a peak in size after 6–12 months, when the lobulated red nodule may resemble a ripe strawberry. Untreated, the naevus disappears spontaneously over several years. It may occur anywhere and may be very troublesome when occurring around an eye or on the 'nappy' area.

Spider naevus is due to a dilated arteriole causing a minute red papule in the skin, the small branching vessels resembling spider legs. A few spider naevi are common in young people but multiple naevi are common in pregnancy and may also be a warning sign of chronic liver disease.

NAIL-BITING A common practice in schoolchildren, most of whom gradually give it up as they approach adolescence. Too much significance should therefore not be attached to it. In itself it does no harm, and punishment or restraining devices do nothing but harm. It is a manifestation of tension or insecurity, the cause of which should be removed. In some people the habit is carried into adulthood.

NAILS (see SKIN).

NAILS, DISEASES OF Disease may affect the nail fold, nail plate or nail bed. Inflammation of the nail fold is called paronychia. Acute paronychia is usually bacterial and caused by trauma. Chronic paronychia is often occupational, due to constant exposure of the hands to water in barmaids, kitchen workers and housewives, but may also be caused by impaired circulation in the fingers.

PSORIASIS is a common cause of disease of the nail plate, as are ECZEMA and FUNGAL INFECTION. Deformity of the nail may point to systemic disease as in clubbing or the spoon-shaped concave nails (koilonychia) of severe iron deficiency. Acute toxic illnesses may temporarily disturb nail growth causing horizontal ridges (Beau's lines) which grow out slowly.

Onycholysis is separation of the nail plate from its bed. It may be due to psoriasis of the nail bed and trauma or may occur spontaneously. Gross thickening of nails is common in the toes, caused by psoriasis or fungal infection.

NALIDIXIC ACID An antibiotic drug, active against gram-negative micro-organisms, used to treat and prevent infections of the URINARY tract.

NALORPHINE reduces or abolishes most of the actions of morphine and similarly acting narcotics, such as pethidine. It was used as an antidote in the treatment of over-dosage with these drugs but has now been superseded by NALOXONE.

NALOXONE An effective drug in the treatment of opioid POISONING. It blocks the effects of most opiates. Administration by mouth is unreliable but, when given intravenously, it acts within two or three minutes. The drug is also given to new-born babies affected by narcotic drugs given to their mothers to relieve pain during childbirth.

NANOMETRE is a millionth of a millimetre. The approved abbreviation is nm.

NAPPY RASH A common form of irritant contact DERMATITIS in the nappy area in babies under one year old. Wetting of the skin by urine, abrasion and chemical changes due to faecal contamination all play a part. Good hygiene and use of disposable absorbent nappies have much reduced its incidence. An ointment containing a mild CORTICOSTEROID drug will usually suppress any inflammation that does occur.

NAPRAPATHY A system of healing which attributes disease to disorder in the ligaments and connective tissues.

NAPROXEN (see NON-STEROIDAL ANTI-INFLAMMATORY DRUGS).

NARCISSISM An abnormal mental state characterized by excessive admiration of self.

NARCOLEPSY A condition in which uncontrollable episodes of sleep occur two or three times a day. It starts at any age and persists for life. The attacks, which usually last for 10 to 15 minutes, come on at times normally conducive to sleep, such as after a meal, or sitting in a bus, but they may occur when walking in the street. In due course, usually after some years, they are associated with cataplectic attacks when for a few seconds there is sudden muscular weakness affecting the whole body. The cataplectic attacks are controlled by imipramine or clomipramine.

Familial narcolepsy is well recognized and recently a near-100-per-cent association between narcolepsy and the histocompatability ANTIGEN HLA-DR2 has been discovered. This has given rise to the notion that narcolepsy is an immune-related disease. The Narcolepsy Association (UK) has been founded to help patients with this strange disorder. (See APPENDIX 2: ADDRESSES.)

NARCOSIS A condition of stupor, resembling sleep, that is usually caused by a drug. It may also occur as a result of liver or kidney failure which causes URAEMIA. The affected person has significantly reduced awareness and is hard to arouse. Treatment is of the underlying cause and the normal precautions for caring for an unconscious or semiconscious subject should be taken. (See APPENDIX 1: BASIC FIRST AID.).

NARCOTICS (see HYPNOTICS).

NASOGASTRIC TUBE A small-bore plastic or rubber tube passed into the stomach through the nose, pharynx and then the oesophagus. It is used either to aspirate gas and liquid from the stomach or to pass food or drugs into it.

NASOPHARYNX is the upper part of the throat, lying behind the nasal cavity. (See NOSE.)

NATIONAL BLOOD AUTHORITY This body was created in 1993 to manage all blood services in England, replacing the Central Blood Laboratories and the National Directorate of the National Blood Transfusion Service. The new authority manages regional transfusion centres, and among its aims are the maintenance and promotion of blood and blood products based on a system of voluntary donors; implementing a cost-effective national strategy for ensuring adequate supplies of blood and its products to meet national needs; and ensuring high standards of safety and quality.

NATIONAL HEALTH SERVICE (NHS) The United Kingdom's National Health Service was created by Act of Parliament and inaugurated on 5 July 1948. Its original aim was to provide a comprehensive system of health care to everyone, free at the point of delivery. Scotland had its own, similar legislation, as did Northern Ireland. The service is funded by National Insurance contributions and from general taxation, with a small amount from patient charges. Approximately £42 billion, excluding patient charges, or under 6 per cent of gross domestic product was spent on the NHS in 1997/1998.

The system has been reformed several times. The latest occurring as this text goes to press. The previous radical change was in 1991 when the 1990 National Health Services and Community Health Act came into force. The aim of the 1990 Act was to improve efficiency and accountability within all branches of the health service by introducing competition and 'market forces'. There has also been some separation between those branches of the health service which 'provide' health care and those which 'purchase' it. Hospital groups and community health services were allowed to become NHS trusts, independent providers of services, and general practitioners (GPs) to hold funds with which to buy certain services from the 'providers'. Legislation planned for 1999 will abolish fund holding and introduce primary care groups to supervise general practice (see below).

The Secretary of State for Health is responsible to Parliament for the provision of health services in England and Wales. The Secretaries of State for Scotland and for Northern Ireland had similar responsibilities. Within the Department of Health the Policy Board (chaired by the Secretary of State) makes the strategic plans for the health service and the NHS Executive deals with the implementation of strategy and operational management. Below the Department of Health in the management structure are eight regional offices, 13 special health authorities, 100 health authorities and over 400 NHS trusts. Community health councils are outside the management structure but at local level are statutory bodies which represent the interests of their communities within the NHS. In Scotland the Department of Health is responsible for health issues; the administration of health has been restructured (1996) and further changes may result from the setting up of elected assemblies for Scotland and Wales.

In England regional offices develop services within the national guidelines, allocate resources to the health authorities (HAs) and primary care groups and monitor their performances. The revenue of HAs is decided on a weighted capitation basis and they are responsible for purchasing hospital and community services for their residents. (They are also responsible for managing the small number of units that are not NHS trusts.) In England HAs are responsible for managing the services provided by GPs, dentists, opticians and retail pharmacists (who are all independent practitioners under contract to the NHS). In 1997 about 70 per cent of the population was cared for by fundholding GPs but the incoming Labour Government (May 1997) intends to replace fundholding with a system of commissioning groups which will collaborate to 'commission' services from trusts.

NHS trusts are hospitals and other units providing patient care which are self governing and are directly accountable to the Secretary of State. They are run by small directly appointed executive boards and their revenue is generated by 'winning' contracts from the various 'purchasers'. Within centrally decided guidelines they are free to control their own assets, management structure and the terms of employment of their staff. Special health authorities which provide highly specialized services, including psychiatric care for mentally ill patients who may be a public danger, are also directly responsible to the Secretary of State.

Scotland, Wales and Northern Ireland have had broadly similar structures, responsibility being held by the Scottish, Welsh and Northern Ireland Offices. Legislation in Northern Ireland is introduced by Orders in Council. In 1972 the country's health and personal social services were reorganized and an integrated management structure introduced.

NATIONAL LISTENING LIBRARY is a charity which produces recorded books for handicapped people who cannot read, with the exception of the blind who have their own separate organization, the Royal National Institute for the Blind. (See APPENDIX 2: ADDRESSES.). (See also CALIBRE.)

NAUSEA The sensation that vomiting is about to occur. Nausea does not always lead to vomiting. (See VOMITING.)

NAVEL, or UMBILICUS The scar on the abdomen marking the point where the umbilical cord joined the body in embryonic life. (See PLACENTA.)

NEAR SIGHT (see REFRACTION).

NEBULA The term applied to a slight opacity on the cornea producing a haze in the field of vision, and also to any oily preparation to be sprayed from a nebulizer, an apparatus for splitting up a fluid into fine droplets.

NEBULIZERS A nebulizer makes an aerosol by blowing air or oxygen through a solution of a drug. Many inhaled drugs such as SALBUTAMOL, ipratropium and beclomethasone can be given in this way. It has the advantage over a medihaler in that no special effort is required to co-ordinate breathing and a nebulizer allows a much greater concentration of the drug to be delivered compared with that of a medihaler. The use of higher doses of bronchodilator drugs made possible by the nebulizer means that the risk of unwanted side-effects is also increased.

NECATOR AMERICANUS A hookworm, closely resembling but smaller than the *Ancylostoma duodenale*. (See ANCYLOSTOMIASIS.)

NECK That portion of the body which extends from the upper limit of the chest to the base of the skull. Its main function is to support the head. Through its front part run the passages for the air and the food. The neck is mainly composed of seven cervical vertebrae with the muscles attached thereto, in front and behind. (See MUSCLE.) Within the canal formed by the rings of these vertebrae lies the cervical part of the spinal cord, from which come the nerves that control the movements of the neck and arms.

In front of the spinal column lies the PHARYNX, or throat-cavity, extending from the base of the skull above down to the lower edge of the sixth vertebra, where the oesophagus continues it directly downwards, while the LARYNX or voice box is positioned in front. The larynx is close to the surface of the front of the neck, and the thyroid cartilage lies beneath the skin. (See LARYNX.) The larynx is continued downwards by the trachea or windpipe, and just beneath the larynx the isthmus of the THYROID GLAND crosses the windpipe, connecting the two lobes of the gland which lie one on either side of the larynx. The strong sterno-cleidomastoid muscle is prominent on each side of the neck, running from the mastoid process of the skull down to the STERNUM and inner end of the clavicle; under cover of it lies a fibrous sheath containing the carotid artery, internal jugular vein and vagus nerve. The sternocleidomastoid muscle divides each side of the neck into two triangular areas, in which lie important nerves and branches of these blood-vessels, as well as chains of LYMPHATIC GLANDS. Several large superficial veins run down the neck, being the external and internal jugular veins. At the root of the neck the apex of each lung projects a short distance from the chest into the neck.

NECROPSY A traditional term for an autopsy or post-mortem examination (see POST-MORTEM EXAMINATION).

NECROSIS Death of a limited portion of tissue, the term being most commonly applied to bones when, as the result of disease or injury, a fragment dies and separates. (See BONE, DISEASES OF.)

NECROTIZING FASCIITIS or CELLULITIS A potentially lethal infection caused by the gram-positive bacterium *STREPTOCOCCUS PYOGENES* which has the property of producing dangerous exotoxins. The infection may spread very rapidly, destroying tissue as it spreads. Urgent antibiotic treatment may check the infection, and surgery is sometimes required, but even with treatment patients may die (see STREPTOCOCCUS).

NEEDLING An operation performed in the treatment of CATARACTS, in which the anterior lens capsule is torn open with a needle, allowing the aqueous fluid to dissolve the opaque soft lens matter, which is gradually washed away into the bloodstream. This 'extra-capsular extraction' may need to be repeated several times before all the opaque lens matter disperses. Although a relatively simple procedure, it is unsuitable for patients over the age of 35 (when the nucleus of the lens becomes increasingly hard), and CRYOSURGERY and LASER THERAPY have become the preferred methods of treatment.

Needling is also used for certain minor dermatological procedures, such as removal of small facial cysts and scabies mites.

NEFOPAM HYDROCHLORIDE A non-opioid analgesic drug of use in the relief of pain that fails to respond to other non-opioid analgesics. It causes little depression of respiration but side-effects may be a problem.

NEGATIVISM means a morbid tendency in a person to do the opposite of what he is desired or directed to do. It is specially characteristic of SCHIZOPHRENIA, but is not uncommon in non-psychotic persons.

NEISSERIA A group, or genus, of rounded bacteria that occur in pairs and are therefore known as diplococci (see MICROBIOLOGY). They are named after Albert Neisser, the German physician who discovered the gonococcus, the causative organism of GONORRHOEA, which is now known as *Neisseria gonorrhoeae*. The group also includes the causative organism of cerebrospinal meningitis (see MENINGITIS): *Neisseria meningitidis*.

NEMATODE A roundworm. (See ASCARIASIS.)

NEOMYCIN is an AMINOGLYCOSIDE antibiotic derived from *Streptomyces fradiae*. It has a wide antibacterial spectrum, being effective against the majority of gram-negative bacilli. Its use is limited by the fact that it is liable to cause deafness and kidney damage. Its main use is for application to the skin, either in solution or as an ointment, for the treatment of infection of the skin. It is also given by mouth for the treatment of certain forms of enteritis due to *E. coli*.

NEONATAL Pertaining to the first month of life.

NEONATAL MORTALITY is the mortality of infants under one month of age. In England and Wales this has fallen markedly in recent decades: from over 28 per 1000 related live births in 1939 to around 6 in 1995. This improvement can be attributed to various factors: better antenatal supervision of expectant mothers; care to ensure that expectant mothers receive adequate nourishing food; improvements in the management of the complications of pregnancy and of labour. Nearly three-quarters of neonatal deaths occur during the first week of life. For this reason, increasing emphasis is being laid on this initial period of life. Between 1960 and 1995, in England, the number of deaths in the first week fell from 9,772 to 1,980, representing a fall in the rate per 1000 live births from 13·2 to 3·2. The chief causes of deaths in this period are immaturity of the infant, birth injuries, congenital abnormalities and asphyxia. After the first week the commonest cause is infection.

NEONATOLOGY The branch of paediatrics responsible for the medical care of newborn babies. Problems may be short term – for example, those linked to prematurity – or life long such as CEREBRAL PALSY. After the first few weeks of life, paediatricians take over the responsibility for any specialist medical care required, with general practitioners looking after the infants' primary-care needs.

NEOPLASM This means literally a 'new formation' and is another word for tumour.

NEPHRECTOMY The operation for removal of the kidney. (See KIDNEYS, DISEASES OF.)

NEPHRITIS Inflammation of the kidneys. (See KIDNEYS, DISEASES OF: glomerulonephritis.)

NEPHROBLASTOMA (WILM'S TUMOUR), or NEPHROBLASTOMA, is the commonest kidney tumour in infancy. It is a malignant tumour, which occurs in around 1 per 10,000 live births. The survival rate with modern treatment (removal of the kidney followed by radiotherapy and chemotherapy) is now around 80 per cent.

NEPHROLITHIASIS A condition in which calculi are present in the kidney.

NEPHROLOGY The branch of medicine concerned with the study and management of kidney disease. A specialist in these diseases is called a nephrologist.

NEPHRON Each kidney comprises over a million of these microscopic units which regulate and control the formation of urine. A tuft of capillaries invaginates the Bowmans capsule which is the blind-ending tube (glomerulus) of each nephron. Plasma is filtered out of blood and through the Bowmans capsule into the renal tubule. As the filtrate passes along the tubule most of the water and electrolytes are reabsorbed. The composition is regulated with the retention or addition of certain molecules (e.g. urea, drugs, etc.). The tubules eventually empty the filtrate, which by now is urine, into the renal pelvis from where it flows down the ureters into the bladder. (See KIDNEYS.)

NEPHROPATHY A description of any damage or disease to the kidneys (see KIDNEYS, DISEASES OF).

NEPHROPEXY Surgical fixation (to the twelfth rib and posterior abdominal wall) of a mobile kidney; this prevents the kidney from descending in the abdomen when the affected person stands up.

NEPHROPTOSIS The condition in which a kidney is mobile or 'floating'.

NEPHRORRHAPHY (see NEPHROPEXY).

NEPHROSTOMY is the operation of making an opening into the kidney to drain it.

NEPHROTIC SYNDROME is one of PROTEINURIA, hypo-albuminaemia and gross OEDEMA. The primary cause is the leak of albumin through the glomerulus. When this exceeds the liver's ability to synthesise albumin the plasma level falls and oedema results. The nephrotic syndrome is commonly the result of primary renal glomerular disease (see KIDNEYS, DISEASES OF: glomerulonephritis). It may also be a result of metabolic diseases such as diabetic glomerular sclerosis and AMYLOIDOSIS. It may be the result of systemic auto-immune diseases such as SYSTEMIC LUPUS ERYTHEMATOSUS and POLYARTERITIS. It may complicate malignant diseases such as myelomatosis, HODGKIN'S DISEASE and LYMPHOCYTIC LEUKAEMIA. It is sometimes caused by nephrotoxins such as gold or mercury and certain drugs, and it may be the result of certain infections such as malaria and Crohn's disease.

NEPHROTOMY means the operation of cutting into the kidney, in search of calculi or for other reasons.

NERVE BLOCK (see ANAESTHESIA, local anaesthetics).

NERVES The nervous system detects and interprets changing events in and outside the body and reacts to them. It is traditionally divided into two parts: the central nervous system, consisting of the brain and spinal cord, which analyses information and initiates responses; and the cerebrospinal, or peripheral nervous system, consisting of the 43 nerves on each side proceeding from them. The peripheral system collects information and returns the response signals. The third major division, the autonomic nervous system, is largely independent of the brain and spinal cord.

Efferent nerves convey impulses originating at, or received by, the nerve cells to the muscles and blood vessels, while afferent nerves receive impulses from the skin, joints and other sense organs. The autonomic nervous system largely concerns the functions of the internal organs, secreting glands, blood vessels, activities which proceed independently of the will.

Structure
NERVE-FIBRES Nerves vary in size from the large pencil-sized sciatic nerve in the back of the thigh muscles to the single, hair-sized fibres distributed to the skin. A nerve, such as the sciatic, possesses a strong, outer fibrous sheath, called the epineurium, within which lie bundles of nerve-fibres, divided from one another by partitions of fibrous tissue, in which run bloodvessels that nourish the nerve. Each of these bundles is surrounded by its own sheath, known as the perineurium, and within the bundle fine partitions of fibrous tissue, known as endoneurium, divide up the bundle into groups of fibres. The finest subdivisions of the nerves are the fibres, and these are of two kinds: medullated and non-medullated fibres. The medullated

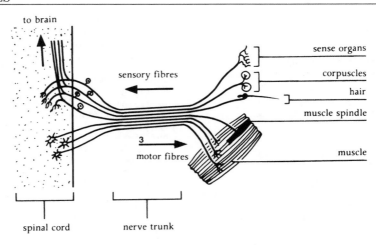

Diagram showing nervous connections between the central nervous system
and muscle and skin.

fibres vary in thickness from 2 to 15 micrometres, some nerves containing a greater proportion of the small fibres than others. Each has an outer membranous sheath, the neurilemma, within which is a clear white material, the medullary (or myelin) sheath, in the centre of which runs

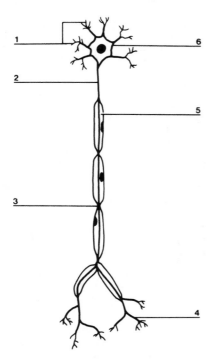

1 dendrites	4 bare axons
2 axon	5 myelin sheath
3 node of Ranvier	6 cell body

Diagram of a nerve.

the axis-cylinder or nerve-fibre proper. The neurilemma is a strong but thin sheath with nuclei at regular intervals on its inner surface. The white medullary sheath is composed of fatty material containing lecithin and cholesterin. It is divided at regular intervals by short gaps, situated about 1 mm apart, known as the nodes of Ranvier, but across these gaps the neurilemma and axis-cylinder are continuous. This medullary, or myelin, sheath acts as an insulation, preventing nerve impulses from passing beyond the nerve-fibre by which they are conveyed. The axis-cylinder, or axon, is the conducting part of the nerve. The non-medullated fibres are very much thinner than the average of medullated fibres, but they do not have a medullary sheath so are greyish in colour.

NERVE-CELLS, from one of which each nerve-fibre originates, are found in the grey matter of the brain and spinal cord. The brain alone contains some 600,000,000 of these cells. They also exist in the ganglia of the sympathetic system, in connection with some of the nerves of special sense, and on the posterior roots of the spinal nerves. The shape of these nerve-cells varies. The most common appearance is that of a large clear cell, containing an oval nucleus, and running out at various points into long processes, which, as a rule, branch repeatedly. These dendritic processes, as they are called, meet with similar processes from neighbouring cells in SYNAPSES.

NERVE-ENDINGS Each nerve-fibre proceeds from a nerve-cell to end in a definite organ, to or from which it carries a special form of nerve impulse. The manner in which the fibre ends in the organ to which it proceeds varies in different cases.

Development The whole nervous system is developed from the ectoderm or outer layer of the embryo, the brain and spinal cord arising from

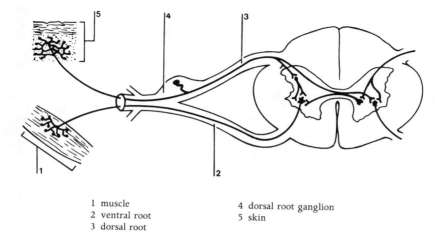

1 muscle
2 ventral root
3 dorsal root

4 dorsal root ganglion
5 skin

Diagram of a reflex arc.

an infolding of the surface along the back to form a tube, and all the nerves being formed directly or indirectly as out-growths from this tube.

Functions of nerves The greater part of the bodily activity originates in the nerve-cells. Impulses are sent down the nerves, which act simply as transmitters. The impulse causes sudden chemical changes in the muscles as the latter contract. (See MUSCLE.) The impulses from a sensory ending in the skin pass along a nerve-fibre to affect nerve-cells in the spinal cord and brain, where it is perceived as a sensation. The impulse travels at a rate of about 30 metres (100 feet) per second. (See NERVOUS IMPULSE.)

The anterior roots of spinal nerves consist of motor fibres to muscles, the posterior roots of sensory fibres from the skin. The terms, efferent and afferent, are applied to these roots, because, in addition to motor fibres, fibres controlling blood vessels and secretory glands leave the cord in the anterior roots. The posterior roots contain, in addition to sensory fibres, the nerve fibres that transmit impulses from muscles, joints and other organs, which among other neurological functions provide the individual with his proprioceptive faculties – the ability to know how various parts of the body are positioned.

The connection between the sensory and motor systems of nerves is important. The simplest form of nerve action is that known as automatic action. In this a part of the nervous system, controlling, for example, the lungs, makes rhythmic discharges to maintain the regular action of the respiratory muscles. This controlling mechanism may be modified by occasional sensory impressions and chemical changes from various sources.

REFLEX ACTION This is an automatic or involuntary activity, prompted by fairly simple neurological circuits, without the subject's consciousness necessarily being involved. Thus a painful pinprick will result in a reflex with-

drawal of the affected finger before the brain has time to send a 'voluntary' instruction to the muscles involved (see diagram of a reflex arc).

VOLUNTARY ACTIONS are more complicated than reflex ones. The same mechanism is involved, but, the brain initially exerts an inhibitory or blocking effect, which prevents immediate reflex action. Then the impulse, passing up to the cerebral hemispheres, stimulates cellular activity, the complexity of these processes depending upon the intellectual processes involved. Finally, the inhibition is removed and an impulse passes down to motor cells in the spinal cord, and a muscle or set of muscles is activated by the motor nerves.

TROPHIC FUNCTION This function of nerves is important. If sensory nerves are diseased or injured, ulceration of the skin, bed sores and other changes are liable to occur, while muscles waste and disappear if their motor nerves are permanently destroyed.

Nervous system The brain and its twelve pairs of cranial nerves are described under BRAIN; the spinal cord and the origin of its thirty-one pairs of nerves are treated under SPINAL CORD.

Each of these spinal nerves arises by two roots, the posterior root being larger than the anterior, and being furnished with a ganglion. The upper four cervical nerves unite to produce the cervical plexus. From this the muscles and skin of the neck are mainly supplied, and the phrenic nerve, which runs down through the lower part of the neck and the chest to innervate the diaphragm, is given off. The brachial plexus is formed by the union of the lower four cervical and first dorsal nerves. In addition to nerves to some of the muscles in the shoulder region, and others to the skin about the shoulder and inner side of the arm, the plexus gives off large nerves that proceed down the arm.

The thoracic or dorsal nerves, with the exception of the first, do not form a plexus, but each runs round the chest along the lower margin of the rib to which it corresponds, whilst the lower six extend on to the abdomen.

The lumbar plexus is formed by the upper four lumbar nerves, and its branches are distributed to the lower part of the abdomen, and front and inner side of the thigh.

The sacral plexus is formed by parts of the fourth and fifth lumbar nerves, and the upper three and part of the fourth sacral nerves. Much of the plexus is collected into the sciatic nerves, the largest in the body, which go to the legs.

The sympathetic system is joined by a pair of small branches given off from each spinal nerve, close to the spine. This system consists of two parts, first, a pair of cords running down on the side and front of the spine, and containing on each side three ganglia in the neck, and beneath this a ganglion opposite each vertebra. From these two ganglionated cords numerous branches are given off, and these unite to form the second part, namely, plexuses connected with various internal organs, and provided with numerous large and irregularly placed ganglia. The chief of these plexuses are the cardiac plexus, the solar or epigastric plexus, the diaphragmatic, suprarenal, renal, spermatic, or ovarian, aortic, hypogastric and pelvic plexuses.

NERVES, INJURIES TO These have several causes. Continued or repeated severe pressure may damage a nerve seriously, as in the case of a crutch pressing into the armpit and causing drop-wrist. Bruising due to a blow which drives a superficially placed nerve against a bone may damage, say, the radial nerve behind the upper arm. A wound may sever nerves, along with other structures; this accident is specially liable to occur to the ulnar nerve in front of the wrist when a person accidentally puts a hand and arm through a pane of glass.

Symptoms When a sensory nerve is injured, sensation is immediately more or less impaired in the part supplied by the nerve. When the nerve in question is a motor one the muscles governed through it are instantly paralysed. In the latter case, the portion of nerve beyond the injury degenerates and the muscles gradually waste, and lose their power of contraction in response to electrical applications. Finally, deformities result and the joints become fixed. This is particularly noticeable when the ulnar nerve is injured, the hand and fingers taking up a claw-like position. The skin may also be affected.

Treatment Damaged or severed (peripheral) nerve fibres should be sewn together, using microsurgery. Careful realignment of the nerve endings gives the fibres an excellent chance of regenerating along the right channels. Full recovery is rare but, with regular physiotherapy to keep paralysed muscles in good shape and to prevent their shortening, the patient can expect to obtain a reasonable return of function after a few weeks, with improvement continuing over several months.

NERVOUS BREAKDOWN A traditional description of a variety of emotional crises ranging from an outburst of hysterical behaviour to a major neurotic illness that may have a lasting effect on an individual's life. Sometimes the term is used to describe an overt psychotic illness – for example, schizophrenia (see MENTAL ILLNESS; NEUROSIS).

1 Schwann cell   4 myelin
2 node of Ranvier   5 neurilemma
3 axon

Diagram of (left) a healthy nerve, (centre) degenerating nerve cell after two days, (right) and after a week.

NERVOUS DISEASES The following conditions are discussed under their individual headings: APHASIA; BRAIN, DISEASES AND INJURIES OF; CATALEPSY; CHOREA; CRAMP; EPILEPSY; HYSTERIA; LEARNING DISABILITY; MEMORY; MENTAL ILLNESS; MULTIPLE SCLEROSIS; NERVE INJURIES; NEURALGIA; NEURITIS; PARALYSIS; PSYCHOSOMATIC DISEASES; SPINE AND SPINAL CORD, DISEASES AND INJURIES OF; STROKE; TABES.

NERVOUS IMPULSE The effects of nervous activity are now believed in all cases to be transmitted chemically, by the formation at nerve-endings of chemical substances. When, for example, a nerve to a muscle is stimulated, there appears at the NEUROMUSCULAR JUNCTION the chemical substance, ACETYLCHOLINE. Acetylcholine also appears at endings of the PARASYMPATHETIC NERVES and transmits the effect of the parasympathetic impulse. When an impulse passes down a sympathetic nerve, the effect of it is transmitted at the nerve-ending by the chemical liberated there: ADRENALINE or an adrenaline-like substance.

NETTLE-RASH (see URTICARIA).

NEURALGIA Pain which is the result of damage to or irritation of a NERVE. The pain tends to be intermittent, occurring in short bursts. It may be very severe and be located along an identifiable nerve. A particular disorder may give rise to neuralgia, MIGRAINE being an example, and HERPES ZOSTER (shingles) another. Neuralgia may also be caused by disturbance to a particular nerve, for instance, trigeminal neuralgia which affects the sensory nerve supplying most of the face.

Treatment Any obvious underlying cause should be dealt with. Neuralgia may be symptomatically relieved with ANALGESICS. Severe pain may be helped by the analgesic carbamazepine or by destroying (freezing, local alcohol injection or surgery) the affected nerve.

NEURASTHENIA A traditional term that described an ill-defined state of nervous exhaustion in which, although the patient suffers from no definite disease, he or she becomes incapable of sustained exertion. The condition which it represented is now recognized to be a form of NEUROSIS or PSYCHOSOMATIC DISEASE.

NEURECTOMY An operation in which part of a nerve is excised: for example, for the relief of neuralgia.

NEURILEMMA The thin membranous covering which surrounds every nerve-fibre. (See NERVES.)

NEURITIS Inflammation affecting a nerve or nerves which may be localized to one part of the body, as, for instance, in sciatica, or which may be general, being then known as multiple neuritis, or polyneuritis. Owing to the fact that the most peripheral parts of the nerves are usually affected in the latter condition, i.e. the fine subdivisions in the substance of the muscles, it is also known as peripheral neuritis.

Causes In cases of localized neuritis the fibrous sheath of the nerve is usually at fault, the actual nerve-fibres being only secondarily affected. This condition may be due to inflammation spreading into the nerve from surrounding tissues, to cold or to long-continued irritation by pressure on the nerve, and the symptoms produced vary according to the function of the nerve, in the case of sensory nerves being usually neuralgic pain (see NEURALGIA), in the case of motor nerves some degree of paralysis in the muscles to which they pass.

In polyneuritis, usually due to some general or constitutional cause, the nerve-fibres themselves in the small nerves degenerate and break down. The condition is protracted because for recovery to occur, the growth of new nerve-fibres from the healthy part of the nerve has to take place. The cause of polyneuritis may be infection by a virus – for example, HERPES ZOSTER – or a bacterium, as in Hansen's disease. Neuritis may also be the result of agents such as alcohol, lead or products from industrial or agricultural activities. ORGANO-PHOSPHORUS INSECTICIDES are believed by some experts to be a factor in neuritis and other neurological conditions.

NEURODERMATOSES (see DERMATITIS).

NEUROFIBRILS A microscopic strand of CYTOPLASM that occurs in the cell body of a NEURONE as well as in the semifluid content of the AXON of a nerve cell.

NEUROFIBROMATOSIS (see VON RECKLINGHAUSEN'S DISEASE).

NEUROGLIA The fine web of tissue and branching cells which supports the nerve fibres and cells of the nervous system. (See NERVES.)

NEUROLEPTICS Although many of these drugs have sedative properties they should not be regarded as tranquillizers. They are used to quieten disturbed patients, whether this is the result of brain damage, mania, delirium, agitated depression or an acute behavioural disturbance. They relieve the florid psychotic symptoms such as hallucinations and thought disorder in schizophrenia and prevent relapse of this disorder when it is in remission.

Most of these drugs are dopamine antagonists (see DOPAMINE) and act by blocking dopamine receptors. As a result they can give rise to the extra pyramidal effects of PARKINSONISM and they may also cause hyperprolactinaemia. The extrapyramidal symptoms are the most troublesome side-effects and they can usually be controlled by ANTICHOLINERGIC drugs. The main anti-psychotic drugs are: (i) chlorpromazine, methotrimeprazine, and promazine. These drugs are characterized by pronounced sedative effects and a moderate anticholinergic and extrapyramidal effect. (ii) pericyazine, pipothiazine and thioridazine. These drugs have moderate sedative effects, marked anticholinergic effects but less extrapyramidal effects than the other groups. (iii) fluphenazine, perphenazine, prochlorperazine, sulpiride and trifluoperazine. These drugs have fewer sedative effects, fewer anticholinergic effects but more pronounced extrapyramidal effects.

NEUROLOGY The branch of medical practice and science which deals with the nervous system and its diseases.

NEUROMA means a tumour connected with a nerve, such tumours being generally composed of fibrous tissue, and of a painful nature.

NEUROMUSCULAR BLOCKADE In clinical practice the transmission of impulses at the NEUROMUSCULAR JUNCTION may be competitively blocked in order to paralyse reversibly a patient for a surgical procedure or to assist treatment on the intensive care unit. There are two main types of drug, both of which competitively block the acetylcholine receptors on the motor end plates: (1) Depolarizing neuromuscular blocking agents: these act by first producing stimulation at the receptor and then blocking it. There are characteristic muscle fasciculations before the rapid onset of paralysis which is of short duration (less than five minutes with the commonly used drug, suxamethonium). The drug is removed from the receptor by the enzyme, cholinesterase. (2) Non-depolarizing neuromuscular blocking agents: these drugs occupy the receptor and prevent acetylcholine from becoming attached to it. However, in sufficiently high concentrations acetylcholine will compete with the drug and dislodge it from the receptor and the effect of these drugs is reversed by giving an anticholinesterase, which allows the amount of acetylcholine at the neuromuscular junction to build up. These drugs have varying durations of action but all are slower in onset and of longer duration than the depolarizers.

NEUROMUSCULAR JUNCTION The specialized area where a motor nerve ends in close proximity to the muscle membrane and is able to initiate muscle contraction. The motor nerve ending is separated from the motor end plate by the synaptic cleft which is only 50–70 nm wide. When a nerve impulse arrives at the motor nerve ending molecules of acetylcholine are released which cross the synaptic cleft and attach to receptors on the motor end plate. This initiates depolarization of the muscle which in turn initiates the process of contraction. Acetylcholinesterase (an enzyme) rapidly breaks

down the molecules of acetylcholine, thus ending their action and freeing the receptor in preparation for the next impulse.

NEURON The single unit of the nervous system, consisting of a nerve cell with its various processes and the nerve fibre or fibres to which it gives origin. As applied to the motor part of the nervous system, two neurons are specially recognized: the upper neuron, which includes a cell on the surface of the brain and a fibre extending down into the spinal cord; the lower neuron, which consists of a cell in the grey matter of the cord with a nerve fibre extending outwards to end in a fibre of the muscle with which it is connected. The former has a controlling influence over the latter, whilst the latter is more directly concerned with the changes that result in the contraction of the muscle fibre and with nutritional influences over it. (See NERVES.)

NEUROPATHIC BLADDER A bladder with complete or partial loss of sensation. As there is no sensation of fullness, the individual either develops complete retention of urine or the bladder empties reflexly. The condition predisposes affected individuals to urinary-tract infections and back pressure on the kidneys, leading to renal failure. It may be caused by spinal injury, SPINA BIFIDA or any disorder which produces NEUROPATHY.

NEUROPATHOLOGY The branch of pathology that covers the reasons for and consequences of the nervous system (see NEUROLOGY).

NEUROPATHY A disease affecting nerves. It may affect a single nerve (mononeuropathy) or be a generalized disorder (polyneuropathy). Symptoms will depend on whether motor, sensory, or autonomic nerves are affected. Trauma or entrapment of a nerve is a common cause of mononeuropathy, pressure or stretching of a nerve occurring in various situations. Complete recovery in four to six weeks is usual. Common causes of polyneuropathy include DIABETES MELLITUS, B vitamin deficiency (often alcohol associated), some viral infections, and carcinomatous. Genetic and toxic neuropathies are also seen.

NEUROSIS A general term applied to mental or emotional disturbance in which, as opposed to PSYCHOSIS, there is no serious disturbance in the perception or understanding of external reality. However, the boundaries between neurosis and psychosis are not always clearly defined. Neuroses are usually classified into anxiety neuroses, depressive neuroses, PHOBIAS, HYPOCHONDRIASIS, HYSTERIA and obsessional neuroses.

Anxiety neurosis, or ANXIETY STATE, constitutes the commonest form of neurosis. Fortunately it is also almost the most responsive to treatment. Once the neurosis develops, sufferers are in a state of persistent anxiety and worry, 'tensed up', always fatigued and unable to sleep at night. In addition, there are often physical complaints, e.g. palpitations or headache.

Obsessional neuroses are much less common and constitute only about 5 per cent of all neuroses. Like other neuroses, they usually develop in early adult life. (See MENTAL ILLNESS.)

NEUROSURGERY Surgery performed on some part of the nervous system, whether brain, spinal cord or nerves. Disorders treated by neurosurgeons include damage to the brain, spinal cord and nerves as a result of injury; tumours in the central nervous system; abnormalities of blood vessels in or supplying blood to the brain – for example, ANEURYSM; brain abscess; bleeding inside the skull and certain birth defects such as HYDROCEPHALUS and SPINA BIFIDA.

NEUROTIC A vague term applied to a person of nervous temperament, whose actions are largely determined by emotions or instincts rather than by reason.

NEUROTOXIN A chemical substance that harms nervous tissue, causing symptoms of numbness or weakness of the body part supplied by the damaged nerve. The venom of some snakes contains neurotoxic substances and bacteria may produce neurotoxins: examples are those that cause DIPHTHERIA and TETANUS. Arsenic and lead are examples of inorganic neurotoxins.

NEUROTRANSMITTER A chemical substance which transmits the action of a nerve to a cell. It is released from nerve endings and transmits the impulse across SYNAPSES to other nerves. In the central nervous system the substances acting as neurotransmitters include ACETYLCHOLINE, NORADRENALINE, DOPAMINE and SEROTONIN. The main transmitter in the peripheral system is acetylcholine, while for the SYMPATHETIC NERVOUS SYSTEM it is noradrenaline. In recent years a new group of neuro-transmitters called neuropeptides has been identified, comprising large protein molecules. One of the best known is that of endorphins which the brain uses to control pain.

NEUTRON is one of the particles that enter into the structure of the atomic nucleus. (See ISOTOPES.)

NEUTROPENIA A reduction in the number of neutrophil LEUCOCYTES per cubic millimetre of circulating blood to a figure below that found in health. There is still some disagreement over the precise limits of normality, but a count of less than 2500 per mm³ would be generally accepted as constituting neutropenia. Several infective diseases are characterized by neutropenia, including TYPHOID FEVER, INFLUENZA and MEASLES. It may also be induced by certain drugs, including chloramphenicol, phenylbutazone, the sulphonamides and chlorpromazine.

NEUTROPHIL A type of LEUCOCYTE or white blood cell (see BLOOD).

NICLOSAMIDE A widely used antihelminthic drug for treating TAENIASIS or tapeworm infection.

NICOTINAMIDE, the amide of nicotinic acid, is usually used instead of NICOTINIC ACID in the treatment of vitamin B deficiency.

NICOTINE The active principle in tobacco. (See TOBACCO.)

NICOTINIC ACID, or NIACIN, is a member of the vitamin B complex. It is essential for human nutrition, the normal daily requirement for an adult being about 15 to 20 mg. A deficiency of nicotinic acid is one of the factors in the etiology of PELLAGRA, and either nicotine acid or nicotinamide is used in the treatment of this condition. Nicotinic acid also reduces the concentration of blood lipids. (See HYPERLIPIDAEMIA.)

NIDUS A site of infection within the body from which it can spread to other tissues.

NIFEDIPINE A member of the CALCIUM-CHANNEL BLOCKERS group of cardiovascular drugs. It relaxes vascular smooth muscle and dilates coronary and peripheral arteries. Nifedipine has been used to prevent and treat ANGINA PECTORIS and certain types of hypertension but is now less popular.

NIGHT BLINDNESS (see BLINDNESS).

NIGHTMARE (see SLEEP).

NIGHT SWEATS Copious perspiration occurring in bed at night and found in conditions such as tuberculosis, brucellosis and lymphomas.

NIPPLE The small sensitive prominence at the tip of each BREAST containing (in women) the small openings through which milk can pass from the milk glands in the breast tissue. The nipple and its surrounding area (the areola) are darker than the adjacent skin. The area becomes darker during pregnancy.

NIPPLES, DISEASES OF (see BREASTS, DISEASES OF).

NITRATES Salts of nitrous acid which have a powerful effect in paralysing the action of involuntary muscle, and they therefore dilate the blood-vessels, and check spasm of all sorts. The most commonly used are glyceryl trinitrate and isosorbide mono- and dinitrates which are used to prevent and treat angina and as supportive treatment for other drugs used to combat heart failure. (See GLYCERYL TRINITRATE.)

NITRAZEPAM A tranquillizer introduced as a hypnotic. It is long acting and may produce drowsiness next day. Addiction can occur. (See TRANQUILLIZERS, BENZODIAZEPINES.)

NITRIC ACID A strong mineral acid, it is a clear, heavy liquid, becoming brownish with age. It is kept in dark, stoppered bottles, and immediately the stopper is removed from the bottle, irritating white fumes are given off.

Action In its pure state, nitric acid acts as a powerful caustic. In weaker solution it is, like all acids, an antiseptic, but is very irritating.

Uses Although a powerful antiseptic and caustic, nitric acid is rarely used now in Britain for the removal of warts (where it has been superseded by cryotherapy).

NITRIC OXIDE (NO) A naturally occurring chemical that performs a wide range of biological roles. It is involved in the laying down of memories in the brain, killing viruses, bacteria and cancer cells, and helping to control blood pressure. NO, comprising a nitrogen atom attached to an oxygen one, is one of the smallest of biologically active compounds as well as having such diverse functions. The chemical is a muscle relaxant and is important in maintaining the heart and circulation in good condition. NO is the toxic agent released by MACROPHAGES to kill invading germs and spreading cancer cells. It acts as an essential neurotransmitter and protects nerve cells against stress. Researchers are studying how it might be used to treat diseases.

NITROFURANTOIN A synthetic nitrofuran derivative which has a wide range of antibacterial activity and is effective against many gram-positive and gram-negative micro-organisms. It is used mainly in the treatment of infections of the lower urinary tract.

NITROGEN MUSTARDS The nitrogen analogues of mustard gas are among the most important ALKYLATING AGENTS used in the treatment of various forms of malignant disease. They include mustine, trimustine, ura-mustine, busulphan, chlorambucil and melphalan.

NITROUS OXIDE GAS Also known as LAUGHING GAS, this is, at ordinary pressures, a colourless sweetish-smelling gas. It is used with oxygen to provide ANALGESIA and mild anaesthesia during childbirth and painful dental procedures and at the site of major accidents. It has a rapid action and the effects do not last for long (see ANAESTHESIA.)

NOCICEPTORS Nerve endings which detect and respond to painful or unpleasant stimuli.

NOCTURIA Excess passing of urine during the night. Among its many causes are glomerulonephritis (see KIDNEY, DISEASES OF) and enlargement of the prostate. (See also URINE.)

NOCTURNAL ENURESIS The involuntary passing of urine during sleep. It is a condition predominantly of childhood. In a small minority of cases it is due to some organic cause such as infection of the genito-urinary tract, but in most affected children it is due to inadequate or improper training.

The age at which a child achieves full control of bladder function varies considerably. Such control is sometimes achieved in the second year, but more commonly in the third year of life, and there are some children who do not normally achieve such control until the fourth, or even fifth, year.

It is a difficult condition to cure in the absence of an organic cause. If there should be an organic cause, it requires treatment. Otherwise the approach consists essentially of reassurance and firm but kindly and understanding training. In quite a number of cases the use of a buzzer alarm which wakens the child should he start passing water is helpful provided that it is backed up by psychological support from the parents and health workers.

NODE The term node is widely used in medicine. For instance, the smaller lymphatic glands are often termed lymph nodes. It is also applied to a collection of nerve cells forming a subsidiary nerve centre found in various places in the sympathetic nervous system, such as the sinuatrial node and the atrio-ventricular node which control the beating of the heart.

NOISE (see DEAFNESS; OCCUPATIONAL DISEASES).

NOMA Another name for cancrum oris. (See CANCRUM ORIS.)

NOMIFENSINE (see ANTIDEPRESSANTS).

NON-ACCIDENTAL INJURY (see CHILD ABUSE).

NON-CONVENTIONAL MEDICINE An umbrella term to describe alternative, complementary, folk and other types of healing practices that are outside the definition of conventional Western-type medical practice. (See COMPLEMENTARY MEDICINE.)

NON-SPECIFIC GENITAL INFECTION, or NON-SPECIFIC URETHRITIS, is an inflammatory condition of the URETHRA due to a cause or causes other than gonorrhoea. The most common is CHLAMYDIA trachomatis – over 39,000 cases were identified by laboratories in England and Wales in 1995. It produces pelvic inflammatory disease in women, which often results in sterility, the risk of ectopic pregnancy (see ECTOPIC), and recurrent pelvic pain. Most cases respond well to TETRACYCLINE. Abstinence from sexual intercourse should be observed during treatment and until cure is complete. Children born to infected mothers may have their eyes infected during birth, producing the condition known as ophthalmia neonatorum. This is treated by the application to the eye of chlortetracycline eye ointment. The lungs of such a child may also be infected, resulting in pneumonia.

NON-STEROIDAL ANTI-INFLAMMATORY DRUGS These act by inhibiting the formation of PROSTAGLANDINS which are mediators of inflammation. They act both as ANALGESICS to relieve pain and as inhibitors of inflammation. Aspirin is a classic example of such a compound. Newer compounds have been synthesized with the aim of producing fewer and less severe side-effects. They are sometimes preferred to aspirin for the treatment of conditions such as RHEUMATOID ARTHRITIS, OSTEOARTHRITIS, sprains, strains and sports injuries. Their main side-effects are gastro-intestinal. Gastric ulcers and gastric haemorrhage may result. This is because prostaglandins are necessary for the production of the mucous protective coat in the stomach and, when the production of prostaglandin is inhibited, the protection of the stomach is compromised. They should therefore be used with caution in patients with dyspepsia and gastric ulceration. The various non-steroidal anti-inflammatory drugs differ little from each other in efficacy though there is considerable variation in patient response. Ibuprofen is one of the first choices in this group of drugs as it combines good efficacy with a low incidence of side-effects and administration is only required twice daily. Other drugs in this series include azapropazone, fenbufen, fenclofenac, fenoprofen, feprazone, flurbiprofen, indomethacin, indoprofen, ketoprofen, naproxen, piroxicam, sulindac, tiaprofenic acid and tolmetin.

NORADRENALINE A precursor of ADRENALINE in the medulla of the suprarenal glands. It is also present in the brain. Its main function is to mediate the transmission of impulses in the SYMPATHETIC NERVOUS SYSTEM. It also has a transmitter function in the brain.

NOREPINEPHRINE (see NORADRENALINE).

NORETHISTERONE A synthetic preparation that has the action of PROGESTERONE, but is active when given by mouth.

NORMAL A term used in several different senses. Generally speaking, it is applied to anything which agrees with the regular and established type. In chemistry the term is applied to solutions of acids or bases of such strength that each litre contains the number of grams corresponding to the molecular weight of the substance in question. In physiology the term normal is applied to solutions of such strength that, when mixed with a body fluid, they are isotonic and cause no disturbance: e.g. normal saline solution. (See ISOTONIC.)

NORMOBLAST The precursor of an ERYTHROCYTE which still contains the remnant of a nucleus.

NORMOTENSIVE Having a BLOOD PRESSURE within the normal range for an individual's age and sex.

NORTRIPTYLINE An antidepressant drug which is also a sedative. (See ANTIDEPRESSANTS.)

NOSE In the course of RESPIRATION incoming air enters via the nose and is here warmed, moistened, and filtered before entering the lungs. It has a protective function, irritant air being expelled by SNEEZING. It is also the organ of SMELL.

The external nose is formed partly of bone and partly of cartilage, covered by skin. In its upper part, the two nasal bones, one on each side, project downwards from the frontal bone for about 25 mm (1 inch), and, supported by a process of the upper jaw-bone, form the hard bridge of the nose between the eyes.

The lower part, including the nostrils, are comprised of cartilage covered by skin. In its interior, the nose is completely divided into two narrow cavities, one on each side, by a septum or partition running from front to back. This septum is a thin plate composed partly of bone, partly of cartilage. On both surfaces this septum is covered by the general mucous membrane that lines the nose. The accompanying diagram shows the structure of the nose.

Several sinuses lie concealed in the bones of the skull, into which air enters freely by apertures connecting them with the nose. These

1 frontal sinus	10 tongue
2 atrium of middle meatus	11 uvula
3 middle nasal concha	12 soft palate
4 middle meatus	13 auditory tube
5 vestibule	14 inferior nasal concha
6 inferior meatus	15 spenoidal sinus
7 maxilla	16 spenoethmoidal recess
8 mandible	and higher nasal concha
9 pharynx	17 superior nasal concha
	18 superior meatus

The lateral wall of the right half of the nasal cavity.

cavities occupy spaces in the frontal bone over the eyebrow (frontal sinus), in the upper jawbone, filling in the angle between the eye and the nose (maxillary sinus), in the sphenoid bone (sphenoidal sinus), and in the lateral part of the ethmoid bone (ethmoidal sinus). The sinuses drain into the interior of the nose, as does the Eustachian or auditory tube from the middle ear (see EAR).

NOSE, DISEASES OF Certain skin diseases, particularly CHILBLAIN, ACNE, LUPUS, and ERYSIPELAS, tend to affect the nose, and may be very annoying. Redness of the skin may be caused by poor circulation in cold weather.

Acute inflammation is generally the result of a viral infection (see CHILLS AND COLDS) affecting the mucous membrane and paranasal SINUSES (see SINUSITIS); less commonly it results from the inhalation of irritant gases. BOILS may develop just inside the entrance to the nose, causing

pain; these are potentially troublesome as infection can spread to the sinuses. DIPHTHERIA is now rare, but HAY FEVER is a distressing form of acute rhinitis.

Malformations are of various kinds. Racial and familial variations in the external nose occur and may be a reason for RHINOPLASTY. Differences in the size and shape of the nose occur, often forming the starting point for chronic inflammation of the nose, hay fever, or asthma. More commonly, obstruction results from nasal polyps or adenoids, leading to inhalation through the mouth. Adenoids are an overgrowth of glandular tissue at the back of the throat, into which the nose opens. Children with enlarged adenoids often have secretory otitis media (glue ear) (see EAR, DISEASES OF), and specialist opinion should be sought. Polyps are growths of soft jellylike character: they arise from chronic inflammation associated with allergic rhinitis, chronic sinusitis, asthma, and aspirin abuse. Large polyps can cause erosion of the nasal bones and should be surgically removed.

Bleeding (see HAEMORRHAGE).

Foreign bodies At first these may not cause any symptoms, but in time they can cause obstruction of the affected nostril with a foul-smelling bloody discharge. The problem is common with small children who tend to push small objects into their noses. Foreign bodies require removal, sometimes in hospital. Anyone attempting to remove a foreign body should take care not to push it further into the nose.

Loss of sense of smell, or ANOSMIA may be temporary or permanent. Temporary anosmia is caused by conditions of the nose which are reversible, whereas permanent anosmia is caused by conditions which destroy the olfactory nerves. Temporary conditions are those such as the common cold, or other inflammatory conditions of the nasal mucosa or the presence of nasal polyps. Permanent anosmia may follow and influenzal neuritis or it may also follow injuries to the brain and fractures of the skull involving the olfactory nerves.

Injury to nose The commonest injury is a fracture of the nasal bones or displacement of the cartilage that forms the bridge of the nose. The nasal septum may also be displaced sideways by a lateral blow. Sporting activities, especially boxing and rugby football, are commonly a cause of nasal injury. If a fracture is suspected or there is substantial tissue swelling, an X-ray examination is necessary. Resetting a damaged bone should be done either immediately, before swelling makes surgery difficult, or 10 days or so later when the swelling has subsided. Results are usually good, ensuring a clear airway as well as a restored profile. It is not unusual for the cheek bone to sustain a depressed fracture at the same time as the nose is broken. Careful assessment and prompt surgery are called for.

NOSOLOGY The term applied to scientific classification of diseases.

NOTIFIABLE DISEASES are diseases, usually of an infectious nature, which are required by law to be made known to a health officer or local authority. (See INFECTION.) Certain occupational diseases are also notifiable.

Notifiable Diseases in the UK as at 1 June 1998

Acute encephalitis
Acute poliomyelitis
Anthrax
Cholera
Diphtheria
Dysentery (amoebic or bacillary)
Ebola virus disease
Food poisoning
Lassa fever
Leprosy (reported to Chief Medical Officer at the Department of Health)
Leptospirosis
Malaria
Marburg disease
Measles
Meningitis
Meningococcal septicaemia (without meningitis)
Mumps
Ophthalmia neonatorum
Paratyphoid fever
Plague
Rabies
Relapsing fever
Rubella
Scarlet fever
Smallpox
Tetanus
Tuberculosis
Typhoid fever
Typhus
Viral haemorrhagic fever (including Lassa fever)
Viral hepatitis
Whooping cough
Yellow fever

Reporting AIDS is voluntary (and in confidence) to the Director, Communicable Diseases Surveillance Centre (PHLS) (see APPENDIX 2: ADDRESSES).

NOVOBIOCIN An antibiotic derived from cultures of *Streptomyces spheroides* or *Streptomyces niveus*. It is particularly active against STAPHYLOCOCCI, and has proved especially useful in the treatment of staphylococcal infections which have not responded to treatment with other antibiotics, or in which the causative micro-organism is resistant to such antibiotics.

NSAID (see NON-STEROIDAL ANTI-INFLAMMATORY DRUGS).

NUCHA The Latin name for the back of the neck.

NUCLEAR MAGNETIC RESONANCE (see MAGNETIC RESONANCE IMAGING (MRI)).

NUCLEAR MEDICINE The branch of medicine concerned with the use of radioactive material in the diagnosis, investigation and treatment of disease.

NUCLEIC ACID A substance constructed out of units known as nucleotides which consist of a purine or pyrimidine base linked to a pentose sugar which in turn is esterified with phosphoric acid. Two types of nucleic acid occur in nature: deoxyribonucleic acid (DNA) and ribonucleic acid (RNA). (See DNA; RNA.)

NUCLEUS The central body in a cell, which controls the activities of the latter. (See CELLS.)

NUCLEUS PULPOSUS The inner core of an intervertebral disc. (See SPINAL COLUMN.)

NULLIPARA The term applied to a woman who has never borne a child.

NUMBNESS (see TOUCH).

NURSING The single largest health profession. Nurses require an elaborate training, although people are often called upon to nurse relatives and friends without any previous experience of the subject. The functions and skills required in nursing range from nursing assistants, who provide basic 'bedside' services, through ward and outpatient nurses registered with the UKCC (see below) who are authorized to give (and sometimes prescribe) drugs and technical treatment to nurses working in operating theatres and intensive-care units. Nurses can also become managers, teach students or do research. The basic registration course is also required for those wanting to become midwives, health visitors or district nurses – all of which require extra training. Changes are taking place in the organization and training of nurses aiming for registration, with greater emphais on an academic and vocational approach in place of the traditional 'apprenticeship' type training. Registered nurses in the United Kingdom now have to complete a recognized three-year university-style course during which they spend time in hospitals. Full details about openings in nursing, details of training and of training schools can be obtained from the Royal College of Nursing (see APPENDIX 2: ADDRESSES). The Nurses, Midwives and Health Visitors Act 1979 led to the establishment of a United Kingdom Central Council and four National Boards for nursing, midwifery and health visiting. The Central Council, supported by the Boards, has responsibility for registration and the setting and maintaining of standards of education and of conduct of nurses, midwives and health visitors throughout the United Kingdom. Over 340,000 nurses and midwives were employed in NHS hospitals, community health services and primary care in England in 1996.

NUTRITION The process by which the living organism physiologically absorbs and used food to ensure growth, energy production and repair of tissues. The science of nutrition includes the study of diets and deficiency diseases (see DIET).

NUX VOMICA The seed of *Strychnos nux-vomica*, an East Indian tree. It has an intensely bitter taste. The medicinal properties of the plant are almost entirely due to two alkaloids, strychnine and brucine, which it contains. (See STRYCHNINE.)

NYSTAGMUS (see EYE DISEASES).

NYSTATIN An antibiotic, isolated from *Streptomyces noursei*, active against *Candida*

albicans. It is not absorbed from the gut but is useful in gastrointestinal and skin candidosis.

O

OAT CELL or SMALL CELL CARCINOMA A type of cell found in one highly malignant form of lung cancer. The cell is small and either oval or round. The nucleus stains darkly and the cytoplasm is sparse and difficult to identify. Oat-cell carcinoma of the bronchus is usually caused by smoking and comprises around 30 per cent of all bronchial cancers. It responds to radiotherapy and chemotherapy but, because the growth has usually spread widely by the time it is diagnosed, the prognosis is poor. Results of surgery are unsatisfactory.

OBESITY A condition in which the energy stores of the body (mainly fat) are too large. It is a prevalent nutritional disorder in prosperous countries. The Quetelet Index or Body Mass Index (BMI), which relates weight in kilograms (W) to height^2 in metres (H^2), is a widely accepted way of classifying obesity in adults according to severity, e.g.

Grade of obseity	BMI (W/H^2)
III	>40
II	30–40
I	25–29·9
not obese	<25

There is no advantage in further classifying obesity according to frame size since this does not improve the accuracy with which levels of body fat are predicted. (See APPENDIX 6: section C.)

Causes For obesity to occur, energy intake must exceed energy output over a sufficiently long period of time. All aetiological factors must ultimately act by reducing energy output or increasing energy intake or both.

Obesity tends to aggregate in families. This has led to the suggestion that some people inherit a 'thrifty' gene which predisposes them to obesity in later life by lowering their energy output. Indeed patients often attribute their obesity to such a metabolic defect. Total energy output is made up of the resting metabolic rate (RMR), which represents about 70 per cent of the total, the energy cost of physical activity and thermogenesis, i.e. the increase in energy output in response to food intake, cold exposure, some drugs and psychological influences. In general, obese people are consistently found to have a higher RMR and total energy output, per person and also when expressed against fat-free mass, than do their lean counterparts. Most obese people do not appear to have a reduced capacity for thermogenesis. Although a genetic component to obesity remains a possibility, it is unlikely to be great or to prevent weight loss from being possible in most patients by reducing energy intake. Environmental influences are believed to be more important in explaining the familial association in obesity.

An inactive lifestyle is thought to play a minor role in the development of obesity, but it remains unclear if people are obese because they are inactive or are inactive because they are obese.

For the majority of obese people a reduction in energy output does not appear to be the main aetiological factor. It follows then that the explanation must lie in an excessive energy intake. Unfortunately, it is difficult to demonstrate this directly since the methods used to assess habitual energy intake are unreliable. For most obese people it seems likely that the defect lies in their failure to regulate energy intake in response to a variety of cognitive factors (i.e. ease of fitting of clothes) in the long term.

Rarely, obesity has an endocrine basis and is caused by HYPOTHYROIDISM, HYPOPITUITARISM, HYPOGONADISM or CUSHING'S SYNDROME.

Symptoms Obesity has adverse effects on morbidity and mortality which are greatest in young adults and increase with the severity of obesity. It is associated with an increased mortality and/or morbidity from cardiovascular disease, non-insulin-dependent DIABETES MELLITUS, diseases of the gall bladder, osteoarthritis, hernia, gout and possibly certain cancers (i.e. colon, rectum and prostate in men, and breast, ovary, endometrium and cervix in women). Menstrual irregularities and ovulatory failure are often experienced by obese women. Obese people are also at greater risk when they undergo surgery. With the exception of gall-stone formation, weight loss will reduce these health risks.

Treatment Creation of an energy deficit is essential for weight loss to occur so the initial line of treatment is a slimming diet. An average deficit of 1000 kcal/day will produce a loss of 1 kg of fat/week and should be aimed for. Theoretically, this can be achieved by increasing energy expenditure or reducing energy intake. In practice, a low-energy diet is the usual form of treatment since attempts to increase energy expenditure, either by physical exercise or a thermogenic drug, are relatively ineffective.

Anorectic drugs, gastric stapling and jaw wiring are sometimes used to treat severe obesity. They are said to aid compliance with a low-energy diet by either reducing hunger (anorectic drugs) or limiting the amount of food the patient can eat. Unfortunately, the long-term effectiveness of gastric stapling is not known and it is debatable if the modest reduction in weight achieved by use of anorectic drugs is worthwhile, though a new drug is becoming available that reduces the amount of fat absorbed from food in the gastrointestinal tract. For some grossly obese patients jaw wiring can be helpful but a regain of weight once the wires are removed must be prevented. These procedures carry a risk, so should be done only if an individual's health is in danger.

OBSESSIVE COMPULSIVE DISORDER A NEUROSIS in which an individual's mind is dominated by a particular idea or emotion. This can lead to repetitive, often ritualized impulsive acts which are beyond the control of the will, the power of judgment being for a time lost. Environmental and hereditary factors play a part in the disorder. (See MENTAL ILLNESS.)

OBSTETRICS The branch of medicine dealing with pregnancy and giving birth. Derived from the Latin word for midwifery, it is closely allied to GYNAECOLOGY. It is concerned with the health of the woman and fetus, from early in pregnancy through to a successful LABOUR. Pregnancy and childbirth are, however, normal physiological events and for most women they take place without complications. So it is important not to 'medicalize' this natural process and, where possible, to allow a woman to have her baby where she wishes. The importance of identifying and, if possible, preventing adverse developments in pregnancy and labour has led to an overemphasis on medical intervention. Nevertheless, if something does go wrong, skilled medical care should help the mother and baby achieve a successful outcome. Routine monitoring of pregnancies by midwives and, where necessary, general practitioners or obstetricians is well recognized as a significant contribution to a successful pregnancy and delivery. Such monitoring has been greatly facilitated by advances in ULTRASOUND, AMNIOSCOPY, amnio- and cordocentesis (see PRENATAL DIAGNOSIS). Numerous problems may occur at all stages, and early detection, followed rapidly by sensitive and appropriate treatment, is vital. Doctors and nurses can specialize in obstetrics after suitable training.

OBSTIPATION Severe CONSTIPATION.

OBSTRUCTION OF THE BOWELS (see INTESTINE, DISEASES OF).

OCCIPUT The lower and hinder part of the head where it merges into the neck.

OCCLUSION The way that the teeth fit together when the jaws close. Also the closing or obstruction of a duct, hollow organ, or blood vessel.

OCCULT Describing something that is not easily seen. Occult blood in the faeces is present in very small amounts and can be identified only by a chemical test or under the microscope.

Cause	Occupation	Disease
Coal dust	Coal mining	Coal-workers' pneumoconiosis
Silica	Gold mining	Silicosis
	Iron and steel industries (metal casting)	
	Metal grinding	
	Stone dressing	
	Pottery	
Asbestos	Asbestos mining	Asbestosis
	Manufacturer of fireproof and insulating materials	
Iron oxide	Arc welding	Siderosis
Tin dioxide	Tin ore mining	Stannosis
Beryllium	Aircraft and atomic energy industries	Berylliosis
Cotton, flax or hemp dust	Textile industries	Byssinosis
Fungal spores from mouldy hay, straw or grain, bagasse, mushroom compost	Agriculture and related industries	Farmer's lung
		Metalworker's lung
		Bagassosis
		Mushroom worker's lung

Some occupational lung diseases. Davidson and Macleod.

OCCUPATIONAL DISEASES Work has been the cause of human illness and injury for centuries. The earliest accounts concentrated on the rigours of underground mining where, in earliest times, the risks to health were severe enough to relegate such 'occupations' to slaves and criminals. Such activities are inherently dangerous but the advent of industrialization widened and broadened the range of health risks to which employed people could be exposed. Control of workplace exposures in modern industrialized society has limited the toll of disease and injury but cannot abolish it entirely.

In the country such as Britain with 30 million employable people, over 400 are killed and another 150,000 injured each year as a direct result of work. One in 4,500 develops an occupational disease annually. By contrast, the Scandinavian figures for occupational disease are ten time 'worse'. Such differences are more to do with reporting criteria than true differences in occupational health. Whilst compensation for such disease rests with government social-security departments, the control of workplace hazards is in the hands of labour inspectorates. In Britain, this responsibility lies in the Department of Employment with the Health and Safety Commission and its Executive. The Executive includes both inspectorates and a medical division staffed by doctors and nurses who have responsibility for giving advise to employers and employees on workplace risk to health in relation to health and safety legislation. Increasingly the laws governing health and safety at work are moving into a European arena as the European Commission promulgates directives which are binding on member states. Although a new European list of compensatable occupational diseases is currently being drafted, member states have widely differing criteria. What follows are brief notes on the numerically more important compen-satable occupational diseases in the United Kingdom.

Inhaled materials

PNEUMOCONIOSIS covers a group of diseases which cause fibrotic lung disease following the inhalation of dust. Around 500 new cases receive benefit each year – mostly due to coal dust with or without silica contamination. Silicosis is the more severe disease. The contraction in the size of the coal-mining industry as well as improved dust suppression in the mines have diminished the importance of this disease, whereas asbestos-related diseases now exceed 1,000 per year. Asbestos fibres cause a restrictive lung disease but also are responsible for certain malignant conditions such as pleural and peritoneal mesothelioma and lung cancer. The lung-cancer risk is ex-acerbated by cigarette smoking.

OCCUPATIONAL ASTHMA is of increasing importance – not only because of the recognition of new allergic agents but also in the number of reported cases. Twenty-two specific agents are listed at present of which the most common offending agents are isocyanates, flour and other grain dusts, soldering flux, epoxy resins and wood dusts. Other notable allergens are platinum salts, proteolytic enzymes, arthropods and crustaceans, antibiotics and reactive dyes. The disease develops after a short symptomless period of exposure and symptoms are temporally related to work exposures and relieved by absences from work. Removal of the worker from exposure does not necessarily lead to complete cessation of symptoms. For many agents, there is no relationship with a previous history of ATOPY. Occupational asthma now accounts for about 10 per cent of all asthma cases.

BYSSINOSIS is considered by many authorities to be a variant of occupational asthma. The condition is, however, broader and more complex than this. In susceptible individuals, exposure to the dusts of cotton, sisal, hemp, or flax can cause acute dyspnoea with cough and reversible airways obstruction. It is first noticed on the first day of the working week and then subsides. Later, with continued exposure, symptoms recur on subsequent days of the week until even weekends and holidays are not free of symptoms.

Other organic dusts can produce extrinsic allergic alveolitis with resultant lowering of respiratory gas transfer in the alveoli. Most of the agents causing this condition are fungal spores and the most common condition in Britain is farmer's lung (see ALVEOLITIS). These diseases frequently start as an influenza-like illness and, if exposure is continued, lead to subacute and chronic pulmonary fibrotic disease.

Dermatitis The risk of dermatitis caused by an allergic or irritant reaction to substances used or handled at work is present in a wide variety of jobs. This condition is the commonest of all the occupational diseases. Whilst changes in the compensation criteria over the last twenty years have reduced successful claims from 11,000 a year to a few hundred, general-practice-based surveys suggest that over 50,000 new cases are diagnosed each year. About three-quarters of these cases are irritant-contact dermatitis due to such agents as acids, alkalis and even soap and water. Allergic contact dermatitis is a more specific response by susceptible individuals to a range of allergens. The main occupational contact allergens include chromates, nickel, epoxy resins, rubber additives, germicidal agents, dyes, topical anaesthetics and antibiotics as well as certain plants and woods. (See SKIN DISEASES.)

Musculo-skeletal disorders Apart from the commonest problems of injured backs from manual handling, there are two groups of disorders caused by repeated injury – the 'beat' conditions and work-related upper-limb disorders. The beat conditions such as beat knee and beat elbow are caused by repeated damage to a joint from kneeling or crawling – problems associated with mining and carpet-laying, for example. The work-related upper-limb disorders range from clear-cut occupationally induced repetitive movement conditions such as tendinitis, TENOSYNOVITIS, CARPAL TUNNEL SYNDROME and epicondylitis to less well-defined disorders of prolonged or repetitive posture disturbances which may lead to shoulder or cervical spine discomfort. These disorders are common in the general population and their occupational attribution is frequently controversial. Particular high-risk occupations include poultry processors, packers, electronic assembly workers, data processors, supermarket check-out operators and telephonists. These jobs often contain a number of the relevant exposures of dynamic load, static load, a full or excessive range of movements and awkward postures. (See UPPER LIMB DISORDERS.)

Physical agents A number of physical agents cause occupational ill health of which most important is occupational deafness. Workplace noise exposures in excess of 85 decibels for a working day are likely to cause damage to hearing which is initially restricted to the vital frequencies associated with speech – around 3–4 KHz. Protection from such noise is imperative as hearing aids do nothing to ameliorate the neural damage once it has occurred.

Hand–arm vibration syndrome is a disorder of the vascular and/or neural endings in the hands leading to episodic blanching and numbness which is exacerbated by low temperature. The condition, which is caused by vibrating tools such as chain saws and pneumatic hammers, is akin to RAYNAUD'S DISEASE and can be disabling.

Decompression sickness is caused by a rapid change in ambient pressure and is a disease associated with deep-sea divers, tunnel workers and high-flying aviators. Apart from the direct effects of pressure change such as ruptured tympanic membrane or sinus pain, the more serious damage is indirectly due to nitrogen bubbles appearing in the blood and blocking small vessels. Central and peripheral nervous-system damage and bone necrosis are the most dangerous sequelae.

Radiation Non-ionizing radiation from lasers or microwaves can cause severe localized heating leading to tissue damage of which cataracts are a particular variety. Ionizing radiation from radioactive sources can cause similar acute tissue damage to the eyes as well as cell damage to rapidly dividing cells in the gut and bone marrow. Longer-term effects include genetic damage and various malignant disorders of which leukaemia and aplastic anaemia are notable. Particular radioactive isotopes may destroy or induce malignant change in target organs, for example, I^{131} (thyroid), Sr^{90} (bone).

Other occupational cancers Occupation is directly responsible for about 5 per cent of all cancers and contributes to a further 5 per cent. Apart from the cancers caused by asbestos and ionising radiation, a number of other occupational exposures can cause human cancer. The International Agency for Research on Cancer lists 50 agents or processes of which occupational agents or processes account for 31. The more important of these are polynuclear aromatic hydrocarbons such as mineral oils, soots, tars (skin and lung cancer), the aromatic amines in dyestuffs (bladder cancer), certain hexavalent chromates, arsenic and nickel refining (lung cancer), wood and leather dust (nasal sinus cancer), benzene (leukaemia) and vinyl chloride monomer (angiosarcoma of the liver). Elimination of all known occupational carcinogens, if possible, would lead to an annual saving of 5,000 premature deaths in Britain.

Infections Two broad categories of job carry an occupational risk. These are workers in contact with animals (farmers, veterinary surgeons and slaughtermen) and those in contact with human sources of infection (health care staff and sewage workers). Estimates of current annual incidences of work related cases are LEPTOSPIROSIS (40 cases), TUBERCULOSIS (30 cases), HEPATITIS B (25 cases), chlamydiosis (see CHLAMYDIA) (16 cases), Q fever (12 cases),

BRUCELLOSIS (10 cases). The less severe ORF accounts for at least 50 cases but this is even more of an underestimate than the figures for the other diseases. Other compensatable infections are ANTHRAX, GLANDERS, ANCYLOSTOMIASIS, streptococcus suis, and hydatidosis.

Poisonings In earlier decades, chemical poisonings by lead, phosphorus, arsenic, mercury, cadmium and a number of organic solvents were much more common. Today, around 2,000 poisonings are reported annually with 20–30 fatalities. The commonest agents are now solvents, gases, acids, alkalis and irritant vapours. The lead regulations specify that persons with blood lead levels above 69μg/100 ml (above 39 for females of reproductive age) should be suspended from working with lead. The success in diminishing morbidity is largely one of prevention.

Prevention There are certain principles of prevention which, if followed, can significantly diminish the risk of occupationally induced diseases. Indeed as these diseases cannot be eliminated from the world – in comparison with smallpox – prevention is the utmost importance. This is a hierachy of control measures. The ideal solution is elimination of the offending substance or process. Failing this, substitution by a less hazardous material or process could be undertaken and/or more effective enclosure or exhaust ventilation, thereby diminishing exposure of the worker. The least satisfactory method is personal protection for the worker.

OCCUPATIONAL THERAPY The treatment of physical and psychiatric conditions through specific selected activities in order to help people reach their maximum level of function and independence in all aspects of daily life.

Occupational therapists work from hospital and community bases. They do much more than keep patients occupied with diverting hobbies. The arts and crafts still have a place in modern therapy techniques but these now also include household chores, industrial work, communication techniques, social activities, sports and educational programmes. An Occupational Therapy Department may have facilities for woodwork, metalwork, printing, gardening, cooking, art and drama. Occupational therapists will use any combination of activities to strengthen muscles, increase movement and restore co-ordination and balance. With mentally ill people similar activies are used. They help provide order, comfort and support and aim to build up self-confidence. Occupational therapists plan courses of treatment which are individually tailored to the needs of the patient. The aim is to help the patient practise all the activites involved in daily life. The therapists are part of a team including doctors, nurses, social workers, home helps, housing officers, physiotherapists, speech therapists and psychologists. Occupational therapists are mainly employed by the National Health Service and by Local Authority Social Services and they work in hospitals, special centres and in the handicapped person's own home. State Registration is essential for employment as an occupational therapists. There are 15 occupational therapy schools in the United Kingdom where the course leading to the diploma of the College of Occupational Therapists can be followed. The course lasts three academic years. (See REHABILITATION.)

OCHRONOSIS A rare condition in which the ligaments and cartilages of the body, and sometimes the conjunctiva, become stained by dark brown or black pigment. This may occur in chronic carbolic poisoning, or in a congenital disorder of metabolism in which the individual is unable to break down completely the tyrosine of the protein molecule, the intermediate product, homogentisic acid, appearing in the urine – this being known as alkaptonuria.

OEDEMA An abnormal accumulation of fluid beneath the skin, or in one or more of the cavities of the body.

Causes Oedema is not a disease, it is a sign, usually of underlying local or systemic disease. Oedema may sometimes be visible as a swelling. Oedema occurs when the normal mechanisms for maintaining a balance between fluid in the tissues and in the blood are upset. That balance depends mainly on the blood pressure that keeps the blood flowing through the circulatory system – thus forcing fluid out of the capillaries – and the osmotic drawing force of the blood proteins which pulls water into the blood stream. The KIDNEYS also have an essential role in maintaining this balance.

Among the disorders that may disturb this balance are HEART failure, NEPHROTIC SYNDROME, kidney failure, CIRRHOSIS of the liver and a diet deficient in protein. Injury may also cause oedema and ascites (fluid in the abdominal cavity) can occur as a result of cirrhosis of the liver or cancer in the abdominal organs.

Treatment The underlying cause of oedema should be treated and, if this is not feasible or effective, the excess fluid should be excreted by boosting the output of the kidney. Restriction of sodium in the diet and the administration of DIURETIC drugs are effective methods of achieving this.

OEDEMA OF THE LUNGS This occurs as a result of left ventricular failure (see HEART DISEASES). There is an abrupt increase in the venous and capillary pressure in the pulmonary vessels followed by flooding of fluid into the interstitial spaces and alveoli. The commonest cause of acute pulmonary oedema is MYOCARDIAL INFARCTION which reduces the ability of the left ventricular myocardial muscle to handle the blood delivered to it. Pulmonary oedema may result from other causes of left ventricular failure such as HYPERTENSION or valvular disease of the MITRAL and AORTIC valves. The initial symptoms are cough with breathlessness and occasionally with wheezing. The patient becomes extremely short of breath and in a severe attack the patient is pale, sweating and cyanosed and obviously gasping for breath. Frequently frothy sputum is produced which may be blood stained. Treatment is with diuretics and measures to deal with the myocardial infarction or other underlying cause.

OEDIPUS COMPLEX A description used by psychoanalysts of the subconscious attraction of a child for its parent of the opposite sex. This is accompanied by a wish to get rid of the parent of the same sex. The origin of the phrase lies in the Greek story in which Oedipus kills his father without realizing who he is and then marries his mother.

OESOPHAGOSCOPE An endoscopic instrument for observing the lining of the oesophagus. (See ENDOSCOPE.)

OESOPHAGUS, or GULLET The tube passing from the throat into the stomach, down which passes swallowed food and drink. It consists of three coats: a strong outer coat of muscle fibres in two layers, the outer running lengthwise, the inner being circular; inside this a loose connective tissue coat containing blood-vessels, glands, and nerves; and finally a strong mucous membrane lined by epithelium, which closely re-sembles that of the mouth and skin.

OESOPHAGUS, DISEASES OF Oesophagitis is inflammation of the oesophagus and may be due to swallowing a corrosive chemical (corrosive oesophagitis) or because the muscles of the lower part of the oesophagus do not work properly (ACHALASIA), allowing the stomach's acidic contents to regurgitate (reflux oesophagitis). HIATUS HERNIA is sometimes associated with the latter condition. Diagnosis can be made by ENDOSCOPY of the oesophagus and/or an X-ray examination using a barium swallow. Treatment of reflux oesophagitis is by an appropriate diet and weight loss. Stricture of the oesophagus can result from swallowing a corrosive fluid and may produce severe narrowing. Such strictures may sometimes be dilated by the use of suitable instruments or surgery may be necessary.

A still more serious and frequent cause of oesophageal stricture is that due to cancer, which may occur at any part, but is most common at the lower end, near the entrance into the stomach. The chief symptoms of this condition are increasing difficulty in swallowing, increasing debility, together with enlargement of the glands in the neck. The condition usually occurs in middle age or beyond and around 5,000 people are diagnosed with cancer every year in the United Kingdom. The incidence is higher in men than in women and is

high in Iran and some areas of East Asia, probably due to local diets. In many cases treatment can only be palliative, but recent advances in surgery are producing promising results. In some cases treatment with irradiation or anti-cancer drugs produces relief, if not cure. In those in whom neither operation nor radiation can be performed life may be prolonged and freedom from pain obtained by fluid food which is either swallowed or passed down a tube. In cases of achalasia the passage of a special bougie down the oesophagus to dilate the sphincter may be effective.

Strictures of the oesophagus may also be produced by the pressure of tumours or aneurysms within the cavity of the chest but external to the gullet.

Finally, difficulty in swallowing sometimes occurs in certain serious nervous diseases from paralysis affecting the nerves supplying the muscular coats of the pharynx, which thus loses its propulsive power (bulbar paralysis).

Foreign bodies which lodge in the respiratory part of the throat, i.e. at the entrance to, or in the cavity of, the larynx, set up immediate symptoms of choking. (See CHOKING.) Those which lodge in the gullet, on the contrary, do not usually set up any immediately serious symptoms, although their presence causes considerable discomfort. Medical attention is usually required.

OESTRADIOL The name given to the oestrogenic hormone secreted by the ovarian follicle. Oestradiol is responsible for the development of the female sexual characteristics, of the breasts, and of part of the changes that take place in the uterus before menstruation.

OESTRADIOL VALERATE (see OESTROGEN).

OESTRIOL (see OESTROGEN).

OESTROGEN Natural or synthetic substances that induce the changes in the uterus that precede ovulation. They are also responsible for the development of the secondary sex characteristics in women: that is the physical changes that take place in a girl at puberty, such as enlargement of the breasts, appearance of pubic and axillary hair and the deposition of fat on the thighs and hips. They are used in the management of disturbances of the menopause, and also in the treatment of cancer of the prostate and certain cases of cancer of the breast.

The oestrogenic hormones of the ovary are oestradiol and oestrone and they are interconvertible. The natural oestrogens, like the hormones of the testis and the adrenal cortex, are steroids. They are rapidly metabolized in the body and excreted in the urine as inactive conjugates. The rapid degradation of natural oestrogens limits their use as therapeutic agents. Chemical substitution of the steroid molecule, as in ethinyl oestradiol, or the use of a non-steroidal synthetic oestrogen such as STILBOESTROL, greatly reduces the rate of degradation and enhances the therapeutic action. A further development has been the use of compounds which are not actually oestrogenic themselves, but which are slowly metabolized to oestrogenic substances, or substances such as chlorotrianisene, which are taken up in the body fat and then slowly released into the circulation. There is in fact little to choose between the various synthetic oestrogens. Ethinyl oestradiol is the most potent oral oestrogen, being twenty times more active than stilboestrol.

Other commonly used oestrogen drugs are dienoestrol, oestradiol and oestrol. The use of oestrogens in hormone replacement therapy (HRT) is dealt with in the entry on the MENO-PAUSE.

OESTRONE (see OESTROGEN).

OFFICE FOR NATIONAL STATISTICS (ONS) This is an executive agency of the UK government formed by an amalgamation in 1990 of the Central Statistical Office and the Office of Population Censuses and Surveys (OPCS). The ONS compiles and publishes statistics on national and local populations including their social and economic situation and contributions to the country's economy. It also records the demographic patterns of births, marriages and deaths, including the medical cause of death. The former OPCS organized a national 10-yearly census and ONS is carrying on this activity. The census is based on the actual presence of individuals in a house or institutions on a given night. The figures provide government departments and local authorities with information for planning services.

OINTMENTS Semi-solid, anhydrous, greasy substances used as emollients, protectants and as vehicles for topical drug delivery, ointments may be hydrophylic or hydrophobic. The former are water soluble and usually contain polyethylene glycols. Hydrophobic ointments are not miscible with water and are paraffin based. Mixing hard and soft paraffins allows stiffness and greasiness to be modified. Pastes are ointments containing a high proportion of inert powder such as starch or zinc oxide which confers stiffness. Pastes are protective and allow precise aplication of drugs to the skin.

OLD AGE (see AGEING).

OLEIC ACID The commonest of naturally occurring fatty acids, being present in most fats and oils in the form of triglyceride. It is used in the preparation of ointments, but not eye ointments.

OLFACTORY NERVES The nerves of smell, which is the first cranial nerve. Each nerve detects smell by means of hairlike receptors positioned in the mucous membrane lining the roof of the nasal cavity (see NOSE).

OLIGAEMIA A diminution of the quantity of blood in the circulation.

OLIG(O)- A prefix which means little or scanty: for example, oliguria, excretion of smaller than normal quantities of urine.

OLIGOMENORRHOEA Infrequent menstruation.

OLIGOSPERMIA A less than normal number of SPERMATOZOA present in each unit volume of seminal fluid. Each ml of semen usually contains 20 million sperm. The condition may be permanent or temporary and is a major cause of INFERTILITY in men. The condition, which may be caused by ORCHITIS, undescended TESTIS or VARIOCOCOELE, should be investigated.

OLIGURIA An abnormally low excretion of urine, such as occurs in acute nephritis.

OLIVE OIL The oil obtained by pressure from the fruit of *Olea europaea*. It is practically a pure fat. It has become increasingly popular over the past decade for its important role in the prevention of heart disease. It owes this popularity to two factors. First, that it is almost entirely a monounsaturated fat, and second, the Mediterraneans, who take a great deal of olive oil in their diet, are reputed to avoid artery problems.

OMENTUM A long fold of peritoneal membrane, generally loaded with more or less fat, which hangs down within the abdominal cavity in front of the bowels. It is formed by the layers of peritoneum that cover the front and back surfaces of the stomach in their passage from the lower margin of this organ to cover the back and front surfaces of the large intestine. Instead of passing straight from one organ to the other, these layers dip down and form a sort of fourfold apron. This omentum is known as the greater omentum, to distinguish it from two smaller peritoneal folds, one of which passes between the liver and stomach (the hepatogastric omentum), and the other between the liver and duodenum (the hepato-duodenal omentum). Together they are known as the lesser omentum.

OMEPRAZOLE This is a PROTON PUMP IN-HIBITOR drug which inhibits gastric acid secretion by blocking a key enzyme system in the parietal cells of the STOMACH. The drug is used to treat (short term) gastric and duodenal ulcers and strictures and inflammatory erosion of the oesophagus. It has a range of side-effects.

OMPHALOCELE Another name for exomphalos – a hernia of abdominal organs through the umbilicus.

ONCHOCERCIASIS Infestation with the filarial worm, *Onchocerca volvulus*. It is found in many parts of tropical Africa south of the Sahara, in Central and South America, and in the Yemen and Saudi Arabia. It is estimated that there are more than 20 million victims of it. It is transmitted by gnats of the genus Simulium. After a period of nine to eighteen months, the young filarial worms, injected into the body by the bite of an infected Simulium, mature, mate and start producing young microfilariae. The females live for up to fifteen years and during this period each may produce several thousand microfilariae a day. It is these microfilariae, which have a life-span of up to two years, that produce the characteristic features of the disease: an itching rash of the skin and the appearance of nodules in different parts of the body. There may also be involvement of the eyes and the worm may invade the optic nerve and so cause blindness; hence the name of African river blindness. Treatment consists of diethylcarbamazine and suramin. An international campaign is now under way in an attempt to destroy Simulium in the affected zones. Meanwhile the only means of prevention is to avoid so far as possible being bitten by the gnat. One means of achieving this is by wearing long trousers, shoes and socks.

ONCOGENE is a GENE found in mammalian cells and viruses that can cause cancer. It is believed to manufacture the proteins that control the division of cells. In certain circumstances this control malfunctions and a normal cell may be changed into one with malignant properties. Extensive research is being done with oncogens with the aim of finding ways to prevent or control cancers.

ONCOLOGY The management of malignant disease, a major health problem since successful management requires close liaison between the patient, surgeons, physicians, oncologists, HAEMATOLOGISTS, PAEDIATRICIANS and other specialists. Diagnosis may involve various investigations and often requires a biopsy. Once a diagnosis has been established, treatment may be divided into two aspects. Curative treatments, involving surgery, radiotherapy or chemotherapy (or various combinations as required).

Surgery may be most common, and is often the only treatment, for some gastrointestinal tumours, soft-tissue tumours, gynaecological tumours and advanced cancers of the head and neck.

Radiotherapy used ionizing radiation to kill tumour cells. Radiation is by naturally occurring isotopes or artificially produced X-rays. Germ-cell tumours, particularly SEMINOMAS and TERATOMAS, and malignant LYMPHOMAS appear to be particularly sensitive to irradiation, and many head and neck tumours, gynaecological cancers and localized PROSTATE and BLADDER cancers are curable with radiotherapy. It is also a valuable means of reducing pain from bone METASTASES. Unpleasant side-effects are common: chiefly lethargy, loss of appetite and dry, itchy skin symptoms.

Chemotherapy is also an important treatment in germ-cell tumours and some leukaemias and lymphomas; ovarian cancer (following surgery); and small-cell lung cancer (although most patients die within 18 months). It is also used in some breast cancers; advanced myeloma; sarcomas; and some childhood cancers (such as Wilms' tumour). Over 20 substances are in common use, the major classes being ALKYLATING AGENTS (e.g. CYCLOPHOSPHAMIDE, CHLORAMBUCIL, BUSULPHAN); ANTIMETABOLITES (e.g. METHOTREXATE); VINCA alkaloids (e.g. VINCRISTINE, VINBLASTINE); antitumour antibiotics (e.g. ACTINOMYCIN D). Choice of agent and the appropriate regimen requires expert guidance. Common side-effects include nausea and vomiting, BONE-MARROW suppression and ALOPECIA, with each substance having its own spectrum of unwanted effects.

Good doctor–patient communication, with the sharing of information and bringing the patient into the decision-making process, is vital. Although it may be time consuming and exhausting, it has been shown to reduce treatment MORBIDITY. Videoing of consultations for repeated viewing by the patient is often helpful; much information may be forgotten or fails to register when the doctor first explains the diagnosis and treatment.

The other chief aspect of treatment is the palliative; good doctor–patient communication is essential for ensuring effective pain control. Common sources of pain in cancer may involve bone, nerve compression, soft tissue, visceral, myofascial, constipation, muscle spasm, low back pain, joint pain (e.g. capsulitis) and chronic post-operative pain. Patients may be suffering from more than one pain, all of which should be identified. The aim should be to eliminate pain.

There are three rungs of the analgesic ladder; if one rung fails, the next one should be tried: (1) non-opioid drugs, e.g. aspirin, PARACETAMOL, NSAID; (2) weak opioids, e.g. CODEINE, DIHYDROCODEINE, dextropropoxyphene; (3) strong opioids, e.g. MORPHINE, DIAMORPHINE, buprenorphine. Oral treatment is always preferable, unless prevented by severe vomiting.

ONYCHIA Disease of the nails. (See NAILS, DISEASES OF.)

ONYCHOGRYPHOSIS A distortion of the nail in which it is much thickened, overgrown and twisted on itself. This usually affects a toenail and is the result of chronic irritation and inflammation.

ONYCHOLYSIS Separation of the nail from the nail-bed.

OÖCYTE An immature OVUM. When the cell undergoes meiosis in the ovary it becomes an ovum and is ready for fertilization by the spermatozoa. Only a small number of the many oöcytes produced survive until PUBERTY, and not all of them will become ova and be ejected into the FALLOPIAN TUBES.

OÖPHORECTOMY Removal, by operation, of an ovary. When the ovary is removed for the presence of a cyst, the term ovariotomy is usually employed.

OÖPHORITIS Another name for ovaritis or inflammation of an ovary.

OÖPHORON Another name for the ovary.

OPERATION A surgical procedure using instruments – or sometimes just the hands, for example, when manipulating a joint or setting a simple fracture. Operations range from simple removal of a small skin lesion under local anaesthetic to a major event such as transplanting a heart which takes several hours and involves many doctors, nurses and technical staff. Increasingly, operations are done on an outpatient or day-bed basis, thus enabling many more patients to be treated than was the case 25 years ago, and permitting them to resume a normal life, often within 24 hours. (See MINIMALLY INVASIVE SURGERY.)

OPHTHALMOLOGIST A doctor with specialist training in OPHTHALMOLOGY.

OPHTHALMOLOGY The study of the structure and function of the eye and the diagnosis and treatment of the diseases that affect it.

OPHTHALMOPLEGIA Paralysis of the muscles of the eye. Internal ophthalmoplegia refers to paralysis of the iris and ciliary body, external ophthalmoplegia refers to paralysis of one or all of the muscles that move the eyes.

OPHTHALMOSCOPE An instrument for examining the interior of the eye. There are different types of ophthalmoscope, all have a light source to illuminate the inside of the eye and a magnifying lens to make examination easier.

OPIATE A preparation of OPIUM.

OPIOID A substance with a pharmacological action that is like that of opium or its derivatives.

OPIOID POISONING Morphine and codeine are natural opium alkaloids found in the opium poppy (*Papaver somniferum*). The other opioids are either synthetic or semi-synthetic analogues of these. Their main use is in the treatment of moderate to severe pain, but they are also used as antidiarrhoeal and antitussive agents. As a result of induced tolerance (see DRUG ADDICTION) and great individual variability the amount of opioid substances required to cause serious consequences varies enormously.

The most common effects of opioid overdose are vomiting, drowsiness, pinpoint pupils, BRADYCARDIA, CONVULSIONS and COMA. Respiratory depression is common and may lead to CYANOSIS and respiratory arrest. HYPOTENSION occurs occasionally and in severe cases noncardiogenic pulmonary oedema and cardiovascular collapse may occur. Cardiac ARRHYTHMIAS may occur with some opioids. Some opioids have a HISTAMINE-releasing effect which may result in an URTICARIAL rash, PRURITUS, flushing and hypotension. Activated CHARCOAL should be given following overdose and NAXOLONE administered to reverse respiratory depression and deep coma.

OPISTHOTONOS The name for a position assumed by the body during one of the convulsive seizures of tetanus. The muscles of the back, by their spasmodic contraction, arch the body in such a way that the person for a time may rest upon the bed only by his heels and head.

OPIUM The dried juice of the unripe seed-capsules of the white Indian poppy, *Papaver somniferum*. It is cultivated mainly in India, but it is also produced in Iran, China, and the Asiatic provinces of Turkey. Opium possesses its medicinal properties only when produced under favourable conditions of soil and climate, and the juice of other species of poppies grown in temperate climates is almost useless. It is a brown, resinous-looking substance, or brown powder, with characteristic smell and bitter taste. The action of opium depends upon the twenty to twenty-five alkaloids it contains. Of these, the chief is morphine, the amount of which varies from around 9 to 17 per cent. Other alkaloids include codeine, narcotine, thebaine, papaverine, and naceine, and as the action of these differs considerably, the effect of the opium naturally varies according to the proportion of each that it contains.

The importation into Britain of opium is strictly regulated under the *Dangerous Drugs Acts*. Similar regulations govern the sale and distribution of any preparation of morphine or diamorphine (heroin) stronger than 1 part in 500. Unfortunately international drug rings manage to smuggle significant quantities of opium, and especially heroin, illegally into the UK. (See DRUG ADDICTION.)

The alkaloids, morphine and codeine, are administered in various forms. Morphine hydrochloride and morphine sulphate are given in doses from 7·5 to 20 mg; codeine phosphate in doses from 10 to 60 mg. Morphine hydrochloride solution (containing 1 per cent of morphine) is used in doses from 0·5 to 2 ml.

Action The action of opium varies considerably, according to the source of the drug and the preparation used.

In small doses, opium produces a state of gentle excitement, the person finding his imagination more vivid, his thoughts more brilliant, and his power of expression greater than usual. This stage lasts for some hours, and is succeeded by languor. In medicinal doses this stage of excitement is short and is followed by deep sleep. When potentially poisonous doses are taken, sleep comes on quickly, and passes into coma and death (see OPIOID POISONING). The habitual use of opium produces great tolerance, so that opium users require to take large quantities daily before experiencing its pleasurable effects. The need for opium also confers tolerance, so that people suffering great pain may take, with apparently little effect beyond dulling the pain, quantities which at another time would be dangerous.

OPPORTUNISTIC A description usually applied to infection resulting from an organism that does not normally cause disease in a healthy individual. It is also used to describe widespread infection by an organism that usually causes local infection. The body's defence mechanism can usually combat these organisms but if it is impaired – as happens in AIDS – opportunistic infection, such as PNEUMONIA, may develop. Some viral and fungal infections behave in this way. Antimicrobial treatment is often effective, even though the weakness in the body's defence mechanism cannot be rectified.

OPSONINS Substances present in the serum of the blood which act upon bacteria, so as to prepare them for destruction by the white cells of the blood.

OPTIC ATROPHY A deterioration in the fibres of the optic nerve resulting in partial or complete loss of vision. It may be caused by damage to the nerve from inflammation or injury, or the atrophy may be secondary to disease in the eye.

OPTIC CHIASMA This is formed by a crossing over of the two optic nerves which run from the back of the eyeballs to meet in the midline beneath the brain. Nerve fibres from the nasal part of the retina cross to link up with fibres from the outer part of the retina of the opposite eye. The linked nerves form two separate optic tracts which travel back to the occipital lobes of the brain.

OPTIC DISC Otherwise known as the blind spot of the eye, the disc is the beginning of the optic nerve, the point where nerve fibres from

the retina's rods and cones – the light- and colour-sensitive cells – leave the eyeball.

OPTICIAN Someone who fits and sells glasses or contact lenses. An ophthalmic optician is trained to perform eye examinations to test for long and short sightedness but they do not treat disorders of the eye.

OPTIC NERVE (see EYE).

OPTIC NEUTRITIS Inflammation of the optic nerve (see EYE) which may result in sudden loss of part of a person's vision. It is usually accompanied with pain and tenderness on touch. The cause is uncertain: CORTICOSTEROID drugs may help by improving the loss of visual acuity but seems not to check the long-term inflammatory activity.

ORAL An adjective referring to the mouth or to substances taken by mouth.

ORAL CONTRACEPTIVES A contraceptive taken by mouth. It comprises one or more synthetic female hormones, usually an oestrogen, which blocks normal ovulation, and a progestogen which influences the pituitary gland and thus blocks normal control of the woman's menstrual cycle. Progestogens also make the uterus less congenial for the fertilization of an ovum by the sperm. (See CONTRACEPTION.)

ORAL REHYDRATION THERAPY (ORT) This is the essential initial treatment for diarrhoea and is particularly valuable for dehydrated children in developing countries. Since it was introduced 25 years ago, it has transformed the prognosis for those ill with diseases such as CHOLERA. A litre of water containing one teaspoonful of salt and eight of sugar, taken by mouth, is readily absorbed. It replaces salts and water lost because of the diarrhoea and usually no other treatment is required.

ORAL SURGERY A branch of surgery that treats deformities, injuries or diseases of the teeth and jaws, as well as other areas of the face and mouth. Surgeons doing this work are usually qualified dentists who have done further training in oral and maxillofacial surgery.

ORANGE An excellent source of vitamin C: 100 millilitres of orange juice contain 50 mg of ascorbic acid (ie. vitamin C). It is also used as a flavouring agent in the form of infusion, tincture and syrup of the peel. Fresh orange is also employed, often mixed with glucose, in feverish conditions for the action of the citric acid it contains. (See CITRIC ACID.)

ORBIT (see EYE).

ORCHIDECTOMY Operation for the removal of the testicles (one or both).

ORCHIDOPEXY When testes do not descend into the scrotum normally in young children (cryptorchidism) an operation is necessary to bring the testes in to the scrotum. This is called surgical orchidopexy.

ORCHITIS Inflammation of the testicle. (See TESTICLE, DISEASES OF.)

ORF A virus infection of sheep and goats commonly transmitted to farm workers. Red papules on the hands or wrists become vesicular or pustular and resolve spontaneously in a few weeks.

ORGAN A collection of different tissues that form a distinct structure in the body with a particular function or functions. The LIVER, for example, comprises a collection of different metabolic cells bound together with connective tissue and liberally supplied with blood vessels that performs vital functions in the breakdown of substances absorbed from the gastrointestinal tract. Other examples of organs are the KIDNEYS, BRAIN and HEART.

ORGANIC DISEASE A term used in contradistinction to the word functional, to indicate that some structural change is responsible for the faulty action of an organ or other part of the body.

ORGANIC SUBSTANCES Those which are obtained from animal or vegetable bodies, or which resemble in chemical composition those derived from this source. Organic chemistry has come to mean the chemistry of the carbon compounds.

ORGANOPHOSPHORUS INSECTICIDES are a group of insecticides which act by inhibiting the action of cholinesterase. (See ACETYLCHOLINE.) For this reason they are also toxic to man and must therefore be handled with great care. The most widely used are PARATHION and MALATHION.

Some of them are of value in agriculture because, when applied to plants, they are absorbed, and distributed to all parts of the plant, where they may kill sucking insects such as aphids.

Treatment After contamination with insecticides, decontaminate (remove clothes, wash skin). Those treating should wear gloves, mask, apron and goggles. For symptoms give 2 mg of atropine IV every 30 minutes until full atropinization (dry mouth, pulse >70). Up to three days' treatment may be needed. Severe poisoning may require pralidoxine mysalate: available from designated centres, this drug should be given intravenously within 24 hours of exposure.

ORGANOPHOSPHORUS NERVE GASES Organophosphates cause damage to the human nervous system and compounds have been developed for use in warfare. After the 1991 Gulf War it was believed that some nerve gases may have been accidentally released during the disposal of stocks stored in Iraq. Soldiers who served in the war and subsequently developed debilitating but unidentifiable illness believe that contamination with organophosphorus gases may have caused or contributed to their condition. An official inquiry is being held about this issue. For the immediate treatment of individuals contaminated with these gases, see ORGANOPHOSPHORUS INSECTICIDES.

ORGASM The climax of sexual intercourse. In men this coincides with ejaculation of the semen when the muscles of the pelvis force the seminal fluid from the prostate into the urethra and out through the urethral orifice. In women orgasm is typified by irregular contractions of the muscular walls of the vagina followed by relaxation. The sensation is more diffuse in women than men and tends to last longer with successive orgasms sometimes occurring.

ORIENTAL SORE This term is a synonym for cutaneous leishmaniasis (see LEISHMANIASIS); others include: Cochin, Delhi, Kandahar, Lahore, Madagascar, Natal, Old World tropical, tropical sore, etc. As with many of the local names for this infection, it is now rarely used.

ORNITHOSIS is an infection of birds with the micro-organism known as *Chlamydia psittaci*, which is transmissible to man.

ORPHENADRINE A drug used in the treatment of PARKINSONISM.

ORTHODONTICS is the branch of dentistry concerned with the prevention and treatment of dental irregularities and malocclusion.

ORTHOPAEDICS Originally the general measures, surgical and mechanical, which can be used for the correction or prevention of deformities in children. Now, that branch of medical science dealing with skeletal deformity (congenital or acquired), fractures and infections of bones, replacement of arthritic joints (hips, knees and fingers, see ARTHROPLASTY) and the treatment of bone tumours.

ORTHOPNOEA A form of difficulty in breathing so severe that the patient cannot bear to lie down, but must sit or stand up. As a rule, it occurs only in serious affections of the heart or lungs.

ORTHOPTIC TREATMENT The examination and treatment by exercises of squints and their sequelae.

OSGOOD-SCHLATTER'S DISEASE The form of OSTEOCHONDROSIS involving the tibial tubercle – the growing point of the TIBIA. It occurs around puberty, mainly in boys, and first manifests itself by a painful swelling over the tibial tubercle at the upper end of the tibia. The pain is worst during and after exercise. A limp with increasing limitation of movement of the knee joint develops. Treatment consists of immobilization of the knee joint in plaster of Paris for six to eight weeks, with gradual return to activity over the next few months.

OSMOLARITY The osmotic pressure of a particular concentration of an osmotic solute dissolved in water. It is defined by the number of active particles in a set volume.

OSMOSIS The passage of fluids through a membrane, which separates them, so as to become mixed with one another. Osmotic pressure is a term applied to the strength of the tendency which a fluid shows to do this, and depends largely upon the amount of solid which it holds in solution.

OSSICLE A small bone, the term is usually applied to the three small bones of the middle ear – malleus, incus, and stapes – that conduct sound from the eardrum to the inner ear. (See EAR.)

OSSIFICATION The formation of bone. In early life, centres appear in the bones previously represented by cartilage or fibrous tissue, and from these the formation of true bone and deposit of lime salts proceed. When a fracture occurs, the bone mends by ossification of the clot which forms between the fragments. (See FRACTURES.) In old age an unnatural process of ossification often takes place in parts which should remain cartilaginous, e.g. in the cartilages of the larynx and of the ribs, making these parts unusually brittle.

OSTEITIS means inflammation in the substance of a bone. Traumatic osteitis is a condition particularly common in footballers, in which the victim complains of pain in the groin following exercise, particularly if this has involved much hip rotation. Examination reveals difficulty in spreading the legs and marked tenderness over the symphysis pubis. It responds well to rest and the administration of non-steroidal anti-inflammatory drugs (NSAIDS) such as ibuprofen or indomethacin.

OSTEITIS DEFORMANS (see PAGET'S DISEASE OF BONE).

OSTEITIS FIBROSA CYSTICA A pathological rather than a clinical entity. The term refers to the replacement of bone by a highly cellular and vascular connective tissue. It is the result of osteoclastic and osteoblastic activity and is due to excessive parathyroid activity. It is thus seen in a proportion of patients with primary hyperparathyroidism and in patients with uraemic osteodystrophy; that is, the secondary hyperparathyroidism that occurs in patients with chronic renal disease.

OSTEOARTHRITIS A term used for joint problems where the primary problem is seen as a change in structure of CARTILAGE and BONE, rather than an inflammatory SYNOVITIS. Osteoarthritis usually implies a loss of the central load-bearing area of articular hyaline cartilage by a process of fibrillation, fissuring and fragmentation. This is usually associated with outgrowth of cartilage at the articular margin with subsequent ossification to form bony outgrowths known as osteophytes. Unfortunately there is confusion because the term is also used to cover joint pain that appears to have a mechanical basis in the absence of clinical or radiographic evidence of cartilage loss. Osteophytes form with increasing age, whether or not there is significant cartilage loss, and in the elderly osteophytes may lead to local frictional symptoms, and in the spine nerve compression. Despite major efforts, it has proved impossible to produce a single clear definition of osteoarthritis and this probably reflects the muddled nature of a concept which will need replacing.

The important problem of loss of central load-bearing articular cartilage occurs increasingly with age but is by no means inevitable. It has a wide range of causes, of which some, like dysplasia and trauma, are known and others have yet to be identified. The main clinical problems occur in the hip and knee. The cartilage loss in the hip usually occurs in the sixth or seventh decade. It may affect both hips in fairly rapid succession, or only one hip and such patients often have no problems in other joints. Cartilage loss in the knee occurs from the fifth decade onwards and is often associated with cartilage loss in small joints in the hand and elsewhere. Cartilage loss in the distal interphalangeal joints of the hand is associated with the formation of bony swellings known as Heberden's nodes.

Treatment Management is largely directed at maintaining activity, with physical and social support as necessary. Analgesics may be of some value, particularly in the management of night pain. Non-steroidal anti-inflammatory agents may help patients with early morning stiffness and may also reduce pain on movement and night pain. Their benefit, however, tends to be less marked than in rheumatoid ARTHRITIS and their long-term usage has considerable toxicity problems. Advanced cartilage loss is best treated by joint replacement. Hip and knee-joint replacements – with a wide variety of artificial joints – are now common surgical procedures which greatly improve the mobility of affected individuals.

People with arthritis and their relatives can

obtain help and advice from Arthritis Care (see APPENDIX 2: ADDRESSES).

OSTEOCHONDRITIS Inflammation of both bone and cartilage. It is a not uncommon cause of backache in young people, particularly gymnasts.

OSTEOCHONDROSIS This includes a group of diseases involving degeneration of the centre of ossification (see BONE) in the growing bones of children and adolescents. They include Kohler's disease, OSGOOD-SCHLATTER'S DISEASE, and PERTHES' DISEASE.

OSTEOCYTE A bone cell formed from an osteoblast or bone-forming cell that has stopped its activity. The cell is embedded in the matrix of the bone.

OSTEOGENESIS IMPERFECTA A hereditary disease due to an inherited abnormality of COLLAGEN. It is characterized by extreme fragility of the skeleton, resulting in fractures and deformities. It may be accompanied by blue sclera (the outermost, normally white coat of the eyeball), transparent teeth, hypermobility (excessive range of movement) of the joints, deafness, and dwarfism (shortness of stature). The cause is not known, though there is some evidence that it may be associated with collagen formation (see COLLAGEN). Parents of affected children can obtain help and advice from the Brittle Bone Society (see APPENDIX 2: ADDRESSES).

OSTEOMALACIA is the adult form of RICKETS. It is due to inadequate mineralization of osteoid tissue caused by a deficiency of vitamin D. This deficiency may arise because of inadequate intake or it may be due to impaired absorption such as occurs in intestinal malabsorption. It may also be due to renal disease as the kidney is responsible for the hydroxylation of cholecalciferol, which has virtually no metabolic action, to dihydroxy-cholecalciferol, the metabolically active form of the vitamin. (See APPENDIX 5: VITAMINS.)

OSTEOMYELITIS Inflammation of the bone as a result of infection (see BONE, DISEASES OF).

OSTEOPATHY A system of healing in which diseases are treated by manipulating bones and other parts with the idea of thereby restoring functions in the bodily mechanism that have become deranged. Properly qualified osteopaths are included on the General Council and Register of Osteopaths (see APPENDIX 13: COMPLEMENTARY MEDICINE).

OSTEOPHYTES Bony spurs or projections. They occur most commonly at the margins of points involved in OSTEOARTHRITIS.

OSTEOPOROSIS A metabolic bone disease resulting from low bone mass (osteopenia) due to excessive bone resorption. Sufferers are prone to bone fractures from relatively minor trauma. Typical examples are the vertebral bodies, distal forearm and proximal femur. With bone densitometry it is now possible to determine individuals' risk of osteoporosis and monitor their response to treatment.

By the age of 90 one in two women and one in six men are likely to sustain an osteoporosis-related fracture. The incidence of fractures is increasing more than would be expected from the ageing of the population, which may reflect changing patterns of exercise or diet.

Osteoporosis may be classified as primary or secondary. Primary consists of type 1 osteoporosis, due to accelerated trabecular bone loss, probably as a result of OESTROGEN deficiency. This typically leads to crush fractures of vertebral bodies and fractures of the distal forearm in women in their 60s and 70s. Type 2 osteoporosis, by contrast, results from the slower age-related cortical and travecular bone loss that occurs in both sexes. It typically leads to fractures of the proximal femur in elderly people.

Secondary osteoporosis accounts for about 20 per cent of cases in women and 40 per cent of cases in men. Subgroups include endocrine (THYROTOXICOSIS, primary HYPERPARATHYROIDISM, CUSHING'S SYNDROME and HYPOGONADISM); gastrointestinal (malabsorption syndrome, e.g., COELIAC DISEASE, or liver disease, e.g., primary biliary CIRRHOSIS); rheumatological (RHEUMATOID ARTHRITIS or ANKYLOSING SPONDYLITIS); malignancy (multiple MYELOMA or metastatic CARCINOMA) and drugs (CORTICOSTEROIDS, HEPARIN). Additional risk factors for osteoporosis include smoking, high alcohol intake, physical inactivity, thin body type and heredity.

Individuals at risk of osteopenia, or with an osteoporosis-related fracture, need investigation with spinal radiography and bone densitometry. A small fall in bone density results in a large increase in the risk of fracture, which has important implications for preventing and treating osteoporosis.

Treatment Antiresorptive drugs: hormone replacement therapy – also valuable in treating menopausal symptoms and cardiovascular morbidity; treatment for at least five years is necessary, and prolonged use may increase risk of breast cancer. Cyclical oral administration of disodium etidronate – one of the biphosphonate group of drugs – with calcium carbonate is also used (poor absorption means the etidronate must be taken on an empty stomach). Calcitonin – currently available as a subcutaneous injection; a nasal preparation with better tolerance is being developed. Calcium (1000 mg daily) seems useful in older patients, although probably ineffective in perimenopausal women, and it is a safe preparation. Vitamin D and calcium – recent evidence suggests value for elderly patients. Anabolic steroids, though androgenic side-effects (masculinization) make these unacceptable for most women.

With established osteoporosis, the aim of treatment is to relieve pain (with analgesics and physical measures, e.g., lumbar support) and reduce the risk of further fractures: improvement of bone mass, the prevention of falls, and general physiotherapy, encouraging a healthier lifestyle with more daily exercise.

Further information is available from the National Osteoporosis Society (see APPENDIX 2: ADDRESSES).

OSTEOSARCOMA or OSTEOGENIC SARCOMA The most common, and most malignant, tumour of bone. It occurs predominantly in older children and young adults. The commonest site for it is at the ends of the long bones of the body: i.e. the femur, tibia and humerus. Treatment is by chemotherapy and surgical reconstruction or amputation of the affected limb. The 5-year survival rate is over 70 per cent.

OSTEOTOMY The operation of cutting of a bone.

OS TRIGONUM A small accessory bone behind the ankle joint which is present in about 7 per cent of the population. It may be damaged by energetic springing from the toes in ballet, jumping or fast bowling.

OTITIS Inflammation of the ear. (See EAR, DISEASES OF.)

OTOLOGY is that branch of medical science which is concerned with disorders and diseases of the organ of hearing, one practising this branch being called an OTOLOGIST.

OTORHINOLARYNGOLOGY Sometimes called otolaryngology, this is the study and treatment of diseases of the ear, nose and throat (ENT). The relevant specialist is called an otorhinolaryngologist.

OTORRHOEA Discharge from the ear. (See EAR, DISEASES OF.)

OTOSCLEROSIS A condition in which abnormal bone is deposited around the footplate of the stapes in the middle ear (see EAR) resulting in fixation of that bone and causing a progressive conductive hearing loss due to immobility of the ossicular chain. There is an hereditary pattern to the disease and its onset is usually in the third decade. It tends to be slightly commoner in women and is often accelerated in pregnancy. Treatment involves supplying a hearing aid or performing an operation known as stapedectomy. Rarely the deposition of abnormal bone may affect the inner ear as well.

OTOSCOPE (see AURISCOPE).

OUABAIN Also known as strophanthin-G, this is a glycoside obtained from the African tree *Strophanthus gratus*, once used as an arrow poison. It is a heart stimulant used to treat heart failure and other heart conditions. Its action and side-effects are similar to those of DIGITALIS.

OUTPATIENT A patient attending hospital on a day basis. He or she is not admitted to a bed. Most patients attend an outpatients' department after referral for a specialist opinion by their general practitioner. An increasing number of investigations and treatments, including surgery, are being done on an outpatient basis.

OVARIES The main female reproductive organs which produce the ova (egg cells) and steroid HORMONES in a regular cycle (see MENSTRUATION) in response to hormones (see GONADOTROPHINS) from the anterior PITUITARY GLAND. Situated one on each side of the uterus in the lower abdomen, each ovary contains numerous FOLLICLES within which the ova develop. Only a small proportion of them reach maturity, when the ovum is described as a Graafian follicle. Ovulation occurs and, if the ovum is fertilized, a pregnancy may develop (see ENDOCRINE GLANDS and also OESTRADIOL, OESTROGEN, PROGESTERONE).

OVARIES, DISEASES OF Oophoritis (infection of the ovaries) rarely occurs alone, except in viral infections such as mumps. Usually it is associated with infection of the FALLOPIAN TUBES (SALPINGITIS). It may occur as a complication of a miscarriage, a therapeutic abortion, or the birth of a baby. Cases not associated with pregnancy typically result from sexual activity. The most common organisms involved are Chlamydia, *E. coli*, and *Neisseria gonorrhoea*. Cervical swabs should be sent for culture and analgesics given, together with the appropriate antibiotics.

Failure of ovulation is the cause of infertility in around a third of couples seeking help with conception. It may also lead to MENSTRUAL problems, such as an irregular menstrual cycle or menorrhagia. An uncommon cause of failure of ovulation is polycystic ovary syndrome often associated with acne, hirsutism, and obesity. Treatment depends on the symptoms. Early ovarian failure is the cause of premature menopause. Treatment consists of hormone replacement therapy using a combination of oestrogen and progestogen.

Ovarian tumours may be physiological or pathological. Physiological cysts (for example, follicular cysts) result from ovulation. Rupture may lead to transient pain, and no specific treatment is required. Rarely, the ruptured cyst causes extensive bleeding, and the condition may be mistaken for an ectopic pregnancy.

Diagnosis, by laparoscopy, leads to treatment aimed at stopping the bleeding.

Pathological tumours, benign or malignant, may cause pain by putting pressure on the bladder or rectum, or as a result of rupture, torsion, haemorrhage, or infection. In young women the commonest benign tumour is a dermoid cyst, while in older women fibroma (see UTERUS, DISEASES OF) is more common. All benign tumours should be removed surgically in order to exclude malignancy.

Malignant tumours may be primary (arising in the ovary) or secondary (metastases from a cancer developing in another organ). Treatment depends on the site and type of the primary tumour.

Around 5,000 women a year are diagnosed as having ovarian cancer in England and Wales. Unfortunately it is not readily detected in its early stages; around 85 per cent of women present after the tumour has metastasized. Early tumours present with symptoms similar to benign tumours, while late ones present with abdominal distension and vague gastrointestinal symptoms. The disease is most common in menopausal women. Earlier diagnosis and treatment can be achieved by the ultrasound screening test for ovarian cancer which is being developed. Treatment is surgical, aimed at totally removing the tumour mass. Nowadays radiotherapy is only used for palliation. Chemotherapy is often given to patients with ovarian metastases, or who have residual disease after surgery. The most active cytotoxic agents are paclitaxol, especially when it is combined with cisplatin.

OVARIOTOMY or OÖPHORECTOMY The operation of removal of an ovary or an ovarian tumour.

OVULATION The development and release of an OVUM (egg) from the ovary into the FALLOPIAN TUBE. Ovulation is initiated by the secretion of luteinizing hormone by the anterior PITUITARY gland and occurs half way through the menstrual cycle. If the ovum is not fertilized, it is lost during MENSTRUATION.

OVUM The single cell derived from the female, out of which a future individual arises, after its union with the spermatozoon derived from the male. It is about 35 micrometres in diameter. (See FETUS; OVARIES.)

OXALIC ACID This is an irritant poison that is used domestically for cleaning purposes. It is also found in many plants including rhubarb and sorrel. Oxalic acid, when swallowed, produces burning of the mouth and throat, vomiting of blood, breathlessness and circulatory collapse. Calcium salts, lime water or milk should be given by mouth. An injection of calcium gluconate is an antidote.

OXIMETRY The measurement by an oximeter of the proportion of oxygenated HAEMOGLOBIN in the blood.

OXPRENOLOL (see ADRENERGIC RECEPTORS).

OXYCEPHALY, or STEEPLE HEAD A deformity of the skull in which the forehead is high and the top of the head pointed. There is also poor vision and the eyes bulge.

OXYGEN A colourless and odourless gas of molecular weight 32. It constitutes just less than 21 per cent of the Earth's atmosphere. Though not itself flammable, it supports combustion. It was first isolated by Priestley in 1772. Medical and industrial oxygen are manufactured by the fractional distillation of liquid air. In Britain it is supplied as a compressed gas at high pressure (13600 kilopascals (KPa)) in cylinders which are black with white shoulders. In hospitals oxygen is often stored as a liquid in insulated tanks and controlled evaporation allows the gas to be supplied via a pipeline at a much lower pressure.

Oxygen is essential for life. It is absorbed via the lungs and is transported by HAEMOGLOBIN within the ERYTHROCYTES to the tissues. Within the individual cell it is involved in the production of adenosine triphosphate (ATP), a compound that stores chemical energy for muscle cells, by the oxidative metabolism of fats and carbohydrates. HYPOXIA causes anaerobic metabolism with a resulting build-up in lactic acid, the result of muscle cell activity. If severe enough, the lack of ATP causes a breakdown in cellular function and the death of the individual.

When hypoxia occurs, it may be corrected by giving supplemental oxygen. This is usually given via a face mask or nasal prongs or in severe cases during artificial ventilation of the lungs. Some indications for oxygen therapy are high altitude, ventilatory failure, heart failure, ANAEMIA, PULMONARY HYPERTENSION, CARBON MONOXIDE poisoning, anaesthesia and postoperative recovery. In some conditions – e.g. severe infections with anaerobic BACTERIA and CARBON MONOXIDE poisoning – hyperbaric oxygen therapy has been used.

OXYGEN DEFICIT In a resting individual the potential oxygen supply to the tissues is greater than its consumption. During heavy exercise the energy required by the tissues is greater than can be supplied by aerobic cellular metabolism and the additional energy is supplied by a biochemical reaction called anaerobic metabolism. There is a build-up of lactate – a product of lactic acid – from anaerobic metabolism which is ultimately oxidized after conversion to citrate and metabolism via the citric acid cycle. The increased amount of oxygen above resting concentrations which needs to be consumed to perform this metabolism is known as the oxygen debt or deficit.

OXYGEN TOXICITY This occurs when high concentrations of oxygen are breathed for long periods. It is thought that under hyperoxic conditions there is increased production of chemicals called free radicals by cellular metabolism which damages cells and organs. The most susceptible organs are the lungs, eyes (particularly in the neonate), central nervous system and gut. Oxygen toxicity in human lungs causes an acute OEDEMA followed by fibrosis and PULMONARY HYPERTENSION. In the neonate retrolental fibroplasia occurs and central-nervous-system damage may result in the infant having fits. Several factors are involved in toxicity and there is no absolute relationship to time or concentration, though inspired concentrations of under 50 per cent are probably safe for long periods.

OXYTETRACYCLINE is an antibiotic derived from a soil organism, Streptomyces rimosus. Its range of antibacterial activity is comparable to that of TETRACYCLINE.

OXYTOCIN is the extract isolated from the pituitary posterior lobe which stimulates the uterine muscle to contract. Oxytocin produced by the PITUITARY GLAND stimulates the flow of milk in breast-feeding mothers. It can also be synthesized. The synthetic form is used to induce or assist labour in pregnancy and childbirth and also to encourage the expelling of the PLACENTA (afterbirth). Sometimes it is given to a woman who has had an incomplete MISCARRIAGE. There have been criticisms that oxytocin is used too often to induce labour for social reasons or for the convenience of obstetric departments. (See PITUITARY BODY.)

OXYURIASIS Another name for the threadworm.

OZAENA A chronic disease of the nose of an inflammatory nature, combined with atrophy of the mucous membrane and the formation of extremely foul-smelling crusts in the interior of the nose. (See NOSE, DISEASES OF.)

OZONE A specially active and poisonous form of oxygen in which three volumes of the gas are condensed into the space ordinarily occupied by two. It has a characteristic smell and is a strong oxidizing agent. Formed when an electrical charge is passed through oxygen or air, it is found at high altitudes in the atmosphere where it screens out much of the sun's ultraviolet radiation. The ozone layer, as it is called, is being damaged by pollutant gases from earth and, unless this damage is reversed, lethal quantities of ultraviolet radiation could penetrate to the earth's surface and warms the world's climates, with long-term damage to the environment.

P

PACEMAKER A cardiac or artificial pacemaker is a device that helps a faulty heart to maintain normal rhythm. It consists of a battery that stimulates the heart by an electric current passed through an insulated wire which is attached either to the surface of the ventricle (epicardial pacemaker) or to the heart lining (endocardial pacemaker). In a normal heart the regular electrical impulses are initiated by a special area of tissue (sinoatrial node). A cardiac pacemaker is used when a person's sinoatrial node is malfunctioning or when there is an impairment to the passage of normal impulses. Some devices send out signals at a fixed rate, others monitor the rate and, when it falters in any way, stimulate regular contractions. Implantation is carried out under a local anaesthetic, and the lithium batteries can last for several years. People with pacemakers should avoid any source of powerful electromagnetic radiation – radio or radar transmitters or airport security screens. (See CARDIAC PACEMAKER.)

PACHYDERMIA Hypertrophy or thickening of the skin. Pachydermia laryngis is a name applied to thickening of the vocal cords due to chronic inflammation or irritation.

PACHYMENINGITIS Inflammation of the dura mater of the brain and spinal cord. (See MENINGITIS.)

PACINIAN CORPUSCLES, or lamellated corpuscles, are minute bulbs at the ends of the nerves scattered through the skin and subcutaneous tissue, and forming one of the end-organs for sensation (see SKIN).

PACKED CELL VOLUME That fraction of the blood's total volume made up of red cells. The packed cell volume is established by centrifuging blood in a tube and measuring the depth of the column of red cells as a fraction of the whole column of blood. (See HAEMATOCRIT.)

PACLITAXEL A cytotoxic drug that is the first of a new group called taxanes. Given by intravenous transfusion, it is used under specialist supervision for the treatment of primary and secondary treatment of advanced ovarian cancer and for secondary treatment of breast cancer. It can be used with CISPLANTIN. Side-effects include hypersensitivity, myelosuppression, cardiac arrhythmias and peripheral neuropathy. Only a minority of patients respond to paclitaxel but when it works the results are often long lasting.

PAEDIATRICS means the branch of medicine dealing with diseases of children (see also NEONATOLOGY).

PAEDOPHILIA A perverse sexual attraction to children of either sex. Paedophiles are nearly always male and may have heterosexual, homosexual or bisexual orientation. Heterosexual activity with individuals under 16 is illegal in the United Kingdom and the age of consent for homosexual activity is 18. Paedophiles suffer from personality problems rather than overt psychoses and the origins of their behaviour may lie in their own early sexual experiences. Fondling of children occurs more often than sexual intercourse and, although research is sketchy, it is probable that child abuse within families and in child-care homes is commoner than was generally realized. (See CHILD ABUSE.)

PAGET'S DISEASE OF BONE, or OSTEITIS DEFORMANS A chronic disease in which the bones – especially those of the skull, limbs, and spine – gradually become thick and also soft, causing them to bend. It is said to be the commonest bone disease in the world, and it is estimated that some 600,000 people in England may suffer from it. It seldom occurs under the age of 40. Pain is its most unpleasant manifestation. The cause is not known, and there is no known cure, but satisfactory results are being obtained from the use of CALCITONIN and a group of drugs known as BIPHOSPHONATES (e.g. etidronate). Those with the disease can obtain help and advice from the National Association for the Relief of Paget's Disease (see APPENDIX 2: ADDRESSES).

PAIN Pain is an unpleasant sensory and emotional experience associated with actual or potential tissue damage or described in terms of such damage (International Association for the Study of Pain, 1979). Pain is perceived in the cerebral cortex (see BRAIN) and is always subjective. Stimuli which cause pain usually damage tissues. Pain is always unpleasant, and sometimes sensations that would usually be benign can be perceived as painful (e.g. allodynia (extreme tenderness of the skin) or dysaesthesia (unpleasant skin sensations resulting from partial damage to sensory nerve fibres)). Pain may be broadly defined as being acute or chronic.

Acute pain is caused by internal or external injury or disease. It warns the individual that harm or damage is occurring and stimulates them to take avoiding or protective action. With either effective treatment of disease or injury and/or the natural healing process the pain resolves, though some acute pain syndromes may develop into chronic pain. Stimuli which are sufficiently intense potentially to damage tissue will cause the stimulation of specific receptors known as NOCICEPTORS. Damage to tissues releases substances which stimulate the nociceptors. On the surface of the body there is a high density of nociceptors and each area of the body is supplied by nerves from a specifici spinal segment or level. This allows the brain to localize the source of the pain accu-

rately. Pain from internal structures and organs is more difficult to localize and is often felt in some more superficial structure. For example, irritation of the diaphragm is often felt as pain in the shoulder as the nerves from both structures enter the spinal cord at the same level (often the structures have developed from the same parts of the embryo). This is known as referred pain.

The impulses from nociceptors travel along nerves to the SPINAL CORD. Within the SPINAL CORD there is modulation of the pain 'messages' by other incoming sensory modalities and descending input from the brain (Melzack and Walls' gate-control theory). This modulation involves endogenous morphinelike molecules (the ENDORPHINS and ENCEPHALINS) amongst many other pain-transmitting and -modulating substances. The modified input then passes up the spinal cord through the thalamus to the cerebral cortex. Thus the amount of pain 'felt' may be altered by the emotional state of the individual and by other incoming sensations. Once pain is perceived then 'action' is taken. This involves withdrawal of the area being damaged, vocalization, and AUTONOMIC NERVOUS SYSTEM response and examination of the painful area. Analysis of the event using memory will occur and appropriate action taken to reduce pain and treat the damage.

Chronic pain may be defined in several ways. It is often defined as pain resistant to one month's treatment or pain persisting one month beyond the usual course of an acute illness or injury. Some doctors may also arbitrarily choose the figure of six months. Chronic pain differs from acute pain. The physiological response is different and pain may be either caused by stimuli which do not usually cause the perception of pain or pain may arise within nerves or the central nervous system with no apparent external stimulation. It seldom has a physiological protective function in the way acute pain has. Also, chronic pain may be self perpetuating. First, if individuals gain a psychological advantage from having pain, they may continue to do so (e.g. gaining attention from family or health professionals, etc.). The nervous system itself alters when pain is longstanding in such a way that it becomes more sensitive to painful inputs and tends to perpetuate the pain. This is because the pathways within the central nervous system are not constant. They are thought to have some plasticity and may be altered by, for example, chronic painful stimuli.

Treatment The treatment of pain depends on its nature and cause. Acute pain is generally treated by curing the underlying complaint and prescribing analgesics or using local anaesthetic techniques. Many hospitals now have acute pain teams for the management of postoperative and other types of acute pain. Chronic pain is often treated in pain clinics. They consist of doctors (who in Britain are usually anaesthetists), nurses, psychologists and psychiatrists, physiotherapists and complementary therapists. A multidisciplinary approach is taken to the treatment of chronic pain. Patients are usually referred from other hospital specialists (though some may be referred by GPs). They will usually have been given a diagnosis and exhausted the medical and surgical treatment of their underlying condition. In the pain clinic patients are assessed and the type of pain that they are suffering from diagnosed. A course of treatment will then be decided upon and performed.

A variety of pharmacological therapies is used to treat chronic pain. All the usual analgesics may be employed and opioids are often used in the terminal treatment of cancer pain.

ANTICONVULSANT and ANTIDEPRESSANT drugs are also used because they alter the transmission of pain within the central nervous system and may actually treat the chronic pain syndrome.

Many local anaesthetic techniques are used. Myofascial pain – pain affecting muscles and connective tissues – is treated by the injection of local anaesthetic into tender spots and nerves may be blocked either as a diagnostic procedure or as treatment. EPIDURAL anaesthetic injections are also used in the same way and all these treatments may be repeated at intervals over many months in an attempt to cure or at least reduce the pain. For intractable pain, nerves are sometimes destroyed using injections of ALCOHOL or PHENOL or by applying CRYOTHERAPY or radiofrequency waves. Intractable or terminal pain may be treated by destroying nerves surgically, and, rarely, the pain pathways within the spinal cord are severed by cordotomy (though this is generally only used in terminal care).

Acupuncture and TENS (TRANSCUTANEOUS ELECTRICAL NERVE STIMULATION) are used for a variety of pain syndromes, particularly myofascial or musculoskeletal pain. It is thought that they work by increasing the release of endorphins and encephalins. It is possible to implant electrodes within the epidural space to stimulate directly the nerves as they traverse this space before passing into the spinal cord.

Physiotherapy is often used, particularly in the treatment of chronic backache, where pain may be reduced by improving posture and strengthening muscles with careful exercises. Relaxation techniques and psychotherapy are also used both to treat chronic pain and help patients cope better with their disability.

Some types of chronic pain are caused by injury to sympathetic nerves or may be relieved by interrupting conduction in sympathetic nerves. This may be done in several ways. The nerves may be blocked using local anaesthetic or permanently destroyed using alcohol, phenol or by surgery. If a limb is being treated then a GUANETHIDINE block may be used.

Many of these techniques may be used in the management of cancer pain. Opioid drugs are often used by a variety of routes and methods and management of these patients concentrates on the control of symptoms and providing a good quality of life.

PALATE   The partition between the cavity of the mouth, below, and that of the nose, above. It consists of the hard palate towards the front, which is composed of a bony plate covered below by the mucous membrane of the mouth, above by that of the nose; and of the soft palate further back, in which a muscular layer, composed of nine small muscles, is similarly covered. The hard palate extends a little further back than the wisdom teeth, and is formed by the maxillary and palate bones. The soft palate is concave towards the mouth and convex towards the nose, and it ends behind in a free border, at the centre of which is the prolongation known as the uvula. When food or air is passing through the mouth, as in the acts of swallowing, coughing, or vomiting, the soft palate is drawn upwards so as to touch the back wall of the throat and shut off the cavity of the nose. Movements of the soft palate, by changing the shape of the mouth and nose cavities, are important in the production of speech.

PALATE, MALFORMATIONS OF   The commonest deformity of the palate is cleft palate, which is a result of faulty embryonic development in which the two sides of the palate fail to fuse or only fuse in part. If the cleft extends the full length with bilateral clefts at the front of the MAXILLA, it may be accompanied by a cleft lip and disruption in the development of

Cleft lip and palate (front view).

the front teeth. About 1 in 500 babies is born with a cleft lip and 1 in 1,000 have a cleft palate. If the parents are affected, the risk is three times that of the normal population; if one child has a deformity, the risk for a subsequent child is higher. Associated abnormalities include tongue tie, malpositioning of the MANDIBLE and fluid in the middle EAR.

Cleft-palate and hare-lip should, if possible, be rectified by operation, because both are a serious drawback to feeding in early life, while later, hare-lip is a great disfigurement, and the voice may be affected. When there is merely a slight degree of hare-lip, it is usual to operate when the infant is about 10 weeks and weighing

1 nostrils
2 primary palate
3 lips
4 palate
5 uvula

Normal palate viewed from below.

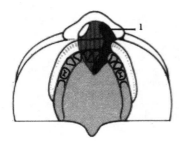

1 Unilateral cleft palate, involving lip and upper jaw

Cleft palate viewed from below.

at least 10 lbs. When the notch is very large, it may be necessary to wait for several months. The closure of a large cleft in the palate, which is a more formidable operation, is usually deferred until 6 to 12 months. The operations performed vary greatly in details, but all consist in paring the edges of the gap and drawing the soft parts together across it.

Further operations may be required to improve the appearance of the nose and lip and to improve speech.

Parents of such children can obtain help and advice from the Cleft Lip and Palate Association, or the Dental and Maxillofacial Department, Hospital for Sick Children, Great Ormond Street (see APPENDIX 2: ADDRESSES).

PALILALIA Also called paliphrasia, this means the involuntary repetition of words or sentences. It is a symptom of GILLES DE LA TOURETTE'S SYNDROME.

PALINDROMIC An adjective describing symptoms or diseases that recur.

PALLIATIVE A term applied to the treatment of incurable diseases, in which the aim is to mitigate the sufferings of the patient, not to effect a cure (see HOSPICE).

PALLOR Unusual paleness of the skin caused by a reduced flow of blood or a deficiency in normal pigments. Pallor may be a sign of fright, shock, anaemia, or other diseases.

PALPATION Examination of the surface of the body and the size, shape, and movements of the internal organs, by laying the flat of the hand upon the skin.

PALPEBRAL Relating to the eyelid.

PALPITATION Forcible and/or irregular beating of the heart such that the person becomes conscious of its action.

Causes As a rule a person is not conscious of the beating of the heart, but when the nervous system is unduly excited its action may become unpleasantly palpable. A disorder of the rhythm of the heart (arrhythmia) may cause palpitations. Sudden emotions, such as fright, and occasionally dyspepsia, may bring it on. Another cause consists in over-use of tobacco, tea, coffee, or alcohol. Sometimes it may appear in people with organic heart disease.

Symptoms There may simply be a fluttering of the heart and a feeling of faintness, or the heart may be felt pounding and the arteries throbbing, causing great distress. The subject may be conscious of the heart missing beats.

Treatment Although these symptoms can be unpleasant, they do not necessarily signify serious disease. Moderate exercise is a good thing. If the person is a smoker, he or she should stop. Tea, coffee, alcohol or other stimulants should be taken sparingly. If symptoms persist or are severe, the individual should see a doctor and any underlying disorder should be investigated and treated. The BETA ADRENORECEPTOR ANTAGONISTS are the most useful drugs in controlling the palpitations of anxiety and those due to some cardiac arrhythmias.

PALSY Another name for paralysis. (See PARALYSIS.)

PALUDRINE (see PROGUANIL HYDROCHLORIDE).

PAN- A prefix meaning all or completely.

PANACEA is a term applied to a remedy for all diseases, or more usually to a remedy which benefits many different diseases.

PANCARDITIS Inflammation of the pericardium, myocardium, and endocardium at the same time.

PANCREAS A long secreting gland situated in the back of the abdomen, at the level of the first and second lumbar vertebrae. It lies behind the lower part of the stomach, an expanded portion, called the head of the pancreas, occupying the bend formed by the duodenum or first part of the small intestine, whilst a long portion known as the body extends to the left, ending in the tail, which rests against the spleen. A duct runs through the whole gland from left to right, joined by many small branches in its course, and, leaving the head of the gland, unites with the bile duct from the liver to open into the side of the small intestine about 7·5 to 10 cm (3 or 4 inches) below the outlet of the stomach.

The gland resembles one of the salivary glands, being composed of tubes of columnar cells bound together by loose connective tissue.

Scattered through the pancreas are collections of cells known as the ISLETS OF LANGERHANS, of which there are around a million in a normal individual. These do not communicate with the duct of the gland, and the internal secretion of the pancreas – INSULIN – is formed by these cells and absorbed directly into the blood.

Functions The most obvious function of the pancreas is the formation of the pancreatic juice, which is poured into the small intestine after the partially digested food has left the stomach. This is the most important of the digestive juices, is alkaline in reaction, and contains, in addition to various salts, four enzymes. These enzymes are: TRYPSIN and CHYMOTRYPSIN, which digest proteins; AMYLASE, which converts starchy foods into the disaccharide maltose; lipase, which breaks up fats. For the action of these see DIGESTION.

Inadequate production of insulin by the islets of Langerhans leads to the condition known as DIABETES MELLITUS. In addition to insulin, another hormone is produced by the pancreas. This is glucagon which has the opposite effect to insulin and raises the blood sugar by promoting the breakdown of liver glycogen.

PANCREAS, DISEASES OF An uncommon but significant disease of the pancreas is acute pancreatitis. This unpredictable disease has a mortality of 5 to 10 per cent. It may start gradually or suddenly, usually accompanied by severe abdominal pain which often radiates through to the back. Biliary tract disease and alcohol account for 80 per cent of patients admitted with acute pancreatitis, while other causes include drugs (see AZATHIPRINE and DIURETICS) and infections such as mumps. Patients are acutely ill with TACHYCARDIA, fever and low blood pressure; many go into shock. The condition may be mistaken for a perforated PEPTIC ULCER, except that in acute pancreatitis the blood concentration of AMYLASE is raised. The main complication is the formation of a PSEUDOCYST. Treatment includes intravenous feeding and ANTICHOLINERGIC and ANALGESIC drugs. Regular measurements of blood GLUCOSE, CALCIUM, amylase, and blood gases are required. Abdominal ULTRASOUND may iden-

tify GALLSTONES and pseudocysts. If the patient deteriorates he or she should be admitted for intensive care as haemorrhagic pancreatic necrosis may be developing. Laparotomy and debridement may be called for.

The incidence of pancreatic cancer is rising: around 7,000 cases are now diagnosed annually in the UK, accounting for 1 to 2 per cent of all malignancies. There is an established association with heavy cigarette smoking, and it is twice as common in patients with DIABETES MELLITUS as compared with the general population. Cancer of the pancreas is hard to diagnose and by the time symptoms occur the tumour may be difficult to treat surgically; palliative bypass surgery may be the only procedure.

Chronic pancreatitis may be painless; it leads to pancreatic failure causing malabsorption and diabetes mellitus, and the pancreas becomes calcified with shadowing on X-RAYS. The malsabsorption is treated by a low fat diet with pancreatic enzyme supplements, the diabetes with insulin and pain is treated appropriately; surgery may be required.

PANCREATIN or PANCREATIC JUICE contains the four powerful enzymes trypsin, chemotrypsin, lipase, and amylase, which continue the digestion of foods started in the stomach (see DIGESTION). It is given by mouth for the relief of pancreatic deficiency in conditions such as pancreatitis (see PANCREAS, DISEASES OF) and fibrocystic disease of the pancreas (see CYSTIC FIBROSIS). It is also used for the preparation of predigested, or so-called peptonized, foods, such as milk and some starchy foods.

PANCYTOPENIA A fall in the number of RED and WHITE BLOOD CELLS as well as of platelets. The condition is found in aplastic ANAEMIA, bone-marrow tumours, enlarged SPLEEN, and other disorders.

PANDEMIC An EPIDEMIC that has spread so widely that very many people in different countries are affected. A well-known example was the Black Death, the epidemic PLAGUE, caused by the bacterium *Yersinia pestis*, that devastated European populations in the Middle Ages, killing more than a third of the people. A modern pandemic is AIDS/HIV.

PANHYSTERECTOMY An operation by which the uterus is completely removed.

PANIC ATTACKS or DISORDERS are recurrent short episodes of acute distress. The sufferer may also be mentally confused and have a fear of impending death. Initially these attacks tend to occur unexpectedly but, if recurrent, they often become associated with certain places such as a confined space (lift) or among crowds. Symptoms include a feeling of breathing difficulties, including overbreathing, PALPITATIONS, dizziness, sweating, faintness and pains in the chest. Attacks are usually short (a few minutes) but not often associated with physical illness, though victims may have an anxiety disorder or PHOBIAS. If troublesome or disabling, they can be treated symptomatically with short-term ANXIOLYTIC DRUGS or on a long-term basis with BEHAVIOUR THERAPY.

PANNICULITIS Inflammation of the subcutaneous fat, and may occur anywhere on the body surface.

PANNUS Blood vessels growing into the cornea beneath its epithelium. Seen in trachoma and to a lesser extent in patients who are long-term soft-contact-lens wearers.

PANTOTHENIC ACID This has now been prepared synthetically and is part of the vitamin B complex. It is known as the chick anti-dermatitis factor because if it is absent from the chick's diet the bird develops dermatitis, and degeneration of nerve-fibres in the spinal cord also occurs. In rats lack of pantothenic acid produces greying of the hair, but there is no evidence that in man greying is due to lack of this vitamin. It plays an important part in the transfer of acetyl groups in the body's METABOLISM and it is one of the essential constituents of the diet. The daily requirement is probably around 10 milligrams. It is widely distributed in foodstuffs, both animal and vegetable. Yeast, liver, and egg-yolk are particularly rich sources. (See APPENDIX 5: VITAMINS.)

PAPANICOLAOU TEST (see CERVICAL SMEAR).

PAPAVERETUM This consists of the hydrochlorides of alkaloids of OPIUM. It relaxes smooth MUSCLE and has the pain-relieving and narcotic effects of MORPHINE, but fewer side-effects. It is largely used to prepare patients for anaesthesia.

PAPILLA A small projection, such as those with which the corium of the skin is covered, and which project into the epidermis and make its union with the corium more intimate; or those covering the tongue and projecting from its surface.

PAPILLITIS Inflammation of any papilla, but especially of the prominence formed by the end of the optic nerve in the retina, also known as optic neuritis.

PAPILLOEDEMA Swelling of the optic disc specifically due to raised intra-cranial pressure.

PAPILLOMA Proliferation of epidermis or epithelium to form a tumour. Benign papillomas are common in the skin and are sometimes viral in origin. BLADDER papilloma may cause HAEMATURIA.

PAPOVA VIRUSES These include the human papilloma viruses (HPV) of which nearly a hundred strains have been identified. HPV cause verrucae on skin and, less often, mucous membranes of mouth, larynx, genitalia and the cervix. Some strains may predispose to eventual cancer.

PAPULE Small (less than 5 mm) solid elevation of the skin or mucous membranes. A larger lesion is called a nodule.

PARA- A prefix meaning near, aside from, or beyond.

PARA-AMINO SALICYLIC ACID One of the early antituberculous antibiotics. It tended to cause dyspepsia and has been replaced by newer antituberculous drugs with fewer side-effects. The first-line drugs for tuberculosis are now rifampicin, isoniazid, and ethambutol. (See TUBERCULOSIS.)

PARACENTESIS The puncture by hollow needle or TROCAR and CANNULA of any body cavity (e.g. abdominal, pleural, pericardial), for tapping or aspirating fluid pathologically accumulated. (See ASPIRATION.)

PARACETAMOL A non-opioid analgesic similar in efficacy to aspirin, but without any demonstrable anti-inflammatory activity. It also has the advantage over aspirin of causing less gastric irritation. It is indicated for mild to moderate pain and pyrexia in a dose of 0.5–1g by mouth (maximum 4 doses every 24 hours).

PARACETAMOL POISONING Paracetamol is one of the safest drugs when taken in the correct dosage but overdose is very common, usually as an intentional overdose or sometimes as an inadvertent overdosage, either because of inadequate pain relief from a therapeutic dose (leading to increased frequency of dosing) or by taking a combination of preparations without realizing that they all contain paracetamol. Susceptibility to paracetamol overdose varies, some patients are more at risk (e.g. alcoholics). Initially there may be no symptoms following an overdose. Alternatively there may be nausea, vomiting, abdominal pain and pallor. Then 16 to 24 hours after ingestion liver damage becomes evident and by 72 to 120 hours the subject may have jaundice, COAGULATION abnormalities, HEPATIC failure, renal failure, ENCEPHALOPATHY and coma. Treatment involves the administration of antidotes such as METHIONINE (within 8 hours) orally or intravenous ACETYLCYSTEINE.

PARAESTHESIA A term applied to unusual feelings, apart from mere increase, or loss, of sensation, experienced by a patient without any external cause: for example, hot flushes, numbness, tingling, itching. Various paraesthesiae form a common symptom in some nervous diseases.

PARAFFIN The general name used to designate a series of saturated hydrocarbon compounds deriviued from petroleum.

Liquid paraffin, it is used in the treatment of constipation. Externally, the hard and soft paraffins are used in various consistencies, being very useful as ointments and lubricants.

PARAGANGLION One of the small ovoid collections of cells occurring in the walls of the ganglia of the SYMPATHETIC NERVOUS SYSTEM adjacent to the SPINAL CORD. They are CHROMAFFIN cells and sometimes secrete ADRENALINE.

PARAGRAPHIA Misplacement of words, or of letters in words, or wrong spelling, or use of wrong words in writing as a result of a lesion in the speech region of the brain.

PARAINFLUENZA VIRUSES These are included in the paramyxovirus (see MYXOVIRUSES) and divided into four types, all of which cause infection of the respiratory system. Infection with type 3 begins in May, reaches a maximum in July or August and returns to baseline level in October. Types 1 and 2 are predominantly winter viruses. Children are commonly affected and the manifestations include CROUP, fever, and a rash.

PARALDEHYDE A clear, colourless liquid with a penetrating ethereal (see ETHER) odour, it may be given by mouth, rectally, or occasionally in intramuscular injection. The drug's prime use is as a hypnotic in mentally unstable patients. It is also indicated as an anticonvulsant in STATUS EPILEPTICUS (after initial intravenous DIAZEPAM) and TETANUS. Its unpleasant taste restricts its use but this has the advantage that it usually prevents the patient from becoming an addict. Nevertheless, it has occasionally been used in the past as a drug of ADDICTION. Caution is important in treating patients with bronchopulmonary disease or hepatic impairment; and intramuscular injection near the sciatic nerve should be avoided, as it may cause severe CAUSALGIA. Adverse effects include rashes; pain and sterile abscess after intramuscular injection; rectal irritation after enema.

PARALYSIS, or PALSY This is loss of muscular power due to some disorder of the nervous system. Weakness, rather than total movement loss, is sometimes described as paresis. Paralysis may be temporary or permanent and may be accompanied by loss of feeling.

Paralysis due to brain disease The most com-

mon form is unilateral palsy, or HEMIPLEGIA, generally arising from cerebral HAEMORRHAGE, THROMBOSIS or EMBOLISM affecting the opposite side of the brain. If all four limbs and trunk are affected, the paralysis is called quadroplegia. If

1 position of haemorrhage causing paralysis of left arm
2 position of haemorrhage causing paralysis of face
3 position of haemorrhage causing complete paralysis of left side
4 position of haemorrhage followed by paralysis of left arm and leg with right side of face (crossed paralysis)
5 cerebellum
6 spinal cord
7 position of disorder causing paralysis of both lower limbs (paraplegia)
8 position of the disease responsible for poliomyelitis in the left leg
9 to leg
10 to arm
11 medulla oblongata
12 seventh nerve (facial)
13 pons
14 lentiform nucleus
15 thalamus
16 cerebral hemisphere
17 leg
18 arm

Brain and spinal cord, showing motor paths and positions of injuries causing various forms of paralysis.

both legs and part of the trunk are affected, it is called paraplegia. Paralysis may also be divided into flaccid (floppy limbs) or spastic (rigid).

In hemiplegia the cause may be an ABSCESS, HAEMORRHAGE, THROMBOSIS or TUMOUR in the brain. CEREBRAL PALSY or ENCEPHALITIS are other possible causes. Sometimes damage occurs in the parts of the nervous system responsible for the fine control of muscle movements: the cerebellum and basal ganglion are such areas, and lack of DOPAMINE in the latter causes Parkinson's disease.

Damage or injury Damage to or pressure on the spinal cord may paralyse muscles supplied by nerves below the site of damage. A fractured spine or pressure from a tumour may have this effect. Disorders affecting the cord which can cause paralysis include osteoarthritis of the cervical vertebrae, MULTIPLE SCLEROSIS, MYELITIS, POLIOMYELITIS and MENINGITIS. Vitamin B_{12} deficiency (see APPENDIX 5: VITAMINS) may also cause deterioration in the spinal cord (see SPINAL CORD, INJURIES AND DISEASES).

Neuropathies are a group of disorders, some inherited, that damage the peripheral nerves, thus affecting their ability to conduct electrical impulses. This, in turn, causes muscle weakness or paralysis. Among the causes of neuropathies are cancers, DIABETES MELLITUS, liver disease, the toxic consequences of some drugs or metals, LEAD being one example.

Disorders of the muscles themselves, for example, MUSCULAR DYSTROPHY, can disturb their normal working and so cause partial or complete paralysis of the part(s) affected.

The diagram shows the effects of lesions of the brain and spinal cord at different sites in the central nervous system.

Treatment The aim of treatment should be to remedy the underlying cause – for example, surgical removal of a displaced intervertebral disc or treating DIABETES MELLITUS. Sometimes the cause cannot be rectified but, whether treatable or not, physiotherapy is essential to prevent joints seizing up and to try to maintain some tone in muscles that may be only partly affected. With temporary paralysis, such as can occur after a stroke, physiotherapy can retrain the sufferers to use their muscles and joints to ensure mobility during and after recovery. Patients with permanent hemiplegia, paraplegia or quadraplegia need highly skilled nursing care, rehabilitative support and resources and expert help to allow them, if possible, to live at home.

PARAMEDICAL A generic title for the professions which work closely with or are reponsible to the medical profession in caring for patients. A paramedical worker has skills, experience and qualifications in certain spheres of health care. Examples are ambulance staff, primarily those trained to deal with emergencies, PHYSIOTHERAPISTS, RADIOGRAPHERS and DIETICIANS.

PARAMETER A measurement of a certain factor – for example, pulse rate, blood pressure, or haemoglobin concentration – that is relevant to a disorder under investigation.

PARAMNESIA A derangement of the memory in which words are used without a comprehension of their meaning; it is also applied to illusions of memory in which a person in good faith imagines and describes experiences which never occurred to him or her.

PARANOIA A form of mental illness characterized by fixed delusions, usually of persecution. Many sufferers are able to go about freely and carry out activities with which their delusions do not interfere. In loose English usage, 'paranoia' means 'subject to any sorts of feelings of persecution'. (See MENTAL ILLNESS).

PARAPHASIA Misplacement of words, or use of wrong words, in speech as a result of a lesion in the speech region of the brain.

PARAPHIMOSIS The constriction of the penis behind the glans by an abnormally tight foreskin that has been retracted. The condition causes swelling and severe pain. Sometimes the foreskin can be returned by manual manipulation after an ice pack has been applied to the glans. Sometimes an operation to cut the foreskin is required to release it.

PARAPHRENIA A form of paranoia. (See also MENTAL ILLNESS.)

PARAPLEGIA Paralysis of the lower limbs, accompanied generally by paralysis of bladder and rectum. (See PARALYSIS.)

PARAPSYCHOLOGY The branch of psychology that studies extrasensory perception. This includes precognition (seeing into the future), psychokinesis (a supposed ability of some people to move or change the state of objects by thinking), telepathy (communicating thoughts from one person to another) and clairvoyance (the ability to visualize events at a distance). These phenomena have no scientific explanation and some of these 'abilities' are sometimes manifestations of mental illness such as SCHIZOPHRENIA.

PARAQUAT A contact herbicide widely used in agriculture and horticulture. A mouthful is enough to kill. Its major misuse has resulted from its being decanted from the professional pack into soft-drink bottles and kept in the domestic kitchen. The resultant potential for accidental and probably fatal ingestion is obvious. It is involved in around 40 cases of suicide every year. The eyes and skin must be carefully protected so as not to come into contact with it. Medical assistance should be obtained as soon as possible as some poisoning victims may require hospital inpatient care, including renal DIALYSIS. Several medical centres have been set up throughout the country to provide treatment in cases of poisoning with it. Details of these can be obtained from the National Poisons Information Service centres (see APPENDIX 2: ADDRESSES).

PARASITE An organism which lives in or on another organism, known as the host. A parasite derives all its nourishment from the host but provides no benefits in return. It may damage the host's bodily functions and in extreme cases cause the death of the host. Human parasites include worms, fungi, bacteria and viruses.

PARASITICIDE A general term applied to agents or substances destructive to parasites.

PARASUICIDE Non-fatal self-poisoning or self-injury, or attempted suicide. It is most common in the 12–15 age-group. The intention is not as a rule to commit suicide, but a cry for help to resolve an acute domestic, social or personal upset.

PARASYMPATHETIC NERVOUS SYSTEM
That part of the AUTONOMIC NERVOUS SYSTEM which is connected with the brain and spinal cord through certain nerve centres in the midbrain, medulla, and lower end of the cord. The nerves from these centres are carried in the 3rd, 7th, 9th, and 10th cranial nerves and the 2nd, 3rd, and 4th sacral nerves. The action of the parasympathetic system is usually antagonistic to that of the sympathetic system. Thus it inhibits the action of the heart and augments the action of the intestine, whereas the sympathetic augments the action of the heart and inhibits that of the intestine. (See diagram of sympathetic and parasympathetic nervous systems under NERVES.)

PARATHION One of the ORGANO-PHOSPHORUS insecticides. It is highly toxic to man and must therefore be handled with the utmost care.

PARATHYROID The grouping of four small glands, about 5 mm in diameter, which lie to the side of and behind the THYROID GLAND. These glands regulate the metabolism of calcium and of phosphorus. If for any reason there is a deficiency of the secretion of the parathyroid glands, the amount of calcium in the blood falls too low and the amount of phosphorus increases. The result is the condition known as TETANY characterized by restlessness and muscle spasms, sometimes severe. The condition is checked by the injection of calcium gluconate – which causes an increase in the amount of calcium in the blood. The commonest cause of this condition, or hypoparathyroidism as it is known, is accidental injury to or removal of the glands during the operation of thyroidectomy for the treatment of GRAVES' DISEASE. If there is over-production of the parathyroids there will be an increase of calcium in the blood. This extra calcium is drawn from the bones, causing cysts to form with resulting bone fragility. This cystic disease of bone is known as OSTEITIS FIBROSA CYSTICA. Tumours of the parathyroid glands result in this overactivity of the parathyroid hormone, and the resulting increase in the amount of calcium in the blood leads to the formation of stones in the kidneys. The only available treatment is surgical removal of the tumour. Increased activity of the parathyroid glands, or hyperparathyroidism, is always considered as a possible cause of stones in the kidneys. (See KIDNEYS, DISEASES OF.)

PARATYPHOID FEVER (see ENTERIC FEVER).

PARENCHYMA A term meaning originally all the soft tissues of internal organs except the muscular flesh, though now reserved for the secreting cells of the glandular organs.

PARENTERAL Administration of drugs by any route other than by the mouth or by the bowel.

PARENTERAL NUTRITION In severely ill patients, especially those who have had major surgery or with sepsis, burns, acute pancreatitis and renal failure, the body's reserves of protein become exhausted. This results in weight loss, reduction of muscle mass, a fall in the serum albumin and lymphocyte count and an impairment of cellular immunity. Severely ill patients are unable to take adequate food by mouth to repair the body protein loss so that enteral or parenteral nutrition is required. Enteral feeding is through the gastro-intestinal tract with the aid of a naso-gastric tube. Parenteral nutrition involves the provision of carbohydrate, fat and proteins by intravenous administration.

The preferred route for the infusion of hyperosmolar solutions is via a central venous catheter. If parenteral nutrition is required for more than two weeks it is advisable to use a long-term type catheter such as the Broviac, Hickman or extra corporeal type, which is made of silastic material and is inserted via a long subcutaneous tunnel, which not only helps to fix the catheter but minimizes the risk of ascending infection.

Dextrose is considered the best source of carbohydrate and may be used as a 20-per-cent or 50-per-cent solution. AMINO-ACIDS should be in the laevo form and should contain the correct proportion of essential and non-essential amino acids. Preparations are available with or without electrolytes and with or without fat emulsions.

The main hazards of intravenous feeding are blood-borne infections made possible by continued direct access to the circulation, and biochemical abnormalities related to the composition of the solutions infused. The continuous use of hypertonic solutions of glucose can cause HYPERGLYCAEMIA and glycosuria and the resultant POLYURIA may lead to dehydration. Treatment with INSULIN is needed when hyperosmolality occurs, and in addition the water and sodium deficits will require to be corrected.

PARESIS A state of partial paralysis. (See PARALYSIS.)

PARIETAL The term applied to anything pertaining to the wall of a cavity: e.g. parietal pleura, the part of the pleural membrane which lines the wall of the chest.

PARIETAL LOBE A major section of each cerebral hemisphere (see BRAIN). The two lobes lie under the parietal bones and contain the sensory cortex.

PARKINSONISM or PARALYSIS AGITANS is a progressive disease of insidious onset usually occurring in the second half of life; it is much commoner in men than in women. Degenerative changes in the basal ganglia lead to a deficiency in the NEUROTRANSMITTER dopamine – or occasionally to other neurotransmitters – and it is this deficiency of dopamine that is responsible for most cases. Rarely, the disease is a sequel to encephalitis lethargica. The clinical picture is characterized by tremor, rigidity and a poverty of spontaneous movements. The loss of natural play of expression in the face produces a masklike expression. Rigidity of the larynx, tongue and lips produces a flat, expressionless voice. The commonest symptom is tremor, often affecting one hand, spreading to the leg on the same side, then to the other limbs. It is more pronounced in resting limbs, is exaggerated by excitement, stopping during sleep. It may interfere with eating and dressing. Limb rigidity leads to an increasing tendency to stoop. The patient has a shuffling walk with a peculiar running gait.

Treatment Several drugs are used to keep the condition under control. None is curative, all have side-effects, and finding the most suitable one for any individual depends largely on understanding co-operation between family doctor and patient. Dopaminergic and ANTIMUSCARINIC drugs are used in treatment. Levodopa, a precursor of dopamine, is a long-used example of the former; it produces spectacular improvement in one-fifth and moderate improvement in two-fifths of patients. Benzhexol hydrochloride is one of several antimuscarinic drugs used in Parkinson's disease. Selegiline is a monoamine-oxidase-B inhibitor used in severe parkinsonism in conjunction with levodopa to reduce 'end-of-dose' deterioration. It has also been suggested that early treatment with selegiline may delay the need for levodopa therapy and possibly slow the rate of progression of the disease, but this remains to be confirmed. Adverse effects: HYPOTENSION, NAUSEA and VOMITING, confusion, agitation; side-effects of levodopa may be increased and concurrent dosage may need to be reduced by 2–50 per cent.

All drugs used in Parkinsonism have side-effects and require regular medical supervision. Some drugs used to treat other disorders produce Parkinsonian side-effects. Patients seeking further advice and help, together with their relatives, are advised to contact the Parkinson's Disease Society of the UK (see APPENDIX 2: ADDRESSES).

PARONYCHIA The term applied to inflammation near the nail. In the acute form it is usually due to infection with *Staphylococcus aureus*, and is most often seen in nurses and others handling septic material. It usually starts at one corner of the nail-fold and then spreads to the other side and deeply under the base of the nail. There is local pain and tenderness, with swelling of the nail-fold. Treatment in mild cases consists of applying an adhesive dressing and giving penicillin. In more severe cases the swelling has to be opened. A new nail grows in two or three months, displacing the old one in front of it. Chronic paronychia occurs usually in women who have their hands much in water. In men it occurs in fishmongers and chefs. It may affect one or more fingers. Treatment consists of keeping the finger dry and giving a suitable antibiotic. (See WHITLOW.)

PAROSMIA A perverted sense of smell; everything usually smells unpleasant to the affected individual. The most common cause is some septic condition of the nasal passages, but it may occasionally be due to a lesion in the brain involving the centre responsible for the sense of smell.

PAROTID GLAND One of the SALIVARY GLANDS. It is situated just in front of the ear, and its duct runs forwards across the cheek to open into the interior of the mouth on a little projection opposite the second last tooth of the upper row. The parotid gland is generally the first of the salivary glands to become enlarged in mumps.

PAROTITIS Inflammation of the parotid gland. Epidemic parotitis is another name for MUMPS.

PAROXETINE An antidepressant drug in the selective serotonin-reuptake inhibitors (SRRIs) group. (See MENTAL ILLNESS.)

PAROXYSM A sudden temporary attack that may take the form of a convulsion or spasm. It may also occur when a patient with a disease suddenly deteriorates.

PARROT DISEASE A colloquial name for PSITTACOSIS.

PARTHENOGENESIS Non-sexual reproduction. In other words, development of the ovum into an individual without fertilization by a spermatozoon. It is common in plants and has been produced in animals experimentally.

PARTOGRAM A method of recording the degree of dilatation, or opening, of the cervix (or neck) of the UTERUS in LABOUR to assess how labour is progressing.

PARTURITION (see LABOUR).

PARVOVIRUSES (from *parvus*, Latin for small) is a group of viruses responsible for outbreaks of WINTER VOMITING DISEASE. One strain is the cause of erythema infectiosum.

PAS is a commonly used abbreviation for PARA-AMINOSALICYLIC ACID.

PASSIVE MOVEMENT A movement induced by someone other than the patient. Physiotherapists manipulate joints by passive movement in order to retain and encourage function of a nerve or muscle that is not working normally because of injury or disease.

PASTES (see OINTMENTS).

PASTEURELLA A group of bacilli. They are essentially animal parasites that under certain conditions are transmitted to man. They include the micro-organism responsible for PLAGUE and TULARAEMIA.

PASTEURIZATION A method of sterilizing milk. In many parts of the world pasteurization has done away with milk-borne infections, of which the most serious is bovine tuberculosis, affecting the glands, bones, and joints of children. Other infections conveyed by milk are SCARLET FEVER, DIPHTHERIA, enteric fever (TYPHOID and PARATYPHOID), undulant fever (BRUCELLOSIS), and food poisoning (e.g. from SALMONELLAE or the toxins of the STAPHYLOCOCCUS).

High-temperature short-time (HTST) PASTEURIZATION consists in heating the milk at a temperature not less than 71·7 °C (161 °F) for at least fifteen seconds, followed by immediate cooling to a temperature of not more than 10 °C (50 °F).

Low-temperature pasteurization, or 'holder' process, consists in maintaining the milk for at least half-an-hour at a temperature between 63 to 65 °C (145 to 150 °F), followed by immediate cooling to a temperature of not more that 10 °C (50 °F). This has the effect of considerably reducing the number of bacteria contained in the milk and of preventing the diseases conveyed by milk referred to above.

PATCH TEST This is used to identify possible substances that may be causing a patient's allergy. Small amounts of different substances are placed on the skin, usually the back or arm. If the patient is allergic a red flare and swelling will appear, usually within about 15 minutes. Sometimes the reaction may take longer – up to three days – to develop.

PATELLA Also known as the knee-cap, this is a flat bone shaped somewhat like an oyster-shell, lying in the tendon of the extensor muscle of the thigh, and protecting the knee-joint in front. (See BONE; KNEE; FRACTURES.)

PATELLAR REFLEX (see REFLEX ACTION).

PATENT In the medical context, a term meaning open, for example, PATENT DUCTUS ARTERIOSUS. The term is also used for proprietary medicines which, because of the research and cost involved in producing many of them, are protected by a patent. This means that without an agreement no company or organization other than the patent holder can produce the substance.

PATENT DUCTUS ARTERIOSUS (see DUCTUS ARTERIOSUS).

PATHO- A prefix indicating relationship to a disease, for example, PATHOLOGY, a study of disease.

PATHOGENIC This term means disease-producing, and is a term, for example, applied to bacteria, capable of causing disease.

PATHOGENESIS The ways that a disease or disorder starts and develops. The term applies in particular to the physiological and cellular activities that are involved in the mode of origin and development of the condition.

PATHOGNOMONIC A term applied to signs or symptoms which are specially characteristic of certain diseases, and on the presence or absence of which the diagnosis depends. Thus the discovery of the *Mycobacterium tuberculosis* in the expectoration is said to be pathognomonic of pulmonary tuberculosis.

PATHOLOGY The science which deals with the causes of, and changes produced in the body by, disease.

PATIENT-CONTROLLED ANALGESIA A technique whereby a patient can deliver an analgesic substance in amounts related to the extent of the pain he is suffering. For example, to combat postoperative pain some hospitals use devices which allow patients to give themselves small intravenous amounts of opiates when they are needed. Pain is more effectively controlled if it is not allowed to reach a high level, a situation which tends to happen when patients receive analgesics only on ward drug rounds or when they ask the nursing staff for them.

PAUL-BUNNELL TEST A test for MONONUCLEOSIS which is based upon the fact that patients with this disease develop ANTIBODIES which agglutinate sheep red blood cells.

PEAK FLOW METER A device that measures the rate at which an individual can expel air from the lungs. This is an indication of the reserve in the lung's capacity. Narrowed airways (bronchospasm) slow the rate at which air can be expelled and the peak flow meter can assess the severity. ASTHMA causes bronchospasm and the device can measure the effectiveness of treatment with BRONCHODILATOR drugs; this should be done regularly to monitor the progress of the disease.

PECTIN A polysaccharide substance allied to starch, contained in fruits and plants, and forming the basis of vegetable jelly. It has been used as a transfusion fluid in place of blood in cases of haemorrhage and shock.

PECTORAL Anything pertaining to the chest, or a remedy used in treating chest troubles.

PECTORILOQUY The resonance of the voice, when spoken or whispered words can be clearly heard through the stethoscope placed on the chest wall. It is a sign of consolidation, or of a cavity, in the lung.

PEDICLE A narrow tube of tissue formed by folded skin which links a piece of tissue used for surgical grafting to its site of origin. A pedicle graft is used by the surgeon – usually a reconstructive/plastic surgeon – when the site under repair is unsuitable for an independent graft, usually because the blood supply at the recipient site is inadequate. (See PLASTIC AND RECONSTRUCTIVE SURGERY.)

A pedicle is also found occurring between a tumour and its tissue of origin, and the term is used in anatomy to refer to any slim tubular process.

PEDICULOCIDE A substance that kills *Pediculosis capitis.*

PEDICULOSIS Infestation with lice of which three species infect humans:

Pediculus humanus var. capitis (head louse) affects the scalp in children or adults, particu-

larly in females. The adult louse may visit many heads in one day, especially in schoolgirls. It lays its eggs on the scalp hair and the resulting 'nit' grows out with the hair. Secondary infection owing to scratching is common in severe infestations, causing enlarged lymph glands in the posterior neck and some general debility. The lice and nits can be killed by applications of MALATHION 0.5-per-cent lotion or PERMETHRIN 1-per-cent lotion. After the hair is washed, application of a conditioner allows nits to be removed with a fine nit comb.

Pediculus pubis (crab louse) is broader and shorter than the head louse and less mobile. Usually transmitted sexually, it is found in the public area but may infect eyelashes and other body hair. It is easily seen, as are the large nits attached to the public hair: permethrin and malathion lotions are effective.

Pediculus humanus var. corporis (body louse) differs from the head and crab louse in that it lives in clothing and only goes on to the body to feed. Infestation is found in vagabonds, armies in the field, or prisoners in conditions where even minimal hygiene is impossible. The lice are found in the seams of clothing together with multiple eggs. Typically excoriation and pigmentation are seen on the back of the infested person. Replacement of clothing or autoclaving or hot ironing of the clothes is curative.

(For further details, see INSECTS IN RELATION TO DISEASE.)

PEDUNCLE A stalk-like structure that usually acts as a support.

PELLAGRA A potentially fatal nutritional disorder caused by a deficiency of vitamin B complex (niacin). The symptoms are DERMATITIS, diarrhoea and DEMENTIA. The deficiency occurs mainly in poor people in developing countries where maize is a prime constituent of the diet. Nicotinic acid in maize is in a bound form that the consumer cannot utilize. Further, maize is deficient in the amino-acid, tryptophan, from which the human body can make nicotinic acid.

Treatment The disease is prevented or cured by adding to the diet foods such as fresh meat, eggs, milk, liver, and yeast extracts, and nicotinic acid, as well as by improvement of the general conditions of life.

PELVIC INFLAMMATORY DISEASE Acute or chronic infection of the OVARIES, FALLOPIAN TUBE, or UTERUS. The condition is usually caused by infection spreading from the VAGINA or from a nearby infected organ – for example, the APPENDIX. Blood-borne infection may also be the cause. Lower abdominal pain, sometimes severe, is characteristic of the condition. Treatment may be by antibiotics or sometimes surgery.

PELVIMETRY   Measurement of the internal dimensions of the pelvis. The four diameters measured are: transverse, anterioposterior, and left and right oblique. These measurements help to establish whether a fetus can be delivered normally. If the outlet is abnormally small, the mother will have to be delivered by CAESAREAN SECTION.

PELVIS   The bony pelvis consists of the two hip bones, one on each side, with the sacrum and coccyx behind. It connects the lower limbs with the spine. Each hip bone is composed of three originally separate bones, in the adult pelvis firmly fused together: the ilium; the ischium, with a rounded part below, the tuberosity, upon which the body rests in sitting; and the pubis in front. The expanded parts of the iliac bones incompletely surround the lower part of the abdomen, known as the false pelvis, and are separated by a distinct line, known as the brim or inlet, from the true pelvis beneath. The true pelvis, as its name implies, is basin-shaped and ligaments and muscles are attached to it. The soft floor of the pelvis is composed mainly of two muscles, the levators of the anus, whilst the deep notch, between the haunch-bone and sacrum behind, is closed in by a pair of strong sacro-sciatic ligaments.

The pelvis varies considerably in the two sexes. In the female it is shallower and the ilia are more widely separated, giving great breadth to the hips of the woman; the inlet is more circular and the outlet larger; whilst the angle beneath the pubic bones (subpubic angle), which is an acute angle in the male, is obtuse in the female. All these points are of importance in connection with child-bearing.

The contents of the pelvis are the urinary bladder and rectum in both sexes; in addition the male has the seminal vesicles and the prostate gland surrounding the neck of the bladder, whilst the female has the womb, ovaries, and their appendages.

In addition to these sex differences, the pelvis differs between races. It tends to be wider from front to back and longer from top to bottom in black people than in white people: the so-called anthropoid pelvis.

PEMPHIGOID (see PEMPHIGUS).

PEMPHIGUS   Autoimmune disease of the skin in which the cells of the epidermis lose their adhesion to each other resulting in blister formation. There are two main types:

Pemphigus vulgaris is a serious form affecting SKIN and mucous membranes. It affects young and middle-aged people with widespread blistering, erosion and crusting of the skin. Extensive involvement of the lips, mouth and throat interfere with nutrition. Untreated, it is eventually fatal, but the disease can now be controlled by large doses of oral CORTICOSTEROID and other IMMUNOSUPPRESSIVE DRUGS. Morbidity from the adverse effects of steroids is a serious problem, but some patients are eventually cured.

Pemphigus foliaceus is seen in the elderly; the blistering is more superficial in the epidermis. It may be very widespread, but is not life threatening because mucous membranes are not affected. Topical corticosteroids will sometimes control the eruption, but in severe cases treatment is as for pemphigus vulgaris.

Pemphigoid is a variant where the blistering occurs because of separation of the epidermis and dermis. Mucosae are rarely affected and the disease affects mainly the arms and legs in the elderly. Treatment is as for pemphigus but smaller doses of corticosteroids usually suffice.

PENICILLAMINE   A metabolite of penicillin which is a CHELATING AGENT. It is sometimes used in RHEUMATOID ARTHRITIS that has not responded to the first-line remedies and it is particularly useful when the disease is complicated by VASCULITIS. Penicillamine is also used as an antidote to poisoning by heavy metals, particularly copper and lead, as it is able to bind these metals and so remove their toxic effects. Because of its ability to bind copper it is also used in WILSON'S DISEASE where there is a deficiency in the copper-binding protein so that copper is able to become deposited in he brain and liver, damaging these tissues.

PENICILLIN   The name given by Sir Alexander Fleming, in 1929, to an antibacterial substance produced by the mould *Penicillium notatum*. This mould was first described in 1911 in Scandinavia, where it was discovered in decaying hyssop. The story of penicillin is one of the most dramatic in the history of medicine, and its introduction into medicine initiated a new era in therapeutics comparable only to the introduction of ANAESTHESIA by Morton and Simpson and of ANTISEPTICS by Pasteur and Lister. The two names that will always be primarily associated with penicillin are those of Sir Alexander Fleming, of St Mary's Hospital, London, who discovered its anti-bacterial action, and Lord Florey, of Oxford, who did so much to develop its practical use during the 1939–45 War. The two great advantages of penicillin are that it is active against a large range of bacteria and that, even in large doses, it is non-toxic. Penicillin diffuses well into body tissues and fluids and is excreted in the urine, but it penetrates poorly into the cerebrospinal fluid. An important side-effect of penicillins is hypersensitivity which causes rashes and sometimes ANAPHYLAXIS, which can be fatal. Among the organisms against which it is active are: staphylococcus, streptococcus, pneumococcus, meningococcus, gonococcus, and the organisms responsible for syphilis, and for gas gangrene.

Penicillin is a beta-lactam antibiotic, one of a group of drugs that also includes CEPHALOSPORINS. Drugs of this group have a four-part beta-lactam ring in their molecular structure and they act by interfering with the cell-wall growth of mutliplying bacteria.

Forms of penicillin Penicillin has been synthesized in the laboratory, and various forms of penicillin are now available. These include the following broad groups: benzylpenicillin and phenoxymethyl-penicillin; penicillinase-resistant penicillins; broad-spectrum penicillins; antipseudomonal penicillins; and mecillinams. Brief details of some of the commonly used penicillins follow.

BENZYLPENICILLIN is available as the sodium or potassium salt. It is given intramuscularly, and is the form that is used when a rapid action is required. It can also be given by mouth but, as the proportion absorbed varies greatly, it is unreliable in action when given in this way.

PROCAINE PENICILLIN is a relatively insoluble form of penicillin. A single daily intramuscular injection of 600,000 units will maintain a bacteriostatic level in the blood for twenty-four hours.

PHENOXYMETHYLPENICILLIN is given by mouth but is absorbed inconstantly.

AMPICILLIN, a broad-spectrum antibiotic, is another of the penicillins derived by semi-synthesis from the penicillin nucleus. It, too, is active when taken by mouth, but its special feature is that it is active against gram-negative micro-organisms such as *E. coli* and the salmonellae.

CLOXACILLIN is yet another of the semi-synthesized penicillins. It has a relatively weak anti-bacterial action, but has the advantage of being active against penicillin-resistant staphylococci.

METHICILLIN is another penicillin derived from the penicillin nucleus. It is active against penicillin-resistant staphylococci but has to be given by injection as it is destroyed by the acid secretion of the stomach.

CARBENICILLIN, a semi-synthetic penicillin, must be given by injection, which may be painful. Its main use is in dealing with infections due to *Pseudomonas pyocanea*. It is the only penicillin active against this micro-organism.

PIPERACILLIN and TICARCILLIN are carboxypenicillins used to treat infections caused by *Pseudomonas aeruginosa* and *Proteus* spp.

FLUCLOXACILLIN, also a semi-synthetic penicillin, is active against penicillin-resistant staphylococci and has the practical advantage of being active when taken by mouth.

TEMOCILLIN is another penicillinase-resistant penicillin, effective against gram-negative bacteria (except PSEUDOMONAS).

AMOXYCILLIN is an oral semi-synthetic penicillin with the same range of action as ampicillin but less likely to cause side-effects.

MECILLINAM is yet another in this series, though of slightly different chemical origin. It is of value in the treatment of infections with salmonellae (see FOOD POISONING), including typhoid fever, and with *E. coli* (see ESCHERICHIA). It is given by injection. There is a derivative, Pivmecillinam, which can be taken by mouth.

PENICILLINASE A bacterial enzyme capable of neutralizing the antibacterial properties of penicillin and other beta-lactam antibiotics such as the CEPHALOSOPRINS. Most staphylococci are now resistant to benzylpenicillin because they produce this enzyme. Cloxacillin, flucloxacillin and temocillin are not inactivated. (See PENICILLIN.)

PENIS The male organ through which the tubular URETHRA runs from the neck of the BLADDER to the exterior at the MEATUS. URINE and SEMEN are discharged along the urethra, which is surrounded by three cylindrical bodies of erectile tissue, two of which (corpora cavernosa) lie adjacent to each other along the upper length of the penis and one (corpus spongiosum) lies beneath them. Normally the penis hangs down in a flaccid state in front of the scrotum. When a man is sexually aroused the erectile tissue, which is of spongy constituency and well supplied with small blood vessels, becomes engorged with blood. This makes the penis erect and ready for insertion into the woman's vagina in sexual intercourse. The end of the penis, the glans, is covered by a loose fold of skin – the foreskin or PREPUCE – which retracts when the organ is erect. The foreskin is sometimes removed for cultural or medical reasons.

A common congenital disorder of the penis is HYPOSPADIAS, in which the urethra opens somewhere along the under side; it can be repaired surgically. BALANITIS is inflammation of the glans and foreskin (see REPRODUCTIVE ORGANS; EJACULATION; IMPOTENCE and PRIAPISM.)

PENTAMIDINE A drug that is used in the prevention and treatment of African TRYPANSOMIASIS, and in the treatment of LEISHMANIASIS.

PEPPERMINT This is extracted from the leaves and tops of *Mentha piperita*. It has an aromatic odour, due to the presence of an oil from which is obtained menthol, a camphor-like substance. Peppermint water is a useful remedy for flatulence and colic in infants. Oil of peppermint is used like the other volatile oils.

PEP PILLS A colloquial term for stimulant drugs, especially the AMPHETAMINE group.

PEPSIN An enzyme found in the gastric juice which digests proteins, converting them into peptides and amino acids. It is used in the preparation of predigested, or 'PEPTONIZED', FOODS, or, more frequently, it is taken orally after meals. Available as a white powder or liquid, it is prepared from the mucous membrane of cow, sheep, or pig stomachs.

PEPTIC ULCER The term commonly applied to ulcers in the stomach and duodenum. (See DUODENAL ULCER; STOMACH, DISEASES OF.)

PEPTIDE A compound formed by the union of two or more amino-acids.

PEPTONIZED FOODS Foods which have been predigested by PANCREATIN and thereby rendered more digestible.

PERCUSSION An aid to diagnosis practised by striking the body with the fingers, in such a way as to make it give out a note. It was introduced in 1761 by Leopold Auenbrugger (1722–1809) of Vienna, the son of an innkeeper, who derived the idea from the habit of his father tapping casks of wine to ascertain how much wine they contained. According to the degree of dullness or resonance of the note, an opinion can be formed as to the state of consolidation of air-containing organs, the presence of abnormal cavities in organs, and the dimensions of solid and air-containing organs, which happen to lie next to one another. Still more valuable evidence is given by AUSCULTATION.

PERCUTANEOUS Any method of administering remedies by passing them through the skin, as by rubbing in an ointment or applying a patch containing a drug.

PERFORATION The perforation of one of the hollow organs of the abdomen or major blood vessels may occur spontaneously in the case of an ulcer or an advanced tumour or may be secondary to trauma such as a knife wound or penetrating injury from a traffic or industrial accident. Whatever the cause, perforation is a surgical emergency. The intestinal contents, which contain large numbers of bacteria, pass freely out into the abdominal cavity and cause a severe chemical or bacterial PERITONITIS. This is usually accompanied by severe abdominal pain, collapse or even death. There may also be evidence of free fluid or gas within the abdominal cavity. Surgical intervention, to repair the leak and wash out the contamination, is often necessary. Perforation or rupture of major blood vessels, whether from disease or injury, is an acute emergency for which urgent surgical repair is usually necessary. Perforation of hollow structures elsewhere than in the abdomen – for example, the heart or oesophagus – may be caused by congenital weaknesses, disease or injury. Treatment is usually surgical but depends on the cause.

PERFUSION The transfer of fluid through a tissue. For example, when blood passes through the lung tissue, dissolved oxygen perfuses from the moist air in the alveoli to the blood. Fluid may also be deliberately introduced into a tissue by injecting it into the blood vessels supplying the tissue.

PERI- A prefix meaning around.

PERIARTERITIS NODOSA (see POLYARTERITIS NODOSA).

PERICARDITIS Acute or chronic inflammation of the pericardium, the membranous sac that surrounds the heart. It may occur on its own or as part of pancarditis when inflammation also affects the MYOCARDIUM and endocardium (membranous lining of the inside of the heart). Various causes include virus infection, cancer and URAEMIA (see HEART DISEASES).

PERICARDIUM The smooth membrane that surrounds the heart. (See HEART.)

PERICHONDRITIS Inflammation of CARTILAGE and the tissue surrounding it, usually as a result of chronic infection.

PERIMETRITIS A localized inflammation of the peritoneum surrounding the uterus.

PERIMETRY A test of the visual fields of the eye that assesses the extent of peripheral vision. The procedure does not normally form part of a routine test of vision but can be of value in assessing neurological diseases such as tumour of the brain.

PERINATAL A term applied to the period starting a few weeks before birth, the birth itself and the week or two following it.

PERINATAL MORTALITY consists of deaths of the fetus after the 28th week of pregnancy and deaths of the new-born child during the first week of life. Today, more individuals die within a few hours of birth than during the following forty years. It is therefore not surprising that the perinatal mortality rate, which is the number of such deaths per 1000 total births, has come to be looked upon as a valuable indicator of the quality of care provided for the mother and her new-born baby. In 1995, the perinatal mortality rate was 8.9 in the United Kingdom compared with 11.4 in 1982 and over 30 in the early 1960s.

The causes of perinatal mortality include intrapartum anoxia (that is, difficulty in the birth of the baby, resulting in lack of oxygen), congenital abnormalities of the baby, antepartum anoxia (that is, conditions in the terminal stages of pregnancy preventing the fetus getting sufficient oxygen), and injuries to the brain of the baby during birth.

The commonest cause of perinatal death is some complication of placenta, cord or membranes. The next most common is congenital abnormality. Intra-uterine hypoxia and birth asphyxia comprise the third most common cause.

PERINEUM Popularly called the FORK, or CROTCH, it is the region situated between the opening of the bowel behind and of the genital organs in front. In women it becomes stretched in childbirth and the vaginal opening, may tear or need to be cut (see EPISIOTOMY) to facilitate delivery of the baby.

PERIOD (see MENSTRUATION).

PERIODIC PARALYSIS A rare condition characterized by the onset of weakness of the voluntary muscles. It usually occurs in young adults. As a rule the onset is in the morning on awakening. The weakness usually lasts for several hours. Attacks may also be brought on by a heavy meal or severe cold. It is a familial condition of obscure origin. There is one form, probably the most common, which is apparently due to a low level of potassium in the blood and is relieved by the taking of potassium chloride – 10 grams in water. There are other forms, however, in which the blood potassium may be raised or normal.

PERIODONTAL An adjective that relates to the tissues around the teeth.

PERIODONTAL MEMBRANE (see TEETH).

PERIOSTEUM The membrane surrounding a bone. The periosteum carries blood-vessels and nerves for the nutrition and development of the bone. When it is irritated, an increased deposit of bone takes place beneath it; if it is destroyed, the bone may cease to grow and a portion may die and separate as a sequestrum. (See BONE.)

PERIOSTITIS means inflammation on the surface of a bone affecting the periosteum. (See BONE, DISEASES OF.)

PERIPHERAL-BLOOD STEM-CELL TRANSPLANTS Peripheral-blood stem-cell transplants have almost completely replaced BONE MARROW TRANSPLANTS, which have been used to treat malignancies such as LEUKAEMIA and LYMPHOMA for the past twenty years. The high doses of CHEMOTHERAPY or RADIOTHERAPY used to treat these diseases destroy the bone marrow which contains stem cells from which all the blood cells derive. In 1989 stem cells were found in the blood during recovery from chemotherapy. By giving growth factors (cytokines) the number of stem cells in the blood increased for about three to four days. In a peripheral-blood stem-cell transplant, these cells can be separated from the peripheral blood, without a general anaesthetic. The cells taken by either method are then frozen and returned intravenously after the chemotherapy or radiotherapy is completed. Once transplanted, the stem cells usually take less than three weeks to repopulate the blood, compared to a month or more for a bone-marrow transplant. This means that there is less risk of infection or bleeding during the recovery from the transplant. The whole procedure has a mortality risk of less than 5 per cent, half the risk of a bone-marrow transplant.

PERIPHERAL NEURITIS means inflammation of the nerves in the outlying parts of the body. (See NEURITIS.)

PERIPHERAL NERVOUS SYSTEM (see NERVES).

PERIPHERAL VASCULAR DISEASE The narrowing of the blood vessels in the legs and, less commonly, in the arms. Blood flow is restricted, with pain occurring in the affected area. If the blood supply is seriously reduced, GANGRENE of the tissues supplied by the affected vessel(s) may occur and the limb may need to be amputated. The common cause is ATHEROSCLEROSIS which may be brought on by HYPERTENSION, excessively fatty diet, poorly controlled DIABETES or smoking, the latter being the biggest risk factor with 90 per cent of affected patients having been moderate to heavy smokers. Stopping smoking is essential; adequate exercise and a low fat diet are important measures. Surgery may be required.

PERISTALSIS The wormlike movement by which the stomach and bowels propel their contents. It consists of alternate waves of relaxation and contraction in successive parts of the tube. Any obstruction to the movement of the contents causes these contractions to become more forcible and are often accompanied by the severe form of pain known as colic.

PERITONEOSCOPY Viewing of the peritoneal cavity through a tube fitted with mirrors and light. The instrument (see ENDOSCOPE) is inserted via an incision just below the umbilicus. The peritoneal cavity is then inflated with air. This simple operation may obviate a more drastic one: for example, if peritoneoscopy shows deposits of cancer in the peritoneum or the liver. Colour photographs of the liver have been taken through the peritoneoscope.

PERITONEUM The serous membrane of the abdominal cavity. The parietal peritoneum lines the walls of the abdomen and the visceral peritoneum covers the abdominal organs. The two are continuous with one another at the back of the abdomen and form a complicated closed sac (see MESENTERY; OMENTUM). A small amount of fluid is always present to lubricate the membrane, while a large amount collects in conditions associated with OEDEMA or in PERITONITIS.

PERITONITIS Inflammation of the peritoneum. It may be acute or chronic, localized or generally diffused, and its severity and danger may vary according to the cause.

Acute peritonitis generally arises because bacteria enter the peritoneal cavity, from penetrating wounds, e.g. stabs, from the exterior or from the abdominal organs. Hence conditions leading to perforation of the STOMACH, BOWELS, BILE DUCTS, BLADDER, and other hollow organs such as GASTRIC ULCER, TYPHOID FEVER, GALLSTONES, rupture of the bladder, strangulated HERNIA, and obstructions of the bowels, may lead to peritonitis. Numerous bacteria may cause the inflammation, most common being *E. coli*, streptococci and the gonococcus.

The symptoms usually begin with a RIGOR together with fever, vomiting, severe abdominal pain and tenderness. Shock develops and the abdominal wall becomes rigid. If untreated the patient usually dies. Urgent hospital admission is required. X-ray examination may show gas in the peritoneal cavity. Treatment consists of intravenous fluids, antibiotics and surgical repair of the causative condition. Such treatment, together with strong analgesics is usually successful if started soon enough.

PERITONSILLAR ABSCESS   The term applied to a collection of pus or an abscess which occurs complicating an attack of tonsillitis. The collection of pus forms between the tonsil and the superior constrictor muscle of the pharynx. This condition is also known as quinsy. The treatment of this condition involves drainage of the abscess and the administration of appropriate antibiotics.

PERMETHRIN   Along with PHENOTHRIN, it is a largely non-toxic pyrethroid insecticide, effective in SCABIES and lice infestations.

PERNICIOUS ANAEMIA   An auto-immune disease in which the sensitized LYMPHOCYTES destroy the parietal cells of the stomach. These cells normally produce intrinsic factor which is the carrier protein for vitamin B_{12} that permits its absorption in the terminal ileum. Without intrinsic factor, vitamin B_{12} can not be absorbed and this gives rise to a macrocytic ANAEMIA. The skin and mucosa become pale and the tongue smooth and atrophic. A peripheral NEUROPATHY is often present and this is commonly manifest by PARAESTHESIAE and numbness, and even ataxia. The more severe neurological complication of sub-acute combined degeneration of the cord is fortunately more rare. The anaemia gets its name from the fact that before the discovery of vitamin B_{12} it was uniformly fatal. Now a monthly injection of vitamin B_{12} is all that is required to keep the patient healthy.

PERONEAL   The name given to structures, such as the muscles, and nerves, on the outer or fibular side of the leg.

PERPHENAZINE (see PHENOTHIAZINES).

PERSEVERATION is the senseless repetition of words or deeds by a person with a disordered mind.

PERSISTENT VEGETATIVE STATE (PVS) may occur in patients with severe brain damage from HYPOXIA or injury. Patients do not display any awareness of their surroundings, and are unable to communicate. Sleep alternates with apparent wakefulness, when some REFLEXES may be present: for example, patients' eyes may reflexly follow or respond to sound, their limbs can reflexly withdraw from pain, and their hands can reflexly grope or grasp. Patients can breathe spontaneously, and retain normal heart and kidney function, although they are doubly INCONTINENT. For a diagnosis of PVS to be made, the state should have continued for more than a predefined period, usually one month. Half of patients die within 2 to 6 months, but some can survive for longer with artificial feeding.

The ethics of keeping patients alive with artificial support are controversial. In the UK, a legal ruling is usually needed for artificial support to be withdrawn after a diagnosis of PVS has been made. The chances of regaining consciousness after one year are slim and, even if patients do recover, they are usually left with severe neurological disability.

PVS must be distinguished from conditions which appear similar. These include the 'LOCKED-IN SYNDROME' which is the result of damage to the brain stem (see BRAIN). Patients with this syndrome are conscious but unable to speak or move except for certain eye movements and blinking. The psychiatric state of CATATONIA is another condition in which the patient retains consciousness and will usually recover.

PERSONALITY DISORDER   Condition in which the sufferers fail to learn from experience or to adapt to changes. The outcome is impaired social functioning and personal distress. There are three broad overlapping groups. One group is characterized by eccentric behaviour with paranoid or schizoid overtones. The second group shows dramatic and emotional behaviour with self-centredness and antisocial behaviour as typical components of the disorder. In the third group anxiety and fear are the main characteristics, which are accompanied by dependency and compulsive behaviour. These disorders are not classed as illnesses but psychotherapy and behavioural therapy may help. The individuals affected are notoriously resistant to any help that is offered, tending to blame other people, circumstances or bad luck for their persistent difficulties. (See MENTAL ILLNESS; MULTIPLE PERSONALITY DISORDER; MUNCHAUSEN'S SYNDROME.)

PERSPIRATION   Commonly called sweat, it is an excretion from the skin, produced by microscopic sweat-glands, of which there are around 2·5 million, scattered over the surface.

There are two different types of sweat-glands, known as eccrine and apocrine. Insensible perspiration takes place constantly by evaporation from the openings of the sweat-glands, well over a litre a day being produced. Sensible perspiration – to which the term sweat is usually confined – occurs with physical exertion and raised body temperature: up to three litres an hour may be produced for short periods.

Eccrine sweat is a faintly acid, watery fluid containing less than 2 per cent of solids. The eccrine sweat-glands in man are situated in greatest numbers on the soles of the feet and palms of the hands, and with a magnifying glass their minute openings or pores can be seen in rows occupying the summit of each ridge in the skin. Perspiration is most abundant in these regions, though it also occurs all over the body.

The chief object of perspiration is to maintain an even body temperature by regulating the heat lost from the body surface. Sweating is therefore increased by internally produced heat, such as muscular activity, or external heat. It is controlled by two types of nerves: vasomotor, which regulate the local blood flow, and secretory (part of the sympathetic nervous system) which directly influence secretion.

Apocrine sweat-glands These start functioning at puberty and are found in the armpits, the eyelids, around the anus in association with the external genitalia and in the areola and nipple of the breast. (The glands that produce wax in the ear are modified apocrine glands.) The flow of apocrine sweat is evoked by emotional stimuli such as fear, anger, or sexual excitement.

Abnormalities of perspiration Decreased sweating may occur in the early stages of fever, in diabetes, and in some forms of glomerulonephritis. Some people are unable to sweat copiously, and are prone to HEAT-STROKE.
EXCESSIVE SWEATING, or HYPERIDROSIS, may be caused by fever, hyperthyroidism, obesity, diabetes mellitus, or an anxiety state. Offensive perspiration, or bromidrosis, commonly occurs on the feet or in the armpits, and is due to bacterial decomposition of skin secretions.

PERTHES' DISEASE An affection of the hip in children, due to fragmentation of the epiphysis (or spongy extremity) of the head of the femur. It occurs in the age-group, 4 to 10 years, with a peak between 6 and 8. It is ten times more common in boys than girls, and is bilateral in 10 per cent of cases. The initial manifestation is a lurching gait with a limp, accompanied by pain. Treatment consists of bed rest and traction of the affected limb so long as there is pain and spasm. The child is then allowed up and about with a walking CALLIPER SPLINT until the condition has healed. Spontaneous recovery occurs in about two years.

PERTUSSIS Another name for whooping-cough. (See WHOOPING-COUGH.)

PES CAVUS Known popularly as claw foot, this is a deformity in which the foot has an abnormally high arch and the tips of the toes are turned under. Pes cavus may be present at birth or it can be caused by disruption of or damage to the blood and nerve supplies to the foot muscles. The use of a specially made insole in the shoe may help but surgery is sometimes needed.

PES PLANUS The technical name for FLAT-FOOT.

PESSARIES These are instruments designed to support a displaced UTERUS, or solid bodies suitably shaped for insertion into the VAGINA. Made of oil of theobromine or a glycerin basis, they are used for applying local treatment to the vagina.

PESTICIDES Any substance or mixture of substances intended for preventing or controlling any unwanted species of plants and animals. This includes any substances intended for use as plant growth regulators, defoliants or desiccants. The main groups of pesticides are: herbicides to control weeds; insecticides to control insects; fungicides to control or prevent fungal disease.

PETECHIAE Small red MACULES due to haemorrhage in the skin.

PETHIDINE HYDROCHLORIDE A synthetic analgesic and antispasmodic drug, which is used in the treatment of painful and spasmodic conditions in place of morphine and atropine. A prompt but short-lasting analgesic, it has less of a constipating effect than morphine but is less potent. Useful for analgesia during childbirth because it produces less respiratory depression in the baby than other opioids. Pethidine is a CONTROLLED DRUG.

PETIT MAL Less severe type of epileptic seizure that occurs usually in children or adolescents but less often in adults. (See EPILEPSY.)

PETRI DISHES Shallow, circular glass dishes, usually 10 cm in diameter, which are used in bacteriology laboratories for the growth of micro-organisms.

PET SCANNING Positron emission tomography is a nuclear-medicine diagnostic technique that works by identifying positrons – positively charged electrons – given off by substances labelled with radioactive varieties of elements. The result is three-dimensional images that identify metabolic and chemical activities of tissues, especially brain tissues. This provides information about tissue and organ functions, and these can be collated with structural images using COMPUTED TOMOGRAPHY or

MAGNETIC RESONANCE IMAGING. This provides information about tissue and organ functions. The equipment is very expensive and available in only a few hospitals in the United Kingdom. The technique is especially valuable in the assessment of neurological disorders.

PEYER'S PATCHES are conglomerations of lymphoid nodules in the ILEUM, or lower part of the small intestine. They play an important part in the defence of the body against bacterial invasion, as in TYPHOID fever.

PEYRONIES DISEASE Painful and deformed erection of the PENIS caused by the formation of fibrous tissue. The cause is unknown but it may be associated with DUPUYTREN'S CONTRACTURE. The condition may be improved by surgery.

pH A measurement of the concentration of hydrogen ions in a solution that is calculated as a negative logarithm. A neutral solution has a pH of 7·0 and this figure falls for a solution with increasing acidity and rises if the alkalinity increases.

PHAEOCHROMOCYTOMA A disorder in which a vascular tumour of the adrenal medulla develops. The tumour may also affect the structurally similar tissues associated with the chain of sympathetic nerves. There is uncontrolled and irregular secretion of ADRENALINE and NORADRENALINE with the result that the patient suffers from episodes of high blood pressure, raised heart rate, and headache. Surgery to remove the tumour may be possible; if not, drug treatment may help. (See HYPERTENSION.)

PHAGOCYTE Cells, including WHITE BLOOD CELLS and MACROPHAGES, that envelop and digest BACTERIA, cells, cell debris, and other small particles. These cells are a vital part of the body's defence system.

PHAGOCYTOSIS A process by which the attacks of bacteria upon the living body are repelled and the bacteria destroyed through the activity of the white cells of the blood.

PHALANX The name given to any one of the small bones of the fingers and toes. The phalanges are fourteen in number in each hand and foot, the thumb and great toe possessing only two each, whilst each of the other fingers and toes has three.

PHALLUS An alternative name for the PENIS, this word may also be used to describe a penis-like object. In embryology the phallus is the rudimentary penis before the urethral duct has completely developed.

PHANTASY, or FANTASY The term applied to an imaginary appearance or day dream.

PHANTOM LIMB Following the AMPUTATION of a limb it is usual for the patient to experience sensations as if the limb were still present. This condition is referred to as a phantom limb. In most patients the sensation passes off in time.

PHARMACISTS Experts in the preparation and dispensing of medicines, and in Great Britain they are registered by the Royal Pharmaceutical Society. The Pharmaceutical Society of Northern Ireland registers pharmacists in that part of the United Kingdom. Registered pharmacists can dispense P (pharmacy only) and POM (prescription-only medicine) products. Pharmacists also have expertise in the use of drugs, the way one drug affects another and possible adverse effects, and can advise on these matters. Hospital pharmacists are now invited by the COMMITTEE ON SAFETY OF MEDICINES to report suspected adverse drug reactions under the 'Yellow Card' scheme in the same way as doctors.

PHARMACOGENOMICS The use of human genetic variations to optimize the discovery and development of drugs and the treatment of patients. The human race varies much more in its genetic makeup than has previously been realized. These variations in GENES and their PROTEIN products could be utilized to provide safer and more effective drugs. Genes affect drug absorption, distribution, METABOLISM and excretion. Drugs are designed and prescribed on the basis of a population's needs, but patients comprise a diverse range of individuals. For example, nearly one-third of patients fail to respond to the cholesterol-reducing group of drugs, the STATINS. Around half do not respond to the TRICYCLIC ANTIDEPRESSANT drugs. Over 80 per cent of patients' responses to drugs depend on their genetics. This genetic variation needs to be identified and so make the prescription of drugs more effective, and technology for analysing genetic variants is progressing. Assessing drug effectiveness, however, is not simple because the health and diets of individuals are different and this can affect the response to a drug. Even so, the genetic identification of people who would or would not respond to a particular drug should benefit patients by ensuring a more accurately targeted drug and by reducing the risks to a person of side-effects from taking a drug that would not work. There would also be substantial economic savings.

PHARMACOKINETICS The way in which the body deals with a drug. This includes the drug's absorption, distribution in the tissues, metabolism, and excretion.

PHARMACOLOGY That part of medical science dealing with knowledge of the action of drugs.

PHARMACOPOEIA An official publication dealing with the recognized drugs and giving their doses, preparations, sources, and tests. Most countries have a pharmacopoeia of their own. That for Great Britain and Ireland is prepared by the British Pharmacopoeia Commission under the direction of the Medicines Commission. Many hospitals and medical schools have a small pharmacopoeia of their own, giving the prescriptions most commonly dispensed in that particular hospital or school. The *British National Formulary* is a compact authoritative volume for those concerned with the prescribing or dispensing of medicines.

PHARMACY The term applied to the practice of preparing and compounding medicines, or to a place where this is carried out.

PHARYNGITIS An inflammatory condition affecting the wall of the pharynx or throat proper. It is most commonly due to a viral upper respiratory tract infection. It may be confined to the pharynx or may also involve the rest of the upper respiratory tract, i.e. the nose and the larynx. The mucous membrane is red and glazed with enlarged lymph-follicles scattered over it. Only symptomatic treatment such as analgesic drugs or lozenges and gargles is necessary for viral pharyngitis, which usually is a stage in the development of a COLD or, less often, but more seriously, INFLUENZA. MONONUCLEOSIS may also start with pharyngitis. STREPTOCOCCAL bacteria – linked to SCARLET FEVER – also cause the condition. DIPHTHERIA is a rare but potentially dangerous infection that produces severe pharyngitis. If a sore throat persists the sufferer should seek medical advice.

PHARYNX Another name for the throat. The term throat is popularly applied to the region about the front of the neck generally, but in its strict sense it means the irregular cavity into which the nose and mouth open above, from which the larynx and gullet open below, and in which the channel for the air and that for the food cross one another. It extends from the base of the skull down to the 6th cervical vertebra, separated from the upper six vertebrae only by some loose fibrous tissue, and is about 12·5 cm (5 inches) long.

It is completely closed behind by a layer of muscles, and by mucous membrane, but in front it opens into the nose, mouth, and larynx in succession from above down. In its upper part, the EUSTACHIAN TUBES open one on either side, and between them on the back wall grows a mass of glandular tissue known as the third tonsil, which, if enlarged, produces the condition known as adenoids. (See NOSE, DISEASES OF.)

PHENAZOCINE HYDROBROMIDE A powerful analgesic which can be given under the tongue if nausea and vomiting are a problem.

PHENELZINE An example of the widely used antidepressant drugs which are classified as MONOAMINE OXIDASE INHIBITORS (MAOIS). The drug is particularly useful because its stimulant effect is less than most other MAOIs. (See ANTIDEPRESSANTS; MENTAL ILLNESS)

PHENINDIONE A synthetic ANTICOAGULANT. Given by mouth, it is used to prevent the formation of clots in the blood in rheumatic heart disease and atrial fibrillation (see HEART DISEASES); as prophylaxis after insertion of a prosthetic heart valve; prophylaxis and treatment of venous thrombosis and pulmonary embolism. It is slower in action than WARFARIN, not achieving its full anticoagulant effect until up to 48 hours after the initial dose. The drug should be avoided in patients with renal or hepatic impairment, and whenever severe hypersensitivity reactions have previously occurred. Adverse effects include rashes, fever, LEUCOPENIA, AGRANULOCYTOSIS, diarrhoea and pink urine; breast feeding should be avoided.

PHENOBARBITONE The *British Pharmacopoeia* name for one of the most widely used of all the BARBITURATE group of drugs. It is mainly used in combination with PHENYTOIN as an anticonvulsant drug in the control of EPILEPSY.

PHENOL Another name for CARBOLIC ACID .

PHENOLPHTHALEIN A laxative given by mouth. It is an irritant and may cause stomach cramps.

PHENOTHIAZINES A group of major antipsychotic drugs, colloquially called 'tranquillizers', widely used to treat psychoses. They can be divided into three main groups. Chlorpromazine, methotrimeprazine and promazine are examples of group 1, usually characterized by their sedative effects and moderate antimuscarinic and extrapyramidal side-effects. Group 2 includes pericyazine, pipothiazine and thioridazine, which have moderate sedative effects but significant anti-muscarinic action and modest extrapyramidal side-effects. Fluphenazine, perphenazine, prochlorperazine and trifluoperazine comprise group 3. Their sedative effects are less than for the other groups and they have little antimuscarinic action; they have marked extrapyramidal side-effects.

Uses Phenothiazines should be prescribed and used with care. The drugs differ in predominant actions and side-effects and selection depends on the extent of sedation required and the susceptibility of the patient to extrapyramidal side-effects. The differences between the drugs, however, are less important than the variabilities in patients' responses. Patients should not be prescribed more than one antipsychotic drug at a time. In the short term these therapeutically powerful drugs can be used to calm disturbed patients, whatever the underlying condition which might have a physical or psychiatric basis. They also alleviate acute anxiety and some have antidepressant properties, while others worsen depression (SEE MENTAL ILLNESS).

PHENOTHRIN (see PERMETHRIN).

PHENOTYPE An individual's characteristics as determined by the interaction between his genotype – his quota of GENES – and the environment.

PHENOXYBENZAMINE An alpha-adrenoceptor blocking drug (see ADRENERGIC RECEPTORS) used in the treatment of hypertension caused by PHAEOCHROMOCYTOMA.

PHENOXYMETHYLPENICILLIN Otherwise known as pencillin V, this drug, which can be taken orally, is used to treat TONSILLITIS, OTITIS MEDIA and ERYSIPELAS and as a prophylactic for RHEUMATIC FEVER and PNEUMOCOCCAL INFECTION. (See PENICILLIN.)

PHENYLALANINE A natural AMINO-ACID essential for growth in infants and nitrogen metabolism in adults.

PHENYLBUTAZONE A potent NON-STEROIDAL ANTI-INFLAMMATORY DRUG (NSAID). It sometimes has serious side-effects such as hypersensitivity and blood dyscrasias and should not be used for patients with cardiovascular disease or impairment of function in their lungs, kidney and liver or who have peptic ulceration. So use should be limited to patients with ankylosing spondylitis with treatment restricted to hospitals.

PHENYLKETONURIA One of the less common, but very severe, forms of mental deficiency. The incidence in populations of European origin is around 1 in 15,000 births. It is due to the inability of the baby to metabolize the amino-acid, phenylalamine. Its outstanding interest lies in the fact that, if it is diagnosed soon after birth – and this can be done by a simple urine test or by a test carried out on a drop of blood – and the infant is then given a diet low in phenylalamine, the chances are that the infant will grow up mentally normal. Parents of children with phenylketonuria can obtain help and information from the National Society for Phenylketonuria (UK) Ltd. (See APPENDIX 2: ADDRESSES.)

PHENYTOIN SODIUM An effective drug for the treatment of epilepsy. One of its advantages is that it does not make the patient feel particularly sleepy. Its use is not without risk and it must therefore be used only under medical supervision. (See EPILEPSY.)

PHEROMONES Chemicals produced and emitted by an individual which produce changes in the social or sexual behaviour when perceived by other individuals of the same species. The precise role of these odours, for it is by their smell that they are recognized, in man is still not clear, but there is growing evidence of the part they play in the animal kingdom. Thus if a strange male rat is put into a group of female rats, this may cause death of the fetus in any pregnant rats, and this is attributed to the pheromones emitted by the male rat.

PHIMOSIS Tightness of the foreskin (PRE-PUCE) which stops its being pulled back over the underlying head (glans) of the PENIS. Some phimosis is normal in uncircumcised males until they are six months old. The condition may, however, persist, eventually causing problems with urination. BALANITIS may occur because the inside of the foreskin cannot be properly washed. There may be an increased risk of cancer of the penis. In adolescents and adults with phimosis, erection of the penis is painful. CIRCUMCISION is the treatment (see PENIS).

PHLEBITIS Inflammation of a vein. (See VEINS, DISEASES OF.)

PHLEBOGRAPHY The study of the VEINS, particularly by means of X-rays after the veins have been injected with a radio-opaque substance.

PHLEBOLITH The term applied to a small stone formed in a VEIN as a result of calcification of a THROMBUS.

PHLEBOTOMY A traditional name for the operation of blood-letting by opening a vein. (See VENESECTION.)

PHLEGM A popular name for mucus, particularly that secreted in the air passages. (See BRONCHITIS; EXPECTORANTS; MUCUS.)

PHLYCTENULE A hypersensitivity reaction of the CONJUNCTIVA. At the turn of the century the commonest cause was TUBERCULOSIS. Nowadays it is most commonly due to hypersensitivity to STAPHYLOCOCCI.

PHOBIA An irrational fear of particular objects or situations. A well-known American medical dictionary lists over 200 'examples' of phobias, ranging, alphabetically, from air to writing. Included in the list are phobophobia (fear of phobias) and triskaidekaphobia (fear of thirteen at table). It is a form of obsession, and not uncommonly one of the features of the anxiety. Treatment is behavioural therapy complemented in some patients with ANTIDEPRES-

SANT drugs. Care is needed as some sufferers can become psychologically dependent on drugs used to treat them. (See MENTAL ILLNESS.) Those who suffer from what can be a most distressing condition can obtain help and advice from the Phobics Society (see APPENDIX 2: ADDRESSES).

PHOCOMELIA This is a great reduction in the size of the proximal parts of the limbs. In extreme cases the hands and feet may spring directly from the trunk. A rare condition, it occurred most commonly in children whose mothers took THALIDOMIDE in early pregnancy.

PHOLCODINE An OPIOID cough suppressant similar to CODEINE; it is not, however, potent enough to suppress severe coughs and it is also constipating.

PHONATION The production of vocal sounds, in particular, speech.

PHONOCARDIOGRAPH An instrument for the graphic recording of heart sounds and murmurs.

PHOSPHATES Salts of phosphoric acid, and, as this substance is contained in many articles of food as well as in bone, the nuclei of cells, and the nervous system, phosphates are constantly excreted in the URINE. The continued use of an excess of food containing alkalis, such as green vegetables, and still more the presence in the urine of bacteria which lead to its decomposition, produce the necessary change from the natural mild acidity to alkalinity, and lead to the deposit of phosphates and to their collection into stones.

PHOSPHATURIA The presence in the URINE of a large amount of phosphates.

PHOSPHORUS A non-metallic element whose compounds are widely found in plant and animal tissues. In humans, this element is largely concentrated in BONES. Some phosphorus-containing compounds such as ADENOSINE TRIPHOSPHATE (ATP) and creatine phosphate are essential participants in the conversion and storage of energy that are part of the body's metabolism. Pure phosphorus is toxic.

PHOSPHORUS BURNS Phosphorus compounds are used in chemical laboratories, some industrial processes, matches, fireworks and in certain types of aerial bombs and artillery shells. If particles of phosphorus settle on or become embedded in the skin, the resulting burn should be treated with a 2-per-cent sodium bicarbonate solution, followed by application of a 1-per-cent solution of copper sulphate.

PHOSPHORUS POISONING Now rare, this is produced only by the yellow, soluble form of phosphorus found in matches, fireworks, some insecticides and rat poisons.

Signs and symptoms When swallowed, it acts first as an irritant, and on being absorbed, results in acute degeneration of the liver and other abdominal organs. Exposure to phosphorus fumes in chemical works may lead to a chronic form of poisoning, with severe debility. Necrosis of the lower jaw bone (phossy jaw) occurs over months or years; this may be partly due to a secondary infection in the bone. Acute symptoms, most common in children after swallowing a large dose of poison, include pain, vomiting, colic, diarrhoea, and even convulsions. The breath often smells of garlic, and death may occur within a few hours. Partial recovery may occur, but jaundice and blood-stained urine develop after a few days, leading to death.

Treatment Phosphorus is slowly absorbed, so stomach wash-outs using copper sulphate up to two hours after swallowing the poison may succeed. Calcium injections along with treatment for kidney and liver failure are advisable. Chronic poisoning in chemical works is prevented by good ventilation, cleanliness, and regular dental examination of the workers. (See POISONS and APPENDIX 2: ADDRESSES.)

PHOTOCHEMOTHERAPY A form of treatment in which deliberate exposure to a photosensitizing drug and ultraviolet light benefits certain skin diseases, particularly PSORIASIS and T-cell LYMPHOMA. A psoralen is the photoactive agent which reacts with long-wave ultraviolet light (UVA), giving the acronym PUVA therapy.

PHOTOCOAGULATION Coagulation of the tissues of the retina by laser for treatment of diseases of the retina such as diabetic retinopathy (see RETINA, DISORDERS OF).

PHOTODERMATOSES Diseases of the skin for which sunlight is partially or wholly responsible. In sufficient dosage, short-wave ULTRAVIOLET LIGHT (UVB) always causes ERYTHEMA. Higher doses progressively cause OEDEMA and blistering; this is acute sunburn. Graduated exposure to UVB causes pigmentation (tanning). Prolonged chronic exposure to sunlight eventually accelerates ageing of the exposed skin with LENTIGO formation and loss of COLLAGEN and elastic tissue. After decades of such exposure, epidermal DYSPLASIA and CANCER may supervene.

Drugs given orally or topically may induce phototoxic reactions of various types. Thus, TETRACYCLINES exaggerate sunburn reactions. SULPHONAMIDES and the diuretic FRUSEMIDE may cause blistering reactions. Psoralens induce erythema and pigmentation. (See PHOTOCHEMOTHERAPY.) AMIODARONE also induces pigmentation.

Phytophotodermatitis is a streaky blistering photodermatosis typically seen on the limbs of children playing in grassy meadows in summer. The phototoxic reaction is caused by psoralens in weeds.

Berlocque dermatitis is a pattern of streaky pigmentation usually seen on women's necks, caused by a reaction to psoralens in perfumes.

Certain rare metabolic diseases may lead to photosensitization. They include the PORPHYRIAS and PELLAGRA. Other skin diseases such as LUPUS ERYTHEMATOSUS and ROSACEA may be aggravated by light exposure. Sometimes, in the absence of any of these factors, some people spontaneously develop a sensitivity to light causing various patterns of ECZEMA or URTICARIA. The commonest pattern is 'polymorphic light eruption' which typically appears within a day or two of arrival at a sunny holiday destination and persists until departure. Continuously exposed areas, such as the hands and face, may be 'hardened' and unaffected.

Treatment of photodermatoses Appropriate clothing and headgear, sunscreen creams and lotions are the main preventative measures.

PHOTOPHOBIA Sensitivity to light. It can occur in disorders of the eye, or in meningitis.

PHOTOPSIA This is a description of the flashing lights which are a not uncommon aura preceding an attack of migraine.

PHOTOSENSITIVITY Abnormal reaction to sunlight. The condition usually occurs as a skin rash appearing in response to light falling on the skin, and it may be caused by substances that have been eaten or applied to the skin. These are called photosensitizers and may be dyes, chemicals in soaps, or drugs. Sometimes plants act as photosensitizers – for example, buttercups and mustard. The condition may occur in some illnesses such as LUPUS ERYTHEMATOSUS.

PHOTOSYNTHESIS The method by which green plants and some bacteria produce CARBOHYDRATES from water and carbon dioxide. They use energy absorbed from the sun's rays by a green pigment in the organism called chlorophyll. It is one of the earth's fundamental biological processes. As well as converting the carbon dioxide into the essential biological compound carbohydrate, the process removes the gas from the atmosphere where, if it builds to excess, the atmospheric temperature rises, thus contributing to global warming.

PHRENIC NERVE The nerve which chiefly supplies the DIAPHRAGM. A phrenic nerve arises on each side of the spinal cord from the 3rd, 4th, and 5th cervical spinal nerves; both follow a long course down the neck, and through the chest to the diaphragm. They play a key part in respiration through control of the diaphragm. Injury to one nerve paralyses one half of the diaphragm. Occasionally the phrenic nerve may be surgically crushed as part of the treatment to repair a HIATUS HERNIA or, rarely, to stop intractable hiccups.

PHRENOLOGY A traditional term applied to the study of the mind and character of individuals from the shape of the head. As the shape of the head has been shown to depend chiefly upon accidental characteristics, such as the size of the air spaces in the bones, and not upon development of special areas in the contained brain, there is no scientific basis for the practice.

PHTHISIS This traditional term means wasting, and was the general term applied to that progressive enfeeblement and loss of weight that arose from tuberculous disease of all kinds, but especially from the disease as it affects the lungs (see TUBERCULOSIS).

PHYSICAL EXAMINATION That part of a patient's consultation with a doctor in which the doctor looks, palpates (feels) and listens to various parts of the patient's body. Along with the history of the patient's symptoms, this enables the doctor to assess the patient's condition and decide whether an immediate diagnosis is possible or whether laboratory or imaging investigations are needed to reach a diagnosis. A full physical examination may take 30 minutes or more. Physical examination, along with certain standard investigations, is done when a person attends for a 'preventive' check-up of his or her state of health.

PHYSICAL MEDICINE A medical specialty founded in 1931 and recognized by the Royal College of Physicians of London in 1972. Physical-medicine specialists started by treating rheumatic diseases. Subsequently their work developed to include the diagnosis and rehabilitation of people with physical handicaps. The specialty has now been combined with the specialty of RHEUMATOLOGY.

PHYSIOLOGY is the branch of medical science that deals with the healthy functions of different organs, and the changes that the whole body undergoes in the course of its activities. The teaching of physiology is a basic part of the medical student's initial education.

PHYSIOTHERAPY An important treatment involving the use of physical measures, such as exercise, heat, manipulation and remedial exercises in the treatment of disease. An alternative name is PHYSICAL MEDICINE. It is an essential part of the rehabilitation of convalescent or disabled patients. Those who practise physiotherapy – physiotherapists – have a recognized training and, on successful completion of this, they are placed on the profession's official register (see APPENDIX 10: PROFESSIONAL ORGANIZATIONS).

PHYSOSTIGMINE, or ESERINE   An alkaloid obtained from Calabar bean, the seed of *Physostigma venenosum*, a climbing plant of West Africa. Its action depends on the presence of two alkaloids, the one known as physostigmine or eserine, the other as calabarine, the former of these being much the more important.

Action   Physostigmine produces the same effect as stimulation of the PARASYMPATHETIC NERVOUS SYSTEM: i.e. it constricts the pupil, stimulates the gut, increases the secretion of saliva, stimulates the bladder, and increases the irritability of voluntary muscle. In poisonous doses it brings on a general paralysis.

Uses   It is used in medicine in the form of eyedrops or ointment to treat GLAUCOMA.

PHYTOMENADIONE   The *British Pharmacopoeia* name for vitamin K. (See APPENDIX 5: VITAMINS.)

PIA MATER   The membrane closely investing the brain and spinal cord, in which run blood-vessels for the nourishment of these organs. (See BRAIN; SPINAL CORD.)

PICA   This is the Latin for magpie and is a term which means an abnormal craving for unusual foods. It is not uncommon in pregnancy. Among the unusual substances for which pregnant women have developed a craving are soap, clay pipes, bed linen, charcoal, ashes – and almost every imaginable foodstuff taken in excess. In primitive races it is taken to mean that it indicates the growing fetus requires such food. It is also not uncommon in children. (See APPETITE; LEAD POISONING.)

PICORNA VIRUSES   These infectious agents derive their name from pico (small) and RNA (because they contain ribonuleic acid). They are a group of viruses which includes the ENTEROVIRUSES and the RHINOVIRUSES.

PIGEON BREAST (see CHEST, DEFORMITIES OF).

PIGMENT   The term applied to the colouring matter of various secretions, blood, etc.; also to any medicinal preparation of thick consistence intended for painting on the skin or mucous membranes.

PILES (see HAEMORRHOIDS).

PILLS   Small round masses containing active drugs held together by syrup, gum, glycerin, or adhesive vegetable extracts. They are some-times without coating, being merely rolled in French chalk, but often they are covered with sugar or gelatin. Some pills, designed to act upon the bowels only, are coated with keratin, salol or other substances which are insoluble in the gastric juice.

PILOCARPINE   An alkaloid derived from the leaves of *Pilocarpus microphyllus* (jaborandi). It produces the same effects as stimulation of the parasympathetic nervous system: i.e. it has exactly the opposite effect to ATROPINE, but cannot be used in the treatment of atropine poisoning as it does not antagonize the action of poisonous doses of atropine on the brain. Its main use today is in the form of eye-drops to decrease the pressure inside the eyeball in GLAUCOMA.

PILONOIDAL SINUS   A SINUS that contains hairs, usually occurring in the cleft between the buttocks. It may get infected and cause considerable pain. Treatment is by antibiotics and, if necessary, surgical removal.

PIMPLES   Technically known as papules, these are small, raised, and inflamed areas on the skin. On the face the most common cause is ACNE. BOILS start as hard pimples. The eruption of smallpox and that of chickenpox begin also with pimples. (See also SKIN DISEASES.)

PINEAL GLAND   A small reddish structure, 10 mm in length and shaped somewhat like a pine cone (hence its name), situated on the upper part of the mid-brain. Many theories have been expounded as to its function, but there is increasing evidence that, in some animals at least, it is affected by light and plays a part in hibernation and in controlling sexual activity and the colour of the skin. This it seems to do by means of a substance it produces known as melatonin. There is also growing evidence that it may play a part in controlling the circadian rhythms of the body – the natural variations in physiological activities throughout the 24-hour day.

PINNA   The part of the ear, formed of cartilage and skin, that is external to the head. In animals it is an important element in detecting the direction of sound.

PINS AND NEEDLES   A form of PARAESTHESIA, or disturbed sensation, such as may occur, for example, in NEURITIS or POLYNEURITIS.

PINT   A measure of quantity containing 16 fluid ounces (wine measure) or 20 fluid ounces (Imperial measure). The metric equivalent is 568 millilitres. (See APPENDIX 6: MEASUREMENTS IN MEDICINE.)

PINWORM (see ENTEROBIASIS).

PIPERACILLIN A ureidopenicillin with a broad spectrum of antibacterial activity. The drug is active against the serious infective agent *Pseudomonas aeruginosa*. (See PENICILLIN.)

PIPERAZINE A drug used for the treatment of threadworms and ascariasis. (See ASCARIASIS; ENTEROBIASIS.)

PIPOTHIAZINE An antipsychotic drug for maintenance treatment of SCHIZOPHRENIA. It is given as a depot injection that lasts four weeks. (See NEUROLEPTICS; MENTAL ILLNESS.)

PIROXICAM An intermediate risk, oral NON-STEROIDAL ANTI-INFLAMMATORY drug with prolonged action. Used to treat pain and inflammation in rheumatoid arthritis, other musculoskeletal disorders and acute gout.

PITHIATISM A group of disorders in which the patient is subject to cure by persuasion or suggestion, the term being used as an equivalent for hysteria. (See HYSTERIA.)

PITUITARY GLAND Also known as the PITUITARY BODY and the HYPOPHYSIS, this is an ovoid structure, weighing around 0·5 gram in the adult. It is attached to the base of the brain, and lies in the depression in the base of the skull known as the sella turcica. Though physically divided into two by a cleavage, the multiplicity of its functions and its dual origins have resulted in its being 'divided up' according to its origins. The anterior part is derived in the embryo from the ectoderm (see FETUS) of the primitive mouth, and this part of the gland is now known as the adenohypophysis. The posterior part is derived from the brain and is now known as the neurohypophysis. The gland is connected to the HYPOTHALAMUS of the brain by a stalk known as the hypophyseal or pituitary stalk. The adenohypophysis is made up of the anterior lobe which, in turn, is subdivided into a pars distalis and a pars tuberalis, and the pars intermedia of the posterior lobe. The neurohypophysis is also made up of three parts: the infundibular process (or neural lobe) of the posterior lobe, the nervous part of the stalk known as the infundibular or neural stalk, and the median eminence of the tuber cinereum. The pars distalis, which accounts for the greater part of the gland, is composed of masses of cells which fall into three main groups: (1) chromophobe cells (ungranulated cells in the front lobe of the pituitary gland) which do not stain and constitute about 50 per cent of the total; (2) acidophil cells which stain with acid dyes and constitute about 35 per cent of the total; and (3) basophil cells which stain with basic stains and constitute about 15 per cent of the total. The pars intermedia consists only of a few cells, whilst the pars tuberalis contains non-granular cells. The neurohypophysis is composed of nerve fibres and brown granular cells known as pituicytes.

The pituitary gland is the most important ductless, or endocrine, gland in the body. (See ENDOCRINE GLANDS.) It exerts over-all control of the endocrine system through the media of a series of hormones which it produces. The adenohypophysis is the major producer of these, and those it produces will be dealt with first. Those which function through the media of other endocrine glands are known as trophic hormones and have therefore been given names ending with 'trophic' or 'trophin'. The thyrotrophic hormone, or thyroid-stimulating hormone (abbreviated to TSH as it is also known, exerts a powerful influence over the activity of the thyroid gland. The adrenocorticotrophic hormone, also known as corticotrophin (ACTH), stimulates the cortex of the adrenal glands. The growth, or somatotrophic, hormone, also known as somatotrophin (SMH), controls the growth of the body. There are also two gonadotrophic hormones which play a vital part in the control of the gonads: these are the follicle-stimulating hormone (FSH), and the luteinizing hormone (LH) which is also known as the interstitial-cell-stimulating hormone (ICSH). (See GONADOTROPHINS.) The lactogenic hormone, also known as prolactin, mammotrophin and luteotrophin, induces lactation. The neurohypophysis produces two hormones. One is oxytocin which is widely used because of its stimulating effect on contraction of the uterus. The other is vasopressin, or the antidiuretic hormone (ADH), which acts on the renal tubules and the collecting tubules (see KIDNEYS) to increase the amount of water that they normally absorb.

ACROMEGALY or gigantism is the result of the over-activity of, or tumour formation of, the acidophil cells in the adenohypophysis which produce the growth hormone. If this over-activity occurs after growth has ceased, acromegaly arises, in which there is gross over-growth of the ears, nose, jaws, and hands and feet. Dwarfism may be due to lack of the growth hormone. DIABETES INSIPIDUS, a condition characterized by the passing of a large volume of urine every day, is due to lack of the antidiuretic hormone. Enhanced pro-duction of ACTH by the basophil cells of the pituitary leads to CUSHING'S SYNDROME. Excessive production of prolactin by micro or macro adenomas leads to hyperprolactinaemia and consequent AMENORRHOEA and GALACTORRHOEA. Some chromophobe adenomas do not produce any hormone but cause effects by damaging the pituitary cells and inhibiting their hormone production. The most sensitive cells to extrinsic pressure are the gonadotrophin-producing cells and the growth-hormone producing cells, so that if the tumour occurs in childhood growth-hormone will be suppressed and growth will cease. Gonadotrophin hormone suppression will prevent the development of puberty and if the tumour occurs after puberty will result in amenorrhoea in the female and lack of libido in both sexes. The thyroid-stimulating hormone cells are the next to suffer and the pressure effects on these cells will result in hypothyroidism. Fortunately the ACTH-producing cells are the most resistant to extrinsic pressure and this is teleologically sound as ACTH is the one pituitary hormone that is essential to life. However, these cells do suffer damage from intracellular tumours, and adrenocortical insufficiency is not uncommon (see APPENDIX 2: ADDRESSES).

PITYRIASIS Dermatosis typified by a branlike desquamation of the skin. There are several varieties including P. alba, rosea, versicolor (fungal caused) and rubra (exfoliative dermatitis).

Pityriasis alba is a mild form of chronic eczema occurring mainly in children on the face and in young adults on the upper arms. It is characterized by round or oval flaky patches which are paler than the surrounding skin due to partial loss of melanin pigment. The appearance is more dramatic in dark-skinned or suntanned subjects. Moisturizing cream often suffices but 1-per-cent hydrocortisone cream is more effective.

Pityriasis rosea is a common self-limiting eruption seen mainly in young adults. It usually begins as a solitary red flaky patch (often misdiagnosed as ringworm). Within a week this 'herald patch' is followed by a profuse symmetrical eruption of smaller rose-pink, flaky, oval lesions on the trunk and neck but largely sparing the limbs and face. Itching is variable. The eruption usually peaks within 3 weeks and fades away leaving collarettes of scale, disappearing within six or seven weeks. It rarely recurs and a viral cause is suspected but not proved. It is not contagious and there is no specific treatment but crotamiton cream (Eurax) relieves discomfort.

PIVAMPICILLIN A broad-spectrum oral PENICILLIN active against some gram-negative and gram-positive organisms. (See ANTIBIOTIC.)

PLACEBO No treatments of specific value are found in all the pages of Hippocrates. Nevertheless the placebo response occurred with sufficient frequency to enable the physician to command respect. The therapeutic opportunities are now very different. However, man himself has not changed. He still wants and expects to take medicine when he is ill and is still just as subject to persuasion and suggestion. Despite the scientific advances of this century the physician remains a key therapeutic agent.

Placebo is the Latin for 'I will please'. Traditionally, placebos were used to pacify without actually benefiting the patient. They were inactive substances formerly given to please or gratify the patient but now only used in controlled studies to determine the efficacy of drugs. However, pharmacologically inert compounds can relieve symptoms and this is called the placebo effect. The reassurance that is associated with placebo administration is accompanied by measurable changes in body function which are affected through autonomic pathways and humoral mechanisms. Alterations in blood pressure and pulse frequency are especially common. Placebos have the ability to relieve a variety of symptoms in a consistent proportion of the population. Some patients with symptoms such as pain or cough will respond to placebo medications and an even higher proportion of patients with psychological symptoms such as anxiety or insomnia may benefit. Current scientific jargon defines the placebo as any therapy or component of therapy that is deliberately or unknowingly used for its non-specific psychological or psycho-biological effect and that is without specific activity for the condition being treated.

PLACENTA The thick, spongy disc-like mass of tissue which connects the EMBRYO with the inner surface of the UTERUS, the embryo otherwise lying free in the amniotic fluid. (See AMNION.) The placenta is mainly a new structure growing with the embryo, but, when it separates, a portion of the inner surface of the womb, called the maternal placenta, comes away with it. It is mainly composed of loops of veins belonging to the embryo, lying in blood-sinuses, in which circulates maternal blood. Thus, though no mixing of the blood of embryo and mother takes place, there is ample opportunity for the exchange of fluids, gases, and the nutriment brough by the mother's blood. The width of the full-sized placenta is about 20 cm (8 inches), its thickness 2·5 cm (1 inch). One surface is rough and studded with villi, which consist of the loops of foetal veins; the other is smooth, and has implanted in its centre the umbilical cord, or navel string, which is about as thick as a finger and 50 cm (20 inches) long. It contains two arteries and a vein, enters the foetus at the navel, and forms the sole connection between the bodies of mother and foetus. The name 'afterbirth' is given to the structure because it is expelled from the womb in the third stage of labour (see LABOUR).

PLACENTA PRAEVIA Implantation of the placenta in the bottom part of the UTERUS adjacent to or over the CERVIX. The condition may cause few problems during PREGNANCY or labour; it may, however, cause vaginal bleeding late in pregnancy and this requires medical attention.

PLACENTOGRAPHY The procedure of rendering the PLACENTA visible by means of X-rays. This can be done either by using what is known as soft-tissue radiography, or by injecting a radio-opaque substance into the blood-stream or into the amniotic cavity. (See AMNION.) The procedure has some risk to both mother and fetus, and is carried out under expert supervision. It can help to assess the cause of antepartum haemorrhage. The placenta and fetus can now be visualized by the non-invasive and safe method of ULTRASOUND.

PLAGUE This infection – also known as bubonic plague – is caused by the bacterium *Yersinis pestis* (identified by Yersin in Hong Kong in 1894). It has caused millions of deaths in numerous epidemics and pandemics over many centuries. Originating in Asia, it probably caused the Plague of Athens (430 BC), and that of Justinian in AD 542. In the Middle Ages the 'Black Death' (1348) swept through Europe reducing the human population by one third to one half; it had a major impact on the educated classes in Britain. The Great Plague of London (1665) killed some 70,000 people in the capital, out of a total population of approximately 460,000. Small outbreaks have since occurred in Europe, the last in Britain being in Suffolk in the 1920s. Plague remains a major infection in many tropical countries; WHO statistics indicate significant annual mortality from this bacterial infection.

The reservoir for the bacillus in urban infection lies in the black (*Rattus rattus*), and less importantly the brown (sewer) rat (*Rattus norvegicus*). It is conveyed to man by the rat flea, usually *Xenopsylla cheopis*: *Y. pestis* multiplies in the gastrointestinal tract of the flea, which may remain infectious for up to 6 weeks. In the pneumonic form (see below), human-to-human transmission can occur by droplet infection. Many lower mammals (apart from the rat) can also act as a reservoir in sylvatic transmission which remains a major problem in the USA (mostly in the south-western States); ground-squirrels, rock-squirrels, prairie dogs, bobcats, chipmunks, etc., can be affected.

Clinically, symptoms usually begin 2–8 days after infection; disease begins with fever, headache, lassitude, and aching limbs. In over two-thirds of patients, enlarged glands (buboes) appear – usually in the groins, but also in the axillae and cervical neck; this constitutes bubonic plague. Haemorrhages may be present beneath the skin causing gangrenous patches and occasionally ulcers; these lesions led to the epithet 'Black Death'. In a favourable case, fever abates after about a week, and the buboes discharge foul-smelling pus. In a rapidly fatal form (septicaemic plague), haematogenous transmission produces mortality in a high percentage of cases. Pneumonic plague is associated with pneumonic consolidation (person-to-person transmission) and death often ensues on the fourth or fifth day. (The nursery rhyme 'Ring-o-ring o' roses, a pocketful o' posies, atishoo! atishoo!, we all fall down' is considered to have originated in the 17th century and refers to this form of the disease.) In addition, meningitic and pharyngeal forms of the disease can occur; these are unusual. Diagnosis consists of demonstration of the causative organism.

Treatment was revolutionized by the introduction of sulphonamides, followed by streptomycin in 1948. Tetracycline or doxycycline is now frequently used and a range of other antibiotics are also effective. There is no indication of development of antibiotic-resistance in *Y. pestis*, which is a highly sensitive organism. Plague remains (together with cholera and yellow fever) a quarantinable disease. Prevention is dominated by vector control. Contacts should be disinfected with insecticide powder; clothes, skins, soft merchandise, etc., which have been in contact with the infection can remain infectious for several months; suspect items should be destroyed or disinfected with an insecticide. Ships must be carefully checked for presence of rats; the rationale of anchoring a distance from the quay prevents access of vermin. Vaccination is not widely available, although research is in progress.

PLANTAR Describing anything related to the sole of the foot.

PLANTAR DERMATOSIS usually called JUVENILE PLANTAR DERMATITIS, is a common form of eczema of the soles of the feet typically seen in boys with an atopic background who constantly wear trainers.

PLANTAR FASCIITIS (See FASCIITIS.)

PLAQUE A coating of the teeth which forms as a result of poor mouth and dental hygiene. It consists of food debris and bacteria and later calcium salts will be deposited in it to form calculus. It is therefore associated with both caries and periodontal disease.

PLASMA The name applied to the straw-coloured fluid portion of the blood composed of a solution of various inorganic salts of sodium, potassium, calcium, etc., as well as serum and fibrinogen, the material which produces clotting. When the plasma is clotted, the thinner fluid separating from the clot is serum.

PLASMA CELLS These are cells that produce antibodies and occur in bone-forming tissue as well as the lining of the gastrointestinal tract and the lungs. The cells develop in LYMPH nodes, SPLEEN and bone marrow when B-LYMPHOCYTES are stimulated by ANTIGENS to produce the precursor cells from which plasma cells originate.

PLASMA EXCHANGE or PLASMAPHERISIS The removal of the circulating PLASMA from the patient. It is done by removing blood from a patient and returning the red cells with a plasma expander. The plasma exchange is carried out through an in-dwelling cannula in the femoral vein and the red cells and plasma are separated by a hemonetics separator. Usually a sequence of three or four sessions is undertaken, at each of which two to three litres of plasma are removed. The lost plasma can either be replaced by human serum albumin or a plasma expander.

In auto-immune disorders the disease is due to damage wrought by circulating ANTIBODIES or sensitized LYMPHOCYTES. If the disease is due to circulating humoral antibodies, removal of these antibodies from the body should theoretically relieve the disorder. This is the principle on which plasma exchange was used in the management of auto-immune diseases due to circulating antibodies. Such disorders include Goodpasture's syndrome, SYSTEMIC LUPUS ERYTHEMATOSUS and MYASTHENIS GRAVIS. One of the problems in the use of plasma exchange in the treatment of such diseases is that the body responds to the removal of antibody from the circulation by enhanced production of that antibody by the immune system. It is therefore necessary to suppress this homeostatic response with cytotoxic drugs such as AZATHIOPRINE. Nevertheless remissions can be achieved in auto-immune diseases due to circulating antibodies by the process of plasma exchange.

PLASMAPHERISIS   (see PLASMA EXCHANGE).

PLASMA TRANSFUSION This procedure is sometimes used instead of blood transfusion. Plasma, the fluid part of blood from which the cells have been separated, may be dried and in powder form kept almost indefinitely; when wanted it is reconstituted by adding sterile distilled water. In powder form it can be transported easily and over long distances. Transfusion of plasma is especially useful in the treatment of shock. One advantage of plasma transfusion is that it is not necessary to carry out testing of blood groups before using it. (See TRANSFUSION OF BLOOD.)

PLASMIDS A generic description of any discrete agents in cells that have genetic functions. They include plasmagenes (self-reproducing copies of a nuclear gene existing outside the cell nucleus) and viruses.

PLASMINOGEN A precursor of plasmin, an enzyme that digests the protein fibrin, the main constituent of blood clots. When tissue is damaged, activators are released which provoke the conversion of plasminogen into plasmin.

PLASMODIUM The general term applied to minute protoplasmic cells, and particularly to those which cause malaria and allied diseases. (See MALARIA.)

PLASTER OF PARIS A form of calcium sulphate, which, after soaking in water, sets firmly. For this reason it is widely used as a form of splinting in the treatment of fractures, for producing casts to immobilize parts of the body and for dental models. Splints are made with bandages impregnated with plaster and a suitable adhesive. Its great advantage, compared with an ordinary splint, is that it can be moulded to the shape of the limb. This technique was originally introduced by a Dutchman in 1852. A predecessor of it, which seemed to serve its purpose well, was a bandage stiffened by soaking in egg white and flour.

PLASTIC or RECONSTRUCTIVE SURGERY Reconstructive surgery on the skin and underlying tissues that have been damaged or lost as a result of disease or injury. Congenital malformations are also remedied using reconstructive surgery. Surgeons graft healthy skin from another part of the body to repair skin damaged or destroyed by burns or injuries. New techniques are under development for growing new skin in the laboratory to be used in reconstructive surgery. Surgeons also repair damage using skin flaps prepared in another part of the body – for example, a skin flap from the arm may be used to repair a badly injured nose or face. Reconstructive surgery is also used to repair the consequences of an operation for cancer of, say, the neck or the jaw. Plastic surgeons also undertake cosmetic surgery to improve the appearance of noses, breasts, abdomens and faces.

PLATELETS Blood platelets, or thrombocytes. Small spherical bodies in the blood, which play an important part in the process of blood COAGULATION. Normally, there are around 300,000 per cubic millimetre of blood.

PLATING A term used in connection with bacteriological investigation to mean the cultivation of bacteria on flat plates containing nutrient material. The term is also applied in surgery to the method of securing union of fractured bones by screwing to the sides of the fragments narrow metal plates, which hold them firmly together while union is taking place.

PLETHORA A condition of fullness of the blood-vessels in a particular part or in the whole body. This results in a florid, red appearance of the affected area, particularly the face. The volume of blood may be increased (POLYCYTHAEMIA) or the blood vessels beneath the skin may be dilated.

PLETHYSMOGRAPH An apparatus for estimating changes in the size of any part placed in the apparatus; in this way changes in the volume of blood in a part can be measured.

PLEURA, or PLEURAL MEMBRANE The name of the membrane which, on either side of the chest, forms a covering for one lung. The two pleurae are distinct, though they touch one another for a short distance behind the breastbone. (See LUNGS.)

PLEURAL CAVITY The normally restricted space between the parietal and visceral PLEURA, which slide over one another as the individual breathes in and out. If gas or fluid are introduced as a result of injury or infection, the pleural surfaces are separated and the pleural space increases in volume. This usually causes breathing difficulties.

PLEURISY, or PLEURITIS Inflammation of the pleura or serous membrane investing the lung and lining the inner surface of the ribs. It is a common condition, and may be either acute or chronic, the latter being usually tuberculous in origin.

Many cases of pleurisy are associated with only a little effusion, the inflammation consisting chiefly in exudation of fibrin. To this form the term 'dry pleurisy' is applied. Further, pleurisy may be limited to a very small area, or, on the contrary, may affect, throughout a greater or less extent, the pleural surfaces of both lungs.

Causes Pleurisy is often associated with other forms of inflammatory disease within the chest, more particularly PNEUMONIA, BRONCHIECTASIS, and TUBERCULOSIS, and also occasionally accompanies PERICARDITIS. It may also be due to carcinoma of the lung, or be secondary to abdominal infections such as subphrenic abscess. Further, wounds or injuries of the thoracic walls are apt to set up pleurisy.

Symptoms The symptoms of pleurisy vary, being generally well marked, but sometimes obscure.
DRY PLEURISY In the case of dry pleurisy, which is, on the whole, the milder form, the chief symptom is a sharp pain in the side, felt especially on breathing. Fever may or may not be present. There is a slight, dry cough, and breathing is quicker than normal and shallow.
PLEURISY WITH EFFUSION is usually more severe than dry pleurisy, and, although it may in some cases develop insidiously, it is in general ushered in sharply by shivering and fever, like other acute inflammatory diseases. Pain is felt in the side or breast, of a severe cutting or stabbing character. A dry cough usually occurs and breathing is painful and difficult.

Treatment The treatment varies greatly with the form and severity of the attack. Bed rest, antibiotics, analgesics and antipyretics are advisable. A large pleural effusion may need to be drained via an aspiration needle.

PLEURODYNIA A painful condition of the chest-wall. It is usually the result of an infection of coxsackie virus B and may occur in epidemics. Often called Bornholm disease, it commonly affects children. Fever, sore throat, headache and malaise are typical but the condition is self limiting, subsiding within a few days.

PLEXUS A network of nerves or vessels: e.g. the brachial and sacral plexuses of nerves and the choroid plexus of veins within the brain.

PLUMBISM Another name for LEAD POISONING.

PLUMMER-VINSON SYNDROME A syndrome associated with certain cases of hypochromic anaemia. It consists of hyochromic anaemia, and difficulty in swallowing due to an oesophageal web. It is found almost exclusively in women. (See ANAEMIA.)

PNEUMO- A prefix relating to the lungs or to air. Examples are PNEUMONIA, PNEUMONECTOMY and PNEUMOPERITONEUM.

PNEUMOCOCCUS A type of STREPTOCOCCAL bacterium which is associated with PNEUMONIA and other infections of the respiratory tract.

PNEUMOCONIOSIS The general name applied to a chronic form of inflammation of the lungs which is liable to affect workmen who constantly inhale irritating particles at work. It has been defined by the Industrial Injuries Advisory Council as: 'Permanent alteration of lung structure due to the inhalation of mineral dust and the tissue reactions of the lung to its presence but does not include bronchitis and emphysema'. Some of the trades liable to suffer are those of stone-masons, potters, steel-grinders, coal-miners, millers, and workers in cotton, flax, or wool mills. (See OCCUPATIONAL DISEASES; TUBERCULOSIS.)

PNEUMOCYSTIS PNEUMONIA Pneumonia caused by a species of the genus of PROTOZOA, a parasitic micro-organism. *Pneumocystis carinii* causes an opportunistic infection in the lung which is dangerous to people whose immune system is impaired, thus reducing their resistance to infections. People with AIDS or leukaemia have impaired immune systems and *P. carinii* is a major cause of death in the former. Fever, dry cough and breathlessness are among the symptoms. Treatment is with high doses of antibiotic drugs such as CO-TRIMOXAZOLE or PENTAMIDINE.

PNEUMONECTOMY The operation of removing an entire lung in such diseases as bronchiectasis, tuberculosis, and cancer of the lung.

PNEUMONIA Pneumonia is an inflammation of the lung tissue caused by infection. The term ALVEOLITIS is used when the inflammation is the result of an ALLERGIC process and PNEUMONITIS when the provoking agent is chemical or physical. Pneumonia can occur with no underlying lung or general disease or in patients with an underlying condition that makes them susceptible.

Pneumonia with no predisposing cause, community-acquired pneumonia, is caused most often by a gram-positive bacterium, *Streptococcus pneumoniae* or the PNEUMOCOCCUS. The other most common causes are viruses, *Mycoplasma pneumoniae* and *Legionella* species (Legionnaire's disease). *Staphylococcus aureus* is an alternative agent seen in influenza epidemics. Another cause, *Chlamydia psittaci*, may be associated with exposure to perching birds.

In patients with underlying lung disease, such as CHRONIC OBSTRUCTIVE PULMONARY DISEASE (COPD) or bronchiectasis, other organisms such as *Haemophilus influenzae*, Klebsiella, *Escherichia coli* and *Pseudomonas aeruginosa* are more prominent. In patients in hospital with severe underlying disease, pneumonia, often caused by GRAM-NEGATIVE BACTERIA, is commonly the terminal event.

In patients with an immune system suppressed by HIV INFECTION, CHEMOTHERAPY or IMMUNOSUPPRESSIVE drugs after organ transplantation, a wider range of opportunistic organisms needs to be considered. Some of these organisms such as CYTOMEGALOVIRUS or the fungus *Pneumocystis carinii* rarely cause disease in immunocompetent individuals – those whose body's immune (defence) system is effective (see IMMUNITY).

TUBERCULOSIS is another cause of pneumonia, although the pattern of lung involvement and the more chronic course usually differentiate it from other causes of pneumonia.

Symptoms The common symptoms of pneumonia are cough, fever, sometimes with RIGORS, pleuritic chest pain and shortness of breath. Sputum may not be present at first but later may be purulent or reddish (rusty).

Examination of the chest may show the typical signs of consolidation of an area of lung. The solid lung in which the alveoli are filled with inflammatory exudate is dull to percussion but transmits sounds better than air-containing lung, giving rise to the signs of bronchial breathing and increased conduction of voice sounds to the stethoscope or palpating hand.

The chest X-ray in pneumonia shows opacities corresponding to the consolidated lung. This may have a lobar distribution fitting with limitation to one area of the lung or have a less confluent scattered distribution in bronchopneumonia. Blood tests usually show a raised white cell (LEUCOCYTE) count. The organism responsible for the pneumonia can often be identified from culture of the sputum or the blood or from blood tests for the specific ANTIBODIES produced in response to the infection.

Treatment The treatment of pneumonia involves appropriate antibiotics together with oxygen, pain relief and management of any complications that may arise. When treatment is started the causative organism has often not been identified and the antibiotic choice is made on the basis of the clinical features, prevalent organisms and their sensitivities. In severe cases of community-acquired pneumonia this will often be a PENICILLIN or CEPHALOSPORIN to cover *Strep. pneumoniae* together with a MACROLIDE (e.g. ERYTHROMYCIN). Pleuritic pain will need analgesia to allow deep breathing and coughing and oxygen may be needed judged by the oxygen saturation or blood gas measurement.

Possible complications of pneumonia are local changes such as lung abscess, pleural effusion or EMPYEMA and general problems such as cardiovascular collapse and abnormalities of kidney or liver function. Appropriate treatment should result in complete resolution of the lung changes but some FIBROSIS in the lung may remain. Pneumonia can be a severe illness in previously fit people and it may take some months to return to full fitness.

PNEUMONITIS An inflammation of the lung due to chemical or physical agents. When the inflammation of the lung is due to infections it is called pneumonia and when it is caused by allergic reactions it is known as alveolitis.

PNEUMOPERITONEUM A collection of air in the peritoneal cavity. Air introduced into the peritoneal cavity collects under the diaphragm which is thus raised and collapses the lungs. This procedure was sometimes carried out in the treatment of pulmonary tuberculosis in the pre-antibiotic days as an alternative to artificial pneumothorax.

PNEUMOTHORAX A collection of air in the pleural cavity, into which it has gained entrance by a lesion in the lung or a wound in the chest wall. When air enters the chest the lung immediately collapses towards the centre of the chest, but, air being absorbed from the pleural cavity, the lung expands again in a short time. (See LUNGS, DISEASES OF.)

Artificial pneumothorax was an operation often performed in the pre-antibiotic days to treat pulmonary tuberculosis. Air was run into the pleural cavity to cause collapse of one lung, which rested it and allowed cavities in it to heal.

PODAGRA Another name for gout affecting the foot. (See GOUT.)

PODOPHYLLIN A resin derived from podophyllum plants, its active agent, podophyllotoxin, in alcoholic solution is used to treat genital WARTS.

PODOPHYLLUM Preparations that contain the active constituent podophyllotoxin that can be applied as a paint, creams or ointments for the treatment of warts or calluses (hard thick skin caused by pressure or friction). Podophyllum is useful for genital warts but must be applied with care and not during pregnancy.

POIKILOCYTOSIS This is a term used to describe the variation seen in the shape of red blood cells in some bone marrow disorders.

POISONS A poison is any substance which, if absorbed by, introduced into or applied to a living organism may cause illness or death. The term toxin is often used to refer to a poison of biological origin. Toxins are therefore a subgroup of poisons, but often little distinction is made between the terms. The study of the effects of poisons is toxicology and the effects of toxins is toxinology.

The concept of the dose-response is important for understanding the risk of exposure to a particular substance. This is embodied in a statement by Paracelsus (c.1493–1541): 'All substances are poisons; there is none which is not a poison. The right dose differentiates a poison and a remedy.'

Poisoning may occur in a variety of ways: deliberate – suicide, substance abuse or murder; accidental – including accidental overdose of medicines; occupational; environmental – including exposure during fire.

Ingestion is the most common route of exposure but poisoning may also occur through inhalation, absorption through the skin, by injection and through bites and stings of venomous animals. Poisoning may be described as acute, where a single exposure produces clinical effects with a relatively rapid onset, or chronic, where prolonged or repeated exposures may produce clinical effects which may be insidious in onset, cumulative and in some cases permanent.

Diagnosis of poisoning is usually by circumstantial evidence or elimination of other causes of the clinical condition of the patient. Some substances (e.g. OPIOIDS, ANTICHOLINERGIC AGENTS) produce a characteristic clinical picture in overdose that can help with diagnosis. In some patients laboratory analysis of body fluids or the substance taken may be useful to determine or confirm the offending agent. Routine assays are not necessary. For a very small number of poisons, such as paracetamol, aspirin, iron and lead, the management of the patient may depend on measuring the amount of poison in the bloodstream.

Accurate statistics on the incidence of poisoning in the UK are lacking. Mortality figures are more reliable than morbidity statistics. Annually well over 100,000 cases of poisoning are admitted to hospital. The annual number of deaths from poisoning is relatively small, about 300. In most cases patients die before reaching hospital. Currently carbon monoxide is by far the commonest cause of death due to poisoning. The most common agents involved in intentional or accidental poisoning are drugs, particularly analgesics, antidepressants and sedatives. Alcohol is also commonly taken by adults, usually in combination with drugs. Children frequently swallow household cleaners, white spirit, plant material, aftershave and perfume as well as drugs. The use of child-resistant containers has reduced the number of admissions of children to hospital for treatment. Bixtrex® is an intensely bitter-tasting agent which is often added to products to discourage ingestion; however not everybody is able to taste it nor has any beneficial effect been proved.

Treatment of poisoning usually begins with decontamination procedures. For ingested substances this may involve making the patient sick or washing the stomach out (gastric lavage). This is usually only worthwhile if performed soon after ingestion. It should be emphasized that salt (sodium chloride) water must never be given to induce vomiting since this procedure is dangerous and has caused death. For substances spilt on the skin the affected area should immediately be thoroughly washed and all contaminated clothing removed. Following eye exposure, the affected eye/s should be thoroughly irrigated with saline or water. Treatment thereafter is generally symptomatic and supportive with maintenance of the victim's respiratory, neurological and cardiovascular systems and, where appropriate, monitoring their fluid and electrolyte balance and hepatic and renal function. There are specific antidotes for a few substances: the most important of these are PARACETAMOL, iron, CYANIDE, OPIOIDS, DIGOXIN, ANTICOAGULANT AGENTS, ORGANOPHOSPHORUS insecticides and some heavy metals.

When a patient presents with an illness thought to be caused by exposure to substances at work, further exposure should be limited or prevented and investigations undertaken to determine the source and extent of the problem. Acutely poisoned workers will usually go to hospital, but those suffering from chronic exposure may attend their GP with non-specific symptoms.

In recent years legislation has been enacted in the UK to improve safety in the workplace and to ensure that data on the hazardous constituents and effects of chemicals are more readily available. These official controls include the Control of Substances Hazardous to Health (COSHH) and the Chemicals (Hazard Information and Packaging) Regulations (CHIP) and are UK legislation in response to European Union directives.

> The National Poisons Information Service is a 24-hour emergency telephone service available to the medical profession and provides information on the likely effects of numerous agents and advice on the management of the poisoned patient. The telephone numbers are available in the medical literature. In the UK this is not a public access service. People who believe they, or their relatives, have been poisoned should seek medical advice from their GPs or attend their local hospital.

POLIOMYELITIS Once known as infantile paralysis, this disease is caused by a viral infection involving the brain and spinal cord.

After the first recorded epidemic in Sweden in 1881, the disease became increasingly important, but has become relatively rare since the successful introduction of oral polio vaccination. The disease has been notifiable in Great Britain since 1912; the annual number of cases is in single figures, with none being reported in some years. Since the development of effective vaccines in the 1950s, polio has been practically eliminated in most developed countries. People who have not been fully vaccinated, however, may get the disease. Polio remains a serious risk for unvaccinated travellers to Africa, Asia or southern Europe. The World Health Organization has a target to eliminate polio throughout the world by the start of the 21st century.

Pathology There are three types of virus, infection spreading by the stools–contaminated hands–mouth route. Children are most susceptible.

One attack usually produces permanent immunity, and second attacks are rare. The virus typically affects the anterior horn cells of the spinal cord, especially those in the lumbar region, and the grey matter of the brain stem and cortex may also be damaged.

Vaccination is given to infants at two, three and four months: a booster dose is given around the age of five. The vaccine contains all three types of polio virus. Two types of vaccine are available: one, inactivated polio virus (IPV) contains dead virus and is administered by injections; the other, oral polio vaccine (OPV) contains live, harmless strains. The latter is used in the United Kingdom.

Symptoms The incubation period is around 7 to 14 days, the onset being marked by a mild fever and headache which improves after a few days. In around 85 per cent of infected children there is no further progression, but in some – after approximately one week – the symptoms recur, together with neck stiffness and signs of meningeal irritation. Weakness of individual muscle groups is common, and may progress – to a variable extent, depending on the distribution of the virus – to widespread paralysis. Involvement of the diaphragm and intercostal muscles may lead to respiratory failure and rapid death unless artificial respiration is provided. Involvement of the cranial nerves and brain may lead to NYSTAGMUS, hoarseness, and difficulty in swallowing, and convulsions may occur in young children. The CEREBROSPINAL fluid shows an early increase in LYMPHOCYTES, followed by a rise in protein concentration.

Treatment Oral vaccine given in childhood has practically banished the disease in many countries, but a booster dose should be given to adults when travelling outside Europe and the USA. When cases of polio occur, there may be great variation in the proportion of abortive and non-paralytic cases – the latter normally recover completely – and in mortality rate. There is no effective drug treatment for the infection. Paralysis is greatest at the end of the first week of the major illness. Gradual recovery may then take place for several months, but any muscle showing no sign of recovery after a month is unlikely to regain any useful function. Treatment involves early bed rest, followed by PHYSIOTHERAPY and orthopaedic measures as required. At the onset of respiratory difficulties a TRACHEOSTOMY and artificial ventilation should be started. In cases of severe paralysis with persistent wasting of the limbs, surgery may be necessary to minimize the resulting disability.

POLIOSIS Premature greying of the hair. It is also the term applied to whitening of the hair in segments, such as a forelock.

POLLEN Microspores formed in flowering plants and conifers. Between 4 and 7 million tons of it are said to be shed annually throughout the world. From ancient days it has had the reputation of being a specific against old age. It has a bitter taste, which is traditionally disguised by honey – the ambrosia of the Bible, the Koran and the Talmud. The levels of pollen in the atmosphere are of importance to hay-fever sufferers since the pollen is a factor in triggering attacks.

POLLEX A Latin term for thumb.

POLYARTERITIS NODOSA or PERIARTERITIS NODOSA A disease of unknown origin, in which prolonged fever and obscure symptoms referable to any system of the body are associated with local areas of inflammation along the arteries, giving rise to nodules in their walls. Recovery occurs in about 50 per cent of cases.

POLYCHROMASIA and **POLYCHROMATOPHILIA** Terms applied to an abnormal reaction of the red blood cells in severe anaemia. They have a bluish tinge instead of the normal red colour in a blood film stained by the usual method. It is a sign that the cell is not fully developed.

POLYCYSTIC DISEASE OF KIDNEY An inherited disease in which the kidneys contain many cysts. These grow in size until normal kidney tissue is largely destroyed. Cysts may also occur in other organs such as the liver. In adults the disease will cause hypertension and kidney failure. There is also a juvenile form. There is no effective treatment, though symptoms can be alleviated by DIALYSIS and sometimes kidney TRANSPLANT.

POLYCYSTIC OVARY SYNDROME In 1935 Stein and Leventhan described seven hirsute and infertile women with amenorrhoea (absent menstruation) or oligomenorrhoea (scanty menstruation) in whom bilateral cystic ovarian enlargement was found at laparotomy and thereby gave their names to a polycystic ovarian disorder. It is characterized by scanty (or absent) menstruation, infertility, hirsutism (excessive hairiness) and obesity and the sufferers often have multiple cysts in their ovaries. The condition is caused by an imbalance between LUTEINIZING HORMONE (LH) and FOLLICLE-STIMULATING HORMONE (FSH) which stops ovulation and varies the testosterone output of the ovaries. The treatment may be with clomiphene, an oestrogen drug, with progestogen drugs, with luteinizing-hormone-releasing hormone or with oral contraceptives. The treatment chosen depends on the severity of the disease and whether the woman wants to conceive. Rarely a section of ovarian tissue is surgically removed.

POLYCYTHAEMIA An excess in the number of red cells in the blood due to raised production of these cells in the bone marrow. It may be a response to reduced oxygen levels – for example, among people living at high altitudes – or to liver or kidney disease. This type is called secondary polycythaemia. The disorder may, however, occur for no obvious reason and is then called polycythaemia vera. This type develops mainly in people over 40 and about 400 people develop the disorder every year in the United Kingdom. The blood thickens, the sufferer may develop high blood pressure, flushing, headaches, itching and an enlarged spleen. A stroke may occur later in the disease process. Treatment of polycythaemia vera is by regular removal of blood by VENESECTION, sometimes in combination with an anticancer drug. Secondary polycythaemia is treated by remedying the underlying cause.

POLYCYTHAEMIA RUBRA VERA A disorder in which the red blood cells increase in number along with an increase in the number of white blood cells and platelets. The cause is unknown. Severe cases may require treatment with cytotoxic drugs or radiotherapy.

POLYDACTYLY The presence of extra, or supernumerary, fingers or toes.

POLYDIPSIA Excessive thirst, which is a symptom of diabetes mellitus and some other diseases.

POLYMORPH A name applied to certain white corpuscles of the blood which have a nucleus of irregular and varied shape. These form between 70 and 75 per cent of all the white corpuscles. (See BLOOD.)

POLYMYALGIA RHEUMATICA A form of rheumatism characterized by gross early morning stiffness, which tends to ease off during the day, and pain in the shoulders and sometimes round the hips. It affects women more than men, and is rare under the age of 60. The cause is still obscure. It responds well to prednisolone, but treatment may need to be long continued. On the other hand the condition is not progressive and does not lead to crippling.

POLYMYOSITIS A disease of the muscles throughout the body. The disorder may be acute or chronic but it usually affects the muscles of the shoulders or hip areas. The muscles weaken and are tender to the touch. Diffuse inflammatory changes occur and symptomatic relief may be obtained with CORTICOSTEROID DRUGS.

POLYMYXIN A group of antibiotics derived from various species of *Bacillus polymyxa*. One variety, colistin, is used to sterilize the bowels before surgery as it is not absorbed when given by mouth. The drugs are sometimes used in topical applications for infections of the skin, eye and ear.

POLYNEURITIS An inflammatory condition of nerves in various parts of the body. (See NEURITIS.)

POLYPEPTIDE A molecule in which several AMINO-ACIDS are joined together by peptide bonds. PROTEIN molecules are polypeptides.

POLYPHARMACY A term applied to the administration of too many drugs to one person. Sometimes combinations of drugs are an effective means of treatment, reducing the risk of drug resistance. Polypharmacy, however, worsens the risk of drug interactions and of adverse effects, especially in the elderly.

POLYPOSIS The presence of a crop, or large number, of polypi. The most important form of polyposis is that known as familial polyposis coli. This is a hereditary disease characterized by the presence of large numbers of polypoid tumours in the large bowel. Every child born to an affected parent stands a fifty-fifty chance of developing the disease. Its importance is that sooner or later one or more of these tumours undergoes cancerous change. If the affected gut is removed surgically before this occurs, and preferably before the age of 20, the results are excellent.

POLYPUS or POLYP A general name applied to tumours which are attached by a stalk to the surface from which they spring. The term refers only to the shape of the growth and has nothing to do with its structure or nature. Most polypi are of a simple nature, though malignant polypi are also found. The usual structure of a polypus is that of a fine fibrous core covered with epithelium resembling that of the surrounding surface. The sites in which polypi are most usually found are the interior of the nose, the outer meatus of the ear, and the interior of the womb, bladder, or bowels (see POLYPOSIS).

Their removal is generally easy, as they are simply twisted off, or cut off, by some form of snare or ligature. (The tissue removed should be checked for malignant cells.) Those which are situated in the interior of the bladder or bowels, and whose presence is usually recognized because blood appears in the urine or stools, require a more serious operation; usually an endoscopic examination (see ENDOSCOPE).

POLYSACCHARIDE A carbohydrate comprising several monosaccharides linked in long chains. Polysaccharides store energy – as starch in plants and glycogen in animals – and they also form the structural parts of plants (as cellulose) and animals (as mucopolysaccharides).

POLYTHELIA The condition in which extra or supernumerary nipples appear along a line between the armpit and the groin.

POLYURIA The production of excessive amounts of urine (1500 ml or thereabout is the usual daily quantity). It is a symptom of DIABETES MELLITUS, DIABETES INSIPIDUS and chronic renal failure.

POMPHOLYX (see DERMATITIS).

POPLITEAL SPACE The name given to the region behind the knee. The muscles attached to the bones immediately above and below the knee bound a diamond-shaped space through which pass the main artery and vein of the limb (known in this part of their course as the popliteal artery and vein), the tibial and common peroneal nerves (which continue the sciatic nerve from the thigh down to the leg), the external saphenous vein, as well as several small nerves and lymphatic vessels. The muscles, which bound the upper angle of the space and which are attached to the leg bones by strong prominent tendons, are known as the hamstrings. The lower angle of the space lies between the two heads of the gastrocnemius muscle, which makes up the main bulk of the calf of the leg.

POPPY Two species are used in medicine: *Papaver somniferum*, the white opium-poppy (see OPIUM), and *Papaver rhoeas*, the red corn-poppy. The corn-poppy is chiefly used as a colouring agent, its syrup being a brilliant crimson colour.

PORE A small opening. The word is usually used to describe an opening in the skin that releases sweat or sebum, a waxy material secreted by the sebaceous glands in the skin.

PORPHYRIAS Group of rare inherited diseases in which disorders of the metabolic pathways leading to the synthesis of HAEM cause excessive production of haem precursors called PORPHYRINS by the bone marrow or liver. The excess porphyrins in the blood mainly affect the skin, causing PHOTOSENSITIVITY, or the central nervous system, causing various neuropsychiatric disorders. Excess porphyrins can be detected in blood, urine and faeces. Usually porphyrias are genetically determined but one form is due to alcoholic liver disease. The commonest form, porphyria cutanea retarda, affects up to 1 in 5,000 people in some countries.

PORPHYRINS Complex organic compounds which are sensitive to light and form the basis of respiratory pigments, for example, haemoglobin and myoglobin. Porphyrins are crucial to many metabolic oxidation/reduction reactions in animals, plants, and micro-organisms.

PORTAL HYPERTENSION Raised blood pressure in the portal vein. This results in increased pressure in the veins of the oesophagus and upper stomach and these grow in size to form varices – dilated tortuous veins. Sometimes these varices rupture causing bleeding into the oesophagus. The raised pressure also causes fluid to collect in the abdomen and form ascites. The commonest reason for portal hypertension is cirrhosis (fibrosis) of the liver (see LIVER DISEASES). Thrombosis in the portal vein may also be a cause. Treatment requires the cause to be tackled, but bleeding from ruptured vessels may be stopped by injecting a sclerosant or hardening solution into and around the veins. Sometimes a surgical shunt may be done to divert blood from the portal vein to another blood vessel.

PORTAL SYSTEM A vein or collection of veins which finish at both ends in a bed of capillary blood vessels. An important example is the hepatic portal system, comprising the portal vein and its tributaries. Blood from the stomach, pancreas, spleen and intestines drains into the veins that join up to comprise the portal vein into the liver, where it branches into sinusoids.

PORTAL VEIN The vein which carries to the liver blood that has been circulating in many of the abdominal organs. It is peculiar among the veins of the body in that it ends by breaking up into a capillary network instead of carrying the blood directly to the heart, a peculiarity which it shares only with certain small vessels in the kidneys. The portal system begins below in the haemorrhoidal plexus of veins round the lower end of the rectum, and from this point, along the whole length of the intestines, the blood is collected into an inferior mesenteric vein upon the left, and a superior mesenteric vein upon the right side. The inferior mesenteric vein empties into the splenic vein, and the latter, uniting with the superior mesenteric vein immediately above the pancreas, forms the portal vein. The portal vein is joined by veins from the stomach and gall-bladder, and finally divides into two branches which sink into the right and left lobes of the liver. (For their further course, see LIVER.)

The organs from which the portal vein collects the blood are the large and small intestines, the stomach, spleen, pancreas, and gall-bladder.

PORT WINE STAIN (see NAEVUS).

POSITRON-EMISSION TOMOGRAPHY (PET) (see PET SCANNING).

POSSETTING The technical term used to describe the quite common habit of healthy babies to regurgitate, or bring up, small amounts of the meal they have just taken.

POST- A prefix signifying after or behind.

POST-COITAL CONTRACEPTION Action taken to prevent conception after intercourse. The type of contraception may be hormonal or an intrauterine device. Pregnancy after intercourse without contraception – or where contraception has failed as a result, for example, of a leaking condom – may be avoided with a course of 'morning-after' contraceptive pills. Such preparations usually contain an OESTROGEN and a PROGESTOGEN. Two doses should be taken within 72 hours of 'unprotected' intercourse. An alternative for the woman is to take a high dose of oestrogen on its own. The aim is to postpone ovulation and affect the lining of the uterus so that the egg is unable to implant itself. Women are advised not to take such pills regularly because of the high hormone doses involved. There have been suggestions in the UK Parliament to make these morning-after pills available over the counter at pharmacists without prescription, the aim being to reduce the high rate of pregnancy in young single women. Britain has the highest teenage pregnancy incidence in Western Europe.

Intrauterine contraceptive device (IUCD) This is, in effect, a form of post-coital contraception since it prevents conception by a physical device after intercourse. The IUCD is a plastic shape up to 3 cm long around which copper wire is wound, carrying plastic thread from its tail. Colloquially known as a coil, it acts by inhibiting implantation and may also impair migration of sperm. Devices need changing every 3 to 5 years. They have generally replaced the larger, non-copper-bearing 'inert' types, which caused more complications but did not need changing (so are sometimes still found *in situ*). IUCDs tend to be chosen as a method of contraception (6 per cent) by older, parous women in stable relationships, with a generally low problem rate.

Nevertheless, certain problems do occur with IUCDs, the following being the most common:

- They tend to be expelled by the uterus in women who have never conceived or by a uterus distorted by, say, fibroids.
- Ectopic pregnancy is more likely.
- They are associated with pelvic infection and infertility, following sexually transmitted disease, or possibly introduced during insertion.
- They often produce heavy painful periods, and women at high risk of these problems (e.g. HIV positive, or any with WILSON'S DISEASE or cardiac lesions) should generally be excluded (unless the IUCD is inserted under antibiotic cover).

POST-COITAL TEST A test for infertility. A specimen of cervical mucus, taken up to 24 hours after coitus (during the post-ovulatory phase of the menstrual cycle), is examined microscopically to assess the motility of the sperms. If motility is above a certain level then sperms and mucus are not interacting abnormally, thus eliminating one cause of sterility.

POST-MORTEM EXAMINATION Also called an autopsy (and less commonly necropsy), this is an examination of a body to discover the causes of death. Such an examination is sometimes required by law. An unnatural death or one occurring in suspicious circumstances or one when a doctor feels unable to complete a certificate about the cause of death must be reported to the coroner (in Scotland to the procurator fiscal). He or she may order an autopsy to be carried out as part of the inquiry into cause of death. Sometimes doctors may request the permission of relatives to perform a post-mortem so that they may discover something of value for the improvement of medical care. Relatives may refuse consent.

POST-OPERATIVE The period after an operation, the patient's condition after operation or any investigations or treatment during this time.

POST-PARTUM The term applied to anything happening immediately after child-birth: for example, post-partum haemorrhage.

POST-TRAUMATIC STRESS DISORDER (PTSD) An individual who has suffered great personal stress arising from an alarming event may develop this severe anxiety disorder. The event may be an injury, exposure to disaster resulting in casualties, participation in warfare as combatant or refugee, an assault or a rape or witnessing an assault or rape. Any reaction may occur months or even years after the causative event. Someone with PTSD has regular recurrences of memories or images of the stressful event. Insomnia, nightmares, feelings of guilt and isolation, an inability to concentrate and irritability may develop. The affected individual often becomes very depressed.

Support from friends and family and skilled counselling help to resolve the condition, which usually – but not always – settles with time.

POST-VIRAL FATIGUE SYNDROME (see MYALGIC ENCEPHALOMYELITIS).

POSTURAL DRAINAGE Facilitation of the drainage of secretions from dilated bronchi of the lungs. The patient lies on an inclined plane head downwards and is encouraged to cough up as much secretion from the lungs as possible. The precise position depends on which part of the lungs is affected. It may need to be carried out for up to three hours daily in divided periods. It is of particular value in BRONCHIECTASIS and lung abscess (see LUNGS, DISEASES OF).

POTASSIUM A metal which, on account of its great affinity for other substances, is not found in a pure state in nature. Its salts are widely used in medicine but, as their action depends in general not on their metallic radicle but upon the acid with which it is combined, their uses vary greatly and are described elsewhere. All salts of potassium depress the heart's action as a result of action by the potassium ion.

POTASSIUM PERMANGANATE A salt of the metallic element POTASSIUM. It is used as a skin ANTISEPTIC and for cleaning wounds; its astringent effect is useful in the treatment of dermatitis. It should not be taken internally because the compound is poisonous.

POTT'S DISEASE A traditional name often applied to the angular curvature of the spine which results from tuberculous disease. (See SPINE AND SPINAL CORD, DISEASES AND INJURIES OF.) The disease is named after Percivall Pott, an English surgeon (1714–88), who first described the condition.

POTT'S FRACTURE A variety of fractures around the ankle, accompanied by a varying degree of dislocation of the ankle. In all cases the fibula is fractured. Named after Percivall Pott, who suffered from this fracture and was the first to describe it (see FRACTURES), it is often mistaken for a simple sprain of the ankle.

POULTICES (see also FOMENTATION) Soft moist applications to the surface of the body, generally used hot to soothe pain due to inflammation and promote resolution.

POUPART'S LIGAMENT Also known as the inguinal ligament, it is the strong ligament lying in the boundary between the anterior abdominal wall and the front of the thigh.

PRAZIQUANTEL An effective drug against all human schistosomes which has a broad spectrum of activity and low toxicity (see SCHISTOSOMIASIS).

PRE- A prefix meaning before.

PRECIPITIN An antibody that combines with an antigen and forms the immune complex as a precipitate. The reaction is used in some diagnostic serological tests to indentify antigens in the serum.

PRECORDIAL REGION The area on the centre and towards the left side of the chest, lying in front of the heart.

PREDNISOLONE A derivative of cortisone, which is five or six times as active as cortisone and has less of the salt- and water-retaining properties of cortisone. It is given by mouth.

PREDNISONE This CORTICOSTEROID drug has a similar level of GLUCOCORTICOID activity as PREDNISOLONE and is converted to prednisolone in the liver. Though prednisone is still in use, prednisolone is the most commonly used oral corticosteroid for long-term anti-inflammatory treatment.

PRE-ECLAMPSIA A complication of pregnancy, of unknown cause, which in severe cases may proceed to ECLAMPSIA. It is characterized by HYPERTENSION, renal impairment, OEDEMA, often with PROTEINURIA and disseminated intravascular coagulation. It usually occurs in the second half of pregnancy, mild cases (without proteinuria) occurring in about 10 per cent of pregnancies, severe cases in about 2 per cent. Predisposing factors include a first pregnancy, or pregnancy by a new partner; a family history of pre-eclampsia, HYPERTENSION, or other cardiovascular disorders; and pre-existing hypertension or DIABETES MELLITUS. Increased incidence with lower socio-economic class may be linked to diet or to failure to attend for antenatal care. Although less common in smokers, fetal outlook is worse. Multiple pregnancy and HYDATIFORM MOLE, together with HYDROPS FETALIS, predispose to early and severe pre-eclampsia.

Treatment Severe pre-eclampsia is an emergency. Urgent admission to hospital should be arranged. Treatment should be given to control the hypertension, the fetal heart rate carefully monitored, and in very severe cases urgent CAESAREAN SECTION may be necessary.

PREGNANCY The time during which a woman carries a developing fetus in the uterus. (Occasional ECTOPIC PREGNANCY occurs outside the uterus.)

Pregnancy lasts about 280 days from the first day of the last menstrual period. In exceptional cases there may be considerable variation. For the purpose of calculating the probable date of confinement, it is usual to take the first day of the last period that occurred, to allow seven days for the duration of this and then to add 273 days for the duration of gestation, making in all 280 days from the beginning of the last menstruation.

Signs of pregnancy

- The sudden stoppage of the menstrual flow is the first sign. This symptom may, however, be due to many other causes (see MENSTRUATION).
- Swelling of the BREASTS may start as soon as the second or third month of pregnancy. A thin fluid, known as colostrum, can, even at this early stage, be pressed from the nipples. The veins on the breasts become enlarged and visible, and the pigmented ring round the nipple (areola) becomes much darker than before, as well as showing small nodules (Montgomery's tubercles) round its edge.
- Morning sickness is also a common sign, occurring in about two-thirds of all women.
- Quickening, or the fluttering sensation felt by the mother in consequence of the child's rapid movements, is an important sign usually occurring during the fifth month of pregnancy or even later.
- Enlargement of the abdomen, though for the first three months the enlargement is not apparent.
- One certain sign of pregnancy is the beating of the fetal heart which can be heard by auscultation over the lower part of the abdomen from the middle of the fifth month onwards.
- Other minor signs which are sometimes present include varicose veins, mucous discharge from the vagina, changes in the neck of the womb.

Pregnancy is a normal state and most women have few major problems and are delivered normally. All women should, however, attend regular antenatal clinics and be supervised by a doctor and/or a midwife. This ensures that any complications can be diagnosed early and dealt with appropriately.

PREGNANCY TESTS There are several tests for pregnancy in its early stages, and these can be done on blood or urine; some of the urine tests may be carried out at home. Most tests are based on the detection of human chorionic GONADOTROPHIN (HCG) in the woman's urine. They are nearly 100-per-cent accurate and may show positive as early as 30 days after the first day of the last normal period.

The haemagglutination inhibition test This, and the subsequent tests to be mentioned, are known as immunological tests. They are based upon the effect of the urine from a pregnant woman upon the interaction of red-blood cells, which have been sensitized to human GONADOTROPHIN, and anti-gonadotrophin serum. They have the great practical advantage of being performed in a test-tube or even on a slide.

Because of their ease and speed of performance, a result can be obtained in two hours.

Enzyme-linked immuno assay (ELISA) is the basis of many of the pregnancy-testing kits obtainable from pharmacies. It is a highly sensitive antibody test and can detect very low concentrations of human chorionic gonadotrophin. Positive results show up as early as 10 days after fertilization – namely 4 days before the first missed period.

Ultrasound The fetal sac can be detected by ULTRASOUND from five weeks and a fetal echo around six or seven weeks. (See also PRENATAL DIAGNOSIS.)

PREGNANDIOL The excretion product of the hormone, PROGESTERONE, manufactured by the corpus luteum of the ovary. Pregnandiol is excreted in the urine during the second half of the menstrual period, and its excretion rises steadily throughout pregnancy.

PREMATURE BEAT (see ECTOPIC BEAT).

PREMATURE BIRTH (see ABORTION; FETUS) This is a birth that takes place before the end of the normal period of gestation, usually before 37 weeks. In practice, however, it is defined as a birth that takes place when the baby weighs less than 2·5 kilograms (5½ pounds). Between 5 and 10 per cent of babies are born prematurely and in around 40 per cent of premature births the cause is unknown. Pre-eclampsia is the commonest known cause; others include hypertension, chronic kidney disease, heart disease and diabetes mellitus. Multiple pregnancy is another cause. In the vast majority of cases the aim of management is to prolong the pregnancy and so improve the outlook for the unborn child. This consists essentially of rest in bed and sedation, but there are now several drugs, such as RITODRINE, that may be used to suppress the activity of the uterus and so help to delay premature labour. Prematurity was once a prime cause of infant mortality but modern medical care has greatly improved survival rates in development countries.

PREMATURE EJACULATION A disorder in which ejaculation of semen occurs before or immediately after the penis penetrates the vagina. The commonest sexual problem in men, persistent premature ejaculation, may have psychological causes, although many adolescents and some adults experience it occasionally. Sexual counselling may help to alleviate the condition.

PREMEDICATION A drug or drugs given to a patient to produce sedation before an operation, whether this is done under a local or general anaesthetic. A narcotic analgesic drug is usually used as this relieves pain as well as anxiety. An antisecretory drug is often added to reduce the secretions in the airways and thus lessen the risk of general anaesthesia. Premedication reduces the amount of anaesthetic needed to make the patient unconscious.

PREMENSTRUAL SYNDROME This has been defined as 'any combination of emotional or physical features which occur cyclically in a woman before menstruation and which regress or disappear during menstruation'. It is characterized by mood changes, discomfort, swelling and tenderness in the breasts, swelling of the legs, a bloated feeling in the abdomen, headache, fatigue and constipation. The mood changes range from irritability and mild depression to outbursts of violence. It may last for three up to 14 days. How common it is is not known, as only the more severe cases are seen by doctors, but it has been estimated that 1 in 10 of all menstruating women suffer from it severely enough to require treatment. The cause is not known, but it is probably due to some upset of the hormonal balance of the body. In view of the multiplicity of causes that have been put forward, it is not surprising that there is an equal multiplicity of treatments. Among these one of the most widely used is PROGESTERONE. Others include PYRIDOXINE, DANAZOL, and gamma linolenic acid available in the form of oil of evening primrose. Whatever drug may be prescribed, psychological treatment is equally essential and, in many cases, is all that is required.

PREMOLAR The two teeth on each side of the jaw positioned between the canines and the molars in the adult. The teeth are used with the molars for holding and grinding food.

PRENATAL DIAGNOSIS or SCREENING of fetal abnormalities may be the result of screening tests carried out on most or all pregnant women or as the result of specific diagnostic tests performed to detect specific conditions. Prenatal diagnosis is important as it will identify babies who might need medical or surgical treatment before or soon after birth. In addition it might also detect severe abnormalities for which parents might decide to have a therapeutic abortion (see ABORTION).

ULTRASOUND SCANNING is probably the most widely used diagnostic tool in obstetric practice. It can detect structural abnormalities such as SPINA BIFIDA and CLEFT PALATE and even cardiac and renal problems. A series of scans can assess whether the baby is growing at a normal rate and it may also be used to assist with other diagnostic tests (e.g. AMNIOCENTESIS).

Tests on the mother's blood can also diagnose fetal abnormalities. Alphafetoprotein (AFP) is produced by babies and 'leaks' into the AMNIOTIC FLUID and is absorbed by the mother. In SPINA BIFIDA and other neural tube defects there is increased leakage of AFP and a blood test at 16 weeks' gestation can detect a raised level which suggests the presence of these abnormalities.

The triple test, also performed at 16 weeks, measures AFP, and two hormones – human chorionic gonadotrophin and unconjugated oestradiol – and is used in diagnosing DOWN'S SYNDROME.

Amniocentesis involves inserting a needle through the mother's abdominal wall into the uterus to remove a sample of amniotic fluid at 16–18 weeks. Examination of the fluid and cells it contains is used in the diagnosis of Down's syndrome and other inherited disorders. The test carries a small risk of miscarriage.

Chorionic villus sampling may be used to diagnose various inherited conditions. A small amount of tissue from the developing placenta is removed for analysis and this test has the advantages of having a lower incidence of miscarriage than amniocentesis and is carried out at an earlier stage (9–13 weeks).

Analysis of a blood sample removed from the umbilical cord (cordocentesis) may diagnose infections in the uterus, blood disorders or inherited conditions.

Direct observation of the fetus via a viewing instrument called a fetoscope is also used diagnostically and will detect structural abnormalities.

Most tests have a recognized incidence of false positive and negative results and are therefore usually cross-checked with another test. Counselling of the parents about prenatal tests is important. This allows them to make an informed choice which may not necessarily involve terminating the pregnancy if an abnormality is found.

PREPUCE Also known as the foreskin, this is the free fold of skin that overlaps the glans PENIS and retracts when the penis becomes erect. It is the part that is removed at CIRCUMCISION.

PRESBYACUSIS Deafness that comes on with increasing years. It is caused by increasing loss of elasticity in the hearing mechanism, combined with the slowing down of the mental processes that accompanies old age. It is characterized by particular difficulty in hearing high notes such as the telephone and the voices of women and children. Hearing in a background of noise, is also early affected. Modern, miniaturized, transistor 'within-the-ear' hearing aids are now available that are proving helpful in making life more bearable for the elderly in this respect. (See also DEAFNESS; HEARING AIDS.)

PRESBYOPIA (see ACCOMMODATION; REFRACTION).

PRESCRIBED DISEASES A collection of industrial diseases which provide those with a disease legal entitlement to welfare benefits. Examples are deafness from excessive noise in the workplace, anthrax from farming, pneumoconiosis from industrially generated dust (coalmining) and lead poisoning from chemicals handling. (See OCCUPATIONAL HEALTH).

PRESCRIPTION The written direction for drugs for medicinal use, given by the doctor, dentist and (for some drugs) nurse to the patient, for dispensation by the pharmacist. Drugs should only be prescribed when essential for treatment, and when any possible risks involved to the patient (and fetus in cases of pregnancy) are outweighed by the potential benefits of giving the drug. When possible, non-proprietary, or generic, titles should be prescribed; by allowing the pharmacist to dispense any equivalent drug this avoids delay for the patient, as well as reducing the cost to the Health Service. Dosage is generally stated in metric units, and both the amount and frequency should be carefully explained to the patient by the doctor, and clearly written when the drug is dispensed (see also DOSAGE; DRUGS). Strict adherence to the Misuse of Drugs Act 1973 is necessary to restrict the inappropriate prescription and abuse of drugs, particularly CONTROLLED DRUGS. Full details of drugs available on NHS prescription are given in the *British National Formulary*, which is published by the British Medical Association and the Royal Pharmaceutical Society of Great Britain twice a year and distributed to all NHS doctors by the government. Careful monitoring of prescribing in the UK is carried out by a government-appointed agency.

PRESENILE Describing the condition of premature ageing. The mental and physical faculties are adversely affected in presenility to an extent that does not usually occur until old age (see DEMENTIA).

PRESENTATION The appearance in labour of some particular part of the child's body at the mouth of the uterus. This is a head presentation in 96 per cent of cases, but in a certain number the breech (or buttocks) may present, or the face, or foot, or even a part of the trunk in cases of cross-birth.

PRESSOR An agent that raises the blood pressure.

PRESSURE SORES (see DECUBITUS ULCERS).

PREVALENCE An epidemiological term describing the proportion of a defined group in the population having a condition at one point in time. It is an appropriate measure only in relatively stable conditions for example, chronic bronchitis – and is not suitable for measuring acute illnesses.

PREVENTIVE MEDICINE The term 'preventive medicine' may be used both in a general lay sense and to cover a specific range of activities carried out by health professionals. The definition and scope vary from country to country. Some people use the term widely and almost synonymously with 'public health'. Others limit its use to specific measures directed at individuals, such as an immunization against an infectious disease, preferring other terms such as 'health promotion' for educational activities and 'health protection' to cover consumer-protection regulations such as food inspection. The preventive approach is an essential component of a broader public-health strategy, and, for example, in relation to diet and physical activity a normal part of the lifestyle of many in the population.

In Britain, for example, preventive medicine is usually taken to encompass a range of activities whose purpose is:

- to reduce the chance of a person's contracting a disease or becoming disabled.
- to identify either an increased susceptibility to develop a disease or an early manifestation of a disease at a stage which will still allow treatment to be effective.

The American College of Preventive Medicine (1983) defined it as 'a specialized field of medical practice composed of distinct disciplines which utilize skills focusing on the health of defined populations in order to promote and maintain health and well-being and prevent disease, disability and premature death.'

However defined, the spectrum of activities encompassed by preventive medicine is wide and includes actions, such as counselling about lifestyle, where there may not be a clear cut-off between a preventive and a curative act. For example, advice about smoking and exercise to a recent victim of a myocardial infarction is both essential to treatment and preventive against a future attack. Action aimed at a whole population such as the addition of fluoride to drinking water to protect against dental caries is part of a population-based public-health strategy but it would also be widely regarded as preventive medicine!

A common and widely accepted classification of preventive medicine is:

Primary prevention which aims at the complete avoidance of a disease (for example, by immunizing a child against an infectious disease).

Secondary prevention which aims at detecting and curing a disease at an early stage before it has caused any symptoms. This requires 'screening' procedures to detect either the early presymptomatic condition or a risk factor which may lead to it. (An example of the former is cervical cytology where a sample of cells is scraped from the CERVIX and examined microscopically for abnormality. An example of the latter is CHOLESTEROL measurement as part of assessing an individual's risk of developing ISCHAEMIC HEART DISEASE. If it is significantly raised dietary or drug treatment can be advised.)

Tertiary prevention aims at minimizing the consequences for a patient who already has the disease (e.g. advising people to take more exercise and stop smoking after a heart attack).

Many prefer to limit the term 'preventive medicine' to primary and secondary prevention emphasizing the focus on risk-reducing interventions targeted at 'well' individuals. Others prefer the wider emphasis because of the importance of a preventive approach in reducing further disability by recognizing and treating symptoms early. This can be particularly important in older people, where, for example, vigorous treatment of an orthopaedic problem can enable the patient to maintain physical mobility with all the benefits to health that brings. Whether primary, secondary or tertiary prevention some form of screening question or test is normally necessary to identify a problem.

The range and extent of opportunities for prevention are expanding as research identifies the causes of diseases and more effective treatment becomes feasible. Inevitably there is economic and political debate about the cost-effectiveness of prevention versus cure and about the ethics. The situation varies in relation to the natural history of the specific disease. Some conditions can easily be prevented but once contracted cannot be cured (e.g. rabies). Others are easily cured but are not yet preventable. Geoffrey Rose has pointed out that the best argument for prevention is the humanitarian argument 'It is better to be healthy than ill or dead. That is the beginning and the end of the only real argument for preventive medicine. It is sufficient.' (Geoffrey Rose, *The Strategy of Preventive Medicine*, Oxford Medical Publications, 1992.)

Screening Screening involves carrying out tests either to identify a treatable disease at a very early stage before it has caused symptoms or damage, or, to identify a risk factor which can lead to a disease. The tests might be by simple questioning (e.g. 'Do you smoke cigarettes?' This predicts a considerable increase in the risk of chronic bronchitis, heart disease, bronchial cancer and many other diseases and enables targeted advice and help to stop smoking to be given). Other screening tests involve carrying out complex special investigations such as blood tests or the microscopic investigations of cells, for example, for precancerous changes.

Many conditions can be identified at an early stage before they cause symptoms or signs of disease and in time for effective treatment to be carried out. Inevitably some of the screening tests proposed can be expensive (particularly if used in large populations), painful or inaccurate and may not improve the results of treatment. Screening can also provoke considerable anxiety in those waiting for tests or results. Therefore over the years considerable research has been carried out into the appropriateness and ethics of screening and the World Health Organization in 1968 identified a set of rules for evaluating screening tests.

- The condition sought should be an important health problem, for which there should be an accepted treatment for patients with recognized disease.
- Facilities for diagnosis and treatment should be available if a case is found.
- The screening test or examination must be suitable and valid. A false positive test will cause massive anxiety and also considerable expense in proving there is no disease. Similarly false negatives can lead people to be reassured and to ignore serious symptoms until too late. If large numbers of positive tests or false positives occur during a screening programme, health services can be swamped.
- The test and any treatment as a possible result should be acceptable. For example, there is little point in screening for a fetal abnormality which, if found, would lead to a recommendation for termination if the mother will refuse it on religious or moral grounds.
- Screening tests also need to be considered from an economic perspective and the cost of case-finding (including diagnosis and treatment of patients diagnosed) balanced in relation to possible expenditure on medical care as a whole.
- Finally the programme should reflect the natural history of the disease and case-finding should normally be a continuing process and not a 'once for all' project.

If these rules are followed, considerable benefits can result from well-planned and managed screening programmes and they form an important part of any health-care system. The extent to which manipulation of genetic material will be added to more traditional approaches such as counselling, IMMUNIZATION and drug treatment cannot yet be predicted but, as time goes by, it is often likely to be ethical and social controls which limit developments rather than technical and scientific limits.

PRIAPISM A persisting painful erection of the PENIS occurring without sexual stimulation. It is a rare but acute condition that requires immediate treatment. The cause is the failure of blood to drain from the spongy corpus caversonum tissues of the penis, thus maintaining an erection. This may happen because of infection, damage to the nerves controlling the blood vessels, or a clotting defect in the blood.

PRICKLY HEAT (see MILIARIA RUBRA).

PRIMARY HEALTH CARE Sometimes called primary medical care, this is the care provided by general medical practitioners (traditionally titled the family doctor) or other health professional who has first contact with a patient needing or wanting medical attention. In the NHS the primary health-care services include those provided by the general, dental, opthalmic and pharmaceutical services as well as the family doctor service. Community health services provided outside the hospitals also offer some primary health care (see NATIONAL HEALTH SERVICE).

PRIMIDONE   A barbiturate-related drug used to treat all forms of EPILEPSY except in sufferers who do not have seizures.

PRIMIGRAVIDA   A woman who is undergoing her first PREGNANCY.

PRIMIPARA   The term applied to a woman who has given birth, or is giving birth, to her first child.

PRION   An aberrant variety of one of the proteins called PrP in a brain cell. The result of a gene mutation, prions are stable, resistant to radiation and impervious to the normal cellular processes of degradation. They seem to react with normal PrP, turning it into an abnormal type that then accumulates in brain tissue. Prions are believed to be the infectious agents that cause a group of serious neurological disorders called spongiform encephapalothies. CREUTZFELDT-JAKOB DISEASE (CJD), the new variant of CJD linked with BOVINE SPONGIFORM ENCEPHALOPATHY (BSE) and kuru, a neurological disorder found in a cannibal tribe in New Guinea, are all diseases in this group that occur in humans. The prion disorders have a long latent period between infection and manifestation of symptoms; they are hard to diagnose until autopsy and there is no cure as yet.

PRO-   A prefix meaning forwards.

PROBE   A slender, flexible instrument usually made of metal designed for introduction into a wound or cavity either to explore its depth and direction, to discover the presence of foreign bodies, or to introduce medicinal substances.

PROBENECID   A benzoic acid derivative which interferes with the excretion by the kidney of certain compounds, including PENICILLIN and PARA-AMINOSALICYLIC ACID, and was originally introduced into medicine for this reason, as a means of increasing and maintaining the concentration of penicillin in the body. It is also used to treat chronic gout.

PROCAINAMIDE HYDROCHLORIDE is a derivative of procaine, used to treat certain cardiac arrythmias (irregularities in the heart beat).

PROCAINE, or PROCAINE HYDROCHLORIDE, once used widely as a local anaesthetic but rarely so now.

PROCAINE PENICILLIN   An intramuscular depot preparation which is the preferred choice for the treatment of SYPHILIS and YAWS (see PENICILLIN).

PROCARBAZINE   An antineoplastic drug used mainly to treat HODGKIN'S DISEASE. It acts by interfering with the process of MITOSIS, the method by which the cells of the body, including tumours, reproduce themselves.

PROCHLORPERAZINE is an anti-psychotic phenothiazine drug. It is also an effective drug for the prevention or treatment of vomiting, and has therefore been used in the treatment of MENIÈRE'S DISEASE. (See NEUROLEPTICS.)

PROCIDENTIA   Another term for PROLAPSE.

PROCTALGIA   'Nerve pain' in the anus or rectum, without any local disease to account for it. Proctalgia fugax is a condition more common in men, characterized by cramplike pains in the rectum, occasionally accompanied by a feeling of faintness. Occurring at night and lasting up to 15 minutes, the cause is unknown, but is probably due to muscle spasm. Rapid relief may be achieved by food or drink, perineal pressure (including inserting a finger into the rectum), or sucking a 1 mg tablet of GLYCERYL TRINITRATE. The attacks usually stop after the age of 50.

PROCTITIS   Inflammation situated about the rectum or anus.

PRODROMATA   A term applied to the earliest symptoms of a disease, or those which give warning of its presence.

PROGERIA   Premature old age.

PROGESTERONE   The hormone of the CORPUS LUTEUM. After the escape of the OVUM from the ruptured follicle, the corpus luteum secretes progesterone, which stimulates the growth and secretion of the endometrial glands of the UTERUS during the fourteen days before menstruation. In the event of pregnancy, the secretion of progesterone continues until the baby's birth. (See also ETHISTERONE; NORETHISTERONE; PREGNANDIOL; CONTRACEPTION; MENSTRUATION.)

PROGESTOGEN   A preparation with an action like that of PROGESTERONE.

PROGLOTTIS   A segment of a tapeworm.

PROGNATHISM   Abnormal protusion of the lower jaw or sometimes of both jaws. The condition may make biting and chewing difficult, in which case corrective surgery is necessary.

PROGNOSIS   The term applied to a forecast as to the probable result of an illness or disease, particularly with regard to the prospect of recovery.

PROGRESSIVE MUSCULAR ATROPHY
(see PARALYSIS).

PROGUANIL HYDROCHLORIDE A synthetic antimalarial drug usually used with CHLOROQUINE to prevent infection with MALARIA. Occasionally the drug is used to treat uncomplicated falciparum malaria in combination with atovaquone.

PROLACTIN is the PITUITARY hormone which initiates lactation. The development of the breasts during pregnancy is ascribed to the action of OESTROGENS. Prolactin starts them secreting. If lactation does not occur or fails, it may be started by injection of prolactin.

The secretion of prolactin is normally kept under tonic inhibition by the secretion of DOPAMINE which inhibits prolactin. This is formed in the HYPOTHALAMUS and secreted into the portal capillaries of the pituitary stalk to reach the anterior pituitary cells. Drugs that deplete the brain stores of dopamine or antagonize dopamine at receptor level will cause hyperprolactinaemia and hence the secretion of milk from the breast and amenorrhoea. METHYLDOPA and RESERPINE deplete brain stores of dopamine and the PHENOTHIAZINES act as DOPAMINE ANTAGONISTS at receptor level. Other causes of excess secretion of prolactin are pituitary tumours, which may be minute and are then called microadenomas, or may actually enlarge the pituitary fossa and are then called macroadenomas. The commonest cause of hyperprolactinaemia is a pituitary tumour. The patient may present with infertility, because patients with hyperprolactinaemia do not ovulate, or the patient may present with amenorrhea and even galactorrhoea.

BROMOCRIPTINE is a dopamine agonist. Treatment with bromocriptine will therefore control hyperprolactinaemia and restore normal menstruation and ovulation and suppress GALACTORRHOEA. If the cause of hyperprolactinaemia is an adenomatous growth in the pituitary gland, surgical treatment should be considered.

PROLAPSE Displacement of an organ or structure from its normal position. The term is applied chiefly to downward displacements of the rectum and uterus.

PROLAPSED INTERVERTEBRAL DISC
The SPINAL COLUMN is built up of a series of bones, known as VERTEBRAE, placed one upon the other. Between these vertebrae lies a series of thick discs of fibro-cartilage known as intervertebral discs. Each disc consists of an outer portion known as the anulus fibrosus, and an inner core known as the nucleus pulposus. The function of these discs is to give flexibility and resiliency to the spinal column and to act as buffers against undue jarring. In other words, they are most efficient shock absorbers. They may, however, prolapse, or protrude, between the two adjacent vertebrae. If this should happen they press on the neighbouring spinal nerve and cause pain. As the most common sites of protrusion, or prolapse, are between the last two lumbar vertebrae and between the last lumbar vertebra and the sacrum, this means that the pain occurs in the back, causing LUMBAGO, or down the course of the sciatic nerve causing SCIATICA. The prolapse is most likely to occur in middle age, which suggests that it may be associated with degeneration of the disc involved, but it can occur in early adult life as well. It usually occurs when the individual is performing some form of exercise which involves bending or twisting, as in gardening. The onset of pain may be acute and sudden, or gradual and more chronic in intensity. (See INTERVERTEBRAL DISC.)

Treatment varies, depending, amongst other things, on the severity of the condition. In the acute phase rest in bed is advisable along with analgesic drugs. Later, exercise and physiotherapy are helpful, and in some cases manipulation of the spine brings relief by allowing the herniated, or prolapsed, disc to slip back into position. The injection of a local anaesthetic into the spine (epidural ANAESTHESIA) is yet another measure that often helps the more chronic cases. If those measures fail, surgery to remove the prolapsed disc may be necessary, but the patient's condition should be carefully reviewed before surgery is considered since success is not certain. An alternative form of treatment is the injection into the disc of chymopapain, an ENZYME obtained from the paw-paw, which dissolves the disc.

PROMAZINE A phenothiazine drug used to tranquillize disturbed patients (see NEUROLEPTICS).

PROMETHAZINE HYDROCHLORIDE A widely used antihistamine drug with a prolonged action and a pronounced sedative effect. (See ANTIHISTAMINE DRUGS.)

PROMETHAZINE THEOCLATE, or AVOMINE A drug that is widely used in the alleviation or prevention of sea-sickness.

PRONATION The movement whereby the bones of the forearm are crossed and the palm of the hand faces downwards.

PRONE Lying with the face down, or positioning the arm and hand so that the palm faces downwards.

PROPHYLAXIS Treatment or action adopted with the view of warding off disease.

PROPOFOL A drug used intravenously to induce general anaesthesia. Propofol may be used by intravenous infusion to maintain anaesthesia. It is also useful for sedating patients in intensive care.

PROPRANOLOL HYDROCHLORIDE
This is a BETA-ADRENOCEPTOR-BLOCKING DRUG that is used in the treatment of ANGINA PECTORIS, myocardial infarction, certain abnormal rhythms of the heart, and high blood-pressure. It also prevents attacks of MIGRAINE, and is used for certain anxiety states, particularly those associated with unpleasant bodily sensations, such as palpitations. (See ADRENERGIC RECEPTORS.)

PROPRIETARY NAME
The trade name of a drug registered by the pharmaceutical company which has developed and patented it. This protects the name, ingredients and manufacturing technique for a set period of time and helps the company to recoup the often costly research and development needed to produce and test the drug. Doctors may prescribe a drug by its trade name or by its official, approved name, though the NHS encourages the latter. (See GENERIC DRUG; PATENT.)

PROPRIOCEPTORS
Sensory nerve endings in the muscles, tendons and joints which signal to the brain their position relative to the outside world and the state of contraction of the muscle. During movement of a regular flow of information to the brain from the proprioceptors, the eyes and ears ensure that actions are co-ordinated and the body's balance maintained.

PROPTOSIS
A condition in which the EYE protrudes from the orbit. Some causes include thyroid disorders, tumours within the orbit, inflammation or infection of the orbit. Proptosis due to endocrine abnormality, e.g. thyroid problems, is known as EXOPHTHALMOS.

PROPYLTHIOURACIL
An oral antithyroid drug given daily to a person with HYPERTHYROIDISM. It interferes with the body's production of thyroid hormones.

PROSTACYCLIN
A PROSTAGLANDIN produced by the endothelial lining of the blood vessels. It inhibits the aggregation of PLATELETS, and thereby reduces the likelihood of the blood clotting. It is also a strong vasodilator.

PROSTAGLANDINS
Those natural substances, so called because they were first discovered in the semen and thought to arise in the prostate gland, are a group of fatty-acid substances with a wide range of activity. The richest known source is semen, but they are also present in many other parts of the body. Their precise mode of action is not yet clear, but they are potent stimulators of muscle contraction and they are also potent VASODILATORS. They

cause contraction of the UTERUS and have been used to induce labour. They are also being used as a means of inducing therapeutic abortions. They play an important part in the production of pain, and it is now known that aspirin relieves pain by virtue of the fact that it prevents, or antagonizes, the formation of certain prostaglandins. In addition, they play some, though as yet incompletely defined, part in producing inflammatory changes. (See INFLAMMATION; NON-STEROIDAL ANTI-INFLAMMATORY DRUGS.)

Thus prostaglandins have potent biological effects but their instability and rapid metabolism make them short acting. They are produced but not stored by most living cells and act locally. The two most important prostaglandins are prostacycline and thromboxane. Prostacycline is a vaso-dilator and an inhibitor of platelet aggregation and may cause relaxation of the myometrium. Thromboxanes have the opposite effects and cause vaso-constriction and platelet aggregation. The NON-STEROIDAL ANTI-INFLAMMATORY DRUGS act by blocking an enzyme called cyclo-oxygenase which converts arachidonic acid to the precursors of the various prostaglandins. Despite their potent pharmacological properties, the role of prostaglandins in current therapeutics is limited and controversial. They have been used most successfully as an inhibitor of platelet aggregation in extra-corporeal haemoperfusion systems. The problems with the prostacyclines is that they have to be given intravenously as they are inactive by mouth, and continuous infusion is required because the drug is rapidly eliminated with a half-life of minutes. Side-effects tend to be severe because the drug is usually given at the highest dose the patient can tolerate. The hope for the future lies in the exploitation of the compound to generate, synthetically, stable orally active prostacycline analogues which will inhibit platelet aggregation and hence thrombotic events, and yet have minimal effects on the heart and blood vessels.

PROSTATE, DISEASES OF
Disease of the prostate can affect the flow of urine so that patients present with urological symptoms.

Prostatitis This can be either acute or chronic. Acute prostatitis is caused by a bacterial infection, while chronic prostatitis may follow on from an acute attack, arise insidiously, or be non-bacterial in origin.
SYMPTOMS Typically the patient has pain in the PERINEUM, groins, or supra pubic region, and pain on EJACULATION. He may also have urinary frequency, and urgency.
TREATMENT Acute and chronic prostatitis are treated with a prolonged course of antibiotics. Patients with chronic prostatitis may also require anti-inflammatory drugs, and anti-depressants.

Prostatic enlargement This is the result of benign prostatic hyperplasia (BPH), causing enlargement of the prostate. The exact cause of this enlargement is unknown, but affects 50 per cent of men between 40 and 59 years and 95 per cent of men over 70 years.

SYMPTOMS These are urinary hesitancy, poor urinary stream, terminal dribbling, frequency and urgency of urination and the need to pass urine at night (nocturia). The diagnosis is made from the history, a digital examination of the prostate gland via the rectum to assess enlargement, and analysis of the urinary flow rate.

TREATMENT This can be with tablets, which either shrink the prostate – an anti-androgen drug such as finasteride – or relax the urinary sphincter muscle during urination. For more severe symptoms the prostate can be removed surgically, by trans-urethral resection of prostate (TURP), using either electrocautery or laser energy. An experimental treatment is the use of microwaves to heat up and shrink the enlarged gland.

Cancer Cancer of the prostate is the fourth commonest cause of death from cancer in UK males: over 10,000 cases are diagnosed every year. Little is known about the cause, but the majority of prostate cancers require the male hormones, androgens, to grow.

SYMPTOMS These are similar to those resulting from benign prostatic hypertrophy. Spread of the cancer to bones can cause pain. The use of a blood test measuring the amount of an ANTIGEN, PROSTATE SPECIFIC ANTIGEN (PSA), can be helpful in making the diagnosis, as can an ULTRASOUND scan of the prostate.

TREATMENT This could be surgical, with removal of the prostate, either via an abdominal incision, total prostatectomy, or trans-urethrally, or could be by radiotherapy. In more advanced cancers treatment with anti-androgen drugs, such as cyprotexone acetate or certain oestrogens, is used to inhibit the growth of the cancer.

PROSTATECTOMY An operation to remove part or all of the PROSTATE gland. The commonest method is transurethral prostatectomy (TURP) carried out during CYSTOSCOPY. A very enlarged prostate may need to be removed by a retropubic prostatectomy. After several weeks most patients are able to resume normal activity including sexual intercourse.

PROSTATE GLAND This is an accessory sex gland in males which is wrapped round the urethra as this tube leaves the bladder. Opening into the urethra, the gland secretes an alkaline fluid during ejaculation and is a constituent of SEMEN. The gland grows during adolescence and is sensitive to the concentrations of sex hormones.

PROSTATE SPECIFIC ANTIGEN (PSA) An ENZYME produced by glandular tissue in the PROSTATE. When the gland enlarges (see PROSTATE, DISEASES OF) greater amounts of PSA are secreted, raising the concentration of the enzyme in the blood. This is especially so in cancer of the prostate, and testing the level of PSA is an indicator that the disease may be present.

PROSTATISM The condition induced by benign enlargement of the PROSTATE GLAND.

PROSTHESIS A prosthesis is an artificial replacement, such as an artificial limb, eye, hip joint or a denture. It is often necessary, for aesthetic or functional reasons, to replace part of the body, lost by injury or disease, with copies of the original, or PROSTHESES as they are now known. From ancient times this has been the case: Herodotus speaks of a man with a wooden foot; the Romans produced effective limbs. The oldest known artificial limb – a leg – in existence, is neatly formed of thin bronze plates, leather and iron, found in a tomb at Capua and dating from around 300 BC; the Etruscans fashioned gold teeth five centuries before the Christian era; Goetz von Berlichingen (1480–1562), to supply his lost right hand, had one made of iron and thus became known as Goetz of the Iron Hand; and Ambroise Paré, who wrote on surgery in the sixteenth century, has a chapter upon artificial limbs. From then there was little advance until 1800 when James Potts, of London, patented an artificial leg made of two hollow wooden cones with a steel knee joint and a wooden ankle joint. It became known as the Anglesey leg after its owner, the Marquis of Anglesey and, with few modifications, remained the basis of British designs until the 1914–18 War. Since the 1939–45 War there have been striking advances, particularly in artificial hands, as the result of the introduction of electronics and myoelectric means of control.

Artificial limbs are best made to meet the individual's requirements but they can be obtained 'off the shelf'. A mould is taken of the amputated limb and is used to fashion a socket for the top of the prosthesis. This socket is made of leather, plastic or wood and is attached to the stump by suction or straps. The prosthesis has an inner strut which is enclosed in foam rubber to match the missing part of the normal limb. An outer shell of leather, metal or wood is then fitted. Artificial joints normally comprise complex mechanisms to stimulate flexion and rotation movements. Leg prostheses are generally more useful than those for arms because leg movements are easier to duplicate than those of the arm. Modern electronic circuitry that enables nerve impulses to be picked up and converted into appropriate movements is greatly improving the effectiveness of limb prostheses.

Eyes Artificial eyes are worn both for appearance and for psychological reasons. They are made of glass or plastic, and are thin shells of a boat-shape, representing the front half of the eye which has been removed. The stump which is left has still the eye-muscles in it, and so the artificial eye still has the power of moving with the other. A glass eye has to be replaced by a new one every year. Plastic eyes have the advantage of being more comfortable to wear, and more durable and of being unbreakable.

Dental prosthesis is any artificial replacement of a tooth. There are three main types, a crown, a bridge and a denture. A crown is the replacement of the part of a tooth which sticks through the gum. It is fixed to the remaining part of the tooth and may be made of metal, porcelain, plastic or a combination of these. A bridge is the replacement of two or three missing teeth and is usually fixed in place. The replacement teeth are held in position by being joined to one or more crowns on the adjacent teeth. A denture is a removable prosthesis used to replace some or all the teeth. The teeth are made of plastic or porcelain and the base may be of plastic or metal. Removable teeth may be held more firmly by means of implants.

Nose The making of a new nose is the oldest known operation in plastic surgery, Hindu records of such operations dating back to 1000 BC. Loss of a nose may be due to eroding disease, war wounds, gun-shot wounds or dog bites. In essence the operation is the same as that practised a thousand years before Christ: namely the use of a skin graft, brought down from the forehead. Alternative sources of the skin graft today are skin from the arm, chest or abdomen. As a means of support the new nose is built round a graft of bone or of cartilage from the ear.

PROTEIN The term applied to members of a group of non-crystallizable nitrogenous substances widely distributed in the animal and vegetable kingdoms and forming the characteristic materials of their tissues and fluids. They are essentially combinations of AMINO-ACIDS. They mostly dissolve in water and are coagulated by heat and various chemical substances. Typical examples of protein substances are white of egg and gelatin.

Proteins constitute an essential part of the diet as a source of energy and for the replacement of protein lost in the wear and tear of daily life. Their essential constituent from this point of view is the nitrogen they contain. To be absorbed, or digested, proteins have to be broken down into their constituent aminoacids. The adult human body can maintain nitrogenous equilibrium on a mixture of eight amino-acids, which are therefore known as the essential amino-acids. They are isoleucine, leucine, lysine, methionine, phenylalanine, threonine, tryptophan and valine. In addition, infants require histidine.

PROTEINURIA A condition in which proteins, principally ALBUMIN, are present in the urine. It is often a symptom of serious heart or kidney disease, although some normal people have mild and transient proteinuria after exercise.

Causes
KIDNEY DISEASE is the most important cause of proteinuria, and in some cases the discovery of proteinuria may be the first evidence of such disease. This is why an examination of the urine for the presence of albumin constitutes an essential part of every medical examination. Almost any form of kidney disease will cause proteinuria, but the most frequent form to do this is glomerulonephritis. In the subacute (or nephrotic) stage of glomerulo-nephritis the most marked proteinuria of all may be found. Proteinuria is also found in infections of the kidney (pyelitis) as well as in infections of the bladder (cystitis) and of the urethra (urethritis).
PREGNANCY The development of proteinuria in pregnancy requires investigation, as it may be the first sign of one of the most dangerous complications of pregnancy: toxaemia of pregnancy, glomerulonephritis, or ECLAMPSIA. Proteinuria may also result from the contamination of urine with vaginal secretions.
CARDIOVASCULAR DISORDERS are commonly accompanied by proteinuria, particularly when the right side of the heart is failing. In severe cases of failure, accompanied by oedema, the proteinuria may be marked.
FEVER often causes proteinuria, even though there is no actual kidney disease. The proteinuria disappears soon after the temperature becomes normal.
DRUGS AND POISONS These include arsenic, lead, mercury, gold, copaiba, salicylic acid and quinine.
ANAEMIA A trace of albumin may be found in the urine in severe anaemia.
POSTURAL OR ORTHOSTATIC ALBUMINURIA This type is important because, if its true cause is unrecognized, it may be taken as a sign of kidney disease. The significance of postural proteinuria is unclear: it is more common among young people and is absent when the person is recumbent, hence the importance of testing a urine sample that is taken before rising in the morning.

Treatment The treatment is that of the underlying disease. (See KIDNEYS, DISEASES OF.)

PROTHROMBIN An inactive substance in the blood plasma that is the precursor of the enzyme thrombin, which clots the blood. The conversion occurs when a blood vessel is damaged and the process of blood coagulation occurs (see COAGULATION).

PROTON PUMP INHIBITORS These are drugs that inhibit the production of acid in the stomach by blocking a key enzyme system, known as the proton pump, of the parietal cells of the stomach. The drugs include omeprazole, lansoprazole and pantoprazole, and they are the treatment of choice for oesophagitis (erosion and stricture) (see OESOPHAGUS, DISEASES OF) and the short-term treatment for gastric and duodenal ulcers and, in combination with ANTIBIOTICS, for the eradication of HELICOBACTER PYLORI.

PROTOPLASM The viscid, translucent, glue-like material containing fine granules and composed mainly of proteins, which makes up the essential material of plant and animal cells and has the properties of life.

PROTOZOA A simple, primitive animal comprising a single cell. Protozoa are microscopic in size but are much larger than bacteria. Most protozoa live freely but around 30 are parasitic in humans causing disease such as amoebiasis and giardiasis (intestinal infections), malaria, kala-azar and sleeping sickness. Some protozoa are able to excrete, respire, and absorb food particles and they may move around like a mobile jelly or by means of flagellae.

PROTRIPTYLINE A tricyclic antidepressant drug. (See ANTIDEPRESSANTS; MENTAL ILLNESS.)

PROXIMAL A term of comparison applied to structures which are nearer the centre of the body or the median line as opposed to more distal, or distant, structures.

PROZAC (see FLUOXETINE).

PRURIGO An intensely itching form of eczema in which LICHENIFICATION takes a nodular form.

PRURITUS Another name for itching, it is a common symptom with many causes. It may accompany obvious skin disease such as URTI-CARIA, ECZEMA, or SCABIES. Pruritus may be systemic in origin and can be caused by advanced hepatic (liver) or renal (kidney) failure, uncontrolled DIABETES, or HYPERTHYROIDISM. It may be due to drugs and certain forms of malignancy – for example, HODGKIN'S DISEASE. Anxiety or depression may also cause pruritus. Pruritus ani, itching round the ANUS, is a common troublesome condition. It may be caused by obsessive efforts to keep this area clean: soft toilet paper and gentle cleaning once daily should be sufficient. A weak anal sphincter, skin tags, and HAEMORRHOIDS may also cause itching and these conditions should be treated.

Treatment The first aim is to identify and treat the cause whether local or systemic. Once the cause has been dealt with, symptomatic treatment may be required to break the cycle of itching, scratching and itching; topical steroid ointments and occlusive dressings help to prevent scratching. For dry skin, emollients (see OINTMENTS) are useful. Local ANAESTHETICS provide relief but may cause allergic reactions and systemic ANTIHISTAMINES at night can help.

PRUSSIC ACID POISONING (see CYANIDE POISONING).

PSEUDOCYESIS means spurious or false

pregnancy, a condition characterized by enlargement of the abdomen, and even enlargement of the breasts and early morning sickness, the unfortunate woman being quite convinced that she is pregnant.

PSEUDOCYST A space within an organ without a defined lining and which contains fluid. Patients with chronic pancreatitis (see PANCREAS, DISEASES OF) sometimes develop these pseudocysts which fill with pancreatic juice containing ENZYMES produced by the gland. Abdominal pain usually results; treatment is by surgical draining.

PSEUDO HERMAPHRODITE A person in whom the GONADS (testes or ovaries) of only one sex are present in the body but the external GENITALIA may not be obviously male or female. The condition is a result of a hormonal imbalance and can normally be treated by appropriate surgery and hormone drugs. (See HERMAPHRODITE.)

PSEUDOHYPERTROPHIC MUSCULAR DYSTROPHY, or PSEUDOHYPERTROPHIC PARALYSIS, is a condition in which certain muscles enlarge owing to a fatty and fibrous degeneration, giving a false appearance of increased strength.

PSEUDOMONAS AERUGINOSA A pathogenic bacterium of the genus pseudomonas – rodlike, motile GRAM-NEGATIVE bacteria – that occurs in plus from wounds and is associated with urinary tract infections. The bacteria mostly live in soil and decomposing organic matter and help to recycle nitrogen in nature. Most of the bacteria in this genus are harmless to man.

PSEUDOXANTHOMA ELASTICUM This is a hereditary disorder of elastic tissue. Degenerating elastic tissue in the skin produces lesions in the skin which look like soft yellow papules. Elastic tissue in the eye and blood vessels is also involved, giving rise to visual impairment, raised blood pressure and haemorrhages.

PSITTACOSIS (PARROT DISEASE) An infectious disease of parrots and other exotic birds which may be transmitted to man and is caused by the micro-organism *Chlamydia psittaci*. It presents as PNEUMONIA or a systemic illness in which the patient has an enlarged spleen and liver and PNEUMONITIS. TETRACYCLINE is an effective treatment but relapses may occur. In the United Kingdom several hundred cases occur annually.

PSOAS A powerful muscle which arises from the front of the vertebral column in the lumbar region, and passes down, round the pelvis and through the groin, to be attached to the inner side of the thigh-bone not far from its upper end. The act of sitting up from a recumbent posture, or that of bending the thigh on the abdomen, is mainly accomplished by the contraction of this muscle. Disease of the spine in the lumbar region may produce an abscess which lies within the sheath of this muscle and makes its way down to the front of the thigh. Such an abscess is known as a psoas abscess. (See ABSCESS, chronic.)

PSORALENS (see PHOTOCHEMOTHERAPY and PHOTODERMATOSIS).

PSORIASIS This chronic, relapsing inflammatory skin disease is extremely common, affecting about 2 per cent of the UK population. Frequently it is mild and trivial, affecting only the points of the elbows or knees and the scalp, but in a substantial minority of sufferers the disease is much more widespread and causes considerable discomfort and social embarrassment. Rarely, it can be universal and even life threatening.

The predisposition to psoriasis is genetic, multiple genes being involved, but postnatal factors such as acute infection, hormonal epochs, pregnancy and drugs can influence or provoke it. The sexes are equally affected and onset is commonest in the second or third decades of life.

The psoriatic lesion is dull red, scaly and well defined. Scale is shed constantly, either in tiny pieces or as large plaques. The scalp is usually affected but the disease does not cause significant hair loss. The finger nails may be pitted or ridged and the toe nails grossly thickened. Several clinical patterns occur: in guttate psoriasis a sudden explosion of multiple tiny lesions may follow a STREPTOCOCCAL throat infection, especially in children. Larger lesions are characteristic of discoid (plaque) psoriases, the usual adult form. In the elderly the plaques may be mainly in the large body folds, flexural psoriasis. Rarely, psoriasis may be universal (psoriatic erythroderma) or a sterile PUSTULAR eruption may supervene (pustular psoriasis).

Mucous membranes in the mouth and elsewhere are not affected. Psoriasis does not affect internal organs but in about 1 per cent of subjects an inflammatory joint disease (psoriatic arthritis) may be associated with it.

Treatment There is no absolute cure but several agents used topically are of value including coal-tar extracts, DITHRANOL, CORTICOSTEROIDS and synthetic derivatives of Vitamins A and D. Ultraviolet B phototherapy (and natural sunlight) benefits most but not all psoriatics. Systemic therapy, including PHOTOCHEMOTHERAPY, is reserved for severe forms of psoriasis. METHOTREXATE and CYCLOSPORIN A are the most effective drugs but both are potentially dangerous and require expert monitoring.

Patient information may be obtained through the Psoriasis Association (see APPENDIX 2: ADDRESSES).

PSYCHE The mind or soul of an individual and his or her mental, in contrast to the physical, functioning.

PSYCHEDELIC DRUGS Drugs, such as lysergic acid diethylamide (LSD), that expand consciousness and perception. (See DRUG ADDICTION.)

PSYCHIATRY That branch of medical science which treats mental disorder and disease and also helps with the management of people with LEARNING DISABILITIES (see MENTAL ILLNESS).

PSYCHO-ANALYSIS The term applied to the theories and practice of the school of psychology originating with FREUD and developed by JUNG and other psychotherapists (see PSYCHOLOGY). It depends upon the theory that states of disordered mental health have been produced by a repression in the subconscious of painful memories or of conflicting instincts, thus absorbing the individual's mental energy and diverting attention from normal mental activities.

Psycho-analysis aims at discovering these repressed memories which are responsible for the diversion of mental power and of which the affected person usually is only dimly aware or quite unaware. The fundamental method of psycho-analytical treatment is the free expression of thoughts, ideas and fantasies on the part of the patient. To facilitate this, the analyst uses techniques to relax the patient and maintains a neutral attitude to his or her problems. In the course of analysis the patient will re-explore his early emotional attitudes and tensions.

The fundamental conception of psychoanalysis, though hard to prove by orthodox scientific methods and therefore challenged by some psychiatrists, has been widely adopted and developed by other schools of psychology. Freud's work changed the attitudes of the scientific community and the public to the problems of the neurotic, the morbidity anxious, the fearful and to the mental and emotional develoment of the child.

PSYCHOGERIATRICS The branch of psychiatry that investigates, diagnoses and treats the mental health problems of old people. Psychogeriatricians work in close co-operation with physicians for the care of the elderly and other health professionals and social workers in this branch of medicine.

PSYCHOLOGY Scientific study of the mind and its methods of working, particularly in relation to behaviour. Psychology covers such matters as memory, rational and irrational thought, intelligence, learning, personality, perceptions and emotions. There are different schools of psychology, differing both in attitude and methods of working. The main groups consist of the introspectionist FREUDIAN, JUNGIAN and ADLERIAN schools, and the GESTALTIST, BEHAVIOURIST, and COGNITIVE schools. Although many practical psychologists deny belonging to any specific school, contemporary psychology in general favours the cognitive schools, although many are subspecialities based on practical considerations.

PSYCHONEUROSIS A general term applied to various functional disorders of the nervous system. (See NEUROSIS.)

PSYCHOPATHIC Psychopathic disorder is defined by the Mental Health Act 1983 as a persistent disorder or disability of mind (whether or not including significant impairment of intelligence) which results in abnormally aggressive or seriously irresponsible conduct. The cardinal features are as follows: (1) Absence of normal feelings for other people such as love, affection, sympathy and condolence. (2) A tendency to anti-social impulsive acts with no forethought of the consequences. (3) A failure to learn by experience and to be deterred from crime by punishment. (4) Absence of any other form of mental disorder that would explain the unusual behaviour. The corresponding American terminology is 'anti-social personality disorder'. (See MENTAL ILLNESS.)

PSYCHOSIS A term applied to serious disorder of the mind, amounting to insanity. (See MENTAL ILLNESS.)

PSYCHOSOMATIC DISEASES Illnesses resulting from the effects of excessive or repressed emotions upon bodily function or structure. They affect vast numbers of patients who do not have any organic disease to account for their illness. Disorders precipitated by emotional factors may be psychotic, psychoneurotic or psychosomatic. In psychotic and psychoneurotic illnesses the symptoms are predominantly psychological, whilst in psychosomatic disorders the symptoms may be largely or entirely physical (somatic). The concept of emotional disturbances contributing to bodily disease is not new. Over 2400 years ago Socrates stressed that 'as you ought not to attempt to cure the eyes without the head, or the head without the body, so you should not treat body without mind'. The rapid advances of scientific medicine have encouraged a preoccupation with the practical and measurable aspects of people's disorders. It has been estimated that one third of patients attending their doctor have an illness with a psychiatric element. In another third symptoms are largely dependent on an emotional factor even though organic disease is present. Over one quarter of all absence from work due to sickness is estimated to be as a result of an illness with an emotional basis.

The three major problems that lead to psychosomatic disorder are marital relationships; occupation, which includes the frustrations, disappointments and feelings of unfulfilment provoked by the patient's work; and finally, social relationships – the feelings which prevail between friends, neighbours and relations.

The many somatic symptoms due to anxiety result from enhanced activity of the AUTONOMIC nervous system which comprises the SYMPATHETIC and PARASYMPATHETIC divisions. Pain may be a manifestation of psychosomatic disease. Psychogenic factors may produce muscle tension and and cause a pain that is organic. The tension headache is due to the increased tone of the muscles of the neck and scalp.

Autonomic nervous overactivity may be manifest in the various systems as follows:

Central nervous system Headache. Often described as a pressure on the head. Dizziness, feelings of faintness, nervousness, tremors, sleeplessness and physical exhaustion.

Cardiovascular system Tachycardia, arrhythmia and precordial pains.

Respiratory symptoms Sighing respirations and a feeling of an inability to breathe deeply. Vasomotor rhinitis, chronic sore throat and asthma.

Gastro-intestinal system Anorexia, nausea, vomiting, indigestion, wind, heartburn, diarrhoea, constipation and sensations of a lump in the throat.

Skin Itching, sweating, parasthesiae and neurodermatitis.

Functional illness has its own characteristics and the diagnosis is not established by the mere exclusion of organic disease. It is suggested by the existence of emotional disturbance as a precipitating factor, by the presence of certain characteristic symptoms, by a family history of a similar disorder and by a phasic course characterized by remissions and relapses. Organic disease may cause anxiety and may provide the stressful factor needed to precipitate psychosomatic disease.

PSYCHOSURGERY This was introduced in 1936 by Egas Moniz, Professor of Medicine in Lisbon University, for the surgical treatment of certain psychoses. For his work in this field he shared the Nobel prize in 1949. The original operation, known as leucotomy, consisted of cutting white fibres in the frontal lobe of the brain. It was accompanied by certain hazards such as persistent epilepsy and undesirable changes in personality. Pre-frontal leucotomy is now regarded as obsolete. Modern stereotactic surgery may be indicated in certain intractable psychiatric illnesses in which the patient is chronically incapacitated, especially where there is a high suicide risk. Patients are only considered for psychosurgery when they have failed to respond to routine therapies. One contra-indication is marked histrionic or anti-social personality. The conditions in which a favourable response has been obtained are intractable and chronic obsessional neuroses, anxiety states and severe chronic depression.

Psychosurgery is now rare in Britain. The

Mental Health Act 1983 requires not only consent by the patient, confirmed by an independent doctor, and two other representatives of the Mental Health Act Commission, but that the Commission's appointed medical representative must also advise on the likelihood of the treatment's alleviating or preventing a deterioration in the patient's condition.

PSYCHOTHERAPY Psychological rather than physical method for the treatment of PSYCHOLOGICAL and PSYCHIATRIC disorders. Almost every type of disease or injury has a mental aspect, even if this relates only to the pain or discomfort that it causes. In some diseases and with some temperaments, the mental factor is much more pronounced than in others; for such cases psychotherapy is particularly important. The chief methods employed all depend on the client–therapist relationship's being of prime importance.

Suggestion is a commonly employed method, used in almost every department of medicine. It may consist, in its simplest form, merely of emphasizing that the patient's health is better, so that this idea becomes fixed in the patient's mind. A suggestion of efficacy may be conveyed by the physical properties of a medicine or by the appearance of some apparatus used in treatment. Again, suggestion may be conveyed emotionally, as in religious healing. Sometimes a therapeutic suggestion may be made to the patient in a hypnotic state.

Analysis consists in the elucidation of the half-conscious or subconscious repressed memories or instincts that are responsible for some cases of mental disorder or personal conflicts.

Group therapy is a method whereby patients are treated in small groups and encouraged to participate actively in the discussion which ensues amongst themselves and the participating therapists. A modification of group therapy is drama therapy. Large group therapy also exists.

Education and employment may be important factors in rehabilitative psychotherapy.

Supportive therapy consists of sympathetically reviewing the patient's situation with him or her and encouraging the patient to identify and solve problems.

Short-term supportive psychotherapy is aimed at stabilizing and strengthening the psychological defence mechanisms of those patients who are confronted by a crisis which threatens to overwhelm their ability to cope, or who are struggling with the aftermath of major life events.

Long-term supportive psychotherapy is needed for patients with personality disorders or recurrent psychotic states, where the aim of treatment is to prevent deterioration and help the patient to achieve an optimal adaptation, making the most of his psychological assets. Such patients may find more profound and unstructured forms of therapy distressing.

Behavioural therapy and cognitive therapy, often carried out by psychologists, attempt to clarify with the patient specific features of behaviour or mental outlook respectively and identify step-by-step methods the patient can use for controlling the disorder. Behaviour therapy is commonly used for agoraphobia and other phobias, and cognitive therapy has been used for depression and anxiety. (See MENTAL ILLNESS.)

PSYCHOTROPIC Affecting the mind. Psychotropic drugs include HALLUCINOGENS, HYPNOTICS or sleeping drugs, sedatives, TRANQUILLIZERS and NEUROLEPTIC (antipsychotic) drugs.

PTERYGIUM A degenerative disorder of the conjunctiva which grows over the cornea medially and laterally. The overgrowths look like wings. They are commonly seen in people who live in areas of bright sunlight, particularly when reflected from deserts or snowfields. Treatment involves excision of the overgrowth. (See EYE DISEASES.)

PTOSIS (see EYE DISEASES).

PTYALIN The name of the ENZYME contained in the saliva, by which starchy materials are changed into sugar, and so prepared for absorption. It is identical with the AMYLASE of pancreatic juice. (See DIGESTION; PANCREAS.)

PUBERTY The change that takes place when childhood passes into manhood or womanhood. This change is generally a very definite one, taking place at about the age of fourteen years, although it is modified by race, climate, and bodily health, so that it may appear a year or two earlier or several years later. At this time the sexual functions attain their full development, the contour of the body changes from a childish to a more rounded womanly, or sturdy manly form, and great changes take place in the mode of thought and feeling. In girls it is marked by the onset of menstruation and development of the BREASTS. Development of the breasts is usually the first sign of puberty to appear, and may occur from 9 years onwards. Most girls show signs of breast development by the age of 13. The time from the beginning of breast development to the onset of MENSTRUATION is usually around two years but may range from six months to five years. The first sign of puberty in boys is an increase in testicular size between the age of 10 and 14. The larynx enlarges in boys, so that the voice after going through a period of 'breaking', finally assumes the deep manly pitch. Hair appears on the pubis and later in the armpits in both boys and girls, whilst in the former it also begins to grow on the upper lip, and skin eruptions are not uncommon on the face. (See ACNE.)

The period is one of transition from a

physical and mental point of view. Puberty is not to be regarded as a physiological 'coming of age', for full development is not attained till between twenty and thirty years of age. (See also MENARCHE; MENSTRUATION.)

PUBIS is the bone that forms the front part of the pelvis. The pubic bones of opposite sides meet in the symphysis and protect the bladder from the front.

PUBLIC HEALTH 'The science and art of preventing disease, prolonging life and promoting health through organized efforts of society.' (E. D. Acheson (Chairman), *Public Health in England*. Cmd 289, HMSO, London 1988.)

Improvements in health can be gained in many ways. Individuals with health problems go to their doctor, are diagnosed and prescribed treatment. In the same way public-health doctors use epidemiological studies to diagnose the causes of health problems in populations and plan services to treat the health and disease problems identified. Their concern is often focused particularly on those who are disadvantaged or marginalized and on the delivery of safe, effective and accessible health care, but to achieve their goal of better health and well-being for everybody they must also influence decision makers across all of the community.

Central to understanding public health is recognition that public-health practitioners are concerned not just with individuals, but with whole populations and that improving health care plays only a part of public-health improvement. The health of populations (public health) is also dependent on many factors such as the social, economic and physical environment in which the people live and the nutrition and health care available to them.

For thousands of years a fundamental feature of civilizations has been to seek to improve the health of the population and protect it from disease. This has led to the development of legal frameworks which differ widely from country to country, depending on their social and political development. All are concerned to stop the spread of infectious diseases, to maintain the safety of urban food and water supplies and most are also associated with housing standards, some form of poverty relief and basic health care. Some trading standards are often covered, at least in relation to the sale and distribution of poisons and drugs, and controls on industrial and transport safety, for example, in relation to drinking and driving and car design. Although these varied functions protect the public health and were often originally developed to improve it, most are managerially and professionally separated from today's public-health departments. So public-health professionals in the NHS, armed with evidence of the cause of a disease problem, must frequently act as advocates for health across many agencies where they play no formal management part. They must also seek to build alliances and add a health perspective to the policies of other services wherever possible.

Epidemiology is the principal diagnostic method of public health. It is defined as the study of the distribution and determinants of health-related states in specified populations and the application of this study to the control of health problems. Public-health practitioners also draw on many other skills, such as those of statisticians, sociologists, anthropologists, economists and policy analysts in identifying and trying to resolve the health problems of the societies they serve. Treatments proposed are likely to extend well beyond the clinic or hospital and may include recommendations for measures to resolve poverty, improve sanitation or housing, control pollution, change life styles such as smoking, improve nutrition, or change health services. At times of acute epidemics public-health doctors have considerable legal powers granted to enable them to prevent infection spreading. At other times their work may be more concerned with monitoring, reporting, planning and managing services, and advocating policy changes to politicians so that health is promoted.

The term 'the public health' can relate to the state of health of the population, and be represented by measures such as MORTALITY indices (e.g. perinatal or infant mortality and standardized mortality rates), life expectancy, or measures of morbidity (illness). These can be compared across areas and even countries. Sometimes people refer to a pubic health-care system. This is a publicly funded service, the primary aim of which is to improve health by the use of population-based measures. They may include or be separate from private health-care services for which individuals pay. The structure of these systems varies from country to country reflecting different social composition and political priorities. There are, however, some general elements that can be identified:

Surveillance The collection, collation and analysis of data to provide useful information about the distribution and causes of health and disease and related factors in populations. These activities form the basis of epidemiology, which is the diagnostic backbone of public-health practice.

Intervention The design, advocacy and implementation of policies to improve health. This may be through the provison of preventive medical care, environmental measures, influencing the behaviour of individuals or the provision of appropriate services to limit disability and handicap. It will lead to advocacy for health, promoting change in many areas of policy including, for example, taxation and improved housing and employment opportunities.

Evaluation Assessment of the first two steps to assess their impact in terms of effectiveness, efficiency, acceptability, accessibility, value for money or other indicators of quality. This enables the programme to be reviewed and changed as necessary.

The practice of public health   The situation in the United Kingdom will be described as, even though systems vary, it will give a general impression of the type of work covered.

HISTORY   Initially public-health practice related to food, the urban environment and the control of infectious diseases. Early examples include rules in the Bible about avoiding certain foods. These were probably based on practical experience, had gradually been adopted as sensible behaviour, become part of culture and finally been incorporated into religious laws. Other examples are the regulations about quarantine for PLAGUE and LEPROSY in the Middle Ages, vaccination against SMALLPOX introduced by William Jenner, and Lind's use of citrus fruits to prevent scurvy at sea in the 18th century.

It was during the 19th century, in response to the health problems arising from the rapid growth of urban life, that the foundations of a public-health system were created. The 'sanitary' concept was fundamental to these developments. This suggested that overcrowding in insanitary conditions was the cause of most disease epidemics and that improved sanitation measures such as sewerage and clean water supplies would prevent them. Action to introduce such measures were often initiated only after epidemics spread out of the slums and into wealthier and more powerful families. Other problems such as the stench of the River Thames outside the Houses of Parliament also led to a demand for effective sanitary control measures. Successive public health laws were passed by Parliament, initially about sanitation and housing, and then, as scientific knowledge grew, about bacterial infections. In the middle of the 19th century the first medical officers of health were appointed with responsibility to report regularly and advise local government about the measures needed to control disease and improve health. Their scope and responsibility widened as society changed and took on a wider welfare role. After more than a century they changed as part of the reforms of the NHS and local government in the 1960s and became more narrowly focused within the health-care system and its management. Increased recognition of the multi-factorial causes, costs and limitations of treatment of conditions such as cancer and heart disease, and the emergence of new problems such as AIDS and BOVINE SPONGIFORM ENCEPHALOPATHY have again showed the importance of prevention and a broader approach to health. With it has come recognition that, while disease may be the justification for action, a narrow disease-treatment-based approach is not always the most effective or economic solution. The role of the director of public health (the successor to the medical officer of health) is again being expanded and in 1997 for the first time in the UK a government Minister for Public Health was appointed. This reflects not only a greater priority for public health, but, also a concern that the health effects of policy should be considered across all parts of government.

The future public-health department will comprise a broadly based, multi-disciplinary team, working to involve the public and decision makers in evidence-based health-policy development across organizational boundaries. Their aim of improving the health of all in the population will link closely with many others whose particular focus may be in improving education, the economy, the built and natural environment and in achieving a sustainable future. The idealism will be coloured by pragmatic acceptance that not everything is achievable for everybody and that therefore resource and service decisions must be equitable, open and accountable.

PUBLIC HEALTH LABORATORY SERVICE (PHLS)   A statutory organization that is part of the NHS. It comprises ten laboratory groups and two centres in the UK, with central co-ordination from PHLS headquarters. The service provides diagnostic-testing facilities for cases of suspected infectious disease. The remit of the PHLS (which was set up during the Second World War and then absorbed into the NHS) is now based on legislation approved in 1977 and 1979. Its overall purpose is to protect the population from infection by maintaining a national capability of high quality for the detection, diagnosis, surveillance, protection and control of infections and communicable diseases. It provides microbiology services to hospitals, family doctors and local authorities as well as providing national reference facilities.

PUERPERAL SEPSIS   An infection, once called puerperal fever, that starts in the genital tract within ten days after childbirth, miscarriage or abortion. Once a scourge of childbirth, with many women dying from the infection, the past 50 years have seen a dramatic decline in its incidence, with only 1 to 3 per cent of women having babies now being affected. This decline is due to much better maternity care and the advent of antibiotics. Infection usually starts in the VAGINA and is caused by the bacteria that normally live in it. They can cause harm because of the mother's lowered resistance or when part of the PLACENTA has been retained in the genital tract. The infection usually spreads to the UTERUS and sometimes to the FALLOPIAN TUBES. Sometimes bacteria may enter the vagina from other parts of the body.

Fever, an offensive-smelling post-partum vaginal discharge (lochia) and pain in the lower abdomen are the main features. Untreated, the women may develop SALPINGITIS, PERITONITIS and septicaemia. Antibiotics are used to treat the infection and any retained placental tissue must be removed.

PUERPERIUM   The period which elapses after the birth of a child until the mother is again restored to her ordinary health. It is generally regarded as lasting for a month. One of the main changes that occur is the enormous decrease in size that takes place in the muscular wall of the womb. There are often afterpains during the first day in women who have borne several children, less often after a first child. (See AFTERPAINS.) The discharge is blood-stained for the first two or three days, then clearer till the end of the first week, before stopping within two or three weeks. The breasts, which have already enlarged before the birth of the child, secrete milk more copiously, and there should be a plentiful supply on the third day of the puerperium.

Management The mother should start practising exercises to help to ensure that the stretched abdominal muscles regain their normal tone. There is no need for any restriction of diet, but care must be taken to ensure an adequate intake of fluid, including at least 580 ml (a pint) of milk a day.

Milk, as already stated, appears copiously on the third day, but this is preceded by a secretion from the breast, known as colostrum, which is of value to the new-born child. The child should therefore be put to the breasts within six to eight hours of being born. This also stimulates both the breasts and the natural changes taking place during this period. Suckling is beneficial for both child and mother and encourages bonding between the two.

PULMONARY DISEASES (see LUNGS, DISEASES OF).

PULMONARY EMBOLISM The condition in which an embolus (see EMBOLISM), or clot, is lodged in the lungs. The source of the clot is usually the veins of the lower abdomen or legs in which clot formation has occurred as a result of the occurrence of deep-vein thrombosis or DVT (THROMBOPHLEBITIS). (See VEINS, DISEASES OF.) Thrombophlebitis, with or without pulmonary embolism, is a not uncommon complication of surgical operations, especially in older patients. This is one reason why nowadays such patients are got up out of bed as quickly as possible, or, alternatively, are encouraged to move and exercise their legs regularly in bed. The severity of a pulmonary embolism, which is characterized by the sudden onset of pain in the chest, with or without the coughing up of blood, and a varying degree of shock, depends upon the size of the clot. If large enough it may prove immediately fatal. In other cases immediate operation may be needed to remove the clot, whilst in less severe cases anticoagulant treatment, in the form of HEPARIN, is given to prevent extension of the clot. For some operations, such as hip-joint replacements, with a high risk of deep-vein thrombosis in the leg, heparin is given for several days post-operatively.

PULMONARY FIBROSIS A condition which may develop in both lungs (interstitial pulmonary fibrosis) or part of one lung. Scarring and thickening of lung tissues occur as a consequence of previous lung inflammation, which may have been caused by PNEUMONIA or TUBERCULOSIS. Symptoms include cough and breathlessness and diagnosis is confirmed with a chest X-ray. The patient's underlying condition should be treated but the damage already done to lung tissue is usually irreversible. (See ALVEOLITIS.)

PULMONARY FUNCTION TESTS Tests to assess how the lungs are functioning. They range from simple spirometry (measuring breathing capacity) to sophisticated physiological assessments.

Static lung volumes and capacities can be measured: these include vital capacity, the maximum volume of air that can be exhaled slowly and completely after a maximum deep breath; forced vital capacity is a similar manoeuvre using maximal forceful exhalation and can be measured along with expiratory flow rates using simple spirometry; total lung capacity is the total volume of air in the chest after a deep breath in; functional residual capacity is the volume of air in the lungs at the end of a normal expiration, with all respiratory muscles relaxed.

Dynamic lung volumes and flow rates reflect the state of the airways. The forced expiratory volume (FEV) is the amount of air forcefully exhaled during the first second after a full breath – it normally accounts for over 75 per cent of the vital capacity. Maximal voluntary ventilation is calculated by asking the patient to breathe as deeply and quickly as possible for 12 seconds; this test can be used to check the internal consistency of other tests and the extent of cooperation by the patient, important when assessing possible neuromuscular weakness affecting respiration. There are several other more sophisticated tests which may not be necessary when assessing most patients. Measurement of arterial blood gases is also an important part of any assessment of lung function.

PULMONARY HYPERTENSION In this condition increased resistance to the blood flow through the lungs occurs. This is usually the result of lung disease and the consequence is an increase in pulmonary artery pressure and in the pressure in the right side of the heart and in the veins bringing blood to the heart. Chronic BRONCHITIS or EMPHYSEMA commonly constrict the small arteries in the lungs, thus causing pulmonary hypertension.

PULMONARY OEDEMA Collection of water in the lungs caused by left ventricular failure or MITRAL STENOSIS which produces back pressure in the lungs, thus forcing fluid into the tissues.

PULMONARY STENOSIS A disorder of the heart in which obstruction of the outflow of blood from the right ventricle (see HEART) occurs. Narrowing of the pulmonary valve at the exit of the right ventricle and narrowing of the pulmonary artery may cause obstruction. The condition is usually congenital though it may be caused by rheumatic fever. In the congenital condition pulmonary stenosis may occur with other heart defects and is then known as Fallot's tetralogy. Breathlessness and enlargement of the heart and eventual heart failure may be the consequence of pulmonary stenosis. Surgery is usually necessary to remove the obstruction.

PULP (see TEETH).

PULSATION or THROBBING An appearance seen or felt naturally below the fourth and fifth ribs on the left side, where the heart lies, and also at every point where an artery lies close beneath the surface. In other situations, it may be a sign of aneurysm. In thin people, pulsation can often be seen and felt in the upper part of the abdomen, due to the throbbing of the normal abdominal AORTA.

PULSE If the tip of one finger is laid on the front of the forearm, about 2·5 cm (one inch) above the wrist, and about 1 cm (half an inch) from the outer edge, the pulsations of the radial artery can be felt. This is known as the pulse, but a pulse can be felt wherever an artery of large or medium size lies near the surface.

The cause of the pulsation lies in the fact that, at each heart-beat, 80 to 90 millilitres of blood are driven into the aorta, and a fluid wave, distending the vessels as it passes, is transmitted along the arteries all over the body. This pulsation falls away as the arteries grow smaller, and is finally lost in the minute capillaries, where a steady pressure is maintained. For this reason, the blood in the veins flows steadily on without any pulsation. Immediately after the wave has passed, the artery, by virtue of its great elasticity, regains its former size. The nature of this wave helps the doctor to assess the state of the artery and the action of the heart.

The pulse rate is usually about 70 per minute, but it may vary in health from 50 to 100, and is quicker in childhood and slower in old age than in middle life; it is low (at rest) in physically fit athletes or other sports people. Fever causes the rate to rise, sometimes to 120 beats a minute or more.

In childhood and youth the vessel wall is so thin that, when sufficient pressure is made to expel the blood from it, the artery can no longer be felt. In old age, however, and in some degenerative diseases, the vessel wall becomes so thick that it may be felt like a piece of whipcord rolling beneath the finger.

Different types of heart disease have special features of the pulse associated with them. In atrial FIBRILLATION the great character is irregularity. In patients with an incompetent AORTIC VALVE the pulse is characterized by a sharp rise and sudden collapse.

An instrument known as the SPHYGMOGRAPH registers the arterial waves and a polygraph (an instrument that obtains simultaneous tracings from several different sources such as radial and jugular pulse, apex beat of the heart and ELECTROCARDIOGRAM (ECG) enables tracings to be taken from the pulse at the wrist and from the veins in the neck and simultaneous events in the two compared.

The pressure of the blood in various arteries is estimated by a SPHYGMOMANOMETER. (See BLOOD-PRESSURE.)

PULSE OXIMETRY Measurement of OXYGEN saturation of HAEMOGLOBIN in a blood sample using a non-invasive device called a spectrophotometer.

PULSES The seeds of the Leguminosa family. They include peas, beans and lentils and constitute a valuable source of food. Most contain around 20 grams of protein per 100 grams of dry weight but the biological value of this protein requires supplementation to ensure an adequate intake of essential AMINO-ACIDS. They have been described as 'the poor man's protein', and a combination of pulse and cereal proteins may have a nutritive value comparable to that of animal protein. They are a good source of the B group of vitamins with the exception of riboflavine. (See also DIET.)

PUNCTATE BASOPHILIA (see BASOPHILIA.)

PUNCTUM (see EYE).

PUPIL (see EYE).

PURGATIVES Drug or other substances used to treat CONSTIPATION. Also called laxative or aperient, purgatives are classified according to their mode of action. The three main groups are bulk, stimulant, and faecal softeners. The time a purgative takes to act may vary, and determines whether it should be taken in the morning or evening.

Bulk purgatives include bran and most high-fibre foods such as fruit, vegetables, and wholemeal foods. These leave a large indigestible residue that holds water in the gut and produces a large soft stool. Inorganic salts such as magnesium sulphate (Epsom Salt) have a similar effect.

Stimulant purgatives, for example, bisacodyl, and senna and castor oil, stimulate peristalsis, though the action may be accompanied by colicky pains.

Faecal softeners (emollients) There are two groups: surface-active agents such as dioctyl sodium and sulphosuccinate retain water in the stools and are often combined with a stimulant purgative. Liquid paraffin is chemically inert and is said to act by lubrication.

PURPURA A skin rash caused by bleeding into the skin from capillary blood vessels. The discrete purple spots of the rash are called petechiae. The disorder may be caused by capillary defects (non-thrombocytopenic purpura) or be due to a deficiency of PLATELETS in the blood (THROMBOCYTOPENIC purpura). (See HENOCH-SCHÖNLEIN PURPURA; IDIOPATHIC THROMBOCYTOPENIC PURPURA; THROMBOCYTOPENIA.).

PUS is a thick, white, yellow, or greenish fluid, found in abscesses, on ulcers, and on inflamed and discharging surfaces generally. Its colour and consistency are due to the presence of white blood corpuscles, and superficial cells of granulation tissue or of a mucous membrane which die and are shed off in consequence of the inflammatory process. Bacteria that normally produce pus are STREPTOCOCCI, PNEUMOCOCCI and ESCHERICHIA COLI. (See ABSCESS; PHAGOCYTOSIS.)

PUSTULE A small collection of pus. (See ABSCESS.) Malignant pustule is one of the forms of ANTHRAX.

PUTREFACTION The change that takes place in the bodies of plants and animals after death, whereby they are ultimately reduced to carbonic acid gas, ammonia, and other simple substances. The change is almost entirely due to the action of bacteria, and, in the course of the process, various offensive and poisonous intermediate substances are formed. In the case of the human body, putrescine, cadaverine, and other alkaloids are among these intermediate products.

PUTRID FEVER An old name for typhus fever.

PUVA (see PHOTOCHEMOTHERAPY; PSORIASIS).

PYAEMIA A form of blood-poisoning in which abscesses appear in various parts of the body. (See BLOOD-POISONING.)

PYELITIS A term describing inflammation of the pelvis of the kidney. In fact, the inflammation usually affects the whole kidney tissue and the description should be pyelonephritis. (See PYELONEPHRITIS.)

PYELOGRAPHY The process whereby the kidneys are rendered radio-opaque, and therefore visible on an X-ray film. It constitutes a most important part of the examination of a patient with kidney disease. (See SODIUM DIATRIZOATE.)

PYELONEPHRITIS Inflammation of the kidney, usually the result of bacterial infection. The inflammation may be acute or chronic.

Acute pyelonephritis comes on suddenly, is commoner in women and tends to occur when they are pregnant. Infection usually spreads up the ureters from the bladder which has become infected (cystitis). Fevers, chills and backache are the usual presenting symptoms. ANTIBIOTIC drugs should be given and in severe cases the intravenous route may be necessary. SEPTICAEMIA is an occasional complication.

Chronic pyelonephritis may start in childhood and the usual cause is backflow of urine from the bladder into one of the ureters, perhaps because of a congenital deformity of the valve where the ureter drains into the bladder. Constant urine reflux results in recurrent infection of the kidney and damage to its tissue. Full investigation of the urinary tract is essential and, if an abnormality is detected, surgery may well be required to remedy it. HYPERTENSION and RENAL failure may be serious complications of pyelonephritis (see KIDNEYS, DISEASES OF).

PYLEPHLEBITIS Inflammation of the PORTAL vein. A rare but serious disorder, it usually results from the spread of infection within the abdomen – for example, appendicitis. The patient may develop liver abscesses and ASCITES. Treatment is by ANTIBIOTICS and surgery.

PYLORIC STENOSIS: Narrowing of the PYLORUS, the muscular exit from the STOMACH. It is usually the result of a pyloric ulcer or cancer near the exit of the stomach. The result is that food is delayed when passing from the stomach to the duodenum and vomiting occurs. The stomach may become distended and peristalsis (muscular movement) may be seen through the abdominal wall. Unless surgically treated the patient will steadily deteriorate, losing weight, becoming dehydrated and developing alkalosis. Congenital pyloric stenosis occurs in babies (commonly boys) about 3 to 5 weeks old, and surgery produces a complete cure.

PYLOROSPASM Spasm of the pyloric portion of the STOMACH. This interferes with the passage of food in a normal, gentle fashion into the intestine and causes the pain that comes on from half an hour to three hours after meals and is associated with severe disorders of digestion. It is often produced by an ulcer of the stomach or duodenum.

PYLORUS The lower opening of the STOMACH, through which the softened and partially digested food passes into the small INTESTINE.

PYO- A prefix attached to the name of various diseases to indicate cases in which pus is formed, such as pyonephrosis.

PYODERMIA GANGRENOSUM This is a disorder in which large ulcerating lesions appear suddenly and dramatically in the skin. It is the result of underlying VASCULITIS. It is usually the result of inflammatory bowel disease such as ULCERATIVE COLITIS or CROHN'S DISEASE but can be associated with RHEUMATOID ARTHRITIS.

PYOGENIC is a term applied to those bacteria which cause the formation of pus and so lead to the formation of abscesses. Although many bacteria have this property, the most common cause of abscess is one of the rounded forms of bacterium (e.g. streptococcus).

PYORRHOEA Any copious discharge of pus. For pyorrhoea alveolaris see under TEETH, DISEASES OF.

PYRAZINAMIDE An antituberculous drug used in combination, usually with RIFAMPICIN and ISONIAZID, as the treatment regime for TUBERCULOSIS. It penetrates the MENINGES so is valuable in treating tuberculous MENINGITIS. The drug is sometimes associated with liver damage and liver function tests should be done before using the drug.

PYREXIA Fever. (See FEVER.)

PYRIDOXINE or VITAMIN B$_6$ This vitamin plays an important part in the metabolism of a number of amino-acids. Deficiency leads to atrophy of the EPIDERMIS, the hair follicles, and the SEBACEOUS glands, and peripheral NEURITIS may also occur. Young infants are more susceptible to pyridoxine deficiency than adults: they begin to lose weight and develop a hypochromic anaemia; irritability and convulsions may also occur. Liver, yeast, and cereals are relatively rich sources of it. Fish is a moderately rich source, but vegetables and milk contain little. The minimal daily requirement in the diet is probably about 2 mg. (See APPENDIX 5: VITAMINS.)

PYRIMETHAMINE An antimalarial drug used with either sulfadoxine or DAPSONE to treat PLASMODIUM FALCIPARUM MALARIAE. It should not be used for prophylaxis because of potentially severe side-effects when used long term.

PYROSIS (see WATERBRASH).

PYURIA The presence of pus in the URINE, in consequence of inflammation situated in the KIDNEY, BLADDER, or other part of the urinary tract. (See URINE.)

Q

QALY This is an outcome measure of health care devised by some health economists in the 1980s. It has proved controversial but nevertheless is an indication of the likely effectiveness of a particular treatment and can contribute to the assessment of treatment and care a patient should have. The initials stand for Quality Adjusted Life Year. It takes a year of healthy life expectancy to be worth 1 and a year of unhealthy life expectancy to be worth less than 1. The worse the forecast of an unhealthy person's quality of life, the lower will be his or her rating. If someone is expected to live five years in a healthy state, the grading will be 5; ten years of life estimated to be only 25-per-cent healthy will rate as 2·5 QALYs.

Q FEVER A disease of worldwide distribution due to the organism *Coxiella burneti*. It is characterized by fever, severe headache and often pneumonia. It was first described in 1937 amongst abattoir workers in Brisbane. The disease was given the name 'Q' fever, the Q (?) referring to the unknown cause of the disease. The aetiology of the infection was later established by Burnet who cultured a micro-organism from the blood of an infected patient. This rickettsia-like organism was originally called *Rickettsia burneti* but was later renamed *Coxiella burneti* when Cox found that it had certain features which differentiated it from the true rickettsia.

The principal reservoir of human infection in Britain is probably cattle and sheep in which the infection is usually sub-clinical. The diagnosis is confirmed by the detection of serum antibodies to *Coxiella burneti*. The organism is sensitive to tetracycline.

QUADRANTANOPIA Inability to see in one quarter of the visual field. Homonymous quadrantanopia is loss of vision in the same quarter of the field in each eye.

QUADRICEPS The large four-headed muscle occupying the front and sides of the thigh, which straightens the leg at the knee-joint and maintains the body in an upright position.

QUADRIPLEGIA Paralysis of the four limbs of the body (see PARALYSIS).

QUADRUPLETS (see MULTIPLE BIRTHS).

QUARANTINE The principle of preventing the spread of infectious disease by which people, baggage, merchandise, and so forth likely to be infected or coming from an infected locality are isolated at frontiers or ports till their harmlessness has been proved to the satisfaction of the authorities. (See INFECTION.)

Originally quarantine, as its name implies, involved detention for forty days; but the period now covers the incubation period of the disease, the presence of which is suspected.

Numerous international conferences upon the subject have been held with the view of arriving at a uniform practice as regards quarantine in different countries. The diseases to which quarantine applies are CHOLERA, YELLOW FEVER, PLAGUE, SMALLPOX, TYPHUS and RELAPSING FEVER.

The general practice with regard to quarantine is that when a serious disease breaks out in any country, the government of that country notifies surrounding governments as to the ports and other places that have become centres of infection. Any people travelling from these centres and attempting to enter another country, are subject to measures prescribed in the appropriate Regulations. These measures vary with the disease involved.

QUARTAN FEVER Description of intermittent fever with paroxysms developing every fourth day. Usually applied to MALARIA.

QUASSIA The wood of *Picrasma excelsa*, a large West Indian tree. It contains quassin, which is excessively bitter and also irritating. The various preparations of the wood are mainly used as a bitter tonic. Quassia cups were for long to be found in many households. Made of quassia wood, they were filled with hot water. This resulted in a bitter water which was drunk as a 'bitter' to stimulate the appetite.

QUICKENING (see PREGNANCY).

QUINIDINE An alkaloid obtained from cinchona bark and closely related in chemical composition and in action to quinine. It is commonly used in the form of quinidine sulphate to treat cardiac irregularities such as supraventricular tachycardia and ventricular arrhythmias.

QUININE An alkaloid obtained from the bark of various species of cinchona trees. This bark is mainly derived from Peru and neighbouring parts of South America and the East Indies. Other alkaloids and acid substances are also derived from cinchona bark, such as quinidine and cinchonine.

Quinine is generally used in the form of one of its salts, such as the sulphate of quinine, or dihydrochloride of quinine. All are sparingly soluble in water, much more so when taken along with an acid.

Action Quinine is a powerful antiseptic. Its best-known action is in checking the recurrence of attacks of malaria, as it destroys malarial parasites in the blood. In fevers it acts as an ANTIPYRETIC.

Among its side-effects are ringing in the ears,

temporary impairment of vision, and sometimes irritation of the kidneys: all these pass off when the drug is discontinued.

Uses The most important use of quinine is its original one in malaria, attacks of which it quickly cuts short or prevents altogether. It has been largely replaced by the more effective and less toxic anti-malarial drugs that were available. (See MALARIA.) Development of malarial parasites resistant to newer drugs has revived the use of quinine. For intravenous injection, when this is necessary in cases of malaria, a soluble form of quinine, the dihydrochloride, is used. Quinine can also be given in combination with other anti-malarial drugs on medical advice. The drug is sometimes used in the treatment of cramps.

QUINSY A corruption of 'cynanche', this is an old name for a PERITONSILLAR ABSCESS.

QUINTUPLETS (see MULTIPLE BIRTHS).

R

RABIES An acute and fatal disease which affects animals, particularly carnivora, and may be communicated from them to man. Infection from man to man is very rare, but those in attendance on a case should take precautions to avoid being bitten or allowing themselves to be contaminated by the patient's saliva as this contains the causative virus.

Cause The disease is in existence constantly among dogs and wolves in some countries, and epidemics occasionally occur. It also occurs in foxes, coyotes and skunks, as well as vampire bats. Thanks to quarantine measures, it has been rare in Great Britain since 1897. Britain still retains strict measures to prevent the entry of infected animals including a six months' quarantine period and vaccination. This quarantine policy is under review by the government and is likely to be relaxed.

It is highly infectious from the bite of an animal already affected, but the chance of infection from different animals varies. Thus only about one person in every four bitten by rabid dogs contracts rabies, whilst the bites of rabid wolves and cats almost invariably produce the disease. The disease is due to a virus which has a special affinity for attacking the nervous system.

Symptoms In animals there are two types of the disease: mad rabies and dumb rabies. In the former, the dog runs about, snapping at objects and other animals, unable to rest; in the latter, which is also the final stage of the mad type, the limbs become paralysed, and the dog crawls about or lies still.

In man the incubation period is usually six to eight weeks, but may be as short as ten days or as long as two years. The disease begins by mental symptoms, the person becoming irritable, restless, and depressed. Fever and DYS-PHAGIA follow. The irritability passes into a form of mania and the victim has great difficulty in swallowing either food or drink.

Treatment The best treatment is, of course, preventive. Local treatment consists of immediate, thorough, and careful cleansing of the wound surfaces and surrounding skin. This is followed by a course of rabies vaccine therapy. Only people bitten or in certain circumstances licked, either by a rabid animal or by one thought to be infected with rabies need treatment with rabies vaccine and antiserum and IMMUNOGLOBULIN. A person previously vaccinated against rabies who is subsequently bitten by a rabid animal should be given three to four doses of the vaccine. The vaccine is also used to give protection to those liable to infection, such as kennel workers and veterinary surgeons.

RAD A unit of ionizing RADIATION absorbed by an individual. The acronym stands for radiation absorbed dose.

RADIAL ARTERY This artery arises from the brachial artery at the level of the neck of the radius. It passes down the forearm to the wrist where it is easily palpated laterally. It then winds around the wrist to the palm of the hand to supply the fingers.

RADIAL NERVE This nerve arises from the brachial plexus in the axilla. At first descending posteriorly and then anteriorly it ends just above the elbow by dividing into the superficial radial and interosseous nerves. It supplies motor function to the muscles which extend the arm, wrist, and some fingers and supplies sensation to parts of the posterior and lateral aspects of the arm, forearm, and hand.

RADIATION Energy in the form of waves or particles. Radiation is mainly electromagnetic and is broadly classified as ionizing and nonionizing. The former can propel ions from an atom; these have an electrical charge and can combine chemically with each other. Ionization occurring in molecules that have a key function in living tissue can cause biological damage which may affect existing tissue or cause mutations in the genes of germ cell nuclei. Nonionizing radiation agitates the constituent atoms of nuclei but is insufficiently powerful to produce ions.

Ionizing radiation comprimes X-RAYS, GAMMA RAYS and particle radiation. X-rays are part of the continuous electromagnetic-wave spectrum: this also includes gamma rays, infra-red radiation, ultraviolet light and visible light. They have a very short wavelength and very high frequency and their ability to penetrate matter depends on the electrical energy generating them. X-rays that are generated by 100,000 volts can pass through body tissue and are used to produce images – popularly known as X-rays. X-rays, generated at several million volts, can destroy tissue and are used in RADIO-THERAPY for killing cancer cells. Gamma rays are similar to X-rays but are produced by decay of radioactive materials. Particle radiation, which can be produced electrically or by radioactive decay, comprises parts of atoms which have mass as well as (usually) an electrical charge.

Non-ionizing radiation includes ultraviolet light, radio waves, magnetic fields and ULTRA-SOUND. Magnetic fields are used in MAGNETIC RESONANCE IMAGING (MRI) and ultrasound which is inaudible high-frequency sound waves and is used for both diagnoses and treatment in medicine.

RADIATION SICKNESS The term applied to the nausea, vomiting, and loss of appetite which may follow exposure to radiation, say, at work or the use of radiotherapy in the treatment of cancer and other diseases. People exposed to radiation at work should have their exposure carefully monitored so that it does not exceed safety limits. Doses of radiation given during radiotherapy treatment are carefully measured. Even so, patients may suffer side-effects. The phenothiazine group of tranquillizers, such as CHLORPROMAZINE, as well as the ANTIHISTAMINE DRUGS, are of value in its prevention and treatment. (See RADIOTHERAPY.)

RADICULPATHY is damage to the roots of nerves where they enter or leave the SPINAL CORD. Causes include ARTHRITIS of the spine, thickening of the MENINGES and DIABETES MELLITUS. Symptoms include pain, paraesthesia, numbness and wasting of muscles supplied by the nerves. Treatment is of the underlying cause.

RADIOACTIVE ISOTOPES (see ISOTOPES).

RADIOACTIVITY Breakdown of the nuclei of some elements resulting in the emission of energy in the form of alpha, beta and gamma rays. Because of this particle emission, the elements decay into other elements. Radium and uranium are naturally occurring radioactive elements. RADIOTHERAPY treatment utilizes artificially produced isotopes (alternative forms of an element) such as iodine-131 and cobalt-60.

RADIOGRAPHY (see X-RAYS).

RADIO-IMMUNO ASSAY A technique introduced in 1960 which enables the minute quantities of natural substances in the blood such as hormones to be measured. A radio-immuno assay depends on the ability of an unlabelled hormone to inhibit, by simple competition, the binding of isotopically labelled hormone by specific antibodies. The requirements for a radio-immuno assay include adequate amounts of the hormone; a method for labelling the hormone with a radio active isotope; the production of satisfactory antibodies; and a technique for separating antibody-bound from free hormone. Radio-immuno assay is more sensitive than the best bio-assay for a given hormone and most sensitive radio-immuno assays permit the detection of picogram ($pg = 10^{-12}g$) and femtogram ($fg = 10^{-15}g$) amounts of material.

RADIOLOGY (see X-RAYS).

RADIONUCLIDE is another word for a radio-active isotope. (See ISOTOPES.)

RADIO-OPAQUE Substances which absorb X-rays, rather than transmitting them, appear white on X-rays and are known as radio-opaque. This is true of bones, teeth, certain types of gallstones, renal stones and contrast media used to enhance the accuracy of radiographic imaging. (See X-RAYS.)

RADIOTHERAPY The treatment of disease (mainly cancer) with penetrating RADIATION. For many years RADIUM and X-RAYS were the only sources available, but developments in knowledge led to the use of powerful X-rays, beta rays or gamma rays, either produced by linear accelerator machines or given off by radioactive isotopes (see ISOTOPE). The latter is rarely used now. Beams of radiation may be directed at the tumour from a distance or radioactive material, in the form of needles, wires or pellets, may be implanted in the body. Sometimes germ cell tumours (SEMINOMA, TERATOMA) and LYMPHOMAS are particularly sensitive to irradiation which therefore forms a major part of management, particularly for localized disease. Many head and neck tumours, gynaecological cancers, and localized PROSTATE and BLADDER cancers are curable with radiotherapy. Radiotherapy is also valuable in PALLIATION, chiefly the reduction of pain from bone metastases. Side-effects are potentially hazardous and these have to be balanced against the substantial potential benefits. Depending on the type of therapy and doses used, generalized effects include lethargy and loss of appetite, while localized effects – depending on the area treated – include dry, itchy skin; oral infection, e.g. THRUSH; bowel problems and DYSURIA.

RADIUM The radiations of radium consist of: (1) alpha-rays, which are positively charged helium nuclei; (2) beta-rays, negatively charged electrons; (3) gamma-rays, similar to X-rays but of shorter wave-length.

At the present day the use of radium is largely restricted to the treatment of carcinoma of the neck of the womb, the tongue, and the lips.

Neither X-rays nor radium supersede active surgical measures when these are available for the complete removal of a tumour.

RADIUS The outer of the two bones in the forearm. (See BONE.)

RÂLE (see CREPITATIONS).

RANITIDINE An H_2-receptor antagonist drug used in the treatment of DUODENAL ULCER by reducing the hyperacidity of the gastric juice. The drugs blocks the production of histamine produced by mast cells in the stomach lining. Histamine stimulates the acid-secreting cells in the stomach. Ranitidine, like other H_2-blocking drugs, should be used in combination with an antibiotic drug to treat ulcers caused by *HELICOBACTER PYLORI* infection in the stomach. The drug should be given for up to eight weeks with repeat courses if ulcers recur.

RANULA A swelling which occasionally appears beneath the tongue, caused by a collection of saliva in the distended duct of a salivary gland. (See MOUTH, DISEASES OF.)

RAPE A criminal offence in which sexual intercourse takes place with an unwilling partner, female or male, under threat of force or violence. Reported rape cases have increased in number in recent years but it is hard to know whether this is because the incidence of rape has increased or because the victims – women and men– are more willing to report the crime. A more sympathetic and understanding approach by the police, courts and society generally has resulted in the provision of greater support for victims who are usually severely traumatized psychologically as well as physically. It is argued that rape is motivated by a desire to dominate rather than simply an attempt to achieve sexual gratification. The majority of rapes are probably unreported because of the victims' shame, anxiety about publicity and fear that the rapist will take reprisals. There are moves to make court proceedings less traumatic for victims, whose attackers are often known to them.

Anxiety, depression and post-traumatic stress disorder are common after rape. Many victims are now given help by rape crisis counselling. A recent report suggests that at least 50 per cent of reported rapes were what has come to be called 'date rape' because the attacker was or had been a friend of the victim.

RAPHE A ridge or furrow between the halves of an organ.

RAREFACTION Diminution in the density of a bone as a result of withdrawal of calcium salts from it. (See OSTEOPOROSIS.)

RASH (see ERUPTION).

RAT-BITE FEVER An infectious disease following the bite of a rat. There are two causative organisms – *Spirillum minus* and *Actinobacillus muris* – and the incubation period depends upon which is involved. In the case of the former it is 5 to 30 days; in the case of the latter it is 2 to 10 days. The disease is characterized by fever, a characteristic skin rash and often muscular or joint pains. It responds well to penicillin.

RAUWOLFIA A drug that has been used in the treatment of high blood-pressure, and as a tranquillizer. It is a peripheral-acting adrenergic antagonist. It is derived from the root of *Rauwolfia serpentina*, a plant which grows widely in India, Ceylon, Burma, and Malaya. The active medicinal properties, which reside mainly in the root of the plant, have been recognized for centuries in India, where extracts of the root were used for the treatment of fevers, insomnia, and nervousness.

The drug and its alkaloid derivatives have been superseded by more effective antihypertensive agents with fewer side-effects and is no longer included on the *British National Formulary*.

RAYNAUD'S DISEASE So called after Maurice Raynaud (1834–81), the Paris physician who published a thesis on the subject in 1862. This is a condition in which the circulation becomes suddenly obstructed in outlying parts of the body. It is supposed to be due to spasm of the smaller arteries in the affected part, as the result of nervous influences, and its effects are increased both by cold and by various diseases involving the blood-vessels. It is predominantly a disease of women, the majority of cases occurring before the age of 40.

Symptoms The condition is most commonly confined to the occurrence of dead fingers, the fingers or the toes, ears, or nose becoming white, numb, and waxy looking. This condition may last for some minutes, or may not pass off for several hours, or even for a day or two.

Treatment People who are subject to these attacks should be careful in winter to protect the feet and hands from cold, and should always use warm water when washing the hands. In addition, the whole body should be kept warm, as spasm of the arterioles in the feet and hands may be induced by chilling of the body. Sufferers should not smoke. Vasodilator drugs are helpful, especially the CALCIUM ANTAGONISTS. In all patients who do not respond to such medical treatment, surgery should be considered in the form of sympathectomy: i.e. cutting of the sympathetic nerves to the affected part. This results in dilatation of the arterioles and hence an improved blood supply. This operation is more successful in the case of the feet than in the case of the hands.

REACTIVE ARTHRITIS An aseptic arthritis secondary to an episode of infection elsewhere in the body. It often occurs in association with enteritis caused by SALMONELLA and certain SHIGELLA strains and in both YERSINEA and CAMPYLOBACTER enteritis. Non-gonococcal urethritis, usually due to CHLAMYDIA, is another cause of reactive arthritis and Reiter's syndrome is a particularly florid form with mucocutaneous and ocular lesions. The synovitis usually starts acutely and is frequently asymmetrical with the knees and ankles most commonly affected. Often there are inflammatory lesions of tendon sheaths and entheses such as plantar fasciitis. The severity and duration of the acute episode are extremely variable. Individuals with the histocompactibility antigen HLA B27 are particularly prone to severe attacks.

READ CODES These form an agreed UK thesaurus of health-care terminology named after the general practitioner who devised them initially in the 1970s. The coding system provides a basis for computerized clinical records that can be shared across professional and administrative boundaries. Such records have essential safeguards for security and confidentiality. The codes accommodate the different views of specialists but use simple terms without any loss of the fine detail necessary in specialist terminology.

RECEPTOR (1) Organs, which may consist of one cell or a small group of cells, which respond to different forms of external or internal stimuli by conveying impulses down nerves to the central nervous system, alerting it to changes in the internal or external environment.
(2) A small, discrete area on the cell membrane or within the cell with which molecules or molecular complexes (e.g. hormones, drugs, and other chemical messengers) interact. When this interaction takes place it initiates a change in the working of the cell.

RECESSIVE Tending to recede. In genetic terms a recessive gene is one whose expression remains dormant if paired with an unlike allele. The trait will only be manifest in an individual homozygous for the recessive gene. (See GENES.)

RECOMBINANT DNA DNA or deoxy-ribo-nucleic acid containing genes from various sources that have been combined by GENETIC ENGINEERING. (See GENES.)

RECOVERY POSITION If an individual is unconscious – whether as a result of accident or illness or when in the post-operative recovery unit – but is breathing and has a pulse, he or she should be placed in the recovery position. The individual is turned on his or her side to allow the tongue to fall forward and so reduce the likelihood of pharyngeal obstruction. Fluid in the mouth can also drain outwards instead of into the TRACHEA and LUNGS. The person can lie on either side with upper or lower leg flexed. Sometimes the semi-prone position is used which gives better drainage from the mouth and greater stability during transport but makes it more difficult to observe the face, colour or breathing.

RECRUDESCENCE The reappearance of a disease after a period without signs or symptoms of its presence.

RECTUM The last part of the large intestine. It pursues a more or less straight course downwards through the cavity of the pelvis, lying against the sacrum at the back of this cavity. This section of the intestine is about 23 cm (9 inches) long. Its first part is freely movable and corresponds to the upper three pieces of the sacrum, the second part corresponds to the lower two pieces of the sacrum and the coccyx, whilst the third part, known also as the anal canal, is about 25 mm (1 inch) long, runs downwards and backwards, and is kept tightly closed by the internal and external sphincter muscles which surround it. The opening to the exterior is known as the anus. The structure of the rectum is similar to that of the rest of the intestine. (See INTESTINE.)

RECTUM, DISEASES OF STOOLS, HAEMORRHOIDS, FISTULA, DIARRHOEA and CONSTIPATION are described under those headings.

Imperforate anus, or absence of the anus, may occur in newly born children, and the condition is relieved by operation.

Itching at the anal opening, or PRURITUS ANI, is common and can be troublesome. It may be due to slight abrasions, piles, the presence of threadworms, and anal sex. The anal area should be bathed once or twice a day. Clothing should be loose and smooth and local application of soothing preparations containing mild astringents (bismuth subgallate, zinc oxide and hamamelis) and corticosteroids may provide symptomatic relief. Proprietary preparations contain lubricants, vasoconstrictors and mild antiseptics.

Pain on defaecation is commonly caused by a small ulcer of fissure or by an engorged haemorrhoid. Haemorrhoids may also cause an aching pain in the rectum. (See also PROCTALGIA.)

Abscess in the cellular tissue at the side of the rectum, known from its position as an ischiorectal abscess, is fairly common and may produce a fistula. (See FISTULA.)

Prolapse or protrusion of the rectum is sometimes found in children, usually between the ages of 6 months and 2 years. This is generally a temporary disorder. Straining at defaecation by adults can cause the lining of the rectum to protrude outside the anus, resulting in discomfort, discharge and bleeding. Treatment of the underlying constipation is essential as well as local symptomatic measures (see above). Haemorrhoids sometimes prolapse. If a return to normal bowel habits with the production of soft faeces fails to restore the rectum to normal, surgery to remove the haemorrhoids may be necessary. If prolapse of the rectum recurs, despite a return to normal bowel habits, surgery may be required to rectify it.

Tumours of small size situated on the skin near the opening of the bowel, and consisting of nodules, tags of skin, or cauliflower-like excrescences, are common, and may give rise to pain, itching, and watery discharges. These are easily removed if necessary. Polypi occasionally develop within the rectum, and may give rise to no pain, though they may cause frequent discharges of blood. Like polypi elsewhere, they may often be removed by a minor operation. (See POLYPOSIS.)

Cancer of the rectum and colon is the commonest malignancy in the gastrointestinal tract. About 20,000 people a year die from these conditions in the United Kingdom. Rectal cancer is commoner in men than women, colonic cancer is commoner in women. Rectal cancer is a disease of later life, seldom affecting young people, and its appearance is generally insidious. The tumour begins commonly in the mucous membrane, its structure resembling that of the glands with which the membrane is furnished, and it quickly infiltrates the other coats of the intestine and then invades neighbouring organs. Secondary growths in most cases occur soon in the lymphatic glands within the abdomen and in the liver. The symptoms appear gradually and consist of diarrhoea, alternating with attacks of constipation, and, later on, discharges of blood or blood-stained fluid from the bowels, together with weight loss and weakness. A growth can be well advanced before it causes much disturbance. Treatment is surgical and usually this consists of removal of the whole of the rectum and the distal two-thirds of the sigmoid colon, and the establishment of a COLOSTOMY. Depending on the extent of the tumour approximately 50 per cent of the patients who have this operation are alive and well after five years. In some cases in which the growth occurs in the upper part of the rectum it is now possible to remove the growth and preserve the anus so that the patient is saved the discomfort of having a colostomy. RADIOTHERAPY and CHEMOTHERAPY may also be necessary.

RECURRENT LARYNGEAL NERVE A branch of the vagus nerve which leaves the latter low down in its course, and, hooking round the right subclavian artery on the right side and round the arch of the aorta on the left, runs up again into the neck, where it enters the larynx and supplies branches to the muscles which control the vocal cords.

RED BLOOD CELL (see ERYTHROCYTE and BLOOD).

REDUCTION The manipulation of part of the body from an abnormal position to the correct one (e.g. fractures, dislocations or hernias).

REFERRED PAIN Pain felt in one part of the body which is actually arising from a distant site (e.g. pain from the diaphragm is felt at the shoulder tip). This occurs because both sites develop from similar embryological tissue and therefore have common pain pathways in the central nervous system. (See PAIN.)

REFLEX ACTION One of the simplest forms of activity of the nervous system. (For the mechanism upon which it depends, see NERVES.) Reflex acts are divided usually into three classes.

Superficial reflexes comprise the sudden movements which result when the skin is brushed or pricked, such as the movement of the toes that results from stroking the sole of the foot.

Deep reflexes depend upon the state of mild contraction in which muscles are constantly maintained when at rest, and are obtained, as in the case of the knee-jerks, by sharply tapping the tendon of the muscle in question.

Visceral reflexes are those connected with various organs, such as the narrowing of the pupil when a bright light is directed upon the eye, and the contraction of the bladder when distended by urine.
Faults in these reflexes give valuable evidence as to the presence and site of neurological disorders. Thus, absence of the knee-jerk, when the patellar tendon is tapped, means some interference with the sensory nerve, nerve-cells, or motor nerve upon which the act depends, as, for example, in POLIOMYELITIS, or peripheral NEURITIS; whilst an exaggerated jerk implies that the controlling influence exerted by the brain upon this reflex mechanism has been cut off, as, for example, by a tumour high up in the spinal cord, or in the disease known as MULTIPLE SCLEROSIS.

REFLUX Fluid flowing in the opposite direction to normal (e.g. backflow). Often refers to regurgitation of stomach contents into the OESOPHAGUS or of urine from the BLADDER back into the URETERS.

REFRACTION The deviation of rays of light on passing from one transparent medium into another of different density. The refractive surfaces of the eye are the anterior surface of the cornea (which accounts for approximately two-thirds of the focusing or refractive power of the eye) and the lens (one-third of the focusing power of the eye). The refractive power of the lens can change, whereas that of the cornea is fixed.

Errors of refraction (ametropia) will occur when the focusing power of the lens and cornea do not match the length of the eye, so that rays of light parallel to the visual axis are not focused at the fovea centralis (see EYE). There are three types of refractive error:
HYPERMETROPIA or long sightedness: the refractive power of the eye is too weak, or the eye is too short so that rays of light are brought to a focus at a point behind the retina. Long-sighted people can see well in the distance but generally require glasses with convex lenses for reading. Uncorrected long sight can lead to headaches and intermittent blurring of vision following prolonged close work, i.e. eye strain. As a result of ageing the eye becomes gradually long sighted, resulting in many people's needing reading glasses in later life. This normal process is known as presbyopia. A particular form of long sightedness occurs after cataract extraction.
MYOPIA (short sight or near sight): rays of light are brought to a focus in front of the retina because the refractive power of the eye is too great or the eye is too short. Short-sighted people can see close to but need spectacles with concave lenses in order to see in the distance.
ASTIGMATISM The refractive power of the eye is not the same in each meridian. Some rays of light may be focused in front of the retina while others are focused on or behind the retina. Astigmatism can accompany hypermetropia or myopia. It may be corrected by cylindrical lenses (these consist of a slice from the side of a cylinder, i.e. curved in one meridian and flat in the meridian at right angles to it).

REFRACTORY Unresponsive or resistant to treatment.

REGIMEN A course of treatment, possibly combining drugs, exercise, diet, etc., designed to bring about an improvement in health.

REGIONAL ANAESTHESIA (see ANAESTHESIA, Local).

REGIONAL ILEITIS (see under ILEITIS).

REGISTRAR (1) A training grade for NHS doctors. It is divided into registrars, specialist registrars and senior registrars. Some registrars will enter general practice or community medicine, while others will be working towards entry into the specialist registrar grade. Doctors from this latter grade will, if they have appropriate skills and qualifications, become senior registrars who are, in effect, consultants in waiting. In 1996 there were almost 13,000 hospital registrars in the UK, over 1,650 GP trainees and around 300 doctors training to be community physicians. The number of students entering medical schools in the UK is strictly regulated by the government. Registrar numbers are also regulated to achieve a balance between the numbers of doctors in training and the likely number of vacancies for career-grade doctors in the future. (See APPENDIX 8: NATIONAL HEALTH SERVICE.)

(2) A public official responsible for registering births, deaths, and marriages.

REGURGITATION is a term used in various connections in medicine. For instance, in diseases of the heart it is used to indicate a condition in which, as the result of valvular disease, the blood does not entirely pass on from the atria of the heart to the ventricles, or from the ventricles into the arteries. The defective valve is said to be incompetent, and a certain amount of blood leaks past it, or regurgitates back, into the cavity from which it has been driven. (See HEART DISEASES.)

The term is also applied to the return to the mouth of food already swallowed and present in the gullet or stomach.

REHABILITATION The restoration to health and working capacity of a person incapacitated by disease, mental or physical, or by injury. Treatment usually includes occupational therapy, physiotherapy and psychotherapy depending on the type of disease or injury. Rehabilitation is commonly carried out at special centres either on a day or residential bases. This allows different types of specialists to co-operate in the patient's rehabilitation. (See DISABLED PERSONS.)

REITER'S SYNDROME A condition probably caused by an immunological response to a virus in which the patient has URETHRITIS (inflammation of the urethra), ARTHRITIS and conjunctivitis (inflammation of the conjunctiva). The skin may also be affected by horny areas which develop in it. The disorder was first described by a German physician, H. Reiter (1881–1969). The disorder is more common in men than women and is the most common cause of arthritis in young men. It usually develops in people who have a genetic predisposition for it. Around 80 per cent of sufferers have the HLA B27 tissue type. Treatment is symptomatic with analgesics and non-steroidal anti-inflammatory drugs. (See REACTIVE ARTHRITIS.)

REJECTION A term used in TRANSPLANT medicine to describe the body's immunological response to foreign tissue. Various drugs, such as CYCLOSPORIN A, can be used to dampen the host's response to a graft and reduce the risk of rejection.

RELAPSE The return of a disease that a patient has had and apparently recovered from. It may also be a worsening of a disease from which a person is still recovering.

RELAPSING FEVER So-called because of the characteristic temperature chart showing recurring bouts of fever, this is an infectious disease caused by SPIROCHAETES. There are two main forms of the disease.

Louse-borne relapsing fever is an epidemic disease, usually associated with wars and famines, which has occurred in practically every country in the world. For long confused with typhus and typhoid, it was not until the 1870s that the causal organism was described by Obermeier. It is now known as the *Borrelia recurrentis*, a motile spiral organism 10 to 20 micrometres in length. The organism is transmitted from man to man by the louse, Pediculus humanus.
SYMPTOMS The incubation period is up to 12 days, usually 7 days. The onset is sudden, with high temperature, generalized aches and pains, and nose-bleeding. In about half the cases a rash appears at an early stage, beginning in the neck and spreading down over the trunk and arms. JAUNDICE may occur; and both the liver and the SPLEEN are enlarged. The temperature subsides after five or six days, to rise again in about a week. There may be up to four such relapses (see the introductory paragraph above).
TREATMENT Preventive measures are the same as those for typhus. Rest in bed is essential, as are good nursing and a light, nourishing diet. There is usually a quick response to penicillin. The tetracyclines and chloramphenicol are also effective. Following such treatment the incidence of relapse is about 15 per cent. The mortality rate is low, except in a starved population.

Tick-borne relapsing fever is an endemic disease which occurs in most tropical and sub-tropical countries. The causative organism is *Borrelia duttoni*, which is transmitted by a tick, *Ornithodorus moubata*. David Livingstone suggested that it was a tick-borne disease, but it was not until 1905 that Dutton and Todd produced the definite evidence.
SYMPTOMS The main differences from the louse-borne disease are: (*a*) the incubation period is usually shorter, 3 to 6 days, but may be as short as 2 days or as long as 12; (*b*) the febrile period is usually shorter and the afebrile periods are more variable in duration, sometimes only lasting for a day or two; (*c*) relapses are much more numerous.
TREATMENT Preventive measures are more difficult to carry out than in the case of the louse-borne infection. Protective clothing should always be worn in 'tick country'. Old, heavily infected houses should be destroyed. Curative treatment is the same as for the louse-borne infection.

RELATE MARRIAGE GUIDANCE The idea of a marriage guidance council came from a group of doctors, clergy and social workers who were concerned for the welfare of marriage. It is based upon two major concepts: that marriage provides the best possible way for a man and woman to live together and rear their children, and that the counsellors share a basic respect for the unique personality of the individual and his (or her) right to make his (or her) own decisions. The organization consists of between 120 and 130 Marriage Guidance Councils throughout the country,

1 ureter	6 symphysis pubis	11 sacrum
2 Fallopian tube and ovary	7 clitoris	12 rectum
3 peritoneum	8 labia minora	13 coccyx
4 uterus	9 labia majora	14 internal sphincter ani
5 bladder	10 vagina	15 external sphincter ani

Vertical section of female reproductive system viewed from left.

comprising about 1250 counsellors. These Councils are affiliated to Relate National Marriage Guidance, which is responsible for the selection, training and continued supervision of all counsellors. Anyone seeking help can telephone or write for an appointment. No fees are charged, but those receiving help are encouraged to donate what they can. (See APPENDIX 2: ADDRESSES.)

RELAXATION THERAPY This is a treatment in which patients are helped to reduce their levels of anxiety by reducing their muscle tone. It can be used on its own or in conjunction with a broader psychotherapy regime. The technique guides people on how to cope with stressful situations and deal with phobias.

REMITTENT FEVER The term applied to the form of fever in which, during remissions, the temperature falls, but not to normal.

REMISSION A period when a disease has responded to treatment and there are no signs or symptoms present.

REM SLEEP Rapid-eye-movement sleep – a stage during sleep in which the eyes are seen to move rapidly beneath the lids and during which dreaming occurs. It occurs for several minutes at a time approximately every 100 minutes. (See SLEEP.)

RENAL Related to the kidney.

RENAL DISEASES (see KIDNEYS, DISEASES OF).

RENIN An ENZYME produced by the kidney and released into the blood in response to stress. Renin reacts with a compound produced by the liver to produce ANGIOTENSIN. This causes blood vessels to constrict and raises the blood pressure. If too much renin is produced, this results in renal HYPERTENSION.

RENNIN A milk-coagulating enzyme produced by the lining of the stomach. Rennin converts milk protein (caseinogen) into insoluble casein, thus ensuring that milk stays in the stomach for some time, during which it can be digested by various enzymes before passing into the small intestine.

RENOGRAPHY The radiological examination of the kidneys using a gamma camera. This is a device that can follow the course of an injected radioactive (see RADIOACTIVITY) compound which is concentrated and excreted by the kidneys. This provides information on kidney function.

1 ureter	8 efferent ductiles	14 vas (ductus) deferens
2 peritoneum	9 rete testis	15 seminal vesicle
3 bladder	10 convoluted seminiferous	16 ejaculatory duct
4 symphisis pubis	tubule	17 internal sphincter ani
5 prostate utricle	11 canal of the epidydimus	18 external sphincter ani
6 urethra	12 sacrum	19 prostatic follicle
7 penis	13 rectum	20 bulbo-urethral gland

Vertical section of male reproductive system viewed from left.

REPETITIVE STRAIN INJURY (see UPPER LIMB DISORDERS).

REPRESSED MEMORY THERAPY Also called RECOVERED MEMORY THERAPY, this treatment was developed in the wake of the widespread exposure in the 1980s and 90s of the frequency of child sexual abuse. A controversial concept emerged in the USA, picked up later by some experts in the UK, that abused children sometimes suppressed their unpleasant memories and that subsequent psychotherapy could help some victims to recover these memories which might aid their rehabilitation. This recall of 'repressed' memories, however, was believed by some psychiatrists to be, in effect, a false memory implanted into the victim's subconscious by the psychotherapy itself – or perhaps invented by the individual for personal motives. In 1997 the Royal College of Psychiatrists in the UK produced a comprehensive report which was sceptical about the notion that the awareness of recurrent severe sexual abuse in children could be pushed entirely out of consciousness. The authors did not believe that events could remain inaccessible to conscious memory for decades, allegedly provoking vague non-specific symptoms to be recovered during psychotherapy with resolu-

tion of the symptoms. Supporting evidence pointed to the lack of any empirical proof that unconscious dissociation of unpleasant memories from conscious awareness occurred to protect the individual. Furthermore experimental and natural events had shown that false memories, created through suggestion or influence, could be implanted. Many individuals who had claimed to have recovered memories of abuse subsequently withdrew and, often, non-specific symptoms allegedly linked to suppression worsened rather than improved as therapy to unlock memories proceeded. The conclusion is that recovered memory therapy should be viewed with great caution.

REPRODUCTIVE SYSTEM A collective term for all the organs involved in sexual reproduction. In the female these are the OVARIES, FALLOPIAN TUBES, UTERUS, VAGINA and VULVA. In the male these are the TESTES, VASA DEFERENTIA, PROSTATE, SEMINAL VESICLES, URETHRA and PENIS. (See diagrams.)

RESECTION The name of an operation in which a part of some organ is removed, as, for example, the resection of a fragment of dead bone.

RESERPINE   An alkaloid obtained from the root of RAUWOLFIA that has been and is used as an anti-hypertensive and a tranquillizing agent.

RESERVE VOLUME   The additional amount of air that a person could breathe in or out if he or she were not using the full capacity of their lungs.

RESIDUAL VOLUME   The amount of air left in the lungs after an individual has breathed out as much as possible. It is a measure of lung function: for example, in a person with emphysema the residual volume is increased. (See RESPIRATION.)

RESISTANCE   In a medical context resistance has several meanings. The walls of blood vessels exert resistance to the flow of blood and this rises as the diameters of the vessels diminish. This leads to a rise in blood pressure: the phenomenon may be PHYSIOLOGICAL or PATHOLOGICAL.

Resistance may also mean the extent of the body's immunity, an indication of its ability to withstand disease.

Another meaning relates to the development of resistance in a BACTERIUM to the effects on it of ANTIBIOTICS.

In psychoanalysis resistance refers to the blocking off from a person's consciousness of repressed emotions and memories. A psychoanalyst helps the patient to break this resistance and bring the repressed material out into the open.

RESOLUTION   A term applied to infective processes, to indicate a natural subsidence of the inflammation without the formation of pus. Thus a pneumonic lung is said to resolve when the material exuded into it is absorbed into the blood and lymph, so that recovery takes place naturally; an inflamed area is said to resolve when the inflammation diminishes and no abscess forms; a glandular enlargement is said to resolve when it decreases in size without suppuration. Resolution is also used to describe the extent to which individual details – for example, cell structures – can be identified by the eye when using a light microscope.

RESONANCE   The lengthening and intensification of sound produced by striking the body over an air-containing structure. Decrease of resonance is called dullness and increase of resonance is called hyper-resonance. The process of striking the chest or other part of the body to discover its degree of resonance is called percussion, and according to the note obtained, an opinion can be formed as to the state of consolidation of air-containing organs, the presence of abnormal cavities, and the dimensions and relations of solid and air-containing organs lying together. (See also AUSCULTATION.)

RESORCINOL   A white, crystalline, antiseptic substance soluble in water, alcohol, and oils. It can be used in combination with sulphur to treat ACNE.

RESPIRATION   The process in which air passes into and out of the lungs so that the blood can absorb oxygen and give off carbon dioxide and water. This occurs 18 times a minute in a healthy adult at rest and is called the respiratory rate. An individual breathes more than 25,000 times a day and during this time inhales around 16 kg of air.

Mechanism of respiration   For the structure of the respiratory apparatus see AIR PASSAGES; CHEST; LUNGS. The air passes rhythmically into and out of the air passages, and mixes with the air already in the lungs, these two movements being known as inspiration and expiration.

INSPIRATION is due to a muscular effort which enlarges the chest in all three dimensions, so that the lungs have to expand in order to fill up the vacuum that would otherwise be left, the air entering these organs by the air passages. The increase of the chest in size from above downwards is mainly due to the diaphragm, the muscular fibres of which contract and reduce its domed shape and cause it to descend, pushing down the abdominal organs beneath it.

The muscles that produce normal inspiration are the diaphragm, intercostal muscles, and levators of the ribs. Forced inspiration, when a specially deep breath is taken, involves other muscles including the trapezius and pectoral muscles (see MUSCLES).

EXPIRATION is an elastic recoil, the diaphragm rising and the ribs sinking into the position that they naturally occupy, when muscular contraction is finished. Expiration occupies a slightly longer period than inspiration. Occasionally, forced expiration may occur, involving powerful muscles of the abdomen and thorax; this is typically seen in forcible coughing.

Nervous control   Respiration is usually either an automatic or a reflex act, each expiration sending up afferent, sensory impulses to the central nervous system, from which efferent impulses are sent down various other nerves to the muscles that produce inspiration. Several centres govern the rate and force of the breathing, although all are presided over by a chief respiratory centre in the medulla oblongata. This in turn is controlled by the higher centres in the cerebral hemispheres, so that breathing can be voluntarily stopped or quickened.

Quantity of air   The lungs do not completely empty themselves at each expiration and refill at each inspiration. An amount equivalent, in normal respiration, to less than one-tenth of the total air in the lungs passes out and is replaced by the same quantity of fresh air, which mixes with the stale air in the lungs. This renewal, which in quiet breathing amounts to about 500 millilitres, is known as the tidal air. By a special inspiratory effort, an individual can draw in about 3000 millilitres, this amount being known as complemental air. By a special expiratory effort, too, after an ordinary breath one can expel much more than the tidal air from the lungs, this extra amount being known as the supplemental or reserve air, and amounting to about 1300 millilitres. If an individual takes as deep an inspiration as possible and then makes a forced expiration, the amount expired is known as the vital capacity, and amounts to about 4000 millilitres in a healthy adult male of average size. Figures for women are about 25 per cent lower. The vital capacity varies with size, sex, age and ethnic origin.

Over and above the vital capacity, the lungs contain air which cannot be expelled and this is known as residual air, and amounts to another 1500 millilitres.

Tests of respiratory efficiency are used to assess lung function in health and disease. Pulmonary-function tests, as they are known, include SPIROMETRY, peak-flow meter (which measures the rate at which a person can expel air from the lungs, thus testing vital capacity and the extent of bronchospasm) and measurements of the concentration of oxygen and carbon dioxide in the blood.

Abnormal forms of respiration Apart from mere changes in rate and force, respiration is modified in several ways, either involuntarily or voluntarily. SNORING, or stertorous breathing, is due to a flaccid state of the soft palate causing it to vibrate as the air passes into the throat, or simply to sleeping with the mouth open, which has a similar effect. COUGHING is a series of violent expirations, at each of which the larynx is suddenly opened after the pressure of air in the lungs has risen considerably; its object is to expel some irritating substance from the air passages. SNEEZING is a single sudden expiration, which differs from coughing in that the sudden rush of air is directed by the soft palate up into the nose in order to expel some source of irritation from this narrow passage. CHEYNE-STOKES BREATHING is a type of breathing found in persons suffering from stroke, heart disease, and some other conditions, in which death is impending; it consists in an alternate dying away and gradual strengthening of the inspirations. Other disorders of breathing are found in CROUP and in ASTHMA.

RESPIRATORY ARREST Sudden stopage of breathing which results from any process that strongly suppresses the function of the brain's respiratory centre. It leads to lack of oxygen in the tissues and, if not remedied, to CARDIAC ARREST, brain damage, COMA and death. Treatment is artificial respiration (see APPENDIX 1: BASIC FIRST AID) and, if necessary, artificial ventilation. Causes of respiratory arrest include cardiac arrest, electrical injury, overdose of narcotic drugs, prolonged seizures (EPILEPSY), serious head injury, STROKE or inhalation of noxious material that causes respiratory failure.

RESPIRATORY DISTRESS SYNDROME may occur in adults as adult respiratory distress syndrome or in new-born children, when it is also known as HYALINE MEMBRANE DISEASE. The adult syndrome consists of pulmonary oedema of non-cardiac origin. It is a complication of shock, systemic sepsis and viral respiratory infections. It was first described in 1967 and despite advances with assisted ventilation it remains a serious disease with a mortality of more than 50 per cent. The maintenance of adequate circulating blood volume, peripheral perfusion, acid base balance and arterial oxygenation is important and assisted ventilation should be instituted early. The aetiology is not understood though the process begins when tissue damage stimulates the autonomic nervous system, releases vaso-active substances, precipitates complement activation and produces abnormalities of the clotting cascade – the serial process that leads to clotting of the blood. The activation of complement causes white cells to lodge in the pulmonary capillaries where they release substances which damage the pulmonary endothelium.

RESPIRATORY SYNCYTIAL VIRUS Usually known as RS VIRUS, this is one of the MYXOVIRUSES. It is the major cause of bronchiolitis and pneumonia in infants under the age of 6 months and its incidence has been increasing, possibly due to atmospheric pollution.

RESTLESS LEGS SYNDROME: A condition in which the patient experiences unpleasant sensations, and occasionally involuntary movements, in the legs when at rest, especially at night. No pathological changes have been identified. It is sometimes indicative of iron-deficiency anaemia, but in many cases the cause remains a mystery and the variety of cures offered are a testimony to this. Some anti-epileptic drugs are said to help.

RESTRICTION ENZYME An endocuclease ENZYME, extracted from bacteria, that is used to cut DNA into short segments, a process essential in GENETIC ENGINEERING.

RESUSCITATION (see APPENDIX 2: BASIC FIRST AID).

RETARDATION Slowing down; developmental delay. Psychomotor retardation is a significant slowing down of speech and activity which eventually leads to a person's being unable to cope with daily activities or to maintain personal hygiene. It is a symptom of severe DEPRESSION.

RETCHING is an ineffectual form of vomiting. (See VOMITING.)

RETENTION OF URINE (see URINE RETENTION).

RETICULOCYTES These are newly formed red blood corpuscles, in which a fine network can be demonstrated by special staining methods.

RETICULO-ENDOTHELIAL SYSTEM This consists of highly specialized cells scattered throughout the body, but found mainly in the spleen, bone marrow, liver, and lymph glands. Their main function is the ingestion of red blood cells and the conversion of HAEMOGLOBIN to BILIRUBIN. They are also able to ingest bacteria and foreign colloidal particles.

RETINA (see EYE).

RETINA, DISORDERS OF The retina can be damaged by disease that affects the retina alone, or by diseases affecting the whole body.

Retinopathy is a term used to denote an abnormality of the retina without specifying a cause. Some retinal disorders are discussed below.

Diabetic retinopathy Retinal disease occurring in patients with DIABETES MELLITUS. It is the commonest cause of blind registration in Great Britain of people between 20 and 65 years of age. Diabetic retinopathy can be divided into several types. The two main causes of blindness are those that follow, first, development of new blood vessels from the retina, with resultant complications and, second, those following 'water logging' (oedema) of the macula. Treatment is by maintaining rigid control of blood-sugar levels combined with laser treatment for certain forms of the disease – in particular to get rid of new blood vessels.

Hypertensive retinopathy Retinal disease secondary to the development of high blood pressure. Treatment involves control of the blood pressure.

Sickle cell retinopathy People with sickle cell disease can develop a number of retinal problems including new blood vessels from the retina.

Retrolental fibroplasia A disorder affecting low-birth-weight premature babies exposed to high oxygen pressures. Essentially new blood vessels develop which cause extensive traction on the retina with resultant retinal detachment and poor vision.

Retinal artery occlusion, retinal vein occlusion These result in damage to those areas of retina supplied by the affected blood vessel. The blood vessels become blocked. If the peripheral retina is damaged the patient may be completely symptom free, although areas of blindness may be detected on examination of field of vision. If the macula is involved, visual loss may be sudden, profound and permanent. There is no effective treatment once visual loss has occurred.

Senile macular degeneration ('senile' indicates age of onset and has no bearing on mental state)

is the leading cause of blindness in the elderly in the western world. The average age of onset is 65 years. Patients initially notice a disturbance of their vision which gradually progresses over months or years. They lose the ability to recognize fine detail, e.g. they cannot read fine print, cannot sew or recognize people's faces. They always retain the ability to recognize large objects such as doors and chairs. They are therefore able to get around and about reasonably well. There is no effective treatment in the majority of cases.

Retinitis pigmentosa A group of rare, inherited diseases characterized by the development of night blindness and tunnel vision. Symptoms start in childhood and are progressive. Many patients retain good visual acuity, although their peripheral vision is limited. One of the characteristic findings on examination is collections of pigment in the retina which have a characteristic shape and are therefore known as 'bone spicules'. There is no effective treatment.

Retinal detachment usually occurs because of development of a hole in the retina. Holes can occur because of degeneration of the retina, because of traction on the retina by the vitreous, or due to injury. Fluid from the vitreous passes through the hole causing a split within the retina. The inner part of the retina becomes detached from the outer part, the latter remains in contact with the choroid. Detached retina loses its ability to detect light with consequent impairment of vision. Retinal detachments are more common in the short sighted, in the elderly or following cataract extraction. Symptoms include spots before the eyes (floaters), flashing lights and a shadow over the eye with progressive loss of vision. Treatment by laser is very effective if caught early, at the stage when a hole has developed in the retina but the retina has not become detached. The edges of the hole can be 'spot welded' to the underlying choroid. Once a detachment has occurred, laser therapy cannot be used, the retina has to be repositioned. This is usually done by indenting the wall of the eye from the outside to meet the retina, then making the retina stick to the wall of the eye by inducing inflammation in the wall. This is done by freezing the wall. The outcome of surgery depends largely on the extent of the detachment and its duration. Complicated forms of detachment can occur due to diabetic eye disease, injury or tumour. Each requires a specialized form of treatment. (See EYE DISEASES.)

RETINOBLASTOMA A rare malignant growth of the retina which occurs in infants.

RETINOIC ACID is a synthetic vitamin A derivative. (See APPENDIX 5: VITAMINS.)

RETINOID Any one of a collection of drugs that are derived from VITAMIN A. They can be taken orally or applied topically and affect the skin by causing drying and peeling, with a reduction in the production of SEBUM. These properties are useful in the treatment of ACNE, ICTHYOSIS and PSORIASIS.

RETINOL is the official chemical name of vitamin A. (See APPPENDIX 5: VITAMINS.)

RETINOPATHY (see RETINA, DISEASES OF).

RETRACTOR An instrument for pulling apart the edges of an incision to allow better surgical access to the organs and tissues being operated on.

RETRO- A prefix signifying behind or turned backward.

RETROBULBAR NEURITIS Inflammation of the optic nerve behind (rather than within) the eye. It usually occurs in young adults and presents with a rapid deterioration in vision over a few hours. Colour vision is also impaired. Usually vision recovers over a few weeks, but colour vision may be permanently lost. It can be associated with certain viral illnesses and with MULTIPLE SCLEROSIS. (See EYE, DISEASES OF.)

RETROGRADE Movement in a contrary or backward direction from normal (e.g. a retrograde pyelogram introduces dye into the pelvis of the kidney by passing it up the ureters).

RETROPHARYNGEAL ABSCESS An abscess occurring in the cellular tissue behind the throat. It is the result in general of disease in the upper part of the spinal column.

RETROSPECTIVE STUDY A historical review of the characteristics of a collection of people to assess morbidity. The procedure is commonly used in studying the EPIDEMIOLOGY of disease.

RETROVERSION An abnormal position of the UTERUS, occurring in about 20 per cent of women, in which its long axis is pivoted backwards in relation to the CERVIX and VAGINA instead of forwards.

RETROVIRUS A virus containing RIBONU-CLEIC ACID (RNA) which is able to change its genetic material into DEOXYRIBONUCLEIC ACID (DNA) using an ENZYME called reverse transcriptase. This conversion enables the retrovirus to become integrated into the host cell's DNA. Retroviruses are believed to be involved in the development of some cancers and they are also associated with disorders linked with an impaired immune system. HIV is a retrovirus.

Retroviruses are also used in the development of gene therapy (see GENETIC ENGINEER-ING).

REYE'S SYNDROME A condition which occurs predominantly in young children following a virus infection of the upper respiratory tract or a viral infection such as chickenpox or influenza. The cause is not known, but there is some evidence that aspirin may play a part in its causation. Doctors recommend that children should be given PARACETAMOL in place of aspirin. The condition is of worldwide distribution, but relatively rare in Western Europe. The initial feature is severe, persistent vomiting and fever. This is followed by outbursts of wild behaviour, delirium and convulsions terminating in coma and death. The mortality rate is around 23 per cent, and 50 per cent of the survivors may have persistent mental or neurological disturbances. The younger the patient the higher the death rate and the more common the permanent residual effects.

RHABDOVIRUSES A group of viruses which includes the rabies virus.

RHESUS FACTOR (see BLOOD GROUPS).

RHEUMATIC FEVER An acute febrile illness, usually seen in children which may include ARTHRALGIA, ARTHRITIS, CHOREA, carditis and rash. The illness has been shown to follow a STREPTOCOCCAL infection and a streptococcal cause is now implicit in the term.

Rheumatic fever is now extremely uncommon in developed countries, but remains common in developing areas. It is rare before the age of 3, occurring most commonly in mid-childhood and adolescence. If chorea is excluded (commoner in girls), the disease is equally common in the two sexes. Recurrences of the acute illness may occur over a period of years. Long-term consequences include damage to heart valves and less commonly a non-erosive deforming arthritis or persistent neurological problems.

The streptococci responsible are the beta haemolytic type. Their presence may be confirmed by a positive throat swab or a rising anti-streptolysin antibody titre in serum.

Clinical features Fever is marked with attacks of shivering or rigor. Joint pain and swelling affect the knee, ankle, wrist or shoulder and may migrate from one joint to another. Tachycardia may be out of proportion to other constitutional features and indicate cardiac involvement. Subcutaneous nodules may occur, particularly over the back of the wrist or over the elbow or knee. Erythema marginatum is a red rash characteristic of the condition.

Cardiac involvement includes PERICARDITIS, ENDOCARDITIS, and MYOCARDITIS. The main long-term complication is damage to the MITRAL and AORTIC VALVES.

The chief neurological problem is chorea (St Vitus's dance) which may develop after the acute symptoms have subsided.

Treatment Eradication of streptococcal infection is essential. Other features are treated symptomatically. Paracetamol may be preferred to aspirin as an antipyretic in young children. A NON-STEROIDAL ANTI-INFLAMMATORY DRUG may benefit the joint symptoms. CORTICOSTEROIDS may be indicated for more serious complications.

Patients who have developed cardiac valve abnormalities require antibiotic prophylaxis during dental treatment and other procedures where bacteria may enter the bloodstream. Secondary cardiac problems may occur several decades later and require replacement of affected heart valves.

RHEUMATISM An obsolete medical term which no longer has a defined meaning. It remains a lay term covering any painful condition of the muscles and/or joints of the arms, legs or spine.

RHEUMATOID ARTHRITIS A chronic inflammation of the synovial lining of several joints, tendon sheaths or bursae which is not due to sepsis or a reaction to crystals. Most patients show a typical symmetrical pattern, suggesting a single aetiology. However, several atypical patterns occur. It is likely that the problem is of multifactorial origin, and that there is some variation in the genetic and environmental factors involved in individual cases. Rheumatoid arthritis is distinguished from other patterns of inflammatory arthritis by the symmetrical involvement of a large number of peripheral joints, by the common association with serum rheumatoid factor antibody, by the presence of bony erosions around joints and, in a minority, the presence of subcutaneous nodules with necrobiotic (decaying) centres.

Causes There is a major immunogenetic predisposition to rheumatoid arthritis in people carrying the HLA-DR4 antigen. Other minor immunogenetic factors have also been implicated. In addition, there is a degree of familial clustering which suggests other unidentified genetic factors. Genetic factors cannot alone explain aetiology, and environmental and chance factors must be important, but these have yet to be identified. Rheumatoid arthritis appears to be more common in developed countries and in rural populations that have moved to an urban lifestyle. No convincing effect of diet has been demonstrated.

Epidemiology Rheumatoid arthritis most commonly occurs in women from the age of 30 onwards, the sex ratio being approximately 4 to 1. Typical rheumatoid arthritis may occur in adolescence, but in childhood chronic SYNOVITIS usually take one of a number of different patterns, classified under juvenile chronic arthritis.

Pathology The primary lesion is an inflammation of the synovial lining, with an accumulation of macrophages on the lining surface and an infiltration of the deeper tissue with LYMPHOCYTES, plasma cells, MACROPHAGES, and small numbers of NEUTROPHIL polymorphs. The synovial fluid becomes diluted with inflammatory exudate, containing a mixture of leukocytes. If inflammation persists for several months, there is often progressive destruction of articular cartilage and bone. CARTILAGE is replaced by inflammatory tissue known as pannus. A similar tissue invades bone to form erosions. Synovitis also affects tendon sheaths, and may lead to adhesion fibrosis or attrition and rupture of tendons. Subcutaneous and other bursae may be involved. Necrobiotic nodules also occur at sites outside synovium, including the subcutaneous tissues, the lungs, the pericardium and the pleura.

Clinical features Rheumatoid arthritis varies from the very mild to the severely disabling. Many mild cases probably go undiagnosed. At least 50 per cent of known cases continue to lead a reasonably normal life, about 25 per cent are significantly disabled in terms of work and leisure activities and a minority become markedly disabled and are limited in their independence. There is often an early acute phase, followed by substantial remission, but in other patients gradual stepwise deterioration may occur, with progressive involvement of an increasing number of joints.

The diagnosis of rheumatoid arthritis is largely based on clinical symptoms and signs. Approximately 70 per cent of patients have rheumatoid factor antibodies in the serum but, because of the large number of false positives and false negatives, this test cannot be considered diagnostic and has very little value in clinical practice. It may be a useful pointer to a worse prognosis in early cases if the titre is high. The erythrocyte sedimentation rate (see ESR) and plasma viscosity (stickiness) are usually raised during periods when the patient has clinical symptoms. They may remain abnormal during periods of clinical remission. Their value in long-term management is arguable. Joint radiographs will show progressive loss of the cartilage joint space and the development of body erosions in many cases. Radiographs may assist in diagnosis in early cases and are particularly helpful when considering surgery or possible complications such as pathological fracture. Patients commonly develop anaemia, which may be partly due to gastrointestinal blood loss from anti-inflammatory drug treatment.

Treatment involves physical, pharmacological, and surgical measures, together with psychological and social support tailored to the individual patient's needs. Regular activity should be maintained. Resting of certain joints such as the wrist with splints may be helpful at night or to assist prolonged manual activities. Sound footwear is important. Early use of anti-rheumatic drugs reduces long-term disability. Drug treatment includes simple analgesics, NON-STEROIDAL ANTI-INFLAMMATORY AGENTS (NSAIDS) and slow-acting drugs including gold, penicillamine, sulphasalazine and aza-thioprine. The non-steroidal agents are largely effective in reducing pain, and early morning stiffness, and have no effect on the chronic inflammatory process. It is important, especially in the elderly, to explain to patients the adverse effects of NSAIDS. Dosage of NSAIDS can be cut by prescribing paracetamol at the same time. Combinations of antirheumatic drugs seem better than single agents. The slow-acting drugs take approximately three months to act but have a more global effect on chronic inflammation with a greater reduction in swelling and an associated fall in erythrocyte sedimentation rate and rise in the level of haemoglobin. Local corticosteroids are useful, given into individual joints. Systemic corticosteroids carry serious problems if continued long term, but may be useful under special circumstances.

RHEUMATOLOGY The medical speciality concerned with the study and management of diseases of the joints and connective tissues.

RH FACTOR (see BLOOD GROUPS).

RHINITIS Inflammation of the mucous membrane of the nose. (See NOSE, DISEASES OF.)

RHINOPHYMA The condition characterized by swelling of the nose due to enormous enlargement of the sebaceous glands which may develop in the later stages of ROSACEA.

RHINOPLASTY Repair of the nose or modification of its shape by operation. This operation is performed by reconstructive and ENT surgeons alike. It may involve alteration of the bony skeleton of the nose and/or alteration of the septum (septorhinoplasty). It is mostly performed for cosmetic reasons. However, any disease process or injury which has caused defect in the nose may be repaired as well. The latter problem would usually involve the utilization of some form of skin flap, whereas this would not be required for cosmetic surgical purposes.

RHINOVIRUSES A large group of viruses; to date around 80 distinct rhinoviruses have been identified. Their practical importance is that some of them are responsible for around one- quarter of the cases of the common cold.

RHIZOTOMY The surgical operation of cutting a nerve root, as, for example, to relieve the pain of trigeminal neuralgia.

RHONCHI A description of the harsh cooing, hissing, or whistling sounds (wheezing) heard by auscultation over the bronchial tubes when they are the seat of infection. (See BRONCHITIS.)

RHYTHM METHOD A method of contraception which attempts to prevent conception by avoiding intercourse during the fertile part of the menstrual cycle. (See CONTRACEPTION; SAFE PERIOD.)

RIBOFLAVINE The *British Pharmacopoeia* name for what used to be known as vitamin B_2. Riboflavine belongs to a group of animal and plant pigments which give a greenish fluorescence on exposure to ultra-violet rays. It is present especially in milk, and is not destroyed during pasteurization. Other rich sources are eggs, liver, yeast and the green leaves of broccoli and spinach. It is also present in beer. Deficiency of riboflavine in the diet is thought to cause inflammation of the substance of the cornea, sores on the lips, especially at the angles of the mouth (CHEILOSIS), and dermatitis.

The minimal daily requirement for an adult is 1·5 to 3 mg, but is greater during pregnancy and lactation. (See APPENDIX 5: VITAMINS.)

RIBONUCLEIC ACID (see RNA).

RIBOSOME Granules either found free within the CELL or attached to a reticular network within the cell's endoplasm (the inner part of a cell's cytoplasm (see CELLS)). Consisting of approximately 65 per cent RNA and 35 per cent protein, they are the sites where protein is made.

RIBOZYME Sections of deoxyribonucleic acid (DNA) – the principal molecule in a cell carrying genetic information – that act as ENZYMES. The function of a ribozyme is to transform the messages encoded in DNA into proteins, using its property of catalysing chemical reactions in a cell. Most ribozymes act only on other pieces of ribonucleic acid (RNA), editing the messenger type that carries instructions to the parts of the cell that makes proteins. This editing ability is being used by scientists researching ways of correcting faulty genes which can cause inherited disorders. The aim is to persuade the ribozyme to inhibit the messenger RNA to prevent production of the faulty gene. Ribozymes might also be used to disrupt infectious agents, such as viruses, which rely on RNA to invade body cells.

RIBS The bones, twelve on each side, which enclose the cavity of the chest. The upper seven are joined to the breast-bone by their costal cartilages and are therefore known as true ribs. The lower five do not reach the breast-bone, and are therefore known as false ribs. Of the latter, the 8th, 9th and 10th are joined by their costal cartilages, each one to the rib immediately above it, while the 11th and 12th are free from any such connection, and are therefore known as floating ribs. Each rib has a head, by which it is joined to the upper part of the body of the vertebra with which it corresponds, as well as to the vertebra immediately above. The greater part of the bone is made up of the shaft, which runs at first outwards and at the angle turns sharply forwards. On the lower margin of the shaft is a groove, which lodges the corresponding intercostal artery and nerve.

RICE-WATER A useful diluent drink for invalids, similar to barley-water.

RICKETS A disease of childhood characterized chiefly by a softened condition of the bones, and by other evidence of perverted nutrition.

Causes This disease is the result of deficiency of vitamin D in the diet. Healthy bones cannot be built up without calcium (or lime) salts, and the body cannot utilize these salts in the absence of vitamin D. Want of sunlight and fresh air in the dwellings where the children are reared is also of importance. Once a common condition in industrial areas, it had almost disappeared in Great Britain, but there has been some recurrence of it in recent years.

The changes that take place in the bones are due to an irregular process of bone formation. The periosteum, the membrane enveloping the bones, becomes inflamed, and in consequence the bone formed beneath it is defective in lime salts and very soft. Changes also occur at the growing part of the bone, the epiphyseal plate. The disease is most common between 1 and 2 years of age and is increasingly rare after the age of 3.

Symptoms The symptoms of rickets most usually appear towards the end of the first year, and rarely after the age of 5. Early symptoms may include disorders of the digestive and alimentary functions.

Gradually changes in the shape of the bones becomes visible, first chiefly noticed at the ends of the long bones. The softened bones also tend to become distorted, the legs bending outwards and forwards so the child becomes bow-legged or knock-kneed. Changes occur in the chest and cranial bones, while teeth appear late and decay or fall out.

The disease usually ends in recovery with more or less of deformity and dwarfing, the bones, although altered in shape, becoming ultimately ossified.

Treatment The treatment of rickets is more hygienic and dietetic than medicinal. The specific remedy is vitamin D, given as a rule in the form of calciferol (vitamin D_2). A full diet is of course essential, with emphasis upon a sufficient supply of milk. Rickets practically does not occur in breast-fed children but it is a wise precaution to give breast-fed babies supplementary vitamin D. After the child is weaned, the provision of suitable food is vital, supplemented by the administration of some source of vitamin D.

Deficiency of vitamin D in adults results in OSTEOMALACIA.

RICKETTSIA The general term given to a group of micro-organisms, which are intermediate between BACTERIA and VIRUSES. They are the causal agents of TYPHUS and a number of typhus-like diseases, such as ROCKY MOUNTAIN SPOTTED FEVER, Japanese River fever, and scrub typhus. These micro-organisms are usually conveyed to man by lice, fleas, ticks, and mites.

Visceral rickettsia is a disease transmitted by mites from an infected house mouse, which occurs in the USA, South Africa, Korea and USSR. The causal organism is *Rickettsia akari*. The incubation period is 7 to 14 days. The characteristic features are fever, headache, and a non-irritating rash on the face, trunk and extremities. The disease is non-fatal and responds rapidly to tetracyclines.

RIFAMPICIN An antibiotic derived from *Streptomyces mediterranei*, it is a key component of any antituberculous regimen. Like ISONIAZID rifampicin should always be included unless there is a specific contraindication. It is also valuable in the treatment of BRUCELLOSIS, LEGIONNAIRE'S DISEASE, serious STAPHYLOCOCCAL infections and LEPROSY.

It is given by mouth; during the first two months it often causes transient disturbance of liver function, with raised concentrations of serum transaminases, but usually treatment need not be interrupted. In patients with pre-existing liver disease more severe toxicity may occur, and liver function should be carefully monitored both before starting and during rifampicin treatment. It induces hepatic enzymes which accelerate the metabolism of various drugs including ANTICOAGULANTS, SULPHONYLUREAS, PHENYTOIN, CORTICOSTEROIDS and OESTROGENS. The effectiveness of oral contraceptives is reduced and alternative family-planning advice should be offered.

Rifampicin should be avoided during pregnancy and breast feeding and extra caution should be applied if there is renal impairment, JAUNDICE or PORPHYRIA. Adverse effects include gastrointestinal symptoms, influenza-like symptoms, collapse and shock, haemolytic anaemia, acute flushing and urticaria; body secretions may be coloured red.

RIFT VALLEY FEVER A virus disease, caused by a phlebovirus and transmitted by mosquitoes, at one time confined to Sub-Saharan Africa and predominantly found in domestic animals, such as cattle, sheep and goats. The only human beings affected were veterinary surgeons, butchers and others exposed to heavy infection by direct contact with infected animals. These usually recovered. In the 1970s it flared up in Egypt, probably owing to a more virulent virus. The illness in man is characterized by fever, haemorrhages, ENCEPHALITIS and involvement of the eye. An effective vaccine protects both animals and human beings against the disease.

RIGIDITY Stiffness, resistance to movement. The term is often used in neurology, e.g. limb rigidity is a sign of PARKINSON'S DISEASE. Smooth rigidity is described as being 'plastic' and jerky rigidity as 'cogwheel'.

RIGOR Shivering; if prolonged, it is generally accompanied by fever, and may be a sign of the onset of some acute disease, such as influenza, pneumonia, or some internal inflammation. Rigor mortis is the name given to the stiffness that ensues soon after death. (See DEATH, SIGNS OF; MUSCLE.)

RING BLOCK Local ANAESTHETIC agent injected into the circumference of the base of a digit numbs the nerves of the finger or toe and so permits minor surgery to be performed. Care must be taken to avoid damage to local blood vessels which can lead to GANGRENE.

RINGWORM (TINEA) The name given to inflammatory rashes caused by DERMATOPHYTE fungi of the genera microsporum, EPIDERMOPHYTON and TRICHOPHYTON. These fungi can infect skin, hair and nails. The important clinical patterns are:

Tinea capitis Usually seen in children in Britain and caused by microsporum species of human or animal (frequently a kitten) origin. Typically, patches of ALOPECIA are seen with broken-off hair stumps which fluoresce bright green under an ultraviolet (Wood's) lamp. In Asia a chronic, scarring alopecia may be caused by a specific trichophyton (favus).

Tinea corporis is usually due to trichophyton species and forms ringed (hence 'ringworm') patches of redness and scaling on the trunk or limbs.

Tinea pedis (athlete's foot) is caused by epidermophyton or trichophyton species. Its minor form manifests as itching, scaling or blistering in the lateral toe clefts. More severe forms can be extensive on the sole. *Trichophyton rubrum* can cause a chronic, dry, scaling inflammation of the foot, eventually extending into the nails and on to the soles and top of the foot which may persist for years if untreated.

Tinea cruris, typically causing a 'butterfly' rash on the upper inner thighs in young adult males, is usually caused by spread from the feet.

Tinea unguium (onychomycosis) Affecting the nails, especially of the toes, *T. rubrum* is the usual cause and may persist for decades.

Tinea barbae This rash of the face and beard is rare. It may be very inflammatory and is usually contracted from cattle by farm workers.

Treatment Tinea of the toe clefts and groin will usually respond to an anti-fungal cream containing terbinafine (a recently introduced allylamine antifungal agent taken orally) or an azole. Tinea capitis, barbae, extensive tinea corporis and all nail infections require oral treatment with terbinafine or itraconazole (a triazole antifungal agent taken orally and used for candidiasis of the mouth, throat and vulgovaginal area as well as for ringworm) which have largely superseded the earlier treatment with the antiobiotic griseofulvin. (See FUNGAL INFECTIONS.)

RINNES TEST A hearing test in which a vibrating tuning fork is placed on the mastoid process (see EAR). When the subject can no longer hear the ringing, it is placed beside the ear. Normal subjects can then hear the noise once more, but in people with conductive deafness air conduction does not persist after bone conduction has ceased. It can help to distinguish between nerve (sensorineural) and conduction deafness.

RIPPLE BEDS A development of the conventional AIR-BED. Their essential feature is a mattress which is alternately pressurized by a compressor to create a gentle rippling effect along the entire length of the mattress. This provides a continuous massaging motion which stimulates the circulation and helps to maintain the nutrition of the skin, thereby reducing the risk of bed sores (DECUBITAL ULCERS).

RISK FACTOR An environmental or genetic factor which makes the occurrence of a disease in an individual more likely.

RISK MANAGEMENT A predictive technique for identifying potential untoward occurrences. It has been in use in certain high-risk industries (such as nuclear power generation) for many years and was introduced to the NHS in 1991 when self-governing trusts were first set up. The reasons were, firstly, that Crown immunity had been removed from the health service in 1988 so it ceased to be immune from prosecution for non-compliance with health and safety legislation; secondly, because trusts were responsible for their own liabilities and any consequential costs. In 1993 the NHS Executive published guidance, *Risk Management in the NHS*, and strategies for corporate risk control as proposed by the Cadbury report on corporate management are being adopted by some trusts. Risk management starts with three simple questions:
- what can go wrong?
- how likely is it to happen?
- how bad would it be if it happened?

The combined answers allow an estimate to be made of the risk. Given the scope for clinical mishaps in the NHS – let alone staff and corporate risks – the need for a credible, operational risk strategy is substantial.

RISK REGISTER A list of infants whose obstetric and/or perinatal history suggests the possibility of serious abnormality.

Children are also placed on a risk register

whose social or family circumstances render them liable to mental, physical or sexual abuse. Those on a risk register – and they may include vulnerable adults – are subject to additional surveillance by the health and/or social services.

RISUS SARDONICUS is the term used for describing the facial appearance when the muscles of the forehead and the face go into spasm in tetanus, giving the effect of a sardonic grin.

RITODRINE A beta$_2$-adrenoceptor-stimulating drug that relaxes uterine muscle. It is used in selected women close to term to inhibit the onset of labour for at least 48 hours. This allows for the implementation of measures to improve the perinatal health of the infant, including making arrangements for transfer to a neonatal intensive-care facility. (See PREMATURE BIRTH.)

RNA is the abbreviation for ribonucleic acid, one of the two types of NUCLEIC ACID that exist in nature. It is present in both the cytoplasm and nucleus of the cells of the body, but principally in the former. With DNA it is an essential component of the genetic code. It exists in three categories known, respectively, as ribosomal (r), transfer (t), and messenger (m) RNA. Genetic information resides in the linear sequence of nucleotides (see NUCLEIC ACID) in DNA and is transcribed into messenger RNA before protein is synthesized. In the language of the computer, the genetic code consists of 64 three-letter code-words, or codons. The code in DNA is comparable to a tape which contains information written linearly in the form of these codons, each of which is the code for one of the 20 AMINO-ACIDS from which proteins are made. The genetic information encoded in DNA is used to programme the manufacture of proteins in two stages.

In the first the information is transcribed from DNA on to a molecule of mRNA. In the second the messenger RNA-intermediary transports the information to the protein-manufacturing centres of the cell where the information is translated from the linear sequence of codons in the RNA into a linear sequence of aminoacids which are concurrently converted into protein. (See GENES.)

ROCKY MOUNTAIN SPOTTED FEVER is a fever of the TYPHUS group. It received its name from the fact that it was first reported in the Rocky Mountain States of USA. These are still the most heavily infected States, but it is now found in all parts of the United States. The causative organism is *Rickettsia rickettsi*, which is transmitted to man by tics. (See also TYPHUS FEVER.)

RODENT ULCER A chronic form of BASAL CELL CARCINOMA, the commonest form of skin cancer.

ROMBERGISM A term applied to marked unsteadiness when a person stands with the eyes shut. It is found as a symptom in some nervous diseases, such as peripheral NEUROPATHY and tabes dorsalis (neurosyphilis).

ROOT FILLING Also called root-canal therapy, this is the treatment given when the nerve of a tooth has been exposed while the tooth is being prepared for a filling, or if it has died or become infected. The nerve debris is removed and, when the chamber is clear of infection, an inert radio-opaque material is inserted to seal off the root.

RORSCHACH TEST A psychological test for investigating personality and disorders of personality. It was devised by a Swiss psychiatrist, Hermann Rorschach (1884–1922), who determined individuals' reactions to a series of symmetrical ink-blots, ten in number and standardized by him. The person investigated is shown the ink-blots in a defined order and is asked to describe what he sees. His descriptions and ideas about the blots are noted and an elaborate system of scoring is said to afford indications of the kind of personality and psychological make-up of the person investigated. Much work has been done on the test and it is thought highly of by experienced psychiatrists.

ROSACEA Common chronic inflammation of the facial skin, this condition is seen in middle and late life. Redness, obvious dilatation of venules and crops of acnelike papules and pustules affect mainly the central forehead, cheeks, nose and chin. A keratoconjunctivitis (combined inflammation of the CORNEA and CONJUNCTIVA of the eye) may be associated. Subjects flush easily, especially after alcohol or hot drinks. Eventually the affected areas may become thickened and oedematous and in men proliferation of fibrous and sebaceous tissue may lead to gross thickening and enlargement of the nose (RHINOPHYMA).

Treatment Long-term, low-dose, oral tetracycline is the treatment of choice. In mild cases, METRONIDAZOLE gel can be helpful. Potent topical CORTICOSTEROIDS are contra-indicated and make rosacea worse.

ROSEOLA INFANTUM is a transient exanthem of toddlers. Mild malaise is followed by a RUBELLA-like rash. It is caused by HERPESVIRUS 6.

ROSE-WAALER TEST A blood test which is proving of value in the diagnosis of rheumatoid arthritis. It is positive in over 70 per cent of patients with this disease, compared with only 4 per cent of people not suffering from rheumatoid arthritis.

ROTATOR CUFF A musculotendinous structure that helps to stabilize the shoulder joint.

The cuff may be damaged as a result of a fall and complete rupture of it requires surgical treatment and intensive physiotherapy.

ROTAVIRUSES A group of viruses (so-called from their wheel-like structure: *rota* is Latin for wheel) which are a common cause of GASTROENTERITIS in infants (see DIARRHOEA). They are rarely found in children over 6 years of age. They cause from 25 to 80 per cent of childhood diarrhoea in different parts of the world. In the United Kingdom they are responsible for 60 to 65 per cent of cases. They infect only the cells lining the small intestine. In the United Kingdom death from rotavirus is rare.

ROUGHAGE Dietary fibre is that part of food that cannot be digested in the gastrointestinal tract, although it can be metabolized in the colon by the micro-organisms there. Roughage falls into four groups: cellulose, hemicelluloses, lignins and pectins, found in unrefined foods such as wholemeal cereals and flour, root vegetables, nuts and fruit. It has long been known to affect bowel function, probably because of its capacity to hold water in a gel-like form. It plays an important role in the prevention of constipation, DIVERTICULOSIS, IRRITABLE BOWEL SYNDROME, APPENDICITIS, DIABETES MELLITUS and cancer of the colon. At present many Western diets do not contain enough roughage, even if bran is not the universal panacea.

ROULEAUX The term applied to the heaps into which red blood corpuscles collect as seen under the microscope.

ROUNDWORMS (see ASCARIASIS).

ROUS SARCOMA A malignant tumour of fowls which is caused by a virus. This tumour has been the subject of much experimental work on the nature of cancer.

RSI (see UPPER LIMB DISORDER).

RUBELLA or GERMAN MEASLES An acute infectious disease of a mild type, which may sometimes be difficult to differentiate from mild forms of measles and scarlet fever.

Cause The cause of infection is a virus. It is spread by close contact with infected individuals, and is infectious for a week before the rash appears and at least four days afterwards. It occurs in epidemics every three years or so, predominantly in the winter and spring. Children are more likely to be affected than infants. One attack gives permanent immunity. The incubation period is usually 14 to 21 days.

Symptoms are very mild, and the disease is not at all serious. On the day of onset there may be shivering, headache, slight catarrh with sneezing, coughing and sore throat, very slight fever, not above 37·8 °C (100 °F), and at the same time the glands of the neck become enlarged. These symptoms are usually slight. Within 24 hours of the onset a pink, slightly raised eruption appears, first on the face or neck, then on the chest, and the second day spreads all over the body.

An attack of German measles during the early months of pregnancy may be responsible for congenital defects in the fetus. The incidence of such defects is not precisely known, but probably around 20 per cent of children, whose mothers have had German measles in the first three months of the pregnancy, are born with congenital defects. These defects take a variety of forms, but the most important ones are: low birth weight with retarded physical development; malformations of the heart; cataract, and deafness.

Treatment The only treatment necessary is confinement to bed so long as there are any symptoms. Infectivity ceases within four days provided there are no symptoms. Children who develop the disease should not return to school until they have recovered, and in any case not before four days have passed from the onset of the rash. In view of the mildness of the disease, contacts are seldom kept in quarantine, but they should be carefully watched from the tenth to the twenty-first day from exposure to infection.

In view of the possible effect of the disease upon the fetus, particular care should be taken to isolate pregnant mothers from contact with infected subjects. As the risk to the fetus is particularly high during the first sixteen weeks of pregnancy, any pregnant mother exposed to infection during this period should be given an intramuscular injection of GAMMA-GLOBULIN. A vaccine is available to protect an individual against rubella. In the United Kingdom it is official policy for all children to have the combined measles, mumps and rubella (MMR) vaccine, subject to parental consent. All women of childbearing age, who have been shown by a simple laboratory test not to have had the disease, should be vaccinated, provided the woman is not pregnant at the time and has not been exposed to the risk of pregnancy during the previous eight weeks.

RUPTURE A popular name for hernia. (See HERNIA.)

RYLE'S TUBE (see NASOGASTRIC TUBE).

S

SABIN VACCINE Introduced in 1962, the attenuated live oral vaccine (Sabin) against POLIOMYELITIS replaced the previous inactivated vaccine (SALK) introduced in 1956. Since the introduction of vaccine, notifications of paralytic poliomyelitis have dropped substantially in the UK, with occasional outbursts of infection with wild virus among unimmunized people, thus showing the importance of maintaining a high level of uptake of the vaccine in the community (see SALK VACCINE).

SACCHARINE A sweetening agent that is 400 times as sweet as cane sugar, but with no energy content. Apart from its rather bitter aftertaste, it has practically no effect on the tissues, and escapes from the body unchanged. Destroyed by heat, saccharine is not used in cooking, but is an important component of all diabetic and low-calorie diets.

SACCHAROMYCES Another name for yeast.

SACRAL NERVES The five pairs of spinal nerves that leave the spinal column in the sacral area. They carry motor and sensory fibres from the anal and genital regions and from both legs.

SACRAL VERTEBRAE The five fused vertebrae that link the thoracic spine and the coccyx and form the sacrum (see SPINAL COLUMN).

SACROILEITIS Inflammation of one or both of the SACROILIAC JOINTS, which lie between the sacrum and the iliac bones. The condition may be the result of RHEUMATOID ARTHRITIS, ANKYLOSING SPONDYLITIS, REITER'S SYNDROME, or the arthritis that occurs with PSORIASIS or infection. Sacroileitis causes pain in the lower back, buttocks, thighs, and groin. Stiffness may occur with ankylosing spondylitis. NON-STEROIDAL ANTI-INFLAMMATORY DRUGS relieve the symptoms and if the cause is infection antibiotics should be used.

SACROILIAC JOINT One of a pair of joints between each side of the SACRUM and each ILIUM. Strong ligaments between the ilium and the sacrum stabilize the joint, permitting little movement. Childbirth or strenuous sporting activities may strain the joint, causing pain in the lower part of the backs and buttocks. Such strains may take a long time to mend; physiotherapy is the treatment. The joint may become inflamed (see SACROILEITIS).

SACRUM The portion of the SPINAL COLUMN near its lower end. The sacrum consists of five vertebrae fused together to form a broad triangular bone which lies between the two haunch-bones and forms the back wall of the pelvis.

SADISM (Marquis de Sade) The term applied to a form of sexual perversion, in which satisfaction is derived from the infliction of cruelty upon another person. The condition is commoner in men than women and is sometimes linked with masochism (a wish to be hurt or abused).

SAFE PERIOD That period during the menstrual cycle when fertilization of the ovum is unlikely to occur. Ovulation usually occurs about 15 days before the onset of the menstrual period. A woman is commonly believed to be fertile for about 11 days in each menstrual cycle: i.e. on the day of ovulation and for 5 days before and 5 days after this. This would be the eighth to the eighteenth day of the usual 28-day menstrual cycle. Outside this fertile period is the SAFE PERIOD: the first week and the last ten days of the menstrual cycle. On the other hand, there is increasing evidence that the safest period is the last few days before menstruation. In the case of irregular menstruation it is not possible to calculate the safe period. In any event the safety is not absolute.

SAFETY OF DRUGS The Medicines Act of 1968, which came into force in 1971, is a comprehensive measure replacing most of the previous legislation on the control of medicines for human and veterinary use. It is administered by the Health and Agriculture Ministers of the United Kingdom. It decreed the setting up of a Medicines Commission – reorganized in 1993 as the Medicines Control Agency – by the Ministers to give them advice generally relating to the execution of the provisions of the Act. On the advice of the Medicines Commission a series of expert advisory committees was set up. These are Standing Committees of independent experts, and consist of the Committee on Safety of Medicines, the Committee on the Review of Medicines, the Committee on Dental and Surgical Materials, the British Pharmacopoeia Commission which is responsible for the production of the *British Pharmacopoeia*, and the Veterinary Products Committee.

The Committee on Safety of Medicines (CSM) has the function of scrutinizing the efficacy, quality and safety of new drugs before clinical trial and before marketing, as well as the surveillance of each drug after marketing so that adverse reactions are monitored and documented, and warnings issued as required. Early clinical trial for a drug can only be carried out after a clinical trial certificate has been issued by the licensing authority: i.e. all Ministers specified in the Act. In the case of human medicines the Minister acts through the Medicines Control Agency.

The major defect in this carefully worked out system is the difficulty in obtaining reports of adverse reaction. The present evidence suggests that at most about 10 per cent of such reactions are reported. One method of trying to obtain this information is the yellow card system. It is so called because it is based on the distribution of yellow cards to all doctors and dentists, on which they are asked to report any adverse reaction they may encounter to a drug even though initially the evidence may not be 100 per cent certain. Alternatively the CSM has a Freephone line and on-line computer facilities (ADROIT) for practitioners to use. Even though the annual number of adverse reactions reported in this way has risen from around 5,000 in 1975 to over 17,700 in 1997–8; this is probably fewer than the number actually occurring.

Two further committees in this safety screen are the Joint Committee on Vaccination and Immunization and the Adverse Reactions to Vaccines and Immunological Substances Committee. The function of the Committee on Review of Medicines is to review all medicinal products on the British market.

SAGITTAL   The term applied to a structure or section running from front to back in the body.

ST VITUS'S DANCE   An obsolete name for CHOREA.

SALBUTAMOL   A short-acting selective Beta$_2$-adrenoceptor stimulant delivered via an aerosol inhaler to control mild to moderate symptoms of ASTHMA. If stimulant inhalation is needed more than twice a day to control asthma attacks, prophylactic treatment should be considered including in severe cases oral CORTICOSTEROIDS. Salbutamol relaxes the muscles which cause bronchial spasms in the lungs, the prime symptom of asthma.

SALICYLIC ACID   A crystalline substance sparingly soluble in water that is used externally in ointments and pastes. It has antifungal properties and helps to loosen and remove scales. In high concentrations it is useful in treatment of VERRUCAE and CORNS.

SALINE   Normal saline is a solution containing 0·9 per cent of sodium chloride (common salt). Saline is used clinically to dilute drugs given by injection and is also given as an intravenous infusion to restore blood volume if blood loss from accident or operation is not too serious or to tide a patient over until PLASMA or blood for transfusion becomes available.

Saline is also given orally to severely dehydrated children or adults suffering from diarrhoea and, in particular, CHOLERA.

SALIVA   The fluid secreted by the SALIVARY GLANDS into the mouth. The ingestion of food stimulates saliva production. Saliva contains much mucus and an enzyme known as PTYALIN, which changes starch into dextrose and maltose (see DIGESTION); also many cells of different types. About 750 millilitres are produced daily.

The principal function of saliva is to aid in the initial processes of digestion and is essential for the process of mastication, whereby food is reduced to a homogeneous mass before being swallowed. In addition, the ptyalin in the saliva initiates the digestion of starch in the food.

An excessive flow of saliva known as salivation occurs as the result of taking certain drugs. Salivation also occurs as the result of irritation in the mouth, as for instance, in the teething child, and from dyspepsia. Deficiency of saliva is known as XEROSTOMIA.

SALIVARY GLANDS   The glands situated near, and opening into, the cavity of the mouth, by which the SALIVA is manufactured. They include the parotid gland, placed in the deep space that lies between the ear and the angle of the jaw; the submandibular gland, lying beneath the horizontal part of the jaw-bone; and the sublingual gland, which lies beneath the tongue.

Each gland is made up of branching tubes closely packed together, and supported by strong connective tissue. These tubes are lined by large cells that secrete the saliva, and ducts transfer the saliva to openings in the mouth. The parotid gland secretes a clear fluid containing the enzyme, ptyalin; in the sublingual gland they mainly produce mucus, whilst the submandibular gland contains cells of both types.

SALK VACCINE   A vaccine obtained by treating the POLIOMYELITIS VIRUS with formalin. This prevents the virus causing the disease but allows it to stimulate the production of antibodies. Salk vaccine is given by injection and protects the recipient against the disease. The orally given Sabin vaccine is used in the United Kingdom.

SALMONELLA INFECTIONS, or SALMONELLOSIS (see FOOD POISONING, ENTERIC FEVER and DYSENTERY).

SALMON PATCHES (see NAEVUS SIMPLEX).

SALPINGITIS   Inflammation situated in the FALLOPIAN TUBES; these run from the OVARY to the UTERUS and carry the OVA or eggs. The disorder is commonly caused by infection spreading upwards from the VAGINA, cervix or uterus. It is one feature of PELVIC INFLAMMATORY DISEASE. Salpingitis is potentially serious and requires treatment with antibiotics and sometimes surgery to drain any puss or, in persistent infections, to remove the Fallopian tubes.

SALPINGO-   A prefix indicating a connection with either the FALLOPIAN (or uterine) tubes or the EUSTACHIAN (or auditory) tubes.

SALT   The substance produced by the replacement of the acidic hydrogen of an acid by a metal or basic radical. It is also a synonym for common salt or sodium chloride. Sodium chloride is a vital constituent of cells, and a proper balance between it and other salts in the cells is important for their viability.

SANDFLY FEVER Also known as PHLEBO-TOMUS FEVER, THREE-DAY FEVER, and PAPATACI FEVER, this is a short, sharp fever occurring in many parts of the tropics and subtropics, including most of the Mediterranean littoral, due to a virus, called phlebovirus, conveyed by the bite of a small hairy midge or sandfly (*Phlebotomus papatasi*). The incubation period is three to seven days.

Symptoms There are headache, feverishness, general sensations like those of influenza, flushed face and bloodshot eyes, but no signs of catarrh. The fever passes off in three days, but the patient may take some time to convalesce.

Treatment As there is no specific remedy, prophylaxis is important. This consists of the spraying of rooms with an insecticide such as GAMMEXANE; the application of insect repellents such as dimethyl phthalate to the exposed parts of the body (e.g. ankles, wrists and face), particularly at sunset; and the use of sandfly nets at night. Once the infection is acquired, treatment consists of rest in bed, light diet and aspirin and codeine.

SANGUINEOUS This term means containing blood.

SAPHENOUS The name given to the two large superficial veins of the leg. The small saphenous vein which runs up the outside and back of the leg joins the deep veins at the bend of the knee; the great saphenous vein, the longest vein in the body, which has a long course from the inner ankle to the groin, is specially subject, with its branches, to become the site of varicose veins.

SAPROPHYTE An organism which lives usually upon decaying and dead matter and produce its decomposition.

SARCO- A prefix signifying flesh or fleshy.

SARCOIDOSIS An uncommon chronic inflammatory disease of unknown origin which can affect many organs, particularly the SKIN, EYES and LUNGS. Commonly it presents as ERYTHEMA nodosum in association with lymph-gland enlargement within the chest. In the eyes it causes UVEITIS. BIOPSY of affected tissue allows diagnosis, which is confirmed by a KVEIM TEST. Often sarcoidosis is self limiting but in severe cases oral corticosteroids may be needed.

SARCOMA (see CANCER).

SARCOPTES Mites which infest humans and animals. *Sarcoptes scabei hominis* causes human SCABIES. Other species infest dogs (sarcoptic mange), cats and birds.

SAUNA A hot-air, steam or smoke bath, combined with ice-cold water bathing or douching. An old Finnish practice, practically every house or block of flats there has its sauna. The precise therapeutic value of saunas may not be clear, though the Finns claim that they are a well-proven means of maintaining health. There is some evidence that they may be good for the skin, the upper air passages, weight reduction, and for the relief of rheumatic pains.

SCAB The crust which forms on superficial injured areas. It is composed of fibrin, which is exuded from the raw surface, together with blood corpuscles and epithelial cells entangled in its meshes. Healing takes place naturally under this protection, and the scab dries up and falls off when healing is complete. Scabs appearing on the face without any previous abrasion are usually caused by an infection. (See IMPETIGO.)

SCABICIDE A drug that eliminates the mites which cause SCABIES.

SCABIES A common contagious itching disease caused by *SARCOPTES SCABEI HOMINIS* which can live only on human skin. The fertilized female burrows into the skin surface creating a tunnel within the stratum corneum in which she deposits 2 or 3 eggs per day and faecal pellets which contain the allergen which initiates the immune reaction responsible for symptoms. The adult female is just visible. Eggs hatch within 3 or 4 days, producing larvae. After successive moults these become adult mites and the 15-day life cycle restarts. A rapid build-up of mite numbers is not noticed by the host until an immune response induces itching after about 6 weeks. Subsequently scratching reduces the adult mites to a dozen or fewer. Scabies is spread by skin-to-skin contact, usually via the hands. It thus spreads in a family or sexual setting; though commonest in young adults, scabies can affect any age group.

Typically the patient complains of widespread severe itching, worse when the body is warm after a bath or in bed. Burrows are visible as 3–5 mm long wavy black lines in the skin of the hands, wrists or sides of the feet. The intensity of the rash depends on the immune response. PAPULES, PUSTULES, crusts and EXCORIATIONS are seen on the hands and there may be a widespread ECZEMATOUS or URTI-CARIAL rash elsewhere. Papules or even nodules on the PENIS and SCROTUM are characteristic. In infants burrows occur on the palms and soles. Diminished immune response in old age, DOWN'S SYNDROME, etc. lead to a type of scabies which is less itching and more scaly. Rarely, absence of immune response causes a mite-saturated, generalized scaly dermatitis (Norwegian scabies). Admission of such a patient to hospital may result in an outbreak of scabies in other patients, staff and visitors caused by mite-infested airborne scale.

Treatment MALATHION 0·5-per-cent aqueous lotion or PERMETHRIN 5-per-cent cream applied to the whole body, except the head, for 24 hours and then washed off cures the infection. In infants the head and neck should be included. The secondary eruption may take 2–3 weeks to settle completely and 10-per-cent crotamiton cream is used during this period. It is essential that all intimate contacts be treated simultaneously. FOMITES need not be treated.

SCALDED-SKIN SYNDROME In infants certain STAPHYLOCOCCAL bacteria can cause an acute toxic illness in which the subjects develops sheets of bright ERYTHEMA, accompanied by shedding of layers of outer epidermis. The result is similar to a hot-water scald. The condition responds promptly to appropriate antibiotic therapy. Drug reactions, especially from SULPHONAMIDES, may cause a similar syndrome in adults. In drug-induced forms mucosae are also affected and the disease is often fatal.

SCALDS (see BURNS AND SCALDS).

SCALP The soft covering of the skull on the top of the head. It consists of five layers, which from the surface inwards are as follows: the skin, from which grows hair; next a subcutaneous layer of fat; thirdly, a tough fibrous membrane known as the epicranium; fourthly, a loose layer of connective tissue attaching the epicranium to the deepest layer, and permitting the free movement of the scalp; and, finally, another fibrous layer clinging closely to the skull, and known as the pericranium.

SCALPEL A small, straight, surgical knife.

SCANNING SPEECH A speech disorder in which articulated syllables are wrongly spaced and each is given the same vocal emphasis. The condition occurs as a result of disease in the cerebellum or its connecting nerves.

SCAPHOID BONE The outside bone on the thumb side of the hand in the row of carpal (wrist) bones nearest to forearm. Fracture of the scaphoid is a common wrist injury that usually occurs when someone falls on to their outstretched hand. The fracture may be missed in which case pain in and permanent damage to the wrist can occur. (See HAND.)

SCAPULA The scientific name for the shoulder-blade. (See SHOULDER-BLADE.)

SCAR The name applied to a healed wound, ulcer or breach of tissue. A scar consists essentially of fibrous tissue, covered by an imperfect formation of epidermis in the case of scars on the surface of the skin. The fibrous tissue is produced by the connective tissue that migrate to the wound in the course of its repair (see WOUNDS). Gradually this fibrous tissue contracts, becomes more dense, and loses its blood-vessels, leaving a hard white scar. (See KELOID.)

SCARLET FEVER This disorder is caused by the erythrogenic toxin of the STREPTOCOCCUS. The symptoms of PYREXIA, headache, vomiting and a punctate ERYTHEMATOUS RASH follow a streptococcal infection of the throat or even a wound. The rash is symmetrical and does not itch. The skin subsequently peels. In the latter half of the 19th century it was the commonest cause of death in children over the age of one year. The mortality was already decreasing by the year 1900 and by 1965 deaths were rare.

Symptoms The period of incubation (i.e. the time elapsing between the reception of infection and the development of symptoms) varies somewhat. In most cases it lasts only two to three days, but in occasional cases the patient may take a week to develop his first symptoms. The occcurrence of fever is usually short and sharp, with rapid rise of temperature to 40 °C (104 °F), shivering, vomiting, headache, sore throat and marked increase in the rate of the pulse. In young children convulsions or delirium may precede the fever. The rash usually appears within 24 hours of the onset of fever and lasts about a week.

Complications The most common and serious of these is glomerulonephritis, which may arise during any period in the course of the fever, but particularly when desquamation occurs. Occasionally the patient develops chronic glomerulonephritis. (See KIDNEYS, DISEASES OF.) Another complication is infection of the middle ears. (See EAR DISEASES.) Other disorders affecting the heart and lungs occasionally arise in connection with scarlet fever, the chief of these being ENDOCARDITIS, which may lay the foundation of valvular disease of the heart later in life. ARTHRITIS is another complication of the disease, producing swelling and pain in the smaller rather than in the larger joints. This complication usually occurs in the second week of illness. Scarlet fever, which is now a mild disease in most patients, should be treated with PENICILLIN.

SCHISTOSOMIASIS Also known as BILHARZIASIS. This infection results from one of the human *Schistosoma* spp. (identified by Theodore Bilharz in Egypt in 1851). It is common in Africa, South America, the Far East, Middle East, and, to a limited extent, the Caribbean. The life-cycle is dependent on freshwater snails which act as the intermediate host for the fluke; the cercarial stage enters via intact human skin and matures in the portal circulation. Clinically, 'swimmers' itch' may occur at the site of cercarial skin penetration. Acute schistosomiasis (Katayama fever) can result in fever, an urticarial rash, and enlargement of liver and spleen. The adult male is about 12 mm and the female 24 mm in length. *S. haematobium* causes cystitis and haematuria – passage of blood in the urine; bladder cancer and ureteric obstruction, giving rise to hydronephrosis and kidney failure, are long-term sequelae in a severe case. *S. mansoni* can cause colonic symptoms and in a severe case, polyposis of the colon; diarrhoea, which may be bloody, can be a presenting feature. In a heavy infection, eggs surrounded by granulomas are deposited in the liver, giving rise to extensive damage (pipe-stem fibrosis) associated with portal hypertension, oesophageal varices, etc; however, unlike cirrhosis, hepatocellular function is preserved until late in the disease. *S. japonicum* (which is confined to the Far East, especially Indonesia) behaves similarly to *S. mansoni* infection; liver involvement is often more severe.

Diagnosis can be made by microscopic examination of urine or faeces. The characteristic eggs (*S. haematobium* which causes the urinary form has a terminal spine; *S. mansoni*, which causes colonic and liver disease, has a lateral spine; and *S. japonicum* is smooth and oval) are usually detectable. Alternatively, rectal or liver biopsy are of value. Serological tests, including an ELISA, have now largely replaced invasive procedures used in making a parasitological diagnosis. Chemotherapy has been revolutionized by the introduction of praziquantel (administered orally); this compound has no serious side-effects, although its cost may limit its use in developing countries. Oxamniquine is cheaper and effective in *S. mansoni* infection, although evidence of resistance has been recorded in several countries. Metriphonate is also relatively cheap and is of value in *S. haematobium* infection. Compounds formerly used – which included antimonial preparations and niridazole – are now rarely used. Prevention is by complete avoidance of exposure to contaminated water; all travellers to infected areas should know about this disease. It is increasing in frequency as new expanses of fresh water appear as a result of irrigation schemes and dam projects. Mollusciciding can be employed for snail-control.

SCHIZO- A prefix signifying splitting.

SCHIZOGONY An asexual phase in the life cycle of a SPOROZOAN that occurs in red blood cells or liver cells.

SCHIZOPHRENIA An overall title for a group of psychiatric disorders typfied by disturbances in thinking, behaviour and emotional response. Sometimes referred to as split personality – a better description would be split mind – the disorder is one of the most common and serious mental illnesses. Its genesis is ill understood but, despite its colloquial description as split personality, schizophrenia should not be confused with MULTIPLE-PERSONALITY DISORDER. The illness is disabling, running a protracted course that usually results in ill

health and, often, personality change. Schizophrenia is really a collection of symptoms and signs but there is no specific diagnostic test for it. Similarity in the early stages to other mental disorders, such as manic depression, means that the diagnosis may not be confirmed until its response to treatment and its outcome can be assessed and other diseases excluded.

Causes Schizoprenia is a worldwide disease and in developed countries about 1 per cent of the population is affected at some time during life. In less developed countries the disease seems to be less common and not so severe. Onset is usually between 15 and 30 years of age and is on average five years later in women than in men. There is an inherited element: parents, children or siblings of schizophrenic sufferers have a 1 in 10 chance of developing the disorder; a twin has a 50-per-cent chance if the other twin has schizophrenia. Some BRAIN disorders such as temporal lobe EPILEPSY, tumours and ENCEPHALITIS seem to be linked with schizophrenia. Certain drugs – for example, AMPHETAMINES – can precipitate schizophrenia and DOPAMINE-blocking drugs often relieve schizophrenic symptoms. Stress may worsen schizophrenia and recreational drugs may trigger an attack.

Symptoms These usually develop gradually until the individual's behaviour becomes so disturbing or debilitating that work, relationships and basic activities such as eating and sleeping are interrupted with the victim requiring daily practical help. Relatives and friends may try to cope with the affected person at home, but as severe episodes may last several months and require regular administration of powerful drugs – patients are not always good at taking their medication – hospital admission may be necessary. About 25 per cent of individuals who develop schizophrenia recover fully from their initial attack: this is known as the acute, short-lived or transient variety. Another 25 per cent, however, are disabled by chronic (permanent) schizophrenia, never recover and are unable to live independently. The remaining half is ranged between these two extremes. An individual with schizophrenia may have disturbed perception with (usually auditory) hallucinations; illogical thought processes and delusions; low-key emotions; a sense of being invaded or controlled by outside forces; a lack of insight and inability to acknowledge reality; lethargy, agitation, a disregard for personal appearance and hygiene and a tendency to act strangely. Violence is rare.

Treatment So far there is no cure for schizophrenia. Since the 1950s, however, a group of drugs called antipsychotics – also described as neuroleptics or major tranquillizers – have enabled many people to leave psychiatric hospitals and live more independently outside. Only some of these drugs have a tranquillizing effect but their sedative properties can calm patients with an acute attack. Chlorpromazine is one such drug and is commonly used when treatment starts or to deal with an emergency. Halperidol, trifluoperazine and pimozide are other drugs in the group but with less sedative effects, so are useful in treating those whose prominent symptoms are apathy and lethargy. The antipsychotics reduce schizophrenic symptoms, especially the delusions and hallucinations. Their mode of action is by blocking the activity of dopamine, the chemical messenger in the brain that is faulty in schizophrenia. The drugs quicken the onset and prolong the remission of the disorder, and it is very important that patients take the drugs indefinitely. This is easier to ensure when a patient is in hospital or in a stable domestic environment.

Clozapine, a newer atypical antipsychotic drug, is used only for treating schizophrenic patients unresponsive to, or intolerant of, conventional antipsychotic drugs. It may cause AGRANULOCYTOSIS and use is confined to patients registered with the Clorazil (the drug's registered name) Patient Monitoring Service.

The welcome long-term shift of mentally ill patients from large hospitals to community care (often in small units) has, because of a lack of resources, led to some schizophrenic patients not being properly supervised with the result that they fail to take their medication regularly. This leads to a recurrence of symptoms and there have been occasional episodes of such patients in community care becoming a danger to themselves and to the public.

The anti-psychotic drugs are powerful agents and have a range of potentially troubling side-effects. These include blurred vision, constipation, dizziness, dry mouth, limb restlessness, shaking, stiffness, weight gain and in the long term TARDIVE DYSKINESIA (abnormal movements and walking) which affects about 20 per cent of those under treatment. Some drugs can be given by long-term depot injection: these include compounds of flupenthixol, zuclopenthixol and haloperidol (See MENTAL ILLNESS.)

SCHWANN CELL The cells that produce the MYELIN sheath of the AXON of a medullated nerve. They are wrapped around a segment of the axon, forming concentric layers.

SCIATICA Pain in the distribution of the sciatic nerve. It is often accompanied by pain in the back, or lumbago. It may be due to a number of causes, such as a tumour in the spine or spinal column, tuberculosis of the spine, ankylosing spondylitis (see SPINE AND SPINAL CORD, DISEASES AND INJURIES OF) or a tumour in one of the organs in the pelvis such as the uterus. In the majority of cases, however, it is due to a PROLAPSED INTERVERTEBRAL DISC pressing on one or more of the nerve roots issuing from the lower part of the spinal cord that make up the sciatic nerve. The precise distribution of the pain will thus depend on which of the nerve roots are affected. As a rule, the pain is felt in the buttock, the back of the thigh and the outside and front of the leg, sometimes extending on to the top of the foot, the back of the

thigh and the calf, and then along the outer border of the foot towards the little toe. What probably happens is that degenerative changes take place in the annulus fibrosus. (See SPINAL COLUMN.) Ultimately this ruptures, either as a result of some special strain – caused, for example, by heavy lifting – or spontaneously. The cushioning disc between the two neighbouring vertebral bodies slips through the rent in the annulus fibrosus, and presses on the neighbouring roots, thus causing the pain.

The condition usually occurs in adults under the age of 60. The pain may come on suddenly when the person is lifting, and may be so severe that he may be locked in one position. More commonly onset is gradual but the pain recurs.

Treatment consists essentially of rest in bed in the early stages until the acute phase is over. Analgesics, such as aspirin and codeine, are given to relieve the pain. Expert opinion varies as to the desirability of wearing a plaster of Paris jacket or a specially made corset. Opinion also differs as to the desirability of manipulation of the spine and operation. Surgeons are selective about which patients might benefit from a LAMINECTOMY.

SCIRRHUS A hard form of cancer containing fibrous tissue.

SCLERA (see EYE).

SCLERITIS (see EYE DISEASES).

SCLERODERMA A rare autoimmune disease. Scleroderma circumscriptum (morphoea) affects the skin, usually of the trunk, producing indurated plaques which resolve over many years. The more serious systemic form of scleroderma usually begins with RAYNAUD'S DISEASE, eventually producing a deforming hardening and clawing of the hands. Later the face and sometimes the internal organs, particularly the gastrointestinal tract and kidneys, may be affected.

SCLEROSIS This term means literally hardening, and is applied to conditions in which portions of organs harden and lose their function as the result of an excessive production of connective tissue. The term is especially applied to a change of this type taking place in the nervous system. (See MULTIPLE SCLEROSIS.)

SCLEROTHERAPY A treatment that involves injecting varicose veins (see VEINS, DISEASES OF) with a sclerosing fluid. This causes fibrosis of the lining of the vein and its eventual obliteration. Sclerotherapy is also used to treat varicose veins in the legs, anus (HAEMORRHOIDS) and at the junction of the OESOPHAGUS with the stomach.

SCOLIOSIS The name applied to curvature of the spine consisting partly of a bend to one side, partly of a rotary twist. It may result from disease of the spine, but in weakly children it may arise from so slight a cause as a bad habit in standing or in leaning one arm on the table at lessons. It also arises from disease affecting one side of the chest, such as chronic pleurisy or tuberculosis. (See SPINE AND SPINAL CORD, DISEASES OF.)

SCORBUTIC   This is an adjective characterizing scurvy; typically swollen, spongy gums that bleed easily, and spontaneous haemorrhages and bruising anywhere in the body.

SCOTOMA   An area of blindness in the field of vision.

SCREENING TEST   The screening of apparently healthy people to identify those who may have treatable diseases. Cervical smears are done when screening women to detect if they have cancer or precancer of the neck of the womb (cervix). Factors to be assessed when planning screening procedures include the severity, frequency, and distribution of the disease and the availability and effectiveness of treatment. Convenience, safety, sensitivity and cost should also be assessed. In the United Kingdom the government has supported the extension of screening procedures for breast cancer, cervical cancer, hypertension and diabetes. (See PREVENTIVE MEDICINE.)

SCRIVENER'S PALSY   Another name for writer's cramp. (See CRAMP.)

SCROFULA, or STRUMA   This is a traditional term for TUBERCULOSIS of the glands in the neck. It was formerly known in England as 'king's evil', from the belief that the touch of the sovereign could effect a cure. This superstition can be traced back to the time of Edward the Confessor in England, and to a much earlier period in France. The disease, which is treated with antituberculous drugs, is now rare in developed societies and usually affects young children.

SCROMBOTOXIN POISONING   This occurs from eating poorly preserved scromboid fish such as tuna, mackerel and other members of the mackerel family. In such fish, a toxic histamine-like substance is produced by the action of bacteria or histidine, a normal component of fish flesh. This toxin produces nausea, vomiting, headache, upper abdominal pain, difficulty in swallowing, thirst, ITCHING and sometimes URTICARIA. The condition settles as a rule in 12 hours. ANTIHISTAMINE DRUGS sometimes ameliorate the condition.

SCROTUM   The pouch of skin and fibrous tissue within which the TESTICLES are suspended. It consists of a purse-like fold of skin, within which each testicle has a separate investment of muscle fibres, several layers of fibrous tissue, and a serous membrane known as the tunica vaginalis.

SCRUM-POX   A popular name for a contagious affection of the face affecting rugby football players. It is most likely to occur in forwards as a result of face-to-face contact with individuals with the infection in the opposing side of the scrum. Other possible sources of infection are changing rooms and communal baths. The condition may take the form of IMPETIGO or HERPES SIMPLEX.

SCURF, or DANDRUFF   A popular name for the scaly condition that is often found on the scalp, and often precedes baldness. (See SEBORRHOEA.)

SCURVY (SCORBUTUS)   This disease is caused by deficiency of vitamin C (ascorbic acid) (see APPENDIX 5: VITAMINS) and is now rarely seen in developed countries except in people on poor diets, such as homeless down-and-outs. Ascorbic acid is a water-soluble vitamin derived from citrus fruits, potatoes and green vegetables. Nowadays woody haemorrhagic oedema of the legs is the usual way that the disease presents. The former classic disease of sailors living on salt beef and biscuits was characterized by bleeding of the gums, loss of teeth, haemorrhage into joints, anaemia, lethargy and depression. The introduction of fresh lime juice into the seamen's diet in 1795 eliminated scurvy in the Royal Navy. Vitamin C is curative.

SEA-SICKNESS (see MOTION SICKNESS).

SEASONAL AFFECTIVE DISORDER SYNDROME   Known colloquially as SADS, this is a disorder in which an affected individual's mood changes with the seasons. He or she is commonly depressed in winter, picking up again in the spring. The diagnosis is controversial and its prevalence is not known. The mood change is probably related to light, with MELATONIN playing a key role. (See MENTAL ILLNESS.)

SEBACEOUS CYST   A misnomer applied to epidermoid cysts of the skin whose contents are kerateous not sebaceous. The common 'wen' of the scalp arises from follicular epithelium and is similar.

SEBACEOUS GLANDS   The minute glands situated alongside of hairs and opening into the follicles of the latter a short distance below the point at which the hairs emerge on the surface. These glands secrete an oily material, and are especially large upon the nose, where their openings form pits that are easily visible. In the mouth the glands open directly on the mucosal surface. (See SKIN.)

SEBORRHOEA Excessive production of sebum; it occurs in acne vulgaris.

SEBUM The secretion of the SEBACEOUS GLANDS. It acts as a natural lubricant of the hair and skin and protects the skin from the effects of moisture or excessive dryness. It may also have antibacterial action.

SECONDARY PREVENTION The early detection of disease that reduces or prevents its serious outcome. Routine regular examination of particular age groups – for example, children or the elderly – and screening tests are examples of secondary prevention.

SECONDARY SEXUAL CHARACTERISTICS The physical characteristics that develop during puberty as the body matures sexually. Girl's breasts and genitals increase in size and like boys they grow pubic hair. Boys also grow facial hair, their voice breaks and their genitals grow to adult size.

SECRETIN A hormone secreted by the mucous membrane of the duodenum, the first part of the small intestine, when food comes in contact with it. On being carried by the blood to the pancreas, it stimulates the secretion of pancreatic juice.

SECRETION The term applied to the material formed by a gland as the result of its activity. For example, saliva is the secretion of the salivary glands, gastric juice that of the glands in the stomach wall, bile that of the liver. (See GLANDS.) Some secretions consist apparently of waste material which is of no further use in the chemistry of the body. These secretions are often spoken of as excretions: for example, the urine and the sweat. (For further details, see SALIVA; URINE; ENDOCRINE GLANDS, and also under the headings of the various organs.)

SECTION (1) A thin slice of a tissue specimen taken for examination under a microscope. (2) The act of cutting in surgery; for example, an abdominal section is done to explore the abdomen. (3) The issuing of an order under the United Kingdom's Mental Health Act to admit someone compulsorily to a psychiatric hospital.

SECUNDINES Another name for the afterbirth, consisting of the PLACENTA and membranes expelled in the final stage of LABOUR.

SEDATION The production of a calm and peaceful state of mind, especially by the use of SEDATIVE drugs. The aim is to reduce abnormal anxiety and bring aggressive behaviour under control. Sedation is also a part of the preparation of a patient for surgery or for any procedure that may be frightening or uncomfortable.

SEDATIVES Drugs and other measures which have a calming effect, reducing tension and anxiety. They are HYPNOTICS given in smaller doses than is needed to induce sleep.

SEDIMENTATION RATE (see ESR).

SELECTIVE SEROTONIN-REUPTAKE INHIBITORS (SSRIs) These antidepressant drugs have few ANTIMUSCARINIC effects, but do have adverse effects of their own, predominantly gastrointestinal. They are, however, much safer in overdose than tricyclic ANTIDEPRESSANTS which is a major advantage in patients who are potentially suicidal. Examples are citalopram, used to treat panic disorders, as well as depressive illness, FLUOXETINE and PAROXETINE. (See MENTAL ILLNESS.)

SELENIUM SULPHIDE This is used as a shampoo in the treatment of dandruff and seborrhoeic DERMATITIS of the scalp. In view of its potential toxicity it should only be used under medical supervision. It must never be applied to inflamed areas of the scalp, and it must not be allowed to get into the eyes, as it may cause conjunctivitis or keratitis. It is also used in the treatment of tinea versicolor. (See RINGWORM.)

SELF-POISONING (see POISONS).

SELEGILINE A monoamine-oxidase-B-inhibiting drug used in conjunction with LEVODOPA to treat severe Parkinsonism. Early treatment with selegiline may delay the need to give the patient levodopa, but at present there is no firm evidence that it slows down the progression of the disease. Two major clinical trials had to be ended early because of problems, thus evidence of the value and risks of long-term treatment is limited and seems likely to remain so. However, those who have been using levodopa and selegiline for some years and are doing well should be able to continue with the treatment. It would seem unwise to start the combination for newly diagnosed cases of Parkinson's disease.

SELLA TURCICA The deep hollow on the upper surface of the sphenoid bone in which the PITUITARY GLAND is enclosed.

SEMEN Fluid produced by the male on ejaculation from the penis at sexual orgasm. Each ejaculate contains up to 500 million spermatozoa (male germ cells) suspended in a fluid that is secreted by the PROSTATE GLAND, SEMINAL VESICLES and Cowper's glands, a pair of small glands (also called the bulbo-urethral glands) that open into the URETHRA at the base of the penis. Semen, or seminal fluid, contains a form of sugar (fructose) essential for the motility of sperm. The hormone TESTOSTERONE is a key element in the production of sperm and of seminal fluid.

SEMILUNAR CARTILAGES Two crescentic layers of fibro- cartilage on the outer and inner edges of the knee-joint, which form hollows on the upper surface of the tibia in which the condyles at the lower end of the femur rest. The inner cartilage is especially liable to be displaced by a sudden and violent movement at the knee. (See KNEE.)

SEMINAL VESICLE One of the small paired sacs lying on either side of the male URETHRA, which collect and store spermatozoa. (See TESTICLE.)

SEMINOMA A malignant tumour of the testis that appears as an often painless swelling of the testicle. Seminomas usually occur in an older age group of men than TERATOMAS. The treatment is surgical removal. (See TESTICLES, DISEASES OF.)

SENILE DEMENTIA Dementia has traditionally been divided into presenile and senile types. This is increasingly recognized as an arbitrary division of a condition in which there is a general and often slow decline in mental capabilities. Around 10 per cent of people over 65 years of age and 20 per cent over 75 are affected by dementing illness, but people under 65 may also be affected. Treatable causes such as brain tumour, head injury, encephalitis and alcoholism are commoner in younger people. Other causes such as cerebrovascular disease, which is a major factor, especially among older people, or ALZHEIMER'S DISEASE are not readily treatable, although ANTIHYPERTENSIVE treatment for the former disorder may help and symptomatic treatment for both is possible. Individuals with dementia suffer a gradual deterioration of memory and of the ability to grasp what is happening around them. They often cover up their early failings and the condition may first become apparent as a result of emotional outbursts or uncharacteristic behaviour in public. Eventually personal habits and speech deteriorate and they become thoroughly confused and difficult to look after. Treatment is primarily a matter of ameliorating the symptoms, coupled with a sympathetic handling of the sufferer and the relatives. Admission to hospital or nursing home may be necessary if relatives are unable to look after the patient at home. (See MEDICINE OF THE AGEING.)

SENILITY (see AGEING).

SENNA The leaves of various species of *Cassia senna*, being known as Tinnerelly senna and Alexandrian senna, according to its source.

It is one of the most active of the simple laxative drugs. Senna is excreted in the urine, giving it a dark red or yellow colour. In the case of nursing mothers, some of the drug is excreted in the milk and may affect the infant. A standardized preparation of senna, Senokot®, is widely used for the management of constipation in children and old people. A side-effect of senna is HYPOKALAEMIA and, like other purgatives, it should not be used too often.

SENSATION (see PAIN; TOUCH).

SENSITIVITY The extent to which a SCREENING TEST detects the proportion of true cases of the disease being screened.

SENSITIZATION (see ALLERGY; ANAPHYLAXIS).

SENSORY Description applied to the part of the nervous system dedicated to bringing information on sensations affecting the body to the brain. The opposite of sensory nerves is motor nerves which carry instructions for action to the voluntary muscles in the body.

SENSORY CORTEX (see BRAIN).

SENSORY DEPRIVATION A substantial reduction in the volume of sensory information impinging on the body – for instance, sitting in a dark silent room. Prolonged deprivation is potentially harmful as the body needs constant stimulation in order to function normally. The main input organs are the eyes, ears, skin and nose. The absence of sensations disorients a person and results in neurological dysfunction. Some interrogation techniques involve sensory deprivation to 'soften up' the individual being questioned.

SEPSIS Poisoning by the products of the growth of micro-organisms in the body, and the general symptoms which accompany it are those of inflammation. (See INFLAMMATION.) It is prevented by the various procedures mentioned under ASEPSIS, and is treated locally with ANTISEPTICS and systemically with ANTIBIOTICS. (See ANTISEPTICS.)

SEPTAL DEFECT A congenital abnormality of the heart affecting about 260 babies in every 100,000 in which there is a hole in the septum – the dividing wall – between the left and right sides of the heart. The effects of the defect depend on its size and position. A defect in the wall between the atria (upper chambers of the heart) is called an atrial septal defect and that between the ventricles a ventricular septal defect, the commonest form (25 per cent of all defects). Both defects allow blood to circulate from the left side of the heart, where pressures are highest, to the right. This abnormal flow of blood is described as a shunt and the result is that too much blood flows into the lungs. PULMONARY HYPERTENSION occurs and, if the shunt is large, heart failure may develop. A small septal defect may not need treatment but a large one will need to be repaired surgically.

SEPTICAEMIA A serious condition caused by the presence of micro-organisms in the blood stream. A very high temperature may be the only sign, but there is often associated shivering (rigor), profuse sweating and pains in the joints and muscles.

The introduction of aseptic surgery by Lister immensely reduced the frequency of septicaemia and the problem was further improved by the introduction of antibiotics.

SEPTIC ARTHRITIS Infection in a joint which becomes warm, swollen and sore, with restricted movement. The infectious agent may enter the joint as a result of a penetrating wound or via the blood stream. The condition is treated by ARTHROTOMY or ARTHROSCOPY, joint irrigation and ANTIBIOTICS. Unless treated, the articular CARTILAGE of the joint is destroyed, resulting in a painful deformed and sometimes immobile joint. (See ARTHRITIS.)

SEPTIC SHOCK A dangerous disorder characterized by a severe fall in blood pressure and damage to the body tissues as a result of SEPTICAEMIA. The toxins from the septicaemia cause widespread damage to tissue, provoke clotting in small blood vessels and seriously disturb the circulation. The kidneys, lungs, and heart are particularly affected. The condition occurs most commonly in people who already have a chronic disease such as cancer, cirrhosis of the liver or diabetes mellitus. Septic shock may also develop in patients with immunodeficiency illnesses such as AIDS. The symptoms are those of septicaemia, coupled with those of shock, cold, cyanotic limbs, fast thready pulse and a lowered blood pressure. Septic shock requires urgent treatment with antibiotics, intravenous fluids, and oxygen.

SEPTUM A dividing wall within a structure in the body. Examples are the divisions between the chambers of the heart and the layer of bone and cartilage that separates the two nostrils of the nose.

SEQUELAE The term applied to symptoms or effects which are liable to follow certain diseases. For example, BRONCHITIS and other chest complaints may be sequelae of measles; heart disease is often a sequel of RHEUMATIC FEVER; paralysis may follow DIPHTHERIA.

SEQUESTRUM A fragment of dead bone cast off from the living bone in the process of necrosis. (See BONE, DISEASES OF.) A sequestrum often remains in contact with, and partly enveloped by, newly formed bone, so that a

sinus is produced, and a constant discharge goes on, till the dead bone is removed.

SEROCONVERSION The production of specific ANTIBODIES to ANTIGENS present in the body. This may happen as a result of infection by a virus or IMMUNIZATION with a VACCINE.

SEROTONIN A substance widely distributed in the body tissue, but especially in the platelets in the blood, the lining of the gastrointestinal tract and the brain. Serotonin is believed to have a similar function to that of histamine in inflammation. In the gut it inhibits gastric secretion and stimulates smooth (involuntary) muscle in the walls of the intestine. Serotonin participates in the transmission of nerve impulses and may have a function in controlling mood and states of consciousness. (See SELECTIVE SEROTONIN-REUPTAKE INHIBITORS.)

SEROTYPE A classification of a substance according to its serological activity. This is done in the context of the ANTIGENS it contains or the ANTIBODIES it may provoke. Microorganisms of the same species may be classified according to the different antigens that they produce.

SEROUS Relating to, containing or resembling serum.

SEROUS MEMBRANES These are smooth, transparent membranes that line certain large cavities of the body. The chief serous membranes are the peritoneum, lining the cavity of the abdomen; the PLEURAE, one of which lines each side of the chest, surrounding the corresponding lung; the PERICARDIUM, in which the heart lies; and the tunica vaginalis on each side, enclosing a testicle. The name of these membranes is derived from the fact that the surface is moistened by thin fluid derived from the serum of blood or lymph. Every serous membrane consists of a visceral portion, which closely envelops the organs concerned, and a parietal portion, which adheres to the wall of the cavity. These two portions are continuous with one another so as to form a closed sac, and the opposing surfaces are close together, separated only by a little fluid. This arrangement enables the organs in question to move freely within the cavities containing them. For further details see under PERITONEUM.

SERPIGINOUS A term describing a creeping or extending skin lesion such as an ulcer.

SERUM The fluid which separates from blood, LYMPH, and other body fluids when clotting occurs (see HAEMORRHAGE). Plasma is the fluid of the blood, including FIBRIN, which carries the circulating blood cells and PLATELETS.

Serum is a clear, yellowish fluid containing around 7 per cent proteins and globulins, small quantities of salts, fat, sugar, urea, and uric acid, and even smaller quantities of immunoglobulins, essential in the prevention of disease (see IMMUNITY; IMMUNOLOGY). The serum given in the commonly used VACCINES is generally derived from horses' blood, after they have been subjected to a long course of treatment.

SERUM SICKNESS A hypersensitivity reaction due to circulating ANTIGEN ANTIBODY complexes. It got its name because it was a not uncommon reaction to the administration of foreign serum which used to be given as a form of passive IMMUNITY before the days of antibiotics. By definition it is a manifestation of sensitivity to serum but the same clinical and pathological picture can occur one to three weeks after the administration of drugs such as PENICILLIN, STREPTOMYCIN and SULPHONAMIDES. It is characterized by fever, ARTHRALGIA and LYMPHADENOPATHY and is usually self-limiting as it resolves when the supply of antigen is used up.

SERUM THERAPY (see IMMUNOLOGY).

SESAMOID BONES Rounded nodules of bone usually embedded in tendon. They are usually a few millimetres in diameter, but some are larger, such as the PATELLA, or knee-cap.

SESSILE A growth or tumour that has no stalk.

SEX CHROMOSOMES In the human being there are 23 pairs of chromosomes. Male and female differ in respect of one pair. In the nucleus of the female somatic cell the two members of the pair are identical and are called X-chromosomes. In the male nucleus there is one X-chromosome and another, unequal, dissimilar chromosome called the Y-chromosome. In the sex cells, after reduction division, all cells in the female will contain X-chromosomes. In the male, half will contain X-chromosomes and half Y-chromosomes. If, then, a sperm with an X-chromosome fertilizes an ovum (with, of course, an X-chromosome) the offspring will be female. If a sperm with a Y-chromosome fertilizes the ovum the offspring will be male. It is the sex chromosomes which determine the sex of an individual.

Sometimes during cell division chromosomes may be lost or duplicated, or abnormalities in the structure of individual chromosomes may occur. The surprising fact is the infrequency of such errors. About one in two hundred liveborn babies has an abnormality of development caused by a chromosome and two-thirds of these involve the sex chromosomes. There is little doubt that the frequency of these abnormalities in the early embryo is much higher but because of the serious nature of the defect early spontaneous abortion occurs.

Chromosome studies on such early abortions show that half have chromosome abnormalities with errors of autosomes being three times as common as sex chromosome anomalies. Two of the most common abnormalities in such fetuses are triploidy with 69 chromosomes and trisomy of chromosome 16. These two anomalies almost always cause spontaneous abortion. Abnormalities of chromosome structure may arise because of:

Deletion Where a segment of a chromosome is lost.

Inversion Where a segment of a chromosome becomes detached and re-attached the other way around. Genes will then appear in the wrong order and thus will not correspond with their opposite numbers on homologous chromosomes.

Duplication Where a segment of a chromosome is included twice over. One chromosome will have too little nuclear material and one too much. The individual inheriting too little may be non-viable and the one with too much may be abnormal.

Translocation Where chromosomes of different pairs exchange segments.

Errors in division of centromere Sometimes the centromere divides transversely instead of longitudinally. If the centromere is not central, one of the daughter chromosomes will arise from the two short arms of the parent chromosome and the other from the two long arms. These abnormal daughter chromosomes are called isochromosomes.

These changes have important bearings on heredity as the effect of a gene depends not only on its nature but on its position on the chromosome with reference to other genes. Genes do not act in isolation but against the background of other genes. Each gene normally has its own position on the chromosome and this corresponds precisely with the positon of its allene on the homologous chromosome of the pair. Each member of a pair of chromosomes will normally carry precisely the same number of genes in exactly the same order. Characteristic clinical syndromes, due to abnormalities of chromosome structure, are less constant than those due to loss or gain of a complete chromosome. This is because the degree of deletion, inversion and duplication is inconstant. However, translocation between chromosomes 15 and 21 of the parent is associated with a familial form of mongolism in the offspring and deletion of part of an X chromosome may result in TURNER'S SYNDROME.

Non-disjunction Whilst alterations in the structure of chromosomes arise as a result of deletion or translocation, alterations in the number of chromosomes usually arise as a result of non-disjunction occurring during maturation of the parental gametes. The two chromosomes of each pair (homologous chromosomes) may fail to come together at the beginning of meiosis and continue to lie free. If one chromosome then passes to each pole of the spindle, normal gametes may result but if both chromosomes pass to one pole and neither to the other, two kinds of abnormal gametes will be produced. One kind of gamete will contain both chromosomes of the pair and the other gamete will contain neither. Whilst this results in serious disease when the autosomes are involved, the loss or gain of sex chromosomes seems to be well tolerated. The loss of an autosome is incompatible with life and the malformation produced by a gain of an autosome is proportional to the size of the extra chromosome carried.

Only a few instances of a gain of an autosome are known. An additional chromosome 21 (one of the smallest autosomes) results in mongolism and trisomy of chromosome 13 and 18 are associated with severe mental, skeletal and congenital cardiac defects. Diseases resulting from a gain of a sex chromosome are not as severe. A normal ovum contains 22 autosomes and an X sex chromosome. A normal sperm contains 22 autosomes and either an X or a Y sex chromosome. Thus as a result of non-disjunction of the X chromosome at the first meiotic division during the formation of female gametes the ovum may contain two X chromosomes or none at all, whilst in the male the sperm may contain both X and Y chromosomes (XY) or none at all. (See aso CHROMOSOMES, GENES.)

SEX EDUCATION   Information given to children and young adults about sexual relationships. Evidence suggests that young people want more information about the emotional aspects of sexual relationships, and about homosexuality and AIDS/HIV. There is growing concern about sexual risk-taking behaviour among adolescents, many of whom feel that sex education was provided too late for them. Although most parents or guardians provide some guidance by the age of 16, friends, magazines, television and films are a more significant source of information. Schools have been targeted as a place to address and possibly limit risky behaviour because they are geared towards increasing knowledge and improving skills, and have a captive audience of young adults. There are concerns that the conditions in schools may not be ideal: class time is limited, teachers are often not trained in handling sensitive subjects, and considerable controversy surrounds teaching about subjects such as homosexuality.

Sex education in schools is known to be an effective way of reducing teenage pregnancy, especially when linked with contraceptive services. Several studies have shown that it does not cause an increase in sexual activity and may even delay the onset of sexual relationships and lessen the number of partners. Programmes taught by youth agencies may be even more effective than those taught in the classroom. This may be because teaching takes place in small groups of volunteer participants, and the programmes are tailored to their target populations.

Sex education including information about AIDS/HIV and other sexually transmitted infections (STIs) is compulsory in all state-maintained secondary schools in England and Wales. The National Curriculum includes only biological aspects of AIDS/HIV, STIs and human sexual behaviour.

All maintained schools must have a written statement of their policy, which is available to parents. The local education authority, governing body and head teacher should ensure that sex education encourages pupils to have due regard to moral considerations and the value of family life. Sex education policies and practice are monitored by the Office for Standards in Education (OFSTED) and the Office of HM Chief Inspector of Schools (OHMCI) as part of school inspections.

SEX HORMONES   These hormones control the development of primary and secondary sexual characteristics. They also regulate sex-related functions – for example, menstruation and the production of sperm and eggs. The three main types of sex hormone are ANDROGENS, or male sex hormones; OESTROGENS, or female sex hormones; and PROGESTERONES, which are involved in pregnancy.

SEX-LINKED INHERITANCE   The way in which a characteristic or an illness determined by the sex chromosomes in an individual's cells is passed on to the succeeding generation. Men have one X and one Y sex chromosome and women have two X chromosomes. Disorders that result from an abnormal number of sex chromosomes include KLINEFELTER'S SYNDROME, which affects only men, and TURNER'S SYNDROME, which affects mainly women. Recessive genes on the X chromosome cause most other sex-linked characteristics and in women these may well be masked because one of their two X chromosomes carries a normal (dominant) gene. In men, who have but one X chromosome, no such masking occurs, so more men than women are affected by X-linked characteristics or diseases.

SEXUAL ABUSE   (see CHILD ABUSE).

SEXUAL DEVIATION   Any type of pleasurable sexual practice which society regards as abnormal. Deviation may be related to the activity such as exhibitionism or sadomasochistic sex, or to the sexual object, for example, women's shoes or clothes (fetishism). Different cultures have different values, and treatment is probably not required unless the deviation is harmful to the participant(s). Aversion therapy or conditioning a person's behaviour may help if treatment is thought necessary.

SEXUAL DYSFUNCTION   Inadequate sexual response may be due to a lack of sexual desire or to an inadequate performance, or it may be that there is a lack of satisfaction or orgasm. The lack of sexual desire may be due to any generalized illness or endocrine disorder or to the taking of drugs that antagonize endocrine function. Disorders of performance in men can occur during arousal, penetration and ejaculation. In the female DYSPAREUNIA and VAGINISMUS are the main disorders of performance. DIABETES MELLITUS can cause a neuropathy which results in loss of erection. Impotence can follow nerve damage from operations on the prostate and lower bowel and can be the result of neurological diseases affecting the autonomic system. Disorders of satisfaction include, in men, impotence, emission without forceful ejaculation and pleasureless ejaculation. In women such disorders range from the absence of the congestive genital response to absence of orgasm. Erectile dysfunction in men can sometimes be treated with SILDENAFIL CITRATE (Viagra®).

Sexual dysfunction may be due to physical or psychiatric disease, or it may be the result of the administration of drugs. The main group of drugs likely to cause sexual problems are the ANTI-CONVULSANTS, PSYCHOTROPHIC DRUGS, the ANTI-HYPERTENSIVE drugs and drugs such as metoclopramide that induce hyperprolactinaemia. The benzodiazepine TRANQUILLIZERS can reduce libido and cause failure of erection. Tricyclic ANTIDEPRESSIVES may cause failure of erection and clomipramine may delay or abolish ejaculation by blockade of alpha-adrenergic receptors. The MONO-AMINE OXIDASE INHIBITORS often inhibit ejaculation. The PHENOTHIAZIDES reduce sexual desire and arousal and may cause difficulty in maintaining an erection. The anti-hypertensive drug, methyldopa, causes impotence in over 20 per cent of patients on large doses. The beta-adrenoceptor-blockers and the DIURETICS can also cause impotence. The main psychiatric causes of sexual dysfunction include stress, depression and guilt.

SEXUALLY TRANSMITTED DISEASES
(STDs) are infections transmitted by sexual intercourse. In the United Kingdom they are treated in genito-urinary medicine (GUM) clinics. Wart-virus infections (93,300), non-specific infection or URETHRITIS (in males 44,530), CHLAMYDIA (39,280), HERPES SIMPLEX (27,060) and GONORRHOEA (12,350) were the commonest registered STDs in England in 1996. On average, it is estimated that people newly diagnosed with AIDS were infected with HIV 10 years previously. The number of people diagnosed as having AIDS in England in 1995 was over 2,200.

Despite regular health-education campaigns and the ready availability of preventive measures, the incidence of STDs (excluding HIV/ AIDS), especially among young people, had risen to over 404,600 in 1995 in England.

SHELLFISH POISONING In the United
Kingdom this occurs in two main forms. Shellfish may be the cause of typhoid fever (see ENTERIC FEVER) as a result of their contamination by sewage containing the causative organism. They may also be responsible for what is known as paralytic shellfish poisoning. This is caused by a toxin, or poison, known as saxotoxin, which is present in certain planktons which, under unusual conditions, multiply rapidly, giving rise to what are known as 'red tides'. In these circumstances this toxin accumulates in mussels, cockles and scallops which feed by filtering plankton. The manifestations of such poisoning are loss of feeling in the hands, tingling of the tongue, weakness of the arms and legs, and difficulty in breathing. There is also growing evidence that shellfish poisoning may be due to a virus infection. (See FOOD POISONING.)

SHELTERED HOUSING Accommodation
that has been adapted to cater for the special requirements of those elderly people who can largely look after themselves but benefit from some discreet supervision. The accommodation is usually a small flat and a warden will supervise a group of flats. Meals and other services may be provided, and the payment system varies depending on whether the accommodation is privately owned or run by a local social services department.

SHIGELLA The name given to a group of
rod-shaped, GRAM-NEGATIVE bacteria that are the cause of bacillary dysentery. (See DYSENTERY.)

SHINGLES   (see HERPES ZOSTER).

SHIN SPLINTS (see MEDIAL TIBIAL SYNDROME).

SHOCK   A state of acute circulatory failure in
which the cardiac output is inadequate to provide normal perfusion of the major organs. It represents a failure of blood flow rather than a failure of blood pressure. While shock is accompanied by a fall in arterial blood pressure, a fall in blood pressure is not necessarily indicative of shock. Shock can arise from a variety of causes and produce variable clinical signs according to the state of deterioration of the underlying disease. Direct bedside measurements of blood flow are not available so that physicians must usually rely on indirect evidence of inadequate perfusion. Shock is therefore a clinical syndrome and is characterized by systemic arterial hypotension (arterial blood pressure less than 80 mm of mercury) sweating and signs of vasoconstriction. These signs include pallor, cyanosis, a cold clammy skin and a low-volume pulse. These may be associated with clinical evidence of poor tissue perfusion, such as mental apathy, confusion or restlessness and oliguria. In haemodynamic terms shock is a state of circulatory failure associated with a low cardiac output and high peripheral resistance.

Shock results from many situations which give rise to inadequate perfusion of tissues and organs. It may occur because of increased resistance to blood flow, pooling or loss of blood or because of cardiac insufficiency, but the end result of impaired tissue perfusion is the same. As perfusion depends on blood flow and not blood pressure the sphygmomanometer reading is a poor indicator of circulatory failure.

The blood volume is approximately 5 litres. The heart puts out this volume each minute, a stroke volume of 70 ml being ejected 70 times per minute in the resting subject. Only 15 per cent of the blood volume lies in the arterial bed so that variations in arterial calibre have little effect on the vascular capacity. The arterioles are extremely muscular vessels and the tone of the arteriolar muscle varies the blood flow enormously. Because the greatest decline in pressure occurs at this level the arterioles are called resistance vessels. Over two-thirds of the circulating blood volume lies on the venous side of the circulation, particularly in the venules. Hence the venous system is called the capacitance system. The veins are less muscular than the arterioles but are also under autonomic nervous control. The pressure in veins is only about 7 mm of mercury. They have a relatively large diameter and correspondingly low resistance. The tension of venous musculature, although not great, has a critical influence on venous return and on venous pressure. Passive assumption of the erect posture will reduce the cardiac output by 25 per cent. Nervous adjustment through the sympathetic nervous system is intended to prevent pooling in the capacitance system. Failure of venous tone with pooling of blood in venules and capillaries is associated with a large fall in cardiac output and failure of the peripheral circulation. Failure of arteriolar tone, on the other hand, with consequent arteriolar dilatation is associated with hypotension but blood flow remains normal and there is only a transient decrease in the venous return to the heart. The normal regulatory mechanisms for the circulation, that is the Baroreceptors and the autonomic innervation of the arterioles and venules, are geared to cope with the adjustments necessary in postural alterations, physical exercise and acute trauma. The ADRENERGIC system regulates blood pressure, the distribution of blood, the capacity of the venous system and the force and rate of cardiac contraction. The AUTONOMIC NERVOUS SYSTEM can adequately compensate for 10 per cent alterations in blood volume, moderate systemic infections and a good deal of myocardial damage, by shunting away blood from visceral organs into cerebral, coronary and skeletal muscle beds. The haemodynamic response to shock inevitably produces inadequate perfusion of viscera in order to preserve circulation to the brain and coronary vessels. If this is prolonged the effects are disastrous. The ischaemic intestine permits the transfer of toxic bacterial products and proteins across its wall into the blood. Renal ISCHAEMIA prevents the

maintenance of a normal electrolyte and acid base balance.

Shock may result from loss of blood or plasma volume. This may occur as a result of haemorrhage or severe diarrhoea and vomiting. It may also result because of peripheral pooling of blood due to such causes as TOXAEMIA or ANAPHYLAXIS. The toxaemia is commonly the result of a septicaemia. Another form of shock is called cardogenic shock which is due to failure of the heart as a pump. It is most commonly seen as a result of myocardial infarction. The treatment of shock is dependent on its cause. If it is the result of haemorrhage or diarrhoea or vomiting, replacement of blood and lost electrolytes is of prime importance. If it is due to SEPTICAEMIA the treatment of the infection is of paramount importance and in addition intravenous fluids and vasopressor drugs will be required.

SHOCK LUNG (see ADULT RESPIRATORY DISTRESS SYNDROME).

SHOCK THERAPY (see ECT).

SHORT-SIGHT A condition in which objects near at hand are seen clearly, while objects at a distance are blurred. The condition is technically known as myopia. (See REFRACTION; VISION.)

SHOULDER The joint formed by the upper end of the HUMERUS and the shoulder-blade or SCAPULA. The acromion process of the scapula and the outer end of the collar-bone form a protective bony arch above the joint, and from this arch the wide and thick deltoid muscle passes downwards, protecting the outer surface of the joint, and giving to the shoulder its rounded character. The joint itself is of the ball-and-socket variety, the rounded head of the humerus being received into the hollow glenoid cavity of the scapula, which is further deepened by a rim of cartilage. One tendon of the biceps muscle passes through the joint, grooving the humerus deeply, and being attached to the upper edge of the glenoid cavity. The joint is surrounded by a loose fibrous capsule, strengthened at certain places by ligamentous bands. The main strength of the joint comes from the powerful muscles that unite the upper arm with the scapula, clavicle and ribs.

SHOULDER-BLADE or SCAPULA A flat bone, about as large as the flat hand and fingers, placed on the upper and back part of the thorax. Many of the large muscles that move the arm are attached to it. It is not in contact with the ribs, and its only attachment to the trunk of the body is through a joint between its acromion process and the clavicle on the tip of the shoulder and by the powerful muscles which suspend it from the backbone and ribs. With the arm hanging by the side the scapula extends from the second to the seventh rib, but, as the arm is raised and lowered, it slides freely over the back of the chest. On the rear surface of the bone is a strong process, the spine of the scapula. This arches upwards and forwards into the acromion process. The latter forms the bony prominence on the top of the shoulder, where it unites in a joint with the outer end of the clavicle.

SHUNT Passage of blood through a channel that is not its normal one. This may occur as a result of a congenital deformity (see SEPTAL DEFECT) or of surgery – for example, a porto-caval shunt in which the main portal vein is joined up to the inferior vena cava. (See CIRCULATION OF THE BLOOD.)

SIALAGOGUES Substances which produce a copious flow of saliva.

SIALORRHOEA (PTYALISM) is the excessive production of saliva. It occurs in various nervous disorders, such as PARKINSONISM; poisoning by MERCURY, mushrooms or ORGANOPHOSPHATES; or RABIES infection.

SIAMESE TWINS or CONJOINED TWINS Twins who are united bodily but are possessed of separate personalities. Their frequency is not known, but it has been estimated that throughout the world six or more conjoined twins are born every year who are capable of separation. The earliest case on record is that of the 'Biddendon Maids' who were born in England in 1100. The 'Scottish Brothers' lived for 28 years at the court of James III of Scotland. Perhaps the most famous, however, were Chang and Eng, who were born of Chinese parents in Siam in 1811. It was they who were responsible for the introduction of the term, 'Siamese twins', which still remains the popular name for 'conjoined twins'. They were joined together at the lower end of the chest bone, and achieved fame by being shown in Barnum's circus in the United States. They subsequently married English sisters and settled as farmers in North Carolina. They died in 1874.

The earliest attempt at surgical separation is said to have been made by Dr Farius of Basle in 1689. The first successful separation in Great Britain was in 1912. Both twins survived the operation and one survived well into adult life. This is said to be the first occasion in which both twins survived the operation. The success of the operation is largely dependent upon the degree of union between the twins. Thus, if this is only skin, subcutaneous tissue and cartilage, the prospects of survival for both twins are good, but if some vital organ such as the liver is shared the operation is much more hazardous.

SIBLING A brother or sister. Sibling rivalry is the term applied to the intense competition that sometimes occurs between brothers and/or sisters. The birth of a new baby in the family may prompt jealousy and rivalry that can persist throughout life.

SICKLE-CELL ANAEMIA A form of anaemia characteristically found in black people, so-called because of the sickle shape of the red blood cells. It is caused by the presence of the abnormal HAEMOGLOBIN, haemoglobin S, due to AMINO-ACID substitutions in their polypeptide chains, reflecting a genetic mutation. Deoxygenation of haemoglobin S leads to sickling, which increases the blood viscosity and tends to obstruct flow, thereby increasing the sickling of other cells. THROMBOSIS and areas of tissue INFARCTION may follow, causing severe pain, swelling, and tenderness. The resulting sickle cells are more fragile than normal red blood cells, and have a shorter life span, hence the anaemia. Advice is obtainable from the Sickle Cell Society (see APPENDIX 2: ADDRESSES).

SICKNESS (see VOMITING; MOTION-SICKNESS).

SIDE-EFFECTS Details of drugs, including all major adverse effects, are listed in the *British National Formulary* and revised twice yearly. Doctors are expected to report any adverse effects they come across in their patients directly to the Committee on Safety of Medicines (by means of the yellow card report), and the committee will then pass the information to the manufacturer (see MEDICINES: safety of medicines).

SIDEROSIS Chronic FIBROSIS of the lungs occurring in iron-workers and due to the inhalation of fine iron particles. The term is also applied to the condition in which there is an excessive deposit of iron in the tissues of the body.

SIDS (see SUDDEN INFANT DEATH SYNDROME).

SIGHT (see VISION).

SIGMOIDOSCOPY Examination of the rectum and sigmoid colon with an endoscopic viewing device called a sigmoidoscope. The procedure is done to investigate rectal bleeding or persistent diarrhoea with the aim of detecting or excluding cancer of the rectum and colitis. Sigmoidoscopy, which nowadays is performed with a flexible instrument, can usually be performed in the outpatients department. (See ENDOSCOPE.)

SILDENAFIL CITRATE An oral drug for treating erectile dysfunction of the PENIS has been approved for use in the United States of America and is now available in the United Kingdom but its use in the NHS is being limited. Sildenafil citrate was originally developed to treat ANGINA. During clinical trials patients reported that they were having more erections than before taking the drug. Clinical trials were then conducted on 4,000 men and 70 per cent of them found sildenafil effective. The men, whose age averaged 55 years, had experienced erectile problems for around five years before taking part in the trials; the medical conditions associated with their problems included high blood pressure, high concentrations of CHOLESTEROL, DIABETES MELLITUS, PROSTATE surgery and psychological disorders. Among side-effects headache was the most common; others included facial flushing, indigestion and a stuffy nose. The drug is a vasodilator so that blood flow to the penis is enhanced. It works in response to sexual stimulation and has no properties as an aphrodisiac nor does it provoke sexual fantasies. Sildenafil must not be taken with drugs containing nitrates such as GLYCERYL trinitrate or isosorbide trinitrate as the subject may suffer a sudden fall in blood pressure. Nitrates inhaled for recreational use (poppers) have a similar effect.

SILICA A major constituent of the earth's crust. Its main danger to health arises from free silica, present mainly as quartz and flint and as an important constituent of granite, sandstone and slate. (See SILICOSIS.)

SILICONES Organic compounds of silicon, with a structure of alternate atoms of silicon and oxygen with organic groups, such as methyl and phenyl attached to the silicone atoms. As they produce a flexible and stable water-repellent film on the skin, they are used as BARRIER CREAMS.

Silicone is also used to make implants for reconstructive and plastic surgery. Silicone oil in a silicone rubber bag is used in breast reconstruction after surgery for breast cancer and for enlargement of the breast. Although usually an inert substance, silicone has been found to cause side-effects, including possible immunological reactions following leakages, and its use in breast surgery in particular has been restricted. Since 1992 in the United States silicone has been used only for reconstructive surgery and not for cosmetic purposes. The use of silicone and its possible side-effects remain controversial.

SILICOSIS The most important industrial hazard in those industries in which silica is encountered: i.e. the pottery industry, the sandstone industry, sand-blasting, metal grinding, the tin-mining industry, anthracite coal mines. It is a specific form of PNEUMOCONIOSIS caused by the inhalation of free silica. Among pottery workers the condition has for long been known as potter's asthma, whilst in the cutlery industry it was known as grinder's rot. For the production of silicosis the particles of silica must measure 0·5 to 5 micrometres in diameter and they must be inhaled into the alveoli of the lungs, where they produce fibrosis. This diminishes the efficiency of the lungs, which manifests itself by slowly progressive shortness of breath. The main danger of silicosis, however, is that it is liable to be complicated by tuberculosis. The incidence of silicosis is steadily being reduced by various measures which diminish the risk of inhaling silica dust. These include adequate ventilation to draw off the dust; the suppression of dust by the use of water; the wearing of respirators where the risk is particularly great and it is not possible to reduce the amount of dust: e.g. in sand-blasting; periodic medical examination of workpeople exposed to risk. Under 100 new cases a year are diagnosed in the United Kingdom.

SIMMONDS' DISEASE, or PITUITARY CACHEXIA A rare condition in which wasting of the skin and the bones, impotence, and loss of hair occur as a result of destruction of the pituitary gland.

SINGER'S NODULE A small excrescence on the VOCAL CORDS which causes hoarseness. This tends to develop in people who abuse their voices, e.g. singers, people who shout excessively.

SINOATRIAL NODE This is the natural pacemaker of the heart and comprises a collection of specialized muscle cells in the wall of the upper chamber (atrium) of the heart. The cells initiate electrical impulses at a rate of up to 100 a minute. These impulses stimulate the muscles of the heart to contract. The rate is altered by the effects of certain hormones and various impulses from the nervous system. Damage or disease of the node affects the regular beating of the heart.

SINUS A term applied to narrow cavities of various kinds, occurring naturally in the body, or resulting from disease. Thus it is applied to the air-containing cavities which are found in the frontal, ethmoidal, sphenoidal and maxillary bones of the skull, and which communicate with the nose. The function of these paranasal sinuses, as they are known, is doubtful, but they do lighten the skull and add resonance to the voice. They enlarge considerably around puberty and in this way are a factor in the alteration of the size and shape of the face. The term is also used in connection with the wide spaces through which the blood circulates in the membranes of the brain. Cavities which are produced when an abscess has burst but remain unhealed, are also known as sinuses. (See ABSCESS; FISTULA; NOSE.)

SINUSITIS is inflammation of the mucosal lining of a sinus. It is usually applied to inflammation of the sinuses in the face. Most cases occur as a result of infection spreading to the sinuses from the nose along the passages that drain mucus secreted by the linings of the

1 scapula (shoulder blade)
2 humerus
3 ilium (hip bone)
4 radius
5 ulna
6 greater trochanter
7 metacarpals (palm facing forward)
8 phalanges (palm facing forward)
9 skull (for details see diagram: SKULL)
10 cervical vertebrae
11 clavicle (collar bone)
12 sternum (breastbone)
13 eleventh and twelfth thoracic vertebrae
14 lumbar vertebrae
15 sacrum
16 pubis
17 hip joint
18 symphisis pubis
19 ischium
20 carpus (palm facing backwards)
21 femur (thigh bone)
22 patella (knee cap)
23 tibia
24 fibula
25 tarsus
26 metatarsals
27 phalanges

Diagram of human skeleton.

sinuses to the nose. The bacterial infection usually follows a viral infection of the upper respiratory tract. Treatment with ANTIBIOTICS is usually effective but the condition tends to recur. If the episodes are severe, they can be disabling with severe headaches. Surgery is sometimes necessary to drain the sinuses. (See NOSE, DISEASES OF.)

SINUSOID A small blood vessel like an enlarged CAPILLARY occurring, for example, in the LIVER, which contains a large number of them. The sinusoids in the liver are drained by the hepatic veins.

SINUS TACHYCARDIA A regular heart rate of 100 or more beats a minute. It is caused by increased electrical activity in the sinoatrial node (see HEART). This level of tachycardia is normal during and just after exercise and may also be caused by stress or anxiety. If tachycardia persists when the person is resting, it may be due to underlying disease such as THYROTOXICOSIS and investigation is advisable.

SI UNITS The international system of measurement units used throughout the sciences. SI Units, which derive from metres, kilograms, and seconds, comprise seven basic units and two supplementary ones. Among the other base units are ampere (electric current) and mole (amount of a substance). Derived SI units include joule (energy), pascal (pressure), becquerel (activity), and newton (force). (See APPENDIX 6: MEASUREMENTS IN MEDICINE).

SJOGREN'S SYNDROME Sjogren described the association of dryness of the mouth (xerostomia) and dryness of the eye (kerato conjunctivitis sieca) with RHEUMATOID ARTHRITIS. It occurs in approximately 10 per cent of patients with rheumatoid arthritis but it can occur, and frequently does so, independently of rheumatoid disease. The lack of tears gives rise to symptoms of dryness and grittiness of the eyes. The dry mouth can occasionally be so severe as to cause a dysphagia. The disease is due to the autoimmune destruction of the salivary glands and the lacrimal glands. The disorder is usually associated with specific HLA antigen. The treatment is unsatisfactory and is limited to oral and ocular hygiene as well as the provision of artificial tears in the form of cellulose eye drops.

SKELETAL MUSCLE Muscle under a person's voluntary control. (See MUSCLE and VOLUNTARY MUSCLE).

SKELETON is the comprehensive term applied to the hard structures that support or protect the softer tissues of the body. Many animals are possessed of an exoskeleton, consisting of superficial plates of bone, horn, or the like; but in man the skeleton is entirely an endoskeleton, covered everywhere by soft parts, and consisting mainly of bones, but in places also of cartilage. The chief positions in which cartilage is found in place of bone are the larynx and the front of the chest. (For the details of the skeleton, see BONE and diagram on p. 495.)

SKIN The membrane which envelops the outer surface of the body, meeting at the body's various orifices, with the mucous membrane lining the internal cavities. The skin comprises two distinct layers differing in structure. They develop, however, from one cell population of keratinocytes present in the germinative zone (see below); these cells divide, mature, keratinize and die, thus producing the skin's layers.

Structure

CORIUM The foundation layer. It overlies the subcutaneous fat, forming a fibrous layer that is the main part of the bodily covering. Varying in thickness from 0·5–3 mm, it is coarser on the back than on the front of the body and is thicker in men than in women. Many nerves run through the corium: these have key roles in the sensations of touch, pain and temperature (See NERVES). Blood vessels nourish the skin and are primarily responsible for regulating the body temperature. Hairs are bedded in the corium, piercing the epidermis to cover the skin in varying amounts in different parts of the body. The amount, colour and distribution of hair are determined genetically. The sweat glands are also in the corium and their ducts lead to the surface. The fibrous tissue of the corium comprises interlocking white fibrous elastic bundles. The corium contains many folds, especially over joints and on the palms of hands and soles of feet with the epidermis following the contours. These are permanent throughout life and provide unique fingerprinting identification.

HAIR Each one has a root and shaft, and its varying tone originates from pigment scattered throughout it.

GLANDS These occur in great numbers in the skin. SEBACEOUS GLANDS secrete a fatty substance and sweat glands a clear watery fluid. The former are made up of a bunch of small sacs producing fatty material that reaches the surface via the hair follicle. Around three million sweat or sudoriparous glands occur all over the body surface; sited below the sebaceous glands they are unconnected to the hairs.

EPIDERMIS This forms the outer layer of skin and is the cellular layer covering the body surface: it has no blood vessels and its thickness varies from 1 mm on the palms and soles to 0·1 mm on the face. Made up of four strata– the corneum (horny), lucidum (clear), granulosum (granular) and germinative (malphighian), which is subdivided into two strata: the spinosum (prickly cell layer) and basal. The impervious horny layer comprises several thicknesses of flat cells (pierced only by hairs and sweat gland openings) that are constantly rubbed off as small white scales; they are replaced by growing cells from below. The clear layer forms a type of membrane, and in the granular stratum cells are undergoing graduated change from their

1 sweat gland duct
2 tactile corpuscle in corium
3 epidermis
   (a) stratum corneum
   (b) stratum lucidum
   (c) stratum granulosum
   (d) stratum spinosum
   (e) stratum basale
4 fascicular papilla in corium
5 corium
6 blood vessel
7 nerve
8 bulb of hair
9 subcutaneous fat
10 hair
11 sebaceous gland
12 arrector pili muscle
13 medulla of hair
14 papilla of hair
15 pacinian corpuscle
16 body of sweat gland

Vertical section through the skin including hair and sweat gland.

origins as keratinocytes in the germinative zone, where fine sensory nerves also terminate. The basal layer of the germinative zone contains melanocytes which produce the pigment melanin, the cause of skin tanning.

Nail   A modification of skin, being analagous to the horny layer, but its cells are harder and more adherent. Under the horny nail is the nail bed, comprising the well-vascularized corium and the germinative zone. Growth occurs at the nail root at a rate of around 0·5 mm a week, a rate that increases in later years of life.

Skin functions   By its ability to control sweating and open or close dermal blood vessels the skin plays a crucial role in maintaining a constant body temperature. Its toughness protects the body from mechanical injury. The epidermis is a two-way barrier. It prevents the entry of noxious chemicals and microbes and prevents the loss of body contents, especially water, electrolytes and proteins. It restricts electrical conductivity and to a limited extent protects against ultraviolet radiation.

The LANGERHANS' cells in the epidermis are the outposts of the immune system just as the sensory nerves in the skin are the outposts of the nervous system. Skin has a social function in its ability to signal emotions such as fear or anger. Lastly it has a role in the synthesis of vitamin D.

SKIN DISEASES   There are a large number of skin diseases: they may be local to the skin or a manifestation of systemic disorders, inherited or acquired. Some major types are described here, other appear under appropriate alphabetical headings (see list at the end of this entry).

Skin cancer Primary cancer is common and chronic exposure to ultraviolet light is the most important cause. BASAL CELL CARCINOMA is the commonest skin cancer. SQUAMOUS CELL CARCINOMA is less common and presents as a growing, usually painless nodule which may ulcerate. Squamous cancer may spread to regional lymph glands and metastasize, unlike basal cell cancer. Occupational exposure to chemical carcinogens may cause squamous carcinoma – for example, cancer from pitch warts or the scrotal carcinoma of chimney sweeps exposed to coal dust in earlier centuries. Squamous carcinoma of the lip is associated with clay-pipe smoking.

Cancer may arise from the population of MELANOCYTES of the skin (see MALIGNANT MELANOMA).

Apart from these three most frequent forms of skin cancer, various forms of cancer can arise from cells of the dermis of which lymphoma is the most important (see MYCOSIS FUNGOIDES).

Lastly, secondary deposits from internal cancer, particularly from the breast, may metastasize to the skin.

Dermatitis and eczema These are broadly synonymous and the terms are commonly interchangeable. Eczema is a pattern of inflammation with many potential causes. The various types have common histopathology marked by the presence of OEDEMA fluid in and between cells in the epidermis. Dermatitis is commonly used to suggest an eczema caused by external factors and customarily has a conditioning adjective. Here dermatitis is used as the prime description. Dermatitis is a common pattern of inflammation of the skin characterized by redness and swelling, vesiculation, and scaling with intense itching and often exudation (weeping). Fissuring, thickening (lichenification) and secondary bacterial infection may follow. Dermatitis can affect any part of the body. It may be genetically determined or due to other 'internal' factors, such as venous hypertension in a leg or stress. Often it is 'external' in origin, due to strong irritants or chemical allergens.

ATOPIC DERMATITIS is genetic in origin and usually begins in infancy. It may persist for years; and later asthma, allergic rhinitis and conjunctivitis ('hayfever') may be associated. Atopic children tend to have multiple allergies, especially to inhaled allergens such as house dust mite, cat and dog dander and pollens. Allergy to foods is less common but potentially more dangerous, especially if to nuts, when it can cause acute URTICARIA or even ANAPHYLACTIC shock. Atopic subjects are particularly prone to persistent and multiple verrucae and mollusca and to severe herpes simplex infections.

EXFOLIATE DERMATITIS (PITYRIASIS RUBRA) Generalized exfoliation and scaling of the skin, commonly with erythema. Drugs may cause it or the disorder may be linked with other skin diseases such as benign dermatoses and lupus erythematosus.

SUMMER POMPHOLYX is an acute vesicular eczema of the palms and soles recurring every summer. Inhaled allergens are a frequent cause.

VENOUS (STASIS) DERMATITIS begins on a lower calf, often in association with purpura, swelling and sometimes ulceration. Chronic venous hypertension in the leg, consequent on valvular incompetence in the deep leg VEINS owing to previous deep-vein thrombosis, is the usual cause.

NEURODERMATITIS A pattern of well-defined plaques of lichenified eczema particularly seen on the neck, ulnar forearms or sides of the calves in subjects under emotional stress.

IRRITANT CONTACT DERMATITIS Most often seen in an industrial setting (occupational dermatitis), it is due to damage by strong chemicals such as cutting oils, cement, detergents and solvents. In almost all cases the hands are most severely affected.

ALLERGIC CONTACT DERMATITIS in contrast, can affect any part of the body depending on the cause – for example, the face (cosmetics), hands (plants, occupational allergens) or soles (rubber boots). Particularly common allergens include metals (nickel and chromate), rubber additities, and adhesives (epoxy resins).

Treatment Avoidance of irritants and contact allergens, liberal use of emollients and topical application of corticosteroid creams and ointments are central.

Other skin disorders under the following headings: ACNE; ALBINISIN; ALOPECIA; ALOPECIA AREATA; APHTHOUS ULCER; BASAL CELL CARCINOMA; BOILS; BOWEN'S DISEASE; CALLOSITIES; CANDIDA; CARBUNCLE; CHEILOSIS; CHEIRAPOMPHOLYX; CRABLOUSE; DANDRUFF; DERMATOFIBROMA; DERMATOMYOSITIS; DERMATOPHYTES; DERMOGRAPHISM; ECYTHYMA; ERYSIPELAS; ERYTHEMA; ERYTHRASMA; ERYTHRODERMA; ESCHAR; EXANTHEM; FUNGAL INFECTIONS; HAND, FOOT AND MOUTH DISEASE; HERPES GENITALIS; HERPES SIMPLEX; HERPES ZOSTER; ICTHYOSIS; IMPETIGO; INTERTRIGO; KELOID; KERATOSIS; LARVA MIGRANS; LICHEN; LUPUS; MADURA FOOT; MELANOMA; MOLLUSCUM CONTAGIOSUM; MILIARIA; MOLE; MYCOSIS FUNGOIDES; NAEVUS; ORF; PEDICULOSIS; PEMPHIGUS; PHOTOCHEMOTHERAPY; PHOTODERMATOSES; PITYRIASIS; PORPHYRIAS; PRURITUS; PSORIASIS; RINGWORM (TINEA); ROSACEA; SARCOIDOSIS; SCABIES; SCLERODERMA; URTICARIA; VITILIGO; WARTS; XANTHOMATA.

SKIN-GRAFTING An operation in which large breaches of skin surface due to wounding, burns or ulceration are closed by transplantation of skin from other parts. There are three methods by which this is done. Most frequently the epidermis only is transplanted, using a method introduced by Reverdin and by Thiersch, and known by their names. For this purpose, a broad strip of epidermis is shaved off the thigh or upper arm, after the part has been carefully purified, and is transferred bodily to the raw or ulcerated surface,

1 supraorbital foramen
2 nasal spine
3 coronal suture
4 frontal
5 parietal
6 sphenoid
7 nasal
8 zygomatic
9 maxilla
10 mandible
11 lambdoid suture
12 occipital
13 temporal
14 atlas vertebra
15 axis vertebra
16 3rd, 4th and 5th cervical vertebrae

Frontal (left) and left lateral (right) views of the skull. The left lateral view includes the first cervical vertebrae.

or is cut into smaller strips and laid upon it. A second method is for small pieces of the skin in its whole thickness to be removed from the arm and thigh, or even from other people, and then implanted and bound upon the raw surface. This method has the disadvantage that the true skin must contract at the spot from which the graft is taken, leaving an unsightly scar. When very large areas require to be covered, a third method is commonly used. A large flap of skin, amply sufficient to cover the gap, is raised from a neighbouring or distant part of the body, in such a way that it remains attached along one margin, so that blood-vessels can still enter and nourish it. It is then turned so as to cover the gap; or, if it be situated on a distant part, the two parts are brought together and fixed in this position till the flap grows firmly to its new bed. The old connection of the flap is then severed, leaving it growing in its new place.

Researchers are having success in growing human skin in the laboratory for grafting on to people who have been badly burned and have insufficient intact skin surface to provide an autologous graft (one provided by the recipient

of the graft). Another technique being researched is the use of specially treated shark skin.

SKULL This is the collection of 22 flat and irregularly shaped bones which protect the brain and form the face (see BONE).

Arrangement of the bones In childhood, the bones are independent, gradually fusing together by sutures, and in old age fusing completely so that the cranium forms a solid bony case. At the time of birth the growth of several bones of the infant's head has not been quite completed, so that six soft spots, or fontanellas present, where the brain is covered only by skin and membranes, and the pulsations of its blood vessels may be seen. One of these spots, the anterior fontanelle, does not close completely until the child is 2½ years old.

Parts of the skull The cranium, enclosing the brain, consists of eight bones, while the face, which forms a bony framework for the eyes, nose and mouth, consists of 14 bones. These two parts can be detached.

Shape of the skull The development of large central hemispheres of the brain in humans has influenced the skull shape. Unlike other mammals the cranium extends above as well as behind the face which therefore looks forward. Classification of the varying shape of skulls in humans can be done by assessing the cephalic index – namely, the percentage that the skull's breadth forms of its length. Long-headed people, like the Australian aborigines, are called dolichocephalic; those with rounded heads (most European races) mesocephalic; and people with broad heads (some Amerindians) brachycephalic. The skull's proportions change with age: the cranium in children is larger in comparison with the face – one eighth of the whole head – than is the case in adults where sizes are about the same. Old age reduces the size of the face because of the loss of teeth and absorption of their bony sockets. Women's skulls tend to be lighter and smoother with less obvious protuberances than those in men.

SLAPPED CHEEK DISEASE or ERYTHEMA INFECTIOSUM (see ERYTHEMA).

SLE (see SYSTEMIC LUPUS ERYTHEMATOSUS).

SLEEP is a state which alternates with wakefulness and in which awareness and responsiveness to the environment are reduced. It is not, however, uniform and can be divided into two main states which are differentiated according to electrical recordings of brain activity (EEG), of the muscles (EMG), and of the eye movements (EOG).

Non-rapid-eye movement (NREM) sleep This is subdivided into four stages of which stage 1 is the lightest and stage 4 is the deepest. The activity of the cerebral cortex is diminished and the body's functions are mainly regulated by brain-stem activity. The metabolic rate is reduced and in keeping with this the temperature falls, respiration is reduced, cardiac output, heart rate, and blood pressure fall, and activity of the sympathetic nervous system is reduced. NREM sleep normally occurs at the onset of sleep except in neonates. During adult life the duration, particularly of stages 3 and 4, of NREM sleep becomes less and very little of this deep sleep occurs after the age of 60 years.

NREM sleep has been thought to have several functions such as energy conservation and growth. Growth hormone is produced in bursts during stages 3 and 4 NREM sleep and more cell division occurs during this type of sleep than during wakefulness. It has also been proposed that processing of information which has been acquired during wakefulness occurs during NREM sleep.

Rapid-eye-movement (rem) sleep This is characterized by the presence of rapid eye movements and a reduction in muscle tone. Cerebral cortical activity is prominent and its blood flow is increased. This activity is, however, different to wakefulness and may cause irregular movements of the body as well as of the eyes. Most dreams occur in REM sleep. These may represent a process of reorganizing mental associations after the period of wakefulness. The analysis of the content of dreams has been subject to a variety of interpretations but no consensus view has evolved.

Physiological changes, such as a fall in temperature and blood pressure, take place just before sleep and continue during the early stages of NREM sleep. There is an intrinsic rhythm of sleep which in most subjects has a periodicity of around 25 hours. This can be modified by external factors to bring it into line with the 24-hour day. Two peaks of a tendency to sleep have been identified and these usually occur between around 1400 hrs and 1800 hrs and 02.00 and 06.00 hours. There are, however, differences according to age, in that, for instance, infants sleep for most of the 24 hours and during adolescence there is also an increase in the duration of sleep. Sleep requirements fall later in life but there are wide genetic differences in the amount of sleep that people require and also the time at which they fall asleep most readily.

The internal clock can be disturbed by a variety of external factors which include irregular sleeping habits due, for instance, to shift work or jet lag. Sleep is also more likely to occur after physical exertion, reading and social activity. The duration and intensity of exposure to light can also modify sleep profoundly. Light promotes wakefulness and is the main factor that adjusts the 25-hour internal rhythm to the 24-hour daily cycle. Neural connections from the retina act on an area in the brain called the supra-chiasmatic nucleus which stimulates the pineal gland which produces MELATONIN. This is thought to trigger the range of neurological and metabolic processes that characterize sleep.

SLEEP, DISORDERS OF There are three main groups of sleep disorders:

Parasomnias These include medical disorders such as asthma, angina or epilepsy which are exacerbated by sleep and the range of behavioural alterations which are usually related to a specific sleep stage or to a change from one state of sleep to another. Sleep walking, night terrors, and nightmares are examples.

Insomnia Insomnia is defined as a difficulty in initiating or maintaining sleep. It affects around 15 per cent of the population at any one time. It is often due to a poor pre-sleep routine (e.g. taking excessive stimulants such as caffeine), unsatisfactory sleep due to poor environments such as an uncomfortable bed or a cold or noisy bedroom, anxiety, depression or occasionally due to a physical problem, for example, pain or a medical disorder associated with sleep such as obstructive sleep apnoeas or periodic limb movements.

Excessive daytime sleepiness This is usually due to sleep deprivation caused either by inadequate duration of sleep or by poor quality sleep. The individual's lifestyle is often a cause and modification of this may relieve the problem. Other common causes of excessive daytime sleepiness are depression, obstructive sleep apnoeas, periodic limb movements, excessive alcohol intake, and, less commonly, NARCOLEPSY.

SLEEP APNOEAS A sleep apnoea is conventionally defined as the cessation of breathing for ten seconds or more. Apnoeas may occur as frequently as 400 times per night. They can be due to a failure of the physiological drive to breathe (central sleep apnoeas) but much more often are due to a transient obstruction of the airway between the level of the soft PALATE and the LARYNX (obstructive sleep apnoeas) when the airway dilator muscles overrelax. Any factor such as alcohol or sedative drugs that accentuates this, or that makes the airway narrower, such as obesity or large TONSILS, will tend to cause sleep apnoeas.

Vigorous respiratory movements are made to overcome the obstruction during each apnoea. These are associated with snoring and snorting noises. The apnoea ends with a mini-arousal from sleep. As a result sleep becomes fragmented and sleep deprivation, manifested as sleepiness during the day, is common. This may result in accidents, for instance, at work or while driving, and sleep apnoea is also linked with an increased risk of strokes, heart attacks and hypertension.

Initial treatment is directed at correcting the cause, e.g., weight loss, but if the apnoeas persist or are severe a nasal mask and pump which introduces air under slight pressure into the upper airway (continuous positive airway pressure, CPAP) is almost invariably effective. SUDDEN INFANT DEATH SYNDROME (SIDS) may be associated with sleep apnoea.

SLEEPING SICKNESS Also termed African trypanosomiasis, this infection is endemic in west, east, central and South Africa between latitudes 14° N and 25° S. Pioneering work was carried out by David Bruce in Zululand and Uganda in 1894 and 1903, respectively. There are two major forms of the disease: *Trypanosoma brucei gambiense* is confined to west and central Africa, and *T.b. rhodesiense* to central, east, and south-east Africa; there is a significant overlap, and it is probable that the two strains form part of a continuous spectrum. The infection is caused by the bite of tsetse fly (*Glossina* spp.). Clinically, a trypanosomal chancre may develop at the site of the tsetse-fly bite. After introduction into the bloodstream, the protozoan parasite develops in blood and lymphatic glands. After the blood stage, it enters the central nervous system, causing characteristic neurological sequelae (see below). Infection may be followed by a generalized macular papular reaction. In *T.b. gambiense* infection, enlarged glands in the neck (Winterbottom's sign) may be striking. Onset of disease is accompanied by fever, progressive anaemia,

and enlarged glands; these signs and symptoms are followed by increasing lethargy, slowing of mentality, and physical weakness, and give way to headache and an increasing tendency to sleep. These symptoms are caused by proliferation of parasites in the patient's cerebral blood vessels; this is accompanied by inflammatory changes and disorganization of nervous tissue. Patients become emaciated and develop bed sores. Death finally takes place either as a result of gross emaciation or an intercurrent infection.

Diagnosis is by detection of trypanosomes in a blood specimen or, alternatively, a sample of cerebrospinal fluid. Recently introduced serological tests are of great value in diagnosis.

Treatment is with suramine or pentamidine; when cerebral involvement has ensued, melarsoprol – which penetrates the blood-brain barrier – is of value. In *T.b. gambiense* infection, eflornithine has recently given encouraging results; however, this form of chemotherapy is not effective in a *T.b. rhodesiense* infection. From the point of view of prevention, control of the tsetse-fly population is crucial; even so, only a very small percentage of these vectors is infected with Trypanosoma spp.

SLING A hanging bandage for the support of injured or diseased parts. Slings are generally applied for support of the upper limb, in which case the limb is suspended from the neck. The lower limb may also be supported in a sling from an iron cage placed upon the bed on which the patient lies, the object usually being to aid the circulation, and so quicken the healing of ulcers on the leg.

SLIPPED DISC The popular name for a PROLAPSED INTERVERTEBRAL DISC. (See SPINAL COLUMN; SCIATICA.)

SLOUGH Dead tissue separated by natural processes from the living body. The term is applied to hard external parts which the lower animals cast off naturally in the course of growth, like the skin of snakes or the shell of crabs. In man, however, the process is generally associated with disease, and is then known as gangrene. (See GANGRENE.) Sloughs may be of very small size, as in the case of the core of a boil, or they may include a whole limb, but in general a slough involves a limited area of skin or of the underlying tissues. The process of separation of a slough is described under gangrene.

SLOW VIRUSES A group of viruses or virus-like agents, now called PRIONS, whose effects take a long time to show after their initial infection of the nervous system. The diseases may take years to develop during which time gradual but widespread damage of the nerve tissue occurs. The outcome is a loss of brain function and eventually death. Slow-virus disease was many years ago recognized as causing scrapie in sheep, and more recently BOVINE SPONGIFORM ENCEPHALOPATHY (BSE) has been identified in cows, the disease being spread through feedstuffs contaminated with nervous tissue from sheep and cattle. In humans CREUTZFELDT-JAKOB DISEASE (CJD) and a new-type CJD (believed to be caused by the infectious agent that causes BSE) result from infection by prions. KURU or laughing sickness is another prion disease. A form of Alzheimer's disease, subacute sclerosing panencephalitis, which is a complication of measles, may also be a prion disorder.

SMALLPOX So called to distinguish the disease from syphilis, the great pox (pox being the plural of pock, the Old English term for a PUSTULE), is also known as VARIOLA (from *varus*, the Latin for pimple). It is an acute, highly infectious disease due to a virus.

Until recent times it was one of the major killing diseases. In the 1960s the World Health Organization undertook an eradication scheme by means of mass vaccination. As a result, the last naturally occurring case was recorded in October 1977, and on 8 May 1980, the World Health Assembly confirmed that smallpox has finally been eradicated from the world. This was a historic event; the first occasion on which man has attempted to eradicate a disease and has succeeded in so doing. The public lack of interest in it is explained by the fact that so few of those living today have had any experience of it – even doctors. (See VACCINATION.)

SMALL-BOWEL TRANSPLANTANTION
Before the advent of small-bowel transplants, long-term intravenous feeding (total parenteral nutrition or TPN) was the last option for patients with chronic intestinal failure. Now a small group of patients are being considered for this innovative procedure. The first successful small-bowel transplant was performed in Germany in 1989. The number of operations and the success rate of small-bowel transplants have risen and the procedure is now performed all over the world. This success is partly due to experience, but also due to the development of new drugs which suppress the immune system and help to prevent the organ from being rejected by the recipient. Most recipients are children, and small-bowel transplantation is currently reserved for patients unable to continue on long-term parenteral nutrition. The main constraints to small-bowel transplantation are the intensity of rejection (necessitating high levels of immunosuppression), and the lack of donors who are the same size as the recipient (a particular problem for children.

SMEGMA A thick, cheesy secretion formed by the sebaceous glands of the glans penis. A bacillus, closely resembling the tubercle bacillus morphologically, develops readily in this secretion.

SMELL The sense of smell is picked up in what is known as the olfactory areas of the nose. Each of these is about 3 square centimetres in area and contains 50 million olfactory, or smelling, cells. They lie, one on either side, at the highest part of each nasal cavity. This is why we have to sniff if we want to smell anything carefully, as in ordinary quiet breathing only a few eddies of the air we breathe in reaches an olfactory area. From these olfactory cells the olfactory nerves (one on each side) run up to the olfactory bulbs underneath the frontal lobe of the BRAIN, and here the impulse is translated into what we describe as smell.

SMOKE INHALATION Smoke is made up of small particles of carbon in hot air and gases. The particles are covered with organic chemicals and smoke may also contain carbon monoxide and acids. When smoke is inhaled the effects on breathing may be immediate or delayed depending on the density of smoke and its composition. Laryngeal stridor (obstruction of the larynx), lack of oxygen and PULMONARY OEDEMA are life-threatening symptoms that require urgent treatment. Immediate removal of the victim from the smoke is imperative, as is the administration of oxygen. The victim may require admission to an intensive-care unit.

SMOKING (see TOBACCO).

SMOOTH MUSCLE Muscle under the 'involuntary' control of the central nervous system (see MUSCLE).

SNAKE-BITE (see BITES AND STINGS).

SNEEZING A sudden expulsion of air through the nose, designed to expel irritating materials from the upper air passages. In sneezing, a powerful expiratory effort is made, the vocal cords are kept shut till the pressure in the chest has risen high, and air is then suddenly allowed to escape upward, being directed into the back of the nose by the soft palate. One sneeze projects 10,000 to 100,000 droplets a distance of up to 10 metres at a rate of over 60 kilometres an hour. As such droplets may contain micro-organisms, it is clear what an important part sneezing plays in transmitting infections such as the common cold. Though usually transitory, sneezing may persist for days on end – up to 204 days have been recorded.

Sneezing may be caused by the presence of irritating particles in the nose, such as snuff, the pollen of grasses and flowers. It is also an early symptom of COLDS, INFLUENZA, MEASLES, and HAY-FEVER, being then accompanied or followed by running at the nose.

SNELLEN CHART The most commonly used chart for testing the acuity of distant vision. The chart comprises rows of capital letters with the letters in each row being smaller than the one above. The top line of large letters can be seen by a normally sighted person standing 60 metres away. The subject under test sits six metres from the screen and, if he can read the six metre line of letters, his visual acuity is normal at 6/6 (see VISION).

SNORING This is usually attributed to vibrations of the soft PALATE, but there is evidence that the main fault lies in the edge of the posterior pillars of the FAUCES which vibrate noisily. Mouth breathing is necessary for snoring, but not all mouth-breathers snore. The principal cause is blockage of the nose, such as occurs during the course of the common cold or chronic nasal catarrh. Such blockage also occurs in some cases of deviation of the nasal septum or nasal polypi. (See NOSE, DISEASES OF.) In children, mouth-breathing, with resulting snoring, is often due to enlarged TONSILS and ADENOIDS. A further cause of snoring is loss of tone in the soft palate and surrounding tissues due to smoking, overwork, fatigue, obesity, and general poor health. One in eight people are said to snore regularly. The intensity, or loudness, of snoring is in the range, 40 to 69 decibels. (Pneumatic drills register between 70 and 90 decibels.) Snoring sometimes alternates with bouts of sleep APNOEA.

Treatment therefore consists of the removal of any of these causes of mouth-breathing that may be present. Should these not succeed in preventing snoring, then measures should be taken to prevent the victim from sleeping lying on his back, as this is a habit which strongly conduces to snoring. Simple measures include sleeping with several pillows so that the head is raised quite considerably when asleep. Alternatively, a small pillow may be put under the nape of the neck. If all these measures fail it may be worth trying the traditional method of sewing a hair-brush, or some other hard object such as a stone, into the back of the snorer's pyjamas. Thus, if victims turn on their back, they are quickly awakened. (See also STERTOR.)

SNOW BLINDNESS Damage caused to the cornea of an unprotected eye by the reflection of the sun's rays from snow. Ultraviolet light is the damaging agent and people going out in snow and sunlight should wear protective goggles. The condition is painful but resolves if the eyes are covered with pads for a day or two. Prolonged exposure may seriously damage the cornea and impair vision.

SNUFFLES The traditional name applied to noisy breathing in children due to the constant presence of nasal discharge. (For treatment, see NOSE, DISEASES OF.)

SOCIAL CLASSES As factors such as the cause of death and the incidence of diseases vary in different social strata, the Registrar-General evolved the following social classification, which has now been in official use for many years:

Class I Professional occupations, such as lawyers, clergymen, and commissioned officers in the Armed Forces.

Class II Intermediate occupations, such as teachers, managers and nurses.

Class III N Non-manual – for example, clerical workers.

Class III M Skilled manual occupations such as miners and bricklayers.

Class IV Partly skilled occupations, such as agricultural workers.

Class V Unskilled occupations, such as building and dock labourers.

SODIUM A metal, the salts of which are white, crystalline, and very soluble. The fluids of the body contain naturally a considerable quantity of sodium chloride.

Sodium carbonate, commonly known as soda or washing soda, has a powerful softening action upon the tissues.

Sodium bicarbonate, or baking soda, is used as an antacid in relieving indigestion associated with increased acidity of the gastric secretion.

The citrate and the acetate of sodium are used as diuretics.

SODIUM CHLORIDE The chemical name for common salt.

SODIUM CROMOGLYCATE The main drug used in the prophylaxis of asthma. It is administered by inhalation and can reduce the incidence of asthmatic attacks but is of no value in the treatment of an acute attack. It acts by preventing the release of pharmacological mediators of bronchospasm, particularly histamine, by stabilizing mastcell membranes. It is thus of particular use in patients whose asthma has an allergic basis and children over four may respond better than adults. The dose frequency is adjusted to the patient's response but is usually administered by inhalation four times daily. Sodium cromoglycate is also used in the prophylaxis of allergic RHINITIS and to treat allergic conjunctivitis. (See ASTHMA.)

SODIUM DIATRIZOATE An organic iodine salt that is radio- opaque and is therefore used as a contrast medium to outline various organs in the body in X-ray films. It is given intravenously. Its main use is in PYELOGRAPHY, that is in rendering the kidneys radio-opaque, but it is also used to outline the blood-vessels (angiography) and the gall-bladder and bile ducts (cholangiography).

SODIUM HYPOCHLORITE is a disinfectant by virtue of the fact that it gives off chlorine. For domestic use, as, for example, for sterilizing baby feeding bottles, it is available in a variety of proprietary preparations.

SODIUM VALPROATE A drug of first choice for the treatment of several forms of EPILEPSY, including primary generalized epilepsy, generalized absences and myoclonic SEIZURES and may be tried in atypical absence, atonic and tonic seizures. Usually taken orally, the drug has shown promising initial results from controlled trials in partial epilepsy. It probably has similar efficacy to CARBAMAZEPINE and PHENYTOIN. The drug has widespread metabolic effects and may have dose-related side-effects. There has been concern over severe hepatic or pancreatic toxicity, but such adverse effects are rare. Other adverse effects include digestive upsets, drowsiness, muscle incoordination and skin rashes. Rare reports have been given of behavioural disturbances, with occasional aggression. Initiation and withdrawal of treatment should always be slow. Patients should reduce their alcohol intake; and any other drugs they are taking that are metabolized by the liver should be carefully monitored.

SODOMY Sexual intercourse in which the penis penetrates the anus and rectum. Sodomy may occur between men, between a man and a woman or between a man and an animal (bestiality).

SOLAR PLEXUS A large network of sympathetic nerves and ganglia situated in the abdomen behind the stomach, where it surrounds the coeliac artery. Branches of the vagus nerve, the most important part of the parasympathetic system, lead into the solar plexus, which in turn distributes branches to the stomach, intestines and several other abdominal organs. A severe blow in the solar plexus may cause temporary unconsciousness.

SOLUTION A liquid preparation containing one or more soluble drugs, usually dissolved in water.

SOLVENT ABUSE or MISUSE Also known as volatile-substance abuse, this is the deliberate inhalation of intoxicating fumes given off by some volatile liquids. Glue sniffing was the most common type of solvent abuse, but inhalation of fuel gases such as butane, especially in the form of lighter refills, is now the major problem in the United Kingdom. The problem has become common among children, particularly teenagers. Solvents or volatile substances are applied to a piece of cloth or put into a plastic bag and inhaled, sometimes until the person loses consciousness. He or she may become acutely intoxicated; chronic abusers may suffer from ulcers and rashes over the face as well as damage to peripheral nerves. Death can occur, probably as a result of an abnormal rhythm of the heart. Tolerance to the volatile substances may develop over months, but acute intoxication may lead to aggressive and impulsive behaviour. Treatment of addiction is difficult and requires professional counselling.

Victims with acute symptoms require urgent medical attention. In Britain most solvent misusers are males under 20 years of age. Around 150 deaths occur every year. (See ADDICTION; DRUG ADDICTION.)

SOMATIC Relating to the body, as opposed to the mind.

SOMATOSTASIN Also known as the growth-hormone-release-inhibiting factor, this is a hormone secreted by the HYPOTHALAMUS and some non-nervous tissues (including the gastrointestinal tract and pancreas). It stops the pituitary releasing somatotrophin – growth hormone. Somatostasin and growth-hormone-releasing hormone are controlled by complicated neural mechanisms linked to exercise, sleep patterns, stress, NEUROTRANSMITTERS and blood GLUCOSE.

SOMATOTYPE The physical build of a person. Attempts have been made to link body build with personality type but with no great success. One approach is to classify people as endomorphs (heavy physique and sociable personality); mesomorphs (strong, muscular build with well-developed bones linked with a physically adventurous temperament); and ectomorphs (thin and lightly built with an introspective nature).

SOMNAMBULISM Sleep-walking. (See SLEEP.)

SOPORIFICS are measures which induce sleep. (See HYPNOTICS.)

SORE is a popular term for ULCER.

SORE THROAT A raw sensation at the back of the throat. A common symptom, the cause is usually PHARYNGITIS, sometimes TONSILLITIS. It is often the presenting symptom of colds, INFLUENZA, LARYNGITIS and infectious MONONUCLEOSIS. Sore throats caused by STREPTOCOCCAL infection should be treated with antibiotics as should other bacteria-initiated sore throats. Otherwise symptomatic treatment with analgesics and antiseptic gargles is sufficient for this usually self-limiting condition.

SOTALOL (see ADRENERGIC RECEPTORS).

SOUND A rod with a curve at one end used to explore body cavities such as the bladder or to dilate strictures in the urethra or other channels in the body. (See URINARY BLADDER, DISEASES OF.)

SOUTHEY'S TUBES Long, fine tubes for drawing off fluid slowly from the tissues (usually from the legs) in patients with oedema. The procedure, introduced by a Dr Southey in the 19th Century, is rarely used now. (See ASPIRATION.)

SOYA BEAN The bean of *Glycine soja*, a leguminous plant related to peas and beans. The outstanding characteristic of the soya bean is its high protein and fat content. There is an almost complete absence of starch, but a large amount of mineral matter. Soya flour contains 40 per cent of protein and 20 per cent of fat. It yields 470 Calories per 100 grams as compared with 370 Calories for white wheat flour. Soya flour contains 0·2 per cent of calcium (about ten times as much as in white flour). It also contains a variable but large amount of iron: 6·7 to 30 mg per 100 grams of soya flour compared with 1 mg in white flour and 3 mg in 100 grams of wholemeal flour. It is a good source of thiamine and riboflavine, and of vitamin A in the form of carotene.

SPACE MEDICINE A medical specialty dealing with the physiological, PSYCHOLOGICAL and pathological consequences of space flight in which the body has to cope with unusual variations in gravitational forces, including weightlessness, a constricted environment, prolonged close contact with work colleagues in very demanding technical circumstances and sustained periods of emotional pressure including fear. Enormous progress has been made in providing astronauts with as normal environment as possible, and they have to undergo prolonged physical and mental training before embarking on space travel.

SPANISH FLY A popular term for cantharides, which is used as a blistering agent. (See CANTHARIDES.)

SPASM An involuntary, and, in severe cases, painful contraction of a muscle or of a hollow organ with a muscular wall. Spasm may be due to affections in the muscle where the spasm takes place, or it may originate in some disturbance of that part of the nervous system which controls the spasmodically acting muscles. Spasms of a general nature are usually spoken of as convulsions; spasms of a painful nature are known as cramp when they affect the muscles of the limbs, and as colic when they are situated in the STOMACH, INTESTINES, URETERS or BILE DUCT, or other organs of the abdomen. Spasm of the heart is called angina pectoris, and is both a serious and an agonizing condition. When the spasm is a prolonged firm contraction, it is spoken of as tonic spasm; when it consists of a series of twitches or quick alternate contractions and relaxations, it is known as clonic spasm. Spasm is a symptom of many diseases.

SPASMODIC TORTICOLLIS A chronic condition in which the neck is rotated or deviated laterally, forwards, or backwards, often with additional jerking or tremor. It is a form of focal dystonia, and should not be confused with the far commoner transient condition of acute painful wry-neck. (See DYSTONIA.)

SPASTIC A term applied to any condition showing increased muscle tone: e.g. spastic gait. This is specially associated with some disease affecting the upper part of the nervous system connected with movement (upper neuron), so that its controlling influence is lost and the muscles become overexcitable.

SPASTIC COLON (see IRRITABLE BOWEL SYNDROME).

SPATULA A flat, knife-like instrument used for spreading plasters and ointments, and also for depressing the tongue when the throat is being examined.

SPECIALIST A doctor or other health professional who has trained to develop a particular skill such as surgery, cardiac medicine, accident and emergency care, care of the ageing, physiotherapy or radiology. As new medical techniques and treatments ae developed, so new specialties evolve to provide them. Specialists have to pass recognized examinations as well as be certfied that they have undergone appropriate education and hands-on training. Specialists, once qualified, are expected to continue their education and training to ensure that their skills are kept up to date. For doctors, the General Medical Council, which is responsible for overseeing the training and registration of all medical doctors in the UK, also notes in its annual *Medical Register* those doctors who have completed appropriate specialist training. Doctors who have qualified and trained overseas have to pass appropriate GMC tests before they can practise in the UK.

SPECIFICITY An epidemiological term describing the extent to which a SCREENING TEST for the presence of the precursors of disease – e.g. premalignant cells in the cervix – throws up false positives. A specific test has few false positives.

SPECULUM An instrument designed to aid the examination of the various openings on the surface of the body. Many specula are provided with small electric lamps so placed as to light up the cavity.

SPEECH DISORDERS These may be of physical or psychological origin – or a combination of both. Difficulties may arise at various stages of development: due to problems during pregnancy, at birth, childhood illnesses, or delayed development. Congenital defects such as CLEFT PALATE or lip may make speech unintelligible until major surgery is performed, thus discouraging talking and delaying development. Recurrent ear infections may make hearing difficult; the child's experience of speech is thus limited, with similar results. Childhood DYSPHASIA occurs if the language development area of the brain develops abnormally; specialist education and SPEECH THERAPY may then be required.

Dumbness is the inability to pronounce the sounds that make up words. Deafness is the most important cause, being due to a congenital brain defect, or acquired brain disease, such as tertiary SYPHILIS. When hearing is normal or only mildly impaired, dumbness may be due to a structural defect such as tongue-tie or enlarged tonsils and adenoids, or to inefficient voice control, resulting in lisping or lalling. Increased tension is a common cause of STAMMERING; speech disorders may occasionally be a hysterical manifestation.

Normal speech may be lost in adulthood (see DYSPHASIA) as a result of a STROKE or head injury. Excessive use of the voice may be an occupational hazard; and throat cancer may require a LARYNGECTOMY, with subsequent help in communication. Severe psychiatric disturbance may be accompanied by impaired social and communication skills (see VOICE AND SPEECH).

Treatment The underlying cause of the problem should be diagnosed as early as possible; psychological and other specialist investigations should be carried out as required, and any physical defect should be repaired. People who are deaf and unable to speak should start training in lip-reading as soon as possible, and special educational methods aimed at acquiring a modulated voice should similarly be started in early childhood, provided by the local authority, and continued as required. Various types of speech therapy or PSYCHOTHERAPY may be appropriate, alone or in conjunction with other treatments, and often the final result may be highly satisfying, with a good command of language and speech being obtained.

Help and advice may be obtained from AFASIC (Overcoming Speech Impairment) (see APPENDIX 2: ADDRESSES).

SPEECH THERAPY Professionally trained speech therapists assist, diagnose and treat the whole spectrum of acquired or developmental communication disorders. They work in medical and education establishments often in an advisory or consultative capacity. The medical conditions in which speech therapy is employed include: dysgraphia, DYSLEXIA, DYSARTHRIA, DYSPHASIA, DYSPHONIA, DYSPRAXIA, AUTISM, BELL'S PALSY, CEREBRAL PALSY, DEAFNESS, disordered language, delayed speech, disordered speech, DOWN'S SYNDROME, LARYNGECTOMY, LEARNING DISABILITIES, MACROGLOSSIA, MOTOR NEURONE DISEASE, malformations of the palate, PARKINSONISM, PSYCHIATRIC DISORDERS, STAMMERING, STROKE and disorders of voice production.

Speech therapists forms a small independent undergraduate profession, most of whom work for the National Health Service in community clinics, general practices and hospitals. They may also work in schools or in units for the handicapped, paediatric assessment centres, language units attached to primary schools, adult training centres and day centres for the elderly.

A speech therapist undergoes a four-year degree course which covers the study of disorders of communication in children and adults, phonetics and linguistics, anatomy and physiology, psychology and many other related subjects. Further information on training can be obtained from the College of Speech Therapists (see APPENDIX 2: ADDRESSES).

If the parents of a child are concerned about their child's speech, they may approach a speech therapist for assessment and guidance. Their general practitioner will be able to give them local addresses or they should contact the district speech therapist. Adults are usually referred by hospital consultants.

The College of Speech Therapists keeps a register of all those who have passed a recognized degree or equivalent qualification in speech therapy. It will be able to direct you to your nearest NHS or private speech therapist.

SPERMATIC The name applied to the blood-vessels and other structures associated with the testicle.

SPERMATORRHOEA The passage of semen without erection of the PENIS or ORGASM.

SPERMATOZOON (plural: SPERMATOZOA) This is the male sex or germ cell which unites with the OVUM to form the EMBRYO or fetus. It is a highly mobile cell approximately 4 micrometres in length, much smaller than an ovum, which is about 35 micrometres in diameter. Each millilitre of SEMEN contains on average about 100 million spermatozoa, and the average volume of semen discharged during ejaculation in sexual intercourse is between 2 and 4 ml. (Some recent research suggests that male fertility is falling because of a reduction in the production of viable spermatozoa, possibly due to environmental factors including the discharge of hormones used for agricultural purposes.) Once ejaculated during intercourse it travels at a rate of 1·5 to 3 millimetres a minute and remains mobile for several days after insemination, but quickly loses its potency for fertilization. As it takes only about 70 minutes to reach the ovarian end of the uterine tube, it is assumed that there must be factors other than its own mobility, such as contraction of the muscle of the womb and uterine tube, that speed it on its way. (See also FETUS.)

SPERMICIDE Contraceptive preparations that kill sperm. They may be in the form of gels, pessaries, cream, or foam and should be used with a barrier contraceptive such as a diaphragm or a condom.

SPHAGNUM MOSS   Peat or bog moss, has been used as a wound dressing from time immemorial. A skeleton from the Bronze Age in Scotland showed a large pad of sphagnum moss applied to what had been a chest wound. It was used on a large scale as a wound dressing in the 1914–18 War. It is widely distributed in Scotland, Ireland and Western England. Its main value lies in its great absorptive powers: it can absorb up to seven times its weight of water. It is deodorizing and does not allow discharges from wounds to pass through it as does cotton wool.

SPHENOID   A bone lying in the centre of the base of the skull, and supporting the others like a wedge or keystone. (See SKULL.)

SPHINCTER   A circular muscle which surrounds the opening from an organ, and, by maintaining a constant state of moderate contraction, prevents the escape of the contents of the organ. Sphincters close the outlet from the BLADDER and RECTUM, and in certain nervous diseases their action is interfered with, so that the power to relax or to keep moderately contracted is lost, and retention or incontinence of the evacuation results.

SPHYGMOGRAPH   An instrument for recording the pulse. (See PULSE.)

SPHYGMOMANOMETER is the name of an instrument for measuring BLOOD-PRESSURE in the arteries. It usually consists of a pneumatic armlet, the interior of which communicates by a rubber tube with an air-pressure pump and a gauge. The armlet is bound about the upper arm and pumped up sufficiently to obliterate the pulse as felt at the wrist or as heard in the artery at the bend of the elbow. The pressure – measured in mm of mercury – registered on the gauge at this point is regarded as the pressure of the blood at each heart-beat (systolic pressure). The pressure at which the sound heard in the artery suddenly changes its character marks the diastolic pressure.

SPINA BIFIDA   This is one of the commonest of the congenital malformations. It is one of the three types of neural tube anomaly, the other two being anencephaly and cranium bifidum. It takes two main forms, spina bifida occulta – said to affect about one in ten individuals – being much the commoner. There is a deficit in the posterior part of the spinal column, usually in the lumbar region, and it is generally asymptomatic, unless the underlying spinal cord is affected. Occasionally it is associated with a hairy patch or birth mark on the back, and a few children develop a mild spastic gait or bladder problems.

Much more serious is spina bifida cystica, in which the spinal wall defect is accompanied by a protrusion of the spinal cord. This may take two forms: a meningocele, in which the MENINGES, containing CEREBROSPINAL FLUID, protrude through the defect; and a meningomyelocele, in which the protrusion contains spinal cord and nerves. Meningocele is less common and has a good prognosis. HYDROCEPHALUS and neurological problems affecting the legs are rare, though the bladder may be affected. Treatment consists of surgery in the first few days of life; long-term follow-up is necessary to pick up any neurological problems that may develop during subsequent growth of the spine. Meningomyelocele is much more serious and more common, accounting for 90 per cent of all cases. Usually affecting the lumbo-sacral region, the range of severity may vary considerably and, while early surgery with careful attention in a minor case may achieve good mobility, normal bladder function and intellect, a more extensive protrusion may cause complete anaesthesia of the skin, with increased risk of trauma, extensive paralysis of the trunk and limbs, with severe deformities, and paralysis and insensitivity of the bladder and bowel. Involuntary movements may be present, and hydrocephalus occurs in 80 per cent of cases.

The decision to operate can only be made after a full examination of the infant to determine the extent of the defect and any coexistent congenital abnormalities. The child's potential can then be estimated, and appropriate treatment discussed with the parents. Carefully selected patients should receive long-term treatment in a special centre, where full attention can be paid to all their various problems.

There is growing evidence of the value of vitamin supplements before and during pregnancy in reducing the incidence of spina bifida. Parents of affected infants may obtain help, advice, and encouragement from the Association for Spina Bifida and Hydrocephalus which has branches throughout the country, or the Scottish Spina Bifida Association (see APPENDIX 2: ADDRESSES).

SPINAL ANAESTHESIA (see ANAESTHESIA).

SPINAL COLUMN also known as the SPINE, BACKBONE, and VERTEBRAL COLUMN, this forms an important part of the skeleton, acting both as the rigid pillar which supports the upper parts of the body and as a protection to the spinal cord and nerves arising from it. The spinal column is built up of a number of bones placed one upon another, which, in consequence of having a slight degree of turning-movement, are known as the vertebrae. The possession of a spinal cord supported by a vertebral column distinguishes the higher animals from the lower types, and is why they are called vertebrates. Of the vertebrates, man alone stands absolutely erect, and this erect carriage of the body gives to the skull and vertebral column certain distinctive characters.

The human backbone is about 70 cm (28 inches) in length, and varies little in full-grown people; differences in height depend mainly

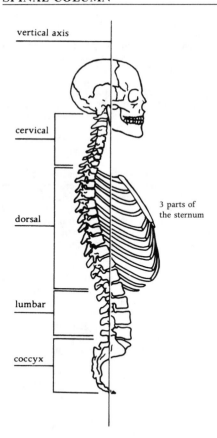

vertical axis

cervical

dorsal

3 parts of
the sternum

lumbar

coccyx

The spinal column.

felt beneath the skin of the back lying in the centre of a groove between the muscular masses of the two sides, and they give to the column its name of the spinal column. One of these spines, that of the 7th cervical vertebra, is especially large and forms a distinct bony prominence, where the neck joins the back. Between the bodies of the vertebrae lies a series of thick discs of fibro-cartilage known as intervertebral discs. Each disc consists of an outer portion, known as the annulus fibrosus, and an inner core, known as the nucleus pulposus. These 23 discs provide the upper part of the spine with pliability and resiliance.

The first and second cervical vertebrae are specially modified. The first vertebra, known as the atlas, is devoid of a body, but has a specially large and strong ring with two hollows upon which the skull rests, thus allowing forward and

upon the length of the lower limbs. The number of vertebrae is 33 in children, although in adult life 5 of these fuse together to form the sacrum, and the lowest 4 unite in the coccyx, so that the number of separate bones is reduced to 26. Of these there are 7 in the neck, known therefore as cervical vertebrae; 12 with ribs attached, in the region of the thorax, and known as thoracic or dorsal vertebrae; 5 in the loins, called lumbar vertebrae; 5 fused to form the sacrum; and 4 joined in the coccyx. These numbers are expressed in a formula thus: C7, D12, L5, S5, Coc4 = 33. Although the vertebrae in each of these regions have distinguishing features, all the vertebrae are constructed on the same general plan. Each has a thick, rounded, bony part in front, known as the body, and these bodies form the main thickness of the column. Behind the body of each is a ring of bone, the neural ring, these rings placed one above another forming the bony canal which lodges the spinal cord. From each side of the ring a short process of bone known as the transverse process stands out, and from the back of the ring a larger process, the spinous process, projects. These processes give attachment to the strong ligaments and muscles which unite, support, and bend the column. The spines can be seen or

1 neural ring
2 articular process
3 transverse process
4 spinous process
5 body of vertebra

The atlas (1st cervical vertebra) and axis (2nd cervical vertebra) vertebrae and a lumbar vertebra seen from above.

backward movements (nodding). The second vertebra, known as the axis, has a pivot on its body which fits into the first vertebra and thus allows free rotation of the head from side to side. The spinal column has four natural curves (see diagram) which help to cushion the shocks of walking and running.

The neural rings of the vertebrae form a canal, which is wide in the neck, smaller and almost round in the dorsal region, and wide again in the lumbar vertebrae. Down the canal runs the spinal cord, and the nerves leaving the cord do so through openings between the vertebrae which are produced by notches on the upper and lower margins of each ring. The intervertebral foramina formed by these notches are so large in comparison with the nerves passing through them that there is no chance of pressure upon the latter, except in very serious injuries which dislocate and fracture the spine.

SPINAL CORD This is the lower portion of the central nervous system which is situated within the spinal column. Above, it forms the direct continuation of the medulla oblongata, this part of the brain changing its name to spinal cord at the foramen magnum, the large opening in the base of the skull through which it passes into the spinal canal. Below, the spinal cord extends to about the upper border of the second lumbar vertebra, where it tapers off into a fine thread, known as the filum terminale,

1 dura mater
2 arachnoid
3 spinal ganglion
4 ventral nerve root
5 dura mater, cut and turned backwards
6 ligamentum denticulatum

The membranes of the spinal cord.

that is attached to the coccyx at the lower end of the spine. The spinal cord is thus considerably shorter than the spinal column, being only 37 to 45 cm (15 to 18 inches) in length, and

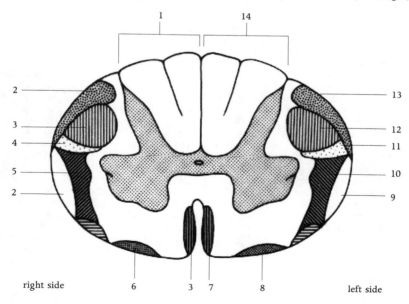

1 conscious muscle sense, direct touch
2 unconscious muscle sense
3 voluntary control of striated muscle
4 involuntary control of striated muscle
5 pain, heat and cold
6 crossed touch
7 ventral corticospinal tract (pyramidal)

8 ventral spinothalamic tract
9 ventral spinocerebellar tract
10 lateral spinothalamic tract
11 rubrospinal tract (extrapyramidal)
12 lateral corticospinal tract (pyramidal)
13 dorsal spinocerebellar tract
14 posterior columns

Cross-section of spinal cord at level of 5th thoracic vertebra.

weighing around 30 grams. In its course from the base of the skull to the lumbar region the cord gives off thirty-one nerves on each side, each of which arises by an anterior and a posterior root that join before the nerve emerges from the spinal canal. The openings for the nerves formed by notches on the ring of each vertebra have been mentioned under SPINAL COLUMN. To reach these openings the upper nerves pass almost directly outwards, whilst lower down their obliquity increases, until below the point where the cord ends there is a sheaf of nerves, known as the cauda equina, running downwards to leave the spinal canal at their appropriate openings. The cord is a cylinder, about the thickness of the little finger. It has two slightly enlarged portions, one in the lower part of the neck, the other at the last dorsal vertebra, and from these thickenings arise the nerves that pass to the upper and lower limbs. (See NERVES.)

The spinal cord, like the brain, is surrounded by three membranes, the dura mater, arachnoid mater, and pia mater, from without inwards. The arrangement of the dura and arachnoid is much looser in the case of the cord than their application to the brain. The dura especially forms a wide tube which is separated from the cord by fluid and from the vertebral canal by blood-vessels and fat, this arrangement protecting the cord from pressure in any ordinary movements of the spine.

In section the spinal cord consists partly of grey, but mainly of white, matter. It differs from the upper parts of the brain in that the white matter in the cord is arranged on the surface, surrounding a mass of grey matter, while in the brain the grey matter is superficial. The arrangement of grey matter, as seen in a section across the cord, resembles the letter H. Each half of the cord possesses an anterior and a posterior horn, and the masses of the two sides being joined by a wide posterior grey commissure. In the middle of this commissure lies the central canal of the cord, a small tube which is the continuation of the ventricles in the brain. The horns of grey matter reach almost to the surface of the cord, and from their ends arise the roots of the nerves that leave the cord. The white matter is divided almost completely into two halves by a posterior septum and anterior fissure and is further split into anterior, lateral and posterior columns.

Functions   The cord is, in part, a receiver and originator of nerve impulses, and in part a conductor of such impulses along fibres which pass through it to and from the brain. The cord contains centres able to receive sensory impressions and initiate motor instructions. These control blood-vessel diameters, eye-pupil size, sweating and breathing. The brain exerts an overall controlling influence and, before any incoming sensation can affect consciousness, it is usually 'filtered' through the brain.

Many of these centres act autonomously. Other cells of the cord are capable of originating movements in response to impulses brought direct to them through sensory nerves, such activity being known as reflex action. (For a fuller description of the activities of the spinal cord, see NERVES.)

The posterior column of the cord consists of the fasciculus gracilis and the fasciculus cuneatus, both conveying sensory impressions upwards. The lateral column contains the ventral and the dorsal spino-cerebellar tracts passing to the cerebellum, the crossed pyramidal tract of motor fibres carrying outgoing impulses downwards together with the rubro-spinal, the spino-thalamic, the spino-tectal, and the postero-lateral tracts. And, finally, the anterior column contains the direct pyramidal tract of motor fibres and an anterior mixed zone. The pyramidal tracts have the best-known course. Starting from cells near the central sulcus on the brain (see BRAIN), the motor nerve-fibres run down through the internal capsule, pons, and medulla, in the lower part of which many of those coming from the right side of the brain cross to the left side of the spinal cord, and vice versa. Thence the fibres run down in the crossed pyramidal tract to end beside nerve-cells in the anterior horn of the cord. From these nerve-cells other fibres pass outwards to form the nerves that go direct to the muscles. Thus the motor nerve path from brain to muscle is divided into two sections of neurons, of which the upper exerts a controlling influence upon the lower, while the lower is concerned in maintaining the muscle in a state of health and good nutrition, and in directly calling it into action.

SPINE AND SPINAL CORD, DISEASES AND INJURIES OF   SCOLIOSIS is a condition where the spine is curved to one side. The spine is normally straight when seen from behind. The deformity may be mobile and reversible or fixed. If fixed, it is accompanied by vertebral rotation and does not disappear with changes in posture. Fixed scoliosis is IDIOPATHIC in 65–80 per cent of cases. There are three main types. The infantile type occurs in boys under three and in 90 per cent of cases resolves spontaneously. The juvenile type affects 4-to-9-year-olds and tends to be progressive. The commonest is adolescent idiopathic scoliosis. Girls are affected in 90 per cent of cases and the incidence is 4 per cent. Treatment may be conservative with a fixed brace, or surgical fusion may be needed if the curve is greater than 45 degrees. Scoliosis can occur as a congenital condition and in neuromuscular diseases where there is muscle imbalance such as FRIEDREICH'S ATAXIA.

Kyphosis is a backward curvature of the spine causing a hump back. It may be postural and reversible in obese people and tall adolescent girls who stoop but it may be fixed. Scheuermann's disease is the term applied to adolescent kyphosis. It is more common in girls. Senile kyphosis occurs in elderly people who probably have OSTEOPOROSIS (bone weakening) and vertebral collapse.

Disc degeneration is a normal consequence of ageing. The disc loses its resilience and becomes unable to withstand pressure. Rupture (prolapse) of the disc may occur with physical stress. The disc between the fourth and fifth lumbar vertebrae is most commonly involved. The jelly-like central nucleus pulposus is usually pushed out backwards, forcing the annulus fibrosus to put pressure on the nerves as they leave the spinal canal. (See PROLAPSED INTERVERTEBRAL DISC.)

Pain is felt in the back and in the distribution of the compressed nerve. If the disc prolapses forwards into the centre of the spinal canal, it may compress the cauda equina.

Treatment is bed rest with traction and pain relief. Rarely removal of the disc is needed. Compression of the cauda equina is a surgical emergency.

Ankylosing spondylitis is a rheumatic disease of young adults, mostly men. It is a familial condition which starts with lumbar pain and stiffness which progresses to involve the whole spine. The discs and ligaments are replaced by fibrous tissue making the spine rigid. Treatment is physiotherapy and anti-inflammatory drugs to try to keep the spine supple for as long as possible.

A National Association for Ankylosing Spondylitis has been formed which is open to those with the disease, their families, friends and doctors. (See APPENDIX 2: ADDRESSES.)

Spondylosis is a term which covers disc degeneration and joint degeneration in the back. Osteoarthritis is usually implicated. Pain is commonly felt in the neck and lumbar regions and in these areas the joints may become unstable. This may put pressure on the nerves leaving the spinal canal and in the lumbar region pain is generally felt in the distribution of the sciatic nerve – down the back of the leg. In the neck the pain may be felt down the arm. Treatment is physiotherapy; often a neck collar or lumbar support helps. Rarely surgery is needed to remove the pressure from the nerves.

Spondylolisthesis means that the spine is shifted forward. This is nearly always in the lower lumbar region and may be familial, or due to degeneration in the joints. Pressure may be put on the cauda equina. The usual complaint is of pain after exercise. Treatment is bed rest in a bad attack with surgery indicated only if there are worrying signs of cord compression.

Spinal stenosis is due to a narrowing of the spinal canal which means that the nerves become squashed together. This causes numbness with pins and needles (paraesthia) in the legs. Computed tomography and nuclear magnetic resonance imaging scans can show the amount of cord compression. If improving posture does not help, surgical decompression may be needed.

Whiplash injuries occur to the neck usually as the result of a car accident when the head and neck are thrown backwards and then forwards rapidly. This causes pain and stiffness in the

neck and the arm and shoulder may feel numb. Often a support collar relieves the pain but recovery commonly takes between 18 months to three years.

Transection of the cord occurs usually as a result of trauma when the vertebral column protecting the spinal cord is fractured and becomes unstable. The cord may be concussed or it may have become sheared by the trauma and not recover (transected). Spinal concussion usually recovers after 12 hours. If the cord is transected the patient remains paralysed.

SPIRAMYCIN A MACROLIDE antibiotic isolated from *Streptomyces ambofaciens* which is useful for some STAPHYLOCOCCAL infections. Although it is not yet on the UK market, there have been encouraging results with spiramycin for the treatment of TOXOPLASMOSIS.

SPIRILLUM A form of micro-organism of wavy or spiral shape. (See MICROBIOLOGY.)

SPIRIT A strong solution of alcohol in water. (See ALCOHOL.) Proof spirit is one containing 57 per cent of alcohol by volume or 49 per cent by weight, and is so named because it can stand the proof of just catching fire. Rectified spirit contains 90 per cent of alcohol by volume or over 85 per cent by weight. Proof spirit is generally used in the preparation of tinctures. Spirits of various drugs contain a solution of any given drug in rectified spirit, examples include aromatic spirit of ammonia (sal volatile), and spirit of ether. Methylated spirit (also known as wood naphtha or wood spirit) is distilled from wood. When taken internally, it is a dangerous poison producing neuritis, especially neuritis of the optic nerves which may result in blindness. Methylated spirit is used to harden the skin for the prevention of bed sores and foot soreness.

SPIRITUAL PAIN Spiritual pain is what may be felt when one of a person's four key spiritual relationships (to other people, to oneself, to the world around or to 'Life' itself) is traumatized or broken. A bad trauma in one of the first three relationships can lead to damage to the last of them, that of the relationships to Life itself. For example, a wife deserted by her husband for another woman may not only feel devastated by the loss of her partner around the place but may also feel a pain caused by the shattering of her beliefs about life (about faithfulness, hope, love, security, etc.). It is as if there is a picture at the centre of each person of what life should be about – whether or not held in a frame by a belief in God – and as if this picture has been smashed by the particular trauma. Nothing makes sense any more. The individual cannot get things together. Everything has lost its meaning. This shattering of someone's picture of life is the source of the deepest pain in any spiritual trauma. The connection is often made between spiritual pain and meaningless-ness. If the shattering of the picture on the other hand is done by the individual, for instance by breaking his or her own moral or religious code, the pain may take the form of guilt and associated feelings. Hence the thera-pist will be intent upon helping a client to recognize and come to terms with this 'pain beneath the pain'.

SPIROCHAETE   An order of bacteria which has a spiral form.

SPIROMETER   A device to test how the lung is working (pulmonary function) to assess the effects of lung disease or the progress of treatment, a procedure called spirometry. The spirometer records the total volume of air breathed out – the forced vital capacity. The machine also records the volume of air breathed out in one second – the forced expiratory volume. In diseases such as asthma, in which the airways are obstructed, the ratio of the forced expiratory volume to the forced vital capacity is reduced. (See RESPIRATION.)

SPIRONOLACTONE   One of the group of substances known as spirolactones. These are steroids similar to ALDOSTERONE in structure which competitively act as inhibitors of it. They can thus antagonize the action of aldosterone in the renal tubules. As there is evidence that there is an increased output of aldosterone in oede-matous conditions, such as congestive heart failure, which accentuates the oedema, spironol-actone is used, along with other diuretics, in

resistant cases of oedema – to antagonize the fluid-retaining action of aldosterone. (See DIURETICS.)

SPLANCHNIC   Anything belonging to the internal organs of the body as distinguished from its framework.

SPLEEN   An organ deeply placed in the abdomen and a major constituent of the RETICULO-ENDOTHELIAL SYSTEM.

Position and size   The spleen lies behind the stomach, high up on the left side of the abdomen, and corresponds to the position of the 9th, 10th, and 11th ribs, from which it is separated by the diaphragm. It is a soft, highly vascular, plum-coloured organ, and has a smooth surface, being almost completely cov-ered by peritoneum. There are two wide perito-neal ligaments that support the spleen, the one attaching it to the stomach, the other to the kidney. Through the latter ligament the large vessels that supply the spleen with blood make their way. The size of the spleen varies widely. It is usually about 12·5 to 15 cm (5 to 6 inches) in length, and weighs about 170 grams or more. In diseased conditions the organ may reach a weight of 8 to 9 kg.

Structure   The spleen is enveloped by perito-neal membrane beneath which is a strong elastic tunic, composed partly of fibrous tissue containing many elastic fibres, and partly of unstriped muscle. This elastic coat allows of the free expansion and contraction of the organ according to the varying amount of blood present in it. From the inner surface of the

1   oesophagus
2   stomach
3   liver
4   spleen
5   pancreas
6   transverse colon

Position of spleen in relation to other abdominal organs.

1   capsule
2   venous sinuses
3   arterial capillaries ending in sinuses
4   small arteries
5   Malphigi corpuscles
6   artery
7   trabecula of capsule
8   central artery of Malphigi corpuscle
9   vein

Cross-section of cone of tissue from spleen.

membrane fibrous partitions known as trabeculae run down into the substance and form a network in which the dark spleen pulp is contained. The pulp consists of delicate connective tissue fibres passing between the various trabeculae and of white and red blood cells lying in this meshwork. The spleen is very vascular and venous blood leaves by the splenic vein and then enters the portal vein from the liver. There are also numerous lymphatics in the organ, which run in the trabeculae or surround the veins.

Functions The organ produces lymphocytes and acts as a reservoir of red blood cells for use in emergencies. It is also one of the sites for the manufacture of red blood cells in the fetus, but not after birth. Useless or worn-out red and white blood cells and blood platelets are broken up by this organ. This results in the production of BILIRUBIN, which is conveyed to the liver, and of iron, which is used in the bone marrow for the production of new red blood cells.

SPLEEN, DISEASES OF In certain diseases associated with marked changes in the blood, such as leukaemia, and malaria, the spleen becomes chronically enlarged. In some of the acute infectious diseases, it becomes congested and acutely enlarged: for example, in TYPHOID FEVER, ANTHRAX, and infectious MONONUCLEOSIS. Rupture of the spleen may occur, like rupture of other internal organs, in consequence of extreme violence, but in malarious countries, where many people have the spleen

greatly enlarged and softened as the result of malaria, rupture of this organ occurs now and then as the result of some quite trivial blow upon the left side. The spleen, in consequence of its structure, bleeds excessively when torn, so that this accident is generally followed by collapse, signs of internal haemorrhage – and death if not dealt with promptly by operation.

SPLENECTOMY Removal of the spleen. This operation may be necessary if the spleen has been severely injured or in the treatment of the severe form of acholuric jaundice or auto-immune thrombocytopenic purpura. (See PURPURA.)

SPLENOMEGALY Enlargement of the spleen beyond its normal size.

SPLINTER HAEMORRHAGES Linear bleeding under the finger nails. Although it may result from injury they are a useful physical sign of infective endocarditis.

SPLINTS Supports for an injured or wounded part. They are most commonly employed in cases in which a bone is fractured, and consist then of some rigid substance designed to take the place of the broken bone in maintaining the shape of the limb, as well as to keep the broken ends at rest and in contact, and thus to ensure their union. Splints are most commonly made of wood either shaped to the limb or consisting merely of strips of wood about the width of the injured limb, and carefully padded with wool or similar soft material. Splints are also made of metal, poroplastic felt, leather, and cotton stiffened with plaster of Paris, as well as other materials. Splints may be improvized for first-aid out of walking-sticks, rifles, broom-handles, branches, folded-up newspapers, and in fact anything of suitable length and rigidity. (See FRACTURES.)

SPONDYLITIS Another name for arthritis of the spine. (See SPINE AND SPINAL CORD, DISEASES AND INJURIES OF.)

SPONDYLOLISTHESIS (see SPINE AND SPINAL CORD, DISEASES AND INJURIES OF).

SPONDYLOSIS (see SPINE AND SPINAL CORD, DISEASES AND INJURIES OF.)

SPONGIFORM ENCEPHALOPATHY A disease of the neurological system caused by SLOW VIRUS or PRION. Spongy degeneration of the brain with progressive dementia occurs. Known examples of the disorder in humans are Creutzfeldt-Jakob disease (CJD) and kuru. Among animals scrapie in sheep and bovine spongiform encephalopathy (BSE) are caused by slow viruses. The latter has occurred as an outbreak in cattle over the past decade or so, probably as a result of cattle being fed processed offal from infected cattle. A few people are though to have developed a form of CJD from eating infected beef (see BOVINE SPONGIFORM ENCEPHALOPATHY).

SPORADIC   The term applied to cases of disease occurring here and there, as opposed to epidemic outbreaks.

SPORE   Part of the life cycle of certain bacteria when the vegetative cell is encapsulated and metabolism falls to a low level. The spore is resistant to changes in the environment and, when these are unfavourable, the spore remains dormant; when they improve, it starts to grow. Certain dangerous bacteria, such as CLOSTRIDIUM, produce resistant ubiquitous spores so sterilization procedures need to be very effective.

SPOROZOA   The name of a group of parasitic PROTOZOA which includes the parasitic Plasmodium that causes MALARIA. The life cycles of sporozoa are complex, often with sexual and asexual stages.

SPOROZOITES is one cell type of the many that are formed during the life cycle of sporozoans. In the case of MALARIA sporozoites pass into the salivary glands of the mosquito and and are the infecting agent of the human host when the insect next feeds on human blood.

SPORTS MEDICINE   The field of medicine concerned with physical fitness and the diagnosis and treatment of both acute and chronic sports injuries sustained during training and competition. Acute injuries are extremely common in contact sports, and their initial treatment is similar to those sustained in other ways, such as falls and road traffic incidents. Tears of the MUSCLES, CONNECTIVE TISSUES, and LIGAMENTS, which are partial (sprains) are initially treated with rest, ice, compression, and elevation (RICE) of the affected part. Complete tears (rupture) of ligaments (see diagrams) or muscles or fractures require more prolonged immobilization, often in plaster, or surgical intervention may be considered. The rehabilitation of injured athletes requires special expertise – an early graded return to activity gives the best long-term results, but doing too much too soon runs the risk of exacerbating the original injury.

Chronic (overuse) injuries affecting the BONES, TENDONS, or BURSAE of the JOINTS are common in many sports. Examples include chronic INFLAMMATION of the common extensor tendon where it attaches to the later EPICONDYLE of the humerus – common in throwers and racquet sports – and stress fractures of the TIBIA or METATARSAL bones of the foot in runners. After an initial period of rest, management often involves coaching that enables the athlete to perform the repetitive movement in a less injury-susceptible manner.

Exercise physiology is the science of measuring athletic performance and physical fitness for exercise. This knowledge is applied to devising and supervising training regimens based on scientific principles. Physical fitness depends on the rate at which the body can deliver oxygen to the muscles, known as the VO_2max, which is technically difficult to measure. The pulse rate during and after a bout of exercise serves as a good proxy of this measurement.

Regulation of sport   Sports medicine's role is to minimize hazard for participants by, for example, framing rule changes which forbid

Torn ankle ligament.

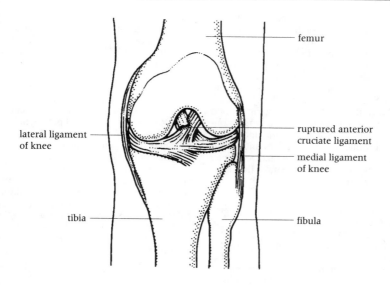

Anterior view of right knee joint.

collapsing the scrum, which has reduced the risk of neck injury in rugby; and in the detection of the use of drugs taken to enhance athletic performance. Such attempts to gain an edge in competition undermine the sporting ideal and are banned by leading sports regulatory bodies. The banned substances include drugs such as the ANABOLIC STEROIDS (TESTOSTERONE and its synthetic derivatives e.g. stanozolol) which increase muscle mass and the body's capacity to withstand more intense training. Stimulant drugs such as AMPHETAMINES have been used to enhance peak performance, and DIURETIC drugs – which deplete the body's water content – may be used in sports such as boxing and weightlifting where competitors must 'make the weight' (fall into a particular weight category).

Drug use can be detected by analysis of the urine, but testing only at the time of competition is unlikely to detect drug use designed to enhance early-season training.

SPOTS BEFORE THE EYES These can arise from a variety of causes including inflammation and bleeding in the eye, or preceding a retina detachment. They may also occur for a variety of totally harmless reasons.

SPOTTED FEVER (see MENINGITIS; EPIDEMIC; TYPHUS FEVER).

SPRAINS Injuries in the neighbourhood of joints, consisting usually in tearing of a ligament with effusion of blood. (See JOINTS, DISEASES OF.)

SPRUE, or PSILOSIS A disease occurring most commonly in patients in or from the tropics, and characterized by diarrhoea with large, fatty stools, anaemia, sore tongue, and weight loss. Its manifestations resemble those of non-tropical sprue, or gluten enteropathy, and COELIAC DISEASE.

Causes Tropical sprue is thought to be due to an inborn error of metabolism, characterized primarily by an inability to absorb fats from the intestines. Its epidemiological pattern suggests that an infection such as DYSENTERY may be the precipitating factor. Subsequently there is interference with the absorption of carbohydrates, vitamins, and minerals, leading to ANAEMIA and HYPOCALCAEMIA.

Symptoms Of gradual or rapid onset, there is initial weakness, soreness of the tongue, difficulty swallowing, indigestion, and diarrhoea with pale frothy stools and poor appetite. Anaemia is typically macrocytic, and mild hypoglycaemia may occur. Untreated, the patient steadily loses weight and, unless appropriate treatment is started early, death may be expected because of exhaustion and some intercurrent infection.

Treatment This consists of bed rest, a high protein diet (initially skimmed milk), and treatment of the anaemia and any other deficiencies present. Minimum fat should be given to sufferers, who should also take folic acid and cyanocobalamin for the anaemia; large vitamin-B-complex supplements (such as Marmite®) are helpful. Vitamins A and D, together with calcium supplements, help to raise the concentration of calcium in the blood. A long convalescence is often required, which may lead to marked depression, and patients should be sent home to a temperate climate.

Non-tropical sprue is the result of GLUTEN hypersensitivty and is treated with a gluten-free diet.

SPUTUM The mucous secretions from the mouth, throat or back of the nose. It is also expectorated by coughing from the lower air passages. Sputum production may be increased by respiratory-tract allergy (asthma) or by breathing in irritants such as tobacco smoke, smoke from a fire or fumes from chemical materials. Sputum is normally white but infection will turn it to yellow or green, and blood from the lungs may produce pink frothy sputum. Treatment is to deal with the underlying disorder. Production of large quantities of sputum, for instance, in BRONCHIECTASIS, may require physiotherapy and postural drainage. (See EXPECTORATION.)

SQUINT or STRABISMUS A condition in which the visual axes of each eye are not directed simultaneously at the same fixation point (i.e. each eye is not pointing at the same object at the same time). Squints may be: (a) Paralytic, where one or more of the muscles, or their nerve supply is damaged; this type usually results in double vision. (b) Non-paralytic, where the muscles and nerves are normal. It is usually found in children. This type of squint can either result in poor vision, or occasionally may result from poor vision. Squints may be convergent (where one eye 'turns in') or divergent (one eye 'turns out'). Vertical squints can also occur but are less common. All squints should be seen by an eye specialist as soon as possible. Some squints can be corrected by exercises or spectacles; others require surgery.

SSRIs (see SELECTIVE SEROTONIN-REUPTAKE INHIBITORS).

STABS (see WOUNDS).

STAGHORN CALCULUS A branched renal stone formed in the image of the collecting system of the KIDNEY. It fills the calyces and pelvis and is commonly associated with an infection of the urine, particularly *Proteus vulgaris*. The calculus may lead to pyonephrosis and an abscess of the kidney.

STAMMERING A disruption of the forward flow of speech. The individual knows what he wants to say but he temporarily loses his ability to execute linguistically formulated speech. Stammering is characterized by a silent or audible involuntary repetition/prolongation of an utterance, be it a sound, syllable or word. Sometimes it is accompanied by accessory behaviours, or speech-related struggle. Usually there are indications or the report of an accompanying emotional state, involving excitement, tension, fear or embarrassment.

Idiopathic stammering begins sometime between the onset of speech and puberty, mostly between 2 and 5 years of age. Acquired stammering at a later age due to brain damage is rare. The prevalence of stammering (the percentage of the population actually stammering at any point in time) is approximately 0·9 per cent. Three times as many boys as girls stammer. About 70 per cent of stammering children recover with little or no therapy. Stammerers have not been shown to demonstrate differences in personality from non-stammerers. There are, however, indications that at least some stammerers show minimal differences from fluent speakers in cerebral processing of verbal material.

There is a genetic predisposition towards stammering. The risk of stammering among first-degree relatives of stammerers is more than three times the population risk. In 77 per cent of identical twins either both stammer or both are fluent. Only 33 per cent of non-identical twins agree in this way. As there are identical twins who differ for stammering, environmental factors must be important for some stammerers. There are relatively large numbers of stammerers in highly competitive societies, where status and prestige are important and high standards of speech competence are valued.

Different treatments have been demonstrated to produce considerable benefit, their basic outline being similar. A long period of time is spent in training stammerers to speak in a different way (fluency-shaping techniques). This may include slowing down the rate of speech, gentle onset of utterance, continuous flow with correct juncturing, etc. When the targets have been achieved within the clinic a series of planned speech assignments outside the clinic is undertaken. In these assignments, and initially in everyday situations, the fluency-enchancing techniques have to be used conscientiously. Gradually speech is shaped towards normality requiring less and less effort. Therapy may also include some work on attitude change (i.e. helping the client to see himself as a fluent speaker) and possibly general communicative skills training.

For information about organizations concerned with stammering, see APPENDIX 2: ADDRESSES.

STANNOSIS The form of PNEUMOCONIOSIS caused by the inhalation of stannous (tin) oxide, which occurs in tin ore mining.

STANOZOLOL (see ANABOLIC STEROIDS).

STAPEDECTOMY An operation on the middle ear to remove the stapes and replace it with an artificial alternative. The procedure is aimed at treating deafness caused by otosclerosis in which the stapes becomes fixed by an overgrowth of bone, preventing it from transmitting sound. Stapedectomy improves hearing in around 90 per cent of those people who have the operation. (See EAR.)

STAPES The innermost of the small trio of bones in the middle ear. It is stirrup shaped and articulates with the incus and is linked to the oval window of the inner ear. (See EAR.)

STAPHYLOCOCCUS is a genus of GRAM-POSITIVE BACTERIUM which under the microscope appears in small masses like bunches of grapes. It is one of the commonest infectious micro-organisms and is found, for example, in the pus discharged from boils (see MICROBIOLOGY).

STARCH A substance belonging to that group of carbohydrates known as the amyloses. It is the form in which utilizable carbohydrate is stored in granules within the seeds and roots of many plants. It is converted into sugar when treated with heat in presence of a dilute acid. It is changed largely into dextrin when exposed to a considerable degree of dry heat, as in toasting bread; and a similar change into dextrin and malt-sugar takes place under the action of various enzymes such as the ptyalin of the saliva. Starch forms a chief constituent of the carbohydrate foods (see DIET), and in the process of digestion the above-mentioned change takes place to prepare it for absorption. It is also slowly broken down in the process of cooking.

Starch is used as a constituent of dusting powders for application to chafed or irritable areas of the skin. (See CHAFING OF THE SKIN.)

STARVATION A condition that results from a lack of food for a long time. The person suffers weight loss and changes in the body's metabolism, with production of potentially harmful chemicals called ketones and acetone. Sometimes starvation may occur as a result of an eating disorder. (See ANOREXIA.) In cases of slow starvation, the vitality of the tissues is reduced and they become more liable to tuberculosis and other diseases. (See also FASTING.)

STASIS A term applied to stoppage of the flow of blood in the vessels or of the food materials down the intestinal canal.

STATUS ASTHMATICUS Repeated attacks of asthma, with no respite between the spasms, usually lasting for more than 24 hours. The patient is seriously distressed and, untreated, the condition may lead to death from respiratory failure and exhaustion. Corticosteroid treatment and other skilled medical care are urgently required. (See ASTHMA.)

STATUS EPILEPTICUS Repeated epileptic fits with no return to consciousness between them. Breathing stops between each fit and the body is deprived of oxygen which causes damage to the brain. Urgent medical attention is required to control the condition or the patient may die. (see EPILEPSY and APPENDIX 1: BASIC FIRST AID.)

STEATOMA A fatty, cystic tumour.

STEATORRHOEA Any condition characterized by the passing of stools containing an excess of fat. (See MALABSORPTION SYNDROME.)

STEM CELL Stem CELLS develop a few days after an egg (ovum) is fertilized by a SPERM and starts developing to form an EMBRYO. These master cells are crucial to the development of a normal embryo. They contain a specialized ENZYME that gives them the facility to divide indefinitely, developing into the many different specialized cells that comprise the various tissues in the body – for example, skin, blood, muscle, glands or nerves.

In a highly significant advance in research, a scientific team in the United States has recently obtained stem cells from newly formed human embryos – donated by women who had become pregnant after successful *in vitro* fertilization – and successfully cultivated these cells in the laboratory. This achievement has opened the way to replicating in the laboratory the various specialized cells that develop naturally in the body. Government legislation constrains the use of human embryos in research (see ETHICS) and the ethical aspects of taking this stem-cell culture technique forward will have to be resolved. Nevertheless, this discovery points the biological way to the use of genetic engineering in selecting differentiated specialized cells from which replacement tissues could be grown for use as transplants to rectify absent or damaged tissues in the human body.

STENOSIS An unnatural narrowing in any passage or orifice of the body. The word is specially used in connection with the four openings of the heart at which the valves are situated. (See HEART DISEASES.)

STENT A surgical device used to assist the healing of an operative anastamosis – a joining up of two structures. A splint is left inside the lumen of a duct and this drains the contents.

STEREOGNOSIS The faculty of recognizing the solidity of objects, and thus their nature, by handling them.

STEREOTAXIS The procedure whereby precise localization in space is achieved. It is applied to that branch of surgery known as stereotactic neurosurgery, in which the surgeon is able to localize precisely those areas of the brain on which he wishes to operate.

STERILITY The state of (1) being free of infectious agents or (2) permanent INFERTILITY.

STERILIZATION means either (1) the process of rendering various objects, such as those which come in contact with wounds, and various foods, free from microbes, or (2) the process of rendering a person incapable of producing children.

The manner of sterilizing bedding, furniture, and the like, after contact with a case of infectious disease, is given under DISINFECTION, whilst the sterilization of instruments, dressings, and skin surfaces, necessary before surgical procedures, is mentioned in the same article and also under ANTISEPTICS, ASEPSIS, and WOUNDS. For general purposes, one of the cheapest and most effective agents is boiling water or steam.

Bacteriological sterilization may be effected in many ways, and different methods are used in different cases.

Sexual sterilization In women it is performed by ligating, or cutting, and then tying the FALLOPIAN TUBES, the tubes that carry the OVUM from the OVARY to the UTERUS. Alternatively the tubes may be sealed off by means of plastic and silicone clips or rings. It is usually performed (by laparoscopy) through a small incision, or cut, in the lower abdominal wall. It has no effect on sexual or menstrual function, and, unlike the comparable operation in men, it is immediately effective. The sterilization is usually permanent (around 0·05 pregnancies occur for every 100 women years of use), but occasionally the two cut ends of the Fallopian tubes reunite, and pregnancy is then again possible. Removal of the uterus and/or the ovaries also sterilizes a woman but such procedures are only used when there is some special reason, such as the presence of a tumour.

The operation for sterilizing men is known as VASECTOMY.

STERNUM The scientific name for the breastbone. This is a long flat bony plate that comprises the central part of the chest. Made up of three parts: an upper triangular piece (manubrium); a middle part (the body); and at the bottom end the small, flexible xiphoid process. The two clavicles articulate to the manubrium. Seven pairs of costal cartilages link the sternum to the ribs. The sternum is very strong and a powerful blow is needed to fracture it: such an injury may damage the underlying heart and lungs. (See diagram on page 508.)

STEROID The group name for compounds that resemble cholesterol chemically. The group includes the sex hormones, the hormones of the adrenal cortex, and bile acids. They have a powerful influence on the normal functioning of the body, and natural and synthetic steroids are used in the treatment of many disorders. (See CORTICOSTEROIDS; ENDOCRINE GLANDS.)

STERTOR is a form of noisy breathing, similar to SNORING, and usually due to flapping of the soft palate. Whereas ordinary snoring results from sleeping with the mouth open, stertor is the result of paralysis of the soft palate, which may be the result of a stroke, suffocation, concussion, drunkenness, or poisoning by OPIUM or chloroform. In severe cases of paralysis, the tongue may loll back against the back of the throat, resulting in a very loud sound. In such cases breathing may be rapidly relieved by pulling the lower jaw forward, pulling the tongue out of the mouth, or turning the person on to one side.

STETHOSCOPE An instrument used for listening to the sounds produced by the action of the lungs, heart, and other internal organs. (See AUSCULTATION.)

STEVENS-JOHNSON SYNDROME (see ERYTHEMA MULTIFORME).

STIFFNESS A condition which may be due to a change in the joints, ligaments, tendons, or muscles, or to the influence of the nervous system over the muscles of the part affected. Stiffness is associated with various forms of rheumatism and with the effects of injuries to joints, tendons and muscles. Stiffness of the neck muscles resulting in bending backward the head, and of the hamstring muscles, causing difficulty in straightening the lower limbs, is a sign of meningitis. Stiffness or spasticity also occurs in certain diseases of the central nervous system.

Treatment is of the underlying disease or injury. Mild stiffness can be treated symptomatically with local warmth and analgesics. Physiotherapy is helpful in relieving stiffness as a result of muscle or joint injuries.

STIGMA Any spot or impression upon the skin. The term, stigmas of degeneration, is applied to physical defects that are found in people with learning disabilities. (See LEARNING DISABILITY.)

STILBOESTROL A synthetic oestrogen. Its physiological actions are closely similar to those of the natural ovarian hormone, and it has the great merit of being active when taken by mouth. The drug may help patients suffering from cancer of the PROSTATE, inducing in some cases regression of the primary tumour and of secondary deposits in bone. (See OESTROGEN.)

STILBOESTROL DIPHOSPHATE (see OESTROGEN).

STILET or STILETTE The delicate probe or the wire used to clear a catheter or hollow needle.

STILLBIRTH A stillborn child is 'any child which has issued forth from its mother after the twenty-eighth week of pregnancy and which did not at any time after being completely expelled from its mother, breathe or show any other sign of life'. In the United Kingdom in 1995 the number of stillbirths was 5·6 per 1,000 live births. (See PERINATAL MORTALITY.)

STILL'S DISEASE or JUVENILE RHEUMATOID ARTHRITIS This is a disease of childhood first described by Sir Frederic Still (1868–1941). The characteristic of the disease is that the arthritis is usually symmetrical. It tends to start in the fingers, which become spindle-shaped due to the swelling of the affected joints. It then spreads to involve other joints, practically always in a symmetrical manner, including the wrists, elbows, knees and ankles. Occasionally, only one joint, such as the knee, may be involved initially. The onset may be abrupt, with high temperature, or gradual. The cervical spine is often involved, leading to stiffness of the neck, and some of these cases go on to ankylosing spondylitis (see SPINE AND SPINAL CORD, DISEASES AND INJURIES OF). As a result of the child's not moving the affected joints because of the pain this causes, there is marked wasting of the muscles. The heart is seldom involved, but there is often a characteristic rash. The age of onset is usually between 2 and 5 years, and the disease is marked by repeated recurrences. The disease is usually self-limiting, but tends to relapse and may persist for several years. Treatment is as for RHEUMATOID ARTHRITIS in the adult.

STIMULANT A drug or other agent that prompts the activity of a body system or function. For example, the sight and smell of food stimulates salivation and the rods and cones in the retina of the eye are stimulated by light. Another example is the use of amphetamines and caffeine to stimulate the central nervous system and make an individual more alert and active or, if taken in excess, hyperactive. In treatment procedures, electrical stimulation may be used to bring muscles into action. Aromatics, spices and bitters are traditional stimulants of digestive processes.

STINGS (see BITES AND STINGS).

STITCH A popular name for a sharp pain in the side. It is generally due to cramp following unusually hard exertion (see CRAMP), but care must be taken that this trivial condition is not taken for pleurisy or for a fractured rib. The word is also used to mean the repair of skin following surgery or any other trauma.

STOKES-ADAMS SYNDROME A term applied to a condition in which slowness of the pulse is associated with attacks of unconsciousness, and which is due to arrhythmia of the cardiac muscle or even complete heart block. Usually the heart returns to normal rhythm after a short period but patients who suffer from the condition are commonly provided

with a PACEMAKER to maintain normal cardiac function.

STOMA A stoma refers to an opening constructed when the bowel has to be brought to the skin surface to convey gastrointestinal contents to the exterior. It is derived from the Greek word meaning mouth. In the United Kingdom there are about 100,000 patients with a colostomy, 10,000 with an ileostomy and some 2,000 with a urostomy in which the ureters are brought to the skin surface. They may be undertaken because of malignancy of the COLON or RECTUM or as a result of inflammatory bowel diseases such as CROHN'S DISEASE. Urostomies usually take the form of an isolated loop of ILIUM into which the URETERS have been implanted and which in its turn is either brought to the skin's surface or converted into an artificial bladder. This is undertaken because of bladder cancer or because of neurological diseases of the bladder. The stomas drain into appliances such as disposable plastic bags. Most of the modern appliances collect the effluent of the stoma without any leak or odour.

Patients with stomas often find explanatory booklets helpful. *Living with your Colostomy* and *Understanding Colostomy* are examples. They are published by the British Colostomy Association (see APPENDIX 2: ADDRESSES).

STOMACH This is a distensible saclike organ with an average adult capacity of 1·5 litres situated in the upper abdomen. It is positioned between the OESOPHAGUS and DUODENUM, lying just beneath the DIAPHRAGM to the right of the SPLEEN and partly under the LIVER (see diagram). The stomach is a part of the gastrointestinal tract with its walls formed of layers of longitudinal and circular muscles and lined by glandular cells that secrete gastric juice. It is well supplied with blood vessels as well as nerves from the autonomic system which enter via the phrenic nerve. The exit of the stomach is guarded by a ring of muscle called the pyloric sphincter which controls the passage of food into the duodenum.

Function As well as the stomach's prime role in physically and physiologically breaking down the food delivered via the oesophagus, it also acts as a storage organ, a function that enables people to eat three or four times a day instead of every 30 minutes or so as their metabolic needs would otherwise demand. Gastric secretion is stimulated by the sight and smell of food and its subsequent arrival in the stomach. The secretions, which contain mucus and hydrochloric acid (the latter produced by parietal cells) sterilize the food; pepsin, a digestive enzyme in the gastric juices, breaks down the protein in food. The juices also contain intrinsic factor, vital for the absorption of vitamin B_{12} when the chyle – as the stomach contents are called – reaches the intestine. This chyle is of creamy consistency and is the end product of

1 oesophagus
2 cardiac orifice of stomach
3 lesser curvature of stomach
4 liver (right lobe)
5 duodenum
6 gall bladder

7 common bile duct entering
   duodenum at ampulla of vater
8 antrum of stomach
9 pylorus
10 fundus of stomach
11 cardia of stomach
12 liver (left lobe)

Interior of stomach.

enzymic action and rhythmic contractions of the stomach's muscles every 30 seconds or so. Food remains in the stomach for varying lengths of time depending on its quantity and nature. At regular intervals a bolus of chyle is forced into the duodenum by contractions of the stomach muscles co-ordinated with relaxation of the pyloric sphincter.

STOMACH, DISEASES OF   Gastritis is the description for several unrelated diseases of the gastric mucosa.

Acute gastritis is an inflammatory reaction of the gastric mucosa to various precipitating factors, ranging from physical and chemical injury to infections. Acute gastrits (especially of the antral mucosas) may well represent a reaction to infection by a bacterium called *Heliobacter pylori*. The inflammatory changes usually go after appropriate antibiotic treatment for the *H. pylori* infection.

Acute and chronic inflammation occurs in response to chemical damage of the gastric mucosa. For example, reflux of duodenal contents may predispose to inflammatory acute and chronic gastritis. Similarly, multiple small erosions or single or multiple ulcers have resulted from consumption of chemicals, especialy aspirin and antirheumatic NON-STEROIDAL ANTI-INFLAMMATORY DRUGS (NSAIDs).

Acute gastritis may cause anorexia, nausea, upper abdominal pain and, if erosive, haemorrhage. Treatment involves removal of the offending cause.

Chronic gastritis   Accumulation of cells called round cells in the gastric mucosal character-izes chronic gastritis. Most patients with chronic gastritis have no symptoms, and treatment of H. pylori infection usually cures the condition.

Atrophic gastritis   A few patients with chronic gastritis may develop atrophic gastritis. With or without inflammatory change, this disorder is common in Western countries. The incidence increases with age, and over 50 per cent of people over 50 may have it. A more complete and uniform type of atrophy, called 'gastric atrophy' characterizes a familial disease called PERNICIOUS ANAEMIA. The cause of the latter disease is not known but it may be an AUTOIMMUNE DISORDER.

Since atrophy of the corpus mucosa results in loss of acid- and pepsin-secreting cells, gastric secretion is reduced or absent. Patients with pernicious anaemia or severe atrophic gastritis of the corpus mucosa may secrete too little intrinsic factor for absorption of vitamin B_{12} and so can develop severe neurological disease (subacute combined degeneration of the spinal cord).

Patients with atrophic gastritis often have bacterial colonization of the upper alimentary tract, with increased concentration of nitrite and carcinogenic N-nitroso compounds. These, coupled with excess growth of mucosal cells, may be linked to cancer. In chronic corpus gastritis, the risk of gastric cancer is about 3–4 times that of the general population.

Postgastrectomy mucosa   The mucosa of the gastric remnant after surgical removal of the distal part of the stomach is usually inflamed and atrophic and is also premalignant, with the risk of gastric cancer being very much greater than for patients with duodenal ulcer who have not had surgery.

Stress gastritis Acute stress gastritis develops, sometimes within hours, in individuals who have undergone severe physical trauma, BURNS (Curling ulcers), severe SEPSIS or major diseases such as heart attacks, STROKES, intracranial trauma or operations (Cushing's ulcers). The disorder presents with multiple superficial erosions or ulcers of the gastric mucosa, with HAEMATEMESIS and MELAENA and sometimes with perforation when the acute ulcers erode through the stomach wall. Treatment involves inhibition of gastric secretion with intravenous infusion of an H$_2$-receptor-antagonist drug such as RANITIDINE or FAMOTIDINE, so that the gastric contents remain at a near neutral pH. Despite treatment a few patients continue to bleed and may then require radical gastric surgery.

Gastric ulcer Gastric ulcers were common in young women during the 19th century, markedly fell in frequency in many Western countries during the first half of the 20th century, but remained common in coastal northern Norway, Japan, in young Australian women, and in some Andean populations. During the latter half of this century, gastric ulcers have again become more frequent in the West, with a peak incidence between 55 and 65 years.

The cause is not known. The two factors most strongly associated with the development of duodenal ulcers – gastric acid production and gastric infection with *H. pylori* bacteria – are not nearly as strongly associated with gastric ulcers. The latter occur with increased frequency in individuals who take aspirin or NSAIDs. In healthy individuals who take NSAIDs, as many as 6 per cent develop a gastric ulcer during the first week of treatment, while in patients with rheumatoid arthritis who are being treated long term with drugs, gastric ulcers occur in 20–40 per cent. The cause is inhibition of the enzyme cyclo-oxygenase which in turn inhibits the production of repair-promoting PROSTAGLANDINS.

Gastric ulcers occur especially on the lesser curve of the stomach. The ulcers may erode through the whole thickness of the gastric wall, perforating into the peritoneal cavity or penetrating into liver, pancreas or colon.

Gastric ulcers usually present with a history of epigastric pain of less than one year. The pain tends to be associated with anorexia and may be aggravated by food, although patients with 'prepyloric' ulcers may obtain relief from eating or taking antacid preparations. Patients with gastric ulcers also complain of nausea and vomiting, and lose weight.

The principal complications of gastric ulcer are haemorrhage from arterial erosion or perforation into the peritoneal cavity resulting in PERITONITIS, abscess or fistula.

Aproximately one in two gastric ulcers heal 'spontaneously' in 2–3 months. However, up to 80 per cent of the patients relapse within 12 months. Repeated recurrence and rehealing results in scar tissue around the ulcer; this may cause a circumferential narrowing, a condition called 'hour-glass stomach'.

The diagnosis of gastric ulcer is confirmed by endoscopy. All patients with gastric ulcers should have multiple biopsies to exclude the presence of malignant cells. Even after healing, gastric ulcers should be endoscopically monitored for a year.

Treatment of gastric ulcers is relatively simple. A course of an H$_2$ RECEPTOR ANTAGONIST heals gastric ulcers in 3 months. In patients who relapse, long-term indefinite treatment with an H$_2$ receptor antagonist such as ranitidine may be necessary since the ulcers tend to recur. Recently it has been claimed that gastric ulcers can be healed with a combination of a bismuth salt or a gastric secretory inhibitor – for example, one of the PROTON PUMP INHIBITORS such as omeprazole or lansoprazole – together with two antibiotics such as AMOXYCILLIN and METRONIDAZOLE. The long-term outcome of such treatment is not known. Partial gastrectomy, which used to be a regular treatment for gastric ulcers, is now much more rarely done unless the ulcer(s) contain precancerous cells.

Cancer of the stomach Cancer of the stomach is common and dangerous and, world-wide, accounts for approximately 1 in 6 of all deaths from cancer. There are marked geographical differences in frequency, with a very high incidence in Japan and low incidence in the USA. In the United Kingdom around 33 cases per 100,000 population are diagnosed annually. Studies have shown that environmental factors, rather than hereditary ones, are mainly responsible for the development of gastric cancer. Diet, including highly salted, pickled and smoked foods, and high concentrations of nitrate in food and drinking water, may well be responsible for the environmental effects.

Most gastric ulcers arise in abnormal gastric mucosa. The three mucosal disorders which especially predispose to gastric cancer include pernicious anaemia, postgastrectomy mucosa, and atrophic gastritis. Around 90 per cent of gastric cancers have the microscopic appearance of abnormal mucosal cells (and are called 'adenocarcinomas'). Most of the remainder look like endocrine cells of lymphoid tissue, although tumours with mixed microscopic appearance are common.

Early gastric cancer may be symptomless and, in countries like Japan with a high frequency of the disease, is often diagnosed during routine screening of the population. In more advanced cancers, upper abdominal pain, loss of appetite and loss of weight occur. Many present with obstructive symptoms, such as vomiting (when the pylorus is obstructed) or difficulty with swallowing. METASTASIS is obvious in up to two-thirds of patients and its presence contraindicates surgical cure. The diagnosis is made by endoscopic examination of the stomach and biopsy of abnormal-looking areas of mucosa. Treatment is surgical, often with additional chemotherapy and radiotherapy.

STOMACH TUBE A soft rubber or plastic tube with rounded end, and usually about 75 cm (30 inches) in length, which is used for washing out the stomach when it contains some poisonous material. (See GASTRIC LAVAGE.) A narrower tube, 90 cm (36 inches) in length, is used to obtain a sample of gastric juice for examination. Such a tube can also be allowed to pass out of the stomach into the duodenum so that the contents of the upper part of the small intestine are similarly obtained for analysis.

STOMACH WASHOUT (see GASTRIC LAVAGE).

STOMATITIS Inflammation or ulceration of the mouth. (See MOUTH, DISEASES OF.)

-STOMY A suffix signifying formation of an opening in an organ by operation: e.g. COLOSTOMY.

STONE (see URINARY BLADDER, DISEASES OF; GALL-BLADDER, DISEASES OF).

STRABISMUS (see SQUINT).

STRAIN Stretching or tearing of muscle fibres caused by subjecting them to sudden pulling. Bleeding into the muscle causes pain and swelling and sometimes muscle spasm. Application of ice packs and strapping, coupled with a day or two's rest and analgesics are usually sufficient to remedy most strains. Sometimes anti-inflammatory drugs or physiotherapy may be required.

STRANGULATION The constriction of a passage or tube in the body that blocks the blood flow and disturbs the working of the affected organ. It is usually caused by compression or twisting. Strangulation customarily occurs when part of the INTESTINE herniates either inside the abdomen or outside as in an inguinal HERNIA. If a section of the intestine twists this may strangulate and is known as a VOLVULUS.

Strangulation of a person's neck either with a ligature or the hands obstructs the jugular veins in the neck preventing the normal outflow of blood from the brain and head. The TRACHEA is also compressed, cutting off the supply of air to the lungs. The combination of these effects leads to HYPOXIA and damage to the brain. If not quickly relieved, unconsciousness and death follow. Strangulation may be deliberate or accidental – the latter being a particular hazard for children, for example, when playing with a rope. Removal of the constriction, artificial respiration, and medical attention are urgently necessary.

STRANGURY A condition in which there is constant desire to pass water, accompanied by a straining sensation, though only a few drops can be voided. It is a symptom of inflammation in the urinary tract.

STRAPPING The application of strips of adhesive plaster, one overlapping the other, so as to cover and exert pressure on an area of the body. This treatment is used in cases of injury or disease when it is desired to keep a part at rest: for example, strapping may be applied to the chest in cases of pleurisy and fracture of the ribs. Also, it is often used to prevent the movement of joints which are sprained or otherwise injured.

STREP THROAT An infection of the throat with STREPTOCOCCUS bacteria: it is most common in children and symptoms range from minor discomfort to sore throat, fever, general malaise and enlarged LYMPH nodes in the neck. If symptoms are severe the infection may lead to SCARLET FEVER. Penicillin is the treatment of choice.

STREPTOCOCCUS is a variety of GRAM-POSITIVE BACTERIUM which under the microscope has much the appearance of a string of beads. Most species are SAPROPHYTIC. A few are PATHOGENIC and these include haemolytic types which can destroy red blood cells in a culture of blood agar. This offers a method of classifying the varying streptococcal strains. Alpha-haeomolytic streptococci are usually associated with bacterial ENDOCARDITIS. SCARLET FEVER is caused by a β-haeomolytic streptococcus called *S. pyogenes*. *S. pneumoniae*, also called PNEUMOCOCCUS, causes respiratory-tract infections, including PNEUMONIA. *S. pyogenes* may on its own, or with other bacteria, cause severe necrotizing fasciitis or cellulitis in which oedema and death of subcutaneous tissues occur. The infection can spread very rapidly and, unless urgently treated with antibiotics and sometimes surgery, death may quickly result. This spread is related to the ability of *S. pyogenes* to produce toxic substances called exotoxins. Although drug-resistant forms are occurring, streptococcal infections usually respond to ANTIBIOTIC treatment.

STREPTOKINASE An enzyme produced by certain STREPTOCOCCI. It acts as a PLASMINOGEN activator, and hence enhances FIBRINOLYSIS. The most important use of streptokinase is in the treatment of myocardial infarction in the first 12 hours after the initial diagnosis. Subsequently, use of this thrombolytic drug should be under hospital supervision. It is given intravenously, in hospital by infusion. It may be given as an infusion to treat severe THROMBOSIS or EMBOLISM, particularly when they occur in a limb, and in deep venous thrombosis. Being antigenic and very expensive it is rarely used for more than two days, and is followed by anticoagulation therapy. The chief risk is haemorrhage, so an antifibrinolytic such as aminocaproic acid should always be available.

STREPTOMYCIN is an anti-bacterial substance obtained from the soil mould, *Streptomyces griseus*. It was first isolated in 1944 by Dr Waksman in the United States of America. It was the first antibiotic to be effective against the tubercle bacillus. It was once routinely used to treat TUBERCULOSIS; then because of resistance to streptomycin it was given in combination with other antituberculous drugs such as ISONIAZIDE. Because of its side-effects and the availability of other drugs it is now rarely used except for tuberculosis resistant to other drugs.

An AMINOGLYCOSIDE, streptomycin has two disadvantages. The most important of these is the tendency of organisms to become resistant to it. This means that the administration of this antibiotic must be carefully supervized to ensure that correct dosage is being used. The other disadvantage is that streptomycin produces toxic effects, especially disturbance of the vestibular and hearing apparatus. This may result in DEAFNESS, VERTIGO, and TINNITUS. Whilst in many cases these toxic manifestations disappear when the antibiotic is withdrawn, they may be permanent. For this reason therefore streptomycin must always be used with special care.

STRESS Any factor or event(s) that threaten a person's health or adversely affect his or her normal functioning. Injury, disease or worry are common examples; others include internal conflicts, emotive life events – such as the death of a close relative or friend, the birth of a baby, separation or divorce – pressures at work or a hostile environment such as war or famine. Some individuals seem to be more prone than others to develop medical problems related to stress.

Stress prompts the body to raise its output of hormones such as ADRENALINE and CORTISOL, causing changes in blood pressure, heart rate and metabolism. These are physiological responses intended to improve a person's physical and mental performance – the 'fight or flight' reaction to fear. Stress may, however, disrupt the ability to cope. Constant or recurrent exposure to stress may produce symptoms such as anxiety, depression, headaches, indigestion, diarrhoea, palpitations and general malaise. (see POST-TRAUMATIC STRESS SYNDROME.) Treatment can be difficult and prolonged; counselling can help as can anxiolytic or antidepressant drugs, but a change in job or life style may be necessary in some circumstances.

STRESS FRACTURES are comparatively common in sportsmen. They tend to occur when an undue amount of exercise is taken: an amount of exercise which an individual is not capable of coping with in his (or her) state of training. The main initial feature is pain over the affected

bone. This is usually insidious in onset, and worse at night and during and after exercise. It is accompanied by tenderness, and a lump may be felt over the affected site. X-ray evidence of them only appears after several weeks. Treatment consists of rest, some form of external support, and in the initial stage ANALGESICS to deaden or kill the pain.

STRIAE Stretch marks seen in the skin, common in adolescent boys and girls owing to stretching of the skin by rapid growth (striae distensae). In boys striae occur around the shoulders and thighs. In girls the breasts and hips are affected. In both sexes horizontal striae on the back may be mistaken for signs of trauma. Striae are common in women in late pregnancy, especially on the lower abdomen (striae gravidarum). Injudicious prolonged use of potent topical CORTICOSTEROIDS can induce striae, particularly about the groins, inner thighs or armpits. Prolonged high-dose oral STEROID therapy may cause widespread striae.

STRICTURE A narrowing in any of the natural passages of the body, such as the gullet, the bowel, or the urethra. It may be due to the development of some growth in the wall of the passage affected, or to pressure upon it by such a growth in some neighbouring organ, but in the majority of cases a stricture is the result of previous ulceration on the inner surface of the passage, followed by contraction of the scar. (See INTESTINE, DISEASES OF; URETHRA, DISEASES OF.)

STRIDOR A noise associated with inspiration due to narrowing of the upper airway, in particular the larynx.

STROKE Stroke or cerebrovascular accident (CVA) is sudden damage to brain tissue caused either by a lack of blood supply or rupture of a blood vessel. The affected brain cells die and the parts of the body they control or receive sensory messages from cease to function.

Causes Blood supply to the brain may be interrupted by arteries furring up with ATHEROSCLEROSIS (which is accelerated by hypertension and diabetes, both of which are associated with a higher incidence of strokes) or being occluded by blood clots arising from distant organs such as infected heart valves or larger clots in the heart. Hearts with an irregular rhythm are especially prone to develop clots. Patients with thick or viscous blood, clotting disorders or those with inflamed arteries, e.g. in systemic lupus erythematosis, are particularly in danger of having strokes. Bleeding into the brain arises from areas of weakened blood vessels, many of which may be congenital.

Symptoms Minor episodes due to temporary lack of blood supply and oxygen (called TRANSIENT ISCHAEMIC ATTACKS (TIAs) or episodes) are manifested by short-lived weakness or numbness in an arm or leg and may precede a major stroke. Strokes cause sudden weakness or complete paralysis of the muscles controlled by the part of the brain affected as well as sensory changes, e.g., numbness or tingling. In the worst cases these symptoms and signs may be accompanied by loss of consciousness. If the stroke affects the area of the brain controlling the larynx and throat, the patient may suffer slurring or loss of speech with difficulty in initiating swallowing. When the face is involved the mouth may droop and the patient dribble. Strokes caused by haemorrhage may be preceded by headaches. Rarely, CVAs are complicated by epileptic fits. If, on the other hand, numerous small clots develop in the brain rather than one major event, this may manifest itself as a gradual deterioration in the patient's mental function, leading to dementia.

Investigations Tests on the heart or computed tomography or ultrasonic scans on arteries in the neck may indicate the original sites of distantly arising clots. Blood tests may show increased thickness or tendency to clotting and the diagnosis of general medical conditions can explain the presence of inflamed arteries which are prone to block. Special brain X-rays, e.g., COMPUTED TOMOGRAPHY, show the position and size of the damaged brain tissue and can usually distinguish between a clot or infarct and a rupture of and haemorrhage from a blood vessel in the brain.

Management It is better to prevent a stroke than try to cure it. The control of a person's diabetes or high blood pressure will reduce the risk of a stroke. ANTICOAGULATION treatment prevents the formation of clots and regular small doses of aspirin stop platelets clumping together to form plugs in blood vessels and both treatments reduce the likelihood of minor transient ischaemic episodes proceeding to a major stroke. Once the latter has occurred, there is no effective treatment to reduce the damage to brain tissue. Function will return to the affected part of the body only if and when the brain recovers and messages are again sent down the appropriate nerves. Simple movements are more likely to recover than delicate ones and sophisticated functions have the worst outlook. Thus, movement of the thigh may improve more easily than fine movements of fingers, and any speech impairment is more likely to be permanent. A rehabilitation team can help to compensate for any disabilities the subject may have. Physiotherapists maintain muscle tone and joint flexibility, whilst waiting for power to return; occupational therapists advise about functional problems and supply equipment to help patients overcome their disabilities; and speech therapists help with difficulties in swallowing, improve the clarity of remaining speech or offer alternative methods of communication. District nurses or home helps can provide support to those caring for victims of stroke at home. Advice about strokes may be obtained from the Stroke Association (see APPENDIX 2: ADDRESSES).

STROMA The name applied to the tissue which forms the framework and covering of an organ.

STRONGYLOIDIASIS This infection is caused by nematode worms of the genus *Strongyloides* spp. – the great majority being from *S. stercoralis*. This helminth is present throughout most tropical and subtropical countries; a single case report has been made in England – about an individual who had not been exposed to such an environment. Larvae usually penetrate intact skin, especially the feet (as with hookworm infection). Unlike hookworm infection, eggs mature and hatch in the lower gastrointestinal tract; thus larvae can immediately re-enter the circulation in the colo-rectum or perianal region, setting up an auto-infection cycle. Therefore, infection can continue for the remaining lifespan of the individual. Severe malnutrition may be a predisposing factor to infection, as was the case in prisoners of war in south-east Asia during World War II (1939–45). Whilst an infected patient is frequently asymptomatic, heavy infection can cause jejunal mucosal abnormalities, and an absorptive defect, with weight loss. During the migratory phase an itchy linear rash (larva currens) may be present on the lower abdomen, buttocks, and groins; this gives rise to recurrent transient itching. In an immunosuppressed individual, the 'hyperinfection syndrome' may ensue; migratory larvae invade all organs and tissues, including the lungs and brain. Associated with this widespread infection, the patient may develop an *Enterobacteriacae* spp. septicaemia; this, together with *S. stercoralis* larvae, produces a meningoencephalitis. There is no evidence that this syndrome is more common in patients with HIV infection.

Diagnosis consists of visualization of *S. stercoralis* (larvae or adults) in a jejunal biopsy-section or aspirate. Larvae may also be demonstrable in a faecal sample, especially following culture. Eosinophilia may be present in peripheral blood, during the invasive stage of infection. Chemotherapy consists of albendazole. The formerly used benzimidazole compound, thiabendazole, is now rarely prescribed in an uncomplicated infection due to unpleasant side-effects. Even so, in the 'hyperinfection syndrome' it probably remains the more effective of the two compounds.

STRYCHNINE An alkaloid derived from *Strychnos nux-vomica*, the seeds of an East Indian tree, as well as from the seeds of several other closely allied trees and shrubs. It is a white crystalline body possessed of an intensely bitter taste, more bitter perhaps than that of any other substance, and it is not very soluble in water. It stimulates all parts of the nervous system, and was at one time widely used for this purpose. Strychnine poisoning is fortunately rare. It shows itself in convulsions, which come on very speedily after the person has taken the poison. The mental faculties remain unaffected, and the symptoms end in death or recovery within a few hours.

Treatment The patient should be kept quiet. Artificial respiration may be necessary and intravenous BENZODIAZEPINE to prevent convulsions may also be needed. (See POISONS and APPENDIX 2: ADDRESSES.)

STUPOR (see UNCONSCIOUSNESS).

STUTTERING (see STAMMERING).

STYE (see EYE DISEASES).

STYPTICS Applications which check bleeding, either by making the blood-vessels contract more fairmly or by causing rapid clotting in the blood. Some possess both modes of action.

SUB- prefix signifying under, near, or moderately.

SUBACUTE The description applied to a disease the duration of which lies between acute and chronic. An example is subacute ENDOCARDITIS, a disorder that may not be diagnosed for several weeks or months, during which time it can severely damage valves in the heart.

SUBACUTE COMBINED DEGENERATION OF THE CORD A degenerative condition of the SPINAL CORD which most commonly occurs as a complication of PERNICIOUS ANAEMIA. The motor and sensory nerves in the cord are damaged, causing spasticity of the limbs and an unsteady gait. Treatment is with vitamin B$_{12}$ (see APPENDIX 5: VITAMINS; ANAEMIA).

SUBACUTE SCLEROSING PANENCEPHALITIS A rare complication of measles due to infection of the brain with the measles virus. It develops two to eighteen years after the onset of the measles, and is characterized by mental deterioration leading on to convulsions, coma and death. The annual incidence in Britain is about 1 per million of the childhood population. The risk of its developing is five to twenty times greater after measles than after measles vaccination.

SUBARACHNOID HAEMORRHAGE A haemorrhage into the subarachnoid space. It is usually the result of rupture of an aneurysm on the CIRCLE OF WILLIS. Head injury or intense physical exercise occasionally causes subarachnoid haemorrhage. The diagnosis is confirmed by CT scan or by identifying blood in the CEREBROSPINAL FLUID at LUMBAR PUNCTURE. Cerebral ANGIOGRAPHY will usually pinpoint the site of bleeding. Treatment is bed rest, lifesupport measures and procedures to reduce blood pressure; sometimes surgery is carried out but not usually until several weeks after the acute episode. About 30 per cent of patients recover fully, some have residual disabilities such as epilepsy, mental deterioration or paralysis. About 50 per cent of those affected die.

SUBARACHNOID SPACE The space between the arachnoid and the pia mater, two of the membranes covering the BRAIN.

SUBCLAVIAN The name applied to a large artery and vein which pass to the upper arm between the collar bone and the first rib.

SUBCLINICAL A description of a disease that is suspected but which has not developed sufficiently or is too mild in form to produce clear signs and symptoms in an individual. Even so, damage may be caused to tissues and organs.

SUBCONSCIOUS A state of being partially conscious, or the condition in which mental processes occur and outside objects and events are perceived with the mind nearly or quite unconscious of them. Such subconscious impressions or events may be forgotten at the time but may nevertheless exert a continued influence over the conscious mind, or may at a subsequent time come fully into consciousness. Much importance is attached to the influence of painful or unpleasant experiences which, though forgotten, continue to influence the mind, and these are held to be largely responsible for neurasthenic and similar states. This injurious influence is removed when the subconscious impressions come fully into consciousness and are then remembered and clearly seen in their relative importance.

SUBCUTANEOUS Anything pertaining to the loose cellular tissue beneath the skin: e.g. a subcutaneous injection. (See HYPODERMIC.)

SUBDURAL Relating to the space between the strong outer layer of the meninges, the membrane which cover the brain, and the arachnoid, which is the middle layer of the meninges. A subdural haemorrhage occurs when bleeding takes place into this space. The trapped blood forms a large blood clot or haematoma within the skull and this causes pressure on the underlying brain. Bleeding may occur slowly as the result of disease or suddenly as the result of injury. Headaches, confusion, and drowsiness result, sometimes with paralysis. Medical attention is required urgently if a serious haematoma occurs soon after injury. (See BRAIN.)

SUBINVOLUTION A term used to indicate that the womb has failed to undergo the usual involution, or decrease in size, which naturally takes place within one month after a child is born.

SUBJECTIVE A term applied to symptoms, and sensations, perceived only by the affected individual. For example, numbness is a purely subjective sensation, whilst the jerk given by the leg on tapping the tendon of the knee is an objective sign.

SUBLIMATION The conversion of a solid substance into a vapour and its recondensation. The term is also used in a mental sense for the process of converting instinctive sexual desires to new aims and objects devoid of sexual significance.

SUBLUXATION A partial dislocation of a joint; the term is sometimes applied to a sprain.

SUBMUCOSA The layer of connective tissue that occurs under a mucous membrane – for example, in the intestinal wall.

SUBPHRENIC ABSCESS An abcess that develops under the diaphragm, usually on the right side of the abdomen between the liver and the diaphragm. The cause may be an organ that has perforated – for instance, a peptic ulcer in the stomach or intestine. An abscess may also occur after an abdominal operation, usually when the bowel or stomach has been operated on. Antibiotics and sometimes surgery are the method of treatment.

SUBSTRATE A compound on which an enzyme acts: for instance, ribonucleic acid (RNA) is the substrate for ribonuclease (an enzyme that catalyses the breakdown of ribonucleic acid, a cellular compound involved in the synthesis of protein).

SUCCUSSION (see THRILL) A clinical technique in which a patient suspected of having excessive fluid in a body cavity – usually the stomach or pleural cavity – is gently shaken in order to elicit splashing sounds.

SUCKLING (see INFANT FEEDING; BREASTS, DISEASES OF).

SUCROSE, or CANE SUGAR (see SUGAR).

SUCTION The use of a reduction in pressure to clear away fluids or other material through a tube. Suction is used to remove blood from the site of a surgical operation. Suction is commonly necessary to remove secretions from the airways of newly born babies to help them breathe.

SUDDEN INFANT DEATH SYNDROME (SIDS) or COT DEATH This refers to the unexpected death, usually during sleep, of an apparently healthy baby. Well over 1,500 such cases are thought to have occurred in the United

Kingdom each year until 1992 when government advice was issued about laying babies on their backs. The figure was over 400 in 1995 and continues to fall. Boys are affected more than girls, and over half these deaths occur between 2 and 6 months. More common in lower social classes, the incidence is highest in the winter, and most of the infants have been bottle fed.

Causes Unknown, possible multiple aetiology. Prematurity and low birth weight may play a role. The sleeping position of a baby and an over-warm environment may be major factors, since deaths have fallen sharply since mothers were officially advised to place babies on their backs and not to overheat them. Some deaths are probably the result of respiratory infections, usually viral, which may stop breathing in at-risk infants, while others may result from the infant's smothering in a soft pillow. Faults in the baby's central breathing control system (central APNOEA) may be a factor. Milk allergy is a possible factor, as may be a sudden disturbance of fluid balance resulting from bottle feeding. Inhalation of milk is a possible contributory cause. Other possible factors include vitamin E deficiency, or smoking, drug addiction or anaemia in the mother. Help and advice may be obtained from the Foundation for the Study of Infant Deaths (see APPENDIX 2: ADDRESSES).

SUDEK'S ATROPHY OSTEOPOROSIS in the hand or foot which develops quickly as a result of injury, infection or malignant growth.

SUDORIFICS Drugs and other agents which produce copious perspiration.

SUFFOCATION (see ASPHYXIA; CHOKING).

SUGAR is a substance containing carbon, hydrogen, and oxygen, and belonging therefore to the chemical group of carbohydrates. This group includes three subdivisions:

- Monosaccharides ($C_6H_{12}O_6$): e.g. glucose, or dextrose, or grape sugar; fructose, or laevulose, or fruit sugar; galactose.
- Disaccharides ($C_{12}H_{22}O_{11}$): e.g. sucrose, or cane sugar, or beet sugar; lactose or milk sugar; maltose or malt sugar.
- Polysaccharides ($C_6H_{10}O_5$): e.g. starch.; glycogen or animal starch.

Glucose, also known as grape sugar because it is found in various kinds of fruit, including grapes, is the form of sugar produced by the tissues and excreted in large amount by the kidneys in diabetes mellitus.

Sucrose is widely distributed through the vegetable kingdom, though it is specially plentiful in the juice of the sugar-cane, beetroot, and maple. When taken as a food, it is converted by the digestive juices into glucose before it is absorbed, this process being known as inversion. It is a valuable food, being utilized in the production of heat and energy, although it is also to a certain extent a tissue-builder so far as fat is concerned. It is to be avoided by people who tend to get fat as well as by diabetics.

Lactose is found in milk, and it is to the fermentation of this sugar and consequent production of lactic acid by certain bacteria that the souring of milk is due. The extent to which it is present in the milk of different animals is mentioned under INFANT FEEDING. It has little sweetening power compared with cane sugar, but it is used sometimes as a laxative.

Maltose is produced by the action of the enzyme, diastase, upon the starch contained in barley, and also by the ferments of the saliva and pancreatic juice, and is still further changed by the intestinal ferments into glucose before it is absorbed.

Invert sugar is a natural mixture of dextrose and laevulose resulting from a chemical decomposition of cane sugar or of starch.

Starch is mentioned under a separate heading, and its use as a food under DIET and CEREAL.

The energy-producing value of sugars generally is taken as being, on the average, 4 Calories for each gram of sugar.

SUICIDE (see under MENTAL ILLNESS).

SULCUS The term applied to any groove or furrow, but especially to a fissure of the brain.

SULFADOXINE A long-acting SULPHONAMIDE which along with pyrimethamine is used as an adjunct to QUININE to treat *Plasmodium falciparum* malaria. The combination should not be used for PHROPHYLAXIS. In many areas in which the disease is endemic the malaria parasite is resistant to the combination.

SULPHADIAZINE One of the sulphonamides. It is a highly active drug and in moderate dosage produces a high and persistent blood concentration. It is relatively non-toxic and is sometimes used to prevent the recurrence of RHEUMATIC FEVER.

SULPHADIMIDINE A sulphonamide similar to sulphadiazine, it has the advantage of being even more non-toxic and of producing higher blood concentrations. Used for treating urinary infections.

SULPHAEMOGLOBIN An abnormal pigment sometimes found in the blood as a result of the interaction of certain drugs derived from aniline, such as phenacetin and acetanilide.

SULPHAMETHOXAZOLE A long-acting SULPHONAMIDE, it has been used in combination with trimethoprim (as co-trimoxazole) to treat urinary infections. Increasing bacterial resistance to sulphonamides and the incidence of side-effects means that caution is needed in prescribing co-trimoxazole.

SULPHANILAMIDE, or *p*-aminobenzene-sulphonamide, is a drug the discovery of which is one of the most important in medicine in the twentieth century. It was the first of the sulphonamide drugs. The drug is no longer used, having been superseded by more effective sulphonamides.

SULPHASALAZINE A chemical combination of sulphapyridine and 5-aminosalicilic acid. It is used to treat ULCERATIVE COLITIS (valuable as oral therapy for mild symptomatic disease; also available as suppositories for rectal disease) and RHEUMATOID ARTHRITIS. The salicylate part is now available alone in drugs such as mesalazine and olsalazine. Several reports of blood dyscrasias from patients taking these drugs have prompted the Committee for Safety of Medicines to recommend that patients with unexplained blood disorders should stop treatment and be given an immediate blood count.

SULPHINPYRAZONE A derivative of phenylbutazone which is of value in the prophylaxis and treatment of gout.

SULPHONAMIDE A drug having the sulphonamide grouping – SO_2NH_2. In 1935, Gerhard Domagk, a German chemist, announced the discovery of the effect of prontosil on streptococci. Subsequent work showed that this action was due to the conversion in the body of prontosil to sulphanilamide. The action of the sulphonamides is bacteriostatic and not bactericidal: i.e. they do not directly kill the bacteria but so interfere with their growth that they are unable to multiply. This action of the sulphonamides is now believed to be due to the similarity of their chemical structure to that of *p*-aminobenzoic acid. This latter substance is essential for the growth of many bacteria. If the bacteria are surrounded by a sulphonamide in greater concentration than *p*-aminobenzoic acid, then the bacteria take up the sulphonamide. This interferes with their development and they therefore never mature; nor are they able to reproduce themselves. Although the sulphonamides have been largely replaced by other antibiotics in the treatment of infections, they still have a useful role in antibacterial therapy.

SULPHONES A group of drugs allied to the sulphonamides. They are used in the treatment of leprosy. The members of this group include DAPSONE.

SULPHONYLUREAS are sulphonamide derivatives which lower the blood sugar when they are given by mouth by enhancing the production of insulin. They are effective only when some residual pancreatic beta cell function is present. All may lead to a hypoglycaemia if given in overdose and this is particularly common when long-acting SULPHONYLUREAS are given to elderly patients. There is no evidence for any difference in the effectiveness of the various sulphonylureas. TOLBUTAMIDE was the first of the sulphonlyurea drugs. It has a short duration of action and is usually given twice daily. CHLORPROPAMIDE has a more prolonged action and only needs to be given once daily but its prolonged action causes more side-effects including sensitivity reactions. Other oral hypoglycaemic agents of this family include glibenclamide, which has a duration of action intermediate between tolbutamide and chlorpropamide and also produces side-effects (in about 30 per cent of outpatients according to a recent study). Other sulphonlyureas include acetohexamide, glibornuride, gliclazide, glipizide, gliquidone and tolazamide. Glymidine is a related compound with a similar action to the sulphonylureas. It is particularly useful in patients who are hypersensitive to sulphonylureas.

Sulphonylureas are best avoided in patients who are overweight as they tend to stimulate the appetite and aggravate obesity. They should be used with caution in patients with hepatic or renal disease. Side-effects are infrequent and usually not severe, the most common being epigastric discomfort with occasional nausea, vomiting and anorexia. In about 10 per cent of patients chlorpropamide and tolbutamide may cause facial flushing after drinking alcohol (see DIABETES MELLITUS). Some patients are hypersensitive to oral hypoglycaemic agents and develop rashes which may progress to erythema multiforme and exfoliative dermatitis. These reactions usually appear in the first 6 to 8 weeks of treatment.

SULPHUR Chemical combinations of this substance were once applied topically because of their antimicrobial activity; they are no longer used.

SULPHURIC ACID or OIL OF VITRIOL In its undiluted state, this is one of the most powerful of the mineral acids. It is a heavy, colourless liquid of oily consistence and is largely used in various manufacturing operations, so that poisoning by sulphuric acid is not uncommon. It chars any organic substance with which it is brought in contact, and acts as a violent corrosive poison. The treatment of sulphuric acid poisoning is that for corrosive poisons generally: e.g. to administer weak alkalis such as baking soda, milk, egg white or water followed by gastric lavage (see APPENDIX 1: BASIC FIRST AID).

SULPHUROUS ACID is a saturated solution of sulphur dioxide. It has an extremely pungent odour and strong disinfectant power.

SUMMER DIARRHOEA (see DIARRHOEA; INFANT FEEDING).

SUNBURN (see PHOTODERMATOSES).

SUPER- A prefix signifying above or implying excess.

SUPERFICIAL Positioned near the surface: for example, superficial blood vessels or capillaries lie just beneath the skin and by contracting and expanding help to regulate body TEMPERATURE.

SUPINATION means the turning of the forearm and hand so that the palm faces upwards.

SUPINE Lying on the back, face upwards. or the position of the forearm where the hand lies face upwards.

SUPPOSITORY A drug preparation in solid, bullet-like form, which is inserted into the rectum or vagina (when it is called a pessary). This method of using drugs, which is more popular on the Continent than in the United Kingdom, may be chosen for various reasons. For example, the suppository, as in the case of glycerin suppositories, may be used to produce an aperient action. Other suppositories, such as those of morphine, are used to reduce pain and check the action of the bowels.

Method of use The suppository is placed with its pointed end against the anus and with a firm but gentle screwing movement is pushed upwards.

SUPPRESSION (1) The stopping of any physiological activity. (2) A psychological defence mechanism by which an individual intentionally refuses to acknowledge an idea or memory that he finds distasteful or unpleasant. (3) A treatment that stops the visible signs of an illness or holds back its usual progress.

SUPPURATION The process of pus formation. When pus forms on a raw surface the process is called ulceration, whilst a deep-seated collection of pus is known as an abscess. (For more detailed information, see ABSCESS; INFLAMMATION; PHAGOCYTOSIS; ULCER; WOUNDS.)

SUPRA- A prefix signifying above or upon.

SUPRAPUBIC An operation in which the abdomen is opened in its lower part, immediately above the pubic bones. It was a common approach for removal of the prostate gland but is now used less often as transurethral prostatectomy has become the standard procedure. (See LITHOTOMY.)

SUPRARENAL GLANDS, (see ADRENAL GLANDS).

SUPRAVENTRICULAR TACHYCARDIA
An unusually fast but regular beating of the heart occurring for periods that may last several hours or days. In most people with this abnormality the heart rate is between 140 and 180 beats a minute. Rarely, the rate may rise as high as 250–300. The condition occurs when abnormal electrical impulses that arise in the upper chambers (atria) of the heart override the normal control centre – the sinoatrial node – for the heart beat. Symptoms usually include breathlessness, palpitations, pain in the chest and fainting. An ELECTROCARDIOGRAM is taken to help make the diagnosis. An acute episode can sometimes be stopped by VALSAVA'S MANOEUVRE or by drinking cold water. Anti-arrhythmic drugs such as adenosine and digoxin are used to treat recurrent attacks. Occasionally, a severe attack may need to be treated with an electric shock to the heart known as DEFIBRILLATION.

SURAMIN   A drug used to treat trypanosomiasis or SLEEPING SICKNESS. Side-effects vary in frequency and intensity and are sometimes serious. They include nausea, vomiting, shock and occasionally loss of consciousness.

SURFACTANT   A surface-active agent lining the alveoli of the lungs, which plays an essential part in RESPIRATION by preventing the alveoli collapsing at the end of expiration. Absence, or lack, of surfactant is one of the factors responsible for HYALINE MEMBRANE DISEASE , and it is now being used in the treatment of this condition by means of instillation into the trachea.

SURGERY   That branch of medicine involved in the treatment of injuries, deformities or individual diseases by operation or manipulation. It incorporates: general surgery; specialized techniques such as CRYOSURGERY, MICROSURGERY, and MINIMALLY INVASIVE or minimal access (keyhole) surgery; and surgery associated with the main specialties, especially cardiothoracic surgery, gastroenterology, GYNAECOLOGY, NEUROLOGY, OBSTETRICS, ONCOLOGY, OPHTHALMOLOGY, ORTHOPAEDICS, TRANSPLANTATION surgery, reconstructive (PLASTIC) surgery, and UROLOGY. Surgery is carried out in specially designed operating theatres and, whereas it used to necessitate days and sometimes weeks of inpatient hospital care, many patients are now treated as day patients, often under local anaesthesia, being admitted in the morning and discharged later in the day.

More complex surgery, such as transplantation and neurosurgery, usually necessitates patients being nursed postoperatively in high-dependency or intensive-care units before being transferred to ordinary recovery wards. Successful surgery requires close co-operation between surgeons, physicians and RADIOLOGISTS as well as ANAESTHETISTS, whose sophisticated techniques enable surgeons to undertake long and complex operations that were unthinkable 30 or more years ago. Successful surgery is also dependent on the skills of supporting staff comprising nurses and operating-theatre technicians.

SURROGATE   A term applied in medicine to a substance used as a substitute for another.

The term is also applied to a woman who agrees to become pregnant and give birth to a child on the understanding that she will give up the child to the parents who have contracted with her for the surrogacy arrangement. When IN VITRO FERTILIZATION proved successful, it became possible to transfer a fertilized egg to a 'uterus of choice'. Artificial insemination of the potential surrogate mother using sperm from the putative 'father' is also practised. Surrogacy has thrown up a host of ethical and legal problems which have yet to be satisfactorily resolved.

SUSCEPTIBILITY   A reduced ability to combat an illness, usually an infection. The patient may be in poor general health or immunization or disease may have affected his defence mechanisms. For example, a person with AIDS is particularly susceptible to infection.

SUTURE   A word used in both an anatomical and a surgical sense. Anatomically suture is a type of immovable joint, found particularly in the skull, including the coronal suture (between the frontal and parietal bones); the lamboidal suture (between the parietal and occipital bones); and the sagittal suture (between the two parietal bones). Surgically the word refers either to the technique of closing a wound or the material used. Stitching methods have been developed for gastrointestinal, neurological, dermatological and other forms of surgery, and include laser surgery. The material used is generally divided into monofilament, twisted or braided. Absorbable sutures include catgut, Vicryl™ and Dexon™. Non-absorbable sutures include silk, nylon and prolene. The type used and time of suture removal depend on the site and general state of the patient. Those patients on steroids who have a malignant or infective disorder heal slowly and their sutures may need to stay in for 14 days or more instead of the usual five to eight days.

SWAB   A term applied to a small piece of gauze, lint, or similar material used for wiping out the mouth of a patient or for drying out a wound. The term is also applied to a tuft of sterilized cotton-wool wrapped round a wire and enclosed in a sterile glass tube used for obtaining a sample from the throat, from wounds, or the like, for bacteriological examination.

SWAN-GANZ CATHETER   A flexible tube with a double lumen and a small balloon at its distal end. It is introduced into a vein in the arm and advanced until the end of the catheter is in the right atrium. The balloon is then inflated with air through one lumen and this enables the blood stream to propel the catheter through the right ventricle to the pulmonary artery. The balloon is deflated and the catheter can then record the pulmonary artery pressure. When the balloon is inflated the tip is isolated from the pulmonary artery and measures the left atrial pressure. These measurements are important in the management of patients with circulatory failure as under these circumstances the central venous pressure or the right atrial pressure is an unreliable guide to fluid replacement.

SWEAT (see PERSPIRATION).

SWEAT GLANDS (see SKIN).

SWEETBREAD A traditional term applied to several glands used for food, including the thymus gland of young animals (neck sweetbread), the pancreas (stomach sweetbread), and the testis.

SYCOSIS BARBAE (Barber's itch) A chronic staphylococcal folliculitis (infection of the hair follicles with STAPHYLOCOCCI bacteria) of the beard area in males causing a papulo-pustular inflammation clearly centred on hair follicles. It must be distinguished from RINGWORM infection of the face and hair follicles (tinea barbae) and from pseudo-folliculitis due to ingrowing hairs. Topical and oral anti-staphyloccoccal antibiotics are effective.

SYDENHAM'S CHOREA Also called St Vitus dance, this type of CHOREA is a disease of the central nervous system that occurs after RHEUMATIC FEVER – up to six months later – and is probably an inflammatory complication of a β-haemolytic STREPTOCOCCAL infection. The patient presents with jerky, purposeless, involuntary movements of a limb and tongue, similar to the symptoms of cerebral palsy. Chorea is best treated as a transitory reversible form of cerebral palsy. The disorder usually lasts six to eight months and residual symptoms are rare.

SYMPATHETIC A term applied to certain diseases or symptoms which arise in one part of the body in consequence of disease in some distant part. Inflammation may arise in one eye, in consequence of injury to the other, by the spread of organisms along the lymphatic channels connecting the two, and is then known as sympathetic inflammation. Pain also may be of a sympathetic nature. (See PAIN.)

SYMPATHETIC SYSTEM Part of the AUTONOMIC NERVOUS SYSTEM. It consists of scattered collections of grey matter known as ganglia, united by an irregular network of nerve-fibres, those portions where the ganglia are placed most closely and the network of fibres is specially dense being known as plexuses. The chief part of the sympathetic system consists of two ganglionated cords that run through the neck, chest, and abdomen, lying close in front of the spine. In conjunction with the other part of the autonomic nervous system – the parasympathetic – this part controls many of the body's involuntary activities involving glands, organs and other tissues. (For further details, see NERVES.)

SYMPATHOMIMETIC DRUGS Those producing an effect comparable to those produced by stimulation of the sympathetic nervous system: e.g. ADRENALINE.

SYMPHYSIS An anatomical description of a joint in which two bones are connected by strong fibrous cartilage. One example is the joint between the two pubic bones in the front of the pelvis, another the joint between the upper and middle parts of the breast bone.

SYMPTOM A term applied to any evidence of disease. The term, physical sign, is generally applied to evidence of disease of which the patient does not complain but which is elicited upon examination. For the symptoms indicative of the various diseases see under the headings of each disease.

SYN- A prefix signifying union.

SYNAPSE The term applied to the anatomical relation of one nerve-cell with another which is effected at various points by contact of their branching processes. The two neurones do not come directly into contact but the release of a chemical NEUROTRANSMITTER by one neuronal AXON is followed by this chemical travelling across the synapse and firing off the signal along another nerve. A signal can be sent across a synapse in one direction only, from presynaptic or postsynaptic membranes. Synapses are divided into excitatory and inhibitory types. When a neurotransmitter travels across an excitatory synapse it usually provokes the receptor neurone into initiating an electrical impulse. Inhibitory synapses cool down the excitation of the adjacent neurones. Drugs that influence the nervous system usually do so by affecting the release or modification of the neurotransmitters passing across the synapse.

SYNCOPE or fainting A loss of consciousness due to a fall in BLOOD PRESSURE. This may result because the cardiac output has become reduced or because the peripheral resistance provided by the arterioles has decreased. The simple faint or vaso-vagal attack is a result of a failure to maintain an adequate venous return of blood to the heart. This is likely to occur after prolonged periods of standing, particularly if one is standing still or if the climatic conditions are hot. It can also result from an unpleasant or painful experience. Pallor, sweating and a slow pulse are characteristic. Recovery is immediate when the venous return is restored by lying flat. Syncope can also result when the venous return to the heart is impaired as a result of a rise in intra-thoracic pressure. This may happen after prolonged vigorous coughing, the so-called cough syncope, or when elderly men with prostatic hypertrophy strain to empty their bladder. This is known as micturition syncope. Syncope is particularly likely to occur when the arterial blood pressure is unusually low. This may result from overtreatment of hypertension with drugs or it may be the result of diseases, such as Addison's disease, which are associated with low blood pressures. It is important that syncope is distinguished from epilepsy.

SYNDACTYLY A congenital condition in which two or more fingers or toes are fused together to a varying extent. The condition is popularly known as WEBBED FINGERS or toes.

SYNDROME A term applied to a group of symptoms occurring together regularly and thus constituting a disease to which some particular name is given: e.g. Cushing's syndrome comprising obesity, hypertension, purple striae and osteoporosis; Korsakoff's syndrome, of loss of appreciation of time and place combined with talkativeness, forming signs of alcoholic delirium.

SYNECHIAE Adhesions between the iris and adjacent structures, e.g. cornea, lens. They usually arise as a result of inflammation of the iris.

SYNERGIST (1) A muscle that works in concert with an AGONIST muscle to perform a certain movement. (2) An agent, for example a drug, that acts with another to produce a result that is greater than adding together the separate effects of the two agents. Synergism in drug treatment may be beneficial as in the case of combined LEVODOPA and SELEGILINE, a selective monoamine oxidase inhibitor, in the treatment of PARKINSON'S DISEASE. It may be potentially dangerous, however, as when MONOAMINE OXIDASE INHIBITORS boost the effects of BARBITURATES.

SYNOSTOSIS The term applied to a union by bony material of adjacent bones which are normally separate.

SYNOVECTOMY Surgical removal of the SYNOVIUM (see SYNOVIAL MEMBRANE) to treat troublesome SYNOVITIS. The operation is not normally done until other treatments have failed.

SYNOVIAL MEMBRANE forms the lining of the soft parts that enclose the cavity of a joint. (See JOINTS.)

SYNOVITIS Inflammation of the membrane lining a joint. It is usually painful and accompanied by effusion of fluid within the synovial sac of the joint. It is found in acute RHEUMATISM, various injuries and inflammations of joints, and in the chronic form in TUBERCULOSIS. Treatment of synovitis is with rest, splinting, ANALGESIC and NON-STEROIDAL ANTI-INFLAMMATORY DRUGS. Infection should be treated with ANTIBIOTICS. If the joint fails to respond, surgery (SYNOVECTOMY) may be needed. (See JOINTS, DISEASES OF.)

SYNOVIUM   (see SYNOVIAL MEMBRANE).

SYNTHETIC A term applied to substances produced by chemical processes in the laboratory or by artificial building up.

SYPHILIS A sexually transmitted or congenital disease (the latter variety is now rare). Because in most cases the disease is acquired as a result of sexual intercourse with an infected individual, it is classed as a sexually transmitted disease. Syphilis normally affects only human beings.

The disease seems to have first attracted public attention about or soon after the year 1494 in consequence of a severe and widespread outbreak among the French soldiers then occupied in the siege of Naples, hence the description Neapolitan or French pox. It has been thought to have brought to Europe from America as a result of European explorers' crossing the Atlantic. The name syphilis was derived from that of the chief character in a Latin poem published by Fracastoro in 1530. Syphilis may have occurred among the Eastern races in ancient times, although it was most likely often confused with LEPROSY and TUBERCULOSIS. Today, according to the World Health Organization, around 40 million new cases are notified annually in the world, and this is probably an underestimate. In 1996 in England around 1,400 new cases of syphilis were diagnosed in NHS genito-urinary medicine clinics. The infection is most common in homosexual men.

Causes The causative organism is the *Treponema pallidum*, a long, thread-like wavy organism with pointed tapering ends. It is found in large numbers in the sores in the primary stage of the disease and in the skin lesions in the secondary stage.

Syphilis may be acquired from people already suffering from the disease, or it may be congenital. The acquired form is usually got by sexual intercourse, kissing or other intimate bodily contact. The epithelium covering the general surface of the skin seems to be an efficient protection, but the infective material penetrates mucous membranes. The acquired form of the disease is infectious from contact with sores, both in its primary and secondary stages; infants suffering from the congenital form are also highly infectious. Accordingly anyone frequently handling such an infant is at risk of infection, although the mother may handle the baby with impunity.

Symptoms The acquired form of the disease is commonly divided into three stages – primary, secondary, and tertiary, though the latter is much less common than it was 50 years ago. The clinical manifestations are varied and are sometimes confused with those of other diseases.There are several laboratory tests for confirming the diagnosis.

The incubation period ranges from 10 to 90 days, though most frequently it is around four weeks. Then a small persistent ulcer appears at the site of infection, which is accompanied by a typical cartilaginous hardness of the tissues immediately round and beneath it. This, which is known as the primary sore (or chancre), may be very much inflamed, or it may be so small as to pass almost or quite unnoticed. A few days later, the lymphatic glands in its neighbourhood, and then those all over the body, become swollen and hard. This condition lasts for several weeks before the sore slowly heals and the glands subside. After a variable period, usually about two months from the date of infection, the secondary symptoms appear and resemble the symptoms of an ordinary fever, with PYREXIA, loss of appetite, vague pains through the body, and a faint red rash seen best upon the front of the chest. People with syphilis are infectious in the primary and secondary stages but not in the latent or tertiary stages.

In untreated or inadequately treated cases manifestations of the tertiary stage develop after the lapse of some months or even years and this is known as the latent period. These consist in the growth, at various sites throughout the body, of masses of granulation tissue known as gummas. These gummas may appear as hard nodules in the skin, or form tumour-like masses in the muscles, or produce thickening of bones. They may develop in the brain and spinal cord, where their presence causes very serious symptoms. Gummas yield readily, as a rule, to appropriate treatment, and generally disappear speedily.

Still later effects are apt to follow, such as disease of the arteries, leading to aneurysm (see ARTERIES, DISEASES OF; ANEURYSM), to stroke, and to mental deterioration (see MENTAL ILL-NESS); also certain nervous diseases, of which tabes dorsalis and general paralysis are the chief.

The congenital form of syphilis, now rare, may affect the child before birth, leading then as a rule to miscarriage, or to a stillbirth if born at full time. Or he (or she) may show the first symptoms a few weeks after birth, the appearances then corresponding to the secondary manifestations of the acquired form.

Laboratory confirmation of a clinical diagnosis is done by identifying active spirochaetes in a smear taken at the site of the initial chancre and by blood tests such as the treponomal antibody absorption tests. These tests are strongly positive at the secondary stage, and in patients with neurosyphilis the tests may have to be done on cerebrospinal fluid.

Treatment Any person with syphilis is a source of infection, and should take precautions not to spread it. Penicillin is the drug of choice in the disease in all its stages, but resistant strains of the *Treponema pallidum* have emerged and are causing problems, especially in developing countries. Treatment must be instituted as soon as possible after infection is acquired; (1) a full course of treatment is essential in every case, no matter how mild the disease may appear to be; (2) periodic blood examinations must be carried out on every patient for at least two years after he or she has been apparently cured.

Prevention is important and promiscuous hetero- or homosexual intercourse involves a risk of infection. Condoms provide some, but not complete protection. Infection can be avoided by maintaining a monogamous relationship.

SYRINGE An instrument for injecting fluid into, or withdrawing fluid from, a body cavity, tissue or blood. Syringes come in different sizes and some are specially designed for use in a particular site – for example, for withdrawing CEREBROSPINAL fluid. The basic design is the same: a calibrated barrel with a plunger at one end, while the other end has a nozzle to which a hollow needle can be attached. Most syringes are disposable, plastic, presterilized and packed in sealed containers. Injections can be given under the skin, into muscle, into a vein or into the cerebrospinal fluid. The term hypodermic, though literally meaning under the skin, is now used to describe most syringes.

SYRINGOMYELIA A rare disease affecting the spinal cord, in which irregular cavities form, surrounded by an excessive amount of the connective tissue of the central nervous system. These cavities encroach upon the nerve tracts in the cord, producing especially loss of the sense of pain or of that for heat and cold in parts of the limbs, although the sensation of touch is retained. Another occasional symptom is wasting of certain muscles in the limbs. Changes affecting outlying parts like the fingers are also found. Because of their insensitiveness to pain, these are often burnt or injured, and troublesome ulcers, or loss of parts of the fingers, result. The condition of the spinal cord is probably present at birth, though the symptoms do not usually appear till adulthood. The disease is slowly progressive, though sudden exacerbations may occur after a cough, a sneeze, or sudden straining. Treatment is supportive for this progressive disorder.

SYSTEMIC A description of something, for example, a drug, that affects the whole body and not just part of it.

SYSTEMIC LUPUS ERYTHEMATOSUS (SLE) is an autoimmune disease occurring predominantly in women (see LUPUS ERYTHEMATO-SUS) that causes chronic inflammation of the connective tissue which affects the skin and various internal organs. The skin is red and scaly, joints develop inflammatory arthritis, and the kidneys may be damaged. The brain, heart and lungs may also be affected, with affected tissue becoming scarred. Treatment is with CORTICOSTEROIDS or immunosuppressive drugs.

SYSTOLE The contraction of the heart. It alternates with the resting phase, known as diastole. The two occupy, respectively, about one-third and two-thirds of the cycle of heart action.

SYSTOLIC PRESSURE (see BLOOD PRESSURE).

T

TABES this means, literally, a wasting disease, and is an old name applied to various diseases, such as tabes dorsalis (tertiary SYPHILIS) and tuberculosis accompanied by enlargement of glands. For instance, the name tabes dorsalis was used for locomotor ataxia.

TABLET A solid disc-like preparation made by compression and containing drugs mixed usually with sugar and other material. Tablets are widely used because of their convenience and accurate dosage. The word, 'tabloid', indicates a proprietary preparation.

TACHYCARDIA A rapid pulse rate. (See HEART DISEASE.)

TACHYPHYLAXIS Rapidly developing tolerance to a drug (see TOLERANCE.)

TACHYPNOEA Unusually rapid breathing.

TACTILE Perceptible to, pertaining to or related to the sense of touch.

TAENIASIS A parasitic disorder caused by taeniae, or tapeworms. Their shape is modified to present as large an absorbing surface as possible to the digested food passing down the intestine, so that they are flat, white and long (up to 12 metres [40 feet] in length), like a piece of tape, as their name implies. Each consists of a head, the size of a small pin's head, provided with suckers, and sometimes with hooklets, for adhesion to the bowel wall, and from this head segments grow that gradually increase in size and develop ova the further they recede from the head. The mature segments at the extremity of the worm are crammed full of ova, and are constantly splitting off to be discharged in the stools. When these mature segments, or proglottides, are discharged, they fall on the ground, and the ova they contain are afterwards taken via food or drink into the stomach of an intermediate host, which may be a pig, ox or cattle, in the case of different parasites.

The geographical distribution of different tapeworm infestation depends largely upon the eating habits of the inhabitants. Thus *Taenia saginata*, or the beef tapeworm, is found in beef-eating areas, especially in Europe and Muslim countries. *Taenia solium*, the pork tapeworm, is found most commonly in Germany and the Slav countries. *Echinococcus granulosus* is found where dogs are widely used, as in Iceland or sheep-rearing countries such as Australia, New Zealand and Argentina.

When the ova reach the stomach of the intermediate host their capsule is dissolved, the embryos escape and find their way through the wall of stomach or intestine into the blood-vessels, by which they are carried to distant parts of the body. In the case of *Taenia solium* the intermediate host is the pig, in the case of *Taenia saginata* it is cattle. The embryos of the worm become encysted in the muscles and remain so till they die, or till the animal's flesh happens to be eaten by the proper host, when they develop again into a new tapeworm in the intestine. The flesh of a pig thus infected shows plainly the encysted embryo (known as *Cysticercus cellulosae*), and is called measly pork. *DIPHYLLOBOTHRIUM LATUM* is seldom met with, except in the north of Europe and Asia, and the intermediate hosts are several varieties of fish. In the case of the tapeworm known as *Echinococcus granulosus*, relations are reversed, and man plays the rôle of intermediate host, the host of the mature tapeworm being the dog, from which the human being derives the embryo worm by allowing the dog to lick his hands and face, or to contaminate his food. Although the worm in the dog is very small (having only three segments, as a rule), the encysted form in man, known as a hydatid cyst, may reach a large size, situated in the liver, lungs, kidney or brain.

In the case of infestation with *Taenia saginata* there may be no symptoms or signs at all, and the 'host' only becomes aware that he is infested, when he sees the tapeworm, or rather part of it, in the stools. In the case of *Taenia solium*, the outlook is more serious because the eggs, when swallowed, are liable to migrate into the tissues of the body, as they do in the pig, and cause cysts. If these occur in the muscles they may cause little trouble but, if they occur in the brain, they can prove very serious.

Hydatid cysts often grow to a great size, budding off in their interior smaller cysts, which may have still smaller ones within them, the final contents of the smallest cysts being a salt, watery fluid and numerous heads of echinococci, each provided with a circle of hooks, and each capable, under proper conditions, of forming a new worm. The symptoms produced by a hydatid cyst depend mainly upon the effects of its size and consequent pressure. Very small cysts in the brain may produce serious results, like those of a tumour, whilst in the liver a cyst may grow to the size of a man's head before causing much trouble.

Treatment of tapeworm infestation consists of the administration of mepacrine, niclosamide or dichlorophen, followed by a purgative. Castor oil must not be used for this purpose. During treatment the stools must be carefully examined for the head of the tapeworm. Unless the head is passed in the stools, the worm will grow again. The treatment of hydatid cyst is surgical: i.e. the cyst must be removed by operation.

TALC is a soft mineral consisting of magnesium silicate. It is much used as an ingredient of dusting powders.

TALIPES The technical name for club-foot, a deformity in which the foot is permanently twisted at the ankle-joint, so that the sole no longer rests on the ground in standing.

Classification The foot can be twisted in four directions. The heel may be pulled up so that the person walks on his toes (talipes equinus), or the toes may be bent up so that he walks on his heel only (talipes calcaneus), or the sole may look inwards so that he walks on the outer edge of the foot (talipes varus), or outwards so that he walks on the inside of the foot (talipes valgus). These are usually combined, the heel being drawn up and the sole turned inwards (equino-varus) or the heel resting on the ground and the sole looking outwards (talipes calcaneo-valgus). A more important division is into those cases in which the deformity exists at birth, which are generally at first fairly easily rectified; and into those cases which are acquired later in life as the result of some disease which do not yield to such simple treatment.

Causes The cases found at birth are due to some arrest of development resulting in a structural deformity of both the forefoot and hindfoot (talipes equino-varus), or faulty position of the fetus in the womb (talipes calcaneo-valgus). The former occurs in 1-2 per 1000 live births in the UK. It is two to three times as common in boys as in girls, and is frequently bilateral. It tends to run in affected families, with an incidence 20-30 times that in the normal population. Despite numerous theories, its cause remains unknown; it is often associated with other abnormalities or forms part of a specific syndrome. Those cases acquired later may be caused by neurological conditions, with spasm of the muscles on the affected side (cerebral palsy), or paralysis of the muscles on the other side (poliomyelitis), or by rigidity due to the scar following a burn or in inflammation.

Treatment should start as soon as possible after birth. Early treatment involves repeated gentle manipulations, maintaining the correction obtained with adhesive strapping, plaster of Paris or

metal splints. The precise method used depends on the surgeon's preferences and the ability of the parents to bring the patient at frequent intervals for treatment. The response is often excellent, particularly with talipes calcaneo-valgus. A tendency to relapse when the child starts walking may be corrected by a wedge on the heel of the shoe. Surgery is usually indicated in more severe cases, and certainly if the initial conservative treatment has not resulted in full clinical and radiological correction after 12-14 weeks. In those cases resulting from disease or injury after birth, treatment involves splinting, strengthening the weakened muscles by massage and electrical stimulation. In severe cases, surgery involving tendon transplantation may be indicated.

TALUS The square-shaped bone which forms the lower part of the ankle-joint and unites the leg bones to the foot.

TAMOXIFEN An OESTROGEN receptor antagonist – namely, the drug blocks the action of oestrogen – which is the treatment of choice for breast cancer in postmenopausal women in conjunction with LUMPECTOMY or partial or complete MASTECTOMY. Around 30 per cent of patients in whom breast cancer has spread to adjacent glands or beyond respond to this hormonal treatment. In patients with tumours that are oestrogen sensitive, the positive response to tamoxifen is 60 per cent. Those tumours that are not oestrogen sensitive are much less likely to respond to the drug. Tamoxifen increases both survival rates and the period between the diagnosis of the tumour and appearance of metastatic growth in tumours sensitive to it. Tamoxifen has fewer adverse effects than most other drugs used for treating breast cancer. Patients in whom the cancer has spread to the bone(s) may suffer pain with tamoxifen treatment.

Tamoxifen is also used to treat INFERTILITY, being taken on certain days of the menstrual cycle.

TAMPON A plug or compressed gauze or cotton wool inserted into a wound or orifice to arrest haemorrhage. Also inserted into the vagina to absorb the flow of blood during menstruation. Infected tampons may cause TOXIC SHOCK, a potentially dangerous but fortunately uncommon reaction.

TAMPONADE The insertion of a tampon. It also may be used to describe the potentially life-threatening compression of the heart by the accumulation of fluid in the pericardial sac. This is characterized by tachycardia, pulsus paradoxus, low blood pressure, raised pressure in the jugular vein and abnormally quiet heart sounds.

Treatment consists of draining the fluid (which may be blood or an effusion) and treating the underlying cause.

TANNIN or TANNIC ACID   An uncrystallizable white powder, soluble in water or glycerin. It is extracted from oak galls in large amount, but it is also present in almost all vegetable infusions. Tannic acid acts as an astringent.

TAPEWORM (see TAENIASIS).

TAPPING   The popular name for the withdrawal of oedema fluid from the cavities or the subcutaneous tissues of the body. (See ASPIRATION; OEDEMA.)

TARS   Complex oily mixtures derived from coal or wood (pine). Prolonged exposure to some crude tars occupationally may lead to multiple cutaneous warty lesions (pitch warts). Squamous carcinoma may supervene. More refined extracts of tar are used in dermatological therapy, especially in PSORIASIS.

TARDIVE DYSKINESIA   Also known as orofacial DYSKINESIA, this is characterized by involuntary chewing and grimacing, usually the result of years of taking antipsychotic drugs, particularly in the elderly, when these drugs are sometimes used to sedate troublesome patients.

TARGET CELL   Abnormal ERYTHROCYTES which are large and 'floppy' and have a ringed appearance, similar to that of a target, when stained and viewed under the microscope. This change from normal may occur with iron-deficiency ANAEMIA, liver disease, a small SPLEEN, haemoglobinopathies (disorders of haemoglobin) and THALASSAEMIAS.

A target cell is also a cell that is the focus of attack by MACROPHAGES (killer cells) or ANTIBODIES; it may also be the site of action of a specific HORMONE.

TARGET ORGAN   The specific organ (or tissue) at which a HORMONE, drug or other agent is aimed to bring about its physiological or pharmacological effect.

TARSAL   Of or pertaining to the TARSUS of the foot and ankle – this comprises talus, calcaneus navicular, cuboid and three cuneiform bones – or eyelid.

TARSUS   The region of the instep with its seven bones, the chief of which are the TALUS supporting the leg-bones and the CALCANEUS or heel-bone, the others being the navicular, cuboid, and three cuneiform bones.

TARTAR   A concretion that forms on the teeth near the margin of the gum, consisting chiefly of phosphate of lime deposited from the saliva. Mixed with this are food particles, and this is an ideal medium for bacteria to flourish in. Regular brushing of the teeth is a preventive measure. Dentists or dental hygienists routinely remove tartar, because it gives rise to wasting of the gums and loosening of the teeth.

TASTE (see TONGUE).

TATTOOING   This has been a cult, or fashion, since the earliest days of history. Apart from the mixed motives for its use, it has a therapeutic use in matching the colour of skin grafts. It is performed by implanting particles of colour pigment into the deeper layer of the skin known as the corium (see SKIN). This is done by means of a needle or needles. The pigments commonly used are carbon for black, cinnabar (red mercuric sulphide) or cadmium salts for red, chrome salts for greens and yellows, cobalt for blue, ferric (iron) salts for browns, pinks and yellows, and titanium for white. The main medical hazard of tattooing is infection, particularly HEPATITIS, which may be fatal. The tattooed person may also become allergic to one of the pigments used, particularly cinnabar. Removal, which should be done by a plastic surgeon, always leaves a residual scar, and often needs to be followed by a skin graft. Removal is not allowed under the National Health Service unless there is some medical reason: for example, allergic reactions to it. Other methods of removal are by CRYOSURGERY, DERMABRASION and laser surgery. These, too, must only be carried out under skilled medical supervision.

In order to reduce the health hazards, tattooists, along with acupuncturists, cosmetic skin-piercers and hair electrolysers, are required by UK legislation to register their premises with health and local authorities before starting business. The practitioners have to satisfy the authorities that adequate precautions have been taken to prevent the transmission of infections, such as hepatitis.

TAXANES   A recently developed group of cytotoxic drugs administered intravenously for the treatment of advanced OVARIAN cancer and secondary spread of BREAST cancer. Given under specialist supervision in hospital, taxanes are not effective for all patients but results are encouraging when they do respond. Side-effects include HYPERSENSITIVITY, MYELOSUPPRESSION, cardiac ARRHYTHMIAS, and peripheral NEUROPATHY.

TAXIS   The method of pushing back, into the abdominal cavity, a loop of bowel which has passed through the wall in consequence of a rupture.

TAY SACHS DISEASE   Also termed amaurotic familial idiocy, this is an inherited recessive condition in which there is abnormal accumulation of LIPIDS in the BRAIN. The result is blindness, mental retardation and death in early childhood. The disease can usually be prevented by genetic counselling in those communities in which the disease is known to occur.

TEARS (see EYE).

T CELL LYMPHOMA (see LYMPHOMA).

TECHNETIUM-99   An isotope of the artificial element technetium. It emits gamma rays and is used as a tracer in building up a scintigraphic radioactive image of organs such as the brain.

TEETH   Hard organs developed from the mucous membranes of the mouth and embedded in the jawbones. They are used to bite and grind food and to aid clarity of speech. In some animals the teeth may be modified in shape to enable them to be used as weapons.

Structure   Each tooth is composed of enamel, dentine, cement, pulp and periodontal membrane.

ENAMEL is the almost translucent material which covers the crown of a tooth. It is the most highly calcified material in the body, 96–97 per cent being composed of calcified salts. It is arranged from millions of long six-sided prisms set on end on the dentine. It is thickest over the biting

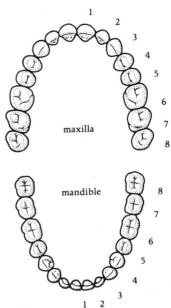

1 central incisor
2 lateral incisor
3 canine
4 1st premolar
5 2nd premolar
6 1st molar
7 2nd molar
8 3rd molar

The permanent teeth of the upper (top) and lower (bottom) jaws.

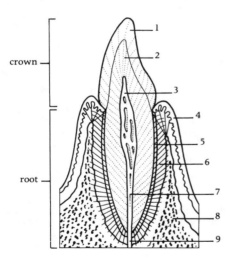

1 enamel
2 dentine
3 pulp (contains blood vessels and nerves)
4 gingiva (gum)
5 cementum
6 periodontal membrane
7 pulp canal
8 bone
9 apical foramen

Vertical section through incisor tooth.

surface of the tooth. With increasing age or the ingestion of abrasive foods the teeth may be worn away on the surface so that the dentine becomes visible. The outer sides of some teeth may be worn away by bad tooth-brushing technique.

DENTINE is a dense yellowish-white material from which the bulk and the basic shape of a tooth are formed. It is like ivory and it is harder than bone but softer than enamel. The crown of the tooth is covered by the hard protective enamel and the root is covered by a bonelike substance called cement. Dentine is formed from cells which produce cylinders of calcified material in the centre of which are tubules which contain protoplasmic processes which are extensions of the cells. These processes can transfer pain from the enamel to the sensitive pulp in the centre of the tooth. Dentine is formed from inorganic and organic matter. The composition is approximately 75 per cent inorganic salts and 25 per cent organic matter and water. Decay can erode dentine faster than enamel.

CEMENT or cementum is a thin bonelike material which covers the roots of teeth and helps hold the teeth in the bone. Fibres of the periodontal membrane are embedded in the cement and the bone. When the gums recede, part of the cement

maxilla

mandible

1 central incisor
2 lateral incisor
3 canine
4 1st premolar
5 2nd premolar
6 1st molar
7 2nd molar
8 3rd molar

8   7   6   5   4   3   2   1

The permanent teeth of the left side of upper and lower jaws.

may be exposed and the cells die. Once this has happened, the periodontal membrane can no longer be attached to the tooth and, if sufficient cement is destroyed, the tooth support will be so weakened that the tooth will become loose. PULP This is the inner core of the tooth and is composed of a highly vascular, delicate fibrous tissue with many fine nerve fibres. The outer layer is formed by the odontoblasts which formed the dentine and are now dormant unless required to lay down a further thickness of dentine in response to a destructive stimulus at the outer edge of the dentine. The pulp is the tissue remaining after the tooth has been formed and may have helped in its eruption. The pulp is very sensitive to temperature variation and touch. If the pulp becomes exposed it will become infected and usually cannot overcome this. Root-canal treatment or extraction of the tooth may be necessary.

PERIODONTAL MEMBRANE This is a layer of fibrous tissue arranged in groups of fibres which surround and support the root of a tooth in a bone socket. The fibres are interspersed with blood-vessels and nerves. Loss of the membrane leads to loss of the tooth. The membrane can release and re-attach the fibres to allow the tooth to move when it erupts or is being moved by orthodontic springs.

Arrangement and form Teeth are present in most mammals and nearly all have two sets: a temporary or milk set followed by a permanent or adult set. In some animals, like the toothed whale, all the teeth are similar, but in man there are four different shapes: incisors, canines (eye-teeth), premolars (bicuspids), and molars. The incisors are chisel shaped and the canine is pointed. Premolars have two cusps on the crown (one medial to the other) and molars have at least four cusps. They are arranged together in an arch in each jaw and the cusps of opposing teeth interdigitate. Some herbivores have no upper anterior teeth but use a pad of gum instead. As each arch is symmetrical, the teeth in an upper and lower quadrant can be used to identify the animal. In man the quadrants are the same, i.e. in the child there are two incisors, one canine and two molars (total teeth 20). In the adult there are two incisors, one canine, two premolars and three molars (total 32). This mixture of tooth form suggests that man is omnivorous. Anatomically the crown of the tooth has mesial and distal surfaces which touch the tooth next to it. The

permanent canine 1   10 premolars

permanent incisors 2   9 first permanent molar

                                     8 second permanent molar

permanent incisors 3   7 second permanent molar

permanent canine 4   6 first permanent molar

                                     5 premolars

Teeth of a six-year-old child. The permanent teeth are coloured black.

mesial surface is the one nearer to the centre line and the distal is the further away. The biting surface is called the incisal edge for the anterior teeth and the occlusal surface for the posteriors.

Development The first stage in the formation of the teeth is the appearance of a downgrowth of EPITHELIUM into the underlying mesoderm. This is the dental lamina, and from it ten smaller swellings in each jaw appear. These become bell shaped and enclose a part of the mesoderm, the cells of which become specialized and are called the dental papillae. The epithelial cells produce enamel and the dental papilla forms the dentine, cement and pulp. At a fixed time the teeth start to erupt and a root is formed. Before the deciduous teeth erupt, the permanent teeth form, medial to them. In due course the deciduous roots resorb and the permanent teeth are then able to push the crowns out and erupt themselves. If this process is disturbed, the permanent teeth may be displaced and appear in an abnormal position or be impacted.

Eruption of teeth is in a definite order and at a fixed time, although there may be a few months leeway in either direction which is of no significance. Excessive delay is found in some congenital disorders such as cretinism. It may also be associated with local abnormalities of the jaws such as cysts, malformed teeth and supernumerary teeth.

The usual order of eruption of deciduous teeth is:

Middle incisors	6–8 months
Lateral incisors	8–10 ,,
First molars	12–16 ,,
Canines (eye-teeth)	16–20 ,,
Second molars	20–30 ,,

The usual order of eruption of permanent teeth is:

First molars	6–7 years
Middle incisors	6–8 ,,
Lateral incisors	7–9 ,,
Canines	9–12 ,,
First and second premolars	10–12 ,,
Second molars	11–13 ,,
Third molars (wisdom teeth)	17–21 ,,

TEETH, DISEASES OF

Teething, or the process of eruption of the teeth in infants may be accompanied by irritability, salivation, loss of sleep and a failure to feed. The child will tend to rub or touch the painful area. Relief may be obtained in the child by allowing it to chew on a hard object such as a toy or rusk. Mild ANALGESICS may be given if the child is restless and wakens in the night.

Toothache is the pain felt when there is inflammation of the pulp or periodontal membrane of a tooth. It can vary in intensity and may be recurring. The commonest cause is CARIES when the cavity is close to the pulp. Once the pulp has become infected, this is likely to spread from the apex of the tooth into the bone to form an

ABSCESS (gumboil). A lesser but more long-lasting pain is felt when the dentine is unprotected. This can occur when the enamel is lost due to decay or trauma or because the gums have receded. This pain is often associated with temperature change or sweet foods. Expert dental advice should be sought early before the decay is extensive. If a large cavity is accessible, temporary relief may be obtained by inserting a small piece of cotton wool soaked, for example, in oil of cloves.

Caries of the teeth or dental decay is very common in the more affluent countries and is commonest in children and young adults. Increasing awareness of the causes has resulted in a considerable improvement in dental health, particularly in recent years. This has coincided with a rise in general health. Now 50 per cent of five-year-old children are caries free and of the others 10 per cent have half of the remaining carious cavities. Since the start of the National Health Service the emphasis has been on preventive dentistry. In south-east England, which has a high ratio of dentists for the population, less than 5 per cent of the people under 45 years have dentures. Now edentulous patients are mainly found among the elderly who had their teeth removed before 1948.

The cause of caries is probably acid produced by oral bacteria from dietary carbohydrates, particularly refined sugar, and this dissolves part of the enamel. The dentine is eroded more quickly as it is softer. The exposed smooth surfaces are usually protected as they are easily cleaned during normal eating and by brushing. Irregular and overcrowded teeth are more at risk from decay as they are difficult to clean. Primitive people who chew coarse foods rarely get caries. Fluoride in the drinking water at the rate of about 1 part per million is associated with a reduction in the caries rate. Prolonged severe disease in infancy is associated with poor calcification of the teeth, making them more vulnerable to decay. As the teeth are formed and partly calcified by the time of birth, the diet and health of the mother are also important to the teeth of the child. Pregnant mothers and children should have a good balanced diet with sufficient calcium and vitamin D. A fibrous diet will also aid cleansing of the teeth and stimulate the circulation in the teeth and jaws. The caries rate can be reduced by regular brushing with a fluoride toothpaste two or three times per day and certainly before going to sleep. The provision of sweet or sugary juices in an infant's bottle should be avoided.

Irregularity of the permanent teeth may be due to an abnormality in the growth of the jaws or to the early or late loss of the deciduous set. Most frequently it is due to an imbalance in the size of the teeth and the length of the jaws. Some improvement may take place with age but many will require the help of an orthodontist (specialist dentist) who can correct many mal-occlusions by removing a few teeth to allow him to move the others into a good position by means of springs and elastics on various appliances which are worn in the mouth.

Loosening of the teeth may be due to an accident or inflammation of the gum. Teeth loosened by trauma may be replaced and splinted in the socket, even if knocked right out. If the loosening is due to periodontal disease the prognosis is less favourable.

Discoloration of the teeth may be intrinsic or extrinsic, i.e. the stain may be in the calcified structure or stuck on to it. Intrinsic staining may be due to jaundice or the antibiotic tetracycline. Extrinsic stain may be due to tea, coffee, tobacco, pan (a mixture of chuna and betel nuts wrapped in a leaf), iron-containing medicines or excess fluoride.

Gingivitis or inflammation of the gums may occur as an acute or chronic condition. In the acute form it is often part of a general infection of the mouth and principally occurs in children or young adults and resolves after ten to fourteen days. The chronic form occurs later in life and tends to be progressive. Various micro-organisms may be found on the lesions including anaerobes. Antiseptic mouthwashes may help and once the painful stage is past, the gums should be thoroughly cleaned and any calculus removed. In severe conditions an antibiotic may be required.

Periodontal disease is the spread of gingivitis to involve the periodontal membrane of the tooth and in its florid form used to be called pyorrhoea. In this, the membrane becomes damaged by the inflammatory process and a space or pocket is formed into which a probe can be easily passed. As the pocket becomes more extensive the tooth loosens. The loss of the periodontal membrane also leads to the loss of supporting bone. Chronic inflammation soon occurs and is difficult to eradicate. Pain is not a feature of the disease but there is often an unpleasant odour (halitosis). The gums bleed easily and there may be dyspepsia. Treatment is largely aimed at stabilizing the condition rather than curing it.

Dental abscess or alveolar abscess is an infection that arises in or round a tooth and spreads to involve the bone. It may occur many years after a blow has killed the pulp of the tooth or more quickly after caries has reached the pulp. At first the pain may be mild and intermittent but eventually it will become severe and a swelling will develop in the gum over the apex of the tooth. A radiograph of the tooth will show a round clear area at the apex of the tooth. Treatment may be by painting the gum with a mild counter-irritant such as a tincture of aconite and iodine in the early stages but later root-canal therapy or apicectomy may be required. If a swelling is present, it may need to be drained or the offending teeth extracted and antibiotics given.

Injuries to teeth are common. The more minor injuries include crazing and the loss of small chips of enamel, and the major ones include a broken root and avulsion of the entire tooth. A specialist dental opinion should be sought as soon as possible. A tooth that has been knocked out can be re-implanted if it is clean and replaced within a few hours. It will then require splinting in place for 4–6 weeks.

Prevention of dental disease As with other matters, prevention is better than cure. Children should be taught at an early age to keep their teeth and gums clean and to avoid refined sugars between meals. It is better to finish a meal with a drink of water rather than a sweetened drink. Fluoride in some of its forms is useful in the reduction of dental caries and a vaccine now being developed may be useful. Overcrowding of the teeth, obvious maldevelopment of the jaw and persistent thumbsucking into the teens are all indications for seeking the advice of an orthodontist. Generally adults have less trouble with decay but more with periodontal disease and, as its onset is insidious, regular dental inspections are desirable.

TEETH GRINDING or BRUXISM In children during sleep, it is of no significance unless really persistent. During the day it may be an attention-seeking device. There is no treatment for it.

In adults it is usually associated with stress or anxiety, but may be due to some local condition in the mouth such as an unsatisfactory filling. It may also be caused by certain drugs, including FENFLURAMINE and LEVODOPA. If not controlled, it produces excessive wear of the enamel covering of the teeth. Treatment consists of alleviation of any condition in the mouth and any anxiety and stress.

TEETHING (see TEETH, DISEASES OF).

TEICHOPSIA This refers to zigzag lines that patients with migraine often experience as an aura preceding an attack.

TEICOPLANIN A glycopeptide ANTIBIOTIC which acts against AEROBIC and ANAEROBIC GRAM-POSITIVE bacteria. Like the similar drugs, VANCOMYCIN, it is given in the PROPHYLAXIS and treatment of ENDOCARDITIS and other serious infections caused by GRAM-POSITIVE cocci, including STAPHYLOCOCCI which have developed resistance to other antibiotics. Its long duration of action means that it need be given only once a day. Teicoplanin can be given intramuscularly or intravenously. Its use should be carefully monitored as there is a range of adverse effects.

TELANGIECTASIS Abnormal dilatation of ARTERIOLES and VENULES. In the skin it is seen in SPIDER NAEVUS and ROSACEA particularly.

TELEMEDICINE A broad term used to describe medicine at a distance through a communications link. Although distance education has been used successfully for some time, more recently distance diagnosis and treatment have been successfully piloted. In teleradiology, radiographic images are transmitted to a distant site for interpretation by a radiologist. A telepathologist can look down, and in some cases control, a microscope located several hundred miles away. In a teleconsultation, the doctor and patient are in different places, joined by a communications link, such as medical videoconferencing. In its simplest form this kind of telemedicine uses the telephone; more recently, full-colour two-way video and audio links have been used.

Telemedicine is useful for remote locations, such as the Antartic, or on board ships, or aeroplanes, where it may be difficult or impossible to get a doctor to the patient. It can also speed up the referral process, reduce unnecessary referrals and improve communication between professionals. Critics of telemedicine believe it represents a threat to the doctor–patient relationship and is risky because it depends on technology which may be unreliable.

TEMAZEPAM A BENZODIAZEPINE ANXIOLYTIC derived from DIAZEPAM. To be used with care for short-term treatment of INSOMNIA, generally associated with difficulty in falling asleep, frequent nocturnal awakening or early morning awakening. Temazepam is a relatively quick-acting hypnotic of short duration, so, although there is little hangover the next morning compared with other hypnotics, there may still be some drowsiness and effect on skilled tasks such as driving. It should be avoided in elderly people who are at risk of becoming ataxic and so liable to falling and injuring themselves. Temazepam is often abused by drug addicts.

TEMPERATURE Body temperature is the result of a balance of heat-generating forces, chiefly METABOLISM and muscular activity, and heat-loss, mainly from blood circulation through and evaporation from the skin and lungs. The physiological process of homeostasis – a neurological and hormonal feedback mechanism – maintains the healthy person's body at the correct temperature. Disturbance of temperature, as in disease, may be caused by impairment of any of these bodily functions, or by malfunction of the controlling centre in the brain.

Animals are divided into two groups: cold-blooded animals, including reptiles, amphibians, fish, and invertebrates generally, whose temperature varies considerably with that of the environment; and warm-blooded animals, and mammals and birds, whose temperature remains almost constant. In man the 'normal' temperature is around 37 °C (98·4 °F). It may rise as high as 43 °C or fall to 32 °C in various conditions, but the risk to life is only serious above 41 °C or below 35 °C.

Fall in temperature may accompany major loss of blood, starvation, and the state of COLLAPSE which may occur in severe fever and other acute conditions. Certain chronic diseases, notably HYPOTHYROIDISM, are generally accompanied by a subnormal temperature. Increased temperature is a characteristic of many acute diseases, particularly infections. Indeed, many diseases have a characteristic pattern that enables a provisional diagnosis to be made or acts as a warning of possible complications. In most cases the temperature gradually abates as the patient recovers, but in others, such as PNEUMONIA and TYPHUS fever, the untreated disease ends rapidly by a crisis in which the temperature falls, perspiration breaks out, the pulse rate falls, and breathing becomes quieter. This crisis is often preceded by an increase in symptoms, including an epicritical rise in temperature.

Temperature in man is usually measured on the Celsius scale, on a thermometer reading from 35 °C to 43·3 °C. Measurement may be taken in the mouth (under the tongue), in the armpit, or (occasionally in infants) in the rectum. (See THERMOMETER.)

Treatment Abnormally low temperatures may be treated by application of external heat, or reduction of heat loss from the body surface. High temperature may be treated in various ways, apart from the primary treatment of the underlying condition. Treatment of hyperthermia or hypothermia should ensure a gradual return to normal temperature (see ANTIPYRETICS; FEVER).

TEMPLE The side of the head above the line between the eye and ear. The term, temporal, is applied to the muscles, nerves, and artery of this region. The hair usually begins to turn grey first at the temples.

TEMPORAL Referring or relating to the temporal region.

TEMPORAL ARTERITIS Inflammation of the temporal artery. Also known as giant cell arteritis, it often affects other arteries too, mainly in the head. It predominantly affects the elderly. The artery becomes tender with reddening of the overlying skin. Headache and blindness may also occur. The diagnosis is confirmed by temporal artery biopsy, and treatment is with STEROIDS.

TEMPORAL ARTERY A branch of the external carotid artery that is the main vessel supplying blood to the temple and scalp. (See CIRCULATION OF THE BLOOD.)

TEMPORAL LOBE Part of the cerebral cortex in each hemisphere of the brain. Areas of the temporal lobe are involved in the understanding of sound and spoken language (see BRAIN).

TEMPORAL LOBE EPILEPSY EPILEPSY in which the abnormal cerebral activity originates in the temporal lobe of the brain. It is characterized by hallucinations of smell and sometimes of taste, hearing, or sight. There may be disturbances of memory, including déjà vu phenomena. AUTOMATISM may occur, but consciousness is seldom lost.

TENDERNESS The term usually applied in medical nomenclature to pain experienced when a diseased part is handled, the term, pain, being reserved for unpleasant sensations felt apart from any manipulation.

TENDINITIS Inflammation of a tendon. Usually caused by unusual or excessive physical activity, it may also be infective in origin or secondary to a connective tissue disorder. The pain and inflammation may be treated with NON-STEROIDAL ANTI-INFLAMMATORY DRUGS, immobilization splinting and steroid injections. Repetitive strain injury, caused by constant use of a keyboard (typewriter, word processor or computer) is tendinitis occurring in the hands and arms. (See UPPER LIMB DISORDER.)

TENDON, SINEW, or LEADER This is the cord of tissue that attaches the end of a muscle to the bone or other structure upon which the muscle acts when it contracts. Tendons are composed of bundles of white fibrous tissue arranged in a very dense manner, and are of great strength. Some are rounded, some flattened bands, whilst others are very short, the muscle-fibres being attached almost directly to the bone. Most tendons are surrounded by sheaths lined with membrane similar to the synovial membrane lining joint-cavities. In this sheath the tendon glides smoothly over surrounding parts. The fibres of a tendon pass into the substance of the bone and blend with the fibres composing it. One of the largest tendons in the body is the Achilles tendon, or tendo calcaneus, which attaches the muscle of the calf to the calcaneus or heel-bone.

Tendon injuries are one of the hazards of sports (see SPORTS MEDICINE). They usually result from indirect violence, or overuse, rather than direct violence.
RUPTURE usually results from the sudden application of an unbalanced load. Thus complete rupture of the Achilles tendon is common in taking an awkward step backwards playing squash. There is sudden pain, the victim is often under the impression that he received a blow. This is accompanied by loss of function, and a gap may be felt in the tendon.
PARTIAL RUPTURE is also accompanied by pain, but there is no breach of continuity or complete loss of function. Treatment of a complete rupture usually means surgical repair followed by immobilization of the tendon in plaster of Paris for six weeks. Partial rupture usually responds to physiotherapy and immobilization, but healing is slow.

TENDON TRANSFER Reconstructive surgery in which the tendon from an unimportant muscle is removed and used to repair or replace a damaged tendon of a major muscle.

TENDOVAGINITIS Inflammation of a tendon and of the sheath enveloping it.

TENESMUS A symptom of disease affecting the lower part of the large intestine, such as dysentery, piles, or tumour. It consists of a constant sense of heavy discomfort about the lower bowel and desire to defaecate, coupled with straining when doing so, with the passage of mucus and often blood.

TENNIS ELBOW (see ELBOW).

TENO- A prefix denoting some relation to a tendon.

TENOSYNOVITIS or TENOSITIS Inflammation of a tendon.

TENOTOMY An operation in which one or more tendons are divided, usually with the object of remedying some deformity.

TENTORIUM A wide flap of dura mater forming a partition between the cerebrum and cerebellum (see BRAIN) and supporting the former.

TERATOGENESIS The production of physical defects in the FETUS. A drug may interfere with a mechanism that is essential for growth and result in arrested or distorted development of the fetus and yet cause no disturbance in adults, in whom these growth processes have ceased. Thus the effect of a drug upon a fetus may differ qualitively as well as quantitively from its effect on the mother. The susceptibility of the embryo will depend on the stage of development it has reached when the drug is given. The age of early differentiation, that is from the beginning of the third week to the end of the tenth week of pregnancy is the time of greatest susceptibility. After this time the likelihood of congenital malformation resulting from drug treatment is less, although the death of the fetus can occur at any time as a result of drugs crossing the placenta or as a result of their effect on the placental circulation. The term teratogenesis was brought into the public arena by the thalidomide disaster.

Thalidomide was an effective non-barbiturate hypnotic which had passed stringent tests before being released for general use. In spite of this it caused several congenital defects, especially of the limbs, in children born to mothers who had taken the drug while pregnant. As soon as this was discovered the drug was withdrawn from use. Subsequently the government set up a statutory body – Committee on

Safety of Medicines – to try and ensure that there was no recurrence of such a distressing episode with subsequent drugs. Even the most stringent precautions, however, cannot ensure the complete elimination of this risk. Although the risk is not great, no drug should be given to a pregnant woman, particularly during the first few months of pregnancy, unless it is absolutely essential for her health or that of her unborn child.

TERATOMA A tumour that consists of partially developed embryonic tissues. The most common sites of this tumour are the ovary and the testicle.

TERBUTALINE A beta-2 adrenoreceptor agonist (see BETA ADRENOCEPTOR-BLOCKING DRUGS). As an AEROSOL it is of particular value in the treatment of mild to moderate attacks of ASTHMA; more severe attacks may need a short course of oral CORTICOSTEROIDS to gain control, and treatment of acute severe cases is usually safer in hospital, where oxygen and resuscitation facilities are immediately available.

Terbutaline is also available in oral and parenteral forms, as well as subcutaneous, intramuscular, or slow intravenous injection, although aerosol inhalation remains a convenient and effective method of administration for moderate airways obstruction.

TERTIAN FEVER is the name applied to that type of malaria in which the fever reappears every other day. (See MALARIA.)

TESTICLE The testes, or testicles, are the two male sexual glands. Each is developed in the corresponding loin, but before birth they descend through openings in the lower part of the front of the abdomen into a fold or pouch of skin known as the SCROTUM. Each testicle has a separate covering, the tunica vaginalis, which is derived from the PERITONEUM while the testicle is within the fetal abdomen. Each testicle consists of up to 1,000 minute tubes and lined by cells from which the spermatozoa are formed. Around 4·5 million spermatozoa are produced per gram of testicle per day. These tubes communicate with one another near the centre of the testicle, and are connected by a much convoluted tube, the epididymis, with the ductus, or vas deferens, which enters the abdomen, and passes on to the base of the bladder. This duct, after joining a reservoir known as the seminal vesicle, opens, close to the duct from the other side of the body, into the urethra where it passes through the PROSTATE gland. Owing to the convolutions of these ducts leading from the testicles to the urethra, and their indirect route, the passage from testicle to urethra is over 6 metres (20 feet) in length. In addition to producing spermatozoa, the testicle also forms the hormone TESTOSTERONE which is responsible for the development of male characteristics.

TESTICLE, DISEASES OF The scrotum may be affected by various skin diseases, particularly exzema, which may be difficult to cure. Chronic irritation of the skin among workers whose clothes may become permeated with dust or dirt containing carcinogenic substances – chimney sweeps and cotton spinners were the traditional occupations – often leads to skin cancer. Hernia may pass into the scrotum (see HERNIA). Defective development of the testicles may lead to their retention within the abdomen.

Hydrocoele is a local dropsy affecting one tunica vaginalis, distending that side of the scrotum with fluid.

Variocoele is distension of the veins of the spermatic cord, especially on the left side, the causes being similar to varicose veins elsewhere. The chief symptom is a painful dragging sensation in the testicle, especially after exertion. Wearing a support provides relief; rarely, an operation may be advisable.

Orchitis or acute inflammation may arise from CYSTITIS, stone in the bladder, and inflammation in the urinary organs, especially GONORRHOEA. It may also follow MUMPS. Intense pain, swelling and redness occur; treatment consists of rest, support of the scrotum, analgesics as appropriate, and the administration of antibiotics if a definitive micro-organism can be identified. In some patients the condition may develop and form an abscess.

Torsion or twisting of the spermatic cord is relatively common in adolescents. About half the cases occur in the early hours of the morning during sleep. Typically felt as pain of varying severity in the lower abdomen or scrotum, the testes become hard and swollen. Treatment consists of immediate undoing of the torsion by manipulation. If done within a few hours no harm should ensue, but it should be followed within six hours by surgical operation to ensure that the torsion has been relieved and to fix the testes.

Tuberculosis may occur in the testicle, especially when the bladder is already affected. Causing little pain, the infection is often far advanced before attracting attention. The condition generally responds well to treatment with a combination of antituberculous drugs (see TUBERCULOSIS).

Tumours of the testes occur in around 600 males annually in the United kingdom, and are the second most common form of malignant growth in young males. There are two types: seminomas and TERATOMAS. When adequately treated the survival rate for seminomas is 95 per cent, while that for teratomas is 50 per cent.

Injuries are relatively rare, though they do occur during some sporting activities. A severe blow may lead to shock and symptoms of severe collapse, usually relieved by rest in bed, but a haematoma may develop. If pain and swelling persist the victim should seek medical attention.

TEST MEAL This is also called a gastric-function test, a term originally applied to a meal given to test digestive function. The original gruel meal has been replaced by the injection of HISTAMINE, a powerful stimulator of gastric juice, or pentagastin. After the stimulant has been injected, the digestive juices are withdrawn through a stomach tube (inserted through the nose and throat) and their volume and chemistry measured. A similar test is used to assess the working of the PANCREAS.

TESTIS (see TESTICLE).

TESTOSTERONE The principal male sex hormone secreted by the testes. It has also been prepared synthetically and has the formula $C_{19}H_{28}O_2$. In true eunuchoid conditions it has the power of restoring male sexual characteristics. (See ANDROGEN.)

TEST-TUBE is a tube of thin glass closed at one end, which is used for observing chemical reactions or for bacterial culture.

'TEST-TUBE BABY' (see EMBRYO TRANSFER).

TETANUS Also called LOCKJAW, this is a bacterial infection of the nervous system. Increased excitability of the spinal cord results in painful and prolonged spasms of the voluntary muscles throughout the body, rapidly leading to death unless treated.

Causes The disease is caused by the bacillus *Clostridium tetani*, found generally in earth and dust, especially in places where animal manure is collected. Infection usually follows a wound, especially a deeply punctured or gunshot wound, with the presence of some foreign body. It is a hazard in war and also among farmers, gardeners and those in the construction industry. The bacillus develops a toxin in the wound, which is absorbed through the motor nerves into the spinal cord. Here it renders the nerves excitable and acutely responsible to mild stimuli.

Symptoms Most commonly appearing within four to five days of the primary wound, the patient's symptoms may be delayed for several weeks – by which time the wound may have healed. Although generally the longer the delay, the better the outlook, a long delay with an acute onset may occasionally be dangerous. Initially appearing as muscle stiffness around the wound, this symptom is followed by stiffness around the jaw, leading to lockjaw, or trismus. This extends to the muscles of the neck, back, chest, abdomen, and limbs, leading to strange, often changing, contorted postures, accompanied by frequent seizures – often provoked by quite minor stimuli. The patient's breathing may be seriously affected, in severe cases leading to ASPHYXIA; the temperature may rise sharply, often with copious sweating; and severe pain is a common feature. Mental clarity

is a characteristic feature of the disease, adding to the patient's anxiety. In severe infections death may rapidly ensue from asphyxia, PNEUMONIA, or general exhaustion. More commonly, the disease takes a more chronic course, leading to a gradual recovery. Outcome depends on several factors, chiefly the patient's immune status and age, and early administration of appropriate treatment.

Tetanus may occur in newborn babies, particularly when birth takes place in an unhygienic environment. It is particularly common in the tropics and Third-World countries, with a high mortality rate. Local tetanus is a rare manifestation, in which only muscles around the wound are affected, though stiffness may last for several months. Strychnine poisoning and rabies, although similar in some respects to tetanus, may be easily distinguished by taking a good history.

Prevention and treatment The incidence of tetanus in the United Kingdom has been substantially reduced by the introduction of antitetanus VACCINE. Children are routinely immunized, and boosters are given later in life to at-risk workers, or those travelling to tropical parts.

Treatment should be started as soon as possible after sustaining a potentially dangerous wound. An intravenous injection of antitoxin should be given immediately, the wound thoroughly cleaned and PENICILLIN administered. Expert nursing is most important. Spasms may be minimized by reducing unexpected stimuli, and DIAZEPAM is helpful. Intravenous feeding should be started immediately if the patient cannot swallow. Aspiration of bronchial secretions and antibiotic treatment of pneumonia may be necessary.

TETANY A condition characterized by spasm of muscle usually caused by a fall in the ionic calcium of the blood. This fall in ionic calcium results in hyperexcitability of the muscles, which are thus liable to go into spasm on the slightest stimulus. This is well demonstrated in two of the classical signs of the disease: Chvostek's sign, in which the muscles of the face contract when the cheek is tapped over the facial nerve as it emerges on the cheek; Erb's sign, in which muscles go into spasm in response to an electrical stimulus which normally causes only a contraction of the muscle. Tetany is most common in infants, in whom it may arise as a result of rickets, excessive vomiting, or certain forms of NEPHRITIS. It may also be due to lack of the active principle of the PARATHYROID glands. Overbreathing may also cause it. Treatment consists of the administration of calcium salts, and in severe cases this is done by giving calcium gluconate intravenously or intramuscularly. High doses of vitamin D are also required.

TETRACYCLINES A group of broad-spectrum ANTIBIOTICS which include oxytetracycline, tetracycline, doxycycline, lymecycline, minocycline, and demeclocycline.

All the preparations are virtually identical, being active against both GRAM-NEGATIVE and GRAM-POSITIVE bacteria. Unfortunately, their value has, lessened owing to increasing resistance to the group among bacteria. They remain the treatment of choice for BRUCELLOSIS, MYCOPLASMA, LYME DISEASE as well as certain RICKETTSIAE and CHLAMYDIA including those causing Q fever, TRACHOMA, PSITTACOSIS, SALPINGITIS, URETHRITIS and LYMPHOGRANULOMA INGUINALE, but must be used with discrimination in young children as they are liable to produce permanent discoloration of the teeth. Tetracyclines must not be used if a woman is pregnant as the infant's deciduous teeth will be stained.

TETRALOGY OF FALLOT The most common form of cyanotic congenital heart disease. The tetralogy consists of stenosis of the pulmonary valve (see PULMONARY STENOSIS); a defect in the septum separating the TWO VENTRICLES; the AORTA over-riding both ventricles; marked hypertrophy of the right ventricle.

THALAMUS One of two masses of grey matter lying on either side of the third ventricle of the brain. It is an important relay and co-ordinating station for sensory impulses such as those for sight. (Plural: Thalami.)

THALASSAEMIA Also known as Cooley's anaemia, this is a condition characterized by severe anaemia, due to the individual's having an abnormal form of HAEMOGLOBIN in his blood. It is an inherited disease which is widely spread across the Mediterranean through the Middle East and into the Far East. It has a particularly high incidence in Greece and in Italy.

THALIDOMIDE A sedative and hypnotic drug now withdrawn from the market because it causes TERATOGENESIS. If taken during the first trimester of pregnancy it may cause an unusual limb deformity in the fetus known as phocomelia ('seal' or 'flipper' extremities).

THALLIUM An element that is toxic to nerve and liver tissues. The radio-isotope thallium-201 is used as a tracer during special imaging studies of blood flow through the heart muscle in the diagnosis of myocardial ischaemia.

THECA A sheathlike structure enclosing an organ or part.

THENAR EMINENCE The projecting mass at the base of the thumb: what is popularly known as the ball of the thumb.

THEOPHYLLINE An alkaloid structurally similar to caffeine, and found in small amounts

in tea. Its main use is for the relief of bronchospasm, where beta-2 adrenoceptor stimulants have failed. It is given intravenously in combination with the stabilizing agent ethylenediamine (as aminophylline) for the treatment of severe ASTHMA or paroxysmal nocturnal DYSPNOEA. Formerly used in the treatment of left ventricular failure, it has been largely superseded by more effective DIURETICS. When indicated, aminophylline should be given by very slow intravenous injection; acute overdose may cause convulsions and cardiac ARRHYTHMIAS.

THERAPEUTICS The general name applied to different methods of treatment and healing.

THERAPY The treatment of disease.

THERIAC An antidote or substance given to neutralize poison. The name was specially given to Venice treacle, a celebrated mixture of 64 drugs prescribed in olden times as an antidote for poisons and a preventive potion.

THERMO- A prefix implying some relation to heat.

THERMOGRAPHY A method of detecting the amount of heat produced by different parts of the body. This is done with an infra-red sensitive photographic film. High blood flow in an area shows up as a heat zone and thus tumours such as breast cancer can be identified. The process records such changes in temperature in a record known as a thermogram. Unfortunately, such hot areas of skin are caused by a number of other conditions. It is therefore a diagnostic method that can be used only as a rough screening procedure.

THERMOMETER An instrument for measuring a person's body temperature. A traditional clinic thermometer comprises a glass capillary tube sealed at one end with a mercury-filled bulb at the other. The mercury expands (rises) and contracts (falls) according to the temperature of the bulb which may be placed under the tongue or arm or in the rectum. Calibration is in degrees Celsius or Fahrenheit. Modern thermometers use an electric probe linked to a digital read-out display, providing an instant reading. Hospitals now have electronic devices that maintain constant monitoring of patients' temperatures, pulse rates and blood pressure.

THERMOMETER SCALES (see TEMPERATURE).

THIABENDAZOLE A drug that was the routine treatment for various parasitic infections, including those due to guinea-worm and certain nematodes, as well as strongyloidiasis. Albendazole is now the preferred treatment with thiabendazole used only in certain circumstances. (See STRONGYLOIDIASIS).

THIAMINE   The *British Pharmacopoeia* name for vitamin B$_1$. Also known as ANEURINE, it is found in the husks of cereal grains. Its deficiency may be produced by too careful milling of rice in the East, or by a diet of white bread to the exclusion of brown bread and other cereal sources of this vitamin. The resulting disease is a form of neuritis with muscular weakness and heart failure, common in Japan and other parts of the East and known as BERIBERI. Vitamin B$_1$ has been isolated in crystalline form, and a minute dose of this rapidly cures the symptoms of beriberi. The best sources of this vitamin are wholemeal flour, bacon, liver, egg-yolk, yeast and the pulses. The daily requirement is dependent, among other things, upon the total food intake, and has been estimated to be in the region of 0·5 mg of thiamine per 1000 Calories, increased during pregnancy to 2 mg daily as a minimum. (See APPENDIX 5: VITAMINS.)

THIAZIDES (see BENZOTHIADIAZINES).

THIERSCH'S GRAFT   The term given to a method of skin-grafting in which strips of skin are shaved from a normal area and placed on a burned, injured or scarred area to be grafted. (See SKIN-GRAFTING.)

THIGH   The portion of the lower limb above the knee. The thigh is supported by the femur or thigh-bone, the longest and strongest bone in the body. This fits by a rounded head at its upper end into the acetabulum, a hollow at the side of the pelvis, and at the lower end two large rounded condyles or knuckles rest upon the head of the tibia, and, along with the patella, or knee-cap, form the knee-joint. A large four-headed muscle, the quadriceps, forms most of the fleshy mass on the front and sides of the thigh and serves to straighten the leg in walking and to maintain the erect posture of the body in standing. At the back of the thigh, lie the hamstring muscles; and on the inner side the adductor muscles, attached above to the pelvis and below to the femur, pull the lower limb inwards. The large femoral vessels emerge from the abdomen in the middle of the groin, the vein lying to the inner side of the artery. These pass downwards and inwards deeply placed between the muscles, and at the knee they lie behind the joint. The great saphenous vein lies near the surface and can be seen towards the inner side of the thigh passing up to the groin, where it joins the femoral vein. The femoral nerve accompanies the large vessels and controls the muscles on the front and inner side of the thigh; while the large sciatic nerve lies close to the back of the femur and supplies the muscles at the back of the thigh and muscles below the knee.

Deep wounds on the inner side of the thigh are dangerous by reason of the risk of damage to the large vessels. Pain in the back of the thigh is often due to inflammation of the sciatic nerve. (See SCIATICA.) The veins on the inner side of the thigh are specially liable to become dilated. (See VEINS, DISEASES OF.)

THIOPENTONE SODIUM   A commonly used intravenous barbiturate anaesthetic. Its main use is for inducing anaesthesia, which it does rapidly and painlessly. (See ANAESTHESIA.)

THIORIDAZINE   A tranquillizer that is a useful anti-psychotic drug. (See NEUROLEPTICS.)

THIOTEPA   One of a dozen or so alkylating agents used to treat malignant disease. It is especially effective for cancer of the bladder. (See CYTOTOXIC.)

THIRST   This, like appetite, is an instinctive craving for something necessary to the continuance of bodily activity. The sensation of thirst is generally referred to the back of the throat, because, when there is a deficiency of water in the system, the throat and mouth especially become parched by evaporation of moisture from their surface. Thirst is increased by heat, and is a constant symptom of fever; it is also present in diseases which remove a considerable amount of fluid from the system, such as diarrhoea, diabetes mellitus, and after great loss of blood by haemorrhage. A demand for water is also a feature of many conditions associated with severe exhaustion and dehydration.

THORACIC DUCT   The large LYMPH-VESSEL which collects the contents of the lymphatics proceeding from the lower limbs, the abdomen, the left arm, and left side of the chest, neck, and head. It is provided with numerous valves, and opens into the veins at the left side of the neck. (See GLANDS; LYMPHATICS.)

THORACOCENTESIS   The withdrawal of fluid from the pleural cavity. (See ASPIRATION.)

THORACOPLASTY   The operation of removing a varying number of ribs so that the underlying lung collapses.

THORAX   Another name for the chest.

THOUGHT DISORDERS   Thought is a mental activity by which people reason, solve problems, form judgements and communicate with each other by speech, writing and behaviour. Disturbances of thought are reflected in how a person communicates. The normal logic of thought is broken up and a person may randomly move from one subject to another. SCHIZOPHRENIA is a mental illness characterized by thought disorder. Confusion, DEMENTIA,

DEPRESSION and MANIA are other conditions in which thought disorders may be a marked feature. (See MENTAL ILLNESS.)

THREADWORM (see ENTEROBIASIS).

THREONINE One of the essential AMINO-ACIDS.

THRESHOLD: The degree of stimulation, or electrical depolarization, necessary to produce an action potential in a nerve fibre (see NERVES). Stimulation below this level elicits no conducted impulse and supramaximal stimulation will elicit the same response as a threshold stimulus (see NERVES).

THRILL A tremor or vibration felt on applying the hand to the surface of the body. It is felt particularly over the region of the heart in conditions in which the valve openings are narrowed or an aneurysm is present.

THROAT In popular language, this is a vague term applied indifferently to the region in front of the neck, to the larynx or organ of voice, and to the cavity at the back of the mouth. The correct use of the word denotes the pharynx or cavity into which the nose, mouth, gullet, and larynx all open. (See PHARYNX. Information will also be found under LARYNX; NECK; TONSILS; NOSE.)

THROMBIN (see COAGULATION).

THROMBOANGIITIS OBLITERANS This disorder is also known as Buerger's disease after the American surgeon who gave the first co-ordinated description of it in 1908. It is an inflammatory disease involving the blood-vessels of the limbs, particularly the lower limbs. The cause is not known, but the use of tobacco is an important factor. It is almost entirely confined to men. Pain is the outstanding symptom, accompanied by pallor of the affected part. Sooner or later ulceration and gangrene tend to develop in the feet or hands. There is no specific treatment, but, if seen in the early stages, considerable relief may be given to the patient.

THROMBOCYTE (see PLATELETS).

THROMBOCYTOPENIA A fall in the number of PLATELETS (thrombocytes) in the blood caused by failure of production or excessive destruction of platelets. The result is bleeding into the skin (PURPURA), serious bleeding after injury and spontaneous bruising. (See IDIOPATHIC THROMBOCYTOPENIC PURPURA; PLATELETS.)

THROMBOCYTOPENIC (see THROMBOCYTOPENIA).

THROMBOEMBOLISM The formation of a thrombus (blood clot) in one part of the circulatory system from which a portion becomes detached and lodges in another blood vessel, partially or completely obstructing the blood flow (an embolism). Most commonly a thrombus is formed in the veins of the leg and the embolism lodges in the pulmonary (lung) circulation. A pulmonary embolus is a potentially fatal condition and requires urgent anti-coagulant treatment and sometimes surgery. Venous thromboses in the legs may occur after surgery and preventive anticoagulant treatment with HEPARIN and warfarin is often used. Similar treatment is needed if a thrombus develops. STREPTOKINASE is also used to treat thromboembolism.

THROMBOLYSIS The breakdown of a blood clot by enzymic activity. Naturally occurring ENZYMES limit the enlargement of clots, and drugs – e.g. STREPTOKINASE – may be given to 'dissolve' clots – e.g., following a coronary THROMBOSIS.

THROMBOPHLEBITIS Inflammation of the veins combined with clot formation. (See VEINS, DISEASES OF.)

THROMBOSIS The formation of a blood-clot within the vessels or heart during life. The process of clotting within the body depends upon the same factors as in clotting of blood outside the body, involving the fibrinogen and calcium salts circulating in the blood, as well as blood platelets. The indirect cause of thrombosis is usually some damage to the smooth lining of the blood-vessels brought about by inflammation, or the result of atheroma, a chronic disease of the vessel walls. The blood is also specially prone to clot in certain general conditions such as anaemia, the ill health of wasting diseases like cancer, and in consequence of the feeble circulation of old age.

Thrombosis may occur in the vessels of the brain and thus causes stroke in people whose arteries are much diseased.

Thrombosis of a coronary artery of the heart is a very serious condition which affects, as a rule, middle-aged or elderly people. (See also ARTERIES, DISEASES OF; CLOT; COAGULATION; CORONARY THROMBOSIS; PULMONARY THROMBOSIS; STROKE; VEINS, DISEASES OF.)

THROMBOXANE A substance produced in the blood PLATELETS which induces aggregation of platelets and thereby THROMBOSIS. It is also a vasoconstrictor (a substance that causes the constriction of blood vessels).

THROMBUS A clot of blood. Usually describing the formation of a clot within a vessel obstructing the flow of blood, but it can also describe blood which has escaped from a damaged vessel and clotted in the surrounding tissue.

THRUSH (see CANDIDA).

THUMB-SUCKING or FINGER-SUCKING A universal and harmless habit in infancy. It is usually gradually given up during the pre-school period, but quite often persists after school age especially if the child is tired, lonely or unhappy. In these cases the remedy is to deal with the cause. Threats should not be used to try to stop the habit.

THYMOCYTE A cell that develops in the THYMUS GLAND, probably from a stem cell of bone marrow. It is a precursor of T lymphocytes originating in the gland (see LYMPHOCYTE).

THYMUS GLAND The thymus gland was given its name by Galen in the second century AD because of its resemblance to a bunch of thyme flowers. It has two lobes and lies in the upper part of the chest. Each lobe is made up of a number of lobules divided into an outer portion, or cortex, and a central portion, or medulla. The cortex resembles lymphoid tissue and is made up of masses of small round cells called THYMOCYTES. It is an area of intense lymphopoiesis and the rate of production of new cells is five times greater than that in lymph nodes and other lymphoid tissues. The medulla is more loosely cellular and consists of a stroma which contains far fewer lymphocytes than in the cortex but also contains epithelial cells and Hassall's corpuscles.

The thymus gland is now established as a vital part of the immunological system. Until 1960 the function of the thymus was completely unknown. Stem cells from the bone marrow come to the thymus where they develop into immunologically competent cells. They are then seeded out to the rest of the lymphoid tissue. There are two distinct populations of lymphocytes. One is dependent on the presence of the thymus (T lymphocytes) and the other is independent of the thymus (B lymphocytes). Both are concerned with immune responses. They differ in their distribution and in their life span. The thymus-dependent lymphocyte is a cell which in the absence of antigenic stimulation circulates through the blood, lymph nodes and back into the circulation again over a period of more than 10 years. It performs a policing role, awaiting recognition of foreign material which it is able to identify as such. It reacts by multiplication and transformation and these are the ingredients of the immune response. B lymphocytes are produced in the bone marrow and are concerned with the production of the circulating humoral anti-bodies.

The most common clinical disorder associated with abnormality of the thymus is MYASTHENIA GRAVIS. Ten per cent of patients with myasthenia gravis will have a tumour of the thymus whilst the remainder will have inflammatory changes in the thymus called thymitis.

THYROID CANCER A rare disease that accounts for around 1 per cent of all cancers, cancer of the thyroid usually presents as an isolated hard nodule in the neck. The rate at which the nodule grows depends on the patient's age and type of cancer cell. Pain is not usually a feature but the increasing size may result in the tumour pressing on vital structures in the neck – for example, the nerves controlling the LARYNX (resulting in hoarseness) and the PHARYNX (causing difficulty in swallowing). If more than one nodule is present, they are likely to be benign, not malignant. Treatment is by surgical removal after which the patient will need to take thyroxine for the rest of his or her life. Radioactive iodine is usually given after surgery to destroy any residual cancerous cells. If treated early, the outlook is good.

THYROID CARTILAGE is the largest cartilage in the larynx and forms the prominence of the Adam's apple in front of the neck. (See LARYNX.)

THYROIDECTOMY Surgical removal of the thyroid gland. Partial thyroidectomy – removal of part of the gland – is sometimes done in patients with hyperthyroidism when drug treatment has failed to control the disorder.

THYROID GLAND is a highly vascular organ situated in front of the neck. It consists of a narrow isthmus crossing the windpipe close to its upper end, and joining together two lateral lobes which run upwards, one on each side of the larynx. The gland is therefore shaped somewhat like a horseshoe, each lateral lobe being about 5 cm (2 inches) long and the isthmus about 12 mm (½ inch) wide, and it is firmly bound to the larynx. The weight of the thyroid gland is about 28·5 grams (1 ounce), but it is larger in females than in males and in some women increases in size during menstruation. It often reaches an enormous size in the condition known as GOITRE.

Structure The gland is enveloped in a layer of fibrous tissue and possesses a rich blood supply. It is composed of multitudes of closed vesicles, each formed by a layer of cubical cells and containing a thick yellow fluid (colloid).

Function The chief function of the thyroid gland is to produce a hormone rich in iodine. The main active ingredient of this hormone is THYROXINE. This hormone, or secretion, which passes directly from the thyroid into the bloodstream, is de-iodinated in the body cells to triiodo-thyronine which exerts the physiological action of the thyroid hormone. The hormone is one of the most important in the body and controls the rate of metabolism. Thus, if it is deficient in children they fail to grow, a condition known as CRETINISM. If the deficiency develops in adult life, the individual becomes obese, lethargic, and develops a coarse skin, a condition known as HYPOTHYROIDISM. Overaction of the thyroid, or HYPERTHYROIDISM, results in loss of weight, rapid heart action, anxiety, overactivity and increased appetite. (See THYROTOXICOSIS.)

The production of the thyroid hormone is controlled by a hormone of the pituitary gland – the thyrotrophic hormone.

THYROID GLAND, DISEASES OF (see CRETINISM; GOITRE; GRAVES' DISEASE; HYPOTHYROIDISM).

THYROIDITIS Inflammation of the THYROID GLAND. The acute form is usually caused by a BACTERIAL infection elsewhere in the body: ANTIBIOTIC treatment is needed. Occasionally a VIRUS may be the infectious agent. Hashimoto's thyroiditis is an autoimmune disorder causing hypothyroidism (reduced activity of the gland). Subacute thyroiditis is inflammation of unknown cause in which the gland becomes painful and the patient suffers fever, weight loss and malaise. It sometimes lasts for several months but is usually self limiting.

THYROTOXIC ADENOMA A variety of THYROTOXICOSIS in which one of the nodules of a multinodular goitre becomes autonomous and secretes excess thyroid hormone. The symptoms that result are similar to those of GRAVES' DISEASE, but there are minor differences.

Treatment The first line of treatment is to render the patient euthyroid by treatment with antithyroid drugs. Then the nodule should be removed surgically or destroyed using radioactive iodine.

THYROTOXICOSIS A disorder of the thyroid gland in which excessive amounts of thyroid hormones are secreted into the bloodstream. Resultant symptoms are TACHYCARDIA, tremor, anxiety, sweating, increased appetite, weight loss and dislike of heat. (See HYPERTHYROIDISM.)

THYROTROPHIN-RELEASING HORMONE (TRH) A hormone produced and released by the HYPOTHALAMUS which stimulates the release of THYROTROPHIN-STIMULATING HORMONE by the PITUITARY GLAND.

THYROTROPHIN-STIMULATING HORMONE (TSH) A hormone manufactured and released by the anterior part of the PITUITARY GLAND which stimulates the THYROID GLAND to manufacture and release thyroid hormones (THYROXINE and TRI-IODOTHYRONINE).

THYROXINE A crystalline substance, containing iodine, isolated from the thyroid gland and possessing the properties of thyroid extract. It has also been synthesized. It is used in patients with defective function of the thyroid, such as CRETINISM, and MYXOEDEMA.

TIA (see TRANSIENT ISCHAEMIC ATTACKS/EPISODES).

TIBIA The larger of the two bones in the leg. One surface of the tibia lies immediately beneath the skin in front, forming the shin. Fractures of this bone are usually compound ones. The thighbone abuts on the larger upper end of the tibia at the knee-joint, whilst below the tibia and fibula together enter into the ankle-joint, the two bosses or malleoli at the ankle belonging, the inner to the tibia, the outer to the fibula.

TIC A repetitive, usually involuntary spasm that varies from being the simple twitch of a muscle – for example, affecting an eyelid – to complex co-ordinated actions. About 20 per cent of children suffer from tic which normally lasts several months. Emotional stress is a common cause (see TOURETTE'S SYNDROME).

TIC DOULOUREUX Another name for TRIGEMINAL NEURALGIA due to some affection of the fifth cranial nerve, and characterized by pain, situated somewhere about the temple, forehead, face, or jaw, and sometimes by spasm in the muscles of the affected region. (See TRIGEMINAL NEURALGIA.)

TICK is the general name given to a group of arachnid insects, some of which act as transmitters of diseases.

Ticks are blood-sucking arthropods which are responsible for transmitting a wide range of diseases to man, including Rocky Mountain spotted fever. African tick typhus and fièvre boutonneuse (see TYPHUS FEVER). Apart from being transmitters of disease, they cause intense itching and may cause quite severe lesions of the skin. The best repellents are dimethyl phthalate and diethyltoluamide. Once bitten, relief from the itching is obtained from the application of calamine lotion. Tick-bites are an occupational hazard of shepherds and gamekeepers. (See BITES AND STINGS.)

TIE (see TRANSIENT ISCHAEMIC ATTACKS/EPISODES).

TIMOLOL MALEATE is a beta-adrenoceptor-blocking drug which of value in the treatment of ANGINA pectoris, myocardial infarction, and HYPERTENSION. It is also used in the treatment of GLAUCOMA. (See ADRENERGIC RECEPTORS.)

TINCTURE An alcoholic solution used in PHARMACY, generally of some vegetable substance.

TINEA (See RINGWORM.)

TINNITUS A noise heard in the ear without any external cause. It is a frequent accompaniment of deafness.

Tinnitus is common, affecting about one in six adults at some time in their life. Only one-third of these consult a doctor and in less than one per cent does the tinnitus interfere with leading a normal life. The cause is damage to the auditory pathway and the most common part of the pathway to be damaged is the cochlea. Tinnitus may be a symptom of general diseases such as ANAEMIA, high blood pressure and arterial disease. It may be the result of drugs, particularly ASPIRIN, CHLOROQUINE, QUININE and certain ANTIBIOTICS. Investigation is necessary to exclude any underlying cause but in most cases no cause can be found, and the management depends on reassurance and psychological support to help relieve the effects of tinnitus on the patient because it is not usually possible to abolish the tinnitus altogether. Drugs such as CARBAMAZEPINE, tocainide amide and mexiletine may help. Avoid using TRANQUILLIZERS but HYPNOTICS may help if the victim's sleep is disturbed. The use of tinnitus maskers and hearing aids can suppress tinnitus by masking it with other sounds which the patient learns to listen to. Hearing aids suppress tinnitus by amplifying background noise.

Under the auspices of the Royal National Institute for Deaf People, the RNID Tinnitus Helpline has been established (see APPENDIX 2: ADDRESSES). Calls are charged at local rates. (See DEAFNESS; MENIÈRE'S DISEASE.)

TISSUES OF THE BODY The simple elements from which the various parts and organs are found to be built. All the body originates from the union of a pair of cells but as growth proceeds the new cells produced from these form tissues of varying character and complexity. (See CELL.) It is customary to divide the tissues into five groups:
- Epithelial tissues, including the cells covering the skin, those lining the alimentary canal, those forming the secretions of internal organs. (See EPITHELIUM.)
- Connective tissues, including fibrous tissue, fat, bone, cartilage. (See these headings.)
- Muscular tissues (see MUSCLE).
- Nervous tissues (see NERVES).
- Wandering corpuscles of the blood and lymph (see BLOOD: LYMPH).

Many of the organs are formed of a single one of these tissues or of one with a very slight admixture of another, such as cartilage, or white fibrous tissue. Other parts of the body that are widely distributed are very simple in structure and consist of two or more simple tissues in varying proportion. Such are blood-vessels (see ARTERIES; VEINS), lymphatic vessels (see LYMPHATICS), lymphatic glands (see GLANDS), serous membranes (see SEROUS MEMBRANES), synovial membranes (see JOINTS), mucous membranes (see MUCOUS MEMBRANE), secreting glands (see GLANDS; SALIVARY GLANDS; THYROID GLAND) and skin (see SKIN).

The structure of the more complex organs of the body is dealt with under the heading of each organ.

TISSUE PLASMINOGEN ACTIVATOR (TPA, tPA) A natural protein that occurs in the body. It has the property of breaking down a THROMBUS in a blood vessel (see THROMBOLYSIS). It is effective only in the presence of FIBRIN and activates plasminogen, which occurs normally on the surface of the fibrin. TPA is an important thrombolytic treatment immediately after a MYOCARDIAL INFARCTION.

TISSUE TYPING The essential procedure for matching the tissue of a recipient in need of transplanted tissue or organ to that of a potential donor. Unless there is a reasonable match the recipient's immune system will reject the donor's organ. The main factors that are relevant to an individual's reaction to donor tissue are called histocompatability ANTIGENS. These are mostly HUMAN LEUCOCYTE ANTIGENS (HLAs) present on the surface of cells. HLAs are inherited and, like fingerprints, unique to an individual, although identical twins have identical HLAs and hence are perfect matches for transplantation procedures.

TITRATION A form of chemical analysis by standard solutions of known strength.

TITRE The strength of a solution as determined by TITRATION. In medicine it is used to describe the amount of ANTIBODY present in a known volume of SERUM.

TITUBATION A regular nodding movement of the head that sometimes involves the trunk. The term can also refer to a staggering or reeling condition, especially due to disease of the spinal cord or cerebellum.

TNM CLASSIFICATION A method of classifying cancers to determine how far they have spread. This helps doctors to determine the best course of treatment and the prognosis; it is useful in research. Originally defined by the American Joint Committee on Cancer, the T applies to the primary tumour, the N to any lymph node involvement and the M to any metastatic spread.

TOBACCO The leaf of several species of Nicotiana, especially of the American plant *Nicotiana tabacum.*

The smoking of tobacco is the major public health hazard in Britain today. It causes a hundred thousand premature deaths per year in the United Kingdom alone. In addition to the deaths caused by cigarette smoking, it is also a major cause of disability and illness in the form of myocardial infarction, peripheral vascular disease, chronic obstructive airways disease and emphysema. Action on Smoking and Health (ASH) is a small charity founded by the Royal College of Physicians in 1971 that attempts to alert and inform the public to the dangers of smoking and to try to prevent the disability and death which it causes (see ASH).

Cigarette smoking is the major cause of chronic obstructive lung disease morbidity and 80 to 90 per cent of chronic obstructive lung disease in the United States is attributable to it. Tobacco's contribution to all cancer deaths is estimated to be 30 per cent. Cigarette smoking is also the most important of the known modifiable risk factors for coronary heart disease.

Composition In addition to vegetable fibre, tobacco leaves contain a large quantity of ash, the nature of this depending predominantly upon the minerals present in the ground where the tobacco plant has been grown. Of the organic constituents the brown fluid alkaloid known as nicotine is the most important. The nicotine content of different tobaccos varies, and the amount absorbed depends upon whether or not the smoker inhales. Nicotine is the substance that causes a person to become addicted to tobacco smoking.

Tobacco smoke also contains some sixteen substances capable of inducing cancer in experimental animals. One of the most important of these is benzpyrene, a strongly carcinogenic hydrocarbon. As this is present in coal-tar pitch, it is commonly referred to in this context as tar. Other constituents of tobacco smoke include pyridine, ammonia and carbon monoxide.

A very small amount of nicotine, such as that derived from a single cigarette, has a stimulating effect upon the mental and bodily powers.

In larger amount, the action is a depressant and narcotic one, which in habitual smokers is modified to a sedative. Recent research suggests that some people may be genetically predisposed to nicotine addiction.

The greatest hazard of smoking, however, is the fact that it is the major cause of lung cancer, coronary artery disease, PERIPHERAL VASCULAR DISEASE, chronic bronchitis and EMPHYSEMA. It also has an adverse effect on the fetus when the pregnant mother smokes.

Another set of symptoms frequently arising in those who smoke is irritable cough and soreness of the throat. These symptoms pass off when smoking is discontinued. There is increasing evidence that passive smoking (inhaling smoke from someone else's cigarette) is also harmful. Children whose parents smoke are at increased risk of pneumonia and glue ear. There is growing pressure under health-and-safety-at-work legislation for employers to provide smoke-free working conditions for their staff.

The giving up of the smoking habit is largely a psychological problem, but self-help groups, acupuncture therapy, hypnosis of nicotine-containing chewing gum may help smokers to stop.

TOBRAMYCIN An AMINOGLYCOSIDE ANTIBIOTIC which has a similar action to gentamycin. It is used to treat serious infections such as MENINGITIS and PERITONITIS as well as those affecting bones, joints and lungs. It is given by injection, sometimes in conjunction with penicillin. It has a range of side-effects including damage to the balance and hearing mechanisms as well as to the kidney.

TOES (see CORNS AND BUNIONS; FOOT; NAILS).

TOLAZOMIDE (see SULPHONYLUREAS).

TOLBUTAMIDE A sulphonamide derivative, or sulphonylurea, which lowers the level of the blood sugar in diabetes mellitus. As it is rapidly excreted from the body, it has to be taken twice daily. Like CHLORPROPAMIDE, it may induce undue sensitivity to alcohol. (See also DIABETES MELLITUS, SULPHONYLUREAS.)

TOLERANCE This occurs when the response to a particular amount of a drug or physiological messenger decreases (i.e. a larger dose must be given to produce the same response as before).

TOLUENE or METHYLBENZENE A product of the distillation of coal tar widely used as a solvent in the manufacture of paint and rubber and plastic cements.

TOMOGRAPHY A technique using X-rays or ultrasound to build up a focused image of a 'slice' through the body at a given level. By producing a series of such slices at different depths a three-dimensional image of the body structures can be built up (see X-RAYS).

-TOMY A suffix indicating an operation by cutting.

TONGUE The tongue is made up of several muscles, is richly supplied with blood-vessels and nerves, and is covered by highly specialized mucous membrane. It consists of a free part known as the tip, a body, and a hinder fixed part or root. The under surface lies upon the floor of the mouth, whilst the upper surface is curved from side to side, and still more from before backwards so as to adapt it to the roof of the mouth. At its root, the tongue is in contact with, and firmly united to, the upper edge of the larynx; so that in some persons who can depress the tongue readily the tip of the epiglottis may be seen projecting upwards at its hinder part.

Structure The substance of the tongue consists almost entirely of muscles running in various directions. The tongue also has numerous outside attachments; one muscle on each side unites it to the lower jaw-bone just behind the chin, and this muscle serves to protrude the

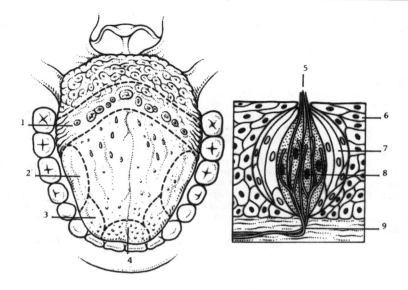

1 bitter
2 sour
3 salt
4 sweet
5 gustatory pore

6 stratified epithelium
7 sustentacular cell
8 gustatory cell with hairlet
9 nerve

(Left) Tongue from above showing different areas of taste discrimination.
(Right) vertical section through surface of tongue showing taste bud (×400).

tongue from the mouth; other muscles, which retract the tongue, attach it to the hyoid bone, the larynx, the palate, and the styloid process on the base of the skull.

The mucous membrane on the under surface of the tongue is very thin. In the middle line a fold of mucous membrane, the frenum, passes from the under surface to the floor of the mouth, and, when this frenum is attached too far forwards towards the tip of the tongue, the movements of the organ are impeded, and the condition is known as tongue-tie. On the upper surface or dorsum of the tongue the mucous membrane is thicker, and in its front two-thirds is studded with projections or papillae most of which are conical. Some of them end in long filaments, and are then known as filiform papillae. On the tip, and towards the edges of the tongue, small red rounded fungiform papillae are seen, which act as end-organs for the sense of taste as do circumvallate papillae, each of which is surrounded by a trench along which open numerous taste buds. These taste-buds are also found in the fungiform papillae, scattered over the throat, fauces, and palate. Five nerves, originating from the 5th, 7th, 9th, 10th and 12th cervical nerves supply the tongue.

Functions   The chief uses of the tongue are:

● to push the food between the teeth for mastication, and then mould it into a bolus preparatory to swallowing;

● as the organ of the sense of taste, and as an organ provided with a delicate sense of touch; and

● to play a part in the production of speech. (See VOICE AND SPEECH.)

It is usual to classify any taste as: sweet, bitter, salt and acid, since finer distinctions are largely dependent upon the sense of smell. The loss of keenness in taste brought about by a cold in the head, or even by holding the nose while swallowing, is well known. Sweet tastes seem to be best appreciated by the tip of the tongue, acids on its edges, and bitters at the back. There are probably different nerve-fibres and end-organs for the different varieties of taste. Many tastes depend upon the ordinary sensations of the tongue.

Like other sensations, taste can be very highly educated for a time, as in tea-tasters and wine-tasters, but this special adaptation is lost after some years.

TONGUE, DISEASES OF (see MOUTH, DISEASES OF).

TONGUE, FURRING OF (see MOUTH, DISEASES OF).

TONICS   These are placebos and may be used in conditions for which there is no known remedy, to strengthen and support the patient.

Available tonics range from rhubarb compound mixture to various mineral and vitamin supplements.

TONSILLITIS is the inflammation of the tonsils. The disorder may be the precurosor of a virus-induced infection of the upper respiratory tract such as COLDS, INFLUENZA or infectious MONONUCLEOSIS, in which case the inflammation usually subsides as other symptoms develop. This section describes tonsillitis caused by bacterial infection.

Acute tonsillitis The infection is never entirely confined to the tonsils; there is always some involvement of the surrounding throat or pharynx. The converse is true that in many cases of 'sore throat' the tonsils are involved in the generalized inflammation of the throat.

CAUSES Most commonly caused by the β-haemolytic STREPTOCOCCUS, its incidence is highest in the winter months. Formerly an important precursor of RHEUMATIC FEVER, early diagnosis and treatment have made this disease rare in developed countries. Occasionally it is the presenting feature of DIPHTHERIA, a disease now rare since the introduction of IMMUNIZATION.

SYMPTOMS The onset is usually fairly sudden with pain on swallowing, fever and malaise. On examination, the tonsils are engorged and covered with a whitish exudate, consisting of a purulent discharge. This may occur at scattered areas over the tonsillar crypts (follicular tonsillitis), or it may be more extensive. The glands under the jaw are enlarged and tender, and there may be pain in the ear on the affected side. Although usually referred pain, it may indicate spread of the infection up the Eustachian tube to the ear, particularly in children. Occasionally an abscess, or quinsy, develops around the affected tonsil. Due to a collection of pus, it usually comes on four to five days after the onset of the disease, and requires specialist surgical treatment.

TREATMENT Penicillin or erythromycin is the drug of choice, together with paracetamol or aspirin, and plenty of fluids.

Removal of tonsils is indicated: when the tonsils and adenoids are permanently so enlarged as to interfere with breathing; in such cases the adenoids are removed as well as the tonsils; when the individual is subject to recurrent attacks of acute tonsillitis which are causing significant debility, absence from school or work on a regular basis; when there is evidence of a tumour of the tonsil.

TONSILS Two almond-shaped glands situated one on each side of the narrow fauces where the mouth joins the throat. Each has a structure resembling that of a LYMPHATIC GLAND, and consists of an elevation of the mucous membrane presenting twelve to fifteen openings, which lead into pits or lacunae. The mucous covering is formed by the ordinary mucous membrane of the mouth, which also lines the pits; and the main substance of the gland is composed of loose connective tissue containing lymph corpuscles in its meshes, and packed here and there into denser nodules or follicles. The tonsils play an important rôle in the protective mechanism of the body against infection.

TOOTH, SUPERNUMERARY Malformed extra teeth are frequently found, particularly in the upper incisor region. They often do not erupt but prevent the eruption of the permanent teeth.

TOOTHACHE (see TEETH, DISEASES OF).

TOPHUS The name given to urate-based deposits which form in connection with joints or tendon sheaths as the result of attacks of gout. At first the tophus is a soft mass, but later becomes quite hard. It is composed of biurate of soda. (See GOUT.)

TOPICAL Pertaining to drugs or other treatment applied locally to the area being treated – e.g. the skin, eye, etc.

TORPOR A condition of bodily and mental inactivity, not amounting to sleep, but interfering greatly with the ordinary habits and pursuits. It is often found in people suffering from fever, and is a common symptom in aged people whose arteries are diseased. It may annoy young people after meals when they are the subjects of constipation or of dyspepsia, due to eating too much indigestible food.

TORSION Twisting. The term is applied to the process in which organs, or tumours, which are attached to the rest of the body by a narrow neck or pedicle, become twisted so as to narrow the blood-vessels or other structures in the pedicle. (See TESTICLES, DISEASES OF.)

Torsion is also the term applied to the twisting of the small arteries severed at an operation, by which bleeding from them is stopped.

TORTICOLLIS This is shortness of the sternomastoid muscle on one side resulting in asymetry and limitation of movement of the neck. (See CRAMP; SPASMODIC TORTICOLLIS; WRY-NECK.)

TOUCH The sense that enables an individual to assess the physical characteristics of objects – for example, their size, shape, temperature and texture. The sense of touch is considered here along with other senses associated with the skin and muscles. The cutaneous senses comprise:

Touch sense proper, by which we perceive a touch or stroke and estimate the size and shape of bodies with which we come in contact, but which we do not see.

Pressure sense, by which we judge the heaviness of weights laid upon the skin, or appreciate the hardness of objects by pressing against them.

Heat sense, by which we perceive that a body is warmer than the skin.

Cold sense, by which we perceive that a body touching the skin is cold.

Pain sense, by which we appreciate pricks, pinches and other painful impressions.

To these we may for convenience add:

Muscular sensitiveness, by which the painfulness of a squeeze is perceived. It is produced probably by direct pressure upon the nerve-fibres in the muscles.

Muscular sense, by which we test the weight of an object held in the hand, or gauge the amount of energy expended on an effort.

Sense of locality, by which we can, without looking, tell the position and attitude of any part of the body.

Common sensation, which is a vague term used to mean composite sensations produced by several of the foregoing, like tickling, or creeping, and the vague sense of well-being or the reverse that the mind receives from internal organs. (See the article on PAIN.)

The structure of the end-organs situated in the skin, which receive impressions from the outer world, and of the nerve-fibres which conduct these impressions to the central nervous system, have been described under NERVES. Touch affects the Meissner's or touch corpuscles placed beneath the epidermis; as these differ in closeness in different parts of the skin, the delicacy of the sense of touch varies greatly. Thus the points of a pair of compasses can be felt as two on the tip of the tongue when separated by only 1 mm; on the tips of the fingers they must be separated to twice that distance, whilst on the arm or leg they cannot be felt as two points unless separated by over 25 mm, and on the back they must be separated by over 50 mm. On the parts covered by hair, the nerves ending round the roots of the hairs also take up impressions of touch.

Pressure is estimated probably through the same nerve-endings and nerves that have to do with touch, but it depends upon a difference in the sensations of parts pressed on and those of surrounding parts. Heat-sense, cold-sense and pain-sense all depend upon different nerve-endings in the skin; by using various tests, the skin may be mapped out into a mosaic of little areas where the different kinds of impressions are registered. Whilst the tongue and finger-tips are the parts most sensitive to touch, they are comparatively insensitive to heat, and can easily bear temperatures which the cheek or elbow could not tolerate. The muscular sense depends on the sensory organs known as muscle-spindles, which are scattered through the substance of the muscles, and the sense of locality is dependent partly upon these and partly upon the nerves which end in tendons, ligaments and joints.

Disorders of the sense of touch occur in various diseases.

HYPERAESTHESIA is a condition in which there is excessive sensitiveness to any stimulus, such as touch. When this reaches the stage when a mere touch or gentle handling causes acute pain it is known as hyperalgesia. It is found in various diseases of the spinal cord immediately above the level of the disease, combined often with loss of sensation below the diseased part. It is also present in neuralgia, the skin of the neuralgic area becoming excessively tender to touch, heat or cold. Heightened sensibility to pain is seen sometimes in drunkards, who wince at a mere touch when not under the influence of alcohol. Heightened sensibility to temperature is a common symptom of neuritis. (See PAIN.)

ANAESTHESIA, or diminution of the sense of touch, causing often a feeling of numbness, is present in many diseases affecting the nerves of sensation or their continuations up the posterior part of the spinal cord. The condition of dissociated analgesia, in which a touch is quite well felt, though there is complete insensibility to pain, is present in the disease of the spinal cord known as SYRINGOMYELIA, and affords a proof that the nerve-fibres for pain and those for touch are quite separate. In tabes dorsalis there is sometimes loss of the sense of touch on feet or arms; but in other cases of this disease there is no loss of the sense of touch, although there is a complete loss of the sense of locality in the lower limbs, thus proving that these two senses are quite distinct.

PARAESTHESIAE are abnormal sensations such as creeping, tingling, pricking or hot flushes.

TOURETTE'S SYNDROME (See GILLES DE LA TOURETTE SYNDROME.)

TOURNIQUET Device, usually a rubber cord or tight bandage, that is bound round a limb to stop temporarily the arterial blood supply and so control severe bleeding. Tourniquets should be applied with caution and, unless untied within 15 minutes, GANGRENE may result, necessitating AMPUTATION. Because of this serious hazard, they are rarely used nowadays; direct pressure on the bleeding points is simpler, safer and equally effective in emergencies. A temporary tourniquet to an arm to increase the distension of veins when taking a sample of blood does no harm.

TOXAEMIA A term applied to forms of blood-poisoning due to the absorption of bacterial products (TOXINS) formed at some local site of infection, such as ABSCESSES. In other cases the toxaemia is due to defective action of some excretory organ, such as the KIDNEY. As regards treatment, the most important consideration is to remove the source of infection.

Toxaemia of PREGNANCY is a term sometimes

used to describe the two complications of pregnancy known as pre-eclampsia and ECLAMPSIA.

TOXIC SHOCK SYNDROME First described in 1978, this disorder is characterized by high fever, diarrhoea, shock and an erythematous rash. It is frequently associated with the use of tampons, but has occasionally been reported in men. The syndrome may also be linked to the use of contraceptives such as the diaphragm, cap and sponge. Skin wounds or infections may also be a cause. The disease is due to a STAPHYLOCOCCAL toxin. The treatment consists of supportive measures to combat shock and eradication of the staphylococcus by antibiotics. The design of tampons has been improved. Recurrence of the disorder has been reported and women who have had an episode should stop using tampons and vaginal contraceptives.

TOXICOLOGY The science dealing with poisons. (See POISONS.)

TOXINS Poisons produced by bacteria. (See IMMUNITY; IMMUNOLOGY; MICROBIOLOGY.) Toxins are usually soluble, easily destroyed by heat, sometimes of the nature of crystalline substances, and sometimes albumins. When injected into animals in carefully graduated doses, they bring about the formation of substances called antitoxins which neutralize the action of the toxin. These antitoxins are generally produced in excessive amount, and the serum of the animal when withdrawn can be used for conferring antitoxic powers upon other animals or human beings to neutralize the disease in question. The best known of these antitoxins are those of DIPHTHERIA and TETANUS. Toxins are also found in many plants and in snake venom.

Some toxins are not set free by bacteria, but remain in the substance of the latter. They are known as endotoxins and are not capable of producing antitoxins.

TOXOCARIASIS A disease acquired by swallowing the ova of a roundworm which lives in the intestine of cats (*Toxocara cati*) or dogs (*Toxocara canis*). In man, the small larval worms produced by these ova migrate to various parts of the body, including the retina of the eye, where they then die, and produce a small GRANULOMA which in turn may produce allergic reactions. In the eye it may cause choroidretinitis. It is said that 2 per cent of apparently healthy people in Britain have been infected in this way. A course of treatment with thiabendazole is recommended, though the drug has side-effects and should be used with caution in the elderly.

TOXOID TOXIN which has been rendered non-toxic by certain chemicals, or by heat, or by being partly neutralized by antitoxin. The best-known example is DIPHTHERIA toxoid. (See IMMUNITY.)

TOXOPLASMOSIS is a disease which is due to infection with protozoa of the genus Toxoplasma. The infection may be acquired from eating raw or undercooked meat, from cats, or from gardening or playing in contaminated soil. It occurs in two forms: an acquired form and a congenital form. The acquired form may run such a benign course that it is not recognized, the patient scarcely feeling ill. In the congenital form the unborn child is infected by the mother. The congenital form, the incidence of which in the United Kingdom is 1 in 5000 pregnancies (1 in 2000 pregnancies in Scotland), may develop in one of two ways. The infant may either appear generally ill, or the brunt of the infection may fall on the nervous system causing HYDROCEPHALUS, mental retardation, or loss of sight. In some cases the infection may be so severe that it kills the fetus, resulting in a miscarriage or stillbirth. In other cases the infection is so mild that it is missed until in later life the child begins to show signs of eye trouble. As the congenital form of the disease, which is most serious, seems to develop only if the mother acquires the infection during pregnancy, it would appear to be a wise precaution that pregnant women should avoid contact with cats and eating raw or undercooked meat foods.

TRACE ELEMENTS are chemical elements that are distributed throughout the tissues of the body in very small amounts and are essential for the nutrition of the body. Nine such elements are now recognized: cobalt, copper, fluorine, iodine, iron, manganese, molybdenum, selenium and zinc.

TRACHEA is another name for the WINDPIPE. (See also AIR PASSAGES.)

TRACHEITIS Inflammation of the trachea. It may occur along with bronchitis, or independently, due to similar causes.

TRACHEOSTOMY or TRACHEOTOMY The operation in which the trachea or WINDPIPE is opened from the front of the neck, so that air may be directly drawn or passed into the lower air passages. The opening is made through the second and third rings of the trachea.

Reasons for operation The cause of laryngeal obstruction should be treated but, if obstruction is acute and endangering the patient's life, urgent intervention is necessary. In most cases the insertion of an endotracheal tube either through the nose or mouth and down the pharynx through the larynx to bypass the obstruction is effective. If not, tracheostomy is performed. The majority of tracheostomies performed nowadays are for patients in intensive-therapy-unit situations. These patients require airway intervention for prolonged periods to facilitate artificial ventilation which is performed by means of a mechanical ventilator. The presence of a tube passing through the larynx for a prolonged period of time is associated with long-term damage to the larynx, and therefore any patients requiring prolonged intubation usually undergo a tracheostomy to prevent further damage to the larynx. Endotracheal intubation is also the preferred method of airway intervention for acute inflammatory disorders of the upper airway as opposed to tracheostomy. Tracheostomy in these cases is performed only in the emergency situation if facilities for endotracheal intubation are not available or if they are unsuccessful. Tracheostomy may also be performed for large tumours which obstruct the larynx until some form of treatment is instituted. Similarly it may be needed in conditions whereby the nerve supply to the larynx has been jeopardized impairing its protective function of the upper airway and its respiratory function.

Tracheostomy tubes When the trachea has been opened it is necessary to introduce a tube in order to keep the opening from closing. The tubes are made either of hard rubber or more often of metal; and there is always an outer tube which is fixed in position by tapes passing round the neck, and an inner tube which slides freely out of and into the other, so that it may be removed at any time for cleansing, and is readily coughed out should it happen to become blocked by mucus.

After-treatment When the operation has been performed for some permanent obstruction, the tube must be worn permanently; and the double metal tube is in such cases replaced after a short time by a soft rubber single one. When the operation has relieved some obstruction caused, say, by diphtheria, the tube is left out now and then for a few hours, and finally, at the end of a week or so, is removed altogether, after which the wound quickly heals up.
(See APPENDIX 2: ADDRESSES.)

TRACHOMA is a severe type of CONJUNCTIVITIS (see EYE DISEASES). This chronic contagious condition is caused by *Chlamydia trachomatis*, a bacterium with virus-like characteristics. Trachoma is common in developing countries, where it is the leading cause of preventable blindness worldwide. The disease may be seen in immigrant populations in developed countries, though it is usually inactive. The bacterium is transmitted by flies and causes inflammation of the conjunctiva and cornea with consequent scarring. The active disease is treated with tetracycline tablets and eye drops and cure is usually satisfactory.

TRACTION The application of a pulling force to the distal part of a fracture in order to allow the fracture to heal with the bone in correct alignment. There are many different methods for applying traction, usually involving weights and pulleys.

TRAINING (see DIET; EXERCISE).

TRANCE A profound sleep from which a person cannot for a time be aroused, but which is not due to organic disease. The power of voluntary movement is lost, though sensibility and even consciousness may remain. It is usually due to hysteria, and may be induced by hypnotism. (See CATALEPSY; ECSTASY; and SLEEP.)

TRANEXAMIC ACID A drug used in the control of bleeding. It inhibits the activation of PLASMINOGEN and FIBRINOLYSIS and may be useful when bleeding cannot be stopped, for instance, dental extraction in HAEMOPHILIA. The drug is also useful in menorrhagia.

TRANQUILLIZERS A tranquillizer is a popular name for a drug which induces a mental state free from agitation and anxiety, and renders the patient calm. Tranquillizers are classified as major and minor. The former are used to treat psychotic illness such as SCHIZOPHRENIA; the latter are sedatives used to treat anxiety and emotional upsets and are called antianxiety drugs or anxiolytics. Major tranquillizers or antipsychotic drugs are given to patients with psychotic disorders which disrupt their normal lives. They do not cure the patient but do help to control his or her symptoms so that they can live in the community and be admitted to hospital only for acute episodes. The drug chosen depends on the type of illness and needs of a particular patient as well as the likely adverse effects. Antisychotic drugs modify the transmission of nerve signals by making brain cells less sensitive to the excitatory neurotransmitter chemical called DOPAMINE. Among the antipsychotic tranquillizers are CHLORPROMAZINE, HALOPERIDOL, CLOZAPINE and flupenthixol.

Anxiety is a consequence of too much stress and may occur without being serious enough to need treatment. Clinically it rises when the balance between certain chemicals in the brain is disturbed. This increases activity in the sympathetic system, thus provoking physical symptoms such as breathlessness, tachycardia, headaches and indigestion. Anxiolytics help to alleviate these symptoms but do not necessarily cure the underlying cause. Two main classes of drug relieve anxiety: BENZODIAZEPINES and beta blockers. The latter, which include atenolol and propanolol, reduce the physical symptoms such as tachycardia and are useful in circumstances – for example, examinations – known to cause anxiety attacks. They block the action of NORADRENALINE, a key chemical of the sympathetic nervous system. Benzodiazepines depress activity in that part of the brain controlling emotion by stimulating the action of a chemical called gamma-aminobutyric acid (GABA). Among the benzodiazepines are CHLORDIAZEPOXIDE and DIAZEPAM. (See MENTAL ILLNESS.)

TRANSCUTANEOUS ELECTRICAL NERVE STIMULATION A method of electrical stimulation that is being used for the relief of pain, including that of migraine, neuralgia and phantom limbs. Known as TENS, its mode of action appears to have some resemblance to that of acupuncture. Several controlled trials suggest that it provides at least a modicum of relief of pain after operations, thereby reducing the amount of analgesics that may be called for.

TRANSFUSION OF BLOOD This has been practised since the 17th century, although with a high mortality rate. The main problems encountered have been the tendency of the transfused blood to clot and the liability of the red blood cells to break up, leading to haematuria and jaundice. Recipients often showed an allergic response, in severe cases leading to anaphylactic shock. It was only when incompatibility of BLOOD GROUPS was considered as a potential cause of this allergy that routine blood testing became standard practice. Since the National Blood Transfusion Service was started, in 1946, in the United Kingdom, blood for transfusion has been collected from voluntary, unpaid donors, screened for infections such as syphilis, HIV and hepatitis, sorted by group, and stored in blood-banks throughout the country. A standard transfusion bottle has been developed, and whole blood may be stored at 2–6 °C for three weeks before use. Transfusions may then be given of whole blood, plasma, blood cells, or platelets, as appropriate. Stored in the dried form at 4–21 °C, away from direct sunlight, human plasma is stable for five years, and is easily reconstituted by adding uninfected distilled water.

Autologous transfusion is the use of an individual's own blood, provided in advance, for transfusion during or after a surgical operation. This is a valuable procedure for operations that may require large transfusions or where a person has a rare blood group. Its use has increased because of the fear of AIDS and hepatitis.

Exchange transfusion is the method of treatment in severe cases of HAEMOLYTIC DISEASE OF THE NEWBORN. It consists of replacing the whole of the baby's blood with Rh-negative blood of the correct blood group for the baby.

TRANSIENT ISCHAEMIC ATTACKS OR EPISODES (TIA, TIE) Episodes of transient ischaemia of some part of the cerebral hemispheres or the brain stem lasting anything from a few minutes to several hours and followed by complete recovery. By definition the ischaemic episode must be less than 24 hours. These episodes may be isolated or they may occur several times in a day. The cause is atheroma of the carotid or vertebral arteries and the embolization of platelets or cholesterol. These attacks present with STROKES that rapidly recover.

TRANSLOCATION The term used to describe an exchange of genetic material between CHROMOSOMES. It is an important factor in the etiology, or causation, of certain congenital abnormalities such as, for example mongolism.

It is one of the main abnormalities sought for in amnioscopy.

TRANSPLANTATION of organs of the body has become a practical possibility within recent years. The major outstanding problem is how to prevent the recipient's body from rejecting and destroying the transplanted organ. Such rejection of a foreign body is part of the normal protective mechanism of the body and is essential for the maintenance of the integrity of the body.

If the transplant comes from another person it is known as an allotransplant. If it comes from the patient himself – for example, a skin graft – it is known as an autotransplant. If it comes from an animal it is known as a xenotransplant.

The pioneering success was achieved with transplantation of the kidney, and this has been most successful when the transplanted kidney has come from an identical twin. Less successful have been live transplants from other blood relatives, while least successful have been transplants from other live donors and cadaver donors. The results, however, are steadily improving. Thus the one-year functional survival of kidneys transplanted from unrelated cadaver donors has risen from around 50 per cent to over 80 per cent, and survival rates of 80 per cent after three years are not uncommon. For a well-matched transplant from a live related donor the survival rate after five years is around 90 per cent. And, of course, if a transplanted kidney fails to function, the patient can always be switched on to some form of DIALYSIS. In the United Kingdom the supply of cadaveric kidneys for transplantation is only about half that necessary to meet the demand.

Other organs that have been transplanted with increasing success are the heart, the lungs, the liver, bone marrow, and the cornea of the eye. Heart, lung, liver and pancreas transplantations are now carried out in specialist centres. It is estimated that in the United Kingdom approximately 200 patients a year between the ages of 15 and 55 would benefit from a liver transplant if an adequate number of donors were available. Over 100 liver transplants are carried out annually in the United Kingdom and one-year-survival rates of up to 80 per cent have been achieved.

Good progress has been made in techniques of tissue typing and immunosuppression to overcome the problems of organ transplantation. Drugs are now available that can suppress the immune reactions of the recipient, which are responsible for the rejection of the transplanted organ. Notable among these are cyclosporin A, which revolutionized the success rate, and tacrolimus, a macrolide immunosuppressant that has been recently introduced. Chemically unrelated to cyclosporin, it has a similar mode of action. The incidence of neurotoxicity and nephrotoxicity appears to be greater, and cardiomyopathy has also been reported.

By these and other means, such as careful

typing of the donor kidney, results are steadily improving. One of the more promising developments is the development of an anti-lymphocytic serum (ALS) which reduces the activity of the LYMPHOCYTES, cells which play an important part in maintaining the integrity of the body against foreign bodies.

Donor cards are now available in all general practitioners' surgeries and pharmacies but, of the millions of cards distributed since 1972, too few have been used. The reasons are complex but include the reluctance of the public and doctors to consider organ donation, poor organization for recovery of donor kidneys and worries about the diagnosis of death. A code of practice for procedures relating to the removal of organs for transplantation was produced in 1978 and this code has been revised in the light of further views expressed by the Conference of Medical Royal Colleges and Faculties of the United Kingdom on the Diagnosis of Brain Death. Under the Human Tissue Act 1961 only the person lawfully in possession of the body or his designate can authorize the removal of organs from a body. This authorization may be given orally. Patients who may become suitable donors after death are those who have suffered severe and irreversible brain damage. Such patients will be dependent on artificial ventilation. Patients with malignant disease or systemic infection and patients with renal disease, including chronic hypertension, are unsuitable. If a patient carries a signed donor card or has otherwise recorded his wishes there is no legal requirement to establish lack of objection on the part of relatives, although it is good practice to take account of the views of close relatives. If a relative objects, despite the known request by the patient, staff will need to judge, according to the circumstances of the case, whether it is wise to proceed with organ removal. If a patient who has died is not known to have requested that his organs be removed for transplantation after his death the designated person may only authorize the removal if, having made such reasonable enquiry as may be practical, he has no reason to believe (*a*) that the deceased had expressed an objection to his body being so dealt with after his death, or (*b*) that the surviving spouse or any surviving relative of the deceased objects to the body being so dealt with. Staff will need to decide who is best qualified to approach the relatives. This should be someone with appropriate experience who is aware how much the relative already knows about the patient's condition. Relatives should not normally be approached before death has occurred but sometimes a relative approaches the hospital staff and suggests sometime in advance that the patient's organs might be used for transplantation after his death. The staff of hospitals and organ exchange organizations must respect the wishes of the donor, the recipient and their families with respect to anonymity.

Relatives who enquire should be told that some post-mortem treatment of the donor's body will be necessary if the organs are to be removed in good condition. It is ethical to maintain artificial ventilation and heart beat until removal of organs has been completed. This is essential in the case of heart and liver transplants and many doctors think it is desirable when removing kidneys. Official criteria have been issued in Britain to recognize when BRAIN-STEM DEATH has occurred. This is an important protection for patients and relatives when someone with a terminal condition – usually as a result of an accident – is considered as a possible organ donor.

TRANS-SEXUALISM The psycho-sexual abnormality characterized by feelings of belonging to the gender opposite to that of the genitalia and the secondary sex characteristics. Trans-sexuals or their families wanting help and guidance should contact the Gender Dysphoria Trust International or the Partner's Group for Partners and Families of Trans-sexuals (see APPENDIX 2: ADDRESSES).

TRANSURETHRAL RESECTION The use of a special CYSTOSCOPE (a resectoscope) inserted through the URETHRA to resect the PROSTATE GLAND or bladder tumours (see RESECTION).

TRANSVERSE An anatomical description of a line, plane or structure at right angles to the long axis of an organ or the body.

TRANSVESTITISM or TRANSVESTISM The term given to a psycho-sexual abnormality in which there is a repetitive compulsion to dress in the clothes of the opposite sex to achieve orgasm.

TRANYLCYPROMINE A monoamine oxidase inhibitor ANTIDEPRESSANT drug.

TRAUMA A term used in a physical sense as a wound or injury – such as a severe blow, maybe leading to a fracture. Physical traumas such as events of birth, severe accidents and any form of childhood or sexual abuse, are considered to be overwhelming stressful events and regarded as psychological traumas. Various scoring techniques have been formed for traumas; generally seen as numerical systems for assessing the severity and prognosis of severe injuries.

TRAUMATOLOGY Branch of surgery specializing in the treatment of wounds and disabilities arising from injuries.

TRAVEL MEDICINE Many countries have reciprocal health arrangements with Britain under which British visitors may receive emergency treatment free or at reduced cost. Information about these arrangements is available in leaflet SA40, available from any local DSS office. General and specific advice for travellers on such matters as immunizations needed can be obtained from their doctor, through travel agents or one of the high street travel 'health shops'. (See APPENDIX 3: TRAVEL AND HEALTH.)

TRAVEL SICKNESS Sickness induced by any form of transport, whether by sea, air, motor-car or train. (See MOTION-SICKNESS.)

Traveller's diarrhoea is an all too common affliction of the traveller, which basks in a multiplicity of names: e.g. Aden gut, Aztec two step, Basra belly, Delhi belly, Gippy tummy, Hong Kong dog, Montezuma's revenge, Tokyo trots, turista. It is caused by a variety of micro-organisms, usually *E. coli*. Some people seem to be more prone to it than others, though for no good cause. Obvious preventive measures include the avoidance of salads, unpeeled fruit and ice cream, and never drinking unboiled or unbottled water. If diarrhoea occurs, co-phenotrope and loperamide are often used to reduce the frequency of bowel movements in adults. Prophylactic antibacterial drugs are not advisable.

TRAZODONE A tricyclic ANTIDEPRESSANT drug.

TREMOR A fine involuntary movement. Tremors may be seen in projecting parts like the hands, head and tongue, or they may involve muscles. Coarse tremors, which prevent a person from drinking a glass of water without spilling it, are found in MULTIPLE SCLEROSIS and in CHOREA; somewhat finer tremors, which produce trembling of the hands or tongue when they are stretched out, are caused by alcoholism (see ALCOHOL), by poisoning with other substances like LEAD, by PARKINSONISM, and by the weakness which follows some acute disease or characterizes old age; a fine tremor of the outstretched fingers is a characteristic of THY-ROTOXICOSIS; very fine tremors, visible in the muscles of face or limbs, and known as fibrillary tremors, are present in general paralysis of the insane, and in progressive muscular atrophy or wasting palsy. Tremors may occur at rest and disappear on movement as in Parkinsonism, or they may occur only on movement (intention tremors) as in cerebellar disease.

TRENCH FEVER An infectious disease caused by *Rickettsia quintana* which is transmitted by the body louse. Large epidemics occurred among troops on active service during the 1914–18 War. It recurred on a smaller scale in the 1939–45 War but is now rare.

TRENCH FOOT or IMMERSION FOOT This is due to prolonged exposure of the feet to water, particularly cold water. Trench warfare is a common precipitating factor, and it was rampant during the 1914–18 War. Cases also occurred during the 1939–45 War and during the Falklands campaign. The less common form due to warm water immersion occurred with some frequency in the Vietnam war. It is characterized by painful swelling of the feet accompanied in due course by blistering and ulceration which, in severe, untreated cases, may go on to gangrene. In mild cases recovery may be complete in a month, but severe cases may drag on for a year.

Treatment Drying of the feet overnight, where practicable, is the best method of prevention, accompanied by avoidance of constrictive clothing and tight boots, and of prolonged immobility. Frequent rest periods and daily changing of socks also help. The application of silicone grease once a day is another useful preventive measure. In the early stages treatment consists of rest in bed and warmth. In more severe cases treatment is as for infected tissues and ulceration. ANALGESICS are usually necessary to ease the pain. Technically, smoking should be forbidden, but the psychological effects in troops on active service may outweigh its advantages.

TRENDELENBERG POSITION First described by Frederick Trendelenberg in 1881, this is a steep head-down tilt so that the patient's pelvis and legs lie above the heart. It is used to improve access and limit blood loss during surgery to the pelvis. It has been used to treat shocked patients, but, as the position increases pressure on the diaphragm and embarrasses breathing, raising the legs by themselves is better.

TREPHINING or TREPANNING An operation in which a portion of the CRANIUM IS removed. Originally the operation was performed with an instrument resembling a carpenter's brace and known as the trephine or trepan, which removes a small circle of bone; but now this instrument is only used, as a rule, for making small openings, whilst, for wider operations, gouge forceps, circular saws driven by electric motor, or wire saws are used.

The operation was one of the commonest major operations of antiquity. Hippocrates describes fully the operation and the conditions that call for it, whilst Galen mentions two varieties of the instrument in common use. Both among the Greeks and Romans, and in the Middle Ages trephining was carried out for conditions believed to arise in the brain.

Nowadays trephining is used in cases of fracture, with splintering of the skull; the operation is performed to remove the fragments of bone and any foreign bodies, like a bullet, which may have entered. In compression of the brain with unconsciousness following an injury, the skull is trephined and any blood-clots removed, or torn vessels ligatured. The operation may also be done for an abscess within the skull and for other conditions where operative access to the brain is required.

TREPONEMA The name of a genus of spirochaetal micro-organisms which consist of slender spirals and which progress by means of bending movements. *Treponema pallidum* (formerly called *Spirochaeta pallida*) is the causative organism of SYPHILIS.

TRIAGE   Derived from French word for 'sorting', a universal term applied to methods of allocating treatment prioritizations for casualties from disasters or in warfare. Triage helps a medical team to treat urgently casualties who, though badly injured, can be saved, to defer those whose treatment is less urgent and to provide care and comfort for those with fatal injuries.

TRIAMCINOLONE   A CORTICOSTEROID, with a potency equivalent to that of prednisone, but is less likely to cause retention of sodium. It is used for the suppression of inflammatory and allergic disorders, and is used particularly for treating the skin and joints by local injection.

TRICHIASIS   A condition in which the eyelashes become ingrown. (See EYE DISEASES.)

TRICEPS   A muscle of the posterior upper arm which acts to extend the forearm. So named because it originates from three heads.

TRICHINOSIS or TRICHINIASIS   A disease caused by eating meat infected with the parasitic nematode worm, *Trichinella spiralis*. Although it infects over 100 animal species, this nematode usually infects humans via pig meat in which the immature *spiralis* is encysted. The full-grown female worm, which inhabits the intestine, is 3 mm in length, and the larvae, to whose movements the disease is due, are much smaller. The disease is acquired by eating raw or underdone pork from pigs that have been infected with the worm. When such a piece of meat is eaten, the embryos contained in it are set free, develop into full-grown trichinellae, and from each pair of these 1000 or more new embryos may arise in a few weeks. These burrow through the walls of the gut, spread throughout the body and settle in voluntary muscle.

Prevention is based on thorough inspection of meat in slaughter-houses, for even cooking, unless the meat is in slices, is not an efficient protection. Pigs should not be fed on unboiled garbage. Rats may be a source of sporadic outbreaks, as infected rats have been found near piggeries. The disease is widely distributed throughout the Americas, Asia, Africa and the Arctic. Sporadic cases and epidemics occur and outbreaks also appear in Europe, though rarely in Britain.

Treatment Thiabendazole or mebendazole are usually effective, while steroids help patients with systemic illness and muscle tenderness.

TRICHO- is a prefix denoting relation to hair.

TRICHOMONAS VAGINALIS   A protozoon normally present in the vagina of about 30 to 40 per cent of women. It sometimes becomes pathogenic and causes inflammation of the genital passages, with vaginal discharge. A man may become infected as a result of sexual intercourse with an infected woman and have a urethral discharge as a result; it may also cause prostatitis. METRONIDAZOLE is usually an effective treatment, and to obtain a satisfactory result it may be necessary to treat both partners. Should metronidazole not work, then tinidazole may be tried.

TRICHOMONIASIS   The disease caused by infection with *TRICHOMONAS VAGINALIS*.

TRICHOPHYTON   (see DERMATOPHYTES).

TRICHORRHOEA   Loss of hair, usually due to some general disease such as scarlet fever or typhoid fever. When there is no obvious cause, such as this, treatment consists of attention to the general hygiene of the scalp.

TRICHOTILLOMANIA   An obsessional impulse to pull out one's own hair.

TRICHURIASIS   A worldwide infection, particularly common in the tropics. It is caused by *Trichuris trichiura*, or whipworm, so called because of its shape, the rear end being stout and the front end hairlike, resembling the lash of a whip. The male measures 5 cm and the female 4 cm in length. Infection results from eating vegetables, or drinking water, polluted with the ova (eggs). These hatch out in the large intestine. The diagnosis is made by finding the eggs in the stools. The worms seldom cause any trouble unless they are present in large numbers when, especially in malnourished children, they may cause bleeding from the bowels, anaemia and prolapse of the rectum. The most effective drug is mebendazole.

TRICUSPID INCOMPETENCE   Failure of the TRICUSPID VALVE in the heart to close fully, thus permitting blood to leak back into the right atrium during contractions of the right ventricle. This reduces the heart's pumping efficiency. Right-sided heart failure usually results. Treatment for heart failure (using DIURETICS and ACE inhibitor drugs) usually restores function but sometimes heart surgery is required to repair or replace the defective valve.

TRICUSPID STENOSIS   Normal working of TRICUSPID VALVE in heart impede by narrowing of opening, often a sequel of rheumatic fever. As with TRICUSPID INCOMPETENCE, heart failure may result and treatment is similar, with surgery to repair or replace faulty valve an option.

TRICUSPID VALVE The valve, with three cusps or flaps, that guards the opening from the right atrium into the right ventricle of the heart. (See HEART.)

TRICYCLIC   ANTIDEPRESSANT DRUGS This group of drugs is one of three main types of drugs used to treat depression and was the first to be introduced (in the 1950s). Tricyclic drugs work by blocking the re-uptake of the NEUROTRANSMITTERS SEROTONIN and NO-RADRENALINE, thus increasing the amount of the neurotransmitters at the nerve cell's receptors. In people with depression fewer neurotransmitters than normal are released, resulting in a slowing down of neural activities. The drugs have a sedative effect, which can be useful for depressives with sleep problems, and an antimuscarinic action which can cause dry mouth and constipation. Overdosage can produce coma, fits and irregular heart rhythm (see MENTAL ILLNESS; ANTIDEPRESSANTS).

TRIFLUOPERAZINE (see NEUROLEPTICS).

TRIGEMINAL NERVE is the fifth cranial nerve. It consists of three divisions: (1) the ophthalmic nerve, which is purely sensory in function, being distributed mainly over the forehead and front part of the scalp; (2) the maxillary nerve, which is also sensory and distributed to the skin of the cheek, the mucous membrane of the mouth and throat, and the upper teeth; and (3) the mandibular nerve, which is the nerve of sensation to the lower part of the face, the tongue and the lower teeth, as well as being the motor nerve to the muscles concerned in chewing. The trigeminal nerve is of special interest, owing to its liability to NEURALGIA, TRIGEMINAL NEURALGIA, or tic douloureux as it is also known, being the most painful form known of neuralgia.

TRIGEMINAL NEURALGIA Also called TIC DOULOUREUX, this is one of the most severe forms of NEURALGIA. It affects the main sensory nerve in the face (trigeminal nerve), and may occur in one or more of the three divisions in which the nerve is distributed. It is usually confined to one side. It is more common in women than men, usually occurring over the age of 50. The attack is often precipitated by movements of the jaw, as in talking or eating, or by tactile stimuli such as a cold wind or washing the face. When the first or upper division of the nerve is involved, the pain is mostly felt in the forehead and side of the head. It is usually of an intensely sharp, cutting, or burning character, either constant or with exacerbations each day while the attack continues. There is also pain in the eyelid, redness of the eye and increased flow of tears. When the second division of the nerve is affected, the pain is chiefly in the cheek and upper jaw. When the third division of the nerve suffers, the pain affects the lower jaw. Attacks may recur for years; and, although interfering with sleeping and eating, they rarely appear to lead to any serious results. Nevertheless, the pain may become intolerable.

Treatment The outlook in trigeminal neuralgia was radically altered by the introduction of the drug CARBAMAZEPINE, which usually relieves the pain. If the side-effects – for example, dizziness, headache, nausea or drowsiness – are unacceptable or pain not relieved, PHENYTOIN may help. Otherwise, surgery is needed in the shape of controlled, radiofrequency heat damage to the appropriate part of the trigeminal nerve.

TRIGGER FINGER or SNAPPING FINGER This is the condition in which when the fingers are straightened on unclenching the fist one finger, usually the ring or middle finger, remains bent. The cause is obscure. In severe cases treatment consists of opening up the sheath surrounding the tendon of the affected finger. When confined to the thumb it is known as TRIGGER THUMB.

TRIGGER THUMB (see TRIGGER FINGER).

TRIGLYCERIDE One of the basic chemical 'building blocks' from which fats are formed. A triglyceride molecules consists of three fatty-acid molecules which have chemically reacted with glycerol.

TRIGONE The base of the BLADDER between the openings of the two URETERS and of the URETHRA.

TRI-IODOTHYRONINE The substance which exerts the physiological action of THYROID hormone. It is formed in the body cells by the de-iodination of THYROXINE (tetra-iodothyronine) which is the active principle secreted by the thyroid gland. It has also been synthesized, and is now available for the treatment of HYPOTHYROIDISM. It is three times as potent as thyroxine. (See also THYROID GLAND.)

TRIMESTER A period of three months. Normal human GESTATION is divided into three trimesters.

TRIMETHOPRIM is an anti-bacterial agent used in the treatment of infections of the URINARY TRACT. It is also a constituent of CO-TRIMOXAZOLE. The drug is also used to treat acute and chronic bronchitis.

TRIMIPRAMINE A tricyclic antidepressant drug which also acts as a sedative. (See ANTIDE-PRESSANTS.)

TRINITRIN (see GLYCERYL TRINITRATE).

TRIPLE VACCINE Also known as DPT vaccine, this is an injection that provides immunity against DIPHTHERIA, PERTUSSIS (whooping-cough) and TETANUS. It is given as a course of three injections at around the ages of two, three and four months. A booster dose of diphtheria and tetanus is given at primary-school age. (See IMMUNIZATION.)

TRIPLETS (see MULTIPLE BIRTHS).

TRISMUS Another name for TETANUS.

TROCAR An instrument provided with a sharp three-sided point fitted inside a tube or cannula, and used for puncturing cavities of the body in which fluid has collected.

TROCHANTER The name given to two bony prominences at the upper end of the thigh-bone. The greater trochanter can be felt on the outer side of the thigh. The lesser trochanter is a small prominence on the inner side of this bone.

TROCHLEAR NERVE The fourth cranial nerve, which acts upon the superior oblique muscle of the eye.

TROPHIC A term applied to the influence that nerves exert with regard to the healthiness and nourishment of the parts to which they run. When the nerves become diseased or injured, this influence is lost and the muscles waste, while the skin loses its healthy appearance and is liable to break down into ulcers. (See NERVOUS DISEASES; BED SORES.)

TROPHOBLAST The outer layer of the fertilized ovum which attaches the ovum to the wall of the UTERUS (or womb) and supplies nutrition to the embryo.

TROPICAL DISEASES Technically, those diseases occurring in the area of the globe situated between the Tropic of Cancer and the Tropic of Capricorn: pertaining to the sun. They include many 'exotic' infections – many of them parasitic in origin – which fall under the umbrella of 'Tropical Medicine'. However, disease in the tropics is far broader than this and includes numerous other infections, many of them with a viral or bacterial basis, e.g. the viral hepatidises, streptococcal and pneumococcal infections, and tuberculosis. The prevalence of other diseases, such as rheumatic cardiac disease, cirrhosis, heptocellular carcinoma ('hepatoma'), and various nutrition-related problems, is also much increased in most areas of the tropics. (See ANCYLOSTOMIASIS; BERIBERI; BLACKWATER FEVER; CHOLERA; DENGUE; DRACONTIASIS; DYSENTERY; ELEPHANTIASIS; FILARIASIS; HEAT STROKE; LEISHMANIASIS; LEPROSY; LIVER DISEASES; MALARIA; ORIENTAL SORE; PLAGUE; PRICKLY HEAT; SCHISTOSOMIASIS; SLEEPING SICKNESS; STRONGYLOIDIASIS; SUNBURN; YAWS; YELLOW FEVER)

TRUNK A major vessel or nerve from which lesser ones arise, or the main part of the body excluding the head, neck and limbs.

TRUSS A device used to support a hernia; or to retain the protruding organ within the cavity from which it tends to pass. Every truss possesses a pad of some sort to cover the opening and a belt or spring to keep it in position.

Before applying a truss the wearer must make certain that the hernia has been reduced. This may mean lying down before applying the truss. A truss will rarely control a hernia satisfactorily, and it should be considered as a temporary measure only until surgical correction is possible. In the past trusses have been supplied to patients considered too frail for surgery, but modern anaesthetic techniques mean that most people can have their hernias surgically repaired. (See HERNIA.)

TRYPANOSOMA A genus of microscopic parasites, several of which are responsible for causing sleeping sickness and some allied diseases. (See SLEEPING SICKNESS.)

TRYPANOSOMIASIS (see SLEEPING SICKNESS.)

TRYPSIN The chief protein ENZYME of the pancreatic secretion. Secreted by the pancreas as trypsinogen (an inactive form), it is converted in the duodenum by another enzyme, enteropeptidase. It changes proteins into peptones and forms the main constituent of pancreatic extracts used for digestion of food. (See PANCREAS; PEPTONIZED FOOD.)

TRYPTOPHAN is an antidepressive drug that has helped some patients with resistant depression. Used as a supporting drug with other treatment, tryptophan was withdrawn because of side-effects. It has, however, been reintroduced for use in hospital for patients for whom no alternative treatment is suitable.

TSETSE FLY An African fly of the genus *Glossina*. One or more of these is responsible for carrying the TRYPANOSOME which causes SLEEPING SICKNESS and thus spreads the disease among cattle and from cattle to men.

TSUTSUGAMUSHI or JAPANESE RIVER FEVER, is a disease of the typhus group. (See TYPHUS FEVER.)

TUBAL PREGNANCY Implantation of the embryo in the FALLOPIAN TUBE rather than in the lining of the UTERUS. The patient usually complains of pain between six and ten weeks' gestation and, if the fallopian tube is not removed, there may be rupture with potentially life-threatening haemorrhage (also known as ectopic pregnancy).

TUBERCLE The term used in two distinct senses. As a descriptive term in anatomy, a tubercle means a small elevation or roughness upon a bone, such as the tubercles of the ribs. In the pathological sense, a tubercle is a small mass, barely visible to the naked eye, formed in some organ as the starting-point of tuberculosis. The name of tubercle bacillus was originally given to the micro-organism that causes this disease but was subsequently changed to *Mycobacterium tuberculosis*. The term 'tubercular' should strictly be applied to anything connected with or resembling tubercles or nodules, and the term 'tuberculous' to anything pertaining to the disease tuberculosis.

TUBERCULIDE The term given to any skin lesion which is the result of infection with the tubercle bacillus, or *Mycobacterium tuberculosis* as it is now known.

TUBERCULIN is the name originally given by Koch in 1890 to a preparation derived from the tubercle bacillus, or *Mycobacterium tuberculosis* as it is now known, and intended for the diagnosis or treatment of tuberculosis.

Varieties
OLD TUBERCULIN (OT) IS the heat-concentrated filtrate from a fluid medium on which the human or bovine type of *Mycobacterium tuberculosis* has been grown for six weeks or more. TUBERCULIN PURIFIED PROTEIN DERIVATIVE (TUBERCULIN PPD) is the active principle of Old Tuberculin, and is prepared from the fluid medium on which the *Mycobacterium tuberculosis* has been grown. It is supplied as a liquid, a powder, or as sterile tablets. The liquid contains 100,000 Units per millilitre, and the dry powder contains 30,000 Units per milligram. It is distributed in sterile containers sealed so as to exclude micro-organisms. It is more constant in composition and potency than Old Tuberculin.

Uses The basis of the tuberculin reaction is that any person who has been infected with the *Mycobacterium tuberculosis* gives a reaction when a small amount of tuberculin is injected into the skin. A negative reaction means that either the individual has never been infected with the tubercle bacillus, or that the infection has been too recent to have allowed of sensitivity developing.

There are various methods of carrying out the test, of which the following are the most commonly used. The Mantoux Test is the most satisfactory of all and has the advantage that the size of the reaction is a guide to the severity of the tuberculous infection. It is performed by injecting the tuberculin into the skin on the forearm. The Heaf Multiple Puncture Test is reliable. It is carried out with the multiple puncture apparatus, or Heaf Gun. The Vollmer Patch Test using an impregnated filter paper, is useful in children because of the ease with which it can be carried out.

TUBERCULOSIS Tuberculosis results form infection with *Mycobacterium tuberculosis*. The lungs are the site most often affected but most organs in the body can be involved in tuberculosis. The other common sites are LYMPH NODES, bones, gastrointestinal tract, kidneys, skin and MENINGES.

The weight loss and wasting associated with tuberculosis before treatment was available led to the popular name of consumption for tuberculosis. Enlargement of the glands in the neck, formerly called scrofula, was known also as the 'king's evil' from the supersition that a touch of the royal hand could cure the condition. LUPUS VULGARIS is another of the skin manifestations of the disease.

The typical pathological change in tuberculosis involves the formation of clusters of cells called GRANULOMAS with death of the cells in the centre producing CASEATION.

It is estimated that there are 7–8 million new cases of tuberculosis world-wide each year with 2–3 million deaths. The incidence of tuberculosis in developed countries has shown a steady decline throughout the 20th century, mainly as a result of improved nutrition and social conditions and accelerated by the development of antituberculous chemotherapy in the 1940s. Since the mid-1980s the decline has stopped and even started to rise again in inner-city areas. In 1996 5,650 cases of tuberculosis were notified in England and Wales compared with under 5,610 in 1995 and 5,590 in 1994; 420 deaths in 1996 were attributed to the disease. Factors involved in this rise are immigration from higher-prevalence areas, poorer social conditions and homelessness in some urban centres and the association with HIV infection and drug abuse. The incidence of tuberculosis is also rising in many developing countries because of the emergence of resistant strains of the tubercle bacillus (see below).

Nature of the disease Tuberculosis has been recognized from earliest times. Evidence of the condition has been found in Egyptian mummies. Hippocrates (460–375BC) called it phthisis because of the lung involvement. In 1882 Koch announced the discovery of the causative organism, the tubercle bacillus or MYCOBACTERIUM TUBERCULOSIS.

The symptoms depend upon the site of the infection. General symptoms such as fever, weight loss and night sweats are common. In the most common form of pulmonary tuberculosis cough and blood-stained sputum (haemoptysis) are common symptoms.

The route of infection is most often by inhalation, although it can be by ingestion of products such as infected milk. The results of contact depend on the extent of the exposure and the susceptibility of the individual. Around

30 per cent of those closely exposed to the organism will be infected but most will contain the infection with no significant clinical illness and only a minority will go on to develop clinical disease. Around 5 per cent of those infected will develop post-primary disease over the next two or three years. The rest are at risk of reactivation of the disease later, particularly if their resistance is reduced by associated disease, poor nutrition or immunosuppression. In developed countries around 5 per cent of those infected will reactivate their healed tuberculosis into a clinical problem.

Immunosuppressed patients such as those infected with HIV are at much greater risk of developing clinical tuberculosis on primary contract or from reactivation. This is a particular problem in many developing countries where there is a high incidence of both HIV and tuberculosis.

Diagnosis This depends on identification of mycobacteria on direct staining of sputum or other secretions or tissue and on culture of the organism. Culture takes 4 to 6 weeks but is necessary for differentiation from other non-tuberculous mycobacteria and for drug-sensitivity testing. Newer techniques involving DNA amplification by polymerase chain reaction (PCR) can detect small numbers of organisms and help with earlier diagnosis.

Treatment This can be preventative or curative. Important elements of prevention are adequate nutrition and social conditions, BCG vaccination, an adequate public-health programme for contact tracing and chemoprophylaxis. Radiological screening with mass miniature radiography is no longer used.

Vaccination with an attenuated organism (BCG – Bacillus Calmette Guerin) is used in the United Kingdom and some other countries at 12–13 years or earlier in high-risk groups. Some studies show 80 per cent protection against tuberculosis for ten years after vaccination.

Cases of open tuberculosis need to be identified and their close contacts reviewed for evidence of disease. Adequate antibiotic chemotherapy removes the infective risk after around two weeks of treatment. Chemoprophylaxis, the use of antituberculous therapy in those without clinical disease, may be used in contacts who develop a strong reaction on tuberculin skin testing or those at high risk because of associated disease.

The major principles of antibiotic chemotherapy for tuberculosis are that a combination of drugs needs to be used and that treatment needs to be continued for a prolonged period, usually six months. Use of single agents or interrupted courses leads to the development of drug resistance. Serious outbreaks of multiply resistant *Mycobacterium tuberculosis* have been seen mainly in AIDS units, where patients have greater susceptibility to the disease, but also in developing countries where maintenance of appropriate antibacterial therapy for six months or more can be difficult.

Streptomycin was the first useful agent identified in 1944. The four drugs used most often now are RIFAMPICIN, ISONIAZID, PYRAZINAMIDE and ETHAMBUTOL. Three to four agents are used for the first two months; then, when sensitivities are known and clinical response observed, two drugs, most often rifampicin and isoniazid, are continued for the rest of the course. Treatment is taken daily, although thrice weekly, directly observed therapy is used when there is doubt about the patient's compliance. All the antituberculous agents have a range of adverse effects that need to be monitored during treatment. Providing the treatment is prescribed and taken appropriately, response to treatment is very good with cure of disease and very low relapse rates.

TUBEROSE SCLEROSIS (EPILOIA) A rare inherited disease transmitted as an autosomal dominant trait. Epilepsy in childhood is often the first manifestation, though ovoid hypopigmented macules ('ash leaf patches') in the skin may be detected in infancy. Later an acne-like eruption of the face (adenoma sebaceum), fibrous outgrowths around the nails and fibrous plaques on the lower back (shagreen patch) can all occur.

Characteristic white streaks appear on the optic fundi (see EYE). Variable degrees of mental handicap is common. Relatives of those with this condition can obtain help and guidance from the Tuberous Sclerosis Association of Great Britain (see APPENDIX 2: ADDRESSES).

TUBOCURARINE The active constituent of CURARE. It is a MUSCLE RELAXANT which is widely used in ANAESTHESIA.

TULARAEMIA A disease of rodents such as rabbits and rats, caused by the bacillus, *Francisella tularense*, and spread either by flies or by direct inoculation, for example, into the hands of a person engaged in skinning rabbits. In man the disease takes the form of a slow fever lasting several weeks, with much malaise and depression, followed by considerable emaciation. It was first described in the district of Tulare in California, and is found widely spread in North America and in Europe, but not in Great Britain. STREPTOMYCIN, the TETRACYCLINES and CHLORAMPHENICOL, offer effective in treatment.

TULLE GRAS A dressing of gauze impregnated with soft paraffin to prevent it sticking to the wound.

TUMOUR This literally means any swelling, but the term does not usually include temporary swellings caused by acute inflammation. The consequences locally, however, of chronic inflammation, like tuberculosis, syphilis, leprosy and glanders, are, however, sometimes classed as tumours, according to their size and appearance.

Varieties Some are of an infective nature, as already stated; some arise, and as the result of injury, and several contributing factors are mentioned under the heading of CANCER.

Traditionally tumours have been divided into benign (simple) and malignant. Even benign tumours can be harmful because their size or position may distort or damage nerves, blood vessels or organs. Usually, however, they are easily removed by surgery. Malignant tumours or cancers are harmful and potentially lethal, not just because they erode tissues locally but because many of them spread, either by direct growth or by 'seeding' to other parts. Malignant tumours arise because of an uncontrolled growth of previously normal cells. Heredity, environmental factors and life-style all play a part in malignancy (see also ONCOGENES). Symptoms are caused by local spread and as a result of metastases – the distant secondary growths caused by the seeding. These metastases cause serious local damage, for example, in the brain or lungs, as well as disturbing the body's metabolism. Unless treated with CHEMOTHERAPY or RADIOTHERAPY or surgery or a combination of these, malignant tumours are ultimately fatal. Many, however, can now be cured. The original site and type of a malignant tumour usually determine the rate and extent of spread. The type of cell and organ site determine the characteristics of a malignant tumour. The prognosis (outlook) for a patient with a malignant tumour depends largely on how soon it is diagnosed. Staging criteria have been developed to assess the local and metastatic spread of a tumour, its size and also likely sensitivity to the types of available treatment. The ability to locate a tumour and its metastases accurately has vastly improved with the introduction of radionucleide and ULTRASOUND scanning, CT scanning and MAGNETIC RESONANCE IMAGING (MRI).

Tumours are now classed according to the tissues of which they are built, somewhat as follows:

- Simple tumours of normal tissue
- Hollow tumours or cysts, generally of simple nature
- Malignant tumours: (*a*) of cellular structure, resembling the cells of skin, mucous membrane, or secreting glands; (*b*) of connective tissue.

TURGOR Being or becoming swollen or engorged.

TURNER'S SYNDROME This occurs in one in 2,500 live female births. It is caused by either the absence of or an abnormality in one of the two X chromosomes. Classical Turner's Syndrome is a complete deletion of one X so that the karyotype is 45XO. Half of the people with Turner's Syndrome have mosaicism with a mixture of Turner cells and normal cells or other abnormalities of the X chromosome such as partial deletions or a ring X. They are females, both phenotypically and sexually; clini-

cal features are variable and include short stature, with final height between 1·295 m and 1·575 m and ovarian failure. However, a few women (fewer than 1 per cent) with Turner's Syndrome do develop ovulatory menstrual cycles. Other clinical features may include a short neck, webbing of the neck, increased carrying angle at the elbow (cubitus valgus), widely spaced nipples, cardiovascular abnormalities of which the commonest is coarctation of the aorta (about 10 per cent), morphological abnormalities of the kidneys, including horseshoe kidney and abnormalities of the pelviureteric tracts, recurrent OTITIS MEDIA, squints, increased incidence of pigmented naevi, HYPOTHYROIDISM and DIABETES MELLITUS. Intelligence is across the normal range, although there are specific learning defects which are related to hand–eye co-ordination and spatial awareness.

Patients with Turner's Syndrome may require therapeutic help throughout their life. In early childhood this may revolve around surgical correction of cardiovascular disease and treatment to improve growth. Usually puberty will need to be induced with oestrogen therapy. In adult life, problems of oestrogen therapy, prevention of osteoporosis, assessment and treatment of hypertension and assisted fertility predominate. For the address of the UK Turner Syndrome Society see APPENDIX 2: ADDRESSES.

TWINS (see MULTIPLE BIRTHS).

TYMPANIC MEMBRANE The ear-drum, which separatees the external and middle ears. (See EAR.)

TYMPANITES Distension of the abdomen due to the presence of gas or air in the intestine or in the peritoneal cavity. The abdomen when struck with the fingers, gives under these conditions a drum-like (tympanitic) note.

TYMPANUM Another name for the middle ear. (See EAR.)

TYPHOID FEVER (see ENTERIC FEVERS).

TYPHUS FEVER An infective disease of world-wide distribution, the manifestations of which vary in different localities. The causative organisms of all forms of typhus fever belong to the genus RICKETTSIA. These are organisms which are intermediate between bacteria and viruses in their properties and measure 0·5 micrometre or less in diameter.

Louse typhus, in which the infecting rickettsia is transmitted by the louse, is of world-wide distribution. More human deaths have been attributed to the louse via typhus, louse-borne RELAPSING FEVER and trench fever, than to any other insect with the exception of the MALARIA mosquito. Louse typhus includes

Louse-borne	Flea-borne	Tick-borne	Mite borne
Epidemic typhus	Murine (endemic) typhus	Rocky Mountain spotted fever	Tsutsugamushi fever
Brill's disease		African tick typhus (Tick-bite fever)	(Scrub typhus)
Trench fever		Fièvre boutonneuse	Rickettsialpox

Classification of the typhus fevers.

epidemic typhus, Brill's disease which is a recrudescent form of epidemic typhus, and TRENCH FEVER.

Epidemic typhus fever, also known as exanthematic typhus, classical typhus, and louse-borne typhus, is an acute infection of abrupt onset which, in the absence of treatment, persists for fourteen days. It is of world-wide distribution, but is largely confined today to parts of Africa. The causative organism is the *Rickettsia prowazeki*, so-called after Ricketts and Prowazek, two brilliant investigators of typhus, both of whom died of the disease. It is transmitted by the human louse, *Pediculus humanus*. The rickettsiae can survive in the dried faeces of lice for 60 days, and these infected faeces are probably the main source of infection of man.
SYMPTOMS The incubation period is usually 10 to 14 days. The onset is preceded by headache, pain in the back and limbs and rigors. On the third day the temperature rises, the headache worsens, and the patient is drowsy or delirious. Subsequently a characteristic rash appears on the abdomen and inner aspect of the arms, to spread over the chest, back and trunk. Death may occur from septicaemia, heart failure (see HEART DISEASES), kidney failure (see KIDNEYS, DISEASES OF) or PNEUMONIA about the fourteenth day. In those who recover, the temperature falls by crisis about this time. In diagnosis the Weil-Felix reaction is helpful. The death-rate is variable, varying from nearly 100 per cent in epidemics among debilitated refugees to about 10 per cent.

Murine typhus fever, also known as flea typhus, is world-wide in its distribution and is found wherever individuals are crowded together in insanitary, rat-infested areas. Hence the old names of jail-fever and ship typhus. The causative organism, *Rickettsia mooseri*, which is closely related to *R. prowazeki*, is transmitted to man by the rat-flea, *Xenopsyalla cheopis*. The rat is the main reservoir of infection. Once man is infected, the human louse may act as a transmitter of the RICKETTSIA from man to man. This explains how the disease may become epidemic under insanitary, crowded conditions. As a rule, however, the disease is only acquired when man comes into close contact with infected rats.
SYMPTOMS These are similar to those of louse-borne typhus, but the disease is usually milder, and the mortality rate is very low (about 1·5 per cent).

Tick typhus, in which the infecting Rickettsia is transmitted by ticks, occurs in various parts of the world. The three best-known conditions in this group are Rocky Mountain Spotted Fever, Fièvre Boutonneuse and Tick-bite Fever.

Mite typhus, in which the infecting Rickettsia is transmitted by mites, includes scrub typhus, or tsutsugamushi disease, and rickettsialpox.

Rickettsialpox is a mild disease caused by *Rickettsia akari*, which is transmitted to man from infected mice by the common mouse mite, *Allodermanyssus sanguineus*. It occurs in USA, West and South Africa and the former Soviet Union.

Treatment The general principles of treatment are the same in all forms of typhus.
PROPHYLAXIS consists of either avoidance of, or destruction of, the vector. In the case of louse typhus and flea typhus, the outlook has been revolutionized by the introduction of efficient insecticides such as DDT and Gammexane. The value of the former was well shown by its use after the Second World War. This resulted in almost complete freedom from the epidemics of typhus which ravaged Eastern Europe after the 1914–18 War being responsible for 30 million cases with a mortality of 10 per cent. Now only 10,000 to 20,000 cases occur a year, with around a few hundred deaths. Efficient rat control is another measure which reduces the risk of typhus very considerably. In areas such as Malaysia, where the mites are infected from a wide variety of rodents scattered over large areas, the wearing of protective clothing is the most practical method of prophylaxis.
CURATIVE TREATMENT was revolutionized by the introduction of chloramphenicol and the tetracyclines. These antibiotics altered the prognosis in typhus fever very considerably.

TYROSINE An AMINO ACID important in the production of CATECHOLAMINES, MELANIN and THYROXINE. .

U

ULCER Destruction of the skin's surface tissues resulting in an open sore. A similar breach may occur in the surface of the mucous membrane lining body cavities – for example, the stomach, duodenum or colon (see COLITIS).

Usually accompanied by pain and local inflammation, ulcers can be shallow or deep, with a craterlike shape. An ulcer may heal naturally but on certain parts of the body – legs (venous ulcers, see below) or bony protuberances (decubitus ulcers, see below) – they can become chronic and difficult to treat. When an ulcer heals granulations (well-vascularized connective tissue) form which become fibrous and draw the edges of the ulcer together. Any damage to the body surface may develop into an ulcer if the causative agent is allowed to persist – for example, contact with a noxious substance or constant pressure on an area of tissue with poor circulation. Treatment of skin ulcers is effected by cleaning the area, regular dry dressings and local or systemic ANTIBIOTICS depending on severity of the ulcer.

Decubitus ulcer (PRESSURE SORE; BEDSORE) occurs when there is constant pressure on and inadequate oxygenation of an area of skin, usually overlying a bony protuberance. Elderly, infirm people or individuals with debilitating, emaciating, or neurological illnesses are vulnerable to the condition. Long-term pressure from a bed, wheelchair, cast or splint is the usual cause. Loss of skin sensation is a contributory factor, and muscle and bone as well as skin may be affected.
TREATMENT The most important treatment is prevention, keeping the patient's back, buttocks, heels and other pressure points clean and dry, and regularly changing his or her position. If ulcers do develop repeated local DEBRIDEMENT, protective dressings and (in serious cases) surgical treatment are required, accompanied by an appropriate antibiotic if infection is persistent.

Venous ulcer (VARICOSE ULCER) This occurs on the lower leg or ankle and is caused by chronic HYPERTENSION in the deep leg VEINS, usually the consequences of previous deep-vein THROMBOSIS which has destroyed the valvular system in the vein(s). The ulcer is usually preceded by chronic OEDEMA, often local ECZEMA, and bleeding into the skin that produces brown staining. Varicose veins may or may not be present. Control of the oedema by compression and encouragement to walk is central to management.

ULCERATIVE COLITIS (see COLITIS).

ULNA The inner of the two bones in the forearem. It is wide at its upper end, and its olecranon process forms the point of the elbow. In its lower part it is more fragile and is liable to be broken by a fall upon the forearm while something is grasped in the hand. Chipping off of the olecranon process is a not uncommon result of falls upon the elbow. (See FRACTURES.)

ULNAR NERVE A major NERVE in the arm, it runs from the brachial plexus to the hand. The nerve controls the muscles that move the fingers and thumb and conveys sensation from the fifth and part of the fourth and from the adjacent palm. Muscle weakness and numbness in the areas supplied by the nerve is usually caused by pressure from an abnormal outgrowth from the epicondyle at the bottom of the humerus (upper arm bone).

ULOGLOSSITIS Inflammation of the gums and of the tongue.

ULTRAFILTRATION Filtration carried out under pressure. Blood undergoes ultrafiltration in the kidneys to remove the waste products, urea and surplus water that constitute urine.

ULTRASOUND or ULTRASONIC WAVES These comprise very high-frequency sound waves above 20,000 Hz that the human ear cannot hear. Ultrasound is widely used for diagnosis and also for some treatments. In obstetrics ultrasound can assess the stage of pregnancy and detect abnormalities in the fetus. It is a valuable adjunct in the investigation of diseases in the bladder, kidneys, liver, ovaries, pancreas and brain. Ultrasound also detects thromboses in blood vessels and enables their extent to be assessed. A non-invasive technique that does not need ionizing radiation, ultrasound is quick, versatile and relatively inexpensive, with scans being done in any plane of the body. There is little danger to the patient or operator and unlike, for example, X-rays, ultrasound investigations can be repeated as needed. A contrast medium is not required. Its reliability is dependent on the skill of the operator. It is replacing isotope scanning in many situations, and also radiography. Ultrasound of the LIVER can separate medical from surgical JAUNDICE in approximately 97 per cent of patients. It is very accurate in detecting and defining cystic lesions of the liver but is less accurate with solid lesions and yet will detect 85 per cent of secondary deposits. This is less than CT scanning. It is very accurate in detecting GALL-STONES and more accurate than the oral CHOLECYSTOGRAM. It is useful as a screening test for pancreatic disease and can differentiate carcinoma of the PANCREAS from chronic pancreatitis with 85 per cent accuracy.

It is the first investigation indicated in patients presenting with renal failure as it can quickly determine the size and shape of the kidney and whether there is any obstruction to the ureter. It is very sensitive to the presence of dilatation of the renal tract and it will detect space-occupying lesions, differentiating cysts and tumours. It can detect obstruction of the ureter due to renal stones by showing dilatations of the collecting system and the presence of the calculus. ADRENAL tumours can be demonstrated by ultrasound though it is less accurate than CT SCANNING. Ultrasound is now the first test for suspected aortic ANEURYSM and it can also show the presence of clot and delineate the true and false lumen. It is good at demonstrating sub-phrenic and sub-hepatic abscesses and will show most intra-abdominal abscesses. CT scanning is however better for the retroperitoneal region. It has a major application in thyroid nodules as it can differentiate cystic from solid lesions and show the multiple lesions characteristic of the nodular goitre. It cannot differentiate between a follicular adenoma and a carcinoma as both these tumours are solid. Ultrasound cannot demonstrate normal parathyroid glands but it can identify adenomas provided they are more than 6 mm in diameter. Ultrasound can differentiate masses in the scrotum into testicular and appendicular and it can demonstrate impalpable testicular tumours. This is important as 15 per cent of testicular tumours metastasize whilst they are still impalpable.

Doppler ultrasound is a technique which shows the presence of vascular disease in the carotid and peripheral vessels as it can detect the reduced blood flow through narrowed vessels.

Ultrasound has particular applications in obstetrics. A fetus can be seen with ultrasound from the seventh week of pregnancy, and the fetal heart can be demonstrated at this stage. Multiple pregnancy can also be diagnosed at this time by the demonstration of more than one gestation sac containing a viable FETUS. A routine obstetric scan is usually performed between the sixteenth and eighteenth week of pregnancy when the fetus is easily demonstrated and most photogenic. The fetus can be measured to assess the gestational age and the anatomy can also be checked. Intra-uterine growth retardation is much more reliably diagnosed by ultrasound than by clinical assessment. The site of the placenta can also be recorded and multiple pregnancies will be diagnosed at this stage. Foetal movements and even the heart beat can be seen. A second scan is often done between the thirty-second and thirty-fourth weeks to assess the position, size and growth rate of the baby. The resolution of equipment now available enables pre-natal diagnosis of a wide range of structural abnormalities to be diagnosed. Spina bifida, hydrocephalus and anencephaly are probably the most important but other anomalies such as multicystic kidney, achondroplasia and certain congenital cardiac anomalies can also be identified. Foetal gender can be determined from twenty weeks of gestation. Ultrasound is also useful as guidance for amniocentesis.

In gynaecology polycystic OVARIES can readily be detected as well as fibroids and ovarian cysts. Ultrasound can monitor follicular growth when patients are being treated with infertility drugs. It is also useful in detecting ectopic pregnancies.

Ultrasonic waves are one of the constituents in the shock treatment of certain types of GALLSTONES and CALCULI in the urinary tract (see LITHOTRIPSY). They are also being used in the treatment of MENIÈRE'S DISEASE and of bruises and strains. In this field of physiotherapy, ultrasonic therapy is proving of particular value in the treatment of acute injuries of soft tissue. If in such cases it is used immediately after the injury, or as soon as possible thereafter, it is claimed, there is no question of delayed, chronic recovery. For this reason it is being widely used in the treatment of sports injuries. The sound waves stimulate the healing process in damaged tissue.

ULTRAVIOLET RAYS (UVR) Invisible light rays of very short wavelength beyond the violet end of the sun's spectrum. Ultraviolet-C (UVC) (wavelength <290 nn (nano metre – see APPENDIX 6: MEASUREMENTS)) is entirely absorbed by the earth's atmosphere and would otherwise be lethally damaging. Ultraviolet-B (UVB) (290–320 nn) intensity increases with altitude. It is greatest in midsummer and at midday and penetrates cirrhus cloud. UVB causes sunburn and also tanning. Ultraviolet-A (UVA) (320–400 nm) penetrates deeper into our skins but does not cause sunburn. UVA is implicated in many photochemical reactions and in PHOTODERMATOSES and in CARCINOGENESIS. UVR helps the skin to synthesize vitamin-D.

Ultraviolet lamps produce UVR and are used to tan skin but, because of the risk of producing skin cancer (see SKIN DISEASES), the lamps must be used with great caution.

UMBILICAL CORD The fleshy tube containing two arteries and a vein through which the mother supplies the fetus with oxygen and nutrients. The cord, which is up to 60cm long, ceases to function after birth and is clamped and cut about 2·5cm from the infant's abdominal wall. The stump shrivels and falls off within two weeks, leaving a scar which forms the umbilicus.

UMBILICUS The scientific name for the navel.

UNCINATE FIT A state in which a patient has a hallucination of smell or of taste; it may be a manifestation of epilepsy, or the result of a tumour pressing on that part of the brain concerned with the appreciation of smell and taste.

UNCONSCIOUS A state of UNCONSCIOUSNESS or a description of mental activities of which an individual is unaware. Unconscious is also used in psychoanalysis to characterize that section of a person's mind in which memories and motives reside. They are normally inaccessible, protected by inbuilt mental resistance. This contrasts with the subconscious where a person's memories and motives, while temporarily suppressed, can usually be recalled.

UNCONSCIOUSNESS The BRAIN is the organ of the mind. Normal conscious alertness depends on its continuous adequate supply with oxygen and glucose, both of which are essential for the brain cells to function normally. If either or both of these are interrupted, altered consciousness results. Interruption may be caused by three broad types of process affecting the brain stem (see BRAIN): the reticular formation (a network of nerve pathways and nuclei-connecting sensory and motor nerves to and from the cerebrum, cerebellum (see BRAIN), SPINAL CORD and cranial nerves) and the cerebral cortex. The three types are diffuse brain dysfunction – for example, generalized metabolic disorders such as URAEMIA or toxic disorders such as SEPTICAEMIA – direct effects on the brain stem as a result of infective, cancerous or traumatic lesions, and indirect effects on the brain stem such as a tumour or OEDEMA in the cerebrum creating pressure within the skull. Within these three divisions are a large number of specific causes of unconsciousness.

Unconsciousness may be temporary, prolonged or indefinite (see PERSISTENT VEGETATIVE STATE), depending on the severity of the initiating incident. The patient's recovery depends on the cause and success of treatment where given. Memory may be affected, as may motor and sensory functions, but short periods of unconsciousness as a result, say, of trauma have little obvious effect on brain function. Repeated bouts of unconsciousness, which can happen in boxing, may, however, have a cumulatively damaging effect, as can be seen on CT scans of the brain.

Poisons such as CARBON MONOXIDE, drug overdose, a fall in the oxygen content of blood (HYPOXIA) in lung or heart disease, or liver or kidney failure harm the normal chemical working or metabolism of nerve cells. Severe blood loss will cause ANOXIA of the brain. Any of these can result in altered brain function in which impairment of consciousness is a vital sign.

Sudden altered consciousness will also result from fainting attacks (syncope) in which the blood pressure falls and the circulation of oxygen is thereby reduced. Similarly an epileptic fit causes partial or complete loss of consciousness by causing an abrupt but temporary disruption of the electrical activity in the nerve cells in the brain (see EPILEPSY).

As the brain's function progressively fails, in these events, drowsiness, stupor and finally COMA ensue. If the cause is removed or, when the patient spontaneously recovers from a fit or faint, normal consciousness is usually quickly regained. STROKES are sometimes accompanied by a loss of consciousness. This may be immediate or come on slowly, depending on the cause or site of the strokes.

Comatose patients are graded according to agreed test scales – for example, the GLASGOW COMA SCALE – in which the patient's response to a series of tests indicate numerically the level of coma.

Treatment of unconscious patients depends on the cause and range from first-aid care for someone who has fainted to hospital intensive-care treatment for a victim of a severe head injury or massive stroke.

UNDULANT FEVER Another name for BRUCELLOSIS.

UNGUAL An adjective relating to the finger nails or toe nails.

UNGUENTUM The Latin name for ointment.

UNIT The term applied to a quantity assumed as a standard for measurement. Thus, the unit of insulin is the specific activity contained in such an amount of the standard preparation as the Medical Research Council may from time to time indicate as the quantity exactly equivalent to the unit accepted for international use. The standard preparation consists of pure, dry, crystalline insulin. (See APPENDIX 6: MEASUREMENTS IN MEDICINE.)

UNITED KINGDOM CENTRAL COUNCIL FOR NURSING, MIDWIFERY AND HEALTH VISITING (See APPENDIX 9: STATUTORY ORGANIZATIONS.)

UPPER LIMB DISORDERS A group of injuries resulting from overuse of a part of the limb. One example is tennis elbow (epicondylitis) caused by inflammation of the tendon attaching the extensor muscles of the forearm to the humerus because of overuse of the muscles. Overuse of the shoulder muscles may cause inflammation and pain around the joint. Perhaps the best-known example is repetitive strain injury affecting keyboard workers and musicians. The result is pain in and weakness of the wrists and fingers. This has affected thousands of people and been the subject of litigation by employees against their employers. Working practices have been improved and the complaint is now being recognized at an early stage. Treatment includes physiotherapy but some sufferers have been obliged to give up their work.

URACHUS is a corded structure which extends from the bladder up to the navel, and represents the remains of the canal which in the fetus joins bladder with allantois.

URAEMIA The clinical state which results from renal failure (see KIDNEY, DISEASES OF). It may be due to disease of the KIDNEYS or it may be the result of pre-renal causes where a lack of circulating blood volume inadequately perfuses the kidneys. It may result from acute necrosis in the tubules of the kidney or it may result from obstruction to the outflow of urine.

The word uraemia means excess UREA in the blood, but the symptoms of renal failure are not due to the abnormal amounts of urea circulating but to the ELECTROLYTE disturbances and acidosis which are associated with impaired renal function. The ACIDOSIS results from a decrease in the ability to filter hydrogen ions from blood into the glomerular fluid and the reduced production of ammonia and phosphate means fewer ions capable of combining with the hydrogen ions so that the total acid elimination is diminished. The fall in glomerular filtration also leads to retention of SODIUM and water with resulting OEDEMA, and to retention of POTASSIUM resulting in HYPERKALAEMIA. The most important causes of uraemia are the primary renal diseases of chronic glomerular NEPHRITIS and chronic PYELONEPHRITIS. It may also result from MALIGNANT HYPERTENSION damaging the kidneys and amyloid disease destroying the kidneys. Analgesic abuse can cause tubular necrosis. DIABETES MELLITUS may cause a nephropathy and lead to uraemia as may MYELOMATOSIS and SYSTEMIC LUPUS ERYTHEMATOSUS. Polycystic kidneys and renal tuberculosis account for a small proportion of cases. (See KIDNEYS, DISEASES OF.)

Symptoms Uraemia is sometimes classed as acute, i.e. those cases in which the symptoms develop in a few hours or days, and chronic, including cases in which the symptoms are less marked and last over weeks, months, or years. There is, however, no dividing line between the two, for in the chronic variety, which may be said to consist of the symptoms of chronic glomerulonephritis, an acute attack is liable to come on at any time.

Headache in the front or back of the head, accompanied often by insomnia and daytime drowsiness, is one of the commonest symptoms. Unconsciousness of a profound type, which may be accompanied by convulsions resembling those of epilepsy, is the most outstanding feature of an acute attack and is a very dangerous condition.

Still another symptom, which often precedes an acute attack, is severe vomiting without apparent cause. The appetite is always poor, and the onset of diarrhoea is a serious sign.

Treatment The treatment of the chronic type of uraemia includes all the measures which should be taken by a person suffering from chronic glomerulonephritis. An increasing number of these patients, especially the younger ones, are treated with dialysis and/or renal transplantation. (See DIALYSIS; TRANSPLANTATION.)

URATES (see URIC ACID).

UREA or CARBAMIDE A crystalline substance of the chemical formula $CO(NH_2)_2$, which is very soluble in water or alcohol. It is the chief waste product discharged from the body in the urine, being formed in the liver and carried to the kidneys in the blood. The amount varies considerably with the quantity and nature of the food taken, rising greatly upon an animal (protein) dietary. It also rises during the continuance of a fever. The average amount excreted daily, during health, on a mixed diet is about 33 to 35 grams.

Urea is usually administered for its DIURETIC action, and also as a test of kidney action, in doses of 5 to 15 grams. It is used, too, as a cream in the treatment of certain skin diseases, characterized by a dry skin, such as ICHTHYOSIS.

Urea is rapidly changed, by a yeast-like micro-organism, into carbonate of ammonia; and to this chemical change the ammoniacal smell of badly kept latrines is due.

UREAPLASMA A group of micro-organisms which plays a larger part in the causation of disease than was at one time suspected. One of them, *Ureaplasma urealyticum*, is now recognized as a cause of chronic prostatitis, non-specific urethritis (see URETHRA, DISEASES OF.) and infertility.

URETER The tube that carries URINE from the KIDNEY to the URINARY BLADDER. There are two ureters, one for each kidney, and they originate from the kidney pelvis and track for 25 to 30 cm (10 to 12 inches) through the loins and pelvis. They open by a narrow slit into the base of the bladder. The lower end of the ureter pierces the wall of the bladder so obliquely (lying embedded in the wall for about 21 mm) that, though urine runs freely into the bladder, it is prevented from returning up the ureter as the bladder becomes distended.

URETHRA The tube which leads from the BLADDER to the exterior, and by which the urine is voided. It is about 20 cm (8 inches) long in the male and 3·5 cm (1½ inches) long in the female. In the male it passes along the PENIS, in the female the urethra opens to the exterior just in front of the VAGINA between the labial folds.

URETHRA, DISEASES OF AND INJURY TO The urethra is the tube that runs from the bladder through which the urine is voided. Disease of or damage to the urethra interferes with the passage of urine.

Trauma Injury to the urethra is often the result of severe trauma to the pelvis – for example, in a car accident or as the result of a fall. Trauma can also result from CATHETER insertion or the insertion of foreign bodies into the urethra. The signs are the inability to pass URINE, and blood at the exit of the urethra. The major complication of trauma is the development of a urethral stricture.

Urethritis is inflammation of the urethra from infection.
CAUSES The sexually transmitted disease GONORRHOEA affects the urethra, mainly in men, and causes severe inflammation and urethritis. Non-specific urethritis (NSU) is an inflammation of the urethra caused by one of many different micro-organisms including BACTERIA, YEAST and CHLAMYDIA.
SYMPTOMS The classic signs and symptoms are a urethral discharge associated with urethral pain, particularly on micturition, and dysuria.

TREATMENT This involves taking urethral swabs, culturing the causative organism and treating it with the appropriate antibiotic. The complications of urethritis include stricture formation.

Stricture This is an abrupt narrowing of the urethra at one or more places. Strictures can be a result of trauma or infection or a congenital abnormality from birth. Rarely tumours can cause strictures.

SYMPTOMS The usual presenting complaint is one of a slow urinary stream. Other symptoms include hesitancy of micturition, variable stream and terminal dribbling. Measurement of the urine flow rate may help in the diagnosis, but often strictures are detected during cystoscopy.

TREATMENT The traditional treatment was the periodic dilation of the strictures with 'sounds' – solid metal rods passed into the urethra. However, a more permanent solution is achieved by cutting the stricture with an endoscopic knife (optical urethrotomy). For more complicated long or multiple strictures an open operation (urethroplasty) is required.

URETHRAL SYNDROME A group of symptoms of unknown cause. It mainly affects women, occasionally men. Pain and discomfort in the lower abdomen, a frequent urge to urinate and, in women, pain in the area of the vulva. Investigation rarely results in any abnormal findings. Post-menopusal women, who are the commonest victims, may have inflammation of the vulva due to thinning of the tissues in that area. Treatment is supportive with the patient being advised to drink a lot of fluid and maintain a high standard of personal hygiene.

URETHRITIS means inflammation of the urethra (see URETHRA, DISEASES OF).

URIC ACID A crystalline substance, very slightly soluble in water, of chemical formula, $C_5N_4H_4O_3$. It is white in the pure state, but when found as a urinary deposit it is reddish-brown, presenting a supposed resemblance to cayenne pepper. The bi-urate of sodium and urate of ammonium occur in considerable amount in the urine during a feverish state or after great exertion, and produce, as the urine cools, a dense pink or yellow sediment. The average daily quantity of uric acid passed by human beings is 0·5 to 1 gram. In the urine of birds and reptiles uric acid is the chief nitrogenous constituent, taking the place of the urea excreted by human beings. Uric acid is formed in the liver and removed by the kidneys from the blood. The amount is increased in the following conditions:

- Excessive consumption of meat, combined with sedentary habits.
- GOUT.
- Diseases in which the white corpuscles of the blood are increased: e.g. leukaemia.

Owing to their insolubility, uric acid and the various urates often produce deposits in the urinary passages, which are known as urinary sand, gravel, or stones according to their size.

URINALYSIS Analysis of the physical and chemical composition of URINE to detect variations in the substances normally present and to identify abnormal constituents such as sugar, drugs, blood, or alcohol.

URINARY BLADDER The urinary bladder is a highly distensible organ for storing urine. It consists of smooth muscle known as the detrusor muscle and is lined with urine-proof cells known as transitional cell EPITHELIUM.

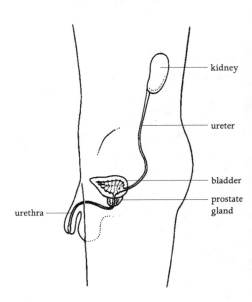

Side view (longitudinal section) of male urinary tract showing prostate.

The bladder lies in the anterior half of the PELVIS, bordered in front by the pubis bone and laterally by the side wall of the pelvis. Superiorly the bladder is covered by the peritoneal lining of the abdomen. The bottom or base of the bladder lies against the PROSTATE gland in the male and the UTERUS and VAGINA in the female.

URINARY BLADDER, DISEASES OF Diseases of the bladder are diagnosed by the patient's symptoms and signs, examination of the urine, and using investigations such as X-rays and ULTRASOUND scans. The interior of the bladder can be examined using a cystoscope, which is a fibreoptic endoscope (see FIBREOPTIC ENDOSCOPY) that is passed into the bladder via the URETHRA.

Cystitis or INFLAMMATION OF THE BLADDER Most cases of cystitis are caused by bacteria

1 right kidney
2 ureter
3 bladder
4 urethra
5 left kidney (section)

Diagram of urinary system: (left) male; (right) female.

which have spread from the bowel, especially *Eschericia coli*, and entered the bladder via the urethra. Females are more prone to cystitis than males owing to their shorter urethra which allows easier entry for bacteria. Chronic or recurrent cystitis may result in infection spreading up the ureter to the kidney (see KIDNEY, DISEASES OF).

SYMPTOMS Typically there is frequency and urgency of micturition, with stinging and burning on passing urine (dysuria) which is often smelly or bloodstained. In severe infection patients develop fever and rigors, or loin pain. Before starting treatment a urine sample should be obtained for laboratory testing, including identification of the invading bacteria.

TREATMENT This includes an increased fluid intake, analgesics, doses of potassium citrate to make the urine alkaline to discourage bacterial growth, and an appropriate course of antibiotics.

Stone or calculus The usual reason for the formation of a bladder stone is an obstruction to the bladder outflow – which results in stagnant residual urine, ideal conditions for the crystallization of the chemicals that form stones – or from long-term indwelling catheters which weaken the natural mechanical protection against bacterial entry and, by bruising the lining tissues, encourage infection.

SYMPTOMS The classic symptom is a stoppage in the flow of urine during urination, associated with severe pain and the passage of blood.

TREATMENT This involves surgical removal of the stone either endoscopically (litholapaxy), by passing a CYSTOSCOPE into the bladder via the urethra and breaking the stone, or by LITHOTRIPSY in which the stone (or stones) is destroyed by applying ultrasonic shock waves. If the stone cannot be destroyed by these methods, the bladder is opened and the stone removed (cystolithotomy).

Cancer Cancer of the bladder accounts for 7 per cent of all cancers in men and 2·5 per cent in women. The incidence increases with age, with smoking and with exposure to the industrial chemicals, beta-napththylamine, and benzidine.

SYMPTOMS The classical presenting symptom of a bladder cancer is the painless passing of blood in the urine, haematuria. All patients with haematuria must be investigated with an X-ray of their kidneys, an INTRAVENOUS UROGRAM (IVU) and a CYSTOSCOPY.

TREATMENT Superficial bladder tumours on the lining of the bladder can be treated by local removal via the cystoscope using diathermy (cystodiathermy). Invasive cancers into the bladder muscle are usually treated with radiotherapy, systemic chemotherapy or surgical removal of the bladder (cystectomy). Local chemotherapy may be useful in some patients with multiple small tumours.

URINE Waste substances resulting from the body's metabolic processes, selected by the kidneys from the blood, dissolved in water, and excreted. Urine is around 96-per-cent water, the chief waste substances being urea (approximately 25 g/1), common salt (approximately 9 g/l), and phosphates and sulphates of potassium, sodium, calcium, and magnesium. There are also small amounts of uric acid, ammonia, creatinine, and various pigments. Poisons, such as morphine, may be excreted in the urine, and in many infections, such as typhoid fever, the causative organism may be excreted.

The daily urine output varies, but averages around 1500 ml in adults, less in children. The fluid intake and fluid output (urine and perspiration) are interdependent, so as to maintain a relatively constant fluid balance. Urine output is increased in certain diseases, notably DIABETES MELLITUS; it is diminished (or even temporarily stopped) in acute glomerulonephritis (see KIDNEY, DISEASES OF), heart failure, and fevers generally. Failure of the kidneys to secrete any urine is known as anuria, while stoppage due to obstruction of the ureters by stones, or of the urethra by a stricture, despite normal urinary secretion, is known as urinary retention.

Normal urine is described as straw to amber coloured, but may be changed by various diseases or drugs. Chronic glomerulonephritis or poorly controlled diabetes may lead to a watery appearance, as may drinking large amounts of water. Consumption of beetroot or rhubarb may lead to an orange or red colour, while passage of blood in the urine (haematuria) results in a pink or bright red appearance, or a smoky tint if just small amounts are passed. A greenish urine is usually due to BILE , or may be produced by taking QUININE.

Healthy urine has a faint aroma, but gives off an unpleasant ammoniacal smell when it begins to decompose, as may occur in urinary infections. Many foods and additives give urine a distinctive odour; garlic is particularly characteristic. The density or specific gravity of urine varies normally from 1015 to 1025. A low value suggests chronic glomerulonephritis, while a high value may occur in uncontrolled DIABETES MELLITUS or during fevers. Urine is normally acidic, which has an important antiseptic action; it may at times become alkaline, however, and in vegetarians, owing to the large dietary consumption of alkaline salts, it is permanently alkaline.

Chemical or microscopical examination of the urine is necessary to reveal abnormal drugs, poisons, or micro-organisms. There are six substances which must be easily detectable for diagnostic purposes. These are ALBUMIN, BLOOD, GLUCOSE, BILE, ACETONE, and pus and tube-casts (casts from the lining of the tubules in the kidneys). Easily used strip tests are available for all of these, except the last.

Excess of urine It is important to distinguish urinary frequency from increase in the total amount of urine passed. Frequency may be due to reduced bladder capacity, such as may be caused by an enlarged prostate, or due to any irritation of the kidneys or bladder, such as

CYSTITIS or the formation of a stone. Increased total urinary output, on the other hand, is often a diagnostic feature of DIABETES MELLITUS. Passage of urine at night may result, leading to bed wetting, or NOCTURNAL ENURESIS in children. Diagnosis of either condition, therefore, means the urine should be tested for glucose, albumin, gravel (fragments of urinary calculi), and pus, with appropriate treatment.

URINE RETENTION This occurs when urine is produced by the kidneys but is not voided by the bladder. It is generally less serious than ANURIA, in which urine is not produced.

Causes Neurological injury, such as trauma to the spinal cord, may cause bladder weakness, leading to retention, although this is rare. Obstruction to outflow is more common: this may be acute and temporary, for example after childbirth or following surgery for PILES, or chronic, for example, with prostatic enlargement (see PROSTATE GLAND). Commonly seen in elderly men, this leads to reduced bladder capacity, with partial emptying every few hours. Total retention is rare, but may result from a stricture, or narrowing, of the URETHRA – usually the result of infection or injury – or to pressure from a large neighbouring tumour.

Retention is generally treated by regular use of a urethral CATHETER, various types of which are available. Tapping of the bladder with a needle passed above the pubis is rarely necessary, but may occasionally be required in cases of severe stricture.

URINOMETER or DENSIMETER A simple instrument designed for estimating the specific gravity of urine.

UROBILINOGEN A chemical compound formed when bacteria in the intestine act on BILIRUBIN. Some is reabsorbed and returns to the liver and some is eliminated in the faeces.

URODYNAMICS The measurement of the pressures within the URINARY BLADDER as well as the pressures of the urethral sphincter. The technique is useful in the investigation of patients with urinary incontinence. Special equipment is needed to carry out the procedure.

UROKINASE is an ENZYME obtained from urine which dissolves blood clots. It is used to treat THROMBOLYSIS in the eye, in arteriovenous shunts and deep-vein THROMBOSIS. It has the advantage over other fibrinolytic drugs of not causing immunological reactions.

UROLOGY The branch of medicine which treats of disorders and diseases of the KIDNEYS, URETERS, BLADDER, PROSTATE, and URETHRA.

URSODEOXYCHOLIC ACID is a preparation used in the treatment of cholesterol gall-stones when laparoscopic CHOLECYSTECTOMY and endoscopic biliary procedures cannot be used. (see GALL-BLADDER, DISEASES OF).

URTICARIA The rash produced by the sudden release of histamine in the skin. It is characterized by acute itching, redness and whealing which subsides within a few minutes or may persist for a day or more. Depending on the cause, it may be localized or widespread and transient or constantly recurrent over years. It has many causes.

External injuries to the skin such as the sting of a nettle ('nettle-rash') or an insect bite cause histamine release from MAST cells in the skin directly. Certain drugs, especially MORPHINE, CODEINE and ASPIRIN, can have the same effect. In other cases, histamine release is caused by an allergic mechanism, mediated by ANTIBODIES of the IMMUNOGLOBULIN E (IgE) class. Thus many foods, food additives and drugs (such as PENICILLIN) can cause urticaria. Massive release of histamine may affect mucous membranes – namely the tongue or throat – and can cause HYPOTENSION and ANAPHYLACTIC shock which can occasionally be fatal.

Physical factors can cause urticaria. Heat, exercise and emotional stress may induce a singular pattern with small pinhead wheals but widespread flares of erythema, activated via the AUTONOMIC NERVOUS SYSTEM (CHOLINERGIC urticaria).

Rarely, exposure to cold may have a smiilar effect ('cold urticaria') and anaphylactic shock following a dive into cold water in winter is occasionally fatal. The diagnosis of cold urticaria can be confirmed by applying a block of ice to the arm which quickly induces a local wheal.

Transient urticaria due to rubbing or even stroking the skin is common in young adults (DERMOGRAPHISM or factitious urticaria). More prolonged deep pressure induces delayed urticaria in other subjects. IgE-mediated urticaria is part of the atopic spectrum (see atopic eczema in SKIN DISEASES). Allergy to peanuts is particularly dangerous in young atopic subjects. Notwithstanding the many known causes, chronic urticaria of unknown cause is common and may have an AUTOIMMUNE basis.

TREATMENT Causative factors must be removed. Topical therapy is ineffective except for the use of calamine lotion, which reduces itching by cooling the skin. Oral antihistamines are the mainstay of treatment and are remarkably safe. Rarely, injection of ADRENALINE is needed as emergency treatment of massive urticaria, especially if the tongue and throat are involved, following by a short course of the oral steroid, prednisolone.

Angio-oedema is a variant of urticaria where massive oedema involves subcutaneous tissues rather than the skin. It may have many causes but bee and wasp stings in sensitized subjects are particularly dangerous. There is also a rare hereditary form of angio-oedema. Acute airway obstruction due to submucosal oedema of the tongue or larynx is best treated with immediate intramuscular adrenaline and antihistamine. Rarely, TRACHEOSTOMY may be lifesaving. Patients who have had two or more episodes can be taught self-injection with a preloaded adrenaline syringe.

UTERUS A hollow, triangular organ, flattened from front to back, the lower angle, or cervix, commincates through a narrow opening (the os uteri) with the VAGINA. The uterus or womb is where the fertilized ovum (egg) normally becomes embedded and in which the EMBRYO and FETUS develop. The normal uterus weighs 30–40 g; during pregnancy, however, enormous growth occurs and muscular thickening (see MUSCLE). The cavity is lined by a thick, soft, mucous membrane, and the wall is chiefly composed of muscle fibres arranged in three layers. The outer surface, like that of other abdominal organs, is covered by a layer of peritoneum. The uterus has a copious supply of blood derived from the uterine and ovarian arteries. It has also many lymphatic vessels, and its nerves establish wide connections with other organs. (See PAIN.) The position of the uterus is in the centre of the pelvis, where it is suspended by several ligaments between the bladder in front and the rectum behind. On each side of the uterus are the broad ligaments passing outwards to the side of the pelvis, the uterosacral ligament passing back to the sacral bone, the utero-vesical ligament passing forwards to the bladder, and the round ligament uniting the uterus to the front of the abdomen.

UTERUS, DISEASES OF

Absence or defects of the uterus Rarely, the uterus may be completely absent as a result of abnormal development. In such patients secondary sexual development is normal but menstru-ation is absent (primary amennorhoea). The chromosomal make-up of the patient must be checked. In a few cases the genotype is male (testicular feminization syndrome). No treatment is available, although the woman should be counselled.

The uterus develops as two halves which fuse together. If the fusion is incomplete, a uterine septum results. Such patients may have fertility problems which can be corrected by surgical removal of the uterine septum. Very rarely there may be two uteri with a double vagina.

Most women have uteri which are pointing forwards (anteversion) and bent forwards (anteflexion). About 25 per cent of women have uteri which are pointed backwards (retroversion) and bent backwards (retroflexion). This is a normal variant and very rarely gives rise to any problems. If it is, the attitude of the uterus can be corrected by an operation called a ventrosuspension.

Endometritis The lining of the uterine cavity is called the endometrium. It is this layer that is partially shed cyclically in women of reproductive age giving rise to menstruation. Infection of the endometrium is called endometritis and usually occurs after a pregnancy or in association with the use of an intrauterine contraceptive device (IUCD). The symptoms are usually of pain, bleeding and a fever. Treatment is with antibiotics. Unless the FALLOPIAN TUBES are involved and damaged, subsequent fertility is unaffected. Very rarely, the infection is caused by tuberculosis. Tuberculous endometritis may destroy the endometrium causing permanent amenorrhoea and sterility.

Menstrual disorders are common. Heavy periods (menorrhagia) are often caused by fibroids (see below) or adenomyosis (see below) or anovulatory cycles. Anovulatory cycles result in the endometrium being subjected to unopposed oestrogen stimulation and occasionally undergoing hyperplasia. Treatment is with cyclical PROGESTOGENS initially. If this form of treatment fails, endoscopic surgery to remove the endometrium may be successful. The endometrium may be removed using the LASER (endometrial laser ablation) or electrocautery (transcervical resection of endometrium). Hysterectomy will cure the problem if endoscopic surgery fails. Adenomyosis is a condition in which endometrial tissue is found in the muscle layer (myometrium) of the uterus. It usually presents as heavy and painful periods, and occasionally pain during intercourse. Hysterectomy is usually required.

Oligomennorhoea (scanty or infrequent periods) may be caused by a variety of conditions including THYROID disease. It is most commonly associated with usage of the combined oral contraceptive pill. Once serious causes have been eliminated, the patient should be reassured. No treatment is necessary unless conception is desired in which case the patient may require induction of ovulation.

Primary amenorrhoea means that the patient has never had a period. She should be investigated, although usually it is only due to an inexplicable delay in the onset of periods (delayed menarche) and not to any serious condition. Secondary amenorrhoea is the cessation of periods after menstruation has started. The most common cause is pregnancy. It may be also caused by endocrinological or hormonal problems, tuberculous endometritis, emotional problems and severe weight loss. The treatment of amenorrhoea depends on the cause.

Dysmenorrhoea, or painful periods, is the most common disorder but in most cases the cause is unknown, though the disorder may be due to excessive production of PROSTAGLANDINS.

Irregular menstruation (variations from the woman's normal menstrual pattern or changes in the duration of bleeding or the amount) can be the result of a disturbance in the balance of OESTROGEN hormones and progesterone hormone which between them regulate the cycle. For some time after the MENARCHE or before the MENOPAUSE menstruation may be irregular. If irregularity occurs in a woman whose periods are normally regular, it may be due to unsus-

pected pregnancy, early miscarriage or to disorders in the uterus, ovaries or pelvic cavity. The woman should seek medical advice.

Fibroids (leiomyomata) are benign tumours arising from the smooth muscle layer (myometrium) of the uterus. They are found in 80 per cent of women but only a small percentage give rise to any problems and may then require treatment. They may cause heavy periods and occasionally pain. Sometimes they present as a mass arising from the pelvis with pressure symptoms from the bladder or rectum. Although they can be shrunk medically using gonadorelin analogues, which raise the plasma concentrations of LUTEINIZING and FOLLICLE-STIMULATING HORMONES, this is not a long-term solution. In any case fibroids only require treatment if they are large or if they are enlarging or if they cause symptoms. Treatment is either myomectomy (surgical removal) if fertility is to be retained or a HYSTERECTOMY.

Uterine cancers tend to present after the age of 40 with abnormal bleeding (intermenstrual or postmenopausal bleeding). They are usually endometrial carcinomas. Eighty per cent present with early (Stage 1) disease. Patients with operable cancers should be treated with total abdominal hysterectomy and bilateral excision of the OVARIES and FALLOPIAN TUBES. Postoperative RADIOTHERAPY is usually given to those patients with adverse prognostic factors. Pre-operative radiotherapy is still given by some centres, although this practice is now regarded as out-dated. PROGESTOGENS may be extremely effective treatment in cases of recurrence but their value remains unproven when used as adjuvant treatment.

Disorders of the cervix The cervix (neck of the womb) may produce an excessive discharge due to the presence of a cervical ectopy or ectropion. In both instances columnar epithelium – the layer of secreting cells – which usually lines the cervical canal is exposed on its surface. Asymptomatic patients do not require treatment. If treatment is required, cryocautery – local freezing of tissue – is usually effective.

Cervical smears are taken and examined in the laboratory to detect abnormal cells shed from the cervix. Its main purpose is to detect cervical intraepithelial neoplasia (CIN) – the presence of malignant cells in the surface tissue lining the cervix – since up to 40 per cent of women with this condition will develop cervical cancer if the CIN is left untreated. Women with abnormal smears should undergo colposcopy, a painless investigation using a low-powered microscope to inspect the cervix. If CIN is found, treatment consists of simply removing the area of abnormal skin, either using a diathermy loop or laser instrument.

Unfortunately cervical cancer remains the most common of gynaecological cancers. Cases diagnosed early may be treated by a radical or Wertheim's hysterectomy. This is a major operation in which the uterus, cervix, upper third of vagina and the tissue surrounding the cervix are removed together with the lymph nodes draining the area. The ovaries may be retained if desired. Most patients with cervical cancer are treated by radiotherapy, either because they present too late for surgery or because the surgical skill to perform a radical hysterectomy is not available. These operations are best performed by gynaecological oncologists who are gynaecological surgeons specializing in the treatment of gynaecological tumours.

In 1991 in England and Wales 3,768 cases of cancer of the cervix were registered and 4,282 cases of cancer of the uterus.

Prolapse of the uterus is a disorder in which the organ drops from its normal situation down into the vagina. First-degree prolapse is a slight displacement of the uterus, second-degree a partial displacement and third-degree when the uterus can be seen outside the VULVA. It may be accompanied by a CYSTOCOELE (the bladder bulges into the front wall of the vagina), urethrocoele (the urethra bulges into the vagina) and rectocoele (the rectal wall bulges into the rear wall of the vagina). Prolapse most commonly occurs in middle-aged women who have had children, but the condition is much less common now than in the past when prenatal and obstetric care was poor, women had more pregnancies and their general health was poor. Treatment is with pelvic exercises, surgical repair of the vagina or HYSTERECTOMY. If the woman does not want or is not fit for surgery, an internal support called a pessary can be fitted – and changed periodically.

UVEA is a term applied to the middle coat of the eye, including the iris, ciliary body and choroid.

UVEITIS An inflammation of the uveal tract. Iritis is inflammation of the iris, cyclitis inflammation of the ciliary body and choroiditis inflammation of the choroid. The symptoms and signs vary according to which part of the uveal tract is involved and tend to be recurrent. The patient may experience varying degrees of discomfort or pain, with or without blurring of vision. In many cases a cause is never found. Some known associations include various types of arthritis, some bowel diseases, virus illnesses, tuberculosis, syphilis, parasites and fungi. Treatment is with anti-inflammatory drops and occasionally tablets (e.g. steroid eye drops and tablets), plus drops to dilate the pupil.

UVULA The small mass of muscle covered by mucous membrane that hangs down from the middle of the soft palate on its posterior aspect. Its function is not certain and it seldom causes problems.

V

VACCINATION Named from vacca, Latin for cow, vaccination means inoculation with the material of cowpox, performed to afford protection to the inoculated person against an attack of smallpox, or to reduce seriousness of, and averting a fatal result from, any such attack. This is the strict sense of the term, but it is used nowadays to describe the process of inoculating with any vaccine to obtain immunity, or protection, against the corresponding disease.

VACCINE The name applied generally to a substance of the nature of dead or attenuated living infectious material introduced into the body with the object of increasing its power to resist or to get rid of a disease. (See also IMMUNITY.)

In cases where healthy people are inoculated with vaccine as a protection against a particular disease, this is done to produce antibodies which will confer immunity against a subsequent attack of the disease. (See IMMUNIZATION for programme of immunization during childhood.)

Vaccines may be divided into two classes: stock vaccines, prepared from micro-organisms known to cause a particular disease and kept in readiness for use against that disease; and autogenous vaccines, prepared from micro-organisms which are already in the patient's body and to which the disease is due. Vaccines intended to protect against the onset of disease are of the former variety.

Autogenous vaccines are prepared from the cultivation of bacteria found in the expectoration, the urine, the faeces, and in areas of inflammation such as boils. This type of vaccine was introduced by Wright about 1903.

Anthrax vaccine was introduced by Pasteur about 1882 for the protection of sheep and cattle against this disease. A safe and effective vaccine for use in human beings has now been evolved.

BCG vaccine is used to provide protection against tuberculosis. BCG vaccination is usually considered for five main groups of people:
(1) Schoolchildren: the routine programme in schools usually covers children aged between 10 and 14
(2) Students including those in teacher training colleges
(3) Children and new-born infants in families of Asian origin because of the high incidence of tuberculosis in this ethnic group
(4) Health service workers and others liable to infection at work
(5) Household contacts of people known to have active tuberculosis and new-born infants in households where there is a history of tuberculosis.
(See BCG VACCINE.)

Cholera vaccine was introduced by Haffkine in India about 1894. Two injections are given at an interval of at least a week; this gives a varying degree of immunity for six months.

Diphtheria vaccine is available in several forms. (See DIPHTHERIA.) It is usually given along with tetanus and pertussis vaccine in what is known as TRIPLE VACCINE. This is given in three doses: the first at the age of 3 or 6 months, the second six to eight weeks later, and the third six months later, with a booster dose at the age of 5 years.

Hay fever vaccine is a vaccine prepared from the pollen of various grasses. It is used in gradually increasing doses for prevention of hay fever in those susceptible to this condition.

Influenza vaccine: a vaccine is now available for protection against influenza due to the influenza viruses A and B. Its use in Britain is customarily based on advice from the health departments according to the type of influenza expected in a particular year.

Measles, mumps and rubella vaccines are given in combination early in the second year of life.

Pertussis (whooping-cough) vaccine is prepared from *Bordetella pertussis*, and is usually given along with diphtheria and tetanus in what is known as Triple Vaccine.

Plague vaccine was introduced by Haffkine, and appears to give useful protection, but the duration of protection is relatively short: from two to twenty months. Two injections are given at an interval of 4 weeks. A reinforcing dose should be given annually to anyone exposed to the disease.

Poliomyelitis vaccine gives a high degree of protection against the disease.

This is given in the form of attenuated Sabin vaccine which is taken by mouth – a few drops on a lump of sugar. Reinforcing doses of polio vaccine are recommended on school entry, on leaving school, and on travel abroad to countries where poliomyelitis is endemic.

Rabies vaccine was introduced by Pasteur in 1885 for administration, during the long incubation period, to people bitten by a mad dog, in order to prevent the disease from developing.

Rubella vaccine, usually given with mumps and measles vaccine in one dose – called MMR vaccine – now provides protection against rubella (German measles). It also provides immunity for adolescent girls who have not had the disease in childhood and so ensures that they will not acquire the disease during any subsequent pregnancy, thus reducing the number of congenitally abnormal children whose abnormality is the result of their being infected with rubella via their mothers before they were born.

Smallpox vaccine was the first introduced. As a result of the World Health Organization's (WHO) successful smallpox eradication campaign – it declared the disease eradicated in 1980 – there is now no medical justification for smallpox vaccination.

Tetanus vaccine is given in two forms: (*a*) In the so-called Triple Vaccine, combined with diphtheria and pertussis (whooping-cough) vaccine for the routine immunization of children. (*b*) By itself to adults who have not been immunized in childhood and who are particularly exposed to the risk of tetanus, such as soldiers and agricultural workers.

Typhoid vaccine was introduced by Wright and Semple for the protection of troops in the South African War and in India. TAB vaccine, containing *Salmonella typhi* (the causative organism of typhoid fever) and *Salmonella paratyphi* A and B (the organisms of paratyphoid fever) has now been replaced by Typhoid Monovalent Vaccine, containing only *S. typhi*. The change has been made because the monovalent vaccine is less likely to produce painful arms and general malaise and there is no evidence that the TAB vaccine gave any protection against paratyphoid fever. Two doses are given at an interval of four to six weeks, and give protection for one to three years.

Yellow fever vaccine is prepared from chick embryos injected with the living, attenuated strain (17D) of pantropic virus. Only one injection is required, and immunity persists for many years. Reinoculation, however, is desirable every ten years.

The hazards of vaccination, or immunization are minimal, compared with its benefits. Complications, however, do occur. Recent publicity about the (small) risk of measles vaccine (contained in the MMR vaccine routinely given to children) causing meningitis has resulted in a slight fall in the number of children receiving MMR.

VACCINIA is another term for cowpox, a disease in which vesicles form on the udders and teats, due to the same virus as is responsible for SMALLPOX in man. It is also the term used to describe the reaction to smallpox vaccination.

VACUOLE A space inside the CYTOPLASM of the CELL. It is formed by a folding in of the cellular membrane when the cell ingests material from the outside – for example, when white blood cells attack bacteria.

VACUUM EXTRACTOR or VENTOUSE The idea of the glass suction cup applied to the emerging head of the baby to assist in delivery was first considered by Younge in 1706, but it was not until 1954 that the modern (ventouse) vacuum extractor was introduced by Malmstrom. The value of the ventouse as against the forceps has been disputed in different clinics, the former being less popular in the UK. Indications are similar for the use of obstetric forceps. Even if the OCCIPUT is not in the anterior position, the extractor may still be applied. Many obstetricians would choose forceps or perform manual rotation of the fetus in such cases. In cases of prolongation of the first stage of labour, the ventouse may be used to accelerate dilatation of the cervix – provided that the cervix is already sufficiently dilated to allow application of the cup. The ventouse cannot be applied to the breech or face; in urgent cases of fetal distress the operation takes too long, and forceps delivery is preferred. There is some doubt on its safety when used on premature babies; many obstetricians feel that forceps delivery reduces the risk of intracranial haemorrhage. The vacuum extractor, while resulting in a slower delivery than when forceps are used, has a lower risk of damage to the mother's birth canal. (See LABOUR.)

VAGINA The lower part of the female reproductive tract (see REPRODUCTIVE SYSTEM) through which a baby is delivered. It is a muscular passage leading from the labial entrance to the UTERUS. It is lined with mucous membrane and receives the erect PENIS during sexual intercourse. The semen is ejaculated into the upper part of the vagina and from there the sperms must pass through the cervix and uterus to fertilize the ovum in the FALLOPIAN TUBE.

VAGINISMUS Spasmodic painful, involuntary contraction of the opening of the vagina on attempted coitus. It is usually psychological in origin, due, for instance, to fear that penetration by the penis will be painful or because of some previous traumatic incident of sexual intercourse such as rape or sexual abuse as a child. It may also be due to some local inflammatory condition.

VAGINITIS Inflammation of the VAGINA. (See LEUCORRHOEA.)

VAGOTOMY The operation of cutting the fibres of the VAGUS nerve to the stomach. It was once performed as part of the surgical treatment of duodenal ulcer, the aim being to reduce the flow or acidity of the gastric juice. The operation is now rarely done.

VAGUS The tenth cranial nerve. Unlike the other cranial nerves, which are concerned with the special senses, or distributed to the skin and muscles of the head and neck, this nerve, as its names imply, passes downwards into the chest and abdomen, supplying branches to the throat, lungs, heart, stomach, and other abdominal organs. It contains motor, secretory, sensory, and vasodilator fibres.

VALGUS This term means literally knock-kneed, and is a bending inward at the knees (genu valgum), or at the ankle, as occurs in flatfoot (pes valgus).

VALINE An essential AMINO-ACID.

VALSALVA'S MANOEUVRE This is carried out by closing the mouth, holding the nose and attempting to blow hard. This raises pressure in the chest – and, indirectly, the abdomen – and forces air from the back of the nose down the EUSTACHIAN TUBE to the middle ear. This latter effect can be used to clear the tube during descent in an aircraft when it sometimes becomes blocked or partially blocked, producing differential pressures on the two sides of each eardrum, usually accompanied by temporary pain and deafness. Valsalva's manoeuvre is involuntarily performed when a person strains to open his or her bowels: in these circumstances the passage of air to the lungs is blocked by instinctive closure of the VOCAL CORDS in the larynx. The resultant raised abdominal pressure helps to expel the bowel contents.

The manoeuvre is also used in the study of cardiovascular PHYSIOLOGY because the rise in pressure in the chest restricts the return of venous blood to the right ATRIUM of the heart. Pressure in the peripheral VEINS is raised and the mount of blood entering and leaving the heart falls. This drop in cardiac output may cause the subject to faint because the supply of oxygenated blood to the brain is reduced.

VALVES These are found in the heart, veins, and lymphatic vessels; they ensure that the circulation of the blood and lymph goes always in one direction. (See HEART; LYMPH; VEINS.)

VALVULAR DISEASE (see HEART DISEASES)

VALVULOPLASTY An operation to repair or reconstruct a defective heart valve. It may be done as an open-heart procedure (with the patient temporarily connected to a heart-lung machine that maintains the circulation of oxygenated blood). Alternatively valvuloplasty can now be performed using a specially designed balloon-ended catheter passed through the skin into a blood vessel and on to the heart. The balloon is inflated and the flaps of a narrowed (stenosed) valve are prised apart.

VALVOTOMY An operation that opens a stenosed heart valve and allows it to function properly again. Various techniques are used including a dilating instrument, a balloon or open-heart surgery.

VANCOMYCIN An antibiotic derived from *streptomyces*, which is active against a wide range of GRAM-POSITIVE organisms, including the STAPHYLOCOCCUS. The drug has a limited use by the intravenous route in the prophylaxis and treatment of endocarditis and other serious infections caused by gram-positive cocci, in particular, METHICILLIN-RESISTANT *STAPHYLOCOCCUS AUREUS* (MRSA). It need be given only every 12 hours, although plasma concentrations should be monitored (especially in patients with renal impairment when the dose may need marked reduction). It can both damage the middle ear and the kidney. A short course of vancomycin is effective in the treatment of antibiotic-associated COLITIS, for which it is given by mouth.

VAN DEN BERGH TEST One performed on a specimen of serum of the blood from patients with jaundice, to decide whether this is due to ordinary bile (immediate or direct reaction) or incompletely formed bile pigment (delayed or indirect reaction).

VAPORIZER A device that turns water or a drug into a fine spray, thus enabling medicine to be taken by inhalation. It is used, for example, in the treatment of ASTHMA.

VARICELLA Another name for CHICKEN-POX.

VARICOCOELE A condition in which the veins of the testicle are distended. (See TESTICLE, DISEASES OF.)

VARICOSE VEINS Veins that have become stretched and dilated. (See VEINS, DISEASES OF.)

VARIOLA Another name for SMALLPOX.

VARIX An enlarged and tortuous vein.

VARUS, meaning bow-legged, is the term applied to a bulging condition at the hip (coxa vara), at the knee (genu varum), or at the ankle (talipes varus).

VAS The Latin term for a vessel, especially a blood-vessel.

VASA EFFERENTIA Efferent seminal ducts of the testis that carry semen from the testis to the head of the epidydimis.

VASCULAR Relating to the blood vessels.

VASCULITIS Inflammation of the blood vessels. This may damage the lining of the vessels and cause narrowing or blockage, thus restricting blood flow. This, in turn, may harm or destroy the tissues supplied by the affected blood vessels. Vasculitis is probably caused by small particles called immune complexes, circulating in the blood, that adhere to the vessel walls and provoke inflammation. Normally these complexes are consumed by the white blood cells.

VASECTOMY The surgical operation performed to render men sterile, or infertile. It consists of ligating, or tying, and then cutting the ductus, or vas, deferens (see TESTICLE). It is quite a simple operation carried out under local anaesthesia, through a small incision, or cut (or sometimes two) in the upper part of the scrotum. It has no effect on sexual drive or ejaculation, and does not cause impotency. It is not immediately effective, and several tests, spread over several months, must be carried out before it is safe to assume that sterility has been achieved. Fertility can sometimes be restored by a further operation, to restore the continuity of the vas, this cannot be guaranteed, and only seems to occur in about 20 per cent of those who have had the operation.

VAS DEFERENS A narrow tube that leads from each TESTIS through the PROSTATE GLAND to join a tube from the SEMINAL VESICLES to form the ejaculatory duct. SPERM and seminal fluid pass through this duct during ejaculation (see TESTICLE).

VASOCONSTRICTION Narrowing of blood vessels which results in the blood flow to a particular part of the body's being reduced. Cold will cause vasoconstriction of the vessels under the skin thus reducing heat loss. Shock due to injury or loss of blood will also provoke vasoconstriction.

VASODILATORS Substances that dilate the blood-vessels. They may be drugs, such as GLYCERYL NITRATE, or natural substances in the body, such as KININS.

VASOMOTOR NERVES Small nerve fibres that lie upon the walls of blood-vessels and connect the muscle fibres of their middle coat with the nervous system. Through these nerves the blood-vessels are retained in a state of moderate contraction. There are vasodilator nerves, through which are transmitted impulses that dilate the vessels, and, in the case of the skin-vessels, produce the condition of blushing. There are also vasoconstrictor nerves which transmit impulses that constrict, or narrow, the blood-vessels, as occurs on exposure to cold. (See HYPOTHERMIA.) Various drugs produce dilatation or contraction of the blood-vessels and several of the substances produced by endocrine glands in the body have these effects: e.g. ADRENALINE.

VASOPRESSIN The fraction isolated from extract of the posterior PITUITARY lobe which stimulates intestinal activity, constricts blood-vessels, and inhibits the secretion of urine. It is also known as the antidiuretic hormone because of this last effect, and its only use in medicine is, on account of this effect, in the treatment of DIABETES INSIPIDUS. (See also PITUITARY BODY.)

VASOVAGAL ATTACK The temporary loss of consciousness caused by an abrupt slowing of the heartbeat. This may happen following shock, acute pain, fear, or stress. A common cause of fainting in normal people, a vasovagal attack may be a consequence of overstimulation of the VAGUS nerve which is involved in the control of breathing and the circulation.

VD The abbreviation for venereal disease, now usually described as a SEXUALLY TRANSMITTED DISEASE (STD), the word 'venereal' is derived from Venus, the Roman goddess of love.

VECTOR An animal that is the carrier of a particular infectious disease (see INFECTION). A vector picks up the infectious agent (bacterium or virus) from an infected person's blood or faeces and carries it in or on its body before depositing the agent on or into a new host. Fleas, lice, mosquitoes and ticks are among common vectors of disease to humans. When a vector is used by the infectious agent to complete part of its life cycle – for example, the malarial agent *PLASMODIUM* conducts part of its life cycle in the mosquito – the vector is described as biological. If the vector simply carries the agent but is not a host for part of its life cycle, the vector is described as mechanical. Flies, for example, may carry an infection such as bacterial dysentery from infected faeces to the fingers of another 'host'.

VEGANISM A strict form of VEGETARIANISM. Vegans do not eat meat, dairy produce, eggs or fish.

VEGETARIANISM Restricting one's diet, for health or humanitarian reasons, to foods of fruit or vegetable origin. Most vegetarians, while excluding meat and fish from their diets, include foods of animal origin, such as milk, cheese, eggs, and butter. Such a diet should supply an adequate balance of nutrients, although people with special dietary requirements, such as pregnant or feeding mothers, and very strict vegetarians, may require dietary supplements (see APPENDIX 5: VITAMINS).

VEGETATIONS Roughenings that appear upon the valves of the heart, usually as the result of acute rheumatism. They lead in time to narrowing of the openings from the cavities of the heart, or to imcompetence of the valves that close these openings. (See HEART DISEASES.)

VEINS The vessels which return the blood to the heart after it has circulated through the tissues; they are both more numerous and more capacious than the ARTERIES.

Structure While of similar structure to an artery, veins have much thinner walls, with much less muscular tissue. Furthermore, most veins have one-way valves to ensure that the blood flows in the right direction. These are most numerous in the legs, then the arms, with few in the internal organs.

Chief veins Four pulmonary veins open into the left atrium of the heart, two from each lung. The superior vena cava returns the blood from the head, neck, and arms; while the inferior vena cava returns blood from the legs and abdomen. The large basilic vein that runs up the inner side of the upper arm is the vein usually opened in blood letting (see VENESECTION). The great saphenous vein is of special interest, because of its liability to become distended or varicose. Within the abdomen, the inferior vena cava receives branches corresponding to several branches of the aorta, its largest branches being the hepatic veins, which return not only the blood that has reached the liver in the hepatic arteries, but also blood which comes from the digestive organs in the portal vein to undergo a second capillary circulation in the liver. (See PORTAL VEIN.)

There are several connections between the superior and inferior cava, the most important being three azygos veins that lie upon the sides of the spinal column, the veins on the front of the abdomen, and some veins that emerge from the abdomen at the navel and connect the portal system with those of the inferior and superior vena cava. (See CIRCULATION OF BLOOD.)

VEINS, DISEASES OF Veins are the blood vessels that convey blood back from the tissues towards the heart. Two common conditions that affect them are thrombosis and varicosities. THROMBOSIS occurs when blood, which is normally a liquid, clots within the vein to form a semisolid thrombus (clot). This occurs through a combination of reduced blood flow and hypercoagulability (a reduced threshold for clotting). The commonest site for this to occur is in the deep veins of the leg where it is known as a deep-vein thrombosis (DVT).

Predisposing factors include immobility (leading to reduced blood flow) such as during long journeys (e.g. plane flights) where there is little opportunity to stretch one's legs, surgery (leading to temporary post-operative immobility and hypercoagulability of blood), oestrogen administration (low-dose oestrogen oral contraceptives carry a very low relative risk) and several medical illnesses such as heart failure, stroke and malignancy.

Deep-vein thrombosis presents as a tender, warm, red swelling of the calf. Diagnosis may be confirmed by venogram (an X-ray taken following injection of contrast medium into the foot veins) or by ultrasound scanning looking for flow within the veins.

Prevention is important. This is why patients are mobilized and/or given leg exercises very soon after an operation, even major surgery. People should avoid sitting for long periods, particularly if the edge of the seat is hard, thus impeding venous return from the legs. Car drivers should stop regularly on a long journey and walk around; airline travellers should, where possible, walk round the aisle(s) and also exercise and massage their leg muscles.

Diagnosis and treatment are important because there is a risk that the clotted blood within the vein becomes dislodged and travels up the venous system to become lodged in the pulmonary arteries. This is known as PULMO-NARY EMBOLISM.

Treatment is directed at thinning the blood with ANTICOAGULANTS, initially with heparin and subsequently with WARFARIN for a period of time while the clot resolves.

Blocked superficial veins are described as superficial THROMBOPHLEBITIS, which produces inflammation over the vein. It responds to anti-inflammatory analgesics. Occasionally heparin and ANTIBIOTICS are required to treat associated thrombosis and infection.

Varicose veins are dilated tortuous veins. They most commonly occur in the legs but may also occur in the anal canal (haemorrhoids) and in the oesophagus (due to liver disease).

Normally blood flows from the subcutaneous tissues to the superficial veins which drain via perforating veins into the deep veins of the leg. This flow, back towards the heart, is aided by valves within the veins. When these valves fail increased pressure is exerted on the blood vessels leading to dilatations known as varicose veins.

Treatment is needed to prevent complications such as ulceration and bleeding, or for cosmetic purposes. Treatment alternatives include injection with sclerosing agents to obliterate the lumen of the veins; surgery; and in the elderly or unfit an elastic stocking may suffice. One operation is the Trendelenburg operation in which the saphenous vein is disconnected from the femoral vein and individual varicose veins are avulsed.

VENA CAVA The name of either of the two large vessels that open into the right atrium of the heart. (See VEINS.)

VENEPUNCTURE The insertion of a needle into a vein, usually for the purpose of injecting a drug or withdrawing blood for haematological or biochemical analysis. The usual site for venepuncture in adults is the median cubital vein in the forearm.

VENEREAL DISEASES (See SEXUALLY TRANSMITTED DISEASES.)

VENESECTION, or BLOOD-LETTING, may be employed for two purposes. Most commonly, small quantities of blood may be required for analysis, as an aid to diagnosis or control of various diseases. For example, knowledge of the plasma glucose concentration is important in the diagnosis and management of DIABETES MELLITUS, or blood may be required in order to test for infections such as HIV or HEPATITIS. Blood may be obtained by pricking a finger tip, or inserting a needle into a vein, depending on the amount required. Controlled bleeding of larger amounts may rarely be used in certain cases of acute heart failure, as a rapid and temporary method of relieving the strain on the heart. It is also used in the treatment of POLYCYTHAEMIA.

Venesection was popular in the 19th century, and was commonly used to avoid the consequences of excessive eating or drinking. Techniques used, such as LEECHES and CUPPING, were generally unhygienic. Many people died from the bleeding, rather than from the original disease, and such techniques are rarely used today.

VENOGRAPHY The study of the veins, particularly by means of X-rays after the veins have been injected with a radio-opaque substance.

VENOUS ULCER (see ULCER).

VENTILATION The process by which air is purified and circulated in domestic, occupational, industrial, and other settings. Ideally, the air we breathe should be of the right temperature and humidity, and free of dust, smoke, pollen, and other contaminants. Ventilation aims to produce such an atmosphere.

Air-conditioning is frequently used in hospitals, offices, and other public places. Special filters may be used to reduce the risk of airborne infections and ALLERGIES, but poorly maintained and contaminated systems may result in outbreaks of serious disorders, such as LEGIONNAIRE'S DISEASE. Sterilization of air is rarely required, but ultraviolet light is sometimes used to kill pathogenic organisms. (See ASTHMA, BRONCHITIS, HUMIDIFICATION.)

VENTILATION, ARTIFICIAL The procedure, usually carried out in an operating theatre or intensive-care unit, in which a device called a ventilator takes over a person's breathing. This is done for someone who is unable to breathe normally. Damage to the respiratory centre of the brain as a result of head injury, disease of the brain, or an overdose of sedative or narcotic drugs may affect the respiratory centre. Chest injuries, disease of the lungs, nerve or muscle disorders or surgery of the chest or abdomen can also affect breathing and require the use of a ventilator to main-tain normal breathing. Artificial ventilation can also be carried out as an emergency by mouth-to-mouth resuscitation (see APPENDIX 1: BASIC FIRST AID and ARTIFICIAL VENTILATION OF LUNGS.)

VENTILATOR Machinery used to provide artificial ventilation. Also called respirator or life-support machine, it is an electric pump linked to a supply of air which it pumps into the patient through an endotracheal tube passed through the nose or mouth into the TRACHEA. Sometimes the air is pumped straight into the trachea through an artificial hole called a TRACHEOSTOMY. During ventilation the patient's blood gases are closely monitored and other bodily activities such as pulse and heart pressure are regularly measured. Some patients need to be kept on a ventilator for several days or even weeks if their medical condition is serious. (See ARTIFICIAL VENTILATION OF LUNGS.)

VENTOUSE (see VACUUM EXTRACTOR).

VENTRAL Positioned or relating to the front of a body or to the front part of an organ.

VENTRICLE The term applied to the two lower cavities of the heart (see HEART), and also to the cavities within the brain.

VENTRICULAR FIBRILLATION A potentially life-threatening and rapid ARRHYTHMIA of the ventricle of the HEART.

VENTRICULOGRAPHY The process of taking an X-ray photograph of the BRAIN after the fluid in the lateral ventricles of the brain has been replaced by air; in this way any alteration in the outline of the ventricles (e.g. from pressure by a tumour) can be detected.

VENULE A very small blood vessel that drains blood from CAPILLARIES. Several venules join up to form a VEIN.

VERAPAMIL is a drug used in the treatment of HYPERTENSION, disordered rhythms of the heart and ANGINA PECTORIS. The drug is one of the CALCIUM-CHANNEL BLOCKERS and acts by reducing cardiac output and slowing the heart rate. It may, however, precipitate heart failure, cause HYPOTENSION and aggravate conduction problems in the heart, so should be prescribed with care. It should not be used with BETA-BLOCKING DRUGS.

VERBIGERATION The pointless repetition of meaningless words and sentences.

VERMICIDES Also called vermifuges, these are substances that kill, or expel, parasitic worms from the intestines.

VERNIX The white, cheesy-like substance that covers the skin of a newly born infant. It consists of dead cells in a fatty secretion, protects the infant's skin and helps lubricate its passage through the cervix and vagina during delivery.

VERRUCA (see WARTS).

VERRUCOSE This term means having a surface resembling verrucae. Certain skin diseases may become verrucose.

VERSION or TURNING The name given to an operation in obstetrics which consists in turning the fetus in the UTERUS in women whose fetus is lying in an abnormal position which may make eventual delivery difficult. In particular, version (which can take place spontaneously) may be done on a fetus between the 34th and 37th weeks of pregnancy when its buttocks rather than its head are positioned at the cervical end of the uterus. The procedure carries a small risk of precipitating premature labour, and it is not always successful, in which case a BREECH delivery is attempted or, in difficult cases, a CAESAREAN SECTION is performed. (See LABOUR.)

VERTEBRA One of the irregularly shaped bones that together form the vertebral column. (See SPINAL COLUMN.)

VERTEBROBASILAR INSUFFIENCY Intermittent incidents of double vision, dizziness, weakness and speaking difficulties caused by a reduced blood supply to parts of the BRAIN. The cause is usually obstruction in the basilar, vertebral and other arteries at the base of the brain. The condition is sometimes the precursor of a STROKE.

VERTIGO or GIDDINESS A condition in which the affected person loses the power of balancing himself, and has a false sensation as to his own movements or as to those of surrounding objects. The power of balancing depends upon sensations derived partly through the sense of touch, partly from the eyes, but mainly from the semicircular canals of the internal ear. In general, vertigo is due to some interference with this mechanism or with the centres in the cerebellum and cerebrum with which it is connected. Giddiness is apt to be associated with headache, nausea, and vomiting.

Causes The simplest cause of vertigo is some mechanical disturbance of the body affecting the fluid in the internal ear; such as that produced by moving in a swing with the eyes shut, the motion of a boat causing sea-sickness, or a sudden fall. (See MOTION-SICKNESS.) The cause which produces a severe and sudden giddiness is MENIÈRE'S DISEASE, a condition in which there is loss of function of the labyrinth of the inner ear. An acute labyrinthitis may result from viral infection and produce a severe vertigo lasting 2 to 5 days. Because it often occurs in epidemics it is often called epidemic vertigo. Vertigo is sometimes produced by the removal of wax from the ear, or even by syringing out the ear. (See EAR, DISEASES OF.) A severe upset in the gastrointestinal tract may cause vertigo. Refractive errors in the eyes, an attack of MIGRAINE, a mild attack of EPILEPSY, and gross diseases of the brain, such as tumours, are other causes acting more directly upon the central nervous system. Finally, giddiness may be due to some disorder of the circulation, e.g. reduced blood supply to the brain produced by fainting, or by disease of the heart.

Treatment while the attack lasts, requires the victim to lie down in a darkened, quiet room. Sedatives have most influence in diminishing giddiness when it is distressing. After the attack is over, the individual should be examined to establish the cause and, if necessary, to be given appropriate treatment.

VESICAL The term applied to structures connected with, or diseases of, the bladder. (See URINARY BLADDER.)

VESICANTS are blistering agents. (See BLISTERS AND COUNTER-IRRITANTS.)

VESICLE A PAPULE containing fluid.

VESICULAR BREATHING Normal breath sounds heard in the lung by means of a stethoscope. These are soft regular sounds which become altered by disease and the changed characteristics may help the physician to diagnose a disease in the lung.

VESTIBULOCOCHLEAR NERVE The eighth cranial nerve. It consists of two sets of fibres, which constitute two separate nerves. One is known as the vestibular nerve, which is the nerve of equilibration or balance. The other is known as the cochlear nerve, which is the nerve of hearing. Disturbance of the former causes giddiness, whilst disturbance of the latter causes deafness.

VESTIBULO-OCULAR REFLEX Eye movement that occurs after or during the slow injection of 20 ml of ice-cold water into each external auditory meatus (see EAR) in turn.

VESTIGIAL An adjective referring to an organ which exists in a rudimentary form and whose function and structure have declined during the course of evolution. An example is the appendix.

VIABLE The ability of an organism to survive on its own. In the UK the legal age of the viability of a fetus is 24 weeks.

VIAGRA (see SILDENAFIL CITRATE).

VIBRATOR An instrument used for vibratory massage to improve the tone of muscles and to relax them. It is of help in speeding the healing process after muscle or ligament strains.

VIBRIO A bacterium with a curved shape, such as the vibrio of CHOLERA.

VILLUS One of the minute processes thickly distributed upon the inner surface of the small intestine, giving it, to the naked eye, a velvety appearance, and greatly assisting absorption of digested food. (See DIGESTION, ABSORPTION AND ASSIMILATION; INTESTINE.)

VINBLASTINE A VINCA ALKALOID CYTOTOXIC drug (first obtained from the periwinkle plant *Vinca rosea* to treat the acute LEUKAEMIAS, LYMPHOMAS and some solid tumours such as breast and lung cancer. (See CYTOTOXIC.)

VINCA ALKALOIDS A group of powerful cytotoxic (anticancer) drugs used to treat the acute LEUKAEMIAS, LYMPHOMAS and some solid tumours such as breast and lung cancers. Originally derived from the periwinkle plant, the latest vinca alkaloid (VINORELBINE) is a semi-synthetic drug. These alkaloids, which are given intravenously, have potentially serious side-effects on the nervous system and also suppress the production of MYELOID cells in the bone marrow.

VINCENT'S ANGINA An ulcerative inflammation of the throat, often foul smelling, and caused by large, spindle-shaped bacilli and spirilla.

VINCRISTINE An alkaloid cytoxic drug (derived from the common periwinkle) with similar properties and uses as VINBLASTINE. (See CYTOTOXIC.)

VINORELBINE A semi-synthetic VINCA ALKALOID cytoxic drug recently introduced for the treatment of advanced breast cancer when anthracycline cytotoxic antibiotics such as DOXORUBIN have failed. Vinorelbine is also used to treat advanced non-small-cell lung cancer (see LUNGS, DISEASES OF). As with all vinca alkaloids, the drug has neurotoxic effects, usually affecting the PERIPHERAL and AUTONOMIC NERVOUS systems. It may also cause (reversible) hair loss. The drug is given intravenously.

VINYL ETHER is an inhalational anaesthetic used in minor surgical procedures of short duration, and for the induction of ANAESTHESIA.

VIRAEMIA A condition occurring at various times in some viral infections in which the infecting VIRUS is present in large amounts in the blood. In other virus infections the organisms are merely transported in the blood on their way to target tissues or organs.

VIRAL HAEMORRHAGIC FEVER or EBOLA VIRUS FEVER, A usually fatal infection caused by a virus related to that of MARBURG DISEASE. Two large outbreaks of it were recorded in 1976 (one in the Sudan and one in Zaïre), with a mortality, respectively, of 50 and 80 per cent, and the disease reappeared in the Sudan in 1979. After an incubation period of 7 to 14 days, the onset is with headache of increasing severity and fever. This is followed by diarrhoea, extensive internal bleeding and vomiting. Death usually occurs on the eighth to ninth day. Infection is by person-to-person contact. Serum from patients convalescent from the disease is a useful source of antibodies to the virus.

VIRILISM The condition in which masculine characteristics develop in the female, and is commonly the result of an overactive SUPRAR-ENAL gland, or of a tumour of its cortex. It may also result from an androgen-secreting OVARIAN TUMOUR (see OVARIES, DISEASES OF) and also from the POLYCYSTIC OVARY syndrome. The overproduction of male sex (androgen) hormones can produce excess growth of hair, male pattern hairline, stopping or disruption of menstruation, enlargement of the clitoris and conversion to a masculine body shape.

VIRULENCE The power of a bacterium or virus to cause disease. Virulence can be measured by how many people the micro-organism infects, how quickly it spreads through the body, and how many people die from it.

VIRUS The term applied to a group of infective agents which are so small that they are able to pass through the pores of collodion filters. They are responsible for some of the most devastating diseases affecting man: e.g. INFLUENZA, POLIOMYELITIS, SMALLPOX, and YEL-LOW FEVER. The virus of influenza measures 80 nanometres, whereas the staphylococcus measures 1000 nanometres. (1 nanometre = one thousand-millionth of a metre.) A single virus particle, known as a virion, comprises an inner core of NUCLEIC ACID which is surrounded by one or two protective coverings (capsid) made of protein. Sometimes the capsid is enclosed by another layer called the viral envelope (also a protein structure). The envelope often disintegrates when the virus invades a cell. Viruses enter cells and then indulge in a complex and variable process of replication using some of the cell's own structure. Viruses may stay in a host's nucleus, being reactivated months or years later. There are over a score of large families of viruses from papoviruses, which cause WARTS, through herpes viruses (cold sores, CHICKENPOX, SHINGLES) and orthomyxoviruses (influenza) to corona viruses (common cold) and retroviruses (AIDS). Virus diseases are more difficult to treat than those caused by bacteria. ANTIBIOTICS are ineffective but INTERFERON, a group of natural substances, show promise. Immunization is the most effective way of combating viral infections and smallpox, poliomyelitis, mumps, measles and rubella are examples of virus diseases which have been successfully combated, while research is progressing to find a vaccine against HIV.

VISCERA The general name given to the larger organs lying within the cavities of the chest and abdomen. The term 'viscus' is also applied individually to these organs.

VISION Broadly speaking, vision is the ability to see.

Pathway of light from the eye to the brain Light enters the eye by passing through the transparent cornea, then through the aqueous humour filling the anterior chamber. It then passes through the pupil, through the lens and the vitreous to reach the retina. In the retina the rod and cone photoreceptors detect light and relay messages in the form of electrochemical impulses through the various layers of the retina to the nerve fibres. The nerve fibres carry messages via the optic nerve, optic chiasm, optic tract, lateral geniculate body and finally the optic radiations to the visual cortex. Here in the visual cortex these messages are interpreted. It is therefore the visual cortex of the brain that 'sees'.

Visual acuity Two points will not be seen as two unless they are separated by a minimum distance. This distance is such that the objects are so far apart that the lines joining them to the eye enclose between them (subtend) an angle of at least one minute of a degree. This amount of separation allows the images of the two points to fall on two separate cones (if the light from two points falls on one cone, the two points would be seen as a single point). There are many tests of visual acuity. One of the more common is the Snellen Test Type. This is made up of many letters of different size. By conventions the chart is placed 6 metres away from the patient. Someone able to see the lowest line at this distance has a visual acuity of 6/4. If they are only able to see the top letter they have 6/60 vision. 'Normal' vision is 6/6.

Colour vision: 'White light' is made up of component colours. These can be separated by a prism, thereby producing a spectrum. The three cardinal colours are red, green, and blue. All other colours can be produced by a varying mixture of these three. Colour vision is a complex subject. The trichromat theory of colour vision suggests that there are three types of cones, each type sensitive to one of the cardinal colours. Colour perception is based on differential stimulation of these cone types. The opponent colour theory suggests that each cone type can generate signals of the opposite kind. Output from some cones can collaborate with the output from others or can inhibit the action of other cones. Colour perception results from these various complex interactions.

Defective colour vision may be hereditary or acquired and can occur in the presence of normal visual acuity.

HEREDITARY DEFECTIVE COLOUR VISION is more common in men (7 per cent of males) than women (0·5 per cent of females). Men are affected, but women convey the abnormal gene to their children. It occurs because one or more of the photopigments of the retina are abnormal, or the cones are damaged. Red–green colour defect is the commonest.

ACQUIRED DEFECTIVE COLOUR VISION is the result of disease of the cones or their connections in the retina, optic nerve or brain, e.g. macular disease, optic neuritis. Colour vision can be impaired but not lost as a result of corneal opacification or cataract formation.

TESTS OF COLOUR VISION   These use specially designed numbers made of coloured dots surrounded by dots of confusing colour (e.g. ISHIHARA plates).

VISION, DISORDERS OF   The list of disorders resulting in poor or dim vision is huge. Disturbance of vision can result from an uncorrected refractive error, disease or injury of the cornea, iris, lens, vitreous, retina, choroid or sclera. It may also result from disease or injury to the structures comprising the visual pathway from the retina to the occipital cortex (see VISION, Pathway of light from the eye to the brain) and from lesions of the structures around the eye, e.g. swollen lids, drooping eyelids. (See EYE DISEASES.)

VISION, FIELD OF   When the eye looks at a specific point or object, that point is seen clearly. Other objects within a large area away from this fixation point can also be seen but less clearly. The area that can be seen around the fixation point, without moving the eye, is known as the field of vision. The extent of the field is limited inwards by the nose, above by the brow and below by the cheek. The visual field thus has its greatest extent outwards from the side of the head. The field of vision of each eye overlaps to a large extent so that objects in the centre and towards the inner part of each field are viewed by both eyes together. Because the eyes are set slightly apart, each eye sees objects in this overlapping part of the field slightly differently. It is because of this slight difference that objects can be perceived as three dimensional. Defects in the visual field (scotomas) can be produced by a variety of disorders. Certain of these produce specific field defects. For example, glaucoma, some types of brain damage and some toxins can produce specific defects in the visual field. This type of field defect may be very useful in diagnosing a particular disorder. The blind spot is that part of the visual field corresponding to the optic disc. There are no rods nor cones on the optic disc and therefore no light perception from this area. The blind spot can be found temporal (i.e. on the outer side) of the fixation point.

VISION TESTS   Most vision tests examine a person's sharpness of VISION (visual acuity) and often of the field of vision (see VISION, FIELD OF). Refraction tests assess whether a person has an error that can be corrected with glasses such as ASTIGMATISM, HYPERMETROPIA or MYOPIA. Visual acuity is tested using a SNELLEN CHART when the patient tries to read letters of differing standard sizes from 6 metres away. The optician will prescribe lenses to correct any defects detected by vision tests. (See VISION.)

VISUAL ACUITY (see VISION).

VISUAL EVOKED RESPONSE   Stimulation of the retina with light causes changes in the electrical activity of the cerebral cortex. These changes can be measured from outside the skull and can give valuable information about the state of the visual pathway from the retinal ganglion cells to the occipital cortex. Not only can it determine that function is normal, it can also help to diagnose some causes of poor vision.

VITAL CAPACITY   The amount of air that can be forcibly exhaled from the lungs after a deep inspiration. (See RESPIRATION.)

VITAL SIGN   An indication that an individual is still alive. Chest movements (resulting from respiration), the existence of a pulse (showing that the heart is still beating) and constriction of the pupil of the eye in response to bright light are all vital signs. Other tests such as assessment of brain activity may also be needed in some circumstances: for example, when a patient is on a life-support machine.

VITAMIN   A term applied to a group of substances which exist in minute quantities in natural foods, and which are necessary to normal nutrition, especially in connection with growth and development. Some, A, D, E and K, are fat soluble and can be stored in the body. The remainder, C, B_{12} and other members of the B complex, are water soluble and are quickly excreted. Most vitamins have now been synthesized. When they are absent from the food, defective growth takes place in young animals and children, and in adults various diseases arise; whilst short of the production of actual disease, persistent deprivation of one or other vitamin is apt to lead to a state of lowered general health. Certain deficiencies in diet have long been known to be the cause of scurvy, beriberi, and rickets. A diet containing foods such as milk, eggs, butter, cheese, fat, fish, wholemeal bread, fresh vegetables and fruit should contain sufficient vitamins. Details of the various vitamins are given in APPENDIX 5: VITAMINS.

VITILIGO   A disease in which small or large areas of skin lose their pigment and become white. The hair may be similarly affected. Probably a consequence of an autoimmune mechanism, vitiligo is associated with other autoimmune diseases such as THYROIDITIS and ADDISON'S DISEASE. There is no cure; the vitiliginous skin must be protected from sunburn.

VITREOUS BODY A semi-fluid, transparent substance which fills most of the globe of the eye behind the lens.

VIVISECTION For over a century the medical profession has aimed at maintaining as high a standard as possible for vivisection. It was the medical profession led by Dr James Paget that was responsible for the passing of the Cruelty to Animals Act 1876, which aimed to eliminate cruelty. The infliction of pain was reduced to a minimum by the use of anaesthetics, and the licensing and surveillance of animal experiments was ensured.

Most experiments are carried out on specially bred mice and rats. Fewer than 1 per cent are done on cats, dogs, non-human primates, farm animals, frogs, fish and birds. Control on experiments have recently been strengthened. The great majority of animal experiments is done without anaesthesia because feeding experiments, taking blood, or giving injection, do not require anaesthetics in animals any more than in man. Universities in Britain are responsible for less than one-fifth of animal experiments; commercial concerns and government institutions are responsible for most of the rest. Tests on cosmetics account for under 1 per cent of all animal work, but are necessary because such materials are often applied with great frequency – and for a long time – to the skin of adults and infants.

The use of tissue cultures and computer models instead of live animals are methods of research and investigation that are being increasingly used. There is, however, a limit to the extent to which infection, cancer, or drugs can be investigated on cultures of tissue cells. Computerized or mathematical modelling of experiments are probably the most promising line of development.

VOCAL CORDS (see LARYNGOSCOPE; LARYNX; VOICE AND SPEECH).

VOCAL RESONANCE The air carrying the voice produced in the larynx passes through the throat, mouth and nose. The shape and size of these structures will influence the timbre of the voice, or vocal resonance. This will vary from person to person and even within an individual; i.e. with a cold.

VOICE AND SPEECH Terms applied to the sounds produced in the upper air passages which form one of the means of communication between human beings. Air passes through the larynx to produce the fundamental notes and tones known as voice. This is then modified during its passage through the mouth so as to form speech or song.

Voice This has three varying characteristics: loudness, pitch and quality or timbre. Loudness depends on the volume of air available and therefore on the size of the chest and the strength of its muscles. Pitch is determined by LARYNX size, the degree of tenseness at which the vocal cords are maintained, and whether the cords vibrate as a whole or merely at their edges. In any given voice, the range of pitch seldom exceeds two and a half octaves. Typically, the small larynx of childhood produces a shrill or treble voice; the rapid growth of the larynx around puberty causes the voice to 'break' in boys. Changes in the voice also occur at other ages as a result of the secondary action of the sex hormones. Generally speaking, the adult voice is bass and tenor in men, contralto or soprano in women. Timbre is due to differences in the larynx, as well as voluntary changes in the shape of the mouth.

Speech Rapid modifications of the voice, produced by movements of the palate, tongue and lips. Infants hear the sounds made by others and mimic them; hence the speech centres in the brain are closely connected with those of hearing.

Defects of speech

MUTISM or absence of the power to speak may be due to various causes. Learning difficulties that prevent the child from mimicking the actions of others is most common. In other cases the child has normal intelligence, but some nervous disorder, or disorder of the speech organs, is responsible. Alternatively, complete deafness or early childhood ear disease may be the cause (see SPEECH DISORDERS).

STAMMERING is a highly individual condition, but is basically a lack of co-ordination between the different parts of the speech mechanism.

DYSPHASIA is the inability to speak or understand speech, most commonly following brain disease, such as stroke.

APHONIA or loss of voice may be caused by laryngitis or, rarely, a symptom of hysteria. It is generally of short duration.

VOLAR A term relating to the palm or sole.

VOLKMANN'S CONTRACTURE The condition in which, as a result of too great a pressure from splint or bandage in the treatment of a broken arm, the flexor muscles of the forearm contract and thus obstruct free flow of blood in the veins; the muscles then swell and ultimately become fibrosed.

VOLUNTARY MUSCLE Also known as skeletal muscle, this forms the muscles which are under a person's conscious control. Muscles that control walking, talking and swallowing are examples of those under such control (see INVOLUNTARY MUSCLE and MUSCLE).

VOLVULUS An obstruction of the bowels produced by the twisting of a loop of bowel round itself. (See INTESTINE, DISEASES OF.)

VOMITING means the expulsion of the stomach contents through the mouth. When the effort of vomiting is made, but nothing is brought up, the process is known as retching. When vomiting occurs, the chief effort is made by the muscles of the abdominal wall and by the diaphragm contracting together and squeezing the stomach. The contraction of the stomach wall is no doubt also a factor, and an important step in the act consists in the opening at the right moment of the cardiac or upper orifice of the stomach. This concerted action of various muscles is brought about by a vomiting centre situated on the floor of the fourth ventricle in the brain.

Causes Vomiting is brought about by some irritation of this nervous centre, but in the great majority of cases this is effected through sensations derived from the STOMACH itself. Thus, of the drugs which cause vomiting some act only after being absorbed into the blood and carried to the brain, although most are irritants to the mucous membrane of the stomach (see EMETICS); various diseases of the stomach, such as cancer, and ulcer, and food poisoning, act in a similar way. Irritation, not only of the nerves of the stomach, but also of those proceeding from other abdominal organs, produces vomiting; thus in obstruction of the bowels, peritonitis, gall-stone colic, renal colic, and even during pregnancy, vomiting is a prominent symptom.

Severe emotional shock may cause vomiting, as may unpleasant experiences such as seeing an accident, suffering severe pain or travel sickness.

Direct disturbance of the brain itself is a cause: for example, a blow on the head, a cerebral tumour, a cerebral abscess, meningitis. Many cases of hysteria also show attacks of vomiting as one of their prominent symptoms.

Nausea and vomiting are common symptoms that may arise from local disease of the gastro-intestinal tract, but they are also associated with systemic illness and also with disturbances of labyrinthine function, such as motion sickness and acute labyrinthitis.

There are two centres in the brain concerned with vomiting. One is the chemo-receptor trigger zone. This centre is in contact with the blood and lies outside the blood-brain barrier. It is the site at which drugs such as apomorphine and toxins act. It is rich in dopamine receptors and hence dopamine antagonists are effective treatment for vomiting. The vomiting centre itself co-ordinates impulses received from the chemo-receptor trigger zone from the vestibular apparatus and the gastro-intestinal tract and also from higher centres in the cerebral cortex. The vomiting centre contains many cholinergic and histamine receptors and this is why anti-cholinergic drugs and anti-histamines are effective drugs in the control of vomiting.

Treatment The cause of the vomiting must be sought and treatment directed towards this. Although sodium bicarbonate and bismuth salts are now rarely used in the treatment of vomiting, bismuth chelate is effective in healing gastric and duodenal ulcers, thought to act by having a direct toxic effect on gastric *Helicobacter pylori*. Granisetron and Ondansetron are 5HT-3 antagonists valuable in the treatment of nausea and vomiting induced by cytotoxic chemotherapy or radiotherapy and prevention and treatment of post-operative nausea and vomiting. Prochlorperazine is valuable in the treatment of severe nausea, vomiting, vertigo and labyrinthine disorders, although extrapyramidal symptoms may occur, particularly in children, elderly and debilitated patients.

Vomiting may occur after surgical operations and this is due to the combined effects of analgesics, anaesthetic agents and the psychological stress of operation. Various drugs can be used to prevent or stop postoperative vomiting.

Nausea and vomiting are common symptoms in pregnancy. Drugs are best avoided in this situation as they may damage the developing fetus. Simple measures, such as the taking of food before getting up in the morning and reassurance, are often all that is necessary.

VON RECKLINGHAUSEN'S DISEASE An inherited disease, also called multiple neurofibromatosis. About one new case occurs every 3,000 live births. The disease is characterized by tumours along the course of nerves which can be felt beneath the skin. Soft tumours may also develop beneath the skin. The condition may have other associated abnormalities such as SCOLIOSIS, decalcification of the bones due to overactivity of the PARATHYROID glands and fibrosis in the lungs. Surgery may be needed for cosmetic reasons or to relieve pressure on the nervous system.

VOYEURISM The regular viewing of people who are naked or part naked or who are taking part in intimate sexual activities. The voyeur's subjects are unaware that they are being watched. The voyeur, nearly always a man, usually becomes sexually excited and may induce orgasm by masturbation.

VULVA is the general term applied to the external female genitals.

VULVO-VAGINITIS Inflammation of the vulva and vagina. It may be due to infection, particularly with *CANDIDA ALBICANS,* and may be a presenting feature of late onset DIABETES MELLITUS. Trauma may sometimes be the cause.

W

WALK (see GAIT).

WARFARIN An ANTICOAGULANT, usually given by mouth on a daily basis. The initial dose depends on the PROTHROMBIN or COAGULATION time, which should be determined before starting treatment, and then at regular treatments during treatment. It is indicated for the prophylaxis of embolization (see EMBOLISM) in rheumatic heart disease and atrial fibrillation (see HEART DISEASES); after prosthetic heart-valve insertion; prophylaxis and treatment of venous thrombosis and pulmonary embolism; and transient ischaemic attacks. When given in tablet form, its maximum effect generally occurs within about 36 hours, wearing off within 48 hours. Special caution is appropriate in patients with disease of the liver or kidneys or who have had recent surgery. Warfarin is contraindicated throughout pregnancy (especially the first and third trimesters), and in cases of PEPTIC ulcers, severe hypertension and bacterial ENDO-CARDITIS. The most important adverse effect is HAEMORRHAGE. Other reported side-effects include HYPERSENSITIVITY, rash, ALOPECIA, diarrhoea, unexplained drop in HAEMATOCRIT readings, purple toes, skin NECROSIS, JAUNDICE, liver dysfunction, nausea, vomiting and pancreatitis (see PANCREAS, DISEASES OF). (See CO-AGULATION.)

WARTS (VERRUCAE) Small solid outgrowths from the skin arising from the epidermis caused by various subtypes of 'human papilloma virus'. The causal viruses are ubiquitous and probably most people harbour them. Whether or not warts develop depends on age, previous infection and natural resistance.

Common warts (verruca vulgaris) are seen mainly in children and young adults on the backs of the fingers and hands and less often on the knees, face or scalp. They may be single or numerous and from 1 mm to 10 mm or more in size. Untreated, they often resolve spontaneously after weeks or months. They may be occupationally contracted by butchers and meat-handlers.

Plane warts (verruca plana) are small, flat-topped, yellowish papules seen mainly on the backs of the hands, wrists and face in young people. They may persist for years.

Digitate warts (verruca digitata) are finger or threadlike warts up to 5 mm or more in length with a dark rough tip. They tend to grow on the eyelids or neck.

Plantar warts (verruca plantaris) occur on the soles of the feet, most commonly in older children, adolescents and young adults. Spread by walking barefoot in swimming pools, changing rooms, etc., these warts may appear as minor epidemics in institutions, such as schools. They are flattened, yellow-white discrete lesions in the sole or heel, tender when squeezed. Multiple black points in the wart are thrombosed capillaries. Occasionally, aggregates of plantar warts form a mosaiclike plaque, especially in chronically warm, moist feet.

Genital warts are sexually transmitted. In the male they occur on the shaft of the penis and on the prepuce or around the anus. In women they occur around the vaginal introitus and labia minora. Genital warts vary from 1–2 mm pink papules to florid cauliflowerlike masses. Pregnancy facilitates their development.

Mucosal warts may develop on the mucous membranes of the mouth.

Laryngeal warts may be found in children whose mothers had genital warts at the time of delivery. Some subtypes of genital wart can infect the uterine cervix, causing changes which may lead eventually to cancer.

Treatment Cryotherapy – freezing with liquid nitrogen – is the principal weapon against all types of warts but CURETTAGE (scraping out the wart with a CURETTE) and cauterization (see ELECTROCAUTERY) or LASER therapy may be required for resistant warts. Genital warts may respond to local application of PODOPHYLLUM preparations. Sexual partners should be examined and treated if necessary. Finally treatment of warts should not be more onerous or painful than the disease itself since spontaneous resolution is so common.

WASHING (see DISINFECTION).

WASHING OUT OF THE STOMACH (see GASTRIC LAVAGE).

WASSERMANN REACTION A test introduced for the diagnosis of SYPHILIS by examination of the blood. It has now been largely supplanted by other more specific tests.

WASTING (see ATROPHY).

WATERBRASH or PYROSIS A symptom of indigestion; during the course of digestion, the mouth fills with tasteless or sour fluid, which is generally saliva, but sometimes brought up from the stomach. This is accompanied by a burning pain often felt at the pit of the stomach or in the chest. The condition is a symptom of excessive acidity of the stomach contents, due sometimes to an injudicious diet, and often characteristic of a DUODENAL ULCER. (See DYS-PEPSIA.)

WATER-HAMMER PULSE The peculiarly sudden pulse that is associated with incompetence of the AORTIC VALVE of the heart. (See PULSE.)

WAX This is used in medicine as an ingredient of ointments, plasters, and suppositories. It is used either as yellow wax derived directly from honeycomb, or as white wax, which is the same substance bleached. It is also used in the form of paraffin wax to apply heat in the relief of rheumatic pains.

For wax in the ear, see EAR, DISEASES OF.

WEAKNESS (see ATROPHY; CACHEXIA; PARALYSIS; TONICS).

WEALS or WHEALS   Raised white areas on the skin with reddened margins, which may result from sharp blows, or may be a symptom of nettle-rash.

WEANING   The process by which a baby is introduced to solid foods after having only had breast milk or artificial milk to drink. The transfer usually starts at around 4 months of age but some infants can start earlier. (See INFANT FEEDING.)

WEBBED FINGERS or TOES or SYNDACTYLY A deformity sometimes present at birth, and which tends to run in families. The web may be quite a thin structure, or the fingers may be closely united by solid tissue. In any case, separation is a matter of considerable difficulty, because, if the web is simply divided, it heals up as before. A special operation is necessary, consisting in turning back a flap of the web upon each of the united fingers, or some other device to produce healing in the new position.

WEBER'S TEST   A test with a tuning fork that is used to assess a person's deafness. (See DEAFNESS.)

WEIGHT AND HEIGHT   Charts relating height to age have been devised and give an indication of the normal rate of growth. (See APPENDIX 6: MEASUREMENTS IN MEDICINE for more details.) The wide variation in normal children is immediately apparent on studying such charts. Deviations from the mean of this wide range are called percentiles. Centile or percentile charts describe the distribution of a characteristic in a population. They are obtained by measuring a specific characteristic in a large population of at least 1,000 of each sex at each age. For each age there will be a height, above and below which 50 per cent of the population lie and this is called the fiftieth centile. The fiftieth centile thus indicates the mean height at a particular age. Such tables are less reliable around the age of puberty because of variation in age of onset.

Minor variations from the mean do not warrant investigation but if the height of an individual falls below the third centile (3 per cent of normal children have a height that falls below the third centile) or above the ninety-seventh centile, investigation is required. Changes in the rate of growth are also important and skeletal proportions may provide useful information. There are many children who are normal but who are small in relation to their parents. The problem is merely growth delay. These children take longer to reach maturity and there is also a proportional delay in their skeletal maturation. The actual height must always be assessed in relation to maturity. The change in skeletal proportions is one manifestation of maturity but other features include the maturing of facial features with the growth of nose and jaw and dental development. Maturity of bone can readily be measured by the radiological bone age.

Failure to gain weight is of more significance. Whilst this may be due to some underlying disease, the commonest cause is a diet containing inadequate calories. Over the last six decades or so there has been quite a striking increase in the heights and weights of European children. Manufacturers of children's clothing, shoes and furniture have had to increase the size of their products. Growth is now completed at 20–21 years, compared with 25 at the turn of the century. This increase, and earlier maturation, it has been suggested, have been due to a combination of genetic mixing as a result of population movements, combined with the whole range of improvement in environmental hygiene, and not merely to better nutrition.

In the case of adults views have changed of recent years concerning 'ideal' weight. Life insurance statistics have shown that maximal life expectancy is obtained if the average weight at ages 25 to 30 years is maintained throughout the rest of life. These insurance statistics also suggest that it is of advantage to be slightly over average weight before the age of 30 years, to be of average weight after the age of 40, and to be under-weight from ages 30 to 40. In the past it has been usual, in assessing the significance of an adult's weight, to allow a 10 per cent range on either side of normal for variations in body build. A closer correlation has been found between thoracic and abdominal measurements and weight.

WEIGHTS AND MEASURES   It is over a hundred years since the metric system was legalized in Britain, but it was not until 1969 that it became illegal to use any system of weights and measures other than the metric system for dispensing prescriptions.

A rationalization of the metric system is now used known as the International System of Units (SI) (see APPENDIX 6: MEASUREMENTS IN MEDICINE).

WEIL'S DISEASE (see LEPTOSPIROSIS).

WERNICKE'S ENCEPHALOPATHY   Also called the Wernicke-Korsakoff syndrome, this uncommon disorder is characterized by mental confusion or delirium that occurs in combination with an unsteady GAIT, nystagmus (see EYE DISEASES), and paralysis of the eye muscles and eventually PSYCHOSIS. It is caused by a deficiency of VITAMIN B₁ (THIAMINE) (see APPENDIX 5: VITAMINS) which affects the brain and nervous system. It occurs in alcoholic individuals and in patients with persistent vomiting. As soon as the condition is diagnosed, it must be treated with large doses of thiamine. Unless the patient has developed symptoms of psychosis, the condition is usually reversible with treatment.

WERTHHEIM'S HYSTERECTOMY A major operation done to remove cancer of the UTERUS or OVARY. The ovaries, FALLOPIAN TUBES, the uterus and its ligaments, the upper vagina, and the regional LYMPH NODES are all excised.

WHEAL A localized area of oedema in the skin, usually evanescent and itching (see URTICARIA).

WHEEZING A popular name applied to the various sounds produced in the chest when the bronchial tubes are narrowed. It is applied particularly to the long-drawn breathing of asthma, and to the whistling or purring noises that accompany breathing in cases of bronchitis. (See ASTHMA; BRONCHITIS.)

WHIPLASH INJURY An injury to the neck region caused by the neck being forcibly bent backwards and forwards (or the other way round). Car accidents are a common cause, when a driver or passenger is suddenly decelerated. The injury usually affects the ligaments, spinal joints and soft tissues of the neck. Subluxation (partial dislocation) of a cervical joint sometimes occurs and cervical vertebra may occasionally be fractured if the forces are severe. Pain and stiffness of the neck result and these may be worse after a day or so. Treatment includes immobilization of the neck in a collar and analgesic and muscle-relaxing drugs. PHYSIOTHERAPY may be necessary. The patient usually recovers fully but may take several weeks to do so.

WHIPWORM A popular name for *Trichuris trichiura*. (See TRICHURIASIS.)

WHITE BLOOD CELL (see LEUCOCYTE).

WHITE HAIR The greying or whitening of hair which takes place with age is due to a loss of its pigment, MELANIN, and the collection of air bubbles in the shaft of the hair. There is no evidence that hair ever goes white overnight, whether in response to shock, strain or any other cause. Rapid whitening may occur patchily in a matter of days, but it is more often a matter of weeks or months. In the more rapid cases the cause is thought to be a form of alopecia areata (see BALDNESS), in which the dark hairs which fall out are replaced by white hairs. An alternative cause is VITILIGO. Certain drugs, including mephenesin and CHLOROQUINE, may also cause whitening of the hair.

WHITEHEAD A common benign blemish of the skin (see MILIA).

WHITES (see LEUCORRHOEA).

WHITLOW A popular term applied to all acute inflammations of the deep-seated tissues in the fingers, whether the structure affected is the root of the nail, the pulp of the finger-tip, the sheaths of the tendons that run along the back and front of the fingers, or the bone. Acute PARONYCHIA is the most common type. The condition is usually very painful. The cause is commonly a bacterial infection and antibiotics are the recommended treatment. If an abscess forms, surgery is sometimes necessary. Whitlows resulting from a virus infection such as herpes simplex will not respond to antibiotics and should be treated with an antiviral drug; surgery should be performed as it may spread the infection.

WHOOPING-COUGH, or PERTUSSIS, is a respiratory-tract infection caused by *Bordetella pertussis* and spread by droplets. It may occur at all ages, but around 90 per cent of cases are children under 5 years, particularly girls. Most common during the winter months, it tends to occur in epidemics, with periods of increased prevalence occurring every three to four years. It is a notifiable disease. The routine vaccination of infants with TRIPLE VACCINE, which includes the vaccine against whooping-cough, has drastically reduced the incidence of this potentially dangerous infection. In 1995-6 94 per cent of children in England had been vaccinated against whooping-cough by their second birthday. In an epidemic of whooping-cough, which extended from the last quarter of 1977 to mid-1979, 102,500 cases of whooping-cough were notified in the United Kingdom, with 36 deaths. This was the biggest outbreak since 1957 and its size was partly attributed to the fall in vaccination acceptance rates. In 1995 under 2,000 cases were notified in England.

Symptoms The first, or catarrhal, stage is characterized by mild, but non-specific, symptoms of sneezing, conjunctivitis (see EYE DISEASES), sore throat, mild fever and cough. Lasting 10 to 14 days, this stage is the most infectious; unfortunately it is almost impossible to make a definite clinical diagnosis, although analysis of a nasal swab may confirm a suspected diagnosis. This is followed by the second, or paroxysmal, stage with irregular bouts of coughing, often prolonged, and typically more severe at night. Each paroxysm consists of a succession of short sharp coughs, increasing in speed and duration, and ending in a deep, crowing inspiration, often with a characteristic 'whoop'. Vomiting is common after the last paroxysm of a series. Lasting two to four weeks, this stage is the most dangerous, with the greatest risk of complications. These may include pneumonia and partial collapse of the lungs, and fits may be induced by cerebral ANOXIA. Less severe complications caused by the stress of coughing include minor bleeding around the eyes, ulceration under the tongue, hernia and prolapse of the rectum. Mortality is greatest in the first year of life, particularly among neonates, infants up to 4 weeks old. Nearly all patients with whooping-cough recover after a few weeks, with a lasting immunity. Very severe cases may leave structural changes in the lungs, such as EMPHYSEMA, with a permanent shortness of breath or liability to ASTHMA .

Treatment Antibiotics, such as erythromycin or tetracyclines, may be helpful if given during the catarrhal stage, but are of no use during the paroxysmal stage. Cough suppressants are helpful, and skilled nursing may be required to maintain nutrition, particularly if the disease is prolonged, with frequent vomiting.

WIDAL REACTION (see AGGLUTINATION).

WILMS' TUMOUR or NEPHROBLASTOMA This is the commonest kidney tumour in infancy. It is a malignant tumour, which occurs in around 1 per 10,000 live births. The survival rate with modern treatment (removal of the kidney followed by radiotherapy and chemotherapy) is now around 80 per cent.

WILSON'S DISEASE or HEPATOLENTICULAR DEGENERATION This is a familial disease in which there is an increased accumulation of copper in the liver, brain, and other tissues including the kidneys. Its main manifestation is the development of tremor and rigidity, with difficulty in speech. In many cases there is improvement following the administration of dimercaprol, penicillamine, or trientine dihydrochloride; these substances cause an increased excretion of copper.

WINDPIPE The popular name for the trachea, which extends from the larynx above to the point in the upper part of the chest where it divides into the two large bronchial tubes, one to each lung. It is about 10 cm (4 inches) in length and consists of a fibrous tube kept permanently open by about twenty strong horizontally placed hoops of cartilage, each of which forms about two-thirds of a circle, the two ends being joined behind by muscle-fibres. This fibrocartilaginous tube is lined by a smooth mucous membrane, richly supplied with mucous glands and covered by a single layer of ciliated epithelium. (See also AIR PASSAGES.)

WINTER VOMITING DISEASE or EPIDEMIC NAUSEA AND VOMITING This condition is characterized by nausea, vomiting, diarrhoea and giddiness, which occurs during the winter. Outbreaks of it usually involve whole families or may affect communities like schools. It is due to PARVOVIRUSES. The incubation period is 24 to 48 hours, and attacks seldom persist for more than 72 hours.

WISDOM TOOTH A popular name for the last molar tooth on either side of each jaw. These teeth are the last to appear and should develop in early adult life, but often they do not cut the gum till the age of 20 or 25 or indeed they may sometimes remain permanently impacted in the jaw-bone. This occurs in up to 25 per cent of individuals. The lower third molar is often impacted against the second because of the direction in which it erupts. (See TEETH.)

WITCH-HAZEL A preparation of the bark, twigs, and dried leaves from *Hamamelis virginiana*, a plant found in the United States. It has strong astringent properties and is used to check haemorrhages and excessive mucous discharges, and also for PILES.

WITHDRAWAL BLEEDING Loss of blood from the UTERUS via the VAGINA occurring when the women's level of oestrogen hormones, progesterone hormone or progestogen drugs falls quickly. The withdrawal bleeding that happens at the end of each month's cycle of combined oral contraceptive pills (see CONTRACEPTION) imitates the woman's menstrual period (see MENSTRUATION) but is normally briefer and less in amount.

WITHDRAWAL SYMPTOMS Unpleasant physical and mental symptoms that occur when a person stops using a drug or substance on which he or she are dependent. The symptoms include tremors, sweating, and vomiting which are reversed if further doses are given. Alcohol and hard drugs, such as morphine, heroin, and cocaine, are among the substances that induce dependence, and therefore withdrawal symptoms, when stopped. Amphetamines and nicotine are other examples.

WOLFFIAN DUCTS The Wolffian ducts and the Mullerian ducts are separate sets of primordia that transiently co-exist in embryos of both sexes. In the male the Wolffian ducts give rise to the vas deferens, the seminal vesicles and the epididymis, while the Mullerian ducts disappear. In female embryos the Mullerian ducts grow and fuse in the midline to produce the Fallopian tubes, the uterus and the upper third of the vagina, whereas the Wolffian ducts regress. The former phase of development requires a functioning testis from which an inducer substance diffuses locally over the primordia to bring about the suppression of the Mullerian duct and the development of the Wolffian duct. In the absence of this substance development proceeds along female lines regardless of the genetic sex.

WOMB (see UTERUS).

WOMB MUSIC The name given to the playing to crying babies of sounds comparable to those by which the unborn babe is surrounded in the womb, such as the beating of the mother's heart, the bowel sounds of the babe and the like. The claim is that the replaying of these brings back the 'peaceful music of the womb', to which they have become conditioned, and thus 'sings' them to sleep.

WOOL-SORTERS' DISEASE Another name for anthrax. (See ANTHRAX.)

WORD BLINDNESS A condition in which, as the result of disease in the brain, a person becomes unable to associate their proper meanings with words, although he may be quite able to spell the letters.

Word deafness is an associated condition in which, though hearing remains perfect, the patient has lost the power of referring the names he hears to the articles they denote. (See DYSPHASIA.)

WORLD HEALTH ORGANIZATION (see APPENDIX 11: SOME INTERNATIONAL HEALTH ORGANIZATIONS).

WORLD MEDICAL ASSOCIATION (see APPENDIX 11: SOME INTERNATIONAL ORGANIZATIONS).

WORMS (see ASCARIASIS, ENTEROBIASIS, TAENIASIS).

WOUNDS A wound is any breach suddenly produced in the tissues of the body by direct violence. An extensive injury of the deeper parts without corresponding injury of the surface is known as a bruise or contusion.

Varieties These are classified according to the immediate effect produced:
INCISED WOUNDS are usually inflicted with some sharp instrument, and are clean cuts, in which the tissues are simply divided without any damage to parts around. The bleeding from such a wound is apt to be very free, but it can be readily controlled.
PUNCTURED WOUNDS, or stabs, are inflicted with a pointed instrument. These wounds are dangerous, partly because their depth involves the danger of wounding vital organs, partly because bleeding from a stab is hard to control, and partly because they are difficult to sterilize. The wound produced by the nickel-nosed bullet is a puncture, much less severe than the ugly lacerated wound caused by an expanding bullet, or by a ricochet, and, if no clothing has been carried in by the bullet, the wound is clean and usually heals at once.
LACERATED WOUNDS are those in which tissues are torn, such as injuries caused by machinery. Little bleeding may occur and a limb can be torn completely away without great loss of blood. Such wounds are, however, specially liable to infection.
CONTUSED WOUNDS are those accompanied by much bruising of surrounding parts, as in the case of a blow from a cudgel or poker. There is little bleeding, but healing is slow on account of damage to the edges of the wound. Any of these varieties may become infected.

First-aid treatment The first aim is to check any bleeding. This may be done by pressure upon the edges of the wound with a clean handkerchief, or, if the bleeding is serious, by putting the finger in the wound and pressing it upon the spot from which the blood is coming.

If medical attention is available within a few hours, it should not be interfered with further than is necessary to stop the bleeding and to cover the wound with a clean dry handkerchief or bandage. When expert assistance is not soon obtainable, the wound should be cleaned with an antiseptic such as CHLORHEXIDINE or boiled water and the injured part fixed so that movement is prevented or minimized. A wounded hand or arm is fixed with a sling (see SLING), a wounded leg with a splint (see SPLINTS). If the victim is in shock he or she must be treated for that (see SHOCK and APPENDIX 1: BASIC FIRST AID).

WRINKLE A natural furrow in the skin commonly associated with ageing. Wrinkles are most prominent on the face and other exposed body parts. Overexposure to sunlight causes premature wrinkling. Cosmetic preparations may temporarily improve excessive wrinkling, but a face lift, which stretches the skin using surgery, can improve a person's face for up to five years.

WRIST The joint situated between the arm above and the hand below. The region of the wrist contains eight small carpal bones, arranged in two rows, each containing four bones. Those in the proximal row, that is the row nearest the forearm, are, from the outside inwards when looking at the palm of the hand, the scaphoid, lunate, triquetrum, and pisiform. Those in the distal row, that is the row nearest the hand, are the trapezium, trapezoid, capitate and hamate. These articulate with the metacarpal bones in the hand are closely bound to one another by short, strong ligaments, and the wrist-joint is the union of the composite mass thus formed with the radius and ulna in the forearm. The wrist and the radius and ulna are united by strong outer and inner lateral ligaments, and by weaker ligaments before and behind, whilst the powerful tendons passing to the hand and fingers strengthen the wrist.

The joint can move in all directions, and its shape and many ligaments mean that it rarely dislocates, although stretching or tearing of some of these ligaments is a common accident, constituting a sprain. (See JOINTS, DISEASES AND INJURIES OF.) Inflammation of the tendon-sheaths may occur as a result of injury or repetitive movement (see UPPER LIMB DISORDERS). A fairly common condition is the presence of a ganglion, in which an elastic swelling full of fluid develops on the back or front of the wrist in connection with the sheaths of the tendons. (See GANGLION.)

WRIST-DROP (see DROP WRIST).

WRITER'S CRAMP A spasm which affects certain muscles when a person is writing, and which may not occur when the same muscles are employed in other acts. Similar symptoms are observed in the case of musicians (guitar, clarinet and piano in particular), typists, word-processor and computer operators and artists.

WRY-NECK A condition in which the head is twisted to one side. It may be caused by the contraction of a scar, such as that resulting from a burn or by paralysis of some of the muscles, but in the great majority of cases it is a spasmodic condition due to excessive tendency of certain muscles to contract. (See CRAMP; SPASMODIC TORTICOLLIS.)

X

XANTHELASMA PALPEBRARUM These yellow smooth nodules of LIPID-laden cells occur in and around the eyelids. Blood lipids are usually normal but there is an association with HYPERCHOLESTEROLAEMIA in a minority of sufferers.

XANTHOMATA Lipid-laden nodules in skin or on tendons, the presence of which generally denotes a disorder of LIPID metabolism.

Tuberose xanthomata are orange-yellow papules, nodules or plaques seen on the points of the elbows or knees and occasionally on the buttocks. They are seen in hypercholesterolaemia.

Tendon xanathomata are firm colourless nodules attached to tendons usually on the knuckles or the back of the heel. They are characteristic of an increase in the amount of low-density lipoprotein in the blood occurring in hypercholesterolaemia (see CHOLESTEROL and HYPER-LIPIDAEMIA).

Eruptive xanthomata are profuse, small yellow papules which erupt widely on skin and mucosal surfaces. They signify hypertriglyceridaemia (raised blood levels of the LIPID TRIGLYCERIDE).

X CHROMOSOME One of two sex CHROMOSOMES. Every normal female body cell has a pair of X chromosomes. Men have only one X chromosome and this is paired with a Y chromosome. The sex cells in men and women each have one X and one Y chromosome. Certain diseases are linked to the presence of an X chromosome: these include HAEMOPHILIA (see GENES).

XENOGRAFT A transplant from one animal to another of a different species. It is also known as a heterograft.

XERODERMA The term means dry skin. Normal skin may become dry when exposed to very low ambient humidity and is then vulnerable to irritation by soaps, detergents and other chemicals which cause 'chapping'. Dryness of the skin may also be a feature of skin disease, especially atopic eczema. Genetically determined xeroderma is called ICHTHYOSIS.

XERODERMA PIGMENTOSUM A rare disease in which DNA repair mechanisms fail, rendering the skin especially vulnerable to damage from ultraviolet light. Extreme photosensitivity begins in infancy. Later marked freckling occurs and premature CARCINOGENESIS in the skin usually leads to early death. There may also be neurological complications.

XEROPHTHALMIA (see EYE DISEASES).

XEROSIS Abnormal dryness, especially of the eye.

XEROSTOMIA Dryness of the mouth due to lack of saliva. Its most extreme form occurs following radiotherapy of the mouth, and in the condition known as Sjögren's syndrome. No satisfactory substitute for natural saliva has been found though some find a methyl-cellulose substitute gives partial relief, as may a glycerin mouth-wash.

XIPHISTERNUM (see XIPHOID PROCESS.)

XIPHOID PROCESS or XIPHOID CARTILAGE: Also known as the xiphisternum, this is the small oval-shaped projection forming the lowest of the three parts of the STERNUM or breast bone.

X-RAYS (RÖNTGEN RAYS) These were discovered in 1895 by Wilhelm Conrad Röntgen. Their use for diagnostic imaging (radiology) and for cancer therapy (see RADIOTHERAPY) is now an integral part of medicine. Many other forms of diagnostic imaging have been developed in recent years, sometimes also loosely called 'radiology'. Similarly the use of chemotherapeutic agents in cancer has led to the term oncology which may be applied to the treatment of cancer by both drugs and X-rays.

The rays are part of the electro-magnetic spectrum; their wavelengths are between 10^{-9} and 10^{-13} metres; in behaviour and energy they are identical to the gamma rays emitted by radioactive isotopes. Diagnostic X-rays are generated in an evacuated tube contining an anode and cathode. Electrons striking the anode cause emission of X-rays of varying energy; the energy is largely dependent on the potential difference (kilovoltage) between anode and cathode. The altered tissue penetration at different kilovoltages is used in radiographing different regions, for example in breast radiography (25–40 kV) or chest radiography (120–150 kV). Most diagnostic examinations use kilovoltages between 60 and 120. The energy of X-rays enbles them to pass through body tissues unless they make contact with the constituent atoms. Tissue attenuation varies with atomic structure, so that air-containing organs such as the lung offer little attenuation, while material such as bone, with abundant calcium, will absorb the majority of incident X-rays. This results in an emerging X-ray pattern which corresponds to the structures in the region examined.

Radiography The recording of the resulting images is achieved in several ways, mostly depending on the use of materials which fluoresce in response to X-rays.

CONTRAST X-RAYS Many body organs are not shown by simple X-ray studies. This led to the development of contrast materials which make particular organs or structures wholly or partly opaque to X-rays. Thus barium-sulphate preparations are largely used for examining the gastro-intestinal tract, i.e. barium swallow, barium meal, barium follow-through (or enteroclysis) and barium enema. Water-soluble iodine-containing contrast agents that ionize in solution have been developed for a range of other studies.

More recently a series of improved contrast molecules, chiefly non-ionizing, has been developed, with fewer side-effects. They can, for example, safely be introduced into the spinal theca for myeloradiculography – contrast X-rays of the spinal cord. Using these agents, it is possible to show many organs and structures mostly by direct introduction, e.g. via a catheter. In urography, however, contrast medium injected intravenously is excreted by the kidneys which are outlined, together with ureters and bladder. A number of other more specialized contrast agents exist, e.g. for cholecystography – radiological assessment of the gall bladder. The use of contrast and the attendant techniques has greatly widened the range of radiology.

IMAGE INTENSIFICATION The relative insensitivity of fluorescent materials when used for observation of moving organs – e.g. the oesophagus – has been overcome by the use of image intensification. A faint fluorographic image produced by X-rays leads to electron emission from a photo-cathode. By applying a high potential difference, the electrons are accelerated across an evacuated tube and are focused on to a small fluorescent screen, giving a bright image. This is viewed by a TV camera and the image shown on a monitor and sometimes recorded on videotape or cine.

TOMOGRAPHY X-rays images are two-dimensional representations of three-dimensional objects. Tomography (Greek *tomos* – a slice) began with X-ray imaging produced by the linked movement of the X-ray tube and the cassette pivoting about a selected plane in the body: over- and underlying structures are blurred out, giving a more detailed image of a particular plane.

In 1975 Godfrey Hounsfield introduced computed tomography (CT). This involves (i) movement of an X-ray tube around the patient, with a narrow fan beam of X-rays; (ii) the corresponding use of sensitive detectors on the opposite side of the patient; (iii) computer analysis of the detector readings at each point on the rotation, with calculation of relative tissue attenuation at each point in the cross-sectional plant. This invention has enormously increased the ability to discriminate tissue composition, even without the use of contrast.

The tomographic effect – imaging of a particular plane – is achieved in many of the newer forms of imaging – ULTRASOUND, magnetic resonance imaging (see NUCLEAR MAGNETIC RESONANCE) and some forms of nuclear medicine, in particular POSITRON EMISSION TOMOGRAPHY (PET). An alternative term for the production of images of a given plane is cross-sectional imaging.

While the production of X-ray and other images has been largely the responsibility of radiographers, the interpretation has been principally carried out by specialist doctors called radiologists. In addition they, and interested clinicians, have developed a number of procedures, such as arteriography (see ANGIOGRAPHY), which involve manipulative access for imaging, e.g. selective coronary or renal arteriography.

The use of X-rays, ultrasound or computerized tomography to control the direction and position of needles has made possible quided biopsies, e.g. of pancreatic, pulmonary or bony lesions, and therapeutic procedures such as drainage of obstructed kidneys (percutaneous nephrostomy), or of abscesses. From these has grown a whole series of therapeutic procedures such as ANGIOPLASTY, STENT insertion and renal-stone track formation. This field of interventional radiology has close affinities with minimally invasive surgery.

Radiotherapy, or treatment by X-rays The two chief sources of the ionizing radiations used in radiotherapy are the gamma rays of RADIUM and the penetrating X-rays generated by apparatus working at various voltages. For superficial lesions energies of around 40 kilovolts are used, but for deep-seated conditions, such as cancer of the internal organs, much higher voltages are required. X-ray machines are now in use which work at two million volts. Even higher voltages are now available through the development of the linear accelerator, which makes use of the frequency magnetron which is the basis of radar. The linear accelerator receives its name from the fact that it accelerates a beam of electrons down a straight tube, 3 metres in length, and in this process a voltage of eight million is attained. The use of these very high voltages has led to the development of a highly specialized technique which has been devised for the treatment of cancer and like diseases.

Protective measures are routinely taken to ensure that the patient's normal tissue is not damaged during radiotherapy. The operators too have to take special precautions, including limits on the time they can work with the equipment in any one period of time.

The greatest value of radiotherapy is in the treatment of malignant disease. In many patients it can be used for the treatment of malignant growths which are not accessible to surgery, whilst in others it is used in conjunction with surgery and chemotherapy. (See RADIOTHERAPY.)

Y

YAWNING An involuntary opening of the mouth, which is accompanied by marked dilatation of the pharynx, a characteristic distortion of the face and usually stretching of the limbs. The cause and function of yawning are quite obscure. It is classically regarded as a sign of drowsiness or boredom, but it it may be the result of raised concentrations of CARBON DIOXIDE (CO_2) in the blood, the physiological aim being to cut the amount of CO_2 and raise the level of oxygen in the blood.

YAWS, known also as FRAMBOESIA and PIAN. A non-venereal spirochaetal infection caused by *Treponema pertenue*; it was formerly widespread in most tropical and subtropical regions amongst the indigenous population, florid disease being more common in children than adults. The term is of Carib-Indian (native to north-eastern South America, the east coast of Central America, and the lesser Antilles) origin. It is directly contagious from person to person; infection is also transmitted by flies, clothing, and living in unclean huts. Clinically, the primary stage is characterized by a granulomatous lesion, or papule (framboesioma or 'mother yaw') at the site of infection – usually the lower leg or foot; this enlarges, crusts, and heals spontaneously. It appears some 2–8 weeks after infection, during which time fever, malaise, pains, and pruritus may be present. In the secondary stage, a granulomatous, papular, macular or squamous eruption occurs; periostitis may also be present. The late, or tertiary stage (which appears 5–10 years later), is characterized by skin plaques, nodules, ulcers, hyperkeratosis (thickening of the skin of the hands and feet) and gummatous lesions affecting bones. Recurrence of infection in individuals suffering from a concurrent infection (e.g., SYPHILIS or TUBERCULOSIS) renders the infection more serious. Diagnosis is by demonstration of

T. pertenue in exudate from a suspected lesion. Treatment is with PENICILLIN, to which *T. pertenue* is highly sensitive. Extensive eradication campaigns (initiated by the WHO in 1949) have been carried out in endemic areas; therefore, the early stages of the infection are rarely counted; only tertiary stages come to the attention of a physician. Failure of surveillance can lead to dramatic local recurrences.

Y CHROMOSOME One of two sex chromosomes that is present in every male body cell where it is paired with an X chromosome. The sex or germ cells in women as well as men contain one X and one Y chromosome (see GENES; SEX CHROMOSOMES).

YEAST This consists of the cells and spores of unicellular fungi belonging to the family of Saccharomycetaceae. The main species of yeast used in medicine is *Saccharomyces cerevisiae*, which is used in the fermentation industries, such as brewing. It is a rich source of the vitamin B complex (see APPENDIX 5: VITAMINS), but its use has largely been given up since the various components of the vitamin B complex became available as separate entities.

YELLOW FEVER, also known as YELLOW JACK and VOMITO AMARILLI. An acute ARBOVIRUS infection caused by a flavivirus of the togavirus family, transmitted from animals to humans by various species of forest mosquito (jungle/sylvan yellow fever), and from human to human by *Aëdes aegypti* (urban yellow fever). Mosquito transmission was shown by Walter Reed and his colleagues in 1900. It is endemic in much of tropical Africa and Central and South America but does not occur in Asia. In the urban cycle, man constitutes the reservoir of infection, and in the jungle/sylvan variety, mammals – especially subhuman primates – are involved in transmission. Historically, yellow fever was enormously important, causing devastating epidemics; it also carried a high mortality rate in travellers and explorers. Differentiation from other infections associated with jaundice was often impossible.

Clinically, yellow fever is characterized by jaundice, fever, chills, headache, gastrointestinal haemorrhage(s), and albuminuria. The incubation period is 3–6 (up to 10) days. Differentiation from viral hepatitides, other viral haemorrhagic fevers, severe *Plasmodium falciparum* malaria, and several other infections is often impossible without sophisticated investigative techniques. Infection carries a high mortality rate. Liver histology (biopsy is contraindicated due to the haemorrhagic diathesis) shows characteristic changes; a fulminating hepatic infection is often present. Acute inflammation of the kidneys and an inflamed, congested gastric mucosa, often accompanied by haemorrhage, are also demonstrable; myocardial involvement often occurs. Diagnosis is primarily based on virological techniques; serological tests are also of value. Yellow fever should be suspected in any travellers from an endemic area. Management consists of instituting techniques for acute hepatocellular (liver-cell) failure. The affected individual should be kept in an isolation unit, away from mosquitoes which could transmit the disease to a healthy individual. Formerly, laboratory infections were occasionally acquired from infected blood samples. Prophylactically, a satisfactory attenuated vaccine (17D) has been available for around 60 years; this is given subcutaneously and provides an individual with excellent protection for 10 years; international certificates are valid for this length of time. Every traveller to an endemic area should be immunized; this is mandatory for entry to countries where the infection is endemic.

YERSINIA A genus of bacteria which includes the causative organism of plague, *Yersinia pestis*. (See PLAGUE.)

YIN AND YANG Basic concepts in traditional Chinese medicine and philosophy. Yang represents active, positive masculine qualities. Yin embodies passive, negative feminine qualities.

YOGA A system of Hindu philosophy and physical discipline involving special breathing techniques and a series of prescribed physical poses. These are intended to relax the body and teach the individual mental and physical control. Yoga is best learned from experienced teachers or those practising it may damage their backs.

YOGHURT Sour milk curdled with one of the lactic-acid producing bacilli, such as *Lactobacillus acidophilus* or *Lactobacillus bulgaricus*. It contains all the protein, fat, calcium, and vitamins of the original milk, and is therefore a nutritious food, but there is no evidence that it has any unique beneficial properties of its own. In countries where standards of hygiene are low it has the advantage of having been sterilized by boiling and is therefore unlikely to be contaminated with dangerous micro-organisms.

YOHIMBINE This substance is derived from the bark of *Pausinystalia yohimbie*, a West African tree. Once widely used as an aphrodisiac, an action for which there is no good evidence, it is now being used in the treatment of certain cases of postural HYPOTENSION and for the treatment of IMPOTENCE. It is an alpha adrenoreceptor agonist.

YTTRIUM-90 An artificially produced isotope of the element Yttrium. The isotope is radioactive and emits beta rays which are utilized for the treatment of tumours.

Z

ZIDOVUDINE An antiviral drug used to treat AIDS and its related conditions, such as pneumocystis PNEUMONIA. The drug slows down the growth of HUMAN IMMUNODEFICIENCY VIRUS (HIV) but does not cure the disease. It may be given intravenously or by mouth. The drug, also called AZT, has been in use since 1987, and it works by blocking the enzyme that simulates HIV to grow and multiply. It may cause anaemia so regular blood tests are necessary.

ZINC A metal, several salts of which are used in medicine for external application. It is essential for growth and development in animals and plants. The average human body contains a total of 1 to 2 grams, and most human diets contain 10 to 15 mg. In human beings, deficiency of zinc results in lack of growth, slow sexual development and anaemia. Deficiency is also associated with a skin disorder known as acrodermatitis enteropathica.

Uses Zinc chloride is a powerful caustic and astringent which, combined with zinc sulphate, is used as an astringent mouth-wash. Zinc sulphate is also used in the form of eye-drops in the treatment of certain forms of conjunctivitis. (See EYE DISEASES.)

Zinc oxide, zinc stearate, and zinc carbonate are made up in dusting powders, in ointments, in paste bandages or suspended in water as lotions for the astringent action they exert upon abraded surfaces of the skin. Zinc and castor oil ointment of the *British Pharmacopoeia* is a well-tried treatment for napkin rash.

Zinc undecenoate is used as an ointment and as a dusting-powder in the treatment of RINGWORM .

ZOLLINGER-ELLISON SYNDROME A rare disorder in which severe PEPTIC ulcers recur in the stomach and duodenum (see DUODENAL ULCER; STOMACH, DISEASES OF). It is caused by a tumour in the pancreas that produces a hormone GASTRIN which stimulates the stomach and duodenum to produce excess acid and this causes ulceration. Treatment is by surgery.

ZONA and **ZOSTER** Two names for the eruption popularly known as shingles. (See HERPES ZOSTER.)

ZONULOLYSIS The process whereby the zonule (see EYE) is dissolved by an enzyme (chymotrypsin) as part of intracapsular cataract surgery. Once the zonule has been dissolved the cataract can be lifted out of the eye (see CATARACT).

ZOONOSES Animal diseases which can be transmitted to man. There are over 150 infections of domestic and wild vertebrates which can be transmitted in this way, including BOVINE

SPONGIFORM ENCEPHALOPATHY, bovine tuberculosis, BRUCELLOSIS, HYDATID CYSTS, RINGWORM, TOXOCARIASIS, TOXOPLASMOSIS, LEPTOSPIROSIS, LISTERIOSIS, and RABIES. (See separate entries for details of these diseases.)

ZYGOMA or ZYGOMATIC BONE The name given to a bridge of bone formed by the union of a process from the temporal bone with one from the malar bone. It lies in the region of the temple, gives attachment to the powerful masseter muscle which moves the lower jaw, and forms a protection to the side of the head.

ZYGOTE This is the cell produced when an OVUM is fertilized by a SPERM. A zygote contains all the hereditary material for a new individual: half comes from the sperm and half from the ovum. After passing down the fallopian tube, when the zygote starts dividing, it becomes implanted in the UTERUS and develops into an embryo.

APPENDIX 1: BASIC FIRST AID

This appendix is designed to cover the basic principles involved in the immediate treatment of some common emergencies. It is not comprehensive, and anyone wishing to become proficient at first aid should attend a course run by a reputable organization such as the British Red Cross, St John Ambulance, and the St Andrew's Ambulance Association (see APPENDIX 2: ADDRESSES)

First-aid treatment in an emergency is intended:
- to preserve life and stop the victim's condition from deteriorating.
- to help recovery and save the victim from further harm.
- to make the casualty as comfortable as possible and reassure him/her and the family.
- to assess the events surrounding the illness or accident so that relevant facts can be given to a doctor, nurse or paramedical staff.

No ill or badly injured person should be moved without skilled assistance – especially if a neck or spinal injury is suspected – unless the individual's life is in immediate danger from the surroundings, for example, a fire. He or she should be kept warm; constricting clothing should be loosened; and a clear airway should be established, with any false teeth removed.

BLEEDING This may occur from arteries, veins or capillary beds. The former is easily recognized as the blood tends to spurt from the wound at the same rate as the pulse. With the latter two types the blood tends to flow from the wound. Minor bleeding is usually treated in the home by the application of bandages, etc. However, the basic principles of treatment for major haemorrhages may be applied. Pressure should be applied to the bleeding point, via gauze or a clean piece of cloth if available, firmly enough to stop the flow of blood. With the pressure applied, the wound should be raised above the level of the heart. The patient should then be transferred to a place where medical care is available. If the loss of blood is severe enough for the victim to have become shocked, he or she should be laid flat with the legs raised, if possible.

BURNS All but the most minor burns should be seen by a doctor as it is difficult to assess the severity of the burn immediately after it occurs. If the person or his or her clothing is actually on fire, then the first move must be to smother the flames by covering them with a blanket or coat, for example, and 'patting out' the flames without sustaining burns yourself. Many burns, however, are caused by hot liquids, hot gases, flashes from explosions or contact with a very hot object so that the person is not actually on fire. The treatment for all these burns is the same – to remove any clothing over the affected area, if possible, and to put the affected area under cold running water until the pain has stopped or the ambulance has arrived (the cold water should be applied for several minutes as cooling of the tissues, particularly the deeper layers of the skin, will limit the extent of the burn). The burn should be left exposed or covered with a piece of clean wet linen, e.g. a pillowcase, for the transfer to hospital. No lotions or potions should be applied to the burn until it has been seen by a doctor or a nurse.

CHOKING Severe life-threatening choking occurs when a piece of food or a foreign object becomes lodged in the LARYNX or TRACHEA causing obstruction. The person may cough, gag, or wheeze and will become cyanosed (blue) as he or she fights to take a breath. Infants or small children should be held along the arm, head down, and several gentle blows with the flat of the hand should be delivered to the back between the shoulder blades. This will usually dislodge the foreign body. In older children or adults the Heimlich Manoeuvre should be employed. Stand behind the victim with your arms wrapped around the waist. Make a fist with one hand with the thumb placed at a point half way between the victim's navel and the bottom of the breastbone. Grasp the fist with your other hand and give a quick inward and upward thrust. This may be repeated several times if necessary. Alternatively, if the person is unconscious, he or she should be placed on the back, face up and the same thrust performed with the heel of the hand whilst kneeling astride the hips. If a choking person is alone, he or she can perform the manoeuvre by placing a fist in the correct position and delivering the thrust by pressing it against a firm surface.

CARDIAC/RESPIRATORY ARREST The measures described here are basic life-support procedures – they can be performed if necessary without any equipment. Before commencing cardiopulmonary resuscitation on a person who has collapsed, it is essential to establish that it is required. Performing artificial ventilation and cardiac massage on a person who is breathing and whose heart is still beating can be dangerous. The person's chest and abdomen should be observed for respiratory movement and the pulse should be checked either at the neck or groin or by feeling directly over the heart.

The technique for simple resuscitation may be remembered by means of the mnemonic 'ABC (Airway, Breathing and Circulation)'. The aim of basic resuscitation is to maintain the flow of oxygenated blood to vital organs until the person's heartbeat and breathing can be restarted, if that is possible.

AIRWAY If the airway is obstructed, no air can enter the lungs; therefore the mouth should be checked for foreign bodies, which can be removed by hooking them out with an index finger. False teeth should be removed. To prevent the tongue from obstructing breathing, the jaw should be pulled forward (using a finger behind the angle or the chin) and the head extended on the neck so that the person looks as if he or she is 'sniffing the morning air'.

> Care must be taken if there is any suspicion of neck injury.

Breathing If clearing the airway does not allow breathing to recommence, then artificial ventilation of the lungs must be started. Mouth-to-mouth ventilation, using the rescuer's expired air to inflate the victim's lungs, is probably the easiest and most satisfactory to use. The victim is positioned as described above. The rescuer uses one hand to obstruct the nose and steady the head and the other to pull the jaw forward and open the mouth. The rescuer then places his or her mouth completely over that of the victim and blows out so as to inflate the victim's lungs, starting with two slow breaths to reinflate the lungs. It is important to observe the victim's chest rise and fall normally before commencing the next breath. If the chest does not rise or there is marked resistance to the inflating breath, then the airway is probably obstructed and the head should be repositioned.

CIRCULATION Ventilating the lungs without any blood's circulating will not provide oxygenated blood to vital organs. Therefore, if there is no pulse or heartbeat, cardiac massage should be started to produce this circulation. The person performing cardiac massage, who should preferably have been trained in the technique, should kneel beside the victim with the heel of one hand over the lower two-thirds of the breastbone and the other hand placed on top. Downward pressure is applied, keeping the arms straight with the elbows locked, so as to depress the breastbone 4–5 cm. Pressure is released slowly so that it takes the same time as compression. The rate of compressions should be 80 per minute. If there are two rescuers, then the person performing cardiac massage should stop after every five compressions to allow the other to perform one cycle of artificial ventilation. A lone rescuer should perform two breaths after every 15 compressions.

Once spontaneous ventilation and cardiac output have returned, the patient should be placed in the recovery, or coma, position. This consists of rolling the person on to his or her side, with the lower arm and leg straight and in line with the body. The upper arm and leg are flexed and brought forward to prevent the patient from rolling on to his or her front.

DROWNING About 500 people die from drowning each year in Britain, and an unknown number survive a near drowning. About a fifth of drownings occur in salt water. Wet drowning (when water is aspirated into the lungs) occurs in 85 per cent of cases. The remaining 15 per cent develop laryngo-spasm so that, although they also die of asphyxia, no water enters the lungs.

There has been some controversy about what type of water carries the worst prognosis, but it is now thought that salt and fresh water are equally bad. The effect of salt water is to draw fluid into the alveoli from the vascular compartment with concomitant damage to the lung. This results in pulmonary oedema and HYPOXIA. Fresh water washes out pulmonary surfactant (causing pulmonary atelectasis and leading to hypoxia) and is absorbed into the vascular compartment causing volume overload and electrolyte disturbances. Both types may result in ACIDOSIS and circulatory collapse and may be complicated by HYPOTHERMIA and trauma (which may have precipitated the drowning).

Treatment Cardiopulmonary resuscitation (see CARDIAC/RESPIRATORY ARREST in this Appendix) should be started as soon as possible and the patient transferred to hospital. This should include people who recover consciousness fairly quickly as pulmonary oedema may develop over the next few hours. If the patient is hypothermic, resuscitation should continue until he or she has been warmed to normal body temperature. Patients may require admission to an intensive care unit for artificial ventilation, circulatory support, or correction of electrolyte imbalance or acidosis.

ELECTROCUTION People may be electrocuted when they touch an object which is live so that a current passes through them to earth. A lightning strike has a similar effect. The severity of the outcome depends on the frequency and amplitude of the current which flows through them. Below 2mA there is only a feeling of strong PARAESTHESIA, 15–100mA will produce muscular contraction in the muscles near the point of contact, which makes letting go of the object impossible, and 50mA–2A is the threshold for producing VENTRICULAR FIBRILLATION. [These thresholds are for the mains electricity supply, which in Britain has a frequency of 50Hz, a frequency that is particularly liable to induce ventricular fibrillation]. Thus electrocution can cause burns to the tissues at the sites where the current enters and leaves the body and may also induce ventricular fibrillation. If a person is seen being electrocuted, no attempt should be made to touch the victim until the power supply is turned off, as the helper may also be electrocuted. If the switch or mains supply cannot be found, then the victim should be knocked away from the power source using a non-conducting object such as wood. Burns should be treated as described above and, if the patient has developed ventricular fibrillation, then cardiopulmonary resuscitation should be started (see CARDIAC/RESPIRATORY ARREST in this Appendix). Any person experiencing significant electrocution should be seen by a doctor.

POISONING The number of substances with which people are poisoned, either deliberately or accidentally, is too great to list individually. This section will merely cover some basic principles to follow on discovering a person who has been poisoned.

If the person is unconscious, he or she should be nursed in the coma position [see CARDIAC/RESPIRATORY ARREST in this Appendix]. Vomiting should never be induced at home except under medical supervision. If corrosive substances have been ingested, then water or milk should be drunk to dilute the effects on the oesophagus and stomach, and any remaining on the skin should be washed away with copious volumes of water. The container from which the tablets or other substance came should be taken to hospital with the patient to help medical staff correctly identify the poison.

Likewise if it is a plant, a leaf or berry should be taken to hospital. (See POISONS.)

SEIZURES A major seizure or fit is known as a Grand Mal convulsion and consists of two phases: the tonic phase when the person may let out a cry, falls to the ground and is observed to be rigid, and the clonic phase when he or she shakes. At the end of the fit there is usually a period of unconsciousness. The most important task in looking after people undergoing a fit is to prevent them from doing any damage to themselves. Any objects which might cause harm, particularly hot food and liquids, should be moved out of their way, but there is no need to try to move them unless they are in danger. It may, however, be necessary to roll the patient on to his or her side to prevent asphyxiation. No attempt should be made to protect the tongue, and a finger should not be inserted to straighten the tongue. Clothing around the patient's neck should be loosened and, if possible, a pillow placed under the neck. At the end of the fit, when the person is unconscious, he or she should be placed in the coma or recovery position (see CARDIAC/RESPIRATORY ARREST).

APPENDIX 2: ADDRESSES: Sources of information, advice, support and self-help

Addresses for other information and support groups can be found in the *Voluntary Agencies Directory* (published by NCVO Publications, National Council for Voluntary Organisations, Regent's Wharf, 8 All Saints Street, London N1 9RL, telephone: 0171–713 6161, distribution: 01536–399016). Telephone helpline numbers can be found in the *Telephone Helplines Directory* (published by the Telephone Helplines Association, 4 Dean's Court, St Paul's Churchyard, London EC4V 5AA, telephone: 0171–248 3388, fax: 0171–248 3399).

Telephone area-code changes From mid-1999 new area codes will come into use for Cardiff, Coventry, Portsmouth, Southampton and London. Northern Ireland numbers will also be affected. In London 0171 numbers will have a new code: 0207, and 0181 numbers: 0208. Helpline numbers which use a special free, national or local rate will also be changing to codes beginning 08–. Details can be obtained from BT help desks on 0808–224 2000 (business) or 0808–731 0202 (residential).

ACCIDENT PREVENTION IN THE HOME Child Accident Prevention Trust, Clarkes Court, 18–20 Farringdon Lane, London EC1R 3HA (0171–608 3828, fax: 0171–608 3674).

Royal Society for the Prevention of Accidents, Edgbaston Park, 353 Bristol Road, Birmingham B5 7ST (0121–248 2000, fax: 0121–248 2001).

ADOPTION See CHILD ADOPTION.

AGEING Age Concern England, Astral House, 1268 London Road, Norbury, London SW16 4ER (0181–765 7200, 0181–679 8000, fax: 0181–765 7211, 0181–679 6069).

AGORAPHOBIA See PHOBIAS.

AIDS National Aids Helpline: 0800–555777. Information leaflets: 0800–567123.

London Lighthouse, 111/117 Lancaster Road, London W11 1QT (0171–792 1200, fax: 0171–229 1258).

Communicable Diseases Surveillance Centre (PHLS), 61 Colindale Avenue, London NW9 5EQ.

ALCOHOL Alcoholics Anonymous, PO Box 1, Stonebow House, Stonebow, York YO1 2NJ (01904–644026, fax: 01904–629091).

Al-Anon Family Groups UK and Eire (including Alateen), 61 Great Dover Street, London SE1 4YF (0171–403 0888, fax: 0171–378 9910).

Alcohol Concern, Waterbridge House, 32–36 Loman Street, London SE1 0EE (0171–928 7377, fax: 0171–928 4644).

Scottish Council on Alcohol, 166 Buchanan Street, Glasgow G1 2NH (0141–333 9677, fax: 0141–333 1606).

Accept (community services for problem drinkers and tranquillizer misusers), 724 Fulham Road, London SW6 5SE (0171–371 7477).

ALZHEIMER'S DISEASE Alzheimer's Disease Society, 2nd floor, Gordon House, 10 Greencoat Place, London SW1P 1PH (0171–306 0606, fax: 0171–308 0808).

ANOREXIA See EATING DISORDERS.

ARTHRITIS Arthritis Care, 18 Stephenson Way, London NW1 2HD (0171–916 1500, helpline 0800–289170 weekdays 12.00–16.00, fax: 0171–916 1505).

ANKYLOSING SPONDYLITIS National Association for Ankylosing Spondylitis, PO Box 179, Mayfield, East Sussex TN20 6ZL (01435–873527, fax: 01435–873027).

ASH (ACTION ON SMOKING AND HEALTH) ASH, 109 Gloucester Place, London W1H 4EJ (0171–935 3519, fax: 0171–935 3463).

ASTHMA National Asthma Campaign, Providence House, Providence Place, London N1 0NT (0171–226 2260, helpline 0345–010203, fax: 0171–704 0740).

ATAXIA Ataxia, Copse Edge, Thursley Road, Elstead, Godalming, Surrey GU8 6DJ (01252–702864, fax: 01252–703715).

AUTISM National Autistic Society, 276 Willesden Lane, London NW2 5RB (0181–451 1114, fax: 0181–451 5865).

BACKACHE National Back Pain Association, 16 Elmtree Road, Teddington, Middlesex TW11 8TD (0181–977 5474, fax: 0181–943 5318).

BACUP See CANCER INFORMATION SERVICE.

BLINDNESS Royal National Institute for the Blind, 224 Great Portland Street, London W1N 6AA (0171–388 1266, fax: 0171–388 2034).

BLOOD TRANSFUSION National Blood Authority, Oak House, Reeds Crescent, Watford, Herts WD1 1QH (01923–486800, fax: 01923–486801). The authority is responsible for 15 regional transfusion centres in England.

BRAIN INJURIES Headway National Head Injuries Association, 4 King Edward Court, King Edward Street, Nottingham NG1 1EW (0115–924 0800, fax: 0115–958 4446).

BREAST CANCER CARE Breast Cancer Care, Kiln House, 210 New Kings Road, London SW6 4NZ (freeline 0500–245 345; administration: 0171–384 2984, fax: 0171–384 3387).

BRITTLE BONE DISEASE Brittle Bone Society, 30 Guthrie Street, Dundee DD1 5BS (01382–204446, fax: 01382–20677).

CALIBRE See TALKING BOOKS.

CANCER CARE Marie Curie Cancer Care, 28 Belgrave Square, London SW1X 8QG (0171–235 3325, fax: 0171–823 2380).

Macmillan Cancer Relief, Anchor House, 15/19 Britten Street, London SW3 3TZ (0171–351 7511, fax: 0171–376 8098).

CANCER INFORMATION SERVICE Cancer BACUP, 3 Bath Place, Rivington Street, London EC2A 3JR (0171–696 9003, fax: 0171–696 9002; information service, from outside London: 0800–181199; London: 0171–613 2121, counselling service: 0171–696 9000).

CARERS Carers National Association, 20–25 Glasshouse Yard, London EC1A 4JS (0171–490 8818, fax: 0171–490 8824).

Women's Royal Voluntary Service, 234–244 Stockwell Road, London SW9 9SP (0171–416 0146, fax: 0171–416 0148).

CARE SERVICES Counsel and Care, Twyman House, 16 Bonny Street, London NW1 9PG (0171–485 1566, fax: 0171–267 6877). See also CARERS.

CEREBRAL PALSY SCOPE, 6 Market Road, London N7 9PW (0171–636 5020, fax: 0171–619 7399).

Capability Scotland, 22 Corstorphine Road, Edinburgh EH12 6HP (0131–337 9876, fax: 0131–346 7864).

CHILD ADOPTION British Agencies for Adoption and Fostering (BAAF), Skyline House, 200 Union Street, London SE1 0LX (0171–593 2000, fax: 0171–593 2001).

Parent to Parent Information on Adoptive Services (PPIAS), Lower Boddington, Daventry, Northamptonshire NN11 6YB (01327–60295, fax: 01327–263 565).

National Organization for Counselling Adoptees and Parents, 3 New High Street, Headington, Oxford OX3 7AJ (01865–875000).

Adoptions Section, Office for National Statistics, Smedley Hydro, Trafalgar Road, Birkdale, Southport PR8 2HH (0151–471 4313, fax: 0151–471 4755).

CHILDBIRTH National Childbirth Trust, Alexandra House, Oldham Terrace, Acton, London W3 6NH (0181–992 8637, fax: 0181–992 5929).

CHILDREN Action for Sick Children (National Association for the Welfare of Children in Hospital), Argyle House, 29–31 Euston Road, London NW1 2SD (0171–833 2041), fax: 0171–837 2110.

National Society for the Prevention of Cruelty to Children (NSPCC), NSPCC National Centre, 42 Curtain Road, London EC2A 3NH (0171–825 2500, fax: 0171–825 2525).

NCH Action for Children, 85 Highbury Park, London N5 1UD (0171–226 2033, fax: 0171–226 2537.

CHIROPODY Society of Chiropodists and Podologists, 53 Welbeck Street, London W1M 7HE (0171–486 3381, fax: 0171–935 6359).

CHIROPRACTIC See APPENDIX 13: COMPLEMENTARY MEDICINE.

CLEFT LIP AND PALATE See PALATE MALFORMATIONS.

COELIAC DISEASE Coeliac Society of the United Kingdom, PO Box 220, High Wycombe, Bucks. HP11 2HY (01494–437278, fax: 01494–474349).

COLITIS AND CROHN'S DISEASE National Association for Colitis and Crohn's Disease, PO Box 205, St Albans, Herts. (01727–844296).

COLOSTOMY British Colostomy Association, 15 Station Road, Reading, Berkshire RG1 1LG (0118–939 1537, fax: 0118–956 9095).

CORONARY HEART DISEASE Coronary Prevention Group, Plantation House, Suite 514 D & M, 31–35 Fenchurch Street, London EC3M 3NN (0171–626 4844, fax: 0171–626 4748).

CYSTIC FIBROSIS Cystic Fibrosis Trust, 11 London Road, Bromley, Kent BR1 1BY (0181–464 7211, fax: 0181–313 0472).

DEAFNESS Royal National Institute for Deaf People, 19–23 Featherstone Street, London EC1Y 8SL (0171–296 8000, fax: 0171–296 8199).

Defeating Deafness (Hearing Research Trust), 330–332 Gray's Inn Road, London WC1X 8EE (0171–833 1733, fax: 0171–278 0404).

Sense (National Deaf Blind and Rubella Association), 11–13 Clifton Terrace, Finsbury Park, London N4 3RS (0171–272 7774, fax: 0171–272 6012).

Sense in Scotland, 5th Floor, 45 Pinnieston Street, Clydeway Centre, Glasgow G3 8JU (0141–564 2444, fax: 0141–564 2443).

National Deaf Children's Society, 15 Dufferin Street, London EC1Y 8UR (0171–490 8656, information and helpline: 0171–250 0123, fax: 0171–251 5020).

DERMATITIS National Eczema Society, 163 Eversholt Street, London NW1 1BU (0171–388 4097, fax: 0171–388 5882).

DIABETES British Diabetic Association, 10 Queen Anne Street, London W1M 0BD (0171–323 1531, fax: 0171–637 3644).

DISABLED LIVING Disabled Living Foundation, 380–384 Harrow Road, London W9 2HU (0171–289 6111, fax: 0171–266 2922).

British Red Cross, 9 Grosvenor Crescent, London SW1X 7EJ (0171–235 5454, fax: 0171–245 6315).

National Demonstration Centre, Department of Postgraduate Education Services, Pinderfields General Hospital, Aberford Road, Wakefield WF1 4DG (01924–814856, fax: 01924–814546).

Disability Scotland, Information Department, Princes House, 5 Shandwick Place, Edinburgh EH2 4RG (0131–229 8632, fax: 0131–229 5168).

Motability, Goodman House, Station Approach, Harlow, Essex CM20 2ET (01279–635666, fax: 01279–632000).

Royal Society for Disability and Rehabilitation (RADAR), 12 City Forum, 250 City Road, London EC1V 8AF (0171–250 3222, fax: 0171–250 0212).

Shaftesbury Society, 16 Kingston Road, London SW19 1JZ (0181–542 5550, fax: 0181–545 0605).

DONORS National Blood Transfusion Service: 0345–711711, fax: 0181–258 8541.

National Blood Authority, Oak House, Reeds Crescent, Watford, Herts. WD1 1QH (01923–486800, fax: 01923–486801).

HM Inspector of Anatomy, Department of Health, Wellington House, 133–155 Waterloo Road, London SE1 8UG.

British Organ Donor Society, Balsham, Cambridge CB1 6DL (tel. and fax: 01223–893636).

DOWN'S SYNDROME Down's Syndrome Association, 155 Mitcham Road, London SW17 9PG (0181–682 4001, fax: 0181–682 4012).

DRUG ADDICTION National Helpline: 0800 776600.

DYSLEXIA British Dyslexia Association, 98 London Road, Reading, Berkshire RG1 5AU (01734–668271, weekdays 10.00–12.00, 14.00–17.00).

DYSPHASIA Action for Dysphasic Adults, 1 Royal Street, London SE1 7LL (0171–261 9572, fax: 0171–928 9542).

Stroke Association, Stroke House, 123–127 Whitecross Street, London EC1Y 8JJ (0171–490 7999, fax: 0171–490 2686).

DYSTONIA Dystonia Society, 46–47 Britton Street, London EC1M 5NA (0171–490 5671, fax: 0171–490 5672).

EATING DISORDERS Eating Disorders Association, 1st Floor, Wensum House, 103 Prince of Wales Road, Norwich NR1 1DW (01603–619090, helpline 01603–621414 Monday–Friday 9.00–18.30; under-18 helpline 01603–765050 Monday–Friday 16.00–18.00; fax: 01603–664915).

ECLAMPSIA AND PRE-ECLAMPSIA Action on Pre-eclampsia (APEC), 31–33 College Road, Harrow, Middlesex HA1 1EJ (0181–863 3271, helpline (Monday to Friday 10.00–13.00, recorded advice at other times): 0181–427 4217, fax: 0181–424 0653).

ECZEMA See DERMATITIS.

EPILEPSY British Epilepsy Association, Anstey House, 40 Hanover Square, Leeds LS3 1BE (0113–243 9393, fax: 0113–242 8804).

Epilepsy Association of Scotland, 48 Govan Road, Glasgow G51 1JL (0141–427 4911, helpline: 0141–427 5225, fax: 0141–427 7414).

FAMILY PLANNING Family Planning Association, 27–35 Mortimer Street, London W1N 7RJ (0171–636 7866, fax: 0171–436 5723.

FIRST AID British Red Cross, 9 Grosvenor Crescent, London SW1X 7EF (0171–235 5454, fax: 0171–245 6315).

St John Ambulance, 1 Grosvenor Crescent, London SW1X 7EF (0171–235 5231, fax: 0171–235 0796).

St Andrew's Ambulance Association, Strachan House, 16 Torphichen Street, Edinburgh EH3 8JB (0131–229 5419, fax: 0131–228 2424).

HAEMOPHILIA Haemophilia Society, Chesterfield House, 385 Euston Road, London NW1 3AU (0171–380 0600, fax: 0171–387 8220).

HEAD INJURIES See BRAIN INJURIES.

HEALTH AND SAFETY Health and Safety Executive, 2 Southwark Bridge, Rose Court, London SE1 9HS (0171–717 6104, fax: 0171–717 6134).

HEALTH EDUCATION Health Education Authority, Trevelyan House, 30 Great St Peter Street, London SW1P 2HW (0171–222 5300, fax: 0171–413 8900).

HEARING AIDS See DEAFNESS.

HOMEOPATHY See APPENDIX 13: COMPLEMENTARY MEDICINE.

HOSPITAL FRIENDS National Association of Leagues of Hospital Friends, 2nd floor, Fairfax House, Causton Road, Colchester, Essex CO1 1RJ (01206–761227, fax: 01206–560244).

HUNTINGTON'S CHOREA Huntington's Disease Association, 108 Battersea High Street, London SW11 3HP (0171–223 7000).

ILEITIS See COLITIS AND CROHN'S DISEASE.

ILEOSTOMY Ileostomy Association of Great Britain and Ireland, PO Box 132, Scunthorpe DN15 9YW (01724–720150, fax: 01724–721601).

LARYNGECTOMY National Association of Laryngectomee Clubs (NALC), Ground Floor, 6 Rickett Street, Fulham, London SW6 1RU (0171–381 9993, fax: 0171–381 0025).

LEARNING DISABILITY Mental Health Foundation, 20–21 Cornwall Terrace, London NW1 4QL (0171–535 7400, fax: 0171–535 7474).

British Institute of Learning Disabilities, Wolverhampton Road, Kidderminster, Worcs. DY10 3PP (01562–850421, switchboard: 01562–850461, fax: 01562–851970).

MENCAP (Royal Society for Mentally Handicapped Children and Adults), 123 Golden Lane, London EC1Y 0RT (0171–454 0454, fax: 0171–608 3254).

ENABLE (Scottish Society for the Mentally Handicapped), 7 Buchanan Street, Glasgow G1 3HL (0141–226 4541, fax: 0141–204 4398).

LUPUS   Lupus UK, St James House, Eastern Road, Romford, Essex RM1 3NH (01708–731251, fax: 01708–731252).

MARRIAGE GUIDANCE   See RELATE.

MASSAGE   Chartered Society of Physiotherapy, 14 Bedford Row, London WC1R 4ED (0171–306 6666, fax: 0171–306 6611).

MASTECTOMY   See BREAST CANCER CARE.

MEDICAL ACCIDENTS   Action for the Victims of Medical Accidents, Bank Chambers, 1 London Road, Forest Hill, London SE23 3TP (0181–291 2793).

MENINGITIS   National Meningitis Trust, Fern House, Bath Road, Stroud, Glos. GL5 3TJ (01453–751738, 24-hour support line: 0345–538118, fax: 01453–753788).

MENTAL HEALTH   MIND (National Association for Mental Health), Granta House, 15–19 Broadway, Stratford, London E15 4BQ (0181–519 2122, fax: 0181–522 1725).

Mental Aftercare Association (MACA), 25 Bedford Square, London WC1B 3HW (0171–436 6194).

Mental Health Foundation, 37 Mortimer Street, London W1N 8JU (0171–535 7400, fax: 0171–535 7474).

Mental Health Act Commission, Maid Marian House, 56 Houndsgate, Nottingham NG1 6BG (0115–943 100, fax: 0115–943 101).

NSF (National Schizophrenia Fellowship), 28 Castle Street, Kingston-upon-Thames, Surrey KT1 1SS (0181–547 3937, fax: 0181–547 3862).

See ALZHEIMER'S DISEASE.

MIGRAINE   Migraine Action Association (British Migraine Association), 178a High Road, Byfleet, West Byfleet, Surrey KT14 7ED (01932–352468, fax: 01932–351257).

MOTOR NEURONE DISEASE   See PARALYSIS.

MULTIPLE BIRTHS   TAMBA (Twins and Multiple Births Association), PO Box 30, Little Sutton, South Wirral L66 1TH (0151–348 0020, TAMBA Twinline: 01732–868000, fax: 0151–348 0765).

MULTIPLE SCLEROSIS   Multiple Sclerosis Society of Great Britain and Northern Ireland, 25 Effie Road, Fulham, London SW6 1EE (0171–610 7171, helpline: 0171–371 8000, fax: 0171–736 9861, counselling service, London: 0171–222 3123, 24 hours; Midlands: 0121–476 4229; Scotland: 0131–226 6573).

Multiple Sclerosis Resource Centre, 4a Chapel Hill, Stansted, Essex CM24 8AG (01279-817101).

SPOD (Association to Aid the Sexual and Personal Relationships of People with a Disability), 286 Camden Road, London N7 0BJ (0171–607 8851, counselling line times Tuesdays and Thursdays 10.30 to 13.30, Wednesdays 13.30 to 16.30, fax: 0171–700 1236).

MUSCULAR DYSTROPHY   Muscular Dystrophy Group of Great Britain, 7/11 Prescott Place, London SW4 6BS (0171–720 8055, fax: 0171–498 0670).

MYALGIC ENCEPHALITIS   ME Association, PO Box 8, 4a Corringham Road, Stanford-le-Hope, Essex SS17 0HA (01375–361479, advice line 01375–361013, fax: 01375–360256).

MYASTHENIA GRAVIS   Myasthenia Gravis Association, Keynes House, Chester Park, Alfreton Road, Derby DE21 4AS (01332–290219, fax: 01332–293641).

MYOPATHY   See MUSCULAR DYSTROPHY.

NARCOLEPSY   Narcolepsy Association (UK), 2 Bishops Close, Hurstpierpoint, Hassocks, West Sussex BN6 9XU (tel. and fax: 01273–832725).

NATIONAL LISTENING LIBRARY   See TALKING BOOKS.

NOTIFIABLE DISEASES   See AIDS.

NURSING   Royal College of Nursing, 20 Cavendish Square, London W1M 0AB (0171–409 3333, fax: 0171–647 3435).

OSTEOARTHRITIS   See ARTHRITIS.

OSTEOGENESIS IMPERFECTA   See BRITTLE BONE DISEASE.

OSTEOPATHY   See APPENDIX 13: COMPLEMENTARY MEDICINE.

OSTEOPOROSIS   National Osteoporosis Society, PO Box 10, Radstock, Bath BA3 3YB (01761–471771, fax: 01761–471104).

PAGET'S DISEASE   National Association for the Relief of Paget's Disease, 1 Church Road, Eccles, Manchester M30 0DL (0161–707 9225, fax: 0161–789 6755).

PALATE MALFORMATIONS   Cleft Lip and Palate Association, 1 Eastwood Gardens, Kenton, Newcastle-upon-Tyne NE3 3DQ (0191–285 9396).

Dental and Maxillofacial Department, Hospital for Sick Children, Great Ormond Street, London WC1N 3JH.

PARALYSIS Spinal Injuries Association, 76 St James's Lane, Muswell Hill, London N10 3DF (0181–444 2121, fax: 0181–444 3761).

Spinal Injuries Scotland, Festival Business Centre, 150 Brand Street, Glasgow G51 1DH (tel. and fax: 0141–314 0056).

Motor Neurone Disease Association, PO Box 246, Northampton NN1 2PR (01604–622269, fax: 01604–624726).

PARKINSONISM Parkinson's Disease Society of the UK, 215 Vauxhall Bridge Road, London SW1V 1EJ (0171–931 8080, fax: 0171–233 9908).

PHENYLKETONURIA National Society for Phenylketonuria (UK) Ltd, 7 Southfield Close, Willen, Milton Keynes MK15 9LL (0845–603 9136).

PHOBIAS National Phobics Society, 407 Wilbraham Road, Chorlton, Manchester M21 0UT (0161–881 1937).

PITUITARY-LINKED CONDITIONS Pituitary Foundation, PO Box 1944, Bristol BS99 2UB (tel. and fax: 0117–927 3355).

POISONS National Poisons Information Service (by telephone):
Belfast 01232–24905
Birmingham 0121–554 3801
Cardiff 01222–709 901
Dublin 00–353 18 379966
Edinburgh 0131–536 2300
Leeds 0113–243 0715
London 0171–635 9191
Newcastle 0191–232 5131

PSORIASIS Psoriasis Association, Milton House, 7 Milton Street, Northampton NN2 7JG (01604–711129, fax: 01604–792894).

RELATE National Relate, Herbert Gray College, Little Church Street, Rugby, Warwickshire CV21 3AP (01788–573241, fax: 01788–535007).

RESTRICTED GROWTH Restricted Growth Association (RGA), PO Box 18, Rugeley, Staffs. WS15 2GH (tel. and fax: 01889–576571).

SICKLE-CELL ANAEMIA Sickle Cell Society, 54 Station Road, Harlesden, London NW10 4UA (0181–961 7795/4006, fax: 0181–961 8346).

SPEECH DISORDERS AFASIC (Unlocking Speech and Language), 347 Central Markets, Smithfield, London EC1A 9NH (0171–236 6487, helpline: 0171–236 3632, fax: 0171–236 8115).

SPEECH THERAPY Royal College of Speech and Language Therapists, 7 Bath Place, Rivington Street, London EC2A 3DR (0171–613 3855, fax: 0171–613 3854).

SPINA BIFIDA Association for Spina Bifida and Hydrocephalus, ASBAH House, 42 Park Road, Peterborough PE1 2UQ (01733–555988, fax: 01733–555985).

Scottish Spina Bifida Association, 190 Queensferry Road, Edinburgh EH4 2BW (0131–332 0743, fax: 0131–343 3651).

SPINE AND SPINAL CORD DISEASES See ANKYLOSING SPONDYLITIS.

STAMMERING BSA (British Stammering Association), 15 Old Ford Road, London E2 9PJ (0181–983 1003, helpline: 0845–603 2001, fax: 0181–983 3591).

STOMA See COLOSTOMY and ILEOSTOMY.

STROKE See DYSPHASIA.

SUDDEN INFANT DEATH SYNDROME Foundation for the Study of Sudden Infant Deaths, 14 Halkin Street, London SW1X 7DP (0171–235 0965, 24-hour helpline: 0171–235 1721, fax: 0171–923 1986).

TALKING BOOKS Calibre, Aylesbury, Bucks. HP22 5XQ (01296–432339, fax: 01296–392599).

Listening Books, 12 Lant Street, London SE1 1QH (0171–407 9417, fax: 0171–403 1377).

TINNITUS See DEAFNESS.

TOY LIBRARIES The National Association of Toy and Leisure Libraries/Playmatters, 68 Churchway, London NW1 1LT (0171–387 9592).

TRAVEL See APPENDIX 3: TRAVEL AND HEALTH.

TUBEROSE SCLEROSIS Tuberous Sclerosis Association of Great Britain, Little Barnsley Farm, Catshill, Bromsgrove, Worcestershire B61 0NQ (01527–71898).

TURNER'S SYNDROME UK Turner Syndrome Society, c/o Child Growth Foundation, 2 Mayfield Avenue, London W4 1PW (0181–995 0257, fax: 0181–995 9075).

VOLUNTARY ORGANIZATIONS National Council for Voluntary Organizations, Regents Wharf, 8 All Saints Street, London N1 9RL (0171–713 6161).

APPENDIX 3: TRAVEL AND HEALTH

INTRODUCTION
Whether a person is travelling abroad for business or pleasure or is going to live in another country, he or she should obtain information about the climate, environment and health risks at their destination (including any stopovers that involve personal contacts with local people). Certain risks to health in another country may always be present; sometimes hazards to health may be temporary because of a local epidemic or sudden adverse environmental circumstance, such as a drought, earthquake or volcanic eruption, any of which can cause problems in obtaining supplies of food, clean water and medicine.

Any intending travellers with an existing illness should find out from their doctors whether they are fit to travel, whether the country of destination will admit them and whether they will be able to obtain appropriate treatment and how it will be paid for.

Healthy travellers are also advised to inquire about health-care arrangements (including payments) in their destination country in case they fall ill while away. Some countries have reciprocal arrangements with the UK. Travellers should take sensible precautions about drinking water and food as hygiene standards vary widely throughout the world. Pharmacists are usually helpful with advice on over-the-counter remedies for travel sickness (q.v.) and traveller's tummy.

Travel agents have a responsibility to advise their clients about health risks, and the travel trade has access to directories giving up-to-date information on visa requirements, recommended immunizations, climate, current health hazards and currency allowances. They cannot, however, be expected to give detailed individual advice, especially if the traveller has an existing medical condition.

There are many publications of help to travellers and authoritative advice is available from organizations listed in this appendix.

Travellers returning home who fall ill – even several months later – should always tell their doctor where they have visited and when in case their illness originated in another country.

USEFUL ADDRESSES
Topical medical advice can be obtained by *those advising travellers* from PHLS Communicable Disease Surveillance Centre, 61 Colindale Avenue, London NW9 5EQ (0181–200 6868); Hospital for Tropical Diseases, 4 St Pancras Way, London NW1 0PE (0171–388 9600); Communicable Diseases (Scotland) Unit, and Department of Tropical Medicine, Ruchill Hospital, Glasgow G20 9NB (0141–946 7120); Department of Infectious and Tropical Diseases, Birmingham Heartlands Hospital, Bordesley Green East, Birmingham B9 5ST (0121–766 6611) (inquiries from doctors and pharmacists only); Department of Infectious

Diseases and Tropical Medicine, North Manchester General Hospital, Delaunays Road, Manchester M8 6RB (0161–795 4567); Liverpool School of Tropical Medicine, Pembroke Place, Liverpool L3 5QA (0151–708 9393).

SOURCES OF 'OFFICIAL' ADVICE
The Department of health produces annually the T4 booklet *Health Advice for Travellers* and this is available free from post offices. It contains information on what compulsory and recommended immunizations apply to countries. Advice is given on reducing health risks and on entitlement to medical treatment at reduced cost. Certificate E111 entitles nationals of European Community countries to care in other member states and the leaflet explains how to get this.

The health departments in Scotland, Wales and Northern Ireland also produce information on immunization against infectious diseases; this is published by HMSO and referred to as the 'green book'.

The World Health Organization in Geneva issues annually *International Travel and Health Vaccination Requirements and Health Advice*, also available from HMSO. It is written primarily for a medical readership. Designated yellow-fever vaccination centres are distributed throughout the UK and details of these can be obtained from local departments of public health and in Scotland and Northern Ireland from health boards.

Most good bookshops contain a range of travel books and specific travel health guides that contain information relating to health. Books may, however, become quickly out of date because of changing circumstances and health regulations in different countries. *The Traveller's Handbook*, published by Wexas Ltd, is a good and comprehensive guide; *The Tropical Traveller*, published by Penguin, is also helpful.

Among several specialist organizations giving travel advice, for instance, to handicapped people, and publishing books and leaflets, are the following: International Association for Medical Assistance to Travellers, Gotthardstrasse 17, 6300 Zug, Switzerland (membership free but voluntary contributions welcome; publishes a directory of English-speaking doctors and leaflets on climate, acclimatization, immunization, etc.); Air Transport Users Council, 103 Kingsway, London WC2B 6QX (0171–242 3882) (*Care in the Air*, advice for handicapped travellers); Intermedic, 77 Third Avenue, New York, United States of America NY 10017 (members may obtain a list of recommended English-speaking doctors in many countries); British Airways Medical Service, Queens Building (N121), Heathrow Airport, Hounslow, Middlesex (0181–562 7070) (*Your Patient and Air Travel* is useful for medical practitioners); British Diabetic Association, 10 Queen Anne Street, London W1M 0BD (0171–323 1531) (leaflets including travel guide concerning the more popular destinations); Royal Association for Disability and Rehabilitation (RADAR), 12 City Forum, 250 City Road, London EC1V 8AF (0171–250 3222) (leaflets available to help the handi-

capped arrange their travels); National Association for Maternal and Child Welfare Ltd, 1st floor, 40–42 Osnaburgh Street, London NW1 3ND (0171–383 4117) (*The Care of Babies and Young Children in the Tropics* by D. Morley, *Travelling with Children*).

APPENDIX 4: COMMON MEDICAL TESTS AND PROCEDURES

ACETONE (URINE)
Aim Detection of diabetic ketoacidosis.
Method Using Acetest tablets, Chemstrip or Multistix.
Normal Negative.

ADRENOCORTICOTROPHIC HORMONE (ACTH) (PLASMA)
Aim Diagnosis of Addison's disease, Cushing's syndrome, etc.
Normal Sleep–wake cycle of ACTH production, with highest levels at 6.00–8.00 (soon after getting up) and lowest levels at 21.00–22.00 (after going to bed). Secretion is increased by pregnancy and stress.

AMNIOCENTESIS
Aim Assessment of fetal maturity and diagnosis of fetal abnormalities.
Method/hazards With ultrasound guidance, a needle is inserted through the mother's abdominal wall and uterus, and a specimen of amniotic fluid withdrawn. There is a small risk to the fetus and the test should only be performed when essential.

AMYLASE (SERUM)
Aim Investigation of pancreatic and hepatic disease.
Normal 25–125 U/1 (units per litre).

APGAR SCORE
Aim Assessment of neonate's physical health.
Method Evaluation at 1 minute and 5 minutes after delivery of skin colour, muscle tone, respiratory effort, heart rate, and response to stimulus. Points are awarded and appropriate action (such as resuscitation) started.

BICARBONATE (WHOLE ARTERIAL BLOOD)
Aim Investigation of acidosis and alkalosis.
Normal 18–23 mmol/l.

BIOPSY OF TUMOURS
Aim Histological diagnosis of type of tumour and malignancy.
Methods Fine-needle and large-needle aspiration biopsy – excision biopsy.

CALCIUM (SERUM)
Aim Diagnosis of hyperparathyroidism, hypoparathyroidism, etc.
Normal See table **B**1 (page 611). Range may be affected by other drugs.

CARDIAC STRESS TEST
Aim Assessment of cardiac efficiency.
Method Heart rate, blood pressure, and electrocardiograph are recorded continuously while the patient performs an incremental work test. The test is stopped whenever requested, e.g. in the presence of excessive dyspnoea, chest pain, etc.

Contraindications include acute infection, recent myocardial infarction, unstable angina, congestive heart failure, uncontrolled dysrhythmia, etc.

CERVICAL CANCER SCREENING
Aim Early detection of changes in cervical cells, allowing earlier treatment.
Method Starting 6 months after first intercourse, then at 3-yearly intervals for rest of life. The test involves a cervical smear with a spatula, the cells then being examined histologically.

CHOLECYSTOGRAM A simple, safe test involving an X-ray of the gall-bladder after the patient has taken a contrast medium by mouth; it is concentrated in the gall-bladder, thus enabling identification of abnormalities such as gall stones, tumours and restricted patency of the cystic duct (which carries the bile from the gall-bladder to the duodenum).

CHORIONIC GONADOTROPHIN (URINE, FIRST MORNING SPECIMEN)
Aim Diagnosis of pregnancy.
Methods Agglutination inhibition assay: positive in pregnancy 8–14 days after first missed period. Monoclonal antibody test: positive in pregnancy 14–18 days from conception.

CHORIONIC 1VILLUS SAMPLING
Aim Ascertainment of fetal chromosome pattern.

Method A small sample of trophoblastic tissue is obtained from the placenta, by ultrasound guidance either transvaginally or transabdominally, taken between the 9th and 11th weeks of pregnancy. There is a small risk of abortion.

CORDOCENTESIS
Aim Investigation of the chromosome pattern and haemoglobinopathies in mid-pregnancy.
Method Blood is withdrawn from the umbilical cord at about the 18th week of pregnancy and extensively analysed.

ENZYME-LINKED IMMUNOSORBENT ASSAY (ELISA) (URINE)
Aim Diagnosis of pregnancy.
Method Measurement of human chorionic gonadotrophin in urine may give a positive result 8–10 days after fertilization. False negative results may be due to testing too early in pregnancy, to excessively dilute urine, or to a urine infection.

ERYTHROCYTE COUNT (WHOLE BLOOD)
Aim Investigation of anaemia.
Normal See table **B1** (page 611).

ERYTHROCYTE SEDIMENTATION RATE (ESR)
Aim Investigation and monitoring of fever, inflammatory, malignant, or autoimmune disease.
Method Anticoagulated whole blood is used. The result obtained may be influenced by numerous factors, notably various conditions and different drugs.

Normal	male	<50	<15 mm/h
		>50	<20 mm/h
	female	<50	<20 mm/h
		>50	<30 mm/h

GLASGOW COMA SCALE (MODIFIED)
Aim To test the depth of coma.
Method Opening of the eyes, best verbal response, and best motor response are scored separately, giving a total quantitative index of the level of cerebral dysfunction.

GLOMERULAR FILTRATION RATE (GFR)
Aim Investigation of renal function.
Method Plasma and urinary creatinine levels are measured and the creatinine clearance rate calculated. This corresponds closely to the GFR, normally 120 ml/min.

GLUCOSE (BLOOD, URINE)
Aim Diagnosis and monitoring of diabetes mellitus.
Method Stick tests available for urine and blood samples.
Normal See tables **B1** and **B4** (pages 580 and 581).

GLUCOSE TOLERANCE TEST (ORAL)
Aim Diagnosis of diabetes mellitus/impaired glucose tolerance.
Method Pretest patient, ensure no recent illness, accident, or surgery. Discontinue non-essential drugs. Patient fasts for 10–16 hours, then takes 75 g glucose over 5 minutes. Serum glucose level is measured at 0, 30, 60, 90 and 120 minutes. The test should be performed in the morning.

Normal	fasting	3.9–5.8 mmol/l
	30 minutes	6.1–9.4 mmol/l
	60 minutes	6.7–9.4 mmol/l
	90 minutes	5.6–7.8 mmol/l
	120 minutes	3.9–6.7 mmol/l

GLYCATED HAEMOGLOBIN (WHOLE BLOOD)
Aim Monitoring of diabetes mellitus.
Method The test reflects the mean blood-glucose concentration over the previous 4–8 weeks. It is a measure of long-term control and should be repeated at around 3-monthly intervals.
Normal (In insulin-dependent diabetic) 7–9 per cent.

HAEMATOCRIT (PACKED RED CELL VOLUME) (WHOLE BLOOD)
Aim Investigation of anaemia and polycythaemia.
Normal See table **B1** (page 611).

HEPATITIS A ANTIGEN (SERUM)
Aim Diagnosis of hepatitis A infection.
Normal Negative.
Anti-HAV IgG appears about four weeks after infection and persists indefinitely.

HEPATITIS B SURFACE ANTIGEN (SERUM)
Aim Diagnosis of active or chronic hepatitis B virus infection.
Normal Negative.

HUMAN IMMUNODEFICIENCY VIRUS (HIV) ANTIBODY (SERUM)
Aim Diagnosis of HIV infection.
Method HIV antibodies are usually detectable from 4 weeks to 4 months after infection, and persist indefinitely. The test is by enzyme-linked immunosorbent assay (ELISA).
Normal Negative.

IRON (SERUM)
Aim Investigation of anaemia.
Normal See table **B1** (page 611).

LIVER FUNCTION TESTS
The liver is a complex organ with metabolic, excretory and protective functions that are interdependent, so there is no single test to assess overall function. Liver biopsy, done under local anaesthetic with entry through the skin, gives helpful diagnostic information with little risk or discomfort to the patient. The procedure enables liver tissue to be examined in the

laboratory for structural changes and the presence of abnormal cells.

Several tests of blood chemistry detect changes in the various functions, as well as assessing the healthiness of liver cells. These include tests on blood serum for the amounts of bilirubin (yellow breakdown products of red blood cells), albumin (a key body protein made in the liver) and alkaline phosphatase (an enzyme in bile) and aminotransferases or transaminases (enzymes entering the blood following liver-cell damage). Prothrombin time (see below) tests how well the blood clots: the process depends on the presence in the blood of vitamin K (see APPENDIX 5: VITAMINS) which is produced by the normal liver; damage to liver cells lengthens the time blood takes to clot. X-ray and ultrasound assessment of liver and gall-bladder structure are valuable, as are radionucleide scanning and computed tomography.

LUMBAR PUNCTURE
Aim To obtain samples of cerebrospinal fluid (CSF) for investigation of central nervous system diseases.
Method With the patient lying on his side, and under local anaesthesia, a long needle is inserted between the third and fourth lumbar vertebrae. When performed correctly, a small volume of fluid should flow out spontaneously; this is collected and analysed (see table **B**2 (page 612) for normal values).

The test should never be carried out in the presence of a raised CSF pressure, since it may precipitate transtentorial or tonsillar herniation.

MYOGLOBIN (SERUM)
Aim Diagnosis of myocardial infarction.
Normal   men   19–92 µg/l
                  women   12–76 µg/l
The increase in value begins 30–60 minutes after onset of myocardial infarction and continues for 2–3 days.

PROSTATE SCREENING TESTS These tests for prostate cancer are still being evaluated. One test is for the protein, prostate-specific antigen (PSA); its drawback is that it detects small areas of cancerous cells which might not necessarily develop and cause symptoms. Ultrasound scanning and biopsy of the gland are useful tests.

PROTHROMBIN TEST This is a quantitative test of the amount of prothrombin in the blood based on the time it takes blood plasma to clot in the presence of thromboplastin and calcium chloride. It measures the integrity of the blood-clotting function. The normal prothrombin time is 10 to 14 seconds. The time is extended in haemophilia, serious liver disorders and when the diet is deficient in vitamin K.

SKIN BIOPSY
Aim Histological or immunofluorescent examination of skin lesions, especially if there is any suspicion of malignancy.
Method Various techniques are used, depending on the amount of skin required and the degree of doubt of the diagnosis.

THYROXINE, FREE (FT4) (SERUM)
Aim Measurement of thyroid function.
Method Various methods are used. The normal value is 10–31 pmol/l, but varies with the technique used.

TUBERCULIN SKIN TESTS
Aim Diagnosis of tuberculosis.
Method Antigens of *Mycobacterium tuberculosis* are injected intradermally. In the Heaf test, six skin punctures are then made through the antigen. The test is read at 3–7 days and a positive result is the appearance of four or more papules.

APPENDIX 5: VITAMINS

INTRODUCTION
A general description of vitamins is in the main text. Vitamins are divided into those that are fat soluble and those that are water soluble. Fat-soluble vitamins are A, D, E and K, the water-soluble ones B group and C.

The water-soluble vitamin B group is complex. Although often found together in similar types of food – cereals, milk, liver, etc. – they are not related chemically. These vitamins are all coenzymes, organic (non-protein) compounds which, when the appropriate enzyme (q.v.) is present, have an essential function in the chemical reaction catalysed by the enzyme. The vitamin B group comprises B_1 (thiamine, aneurine), B_2 (riboflavin), B_3 (niacin, nicotinic acid), B_6 (pyridoxine), B_{12} (cobalamin, cyanocobalamin), biotin, folacin (folic acid) and pantothenic acid.

Unlike fat-soluble vitamins, the water-soluble ones are not stored in large amounts in the body so deficiency of these is more likely.

FAT-SOLUBLE VITAMINS

VITAMIN A (PREFORMED SPECIFIC COMPOUNDS: RETINOL, RETINAL, RETINOIC ACID. PRECURSOR: CAROTENE)
Functions Maintenance of epithelial cells and mucous membranes. Constituent of visual purple (for night vision). Necessary for normal growth, development and reproduction. Maintenance of immune system.
Symptoms of deficiency Keratinized skin, dry mucous membranes, xerophthalmia. Night blindness. Susceptibility to disease.
Symptoms of toxicity Dry skin. Loss of appetite and hair, enlarged spleen and liver, abnormal pigmentation of skin. Fetal malformations.
Food sources *Preformed vitamin A* Liver, especially cod and halibut liver oil; egg yolk; milk and butter. *Carotene* Dark-green, leafy vegetables, especially spinach, broccoli, kale. Deep orange vegetables and fruits, especially carrots, tomatoes, apricots.
Recommended daily amounts (IUs*)

Babies and children	1875–3500
Boys (>11 years) and men	5000
Girls (>11 years) and women	4000
Lactating women	6000–6500

*International Units

VITAMIN D (ERGOCALCIFEROL OR CALCIFEROL (VITAMIN D_2); CHOLECALCIFEROL (VITAMIN D_3); 25-HYDROXYCHOLECALCIFEROL (MAIN CIRCULATING FORM OF VITAMIN D); 1,25-DIHYDROXY-CHOLECALCIFEROL (MAIN ACTIVE FORM OF VITAMIN D). PRECURSOR OF VITAMIN D_2: ERGOSTEROL (PLANTS); OF VITAMIN D_3: 7-DEHYDROCHOLESTEROL (IN SKIN).
Functions Helps in absorption of calcium and phosphorus. Regulates blood concentrations of calcium. Promotes mineralization of teeth and bones.
Symptoms of deficiency Rickets in children. Osteomalacia in adults.
Symptoms of toxicity Calcification of soft tissues, hypercalcaemia, renal stones, loss of weight and appetite, nausea and fatigue, failure of growth.
Sources Cod and halibut liver oils, bony fish, egg yolk, fortified milk, butter and polyunsaturated margarine. Sunlight acts on ergosterol in plants to produce vitamin D_2 and on the skin to produce vitamin D_3.
Recommended daily amounts (IUs)

Babies and children	300–400
Subjects aged 11–25	400
Subjects over 25	200
Pregnant and lactating women	400

VITAMIN E (α-TOCOPHEROL)
Functions Prevents oxidation of vitamin A in gut. Protects red blood cells from haemolysis. Maintains cell membranes by reducing the oxidation of polyunsaturated fats.
Symptoms of deficiency Breakdown of red blood cells.
Symptoms of toxicity Headache, nausea, longer blood-clotting times.

Food sources Wheat germ, vegetable oils, legumes, nuts, whole grains, fish, green, leafy vegetables.
Recommended daily allowances (mg)

Babies and children	3–7
Boys (>11 years) and men	10
Girls (>11 years) and non-pregnant women	8
Pregnant and lactating women	10–12

VITAMIN K (PHYTOMENADIONE, PHYLLOQUINONE)
Functions Necessary for the formation of prothrombin and other factors necessary for blood clotting.
Symptoms of deficiency Haemorrhage.
Symptoms of toxicity Haemolytic anaemia, liver damage.
Sources Dark-green leafy vegetables, especially alfalfa, spinach, cabbage. Cauliflower. Egg yolk. Soybean oil. From synthesis by intestinal bacteria.
Recommended daily amounts (μg)

Babies and children	5–20
Boys (>11 years) and men (increasing with age)	45–80
Girls (>11 years) and women (increasing with age)	45–65
Pregnant and lactating women	65

CHOLINE
The basic compound participates in the synthesis of lecithin (q.v.) and other phospholipids as well as of acetylcholine. Choline, which helps to transport fat in the body, and is essential to life, is sometimes classed as a vitamin, but the body is able to produce the compound.

WATER-SOLUBLE VITAMINS

VITAMIN B_1 (THIAMINE, ANEURINE)
Functions Has role in carbohydrate metabolism. Helps nervous system, heart and muscles to function properly. Promotes appetite and functioning of digestive tract.
Symptoms of deficiency Polyneuritis, beriberi, fatigue, depression, poor appetite and functioning of digestive tract.
Symptoms of toxicity Anaphylactic shock, lethargy, ataxia, nausea, hypotension.
Sources Whole grains, wheat germ, enriched white-flour products, legumes. Brewer's yeast. Heart, liver, kidney; pork.
Recommended daily amounts (mg)

Babies and children	0.3–1.0
Boys (>11 years) and men	1.2–1.5
Girls (>11 years) and women	1.0–1.1
Pregnant women	1.5
Lactating women	1.6

VITAMIN B_2 (RIBOFLAVIN (FORMERLY VITAMIN G))
Functions Essential for certain enzyme systems important in the metabolism of food (carbohydrate, protein and fat).
Symptoms of deficiency Inflamed tongue, scaling and burning skin, sensitive eyes, angular stomatitis and cheilosis, cataracts.

Symptoms of toxicity   None recorded.
Sources   Green, leafy vegetables, peanuts, whole grains. Milk and its products, eggs, liver, kidney, heart.

Recommended daily amounts (mg)

Babies and children	0.4–1.2
Boys (>11 years) and men	1.4–1.8
Girls (>11 years) and women	1.2–1.3
Pregnant women	1.6
Lactating women	1.7–1.8

VITAMIN B₃ (NIACIN, NICOTINIC ACID (A DERIVATIVE OF PYRIDINE))

Functions   Part of two important enzymes regulating energy metabolism. Promotes good physical and mental health and helps maintain the health of the skin, tongue and digestive system.
Symptoms of deficiency   Pellagra, gastrointestinal disturbances, photosensitive dermatitis, depression.
Symptoms of toxicity   Flushing, loss of appetite, nausea and vomiting, abnormal energy metabolism, anaphylaxis, circulatory collapse.
Sources   Whole grain flour, enriched white flour, legumes. Brewer's yeast. Meat; heart, liver, kidney.

Recommended daily amounts (mg)

Babies and children	5–13
Boys (>11 years) and men	15–20
Girls (>11 years) and women	13–15
Pregnant women	17
Lactating women	20

VITAMIN B₆ (PYRIDOXINE (PYRIDOXAL IS A COENZYME DERIVATIVE OF PYRIDOXINE))

Functions   Important in metabolism of proteins, amino-acids, carbohydrate and fat. Essential for growth and health.
Symptoms of deficiency   Not fully known but possibly convulsions, peripheral neuropathy, secondary pellagra, depression and oral symptoms.
Symptoms of toxicity   Reduces prolactin secretion, which is important for milk production. Damage to sensory nerves. Liver damage.
Sources   Whole grains, potatoes, green vegetables, maize. Liver; red meat.

Recommended daily amounts (mg)

Babies and children	0.3–1.4
Boys (>11 years) and men	1.7–2.0
Girls (>11 years) and women	1.4–1.6
Pregnant women	2.2
Lactating women	2.1

VITAMIN B₁₂ (COBALAMIN, CYANOCOBALAMIN)

Functions   Important for haemoglobin synthesis. Essential for normal functioning of all cells, especially of the nervous system, bone marrow, and gastrointestinal tract.
Symptoms of deficiency   Pernicious anaemia, subacute degeneration of the spinal cord, various psychological disorders, possibly loss of appetite (anorexia).

Symptoms of toxicity   Not known.
Sources   Not found in significant amounts in plant foods. Eggs, dry milk and milk products. Meat; liver, kidney, heart.

Recommended daily amounts (µg)

Babies and children	0.3–1.4
Subjects over 11 years	2.0
Pregnant women	2.2
Lactating women	2.6

VITAMIN B COMPLEX (FOLATE, FOLIC ACID)

Functions   Formation of red blood cells. Normal function of gastrointestinal tract. Helps in metabolism of protein.
Symptoms of deficiency   Possible neural tube defect in fetuses, anaemia.
Symptoms of toxicity   Possible hypersensitivity reactions.
Sources   Dark-green, leafy vegetables, legumes, whole grains. Yeast. Glandular meats.

Recommended daily amounts (µg)

Babies and children	25–100
Boys (>11 years) and men	150–200
Girls (>11 years) and women	150–180
Pregnant women	400
Lactating women	260–280

VITAMIN B COMPLEX (BIOTIN)

Functions   Takes part in amino-acid and fatty-acid metabolism.
Symptoms of deficiency   Rare: dermatitis, soreness of the tongue, dependency.
Symptoms of toxicity   Not known.
Sources   Egg yolk, cauliflower, kidney, legumes, liver, nuts, yeasts.
Recommended daily amounts   150–300 µg.

VITAMIN B COMPLEX (PANTOTHENIC ACID)

Functions   An essential component of coenzyme A, which is a key factor in many of the body's metabolic activities.
Symptoms of deficiency   Rare, but in a trial on volunteers malaise, abdominal discomfort and sensory disturbances occurred.
Symptoms of toxicity   Not known.
Sources   Widely distributed in foodstuffs.
Recommended daily amounts   Adults probably need about 4 to 7 mg/day.

VITAMIN C (ASCORBIC ACID, DEHYDROASCORBIC ACID)

Functions   Protects against infection and helps in wound healing. Important for tooth dentine, bones, cartilage, connective tissue and blood vessels.
Symptoms of deficiency   Scurvy, anaemia, swollen and bleeding gums, loose teeth, bruising (from rupture of small blood vessels).
Symptoms of toxicity   Kidney stones.
Sources   Citrus fruits, tomatoes, strawberries, currants, green, leafy vegetables, broccoli, cabbage, potatoes.

Recommended daily amounts (mg)

Babies and children	30–45
Subjects over 11 years	50–60
Pregnant women	70
Lactating women	90–95

APPENDIX 6: MEASUREMENTS IN MEDICINE

INTRODUCTION
This appendix gives a brief description of the System of International Units (SI units) and tables of 'normal' values for the composition of body fluids and body wastes. In addition there are tables of desirable body weights according to age (infants) and height and body build (adults).

Readers should bear in mind that 'normal' values may vary, sometimes quite widely, in healthy individuals. Furthermore, the relationships between height, build and weight are flexible and should not be treated as absolute targets.

A SI UNITS AND MULTIPLES
The International System of Units (*Système International*) usually referred to as SI units, was introduced in the 1970s and has been expanded and developed since. Now the SI units and symbols and certain units derived from the system are used for measurements in most scientific disciplines and are an integral part of scientific language. The units comprise three classes: base units, supplementary units and derived units. The seven base units are the metre (length), kilogram (weight), second (time), ampere (electric current), kelvin (temperature), mole (amount of substance: one mole of a compound has a mass equal to its molecular weight in grams) and candela (luminous intensity). The SI units used commonly in medicine are shown below. Some traditional measurements are still used, one example being millimetres of mercury (Hg) which is the unit for blood pressure.

SI UNITS COMMONLY USED IN MEDICINE

Quantity	SI unit (abbreviation)
Length	metre (m)
Area	square metre (m^2)
Volume	cubic metre (m^3) = 100 litre (l or L)
Mass	kilogram (kg)
Amount of substance	mole (mol)
Energy	joule (J)
Pressure	pascal (Pa)
Force	newton (N)
Time	second (s)
Frequency	hertz (Hz)
Power	watt (w)
Temperature	degree Celsius (°C)

MULTIPLES AND SUBMULTIPLES

Factor	Prefix	Abbreviation
10^6	mega	m
10^3	kilo	k
10^{-1}	deci	d
10^{-2}	centi	c
10^{-3}	milli	m
10^{-6}	micro	μ
10^{-9}	nano	n
10^{-12}	pico	p

B 'NORMAL' BODY VALUES
1 BLOOD (PLASMA, SERUM)
Biochemical values

Substance	Approximate adult range
Ammonium	24–48 μmol/l
Ascorbate	45–80 μmol/l
Base excess	0±2 mmol/l
Bicarbonate (serum)	23–29 mmol/l
Bilirubin, total (plasma)	5–17 μmol/l
Caeruloplasmin (serum)	1.5–2.9 μmol/l
Calcium (serum)	2.1–2.6 mmol/l
Carbon dioxide tension (Pco2)	4.5–6.1 kPa
β-carotene	0.9–5.6 mmol/l
Chloride (serum)	95–105 mmol/l
Cholesterol (serum)	3.9–6.5 mmol/l
Copper (serum)	13–24 mmol/l
Cortisol (plasma)	280–700 nmol/l
Creatine (serum)	15–61 μmol/l
Creatinine (serum)	62–133 μmol/l
Fibrinogen (plasma)	5.9–11.7 μmol/l
Folate (serum)	11–48 nmol/l
Glucose, fasting (serum)	3.9–6.4 mmol/l
Iron (serum)	13–31 μmol/l
Iron binding capacity, total (serum)	45–73 μmol/l
Lactate	0.6–1.8 mmol/l
Lipids, total (plasma)	4.0–10.0 g/l
Osmolality (serum)	280–295 mmol/kg
Oxygen tension (Po2)	11–14 kPa
pH	7.35–7.45
Potassium (serum)	3.5–5.0 mmol/l
Protein (serum)	
total	62–82 g/l
albumin	35–55 g/l
globulin	25–35 g/l
Pyruvate	45–80 μmol/l
Sodium (serum)	135–145 mmol/l
Triglycerides (serum)	0.3–1.7 mmol/l
Urate (serum)	0.1–0.4 mmol/l
Urea (serum)	4.0–8.0 mmol/l

Haematological values

Measurement	Adult daily range
Bleeding time (Ivy)	5 minutes
Cell counts	
Erythrocytes, men	4.6–6.2 × 10 12/l
women	4.2–5.8 × 10 12/l
Leucocytes, total	4.5–11.0 × 10 9/l
Differential:	
Neutrophils	3.0–6.5 × 10 9/l
Lymphocytes	1.5–3.0 × 10 9/l
Monocytes	0.3–0.6 × 10 9/l
Eosinophils	50–300 × 10 6/l
Basophils	15–60 × 10 6/l
Platelets	150–350 × 10 9/l
Reticulocytes	25–75 × 10 9/l
Haemoglobin, men	2.2–2.8 mmol/l
women	1.9–2.5 mmol/l
Haematocrit, men	0.40–0.54
women	0.37–0.47
Mean corpuscular haemoglobin (MCH)	0.42–0.48 fmol

Mean corpuscular volume
(MCV)   80–105 fl
Mean corpuscular
haemoglobin
  concentration (MCHC)   0.32–0.36
Red cell life span (mean)   120 days

2 CEREBROSPINAL FLUID

Measurement	Approximate adult range
Cells	5/µl; all mononuclear
Chloride	120–130 mmol/l
Glucose	2.8–4.2 mmol/l
Pressure	70–180 mm water
Protein, total	0.2–0.5 g/l
IgG	0.14 of total protein

3 FAECES

Measurement	Approximate adult range
Bulk	100–200 g/24 hours
Dry matter	23–32 g/24 hours
Fat, total	6.0 g/24 hours
Nitrogen, total	2.0 g/24 hours
Urobilinogen	40–280 mg/24 hours
Water	0.65 g/24 hours

4 URINE

Measurement	Approximate adult range
Albumin	0.2–1.5 µmol/24 hours
Calcium	2.5–7.5 mmol/24 hours
Catecholamines (adrenalin)	55 nmol/24 hours
Chloride	110–250 mmol/24 hours
Copper	0.8 µmol/24 hours
Creatine, men	300 µmol/24 hours
women	700 µmol/24 hours
Creatinine	9–17 mmol/24 hours
Glucose	11 mmol/l
Magnesium	3.0–4.5 mmol/24 hours
Osmolality	38–1400 mmol/kg water
pH	4.6–8.0
Phosphorus (inorganic)	20–45 mmol/24 hours
Porphyrins:	
Coproporphyrin	77–380 nmol/24 hours
Uroporphyrin	12–36 nmol/24 hours
Potassium	25–100 mmol/24 hours
Protein	10–150 mg/24 hours
Sodium	130–260 mmol/24 hours
Urate	1.2–3.0 mmol/24 hours

5 TEMPERATURE

Normal, adults	36.6–37.2 °C
children	36.5–37.5 °C
infants	37.5–38.5 °C
Hyperpyrexia (q.v.)	41.6 °C
Hypothermia (q.v.)	35.0 °C

NB The temperature in the axilla or groin is about 0.5 °C lower, and in the rectum about 0.5 °C higher, than the oral temperature.

C DESIRABLE BODY WEIGHTS AND HEIGHTS

1 CHILDREN, BIRTH TO 5 YEARS, SEXES COMBINED

Age	Standard weight (kg)	Standard height (cm)
0 (birth)	3.4	55
1 month	4.3	
2 months	5.0	
3 months	5.7	60
4 months	6.3	
5 months	6.9	
6 months	7.4	65
8 months	8.4	
10 months	9.3	
12 months	9.9	75
18 months	11.3	80
2 years	12.4	85
3 years	14.5	95
4 years	16.5	100
5 years	18.4	105

2 ADULTS, ACCORDING TO HEIGHT AND BUILD

Men

Height (m)	Build (weight in kg)		
	Small	Medium	Large
1.550	50.8–54.4	53.5–58.5	57.2–64.0
1.575	52.2–55.8	54.9–60.3	58.5–65.3
1.600	53.5–57.2	56.2–61.7	59.9–67.1
1.625	54.9–58.5	57.6–63.0	61.2–68.9
1.650	56.2–60.3	59.0–64.9	62.6–70.8
1.675	58.1–62.1	60.8–66.7	64.4–73.0
1.700	59.9–64.0	62.6–68.9	66.7–75.3
1.725	61.7–65.8	64.4–70.8	68.5–77.1
1.750	63.5–68.0	66.2–72.6	70.3–78.9
1.775	65.3–69.9	68.0–74.8	72.1–81.2
1.800	67.1–71.7	69.9–77.1	74.4–83.5
1.825	68.9–73.5	71.7–79.4	76.2–85.7
1.850	70.8–75.7	73.5–81.6	78.5–88.0
1.875	72.6–77.6	75.7–83.9	80.7–90.3
1.900	74.4–79.4	78.0–86.2	82.6–92.5

Women

Height (m)	Build (weight in kg)		
	Small	Medium	Large
1.425	41.7–44.5	43.5–48.5	47.2–54.0
1.450	42.6–45.8	44.5–49.9	48.1–55.3
1.475	43.5–47.2	45.8–51.3	49.4–56.7
1.500	44.9–48.5	47.2–52.6	50.8–58.1
1.525	46.3–49.9	48.5–54.0	52.2–59.4
1.550	47.6–51.3	49.9–55.3	53.5–60.8
1.575	49.0–52.6	51.3–57.2	54.9–62.6
1.600	50.3–54.0	52.6–59.0	56.7–64.4
1.625	51.7–55.8	54.4–61.2	58.5–66.2
1.650	53.5–57.7	56.2–63.0	60.3–68.0
1.675	55.3–59.4	58.1–64.9	62.1–69.9
1.700	57.2–61.2	59.9–66.7	64.0–71.7
1.725	59.0–63.5	61.7–68.5	65.8–73.9
1.750	60.8–65.3	63.5–70.3	67.6–76.2
1.775	62.6–67.1	65.3–72.1	69.4–78.5

An individual assessment of a person's size can be made by using the BODY MASS INDEX (BMI). (See also OBESITY.)

APPENDIX 7: UK HEALTH STATISTICS:
a selection

Leading causes of death

DEATH RATES FOR LEADING CAUSES OF DEATH (MALE AND FEMALE) PER **100,000** POPULATION, UK

	1970	1975	1980	1985	1990	1993
All deaths	1,178	1,178	1,174	1,185	1,118	1,123
Ischaemic heart disease	290	315	314	330	295	288
Cerebrovascular disease	165	159	147	148	133	122
Pneumonia	84	92	104	59	57	105*
Malignant neoplasm of trachea[1]	62	66	71	72	68	65
Diseases of pulmonary circulation[2]	57	52	69	47	40	52
Malignant neoplasm of breast	22	23	24	27	27	25
Malignant neoplasm of stomach	26	24	22	20	17	15
Bronchitis, emphysema	59	49	38	27	13	12
Diabetes mellitus	10	10	10	14	15	12
Leukaemia	6	6	7	7	7	7
Nephritis, nephrotic syndrome[3]	5	6	9	10	8	7
Suicide and self-inflicted injury	8	7	9	9	8	7
Ulcer of stomach and duodenum	8	8	9	10	8	7
Chronic liver disease and cirrhosis	3	4	5	5	6	6
Hypertensive disease	20	16	11	9	6	6

Notes: * Part of the increase is due to definition changes.
[1] Including bronchus and lung.
[2] Including other forms of heart disease.
[3] Nephritis, nephrotic syndrome and nephrosis.
Source: Office for National Statistics, *Annual Abstract of Statistics*.

RANKING OF LEADING CAUSES OF DEATH (MALE AND FEMALE), UK

	1970	1975	1980	1985	1990	1993
Ischaemic heart disease	1	1	1	1	1	1
Cerebrovascular disease	2	2	2	2	2	2
Malignant neoplasm of trachea[1]	4	4	4	3	3	3
Pneumonia	3	3	3	4	4	4
Diseases of pulmonary circulation[2]	6	5	5	5	5	5
Malignant neoplasm of breast	8	8	7	7	6	6
Malignant neoplasm of stomach	7	7	8	8	7	7
Diabetes, mellitus	13	12	11	9	8	8
Bronchitis, emphysema	5	6	6	6	9	9
Ulcer of stomach and duodenum	16	13	13	11	11	10

Notes: [1] Including bronchus and lung.
[2] Including other forms of heart disease.
Source: Office for National Statistics, *Annual Abstract of Statistics*.

Incidence rate for all cancers

AVERAGE NUMBER OF CASES PER YEAR SPAN

Year span	Male	Female
1971–74	83,812	78,284
1975–79	90,876	84,533
1980–84	99,509	92,444
1985–87	101,430	95,805

Source: Office of National Statistics, *Health of Adult Britain 1841–1994* (vol. 2), The Stationery Office, London, 1997.

INCIDENCE RATES FOR BREAST CANCER (ENGLAND AND WALES) PER **100,000** POPULATION

Year span	Number	Rate
1971–74	78,389	98.4
1975–79	101,744	101.77
1980–84	106,258	105.33
1985–87	66,225	108.57

Source: Office for National Statistics, *Health of Adult Britain 1841–1994* (vol. 2), The Stationery Office, London, 1997.

INCIDENCE OF CANCER OF THE LUNG (ENGLAND AND WALES) PER **100,000** POPULATION

Year span	Male		Female	
	Number	Rate	Number	Rate
1971–74	103,927	147.07	24,058	30.4
1975–79	134,594	147.51	36,766	36.76
1980–84	134,255	141.45	45,619	45.27
1985–87	73,769	126.19	29,578	48.81

Source: Office for National Statistics, *Health of Adult Britain 1841–1994* (vol. 2), The Stationery Office, London, 1997.

Incidence of AIDS and HIV (England) (cases diagnosed)

Year	1978	1988	1989	1990	1991	1992	1993	1994	1995
HIV	2,134	1,505	1,607	2,024	2,251	2,299	2,154	2,145	2,225
AIDS	605	699	766	1,181	1,264	1,466	1,601	1,662	1,524

Source: Department of Health, *Health and Personal Social Statistics for England 1997*.

Patient consulting (rates per 1,000 population)

Year	Male	Female
1995–56	684	727
1970–71	660	670
1981–82	740	772
1991–92	846	866

Source: Office for National Statistics, *Health of Adult Britain 1841–1994* (vol 2), The Stationery Office, London, 1997.

APPENDIX 8: NATIONAL HEALTH SERVICE (NHS) RESOURCES, STAFFING AND STATISTICS SOURCES

The following tables have been compiled from a range of government statistical sources which have been coded as follows:

A   *The Government's Expenditure Plans* (Department of Helth).
B   *Health and Personal Social Services Statistics for England* (Department of Health).
C   *Community Statistics* (Department of Health and Social Services Northern Ireland).
D   *Annual Abstract of Statistics* (Office for National Statistics).
E   *Economic Trends* (Office for National Statistics).
F   *Family Expenditure Survey* (Office for National Statistics).
G   *UK National Accounts* (Office for National Statistics).
H   *Scottish Health Statistics* (Scottish Office Department of Health).
I   *Health Statistics Wales* (Welsh Office Health Department).

Funding of the NHS

TOTAL HEALTH CARE EXPENDITURE IN THE UK PER CAPITA

Calendar year	Cash £	Constant prices* 1973=100
1973	60	100
1975	100	115
1980	222	127
1985	345	143
1990	554	177
1995	807	220

* Figures have been adjusted by the Gross Domestic Product deflator and hence may include relative price effects.
Sources: A, D, E, G.

SOURCES OF FINANCE UK (£M)

	Taxation	NHS contribution	Patient payments	TOTAL NHS year
1970	1,635	209	61	2,040*
1975	4,675	451	111	5,237
1980	10,215	1,042	264	11,521
1985	15,122	2,032	487	17,641
1990	22,902	4,288	1,146	28,336
1995	35,376	5,112	919	41,407

* includes £135m from local health authorities.
Sources: D, E (Annual Supplement), F, G.

UK HEALTH EXPENDITURE (£M)

	NHS	Private	Other	TOTAL
1975	5,237	134	276	5,647
1980	11,521	355	615	12,491
1985	17,641	738	1,190	19,569
1990	28,336	1,623	1,919	31,878
1995	41,407	2,598	3,271	47,276
1998*	45,305	3,270*	3,551*	52,126*

* Office of Health Economics estimate.
Sources: D, E, F, G.

UK NHS EXPENDITURE (£M)

	Public	Private	TOTAL	TOTAL cost at 1949 prices (1949=37)
1970	1,979	61	2,040	919
1975	5,129˙	111	5,240	1,201
1980	11,257	264	11,521	1,370
1985	17,154	487	17,641	1,517
1990	27,191	1,146	28,337	1,824
1995	40,488	919	41,407	2,203

Sources: D, E, F, G.

UK HEALTH AS PERCENTAGE OF GROSS DOMESTIC PRODUCT (GDP)

	NHS	Private and other	TOTAL
1975	4.9	0.4	5.3
1980	5.0	0.4	5.4
1985	4.9	0.5	5.5
1990	5.1	0.6	5.8
1995	5.9	0.8	6.8

Sources: D, E, F, G.

PROJECTED CASH AND REAL NET NHS EXPENDITURE (ENGLAND) **1998/99** TO **2001/02**

	1998/99 Base	1999/2000	2000/01	2001/02
Net NHS spending (cash) £m	36,509	39,265	40,888	42,511
% increase	5.2	7.5	4.1	4.0
Inflation assumption (%)	3.0	2.5	2.5	2.5
Net NHS spending (real) £m	36,509	38,307	38,917	39,475
% increase	2.2	4.9	1.6	1.4
% increase	2.2	4.9	1.6	1.4
% of money GDP	5.4	5.6	5.5	5.5

Source: *NHS Funding : A Briefing Note*, Health Policy and Economic Research Unit, BMA, June 1998.

NHS staffing

NHS MEDICAL WORKFORCE

	GPs Number	Hospital Medical Staff*	Community Medical Staff*	TOTAL
1970	24,865	26,684	2,415	53,964
1975	26,942	33,922	3,295	65,159
1980	29,336	39,562	3,593	72,491
1985	32,436	44,757	3,678	80,871
1990	34,083	49,314	3,457	86,854
1995	35,628	59,352	3,113	98,093

* The figures relate to whole-time equivalent posts; many medical posts in the NHS are part-time ones.
Sources: B, C, D, H, I.

HOSPITAL MEDICAL STAFF—UK (WHERE AVAILABLE)*

	1980	1982	1984	1986	1988 (GB)	1990	1992	1994	1996 (GB)
Consultant	15,178	15,754	16,467	17,067	17,269	18,899	20,414	21,131	21,066
Associate specialist	1,346	1,330	1,278	1,143	1,018	1,145	1,171	1,216	1,223
Staff grade practitioner	—	—	—	—	—	270	868	1,628	2,440
Registrar grade**	—	—	—	—	—	—	—	—	11,898
Senior registrar	3,509	3,636	3,671	3,931	3,727	4,128	4,490	4,760	—
Registrar	7,318	7,557	7,566	7,603	7,740	7,876	7,622	7,750	—
Senior house officer	11,086	11,540	11,662	11,793	11,714	13,290	14,003	15,658	16,616
House officer	3,540	3,590	3,655	3,649	3,569	3,913	3,972	3,957	4,025

* In years for which Northern Ireland figures not available, Great Britain figures are given for all grades.
** Includes Specialist Registrar/Senior registrar/Registrar grades.
Source: *Manpower Statistics*.

GENERAL MEDICAL PRACTITIONERS IN UK (WHERE AVAILABLE)*

	1980	1982	1984	1986
Unrestricted principals	26,899	28,025	29,536	30,180
Restricted principals	265	234	202	181
Assistants	323	309	307	289
Trainees (GB)	1,704	2,022	2,182	2,127

	1988	1990	1992	1994 (GB)	1996 (GB)
Unrestricted principals	31,177	31,518	31,966	31,767	32,164
Restricted principals (GB)	172	163	152	156	126
Assistants (GB)	277	221	521	626	711
Associates	—	—	—	31	1,605
Trainees (GB)	2,165	2,040	2,067	1,841	1,653

* For years in which Northern Ireland figures are not available for all grades, Great Britain figures are given as indicated.
Sources: B, C, D, H, I.

NUMBER OF STAFF EMPLOYED IN NHS HOSPITALS BY CATEGORY

	1985	1990	1995
Medical and dental staff	47,717	52,733	62,193
Nurses and midwifery	511,191	514,618	441,713
Professional and technical	91,471	103,302	118,503
Administrative and clerical	137,982	165,042	199,913
Domestic and ancillary	221,334	156,995	110,336
Total	1,009,695	992,690	932,658

Sources: B, D, H, I.

UK NHS HOSPITAL STAFFING – **1995**

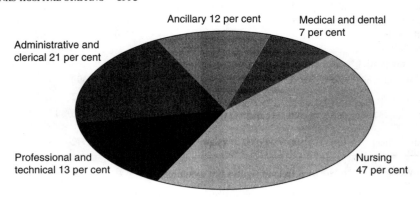

Ancillary 12 per cent

Medical and dental 7 per cent

Administrative and clerical 21 per cent

Professional and technical 13 per cent

Nursing 47 per cent

Sources: B, D, H, I.

NHS statistics

The major sources for UK health statistics are the various health departments in England, Scotland, Wales and Northern Ireland. Each has different methods of collecting data and subsequently selecting what is published. For instance, the English Department of Health collects data quarterly or annually (in some cases bi-annually) via central statistics returns from NHS trusts, health authorities and NHS Executive regional offices.

The central data collections cover a range of areas from financial, manpower, activity and miscellaneous data.* The selection of some of the categories of data is outlined in the table below. In addition to this data, *ad hoc* reviews and studies are also undertaken.

Financial	*Activity*	*Manpower*	*Other*
Statement of financial activities	Hospital episode statistics – reviews inpatient activity and bed occupancy alongside monitoring trends in specific conditions	NHS census of hospital staff	Patient Charter key standards returns
GMS quarterly summary of non-cash-limited expenditure		Annual questionnaire on GP practice staff	HCHS and FHS complaints
Health authority refunds*		Census of GMPs	Screening programme data
HCHS expenditure by activity categories	Summary of NHS trust activity	Collection of non-medical workforce discharges	Monitoring of delayed discharges
GPFH budget and expenditure†	Mental health		
Analysis of expenditure by type	Continuing care		
	Summary of ward attenders		

* not published
† Refer to HSC 1998/054 *Central Data Collections from the NHS* for full list of central data returns and source of publication.

FHS　　Family Health Service
GMP　　General medical practitioner
GMS　　General Medical Service
GPFH　General practitioner fundholders
HCHS　Hospital and community health service

WHERE CAN THE DATA BE FOUND?

Examples of where the data is published is set out below:

	Finance and expenditure	*Activity, manpower and other statistics*	*Comparative health statistics*
Statistical publications	Health Service cost index.	Departmental statistical bulletins Hospital episode statistics	
Other government publications	NHS accounts – National Audit Office. Government expenditure plans Prescriptions Pricing Authority (PPA).	Department of Health submissions to the professional review bodies. Evidence to House of Common Committees on health and public expenditure.	

	Hansard		
		Health and Personal Social Service Statistics	
	Health and Personal Social Service statistics		
	Evidence to House of Common Committees on health and public expenditure.		
Non-government publications	Chartered Institute of Public Finance and Accountancy (CIPFA) health service database.	NHS compendium of statistics – OHE	*OHE: Compendium of Health Statistics*
	Office of Health Economics (OHE)		Organization for Economic Co-operation and Development (OECD) databases and reports
			World Health Organization

In addition there are many databases primarily concerned with clinical data and evaluation of care such as Medline and the Centre for Review and Dissemination at York. The Office of National Statistics also produces some important documents such as the General Household Survey (provides general population health information and some general practice data) and the health survey for England as well as demographic data relating to births, fertility rates and mortality.

In recent years, the data available in the public arena has decreased, due in part to attempts to simplify the data collection and publication but also as a consequence of the 1990 NHS reforms. These reforms saw the introduction of competition between the health bodies which resulted in the withholding of financial information by each NHS body on the grounds of commercial interests.

Confidence in official statistics is clouded by concerns about their integrity and their public use. One commonly cited example is the inappropriate use of Finished Consultant Episodes (FCEs) to illustrate NHS performance in relation to the number of patients treated by the NHS. The use of FCEs to do this is misleading as FCEs merely record each contact by clinicians with a patient, regardless of whether it is part of ongoing treatment or a single episode. They are equally insensitive to patient readmission rates. Publication of league tables comparing hospitals' activity and mortality rates has been criticised as being crude indices, insufficiently adjusted for confounders such as high-risk patients, etc.

Information about the quality of the care and care outcomes provided by the NHS is limited. The government has made clear its intention to judge the NHS on its quality of care, not merely its activity rates, and is consulting widely on clinical and performance indicators which are sensitive to such factors in order to develop appropriate measurements for comparison.

APPENDIX 9: STATUTORY ORGANIZATIONS

Names, addresses and functions of a selection of government-funded bodies whose activities are related to the provision of health care in the United Kingdom.

AUDIT COMMISSION, 1 Vincent Square, London SW1P 2PN (0171–828 1212). Appoints auditors to local authorities, health authorities and NHS trusts and promotes studies to encourage economy, efficiency and effectiveness in the NHS and local government.

CLINICAL STANDARDS ADVISORY GROUP, Room 19, Wellington House, 133–155 Waterloo Road, London SE1 8UG (0171–972 4918). Advises health ministers and the NHS on standards of clinical care for, access to and availability of services to NHS patients

COMMITTEE ON SAFETY OF MEDICINES   See MEDICINES CONTROL AGENCY.

COMMON SERVICES AGENCY FOR THE SCOTTISH HEALTH SERVICE, Trinity Park House, South Trinity Road, Edinburgh EH5 3SE (0131–552 6255). Provides the NHS in Scotland with a range of services and products as directed and ensures they are delivered to customer requirements and to defined standards of quality.

COUNCIL FOR PROFESSIONS SUPPLEMENTARY TO MEDICINE, Park House, 184 Kennington Park Road, London SE11 4BU (0171–582 0866). Supervises the professional education and discipline in chiropody, dietetics, medical laboratory sciences, occupational therapy, orthoptics, physiotherapy and radiography.

GENERAL DENTAL COUNCIL, 37 Wimpole Street, London W1M 8DQ (0171–486 2171). Maintains a register of dentists, promotes high standards of dental education at all stages and of professional conduct among dentists. The council has disciplinary powers in respect of dentists' professional conduct.

GENERAL MEDICAL COUNCIL, 178 Great Portland Street, London W1N 6JE (0171–580 7642). The GMC is the medical profession's regulatory body and also has responsibility for setting educational and ethical standards. The council is a statutory body, set up in 1858, which is responsible to the Privy Council. It has powers under the Medical (Professional Performance) Act 1995 to act in respect of doctors whose professional performance is seriously deficient. The GMC has the authority to investigate and, where appropriate, discipline doctors for professional misconduct.

GENERAL OPTICAL COUNCIL, 41 Harley Street, London W1N 2DJ (0171–580 3898). Registers and regulates the professions of ophthalmic opticians and dispensing opticians.

HEALTH AND SAFETY COMMISSION and **HEALTH AND SAFETY EXECUTIVE (HSE)**, 2 Southwark Bridge Road, London SE1 9HS (0171–717 6000). Both these bodies are dedicated to securing the health, safety and welfare of persons at work and to protect the public generally against risks to health or safety arising from work activities. The HSE has powers to inspect the health and safety arrangements of organizations and, where these fail to meet statutory requirements or where accidents have occurred, it can investigate and prosecute offenders.

HEALTH EDUCATION AUTHORITY, 88 Trevelyan House, 30 Great Peter Street, London SW1P 2HW (0171–222 5300), **HEALTH EDUCATION BOARD FOR SCOTLAND**, Woodburn House, Canaan Lane, Edinburgh EH10 4SG (0131–447 8044) and **HEALTH PROMOTION AUTHORITY FOR WALES**, Ffynnon-las, Ty Glas Avenue, Llanishen, Cardiff CF4 5DZ (01222–752222). These three bodies advise respective UK health departments on matters relating to health education.

HEALTH SERVICE COMMISSIONER (OMBUDSMAN), 11th Floor, Millbank Tower, Millbank, London SW1P 4QP (0171–276 2035). Appointed by the government, the Commissioner investigates complaints about services provided under the

NHS and presents regular reports to Parliament.

HUMAN FERTILIZATION AND EMBRYOLOGY AUTHORITY, Paxton House, 30 Artillery Lane, London E1 7LS (0171–377 5077). A government licensing body concerned with storage of human gametes (sperm and eggs) and embryos, research on human embryos, and any infertility treatment which involves the use of donated gametes or embryos created outside the body.

MEDICAL RESEARCH COUNCIL (MRC), 20 Park Crescent, London W1N 4AL (0171–636 5422). The MRC's main objectives are to promote the balanced development of medical and related biological research so as to improve health care. It employs its own research staff in over 40 research establishments, and also provides grants to individual scientists.

MEDICINES COMMISSION See MEDICINES CONTROL AGENCY.

MEDICINES CONTROL AGENCY (MCA), Market Towers, Nine Elms Lane, London SW8 5NQ (0171–273 0393). The MCA is an executive agency of the Department of Health. Its main function is to safeguard public health by ensuring that branded and non-branded human medicines in the UK meet appropriate criteria of safety, quality and efficiency. It applies standards laid down in the Medicines Act of 1968 and by European Community legislation. The agency seeks advice from expert professional committees such as the Committee on Safety of Medicines and the Medicines Commission, both statutory committees based at the same address as the MCA.

MENTAL HEALTH ACT COMMISSION, Maid Marian House, 56 Houndsgate, Nottingham NG1 6BG (0115–943 7100). Set up in 1983 as a special health authority, the commission is responsible for protecting the interests of patients detained in England and Wales under the Act. Scotland and Northern Ireland have separate legislation.

MENTAL WELFARE COMMISSION FOR SCOTLAND, Argyle House, 3 Lady Lawson Street, Edinburgh EH3 9SH (0131–222 6111). This body has similar responsibilities in Scotland to those of the Mental Health Act Commission in England and Wales (see above).

NATIONAL AUDIT OFFICE (NAO), 157–197 Buckingham Palace Road, Victoria, London SW1W 9SP (0171–798 7000). The NAO audits public expenditure and is accountable to Parliament that money is spent for the purpose intended by Parliament and is properly accounted for.

NATIONAL BLOOD AUTHORITY (NBA), Oak House, Reeds Crescent, Watford, Herts. WD1 1QH (01923–486800, fax: 01923–486801). Created in 1993 to manage all NHS blood services, the NBA manages 15 regional transfusion services. Its objectives are to maintain blood and blood-product supply, based on a system of two million voluntary donors, and to ensure a safe, high-quality, cost-effective supply of blood and blood products for national needs.

NATIONAL RADIOLOGICAL PROTECTION BOARD, Chilton, Didcot, Oxfordshire OX11 0RQ (01235–831600). An independent government body which acts as the national point of authoritative reference for radiological protection.

NHS HEALTH ADVISORY SERVICE (HAS), Sutherland House, 29–37 Brighton Road, Sutton, Surrey SM2 5AN (0181–642 6421). The HAS is an independent advisory body reporting to ministers and is charged with improving the management, organization and delivery of patient care services, especially for the elderly, mentally ill people and those who misuse drug substances.

NORTHERN IRELAND CENTRAL SERVICES AGENCY FOR THE HEALTH AND SOCIAL SERVICES, 25–27 Adelaide Street, Belfast BT2 8FH (01232–324431). Offers a range of services to GPs and the four health and social services boards.

PRESCRIPTION PRICING AUTHORITY, Bridge House, 152 Pilgrim Street, Newcastle upon Tyne NE1 2SN (0191–232 5371). The authority's main functions are to calculate and make payments to dispensing pharmacists and doctors in England for NHS prescriptions and to provide information on prescribing and dispensing to NHS GPs and NHS authorities.

PUBLIC HEALTH LABORATORY SERVICES (PHLS), Headquarters Office, 61 Colindale Avenue, London NW9 5DF (0181–200 1295). The PHLS co-operates with the NHS to provide national facilities for the diagnosis, prevention and control of infectious and communicable diseases. The network of 50 laboratories in England and Wales is led by the headquarters complex at Colindale, where the Central Public Health Laboratory and Communicable Disease Surveillance Centre are sited.

STANDING MEDICAL ADVISORY COMMITTEE, Department of Health, Room 919, Wellington House, 135–155 Waterloo Road, London SE1 8UG (0171–972 4919), **STANDING NURSING AND MIDWIFERY ADVISORY COMMITTEE,** Department of Health, Room 919, Wellington House, 135–155 Waterloo Road, London SE1 8UG (0171–972 4919), and **STANDING PHARMACEUTICAL ADVISORY COMMITTEE,** Department of Health, Room 301, Richmond House, 79 Whitehall, London SW1A 2NS (0171–210 5117). The three standing advisory committees advise health ministers in England and Wales on matters relating to medicine, nursing, midwifery and pharmaceutical services.

STANDING COMMITTEE ON POSTGRADUATE MEDICAL AND DENTAL EDUCATION (SCOPME), One Park Square West, London NW1 4IJ (0171–935 3916). There are separate councils for Scotland, Wales and Northern Ireland. Advises the secretary of state on the delivery of postgraduate and continuing medical and dental education.

UNITED KINGDOM CENTRAL COUNCIL FOR NURSING, MIDWIFERY AND HEALTH VISITING, 23 Portland Place, London W1N 4JT (0171–637 7181). A regulatory body which sets standards for education and conduct of the nursing, midwifery and health visiting professions and maintains the professional registers.

UNITED KINGDOM TRANSPLANT SUPPORT SERVICE AUTHORITY, Fox Den Road, Stoke Gifford, Bristol BS12 6RR (0117–975 7575). A special health authority providing a support service for the matching, allocating and distribution of donor organs for transplant.

APPENDIX 10 : PROFESSIONAL ORGANIZATIONS

A selection of health-related non-statutory professional organizations.

Specialist organizations of the medical profession

The royal colleges and faculties in the list that follows represent the range of recognized specialties in medicine in the United Kingdom. They are responsible for setting the criteria for specialist training, for approving and monitoring training posts in the NHS, for organizing appropriate specialist examinations and admitting successful candidates to membership or fellowship of the relevant institution. This enables doctors to be registered with the General Medical Council (p.626) as specialists. Representatives of the colleges and faculties join with representatives of hospital doctors in the British Medical Association and the British Dental Association to form the Joint Consultants Committee. This Committee meets regularly with ministers and officials from the UK's health departments to discuss the provision and standards of NHS specialist care along with the postgraduate educational requirements of NHS doctors.

The royal colleges and faculties also have an umbrella organization called the Academy of Medical Colleges (1 Wimpole Street, London W1M 4AE) which facilitates co-ordination of their activities.

ROYAL COLLEGE OF ANAESTHETISTS, 48–49 Russell Square, London WC1B 4JP (0171–813 1900).

ROYAL COLLEGE OF GENERAL PRACTITIONERS, 14 Prince's Gate, London SW7 1PU (0171–581 3232).

ROYAL COLLEGE OF OBSTETRICIANS AND GYNAE-COLOGISTS, 27 Sussex Place, Regent's Park, London NW1 4RG (0171–262 5425).

ROYAL COLLEGE OF OPHTHALMOLOGISTS, 17 Cornwall Terrace, London NW1 4QW (0171–935 0702).

ROYAL COLLEGE OF PATHOLOGISTS, 2 Carlton House Terrace, London SW1Y 5AF (0171–930 5861).

ROYAL COLLEGE OF PAEDIATRICS AND CHILD HEALTH, 5 St Andrews Place, Regent's Park, London NW1 4LB.

ROYAL COLLEGE OF PHYSICIANS, 11 St Andrews Place, London NW1 4LE (0171–935 1174).

ROYAL COLLEGE OF PHYSICIANS OF EDINBURGH, 9 Queen Street, Edinburgh EH2 1JQ (0131–235 7324).

ROYAL COLLEGE OF PHYSICIANS AND SURGEONS OF GLASGOW, 234–242 St Vincent Street, Glasgow G2 5RJ (0141–221 6072).

ROYAL COLLEGE OF PHYSICIANS OF IRELAND, 6 Kildare Street, Dublin 2 ([00353] 1–6616677).

ROYAL COLLEGE OF PSYCHIATRISTS, 17 Belgrave Square, London SW1X 8PG (0171–235 2351).

ROYAL COLLEGE OF RADIOLOGISTS, 38 Portland Place, London W1N 3DG (0171–636 4432).

ROYAL COLLEGE OF SURGEONS OF EDINBURGH, 18 Nicolson Street, Edinburgh EH8 9DW.

ROYAL COLLEGE OF SURGEONS OF ENGLAND, 35–43 Lincoln's Inn Fields, London WC2A 3PN (0171–405 3474).

ROYAL COLLEGE OF SURGEONS OF IRELAND, 123 St Stephen's Green, Dublin 2 ([00353] 1–4022100)

FACULTY OF OCCUPATIONAL MEDICINE, 6 St Andrews Place, Regent's Park, London NW1 4LE (0171–487 3414).

FACULTY OF PHARMACEUTICAL MEDICINE, 1 St Andrews Place, Regent's Park, London NW1 4LB (0171–224 0343).

FACULTY OF PUBLIC HEALTH MEDICINE, 4 St Andrews Place, London NW1 4LB (0171–935 0243).

Voluntary organizations

BRITISH MEDICAL ASSOCIATION, BMA House, Tavistock Square, London WC1H 9JP (0171– 387 4499). The BMA is a voluntary professional association of doctors from all branches of medicine with more than 80 per cent of practising doctors in the UK in membership. It is a scientific and educational body, an independent trade union and a publishing house.

BRITISH DENTAL ASSOCIATION, 64 Wimpole Street, London W1M 8AL (0171–935 0875). A voluntary professional body representing the dental profession; it also has scientific and educational responsibilities.

CHARTERED SOCIETY OF PHYSIOTHERAPY, 14 Bedford Row, London WC1R 4ED (0171–306 6666). The professional and educational body and trade union for chartered physiotherapists.

COLLEGE OF HEALTH CARE CHAPLAINS, PO Box 105, Addenbrooke's Hospital, Cambridge CB2 2QQ (01223–245151). Provides educational opportunities for health-care chaplains, sets and maintains high standards of chaplaincy and provides support through a regional branch structure.

THE COLLEGE OF OPTOMETRISTS, 10 Knaresborough Place, London SW5 0TG (0171–373 7765). Members of the college have passed its qualifying examination and met its training requirements. The college's aims are to improve and conserve human vision, to study and research ophthalmic optics and to maintain high professional standards and competence.

MEDICAL WOMEN'S FEDERATION, Tavistock House North, Tavistock Square, London WC1H 9HX (0171–387 7765). The federation promotes equal opportunities for women doctors and patients through a network of local associations in the UK. Membership is open to women doctors and medical students and the federation organizes local and national seminars and conferences.

NHS CONFEDERATION, Birmingham Research Park, Vincent Drive, Birmingham B15 2SQ (0121–471 4444). The NHS Confederation is a representative organization with over 500 trusts, 100 health authorities and health boards as members.

ROYAL COLLEGE OF MIDWIVES, 15 Mansfield Street, London W1M 0BE (0171–872 5100). A professional organization, educational trust and trade union for midwives.

ROYAL COLLEGE OF NURSING OF THE UNITED KING-DOM (RCN), 20 Cavendish Square, London W1M 9AE (0171–409 3333). The RCN is the voluntary professional association for registered, student and pupil nurses, midwives and health visitors. It has a world-wide membership of over 300,000. The college promotes the science and art of nursing, the training of nurses and the professional standing and interests of members and the profession. It represents nurses and negotiates on their behalf with the government and other employers.

ROYAL COLLEGE OF SPEECH AND LANGUAGE THERA-PISTS, 7 Bath Place, Rivington Street, London EC2A 3DR (0171–613 3855). Responsible for the accreditation of courses and examinations leading to qualification to practise as a speech and language therapist and the maintenance of a register.

ROYAL PHARMACEUTICAL SOCIETY OF GREAT BRITAIN, 1 Lambeth High Street, London SE1 7JN (0171–735 9141). A professional body, promoting pharmaceutical education and science and the interests of its members.

ROYAL SOCIETY OF MEDICINE (RSM), 1 Wimpole Street, London W1M 8AE (0171–290 2900). An independent, apolitical society of mainly medical members which provides a neutral forum for the exchange of views on medical,

educational and other health-care issues. It also provides continuing medical education and possesses one of the most comprehensive medical libraries in the world.

Medical defence bodies

The two commercial institutions listed below assist doctors, dentists and other health-care professionals with complaints and negligence claims arising from clinical practice and payments of legal costs and damages. They also provide advice on medicolegal and professional problems associated with clinical practice.

MEDICAL DEFENCE UNION, 3 Devonshire Place, London W1N 2EA (0171–486 6181).

MEDICAL PROTECTION SOCIETY, 50 Hallam Street, London W1N 6DE (0171–637 0541).

APPENDIX 11: INTERNATIONAL ORGANIZATIONS

World Health Organization
Founded in 1948, the World Health Organization (WHO) is a United Nations agency whose self-stated objective is 'the attainment by all people of the highest possible level of health.' WHO aims to do this by setting standards in health care, providing technical assistance on medical issues, and advocating health-policy reform. With its headquarters in Geneva, WHO divides the world up into six regions: Africa, the Americas, Eastern Mediterranean, Europe, South-East Asia and Western Pacific. As well, WHO maintains an office in each member state (166 in 1987), usually in the ministry of health.

Policy is formulated at the annual meeting, the World Health Assembly, attended by delegates from each member state. The assembly elects 32 representatives to the executive board, and at the top of the hierarchical ladder is the director general, who is supported by technical and administrative staff.

WHO's main focus has been primary health care, especially the eradication of infectious diseases through vaccination programmes. WHO has also traditionally worked closely with governments in the fields of maternal and child health, population planning, nutrition, sanitation and the supply and distribution of medicines.

Its greatest success has been the world-wide eradication of smallpox, with the last case occurring in 1977. In the same year, WHO outlined its goal that all of the world's inhabitants should achieve 'a level of health that will permit them to lead a socially and economically productive life: health for all by the year 2000.' An impossible target now.

In the 1990s WHO has seen a waning of its influence as a result of inadequate funding, and a shift in the health-care agenda towards health economics and health policy – both neglected by WHO.

In an attempt to halt the decline, former prime minister of Norway, Dr Gro Harlem Bruntland, was elected director general of WHO in 1998. Many now see WHO's role as continuing to provide excellent technical assistance while other agencies with more financial sway, like the World Bank, influence the health policy of governments.

World Bank
The World Bank was established, along with the International Monetary Fund, at the Bretton Woods Conference in 1944. A United Nations Agency, the World Bank's aim is 'to reduce poverty and improve living standards by promoting sustainable growth and investment in people.'

The World Bank provides low-interest loans to member states (181 in 1998), and the very poorest countries are eligible for interest-free credits. Heavily criticized in the past for lending to poor countries for ill-conceived large-scale projects such as hydroelectric dams, pipelines and transport networks, the World Bank signalled a shift in emphasis with its annual World Development Report of 1993 which focused on health, nutrition and population.

That report was widely seen as the moment the World Bank usurped the World Health Organization as the lead agency in world health. With its volume of lending running into tens of billions for health-related projects, and its powerful influence in ministries of finance, the World Bank is well placed to persuade governments to adopt its health policies, which have, however, been criticized for promoting economic growth rather than health. The World Bank's view is that the two are inseparable.

World Medical Association

The World Medical Association (WMA) is an independent confederation of non-governmental professional medical associations from over 60 countries. The association is apolitical and provides a forum for its 70 or so member associations to communicate with each other, to co-operate actively, and to achieve consensus on high standards of professional competence and medical ethics.

Founded in 1947 at a meeting convened by the British Medical Association at its London headquarters, the WMA is funded by annual contributions from its member associations. Policy is determined by its general assembly, which meets annually and comprises delegations from national medical associations. The executive body is a biennially elected council, with representation from six regions: Africa, Asia, Europe, Latin America, North America and the Pacific. The secretariat is based at Ferney-Voltaire, France, near Geneva, the headquarters of the World Health Organization (see above).

As well as promoting high professional standards, the WMA champions the professional freedom of physicians world-wide, a task the association believes facilitates humane, high-calibre medical care, which, in turn, should enhance the quality of life for everyone. Since its foundation the association has developed, through its declarations and statements, guidance to doctors, national medical associations, governments, and other international bodies. Among the subjects it has covered are patients' rights, research on human subjects, torture of prisoners, the use and misuse of drugs, family-planning measures, pollution, and care of sick and wounded people in times of armed conflict. The association has also published its influential international code of medical ethics.

Commonwealth Medical Association

A non-governmental organization with recognized relationship to United Nations health activities and to the World Health Organization (see above), the CMA is accredited to the Commonwealth Heads of Government meeting. About 40 national medical associations subscribe to the CMA, which is based in the United Kingdom and registered there as a company limited by guarantee.

The association's council meets triennially in different Commonwealth countries. The CMA's main objective is to strengthen the capacity of national medical associations, in collaboration with other health-professional associations and health-concerned non-governmental organizations to improve the health status of vulnerable and disadvantaged groups in developing countries. The association's activities, therefore, are mainly in women's and youth health, sexual and reproductive health, and the ethical and human rights implications of providing health information and services. The CMA provides some technical co-operation and help to its member associations – for example, advice on drafting health-related legislation.

The association's address is: Commonwealth Medical Association, BMA House, Tavistock Square, London, WC1H 9JP (0171–383 6095).

APPENDIX 12: HEALTH-POLICY RESEARCH ORGANIZATIONS

This is a list of some of the bodies involved in health-policy research and consultancy; it is not exhaustive but includes those bodies that publish regularly for a national audience.

CENTRE FOR HEALTH ECONOMICS, University of York, Heslington, York YO1 5DD (01904–433718). Director: Professor Michael Drummond. The centre specializes in health-economics research. Principal areas of research activity include economic evaluation of health technologies, outcome measurement, primary care, community care, the determinants of health.

CENTRE FOR HEALTH SERVICES RESEARCH, University of Newcastle upon Tyne, 21 Claremont Place, Newcastle upon Tyne NE2 4AA (0191–222 7045). A multidisciplinary organization that mainly does research aimed at improving the health status of people in Europe, the United Kingdom and North-East England. Among its research interests are primary-care and outpatient sectors, outcomes of care and medical audit.

CENTRE FOR POLICY ON AGEING, 25/31 Ironmonger Row, London EC1V 3QP (0171–253 1787). Director: Dr Gillian Dalley. Using research and analysis, this organization aims to formulate better policies for older people.

HEALTH ECONOMICS RESEARCH UNIT, University of Aberdeen, Department of Public Health, University Medical Buildings, Foresterhill, Aberdeen AB25 2ZD (01224–681818). Director: Professor John Cairns. The unit receives core funding from the Chief Scientist's Office of the Scottish Office Departments of Health and from competitive research grants and funding.

It has two underlying aims: to develop methods within health economics and to encourage use of the techniques of economic appraisal by clinicians and managers in the NHS. Produces regular discussion papers and undertakes consultancy in the NHS in Scotland.

HEALTH POLICY AND ECONOMIC RESEARCH UNIT, British Medical Association, BMA House, Tavistock Square, London WC1H 9JP (0171–387 4499). Director: Jon Ford. Established in January 1994 to help the BMA make contribution to wider debates about health policy by producing briefing and discussion documents and conducting original research. The documents it produces are not BMA policy as such and are intended to provoke debate inside and outside the association. Some work is 'commissioned' internally, otherwise it is free to determine the topics it studies.

HEALTH SERVICES MANAGEMENT CENTRE, University of Birmingham, Park House, 40 Edgbaston Road, Birmingham, B15 2RT (0121–414 7050). Director: Professor Chris Ham. The aim of the centre is to strengthen the management of health services and so promote better health. Current areas of activity include the development and evaluation of approaches to commissioning in health care, primary-care provision and management, quality management and clinical effectiveness, priority setting and rationing, involving users and the public in health-service decision making.

The centre conducts research, postgraduate programmes, courses and seminars and undertakes consultancy.

INSTITUTE FOR HEALTH POLICY STUDIES, University of Southampton, Faculty of Social Sciences, 129 University Road, The University of Southampton SO17 1BJ (01703–593394). Director: Professor Ray Robinson. A multidisciplinary research and policy-analysis institute aimed at improving understanding about important health-policy issues through the synthesis and analysis of existing data and to conduct research to extend the information used for preparing policy.

INSTITUTE FOR PUBLIC POLICY RESEARCH, 30–32 Southampton Street, London WC2E 7RA (0171–470 6100). Deputy Director (Health): Anna Coote. Independent charity whose purpose is to contribute to public understanding of social, economic and political questions through research, discussion and publications. Established to provide an alternative to the free-market think tanks.

Current interests in health issues include public health, information technology and health care. Also interested in public involvement and in particular citizens' juries.

INSTITUTE OF ECONOMIC AFFAIRS, 2 Lord North Street, London SW1P 3LB (0171–799 3745). Director of Health and Welfare Unit: Dr David Green. Research and educational charity, controlled by managing trustees, independent of any political party or group and financed by sales of publications, conference fees and voluntary contributions from individuals and organizations. Specializes in studies of markets and pricing systems as technical devices for registering preferences and apportioning resources.

KING'S FUND, 11–13 Cavendish Square, London W1M 0AN (0171–307 2400). Chief executive: Rabbi Julia Neuberger. Independent charity which aims to improve the health and health care of Londoners. It recognizes, however, that London cannot be viewed in isolation and therefore carries out research and development, audit and education across the UK.

Undertakes health-policy research and analysis, promotes good practice in health and social care, supports leadership development and offers grants to London projects. Also runs King's Fund organizational audit for hospitals. Comprehensive health-policy library open to researchers.

LSE HEALTH, London School of Economics and Political Science, Houghton Street, London WC2A 2AE (0171–955 7540). Director: Dr Elias Mossialos. Multidisciplinary research centre which brings together members of LSE academic staff from different departments working on health-policy issues. Its fundamental mission is to undertake research consultancy and training in the area of international health policy and to influence thereby international health policies.

NATIONAL PRIMARY CARE RESEARCH AND DEVELOPMENT CENTRE, University of Manchester, Williamson Building, Oxford Road, Manchester M13 9PL (0161–275 7601). Chief executive: Professor David Wilkin. Multidisciplinary centre which brings together academic disciplines, clinical professions and health-service managers to engage in a broad programme of policy-relevant research and to promote research-based service development in primary care.

NUFFIELD INSTITUTE FOR HEALTH, University of Leeds, 71–75 Clarendon Road, Leeds LS2 9PL (0113–233 6633). Director: Professor Gerald Wistow. Interests include health and social policy and management practice, public health, health services, research and community-care research with particular attention to needs assessment and health and social-care outcomes. Also acts as co-ordinating body for UK Clearing House on Health Outcomes and European Clearing House.

Offers courses and undertakes research and consultancy.

NUFFIELD TRUST, 59 New Cavendish Street, London W1M 7RD (0171–631 8450). Secretary: John Wyn Owen, CB. Describes itself as an independent observer of the UK health scene and the NHS. Main areas of activity are invited meetings, workshops and seminars, publications, a grant programme and fellowships. Activities currently centre on two main themes: 'How well is the NHS?' and 'Health policies for the 21st century'.

OFFICE OF HEALTH ECONOMICS, 12 Whitehall, London SW1A 2DY (0171–930 9203). Director: Adrian Towse. Supported from an annual grant from the Association of the British Pharmaceutical Industry. Its terms of reference are to commission and undertake research on the economics of health and health care, collect and analyse health and health-care data from the UK and other countries and to disseminate the results of this work and stimulate discussion of them and their policy implications.

Recent commissioned reports have included topics such as managed care and waiting lists. OHE publishes on a regular basis a comprehensive compendium of UK health statistics.

POLICY STUDIES INSTITUTE, 100 Park Village East, London NW1 3SR (0171–468 0468). Director (interim): Professor Margaret Blunden. Independent research organization undertaking studies of social and economic policy. PSI is a registered charity and, since January 1998, a wholly owned subsidiary company of the University of Westminster.

Among areas of interest in health-related research are doctors' careers. Recent publications include research commissioned by the General Medical Council (the statutory registration body for the medical profession) on handling complaints against doctors, an evaluation of the role of midwives in maternity care and reducing the length of hospital stay.

APPENDIX 13: COMPLEMENTARY MEDICINE

Introduction

This appendix is titled 'complementary medicine' because the term is well recognized by the public. 'Alternative medicine' is another commonly used description. A more accurate description, however, might be 'non-conventional therapy', as proposed in a report on the subject published in 1993 by the British Medical Association.[1] Such therapies may be offered as alternatives to orthodox Western medicine or as complementary to orthodox treatments. Some registered medical practitioners provide complementary treatments as well as orthodox therapies (occasionally under the umbrella of the National Health Service). Most non-conventional health care, however, is provided by practitioners who have received training or who are experienced in the relevant procedures.

Whatever the generic title used, the public's use of non-conventional therapies has been rising in recent years. This probably reflects the findings of a study in 1997 that one quarter of GP consultations and half of outpatient attendances are by people with unexplained physical symptoms and for whom there is little orthodox treatment.[2] In a survey in 1995 by the UK's Consumers' Association (an independent body funded by members' subscriptions) one in three of nearly 9,000 respondents had used 'complementary medicine at some time in their lives [and of those] one in five had done so during the preceding year.'[3] The Association reported that in France 48 per cent of the population regularly visited a complementary therapist, while in Germany 46 per cent did so, in Belgium 31 per cent and in the Netherlands 20 per cent.

A large survey of UK general practitioners done by the BMA in 1992 showed that out of almost 22,500 doctors responding (70 per cent of NHS GPs), 29 per cent supported the provision of acupuncture and osteopathy at their NHS surgeries and 18 per cent wanted homeopathy services provided. Younger GPs supported the inclusion of non-conventional therapies more strongly than GPs overall.

The Consumers' Association's *The Which? Guide to Complementary Medicine*[3] categorized therapies as follows: touch therapies; mind–body medicine; manipulative and structural therapies; postural techniques; medicinal therapies; Oriental medicine; and self-help practices. This appendix offers a framework of information, briefly describing a selection of non-conventional therapies practised in the UK and, where possible, providing a national contact address. The text contains no judgements about the efficacy of any treatments described or on the standards of training of those providing them. Many publications and organizations provide information on non-

[1] British Medical Association, *Complementary Medicine: New Approaches to Good Practice*, Oxford, Oxford University Press, 1997.

[2] R. Mayor and M. Sharpe, 'Treating medically unexplained physical symptoms', *British Medical Journal*, 315: 561–2, 1997.

[3] B Rowlands, *The Which? Guide to Complementary Medicine*, London, Consumers' Association, 1997.

conventional therapies and the *Which?* guide offers practical advice on how to find a reliable practitioner.

Acupuncture

Traditional Chinese medicine dating back 2,000 years or more. Brought to Europe in 19th century.

Chinese acupuncture is a prime component of traditional Chinese medicine. Medical acupuncture (also called Western or scientific acupuncture) is practised by doctors on the *Medical Register*. Acupuncture is a touch technique based on the theory of body meridians, a network of lines of force. The aim is to insert needles along the meridians so as to balance the body's various *yin* and *yang* forces and to restore a person's health. Western practitioners also use acupuncture to achieve anaesthesia.

For Western acupuncture a doctor has to undertake two years of postgraduate study. Nurses and physiotherapists have to do the same. The course ends with an examination. Both organizations listed below keep registers of members.

BRITISH MEDICAL ACUPUNCTURE SOCIETY, Newton House, Newton Lane, Whitley, Warrington WA4 4JA (01925–730727).

BRITISH ACUPUNCTURE COUNCIL, Park House, 206–8 Latimer Road, London W10 6RE (0181–964 0222).

Alexander technique

Founded by an Australian actor whose respiratory problems hindered his acting career, this is a system of postural re-education in which people are taught to stand and move more efficiently.

The main organization is the Society of Teachers of the Alexander Technique, which supervises training, maintains a code of ethics and a register of teachers.

SOCIETY OF TEACHERS OF THE ALEXANDER TECHNIQUE, 20 London House, 266 Fulham Road, London SW10 9EL (0171–351 0828).

Aromatherapy

This therapy originated in the Middle East and was introduced to Europe by the Romans.

A touch technique based on the healing properties of essential plant oils which give plants their distinctive smells. Holistic aromatherapy uses essential oils and massage to treat physical and emotional disorders.

Aromatherapy is not statutorily regulated and any individual may set up as a practitioner, but an Aromatherapy Organizations Council (1991) aims to improve training and set national standards, with 50 hours of clinical training, an examination and entry to the Register of Qualified Aromatherapists.

AROMATHERAPY ORGANIZATIONS COUNCIL, 3 Latymer Close, Braybrooke, Market Harborough LE16 8LN (01858–434242).

Art therapies (art, music, sound, dance, and drama)

Used in most cultures in one form or another for centuries, art therapy was used in Britain in World War II to rehabilitate soldiers.

A mind–body technique that uses art, music, dance, and drama therapies to relieve pain and anxiety and to integrate participants into the community, it is particularly helpful in rehabilitating people with psychiatric and psychological problems.

Art therapies all have professional bodies, many of them well established; practitioners must be graduates in the relevant subject.

ASSOCIATION FOR DANCE MOVEMENT THERAPY, c/o The Art Therapies Department, Springfield Hospital, Glenburnie Road, London SW17 7DJ.

ASSOCIATION OF DRAMA THERAPISTS, 4 Funnydale Villas, Durlstone Road, Swanage, Dorset BN19 2HY.

Chiropractic (manipulative and structural)

This therapy, developed by a Canadian osteopath at the start of the 20th century, uses joint-adjusting procedures, manipulation, massage, and other techniques to treat musculoskeletal complaints. Therapists use spinal X-rays for the diagnosis of mechanical problems.

Education consists of a five years' full-time BSc degree course at the Anglo European College of Chiropractic, plus a postgraduate year in a British Chiropractic Association clinic, to obtain an honorary doctorate of chiropractic.

BRITISH CHIROPRACTIC ASSOCIATION, 29 Whitley Street, Reading, Berkshire RG2 0EG (01734–757557).

BRITISH ASSOCIATION FOR APPLIED CHIROPRACTIC, The Old Post Office, Cherry Street, Stratton Audley, Near Bicester, Oxfordshire OX6 9BA (01869–277111).

CHIROPRACTIC PATIENTS ASSOCIATION, 8 Centre One, Lysander Way, Old Sarum Park, Salisbury, Wilts. SP4 6BU (01722–415027, fax: 01722–415128).

Healing (touch and mind–body)

Its origins lie in religion, magic and shammanism. Healing therapy was established on an organized basis in the UK in 1955 when the National Federation of Spiritual Healers was founded.

Restoration to health is by the laying on of hands and also by distance healing.

There are no academic qualifications; the training course comprises a probationary period of around two years.

CONFEDERATION OF HEALING ORGANIZATIONS, Suite J, 113 High Street, Berkhamsted HP4 2DJ (01442–870660).

NATIONAL FEDERATION OF SPIRITUAL HEALERS, Old Manor Farm Studio, Church Street, Sunbury-on-Thames TW16 6RG (01932–983164).

Herbalism

The use of herbs as medicines is probably as old as man; every culture has its own traditions. Herbalism was formally established in England by an Act of Parliament during Henry VIII's reign. It is a system of treatment in which different parts of a variety of plants are used to restore function and to treat symptoms.

Anyone can set up as a herbalist, but there are two institutes, the School of Phytotherapy and Middlesex University, which offer four-year BSc courses (including at least 500 hours of clinical supervision).

NATIONAL INSTITUTE OF CLINICAL HERBALISTS, 56 Longbrook Street, Exeter, Devon EX4 6AH (01392–426022).

Homeopathy

Hippocrates (4th century BC) suggested that treatment with something that mimics illness might cure it. Samuel Hahnemann treated patients utilizing this principle in Europe in the late 18th century. Homeopathy is now well established with several hundred medically qualified doctors registered as homeopaths.

Patients are treated by the administration of greatly diluted forms of natural substances that in a healthy person would bring on symptoms similar to those which the medicine is prescribed to treat.

The Statutory Faculty of Homeopathy trains and registers medical practitioners in homeopathy. Three years' full-time training equivalent to undergraduate degree requirements. Course assessment and final written and clinical examinations.

BRITISH HOMEOPATHIC ASSOCIATION, 27a Devonshire Street, London W1N 1RJ (0171–935 2163).

FACULTY OF HOMEOPATHY, 2 Powis Place, Great Ormond Street, London WC1N 3HT (0171–837 9469).

SOCIETY OF HOMEOPATHS, 2 Artizan Road, Northampton, Northamptonshire NN1 4HU (01604–214000).

Hypnotherapy (mind–body)

Probably first used in ancient Greece to treat anxiety and hysteria. Primitive societies have often used it in various forms. An 18th-century Viennese physician, Franz Mesurer, treated

people by putting them into a trance. A French doctor, Ambrose Lebeaut, developed the technique and hypnosis arrived in Britain in the late 19th century when it was used by a surgeon, James Braid.

The patient is made to relax with the use of hypnosis, the aim being to reduce pain, bring about changes in mental state and make suggestions for relieving symptoms.

Anyone can set up as a hypnotherapist but about 500 doctors, dentists and pyschologists are clinically trained. There is no regulatory body. Training for lay hypnotherapists may vary from a few days to several months. The National School of Hypnotherapy and Psychotherapy offers training courses.

BRITISH SOCIETY OF MEDICAL AND DENTAL HYPNOSIS, 17 Keppel View Road, Kimberworth, Rotherham, Yorkshire S61 2AR (01709–554558).

NATIONAL SCHOOL OF HYPNOTHERAPY AND PSYCHOTHERAPY, The Central Register of Advanced Hypnotherapists, 28 Finsbury Park Road, London N4 2JX (0171–359 6991).

Massage (touch)

References to massage appear in the Bible and the Koran and it was used in China 5,000 years ago. European massage therapy developed in Sweden in the 19th century and was used in Britain in the first part of this century and formed the basis of physiotherapy.

Therapeutic massage is used mainly for back problems but also for headaches, stiffness and complaints caused by tension. Massage is based on Swedish techniques, oils and aromatherapy.

Massage therapists are unregulated, but physiotherapy has a recognised training structure and statutory registration. There are around 200 training institutions for massage therapy with some 60 massage 'qualifications', training lasting from a few days to two years. The London College of Massage provides courses of up to 72 hours of instruction with supervised clinic attendance.

BRITISH MASSAGE THERAPY COUNCIL, Greenbank House, 65a Adelphi Street, Preston, Lancashire PR1 7BH (01772–881063).

MASSAGE THERAPY INSTITUTE OF GREAT BRITAIN, PO Box 2726, London NW2 4NR (0181–208 1607).

Osteopathy (manipulative and structural)

Founded in the 1870s by an American who was both doctor and engineer, the technique arrived in Britain at the start of the 20th century, and in 1917 the first school was established (in London).

System of diagnosis and treatment dealing primarily with the musculoskeletal system. Practitioners use mainly gentle manual and manipulative methods to restore and maintain biomechanical functions.

Osteopathy was the first complementary therapy to be statutorily regulated. The Osteopaths Act 1993 protects patients from untrained practitioners. After 1999 all osteopaths will have to be registered with the new General Osteopathic Council which will have a list of professional requirements, including a recognized qualification and compulsory preregistration training.

GENERAL COUNCIL AND REGISTER OF OSTEOPATHS, 56 London Street, Reading, Berkshire RG1 4SQ (01734–576585).

COLLEGE OF OSTEOPATHIC PRACTITIONERS ASSOCIATION, 13 Furzehill Road, Borehamwood, Hertfordshire WD6 2DG (0181–905 1937).

Reflexology (touch, oriental)

Over 5,000 years ago hand and foot massage was practised in China and India. Early in the 20th century an American surgeon identified areas of the hand and foot which, if pressurized, could produce partial anaesthesia in the ear, nose, and throat, allowing minor surgery to be performed. The concept was developed and later introduced to Britain.

The therapy comprises compression and massage methods using reflex areas in hands and feet.

The Association of Reflexologists has accredited around 70 courses in the UK. The British Reflexology Association is a representative professional organization. Both have codes of practice and ethics as well as lists of accredited therapists.

ASSOCIATION OF REFLEXOLOGISTS, 27 Old Gloucester Street, London WC1 3XX (0990–673320).

BRITISH REFLEXOLOGY ASSOCIATION, Monks Orchard, Whitbourne, Worcester, Worcestershire WR6 5RB (01886–821207).

T'ai chi (oriental, self-help, postural)

This exercise technique originated in 12th-century China and was introduced in the UK in the 1970s. Influenced by Taoist, Confucian and Buddhist philosophies.

Described as a non-violent martial art, *t'ai chi* consists of a series of postures linked by gentle, graceful movements aimed at stabilizing the interplay of the body's opposing forces, *yin* and *yang*. This self-help technique is best learnt in a class, where movements are demonstrated and which may take many months to perform effectively.

SCHOOL OF T'AI CHI CHUAN CENTRE FOR HEALING, 5 Tavistock Place, London WC1H 9SN (0171–444 6445).

Yoga (oriental, self help, postural)

Probably developed in India 5,000 years ago. Introduced to England in Victorian era.

Yoga postures and breathing exercises are aimed at calming the mind and improving vital energy (*prana*) which flows along invisible channels (*nadis*). Meditation has a central role in yoga.

Most people join a local class. These may be run privately, by employers, or by local community organizations. They should be led by teachers who are members either of the British Wheel of Yoga or the Iyengan Yoga Institute.

BRITISH WHEEL OF YOGA, 1 Hamilton Place, Boston Road, Sleaford NG34 7ES (01529–306851).

IYENGAN YOGA INSTITUTE, 223a Randolph Avenue, London W9 1NL (0171–624 3080).

YOGA THERAPY CENTRE, Royal London Homeopathic Hospital Trust, 60 Great Ormond Street, London WC1N 3HR (0171–833 7267).